ACUTE & CHRONIC WOUNDS

INTRAPROFESSIONALS FROM NOVICE TO EXPERT

RUTH A. BRYANT, PHD, RN, CWOCN, Retired/Emeritus, FAAWC

Principal Research Scientist
Abbott Northwestern Hospital Minneapolis, Minnesota;
Affiliate Faculty, School of Nursing, University of Minnesota,
Minneapolis, Minnesota; Visiting Professor, Universidad Panamericana
Nursing School, Mexico City, Mexico; President and Owner,
Bryant WOC Consulting, St. Paul, Minnesota Immediate Past-President
Association for the Advancement of Wound Care

DENISE P. NIX, RN, MS, CWOCN

WOC Nurse
M Health Fairview Hospitals and Clinics
Minneapolis, Minnesota;
Subject Matter Expert, Patient Safety
Minnesota Hospital Association
St Paul, Minnesota; Consultant
Nix Consulting LLC
Minneapolis, Minnesota

SIXTH EDITION

ELSEVIER

Elsevier
3251 Riverport Lane
St. Louis, Missouri 63043

ACUTE & CHRONIC WOUNDS: INTRAPROFESSIONALS FROM NOVICE
TO EXPERT, SIXTH EDITION

ISBN: 978-0-323-71190-6

Notices

Practitioners and researchers must always rely on their own experience and knowledge in evaluating and using
any information, methods, compounds or experiments described herein. Because of rapid advances in the
medical sciences, in particular, independent verification of diagnoses and drug dosages should be made. To the
fullest extent of the law, no responsibility is assumed by Elsevier, authors, editors or contributors for any injury
and/or damage to persons or property as a matter of products liability, negligence or otherwise, or from any use
or operation of any methods, products, instructions, or ideas contained in the material herein.

Previous editions copyrighted 2016, 2012, 2007, 2000, 1992.

Senior Content Strategist: Sandra Clark
Senior Content Development Manager: Lisa P. Newton
Senior Content Development Specialist: Tina Kaemmerer
Publishing Services Manager: Deepthi Unni
Senior Project Manager: Umarani Natarajan
Design Direction: Ryan Cook

Printed in India

Last digit is the print number: 9   8   7   6   5   4   3   2

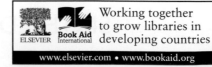

In all of our lives, we have certain individuals who have played a significant role in making our success possible, who enhance our lives and share our dreams. For me, this includes, of course, my Mom and Dad, Dennis Confer, my amazing coworkers as I was starting my career (Joy Boarini, Bonnie Sue Rolstad, and Mary Zink), my tribe of supporters at the WOCN Society, my wound care warriors at Sacred Heart Medical Center (Robin, Teresa, Michelle, Becca, and Beth), and all my diverse AAWC colleagues (Kara, Karen, BBJ, and Greg). There are so many more significant people I should mention, including all the students I have had the pleasure to work with! It is only with friends and colleagues like you that I have been able to achieve what I have achieved. I have to specially acknowledge, however, the contributions of Denise Nix to this textbook, but also in my life personally. The textbook is because of DeeDee's coordination, attention to detail, coaxing, and perseverance!

Ruth Ann Bryant

I'd like to dedicate this book to all the patient's families, nurses, and healthcare workers who were impacted by COVID-19. To my partners at M Health Fairview Southdale Hospital (Julie, Annika, Amanda, Kaitlin, Andrea, and Kathy), I am grateful for the sisterhood; it's the reason I smile all alone in my car on my way to work. To my family, especially my amazing husband John, our sons Ian and Adam, and my mom Barbara Henry for their patience and support my entire career but especially during the creation of this book. Finally, to Ruth, also family, we have shared our lives with each other for decades now, often with intense laughter. I remain in awe of her brilliance, resilience, faith, compassion, and the many accomplishments that have touched the lives of so many. It's been a privilege.

Denise (Dee Dee) Henry Nix

CONTRIBUTORS

Latricia Allen, DPM, MPH, FACPM
Advanced Geriatrics Fellow
Birmingham Atlanta Geriatric Research Education and
    Clinical Center
Atlanta VA Health Care System;
Assistant Professor
Division of Geriatrics & Gerontology
Emory University
Decatur, Georgia

Rex E. Atwood, MD, MBA
Resident
Department of Surgery
Walter Reed National Military Medical Center
Bethesda, Maryland

**Frank Aviles Jr., PT, CWS, FACCWS, CLT-LANA, ALM,
    AWCC, DAPWCA**
Wound Care Clinical Coordinator
Wound Care/Lymphedema Instructor/Educator
Natchitoches Regional Medical Center
Natchitoches, Louisiana

Karen L. Bauer, DNP, APRN-FNP, CWS
Director of Wound Services
Nurse Practitioner
Division of Vascular, Endovascular, and Wound Surgery
University of Toledo
Toledo, Ohio

**Janice M. Beitz, PhD, RN, CS, CNOR, CWOCN-A, CNRP,
    ANEF, FNAP, FAAN**
Professor
WOCNEP Director
School of Nursing
Rutgers University
Camden, New Jersey

Greg Bohn, MD, ABPM/UHM, FACS, FACHM, FAAWC
President Board
American Board of Wound Healing
Onekama, Michigan

Kathleen Borchert, MS, RN, APRN, CNS, CWOCN, CFCN
Program Manager
WOC Departments
M Health Fairview University of Minnesota Hospital,
Minneapolis, Minnesota;
M Health Fairview Southdale Hospital
Edina, Minnesota;
M Health Fairview Ridges Hospital
Burnsville, Minnesota;
Faculty Member

WEB WOC Nursing Education Programs,
Minneapolis, Minnesota

Jacalyn Anne Brace, PhD, ANP-BC, RN-BC, WOC Nurse
Owner & CEO, Advanced Wound Healing Consultants
Affiliate Clinical Faculty, Rowan University and School of
    Nursing & Health Professions, Glassboro, New Jersey

Matthew J. Bradley, MD
Commander, US Navy
Board Certified, General Surgery and Trauma Critical Care
Trauma, Critical Care and General Surgeon
Program Director, General Surgery Residency;
Professor of Surgery, Department of Surgery Uniformed
    Services University of the Health Sciences & the Walter
    Reed National Military Medical Center
Bethesda, Maryland

Ruth A. Bryant, PhD, RN, CWOCN_Retired/Emeritus
Principal Research Scientist
Abbott Northwestern Hospital
Minneapolis, Minnesota;
Affiliate Faculty, School of Nursing, University of Minnesota,
    Minneapolis, Minnesota;
Visiting Professor, Universidad Panamericana Nursing
    School, Mexico City, Mexico;
President and Owner,
Bryant WOC Consulting,
    St. Paul, Minnesota
Immediate Past-President
Association for the Advancement of Wound Care

Lisa Q. Corbett, DNP, APRN, ACNS-BC, CWOCN
Advanced Practice Program Manager
Wound Programs
Hartford Healthcare
Hartford, Connecticut

Renee Cordrey, PT, PhD(c), MSPT, MPH, CWS, FAAWC
Physical Therapist
Enhabit Home Health
Williamsburg, Virginia;
Adjunct Professor
Department of Health
Human Function, and Rehabilitation Sciences
The George Washington University
Washington, District of Columbia

Joshua R. Dilley, MD
Clinical Assistant Professor,
Plastic and Reconstructive Surgery
Wake Forest University School of Medicine Atrium Health
    Wake Forest Baptist
Winston-Salem, North Carolina

Vickie R. Driver, DPM, MS, FACFAS, FAAWC
Chair, Wound Care Collaborative Community;
Professor, University of Virginia, Virginia
Professor, Affiliate Podiatric
Podiatric Medicine and Surgery
Barry University, Miami Shores, Florida;
Honorary Visiting Professor
Medicine, Cardiff University,
Cardiff University
Cardiff, United Kingdom

Scott Ellis, BA, MD
Research Fellow
Vascular Surgery
Mt. Sinai
New York, New York

Eric A. Elster, MD
Professor and Chair
Surgery
Uniformed Services University of the Health Sciences
Bethesda, Maryland

JoAnn Ermer-Seltun, MS, RN, ARNP, FNP-BC, CWOCN, CFCN
President, Co-Director & Faculty
WEB WOC Nursing Education Programs
Minneapolis, Minnesota;
Family Nurse Practitioner & Certified WOC Nurse
Continence & Wound Clinic
Mercy One North Iowa Medical Center
Mason City, Iowa

Brenda Freymiller, RN, BSN, MBA, CWON, CWS, CHRN
Director, Wound Care
Intermountain Healthcare
Salt Lake City, Utah

Tiffany Hamm, BSN, RN, CWS, ACHRN, UHMSADS
Principal Partner
Midwest Hyperbaric, LLC
Overland Park, Kansas

Vicki Haugen, MPH, BSN, RN, CWOCN
WOC Consultant
Boothbay Harbor, Maine

Sheila Howes-Trammel, MSN, APRN, FNP-BC, CWCN, CCCN, CFCN, CLNC
Family Nurse Practitioner
Medicine Department
Hennepin County Medical Center
Instructor, WEB WOC Nursing Education
  Programs
Minneapolis, Minnesota;
Visiting Professor, Universidad Panamericana Nursing
  School, Mexico City, Mexico

Jennifer Hurlow, GNP-BC, CWCN
Wound Nurse Practitioner
Wound Clinic
Advanced Wound Care
Southaven, Tennessee

Lindsay Kalan, BSc, PhD
Associate Professor
Department of Biochemistry & Biomedical Sciences
Michael G. DeGroote Institute for Infectious Disease Research
David Braley Center for Antibiotic Discovery
McMaster University
Hamilton, Ontario, Canada

Geness Koumandakis, BSRT, RRT, CHT
Hyperbaric Respiratory Therapy Coordinator and Safety
  Director
Hyperbaric Medicine
Intermountain Healthcare
Salt Lake City, Utah

John C. Lantis, II, MD
Chief and Professor, Surgery
Mount Sinai West Hospital and Icahn School of Medicine
New York, New York

Marc Robert Matthews, MD, MS, MCG, FACS, FASGS
Staff Surgeon
Surgery
Creighton University
Phoenix, Arizona

Catherine T. Milne, MSN, APRN, ANP/ACNS-BC, CWOCN-AP
Advanced Practice Wound, Ostomy, Continence Nurse
Connecticut Clinical Nursing Associates
Bristol, Connecticut;
Advanced Practice Wound, Ostomy, Continence Nurse
Department of Surgery
Bristol Hospital
Bristol, Connecticut

Jeffrey Mize, RRT CHT, CWCA
Principal Partner
Midwest Hyperbaric, LLC
Overland Park, Kansas

Joseph A. Molnar, MD, PhD
Professor
Plastic and Reconstructive Surgery and Regenerative Medicine
Wake Forest University School of Medicine
Winston-Salem, North Carolina

Victoria Nalls, PhD, GNP-BC, ACHPN, CWS
Director of Learning & Development CareBridge Health
Nashville, TN
Adjunct Faculty
Organizational Systems and Adult Health
University of Maryland School of Nursing
Baltimore, Maryland

Munier Nazzal, MD, MBA, FRCS(UK), FACS, RVT, RPVI, FACC WS
Professor, Surgery
Chief, Division of Vascular Surgery and Endovascular
    Surgery
Heart and Vascular Center
Toledo, Ohio

Debra S. Netsch, DNP, APRN, FNP-BC, CWOCN-AP, CFCN
Co-Director and Faculty
WEB WOC Nurse Education Programs
Minneapolis, Minnesota;
Advanced Practice WOC Nurse
Wound & Hyperbaric Healing Center
Ridgeview Medical Center
Waconia, Minnesota

Ann Marie Nie, PhD, MSN, FNP-BC, CNP, CWOCN
Wound Nurse Practitioner
Dayton Children's Hospital,
    Dayton, Ohio, Board of Directors, National Pressure
    Injury Advisory Panel
Westford, Massachusetts

Denise P. Nix, RN, MS, CWOCN
Wound, Ostomy, Continence Nurse
M Health Fairview Hospitals and Clinics
Minneapolis, Minnesota;
Subject Matter Expert, Patient Safety
Minnesota Hospital Association
St. Paul, Minnesota;
Consultant
Nix Consulting LLC
Minneapolis, Minnesota

Alisha Oropallo, MD, FACS, FSVS, FAPWCA, FABWMS
Professor of Surgery, Zucker
    School of Medicine,
    Hofstra/Northwell;
Program Director, Wound and Burn Fellowship, Northwell
    Health;
Medical Director
Comprehensive Wound Healing Center and Hyperbarics
Northwell Health
New Hyde Park, New York

Nanjin J. Park-McRae, DPM
Podiatry Specialist
Outside In Clinic
Portland, Oregon

Waqaas Quraishi, MD
Board Certified Pain, Physical Medicine & Rehabilitation
    Interventional Pain Management
Orthopedic SpineCare of Long Island
Huntington Station, New York

Catherine R. Ratliff, PhD, GNP-BC, CWOCN, CFCN, FAAN
Nurse Practitioner
Department of Surgery
University of Virginia Health
Charlottesville, Virginia

Gregory S. Schultz, PhD
Emeritus Professor
Obstetrics & Gynecology
University of Florida
Gainesville, Florida

Richard Simman, MD, FACS, FACCWS
Adjunct Professor
Wright State University
Dayton, Ohio;
Wound Care Program Director
Plastic and Reconstructive Surgery
ProMedica Health System
Toledo, Ohio

Elaine Horibe Song, MD, PhD, MBA
CEO
Wound Reference, Inc.
Moraga, California

William H. Tettelbach, MD, FCAP, FIDSA, FUHM, MAPWCA, CWSP
Executive Medical Director, Wound & Hyperbaric Medicine
    Service Line - Mountain Division, HCA Healthcare;
Adjunct Assistant Professor Undersea and Hyperbaric
    Medicine,
Duke University School of Medicine
Durham, North Carolina;
Adjunct Professor Podiatric Medicine & Surgery
Western University of Health Sciences
Pomona, California;
Medical Director Wound Care & Infection Prevention,
    Encompass Health & Rehabilitation Hospital of Utah;
Medical Director of Infectious Diseases & Wound Care,
Western Peaks Specialty Hospital,
Bountiful, Utah;
Former Executive System Director & Founder of the Wound &
    HBO2 Medicine Service Line - Intermountain Healthcare;
Former Program Director of Duke University Undersea &
    Hyperbaric Medicine Fellowship - Salt Lake City, UT

Lucian G. Vlad, MD
Assistant Professor
Plastic & Reconstructive Surgery
Wake Forest School of Medicine
Winston-Salem, North Carolina

Annette B. Wysocki, PhD, RN, FAAN
Dean and Professor
School of Nursing
Stony Brook University
Stony Brook, New York

This sixth edition of our textbook is a testament to the significant improvements we as clinicians and scientists have experienced in wound care over the past 5 years. In this edition, we have made a concerted effort to maintain the excellent content we have provided in the past and embellish it with more diversity in clinical examples and contributors, as well as an expansion of content to include wound care across the healthcare spectrum. In this edition, it was very important for us to emphasize that this text is for the novice as well as the seasoned wound care clinician and that it crosses all disciplines. *Acute and Chronic Wounds: Intraprofessionals From Novice to Expert* includes previous and new authors to reflect the interdisciplinary nature of the wound care discipline, which is so fundamental to providing excellent care to our patients. Our authors are scientists, researchers, and clinical experts; they are leaders in their field with the expertise to convey to you, the reader, the salient aspects of their discipline in a way that can be readily applied to your clinical practice.

Unique additions to this edition are several. First, we added chapters to address billing and reimbursement in the outpatient setting, wound care in the postacute care setting, wound care provided remotely using telehealth technology, the impact of traditional and alternative medications in wound care, and quality metrics and tracking. Second, we consolidated our presentation of pressure injury prevention and management into two chapters to facilitate the readers' ability to easily access content. We also added content to describe the early detection of pressure-induced tissue damage through the adoption of new technologies: early detection that precedes visual cues. Third, we expanded our color plates to include an additional 50 color plates! In this edition, we also grouped many plates to consolidate the variety of examples on a particular topic to assist the reader in appreciating the diversity of manifestations of many complex skin and wound conditions. Last, we are very proud that our textbook does not shy away from presenting tough subjects that may be either controversial (such as the nomenclature for the staging system for pressure injuries/ulcers) or lacking in clarity in definition such as slough.

We are also proud to have maintained the quality attributes for which our textbook is known. We avoid redundancy among the chapters so that a topic presented in one chapter does not overlap in another chapter; we like the "one and done" concept in that regard! We also work to ensure consistency between the chapters. For example, recommendations on the values for ABI will be the same from chapter to chapter. You will also find, as with our previous editions, an integration of all relevant national and international guidelines throughout this textbook. However, this textbook is not a regurgitation of guidelines; rather, it provides insight into the application of guidelines into best practice and the implementation of guidelines in the clinical setting.

Thank you for all that you do to improve the quality of care not only for our patients with a wound but also, more importantly, in the upstream prevention you incorporate into your practice so that we can one day truly succeed in preventing the wounds that are so prevalent in our individual practices today. We are confident that you will find this edition beneficial to enrich the breadth and depth of your clinical practice.

ACKNOWLEDGMENTS

We acknowledge the Elsevier staff—especially Tina Kaemmerer and Uma Natarajan—for navigating through the business challenges during a worldwide pandemic so that we could finally get this book published. Phew! We experienced many unique hurdles during this time but through your commitment, hard work, and patience, we were able to make this sixth edition a reality!

Ruth and DeeDee

CONTENTS

Principles for Practice Development to Facilitate Outcomes and Productivity

Ruth A. Bryant and Denise P. Nix

OBJECTIVES

1. Describe the services provided by the wound specialist.
2. Identify the value in a legally defensible certification process.
3. Describe the data that are collected and used to drive practice and justify the wound specialist position.
4. Provide an example of two stakeholders and why they hold that position in a skin and wound care practice.
5. Cite three examples of how the wound specialist can affect cost savings within a care setting.

A comprehensive wound care program is essential to any organization, agency, or healthcare system offering a full scope of services to its clientele. The wound specialist can provide a multitude of valuable services: state-of-the-art, evidence-based wound management; staff education; control of wound-related costs; quality improvement activities; protocol and formulary development; pressure injury risk reduction; and insight into efficient use of personnel and resources. The wound specialist is instrumental in bringing together many departments to more fully appreciate and manage the condition of the patient with a wound. In addition, the wound specialist can affect the quality of care in an organization or agency through administrative activities, collaboration with materials management personnel, establishment of a skin safety team, and provision of direct and indirect patient care through consultation and staff education.

Many factors contribute to a successful practice as a wound specialist. Obviously, the specialist must have a strong knowledge base in wound care and the relevant pathologies. In addition, the specialist must establish credibility, which is earned by demonstrating clinical competence, critical thinking, organization, self-confidence, and an eagerness to collaborate and share information with colleagues. However, a successful practice also requires the wound specialist to integrate business skills to develop goals that reflect the organization's mission and goals, effectively define services, identify benefits of services, outline a marketing approach to potential referral sources, and draft a conservative but realistic budget. Many

decision-making tools and clinical resources are needed in a wound management program. The wound specialist would be wise to assemble a business plan for new skin/wound care program. Components of a business plan are listed in Chapter 2, Box 2.1. This chapter discusses the application of business skills in terms of qualifications, role development, time management, data collection, marketing, value-added services, and outcomes measurement.

EDUCATIONAL PREPARATION OF THE WOUND SPECIALIST

When an organization is developing a skin and wound management program, it is incumbent upon the administration to demand appropriate educational preparation, qualifications, and credentialing of the healthcare professional who will function as the wound specialist. Appropriate education and certification should not be confused with attendance at individual seminars or continuing education courses. Upon completion of a continuing education course, the attendee receives a certificate of completion. However, in no way should this certificate of completion be misconstrued as an indication of the attendee's expertise, mastery, or competence. The certificate simply denotes the individual's attendance at the educational event. Chapter 6 (Quality tracking) is a must-read for any wound specialist. The value of legally defensible wound certification to any healthcare quality management program is described in greater detail.

NATIONAL CERTIFICATION: VALUE AND ROUTES

National certification yields many benefits to the individual, the employer, and the patient (Box 1.1) (Bonham, 2009; Cary, 2001; Fleck, 2008; Woods, 2002). National certification is the formal recognition of an individual's knowledge and expertise in a defined functional or clinical area of care. National certification is intended to protect the public and should validate an individual's specialty knowledge, experience, and clinical judgment. Not all programs are legally defensible or psychometrically sound. The following components of the organization providing the certification are important to assess national accreditation, eligibility criteria (educational degree, formal wound care education, structured clinical practicum in wound care, prior clinical experience), and recertification requirements. Collectively, these components influence the extent to which the certification designation is legally defensible.

National Accreditation and Testing Standards

Accreditation of the certifying organization by an independent national certifying body is important because accreditation denotes the certifying organization's compliance with national standards relevant to all aspects of the certification process. Additionally, accreditation ensures that the certification credential meets specific criteria consistent with a testing process that is psychometrically sound (i.e., accuracy and effectiveness of each test item). A strong psychometric foundation underlying the certifying process assures candidates of accuracy of content and fairness in the testing process.

Eligibility Criteria

A key distinction among the certification designations is the education and clinical experience criterion for eligibility.

BOX 1.1   Value of Certification

Consumer's (Patient's) Perspective
- Patients are aware that specialty certifications exist
- Patients want to receive care from certified staff
- Patients are more confident when they are cared for by certified staff

Administrator's Perspective
- Certification is associated with job satisfaction and retention
- Certified staff have greater skill competence and less risk for error or harm
- Certified staff have better skill-related knowledge and skill performance than noncertified staff

Certified Individual's Perspective
- Colleagues recognize certified staff as experts
- Certified staff have job satisfaction
- Certified staff have significant positive impact on patient care and safety
- Managers express preference for hiring certified staff
- Certified staff have advancement potential
- Certification provides more effective resource to staff

Eligible disciplines and their educational preparation differ among certifying organizations. For example, the designation CWOCN© (Certified Wound, Ostomy, Continence Nurse) is bestowed only upon eligible baccalaureate-prepared nurses, whereas other certifications are available to all nurses regardless of educational preparation.

Preexamination wound-specific coursework and clinical practicum requirements vary among certifying organizations. Coursework requirements can range from 0 to 5 days to many weeks. Similarly, required clinical experience varies among certifying bodies, ranging from "experience" with care, management, or research related to wounds to a more rigorous competency-based precepted clinical practicum to facilitate integration of new knowledge into an actual patient care setting in the presence of a qualified, experienced expert.

Recertification Requirements

In the ever-changing world of wound care and the need to stay current, recertification requirements are critically important and vary among credentialing organizations. Required frequency of recertification is 5 or 10 years, depending on the organization. Methods of recertification vary significantly and include self-assessment, proof of experience, and retesting.

ROLES, FUNCTIONS, AND RESPONSIBILITIES OF A WOUND SPECIALIST

The wound specialist is not responsible for conducting every wound assessment or dressing change. Clarity in terms of expectations of the wound specialist, staff nurse, and physical therapist (PT) is essential to promote collaboration and deliver comprehensive and effective skin and wound care. This clear delineation of roles is important to foster an empowering environment, avoid duplication of efforts, and maximize the efficient use of resources, including personnel. Table 1.1 provides examples to delineate roles of a wound specialist and a staff nurse.

Participation in staff orientation programs is a key strategy to communicate roles, functions, and responsibilities. This setting offers an opportunity to orient new staff members to their role in maintaining skin health, providing wound care, performing skin assessment and surveillance, performing risk assessment, and preventing pressure injuries. It is critical to provide guidance to staff on when and how to access the wound specialist. Key stakeholders (e.g., physicians, information technology personnel, purchasing director, materials management, director of nursing) should be contacted to describe and clarify the role of the wound specialist. Nurturing a relationship with key stakeholders to highlight the benefits of a skin and wound care program, the role of the wound specialist and the impact on patient safety is critical to enhancing the success of the program and the position. Ultimately, however, the wound specialist will need to demonstrate competence and confidence in his or her practice. Regardless of the healthcare setting in which the wound

TABLE 1.1   Delineation of Roles of Wound Specialist and Staff Nurse

Wound and Skin Specialist	Staff Nurse
Facilitate creation and implementation of pressure injury risk assessment protocol	Conduct risk assessment per protocol
Establish protocol for prevention guidelines to correlate with risk assessment	Implement appropriate risk reduction interventions
Establish protocols for management of minor skin lesions (candidiasis, skin tears, incontinence-associated dermatitis, Stage 1 and 2 pressure injuries)	Implement appropriate care of minor skin lesions
Formulate skin and wound care product formulary to specify indications and parameters for use of products	Use wound products per formulary. Notify wound specialist if product performs poorly or if expected outcome is not achieved
Conduct comprehensive assessment, establish plan of care for complex patients (e.g., leg injuries, Stages 3 and 4 pressure injuries), conduct regular reevaluation of healing	Notify wound specialist of complex patients. Conduct focused wound assessment. Implement appropriate care per wound specialist's direction and facility protocols
Provide competency-based staff education for new employees and annual competency-based education for existing employees	Identify and recommend topics of interest for staff education and updates
Track outcomes and identify skin and wound care issues. Initiate quality improvement activities	Participate in quality improvement activities

BOX 1.2   Roles of the Wound Specialist

Consultant/Expert

- Evaluates patient response to treatment and the progress of wound healing, making adjustments and modifications as indicated
- Where qualified and appropriate, provides conservative sharp debridement of devitalized tissue and applies silver nitrate to epibole, granulation tissue, and areas with minor bleeding
- Provides consultation and follow-up for patients with draining or chronic wounds, fistulas, or percutaneous tubes through outpatient clinic visits and/or phone consultations; initiates appropriate referrals for medical or surgical intervention

Educator

- Provides appropriate education to patient, caregiver, and staff regarding skin care, wound management, percutaneous tubes, and draining wound/fistula management
- Assists staff to maintain current knowledge and competence in the areas of skin and wound care through orientation and regularly scheduled education
- Attends continuing education programs related to skin and wound management

Change Agent (see Tables 1.2 and 1.3)

- Identifies barriers to change
- Provides evidence that persuades staff that change will achieve desired outcome
- Considers all stakeholders when planning change
- Communicates aspects of practice changes that will positively affect key stakeholders (especially the staff expected to implement the change)

Program Coordinator/Leader

- Provides consultation and assistance to staff in developing and implementing protocols used in the identification and management of patients with potential or actual alteration in skin integrity
- Provides guidance to staff in implementation of protocols to identify, control, or eliminate etiologic factors for skin breakdown, including selection of appropriate support surface
- Establishes protocols and guidelines for appropriate and cost-effective use of therapeutic support surfaces
- Maintains records and statistics and submits reports to employer
- Analyzes inventory and recommends appropriate additions and deletions to ensure quality and cost-effectiveness of products used for skin and wound care
- Serves on agency-wide committees and participates in agency-wide projects as requested
- Coordinates wound management teams or committees

Facilitator of EBP and Quality Improvement

- Assists staff to maintain current state-of-the-art practice by reviewing and revising policies and procedures to be consistent with national guidelines and other sources of evidence-based literature
- Provides leadership with prevalence and incidence studies
- Conducts product evaluations or contributes to research studies related to skin and wound care when indicated; submits reports and recommendations based on results
- Participates in public policy through guideline development, consensus statements, advisory panel membership, etc.

specialist will practice, role implementation will share common overlapping components: clinical consultant/expert, leader/coordinator, educator, change agent, and facilitator of evidence-based practice (EBP) and quality improvement to improve outcomes (Box 1.2).

Consultant

Although many wound specialists provide direct care for patients with the most complex wounds, in most settings the wound specialist serves primarily as a consultant. As a consultant, the specialist can better meet the majority of patients' needs by coordinating a skin and wound care program implemented by a multidisciplinary team of healthcare providers. The consultant role builds on the foundations of the wound specialist's clinical expertise in wound-related pathophysiology, physical assessment, wound assessment, appropriate use of interventions, and documentation. A successful consultant must effectively communicate, collaborate, and educate. Clinical decision-making tools and resources, such as protocols, product formularies, and clinical practice guidelines, pave the way for the specialist to adopt a consultative approach within the organization (Murad, 2017; Pasek, Geyser, Sidoni, et al., 2008).

Educator

Knowledge about skin inspection, pressure injury prevention, basic wound care, and comprehensive, accurate documentation is essential to maintaining and restoring skin integrity. Information about wound and skin care is increasingly accessible in print and electronically via webinars. Reimbursement restrictions provide greater incentive for staff to familiarize themselves with basic skin care and pressure injury prevention. However, the wound specialist needs to triage and prioritize the available information so that it best meets the organization's needs and is in a clinically useful and familiar format. Resources typically needed in the clinical setting include (1) a formulary of wound and skin care products, (2) a process and algorithm for selecting and ordering an appropriate support surface, and (3) standard of care to prevent pressure injuries or to manage common situations such as skin tears and perianal denudement. As an educator, the wound specialist will develop routine orientation sessions to introduce new staff to the pressure injury prevention program, addressing, for example, basic wound assessment, support surface selection, and the essential nature of skin inspection and risk assessment.

By auditing chart documentation or surveying the staff's knowledge about specific areas of wound care, the specialist can identify additional needs and target follow-up educational activities to satisfy those needs (Beeckman, Clays, Van Hecke, et al., 2013). Beitz, Fey, and O'Brien (1999) warn that "professional staff who perceive little need for additional wound care education may 'tune out' opportunities for increasing their knowledge base because they consider themselves 'competent'". This information underscores the importance of using pretests and other means of educational needs assessments; however, education does not guarantee practice change.

Change Agent

Staff education is a critical role for the wound specialist and should be viewed as an innovation that will decrease workload and improve patient outcomes. The infusion of innovation adaptation principles can be used to increase the likelihood of success with educational efforts. Rogers' *Diffusion of Innovations* (2003) provides a framework for changing practices in a group, individual, or organization (Rogers, 2003). This theory describes how people adopt innovations using five stages: knowledge, persuasion, decision, implementation, and confirmation (Table 1.2).

TABLE 1.2 Five Stages of Rogers's Innovation-Decision Process

Stage	Description
Knowledge	Individual becomes aware of an innovation and of how it functions. May occur with reading, reviewing posted flyers, attending lectures
Persuasion	Favorable or unfavorable attitude toward an innovation forms. To form a favorable attitude, the individual must be convinced that the innovation has greater value than current practice (e.g., identify patients at risk for pressure injuries or target appropriate interventions)
Decision	Individual receives enough information to form an opinion about innovation. Individual pursues activities that lead to adoption or rejection of the innovation
Implementation	Once an individual makes a decision to adopt the innovation, barriers (structural, process, psychological) to implementation must be overcome (e.g., adequate number of forms is available)
Confirmation	Individual seeks to reinforce his or her decision. Observable and positive results are critical at this stage to prevent a reversal in decision. Careful monitoring is required, and information validating positive effects is important (e.g., decrease in incidence of pressure injuries after adoption of new risk assessment tool)

Adapted from Landrum, B. J. (1998). Marketing innovations to nurses, Part 1: How people adopt innovations. *The Journal of Wound, Ostomy and Continence Nursing, 25*,194–199.

Innovation is more likely to be adopted when it is perceived as relevant and consistent with the individual's attitudes and the attitudes of colleagues. Five attributes of an innovation significantly influence the rate at which it is adopted: relative advantage, compatibility, complexity, trialability, and observability (Table 1.3). To enhance likelihood of successful adaptation, these attributes should be integrated and addressed prior to the persuasion stage.

Facilitator of Evidence-Based Practice and Quality Improvement

The wound specialist serves a pivotal role in facilitating and implementing EBP and quality improvement (QI) studies within the context of skin and wound care for the facility or agency. Examples of QI activities that the wound specialist could participate in are discussed later in this chapter. Many wound specialists have a role in public policy through guideline development, consensus statements, advisory panel membership, and research. These activities have helped shape public policy by strengthening the evidence base and

TABLE 1.3 Attributes that Influence Adoption of Innovation	
Attributes of Innovation	**Description**
Relative advantage	Is this better than an existing practice (e.g., potential decrease in costs, decrease in staff time, ease of use)?
Compatibility	Is this consistent with the individual's existing values, experiences, and needs?
Complexity	Is this innovation difficult to understand or use? For example, when a protocol is developed that links risk assessment scores with nursing interventions, the decision about which preventive nursing intervention to use may be perceived as less complex than before the protocol; therefore, the protocol may be more likely to be adopted
Trialability	Can the individual experiment with the innovation on a limited basis?
Observability	Are the results of an innovation visible to others? Subtle outcomes are harder to communicate to others, so the innovation often is slower to be adopted

Adapted from Landrum, B. J. (1998). Marketing innovations to nurses, Part 1: How people adopt innovations. *Journal of Wound Ostomy & Continence Nursing, 25,* 194–199.

educating lawmakers to help improve outcomes through better access to appropriate supplies, equipment, and services.

Translating and applying these new resources or pieces of knowledge into practice requires an EBP or QI approach. Regardless of the type of project being planned (i.e., EBP, QI, or research), the first step in the process is to formulate and refine a question. PICOT is a common format recommended for phrasing the question. A well-designed PICOT question contains the following pieces of information: P (patient population), I (intervention or issue of interest), C (comparison intervention or group, O (outcome), and T (timeframe). This type of narrowly defined question facilitates the search so as to obtain the most relevant and best evidence (Melnyk & Fineout-Overholt, 2019).

Evidence-Based Care

Integrating evidence into practice is a fundamental expectation of the wound specialist and a key component of an EBP. Defined as "the integration of best research evidence with clinical expertise and patient values to facilitate clinical decision making" (Sackett, Strauss, Richardson, et al., 2000), EBP acknowledges that the care provided to patients should not be based on habit, but rather supported by the best possible evidence of effectiveness. Evidence-based practice requires consideration of the following types of evidence: external evidence (i.e., research, theories, expert panel), internal evidence (i.e., clinical expertise, QI, patient data), and patient

preferences and values (Melnyk & Fineout-Overholt, 2019). Providing evidence-based care requires that we *synthesize* the best available evidence from what is currently known.

Many individual and organizational barriers exist to research utilization and evidence-based care (Melnyk & Fineout-Overholt, 2019). One individual barrier is feeling inadequately prepared to evaluate the quality of research and a lack of knowledgeable colleagues with whom to discuss research. In addition, access to the literature may be a hardship because of workload and time limitations. On an organizational level, barriers may arise from a lack of interest, motivation, vision, and strategy on the part of leadership. Organizational barriers also may be related to library access, the extent of library holdings, and Internet access. Recognizing and overcoming these barriers is important in order to positively impact implementation of EBP.

To embark on the path of evidence-based care, the specialist must keep abreast of relevant healthcare literature to "find the evidence." In the face of a constantly growing body of healthcare literature, remaining current in the literature may seem impossible or all consuming. However, preappraised literature is increasingly available that expedites access to evidence (Fineout-Overholt, Berryman, Hofstetter, et al., 2019).

Preappraised literature are products that have been developed by an individual or group that has reviewed the literature, filtered out the flawed studies, and included only the methodologically strongest studies. A hierarchy of preappraised literature with relevant examples is given in Fig. 1.1. Such sources include practice guidelines, clinical pathways, evidence-based abstract journals, and systematic reviews. These types of pertinent resources are commonly available on the website of professional organizations such as the Wound, Ostomy and Continence Nurses Society™, Wound Healing Society, Association for the Advancement of Wound Care, the Cochrane Collaboration, and the National Pressure Injury Advisory Panel/European Pressure Injury Advisory Panel/Pan Pacific Pressure Injury Alliance.

When appraised literature relative to a particular clinical issue is not available, unprocessed resources are necessary. Unprocessed resources are databases (e.g., CINAHL, MEDLINE, EMBASE) that contain millions of primarily original study citations (Table 1.4). The Web is a source of unprocessed information. There are six criteria that can be used to assess the quality of healthcare information obtained from the Internet (Dalhousie University Libraries, 2020).

Two tools are essential when evaluating research: critical appraisal tools and reporting guidelines. Critical appraisal is an objective structured process used to understand the strengths and weaknesses of a study, specifically the reviewer is guided to appraise the research methods relative to rigor, reliability, and bias (Table 1.5). Similarly, reporting guidelines have been developed that stipulate essential criteria when reporting research as a means of adding clarity and standardizing how research is reported (Table 1.6). Most publishers require authors of research, EBP and QI to adhere to the relevant reporting guideline.

The value of research-based care to the organization and the patient is significant. Results of a metaanalysis of studies have

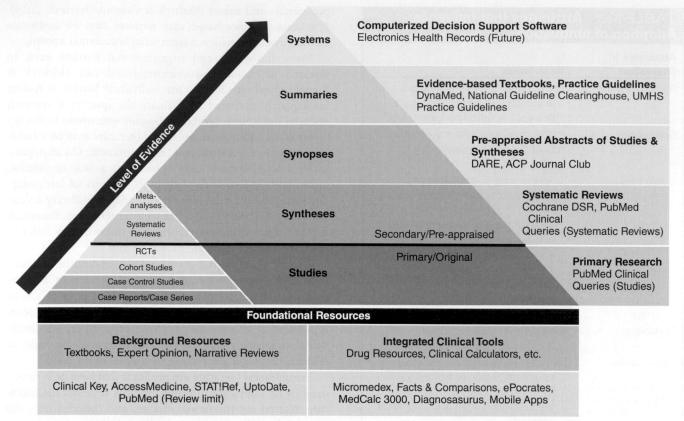

Fig 1.1 Sources for evidence-based research. Modified from Haynes, R. B. (2006). Of studies, syntheses, synopses, summaries and systems: The "5S" evolution of services for evidence-based healthcare decisions. *ACP Journal Club, 145*(3), A8–A9.

TABLE 1.4	Unprocessed Sources of Evidence		
Database	**Maintained by**	**Unique Features**	**Contents**
CINAHL	Information systems and updated quarterly	Largest bibliographic database specifically related to nursing, allied health disciplines, and consumer health	Full text articles Clinical practice guidelines Bibliographies of major articles Research instruments Government publications Comments Book reviews Evaluations of multimedia and computer software and systems Patient education materials
MEDLINE	United States National Library of Medicine	Readily accessible Searching effectively requires thorough knowledge of how database is structured and publications are indexed	Comprehensive coverage of health care journals
EMBASE	Elsevier Science	Comprehensive bibliographic database of worldwide literature Requires thorough knowledge of how database is structured and publications are indexed	Biomedical and pharmaceutical literature fields Indexes large proportion of European biomedical and science literature

TABLE 1.5 Criteria for Evaluating Internet Health Information

Criteria	Description
Credibility	Includes source, currency, relevance/utility, and editorial review process for the information and disclosure of sponsorship and motivation as provider of information
Content	Must be accurate, complete, and provide an appropriate disclaimer
Disclosure	Includes informing the user of the purpose of the site, as well as any profiling or collection of information associated with site use
Links	Critical to quality of the site; should lead users to verify content on the site, lead users to other reliable sources of information
Design	Encompasses accessibility, logical organization (navigability), and internal search capability and content reflects reading level of the user
Interactivity	Includes feedback mechanisms and means for information exchange among users

Adapted from Dalhouseie University Dalhouse Libraries. (2020). Evaluation of health information on the web. https://dal.ca.libguides.com/c.php?g=257155. Accessed December 8, 2020.

demonstrated that research-based care offers patients better outcomes than does routine procedural care. However, the wound specialist not only should *apply* evidence to practice, but also should *generate* evidence from practice (Ehrenberg, Fraser, & Gunningberg, 2004). Evidence can be generated by publishing individual case studies or by partnering with doctoral-prepared researchers to design and conduct basic research that answers clinically relevant questions.

Historically, a gap in healthcare has existed between what is known and what is practiced. The wound specialist has a critical leadership role in making EBP a reality. When leaders not only expect but also promote EBP to staff, quality of care is enhanced, and optimal patient outcomes are achieved. Caregivers are most effective at integrating research into practice when the leader is clinically based, has specific clinical expertise and knowledge, and expresses a positive attitude toward research.

Evidence ranking. Evidence derives from many sources, and each source has its own merits and deficiencies. Clinical observations, expert opinions, and generalizations from physiology constitute the weakest forms of evidence. Systematic studies, such as clinical trials, prospective studies, and case studies, provide a higher level of evidence. Typical classification schemes place the metaanalysis and randomized clinical trial (RCT) as the highest levels of evidence because they are designed to reduce the risk of bias and have less risk of

TABLE 1.6 Guide for Evaluating Intervention-Based Research

Steps	Description	Related Study Design Questions
1. Are the results valid?	The study must be designed and conducted in a valid manner so that the results are believable and credible. A study design that is less than rigorous and contains sources of bias will generate skewed and false conclusions. Only when the study methods are valid and rigorous should the reader continue on to further assess the study results	Did intervention and control groups begin the study with a similar prognosis? Were patients randomized? Was randomization concealed? Were patients analyzed in the groups to which they were randomized? Were groups shown to be similar in all known determinants of outcome, or were analyses adjusted for differences? Did intervention and control groups retain a similar prognosis after the study started? Were patients aware of group allocation? Were clinicians aware of group allocation? Were outcome assessors aware of group allocation? Was follow-up complete?
2. What are the results?	Any difference between the groups in the study will be expressed in terms of a risk measure, such as risk reduction or benefit increase. The accuracy of the risk measure (the effect of the intervention) will be expressed in terms of a confidence interval or p-value. In general, a narrow confidence interval, which does not include zero, suggests more precision and, therefore, greater confidence in the results	How large was the intervention effect? How precise was the estimate of the intervention effect?
3. How can results be applied to patient care?	The patients in the wound care specialist's practice should be similar to the patient population that participated in the study if the research results are to be applied to them	Were the study patients similar to the patients in my clinical setting? Were all of the important outcomes considered? Are the likely intervention benefits worth the potential harm and costs?

systematic errors. However, not all clinical questions can be researched using an RCT design (e.g., rare conditions, ethical concerns). In addition, the RCT is not an appropriate design for a prognosis or diagnosis question. Therefore different specialties and organizations often adopt variations in the classification scheme to best meet the types of questions being posed, yet all share common threads with the goal of providing a consistent method for interpreting the quality of evidence. The Johns Hopkins Nursing EBP (https://hopkinsmedicine.org) and the Centre for Evidence-Based Medicine (CEBM) (http://www.cebm.net) are valuable resources for detailed information about evidence appraisal and levels of evidence).

Quality Improvement

Quality improvement activities incorporate elements of research methods and are a high priority for the wound specialist. Quality improvement initiatives often are initiated to improve processes that will decrease cost, save time, or improve patient or staff satisfaction (Orsted, Rosenthal, & Woodbury, 2009). Evidence demonstrates that a facility's ongoing involvement in QI initiatives (including evidence-based guideline introduction and implementation, regular prevalence surveys, and annual national surveys) is associated with significant reductions in wounds within the facility (Bales & Duvendack, 2011; Bales & Padwojski, 2009; Kelleher, Moorer, & Makic, 2012). Such activities often consist of simple chart audits designed to ascertain the adequacy of documentation of assessment parameters, interventions, and effects or outcomes. These types of QI tools are discussed in more detail in Chapter 6.

Without a QI process, delays, inefficiencies, or harmful interventions may go undetected and thus contribute to staff or patient dissatisfaction, delayed discharge, or increased costs of care. Quality improvement activities that should be central to all wound care programs are prevalence and incidence studies and pressure injury prevention programs. See Chapter 6 for more information about quality tracking.

Program Coordinator

A fundamental need of any practice is a skin safety program consisting of skin and wound care policies, dressing change procedures, decision support tools, skin and wound care product formularies, support surface algorithms, and treatment protocols. Decision support tools enhance the clinician's decision-making capacity (Ehrenberg et al., 2004), thus empowering caregivers to act independently and wisely in a consistent fashion. Specifically, treatment protocols guide staff to (1) address critical assessment parameters, (2) perform steps of assessment and treatment procedures in a proper sequence, (3) learn proper application and utilization of specific products, and (4) assess the effectiveness of interventions (Pasek et al., 2008).

Policies and procedures are essential for guiding the delivery of care and meeting standards required by The Joint Commission and state health departments. Relative to skin and wound care, each facility or healthcare organization should develop policies for skin assessment, pressure injury risk assessment, wound cleansing, wound assessment,

treatment of wounds, documentation and staging, compression therapy, debridement, and culturing. In addition, a policy should exist to delineate appropriate interventions for different levels of pressure injury risk, as well as for high-risk patients. Examples of policies, procedures, and decision-making tools are given in Appendix A.

Skin and wound assessment parameters (see Chapter 10) should be incorporated into the admission database to ensure that the data are collected. Such data can also be incorporated into daily documentation flow sheets. Flow sheets that are dedicated to wound assessment and wound care interventions are particularly useful because they will best reflect changes in wound status over time at a glance. Documentation in multiple places increases the risk of errors, inconsistencies, and omissions and should be avoided. Electronic medical records are becoming more common in the healthcare setting but may not necessarily facilitate appropriate documentation or effective integration of wound- and skin-related EBP guidelines (Milne, Trigilia, Houle, et al., 2009). Therefore, it is critical that the wound specialist serve as content expert when choosing or building an electronic documentation system so that wound- and skin-specific data can be aggregated into relevant clinical information (Golinko, Clark, Rennert, et al., 2009).

Skin Safety Committees and Teams

Wound care is a team effort. Each member of the team has an invaluable and irreplaceable contribution. A team approach to wound care is critical to achieve consistency in care and to provide patient-centered care. The members of a team focus on working together to achieve a mutually agreed-upon goal, and team members are accountable for attaining the desired results. Functioning as a team requires commitment, shared expectations, and leadership (Moore, Butcher, Corbett, et al., 2014). The role of a "wound navigator" has also been proposed to facilitate the integration of the patient's perspective into a wound care plan.

Successful skin safety programs have reported the use of multidisciplinary meetings and interdisciplinary collaboration (Ackerman, 2011; Thomas, 2008; Tippet, 2009). As a leader and program coordinator, the wound specialist will develop programs and projects that reflect the needs of the patient population; are consistent with the priorities of the corporation; and are fiscally responsible, evidence based, and educationally and professionally valuable to the staff. A skin and wound care program is basic and essential to all care settings and facilities. In the United States, the gold standard for a comprehensive wound care program is a system-wide skin safety committee with unit-based skin care teams. Such programs consistently demonstrate enhanced clinical outcomes, reduced liability, increased staff satisfaction, and reduced costs (Andriessen, Polignano, & Abel, 2009; Chicano & Drolshagen, 2009; Hiser, Rochette, Philbin, et al., 2006; Lloyd-Vossen, 2009; McIsaac, 2007; Orsted et al., 2009). Keys to the success of a skin and wound care program are dissemination of information; involvement of all stakeholders; and consistent, intuitive documentation.

From a structural aspect, the program will need a mechanism for oversight of the program and for operationalizing the program at the bedside. Program oversight is provided by a system-wide committee (e.g., skin safety committee) that is responsible for creating policies and procedures, formularies, decision-making guides, documentation tools, and educational resources. This group also facilitates transfer of knowledge and guidelines to the unit and bedside (Lloyd-Vossen, 2009). Members of the skin safety committee providing oversight of the program are representative of all stakeholders and key decision makers, including administration, pharmacy, purchasing, and utilization review/risk management.

The success of the skin safety program ultimately lies in the ability to embed the program into the facilities infrastructure and operationalize the program at the unit level and on to the bedside. Operationalizing or implementing the skin safety program will be dictated by the size of the facility or agency, the magnitude of the existing skin and wound care needs, and the available personnel. The mechanism created for operationalizing the skin safety program requires identifying who will implement the program at the bedside. Small agencies or facilities often provide operationalization of the program and oversight. Larger facilities or agencies often identify unit-based nurse champions (described in the next section) for operationalization to the bedside.

Responsibilities and membership. Responsibilities and membership will vary according to the needs of the patient population, community laws, and the regulating bodies of the various disciplines involved. Membership of the Skin Safety Committee is listed in Box 1.3; responsibilities of this committee are listed in Box 1.4.

Certification in wound care. At least one member of the skin safety team should possess a legally defensible certification in wound care issued by an independent national certification organization that validates specialty knowledge, experience, and clinical judgment. As previously stated, this

---

BOX 1.3 Potential Members of a Skin Safety Committee

- Medical director
- Certified wound specialist
- Certified wound care nurse (CWCN©, CWON©, CWOCN©)
- Physical therapist
- Nursing leader
- Unit-based nurse champions
- Dietician
- Occupational therapist
- Speech therapist
- Quality management representative
- Consultants/ad hoc members
  - Infection control specialist
  - Dermatologist
  - Podiatrist
  - Orthotics specialist
  - Diabetologist
  - Gerontologist
  - Plastic surgeon
  - Information technologist
  - Vascular surgeon
  - Pharmacist

BOX 1.4 Skin Safety Committee Oversight Responsibilities

Protocols and Decision-Making Tools
- Decision-making tools linking risk assessment with preventive interventions
- Offloading (specialty beds, heels, chair cushions)
- Policies or guidelines for pressure injury prevention, assessment, and treatment
- Protocols for care of common clinical conditions (e.g., incontinence, incontinence-associated dermatitis, skin tears)

Formulary
- Skin care and continence products
- Wound care products
- Offloading products

Documentation
- Admission database to incorporate wound and skin assessment
- Ongoing documentation methods for prevention, assessment, and treatment
- Patient education

Education
- Patient education materials
- Staff educational needs assessment
- Staff orientation
- Annual education and competency
- Newsletter for just-in-time updates, announcements, learnings

Quality Management
- Review AHEs and RCA
- Implement infrastructure changes based on AHE and RCA findings
- Analyze unit-based reports for outcomes and trends

Research
- Clinical trials of products using standard evaluation protocols
- Prevalence and incidence studies
- Ongoing review of literature to maintain evidence-based practice

AHE, Adverse health event; *RCA,* root-cause analysis.

---

is particularly important for the delivery of quality outcomes and the ability to legally defend the validity of the certification. This member will serve as content expert specifically related to pressure injury prevention and wound care.

When this member is a certified wound, ostomy, and continence nurse (CWOCN©) or a certified wound care nurse (CWCN©), the committee reaps additional benefits. Wound, ostomy, and continence nursing is a specialty recognized by the American Nurses Association (WOCN®, 2017). Wound, ostomy, and continence nurses have expertise in a full range of skin issues (e.g., incontinence-associated dermatitis, tube site care, ostomy skin issues, complex fistula care) and the nurse's multifaceted role (WOCN®, 2011, 2017). Given the increased incidence of device-related pressure injuries (see Chapter 11), the nurse with this broader skill set is invaluable to the skin safety committee. A productivity survey of WOC nurses showed that two-thirds are prepared at the baccalaureate level and slightly less than one-third are prepared at the master's degree or doctorate level (WOCN®, 2012). The certified WOC nurse often serves as the skin and wound care program coordinator by (1) organizing outcomes measurement studies and prevalence and incidence studies; (2) providing individualized holistic patient assessments; (3) making recommendations for wound care products, adjunctive therapies, and specialty beds or equipment; (4) performing debridements, if within the individual's skill level and scope of practice; (5) providing ongoing assessment and evaluation of healing for patients with complex wounds; and (6) educating staff in the prevention, assessment, and treatment of skin and wound problems. Research has demonstrated faster healing when a WOC nurse is involved in the care of a patient with a wound (Bolton, McNees, van Rijswijk, et al., 2004; Harris & Shannon, 2008).

Director. The director of the skin safety team is ideally a provider. This person oversees ongoing treatment and overall management of patients with complex wounds. The director interacts as needed with primary and consulting providers to facilitate consistent and effective skin and wound management that is in alignment with overall patient goals. Responsibilities include, but are not limited to, assisting the facility in the development and implementation of policies and procedures for prevention and treatment of skin breakdown that are consistent with national guidelines. Ideally, the director of a skin safety team is a certified wound specialist. However, when supported by qualified and competent team members, a provider without certification can be highly effective.

Nursing. The registered nurse directs the development and implementation of an individualized plan of care based on the needs and goals assessed for the patient. Nursing focuses on risk assessment, early problem identification, preventive measures to promote skin integrity, and responses to treatments. The nurse documents and reports condition changes and revises the plan of care as necessary. In the United States, several training pathways for nurses are available, ranging from licensed practical nurses to registered nurse to advanced practice nurses and nurses with doctoral degrees. The nurse is instrumental in providing valuable patient-centered input to the committee.

Unit-based skin champions. As previously discussed, the success of the skin safety program ultimately lies with the ability and commitment of the nurse to operationalize the program at the unit level and on to the bedside. Unit-based champions are a core group of staff nurses with a special interest and additional education in skin health and wound management. This group of nurses becomes the "eyes and ears" of the program oversight committee. In addition, these unit-based skin care members are empowered to identify and problem-solve adverse clinical findings, such as Stage 1 pressure injuries and incontinence-associated dermatitis. Unit-based champions must be provided the information, tools, and resources and education they need to conduct staff education and lead the initiative for skin and wound care. A wound treatment associate (WTA) continuing education program is an example of additional education that can be

provided. The WTA is a credential designated to a registered nurse (RN), licensed practical nurse/licensed vocational nurse (LPN/LVN), or military medic with a certificate of completion from a WOCN®-endorsed WTA© continuing education program that functions under the direction of a supervising advanced practice registered nurse (APRN), WOC nurse, or physician (WOCN®, 2011). Continuing education for the WTA can be obtained onsite.

The process by which the unit-based skin team member functions is dictated by census, patient acuity, length of stay, and realistic staff expectations. In one scenario, the unit-based skin team members make rounds of all patients with a skin-related issue or a Braden scale rating less than 15 once or twice weekly, based on a list of patients to be seen provided by the charge nurse. Between rounds, any Stage 1 or 2 pressure injuries would be reported immediately to a member of the unit-based skin team so that a root-cause analysis can be performed to identify the source and take corrective action. This information is taken back to the program oversight committee to further evaluate and make modifications to the infrastructure (policies, procedures, decision-making tools) as needed so that the situation does not recur.

Physical therapy. The role of the PT can differ widely among care settings and facilities. If involved in wound care, the role of the PT may appear to overlap with that of the certified wound nurse or the WOC nurse. Physical therapists may collaborate during evaluation and care planning, or they may coordinate a team. Physical therapists often are involved throughout the process of care, from preventing breakdown to facilitating healing. Physical therapy interventions address range of motion, strength training, seating and positioning, support surfaces, and functional mobility training. Physical therapists may offer therapeutic intervention for contractures, edema, motor control, muscle weakness, and pain. Other interventions, such as electrical stimulation, pulsed lavage, and sharp debridement, may be within the scope of practice for some PTs. As with nurses, PTs should function within their scope of practice, be regulated by accredited educational programs and curricula, and have certifications with sound practicum experience.

Occupational therapy. The occupational therapist (OT) plays a rehabilitative role, assessing cognitive and functional capabilities and then introducing patient-specific adaptive techniques and equipment. Patient-specific adaptive techniques and equipment promote the patient's optimal performance of activities of daily living, including the patient's ability to take an active role in wound care. The patient with a slow-healing or nonhealing wound may benefit from the expertise of the OT in promoting the patient's overall health maintenance and quality of life by incorporating skin and wound care into the patient's and family's daily routine.

Speech therapy. The speech therapist helps promote optimal nutrition by ensuring that the patient is able to safely swallow. Speech therapy may include strengthening oral and/or pharyngeal musculature, performing swallowing trials for diet advancement, and/or providing compensatory techniques with oral intake to improve the safety of the patient's swallowing and reduce aspiration risk. The speech therapist focuses on improving the patient's ability to effectively communicate to his or her maximum functional level. Cognitively, speech therapy works to improve cognitive-linguistic skills for safe and effective communication upon the patient's transition to the least restrictive environment possible.

Dietitian or nutritionist. The dietitian promotes optimal nutrition through nutritional assessment and intervention. The dietician monitors relevant laboratory values, anthropometric measurements, and food intake or nutrition support parameters. The dietitian collaborates with the team in making recommendations that optimally meet the nutritional needs and goals of the patient.

Social services. The social worker is a key member of the skin safety team. The patient with a wound often is vulnerable and requires astute assessment of the home situation, particularly as it relates to the patient's safety, support, and ability to realistically adhere to wound management goals. The social worker is knowledgeable about financial resources and the barriers to follow-up care that are unique to each individual situation. The social worker obtains prior authorization for supplies and other services needed upon discharge to prevent unexpected costs to the patient. As the key liaison between care settings, the social worker coordinates and leads discharge-planning conferences, which include the patient, skin safety team members, and the family. Representatives from facilities and agencies responsible for future care often are included in discharge-planning meetings for patients who have complex management issues. This collaboration among the patient, the family, and the healthcare team members from both settings helps to establish mutual goals and continuity in care.

Utilization review. In the United States, the utilization review (UR) specialist functions as a critical link among the patient, the physician, and the payer (insurance company, health maintenance organization, state or federal provider). Both nurses and social workers may hold UR positions. In many care settings, UR responsibilities have become incorporated into the case management role. The UR specialist provides information to payers to ensure funding for the most appropriate and cost-effective care.

MARKETING, JUSTIFYING, AND SECURING THE WOUND SPECIALIST ROLE: BENEFITS AND OUTCOMES

Employing a wound specialist yields many benefits to the organization, the value of which is more dramatic in the current climate of cost constraints. Through efficient use of materials, accurate and thorough documentation, prompt reassessment and revisions to the plan of care, and adherence to a formulary, the wound specialist has the potential to positively impact staff retention, physician satisfaction, facility reimbursements, infection rates, and patient satisfaction.

A key factor to a successful skin and wound care practice is effective communication and marketing of the role and the service. Measuring productivity and outcomes and communicating benefits are critical in securing and maintaining the role. Demonstrating and communicating the impact are essential so that the specialist and the services provided remain visible and the administration can justify the budget required to fund the wound specialist's position and program. This goal is accomplished not only through outstanding outcomes but, more importantly, by tracking and communicating outcomes through routine operations reports to key stakeholders and committees. These reports will help remind the administration that a low incidence of wound-related and skin-related problems is a result of having a qualified wound specialist; it is not an indication that staffing for the wound specialist should be reduced. This section outlines the benefits of having a wound specialist and the operations reports that are necessary to market, justify, and secure the role of the wound specialist. Checklist 1.1 provides tips for maintaining program infrastructure and securing the specialist's role. Box 1.5 provides examples of productivity and outcomes that can be communicated through an operations and outcome presentation report. Appendix A contains an example of a patient satisfaction survey.

Increased Accountability

One benefit of the services of a wound specialist is to serve as a content expert to maintain currency with national guidelines and integrate these into workflow, thereby attaining compliance with regulatory statutes. The Centers for Medicare & Medicaid Services (CMS) and The Joint Commission are clear in their intent to encourage all facilities to adopt evidenced-based pressure injury protocols. The surveyor community

---

CHECKLIST 1.1 Checklist to Maintain Infrastructure for Skin Health Committee

✓ Ensure time and staff are available to convert policies, procedures, and formulary with every change in contract, documentation, or technology. New initiatives (e.g., revised documentation forms, conversion to electronic medical records) require adaptations to existing processes and procedures, reorientation of staff.

✓ Network with key stakeholders and committees that can affect infrastructure; be visible and "in the loop" so that decisions that may impact the skin and wound care program are recognized and addressed.

✓ Include the patient as a key stakeholder; conduct patient satisfaction surveys, customized patient education to reflect patient demographics.

✓ Report to a director or vice president, not unit manager.

✓ Ensure program is sustainable, regardless of new technology, changes in staffing, changes in care delivery model.

✓ Position wound specialist as a high-profile change agent, not a technician.

✓ Generate data and reports that justify sufficient staffing without compromise.

✓ Utilize operation reports as tools for monitoring and driving change, not as tasks to complete (Box 1.5).

BOX 1.5   Suggested Items to Include in an Operations and Outcomes Report

Operations
- Number and type of patients (example in Appendix A)
- Number of visits, type of visit, time spent
- Trends (volume, issues, demographics)
- Referral sources and utilization patterns (e.g., physicians, units, facilities)
- Specific activities and scope of practice (e.g., managing patient population, quality improvement activities, committees, projects, education)

Outcomes
- Cost avoidance and cost savings with improved resource utilization processes (i.e., specialty beds and product usage before and after formularies, algorithms, and decision tools are implemented)
- Reduction in preventable skin injury (i.e., concurrent tracking for rates and P&I studies)
- Patient Satisfaction Survey (see example in Appendix A).

---

has a common language that should be used in the medical record when referring to pressure injuries. For example, CMS recognition and definition of the *avoidable* and *unavoidable* pressure injury in long-term care and *present on admission* (POA) criteria (see Chapter 6) highlight the need for incorporation of regulatory updates into practice. Because of their familiarity with national guidelines and consensus documents, the wound specialist is in a position to implement the requisite pressure injury prevention and treatment program. These programs include guidance on clear, concise, and accurate documentation.

Improved Financial Outcomes

Cost-effectiveness is a significant method for acquiring the administration's support. The wound specialist has the opportunity to help prevent costly wounds, use resources more efficiently, and, in some situations, generate revenue. Through ongoing continuing education opportunities, the wound specialist can foster state-of-the-art patient care and EBP by using products that have scientific evidence of their effectiveness. Again, not only do the patients benefit from this expertise, but the facility also benefits financially by cutting expenditures. The wound specialist can work with QI team members to identify select aspects of care that can be monitored and tracked over time and thus obtain outcomes data and clinical effectiveness information.

Reduction of Preventable Wounds

The costs of caring for a patient with a wound range widely across the world. The estimated cost of individual patient care ranges from $20,900 to $151,700 per wound (AHRQ, 2011). In addition, nonhealing chronic wounds predispose the patient to the risk of nontraumatic limb amputations, of which up to 85% can be avoided when an effective care plan for the patient with a diabetic foot injury is followed (International Best Practice Guidelines, 2013). When patients

at risk are identified and interventions are put in place before the wound develops or progresses, morbidity and healthcare costs are decreased (Padula, Mishra, Makic, et al., 2011).

Improved Healing Rates

Studies have shown that patients who were cared for by a WOC nurse specialist had better outcomes in terms of healing rates and/or costs of care compared with patients cared for by nurses who are not trained in wound care (Bolton et al., 2004; Harris & Shannon, 2008).

Efficient Use of Resources

The wound specialist must become cognizant of the implications of the efficient use of resources (both materials and personnel). Information on the cost implications of the skin and wound care practice or the cost savings that have been generated must be gathered and specifically communicated routinely to the supervisor. Wound management is costly; in most situations, wound management is more costly than prevention (Padula et al., 2011). Effective wound management reduces costs by allowing use of fewer supplies and providing more efficient and effective use of dressings, all desirable endpoints for the success of the organization.

The wound specialist should become involved with the discussion of supply contracts in order to sort through the maze of different products and their indications. A successful means of proven cost-effectiveness is limiting the number of similar supplies stocked by the facility. When a formulary for skin and wound care products and support surfaces is created, use of these products can be standardized and simplified. Furthermore, the wound specialist can serve as a resource for materials management, providing clarification on product use. Collaboration with materials management can increase the success of contractual arrangements with manufacturers and increase the facility's ability to maintain compliance with contracts.

Another area with potential for cost savings is standardizing the use of support surfaces. A policy that describes patient indicators for the use of specialty beds should be developed, and compliance with contracts for these specialty beds should be supported. A procedure for "stepping down" from a specialty bed as the patient's condition warrants should be established. In addition, units with a high prevalence of at-risk patient populations might benefit from the implementation of replacement mattresses. Standardizing the products and providing indicators or patient characteristics that guide the use of these products can reduce overuse and enhance appropriate use.

Finally, by incorporating appropriate use of skin and wound care products and state-of-the-art wound care, the wound specialist affects the use of personnel. Decreased frequency of dressing changes, expedient access to the correct dressing supplies, and printed directions for dressing changes will reduce staff frustration and time required for wound care.

Revenue Generation

Depending on payer sources, the level of education of the wound specialist and whether or not the specialist is employed by the institution, the services that are provided may be billable. Working closely with the billing department and fiscal intermediaries may be productive with regard to revenues. Chapters 2 and 4 provide specific details about the development of an outpatient clinical practice and reimbursement.

The skin and wound care program, like all departments, must have a means for tracking productivity. A mechanism for documenting visits and referrals can be formulated with the assistance of the billing department. One possible method is a system of "charge codes" for skin and wound care services based on increments of time or services provided. This is an excellent way to track, document, and justify the value of a wound specialist. However, the specialist should avoid providing services that are considered basic nursing care in order to inflate the number of charges. The specialist should not focus solely on the number of patients or charges, but rather on the types of patients and services provided. This charging system also may assist with the compilation of workload and time management data for the department. Another consideration is whether the wound specialist's interventions are affecting outcomes.

Depending on payer sources, the services that are provided through the skin and wound care program might be billable, for example, if the services are classified as a therapy rather than a nursing service. The availability of skin and wound care services may enable the institution to market itself for managed care contracts. This again defines the value of a skin and wound care program. However, inpatient skin and wound care services will seldom, if ever, be revenue-producing. Working closely with the billing department and fiscal intermediaries may be instructive.

The value of a skin and wound care program is not limited to just providing care to inpatients. The wound specialist can serve as a link to community and outreach programs and provide education that draws attention and referrals to the wound care program and the facility. The wound specialist can provide education within his or her facility in collaboration with colleagues, such as PTs and OTs. Grants to conduct some of these programs may be available from manufacturers. The manufacturers often have established programs that have been approved by licensing boards for continuing education hours, and these programs may be a cost-effective way to provide continuing education to staff. Continuing medical education programs also may be attractive; for example, well-recognized speakers may be invited to conduct an educational session.

When starting the skin and wound care program, the specialist initially may conduct a series of chart audits or a prevalence and incidence study. These activities may provide information that would be helpful in determining whether a certain problem (e.g., pressure injuries, inadequate documentation) exists. From this information, the continuous improvement process can be initiated with involved departments and personnel so that problems can be discussed, and possible solutions identified. As the wound specialist begins an inpatient practice, visibility is essential. Being open to new ideas and opportunities will assist the wound specialist

in creating and maintaining a successful program. Maintaining visibility and an alliance with physicians and staff will reinforce the message that the skin and wound care program is an indispensable service.

Staff Retention and Satisfaction

A key role of the wound specialist is establishing decision-making tools to expedite and standardize delivery of care. These tools help the staff to develop their comfort level in skin and wound care, facilitate utilization of products, and implement appropriate preventive interventions. Recognition and rewards can be provided for program contributions or accomplishments. Establishing skill competencies in wound care can provide a professional objective that the staff can strive for, again targeting the individual's personal satisfaction.

Critical features of a successful, enduring skin and wound care program are routine and regular operations reports, analysis of clinical practice data, and sharing of these data. Clinical practice data become the tool by which workload is measured, trends are identified, outcomes are quantified, and the valuable contribution of the wound specialist is recorded and measured. Data collection should be purposeful and outcomes oriented. In fact, data collection and practice improvement are inseparable because improvement requires measurement. Clinical practice data should include time management and outcomes reports.

Patient Satisfaction and Improved Quality of Life

Having a chronic wound can decrease satisfaction and quality of life by factors that impact physical, psychological, emotional, social, and occupational aspects of life (Herber, Schnepp, & Rieger, 2007). Specific experiences impacting quality of life include intolerable pain, fatigue, embarrassing drainage and odor, depression, shame, isolation, impaired ability to perform activities of daily living (ADL), and job loss (Fagervik-Morton & Price, 2009; Gorecki, Lamping, Brown, et al., 2010; Persoon, Heinen, Vleuten, et al., 2004; Ribu & Wahl, 2004). Patients also report a decrease in satisfaction and frustration with health professionals and service due to lack of explanation, conflicting information related to treatment options, diagnostic tests, and progress reports (Herber et al., 2007).

The wound specialist is uniquely qualified to help prevent or minimize some of these devastating experiences, with expertise in holistic assessment of the patient with a wound (see Chapter 10) and use of appropriate dressings to help manage pain, exudate, and odor with products that consider the patient's needs and lifestyle (see Chapter 21). Quality of life and strategies for improvement are discussed in Chapter 5 and throughout this text. Quality-of-life questionnaires and scales, as well as patient satisfaction surveys, can be used to measure outcomes (Augustin, Herberger, Rustenbach, et al., 2010; Iglesias, Birks, Nelson, et al., 2005; Price & Harding, 2004).

Operations and Outcomes Reports

When cost containment, efficient use of resources, and managed care dominate discussions, information concerning time use is invaluable. This type of data can validate any subjective perception of an increase or change in workload and communicates a strong objective message. Data should be recorded daily and tabulated weekly, monthly, quarterly, and annually. Summary data (e.g., number of patient referrals, number of visits, average length of visits, average number of visits per patient or wound type, reason for referral, number of projects/activities, and time per project) should be submitted to the wound specialist's supervisor on a monthly basis, with trends highlighted. Plots can graphically display time or volume by month. Data collection can be maintained by hand on paper or by computer through one of the many commercially available software packages. Reports can be generated from an electronic medical record system through collaboration with the information technology department. Appendix A contains an example of a simple database created using the Microsoft Excel program.

Benefits of services to the organization become tangible and coherent when they are phrased in terms of outcomes. Outcomes should include specific patient population outcomes and organizational outcomes. Potential outcomes should be discussed relative to behaviors or physical conditions that can be affected by the wound specialist. For example, an outcome of shortened length of stay in the hospital may not be realistic because many variables impact an individual's length of stay and are not necessarily under the control of the wound specialist. However, the outcome could be rephrased to more precisely define the patient population or type of wound for which length of stay will be decreased. Another outcome could address the control of wound care products. However, in order for this outcome to be feasible, tools that will assist the staff in appropriate product use, such as protocols and a formulary, would be required.

CLINICAL CONSULT

Memorandum
To: Medical and Nursing Staff
From: Nursing Administration and Wound Care Department
S: Weekend coverage for new patient referrals for wound consultations.
B: In the past our wound care staff was not available on weekends or holidays for new patient referrals.
A: With an increasingly shorter length of stay for hospitalized patients and the growing number of referrals for wound care, we will pilot a new weekend/holiday coverage policy.

R: For nonemergent new patient consults, please initially refer to the new online wound and skin troubleshooting guidelines. If this is not sufficient, contact the house nursing supervisor and he or she will contact the on-call wound care specialist to determine if a phone call will adequately address the problem or if the wound care specialist will need to make a hospital visit. After 3 months we will ask for feedback on the process and determine our ongoing plan for better coverage of our wound care patients. Thank you all for the great care you consistently give our patients.

SUMMARY

Establishing a skin and wound care practice in any setting requires the skills of an entrepreneur and a strong foundation in pathophysiology and clinical management. The wound specialist must determine how his or her role will be implemented, how his or her relationship with colleagues will be defined, what quality management processes can be implemented, and what type of data is needed. Data should describe how time is spent and what outcomes are being achieved. The wound specialist must stay current in the art and science of wound management by adopting lifelong learning strategies, such as regularly attending continuing education programs, critically reading journals, and monitoring select websites. The time and energy spent in initial and ongoing practice development are critical to a successful, satisfying, and effective skin and wound care practice.

SELF-ASSESSMENT QUESTIONS

1. The resource that provides the highest level of evidence is:
   a. Evidence-based abstract journals
   b. UpToDate
   c. Clinical practice Guidelines
   d. Cochrane Library
2. Which of the following will positively influence the rate that an innovation is adopted?

   a. The innovation is integrated into workflow following approval at the executive leadership level.
   b. The innovation is implemented without a trial.
   c. Results of the innovation are readily apparent to staff and leadership.
   d. Results are so subtle that nobody will notice the change.

3. While role would be most appropriate for a wound specialist rather than a staff nurse?
   a. Conduct a skin and wound assessment on a new admission
   b. Conduct a pressure injury risk assessment and implement appropriate preventive interventions
   c. Change wound dressings as ordered
   d. Establish protocols for management of candidiasis, skin tears and incontinence-associated dermatitis

4. What are the advantages to certification as a wound specialist?
   a. Certified wound specialists receive demonstrate better outcomes than noncertified wound care staff
   b. Certified wound specialists make more money than noncertified wound care staff
   c. Nurses can delegate their wound care to a certified wound specialist and save time for documentation
   d. Certification qualifies the wound specialist to bill for services.

REFERENCES

Ackerman, C. L. (2011). "Not on my watch": Treating and preventing pressure ulcers. *Medsurg Nursing, 20*(2), 86–93.

Agency for Healthcare Research and Quality (AHRQ). (2011). *Are we ready for this change? Preventing pressure ulcers in hospitals: A toolkit for improving quality of care.* Rockville: AHRQ. http://www.ahrq.gov/professionals/systems/long-term-care/resources/pressure-ulcers/pressureulcertoolkit/putool1.html. Accessed January 26, 2014.

Andriessen, A. E., Polignano, R., & Abel, M. (2009). Development and implementation of a clinical pathway to improve venous leg ulcer treatment. *Wounds, 21*(5), 127–133.

Augustin, M., Herberger, K., Rustenbach, S. J., et al. (2010). Quality of life evaluation in wounds: Validation of the Freiburg Life Quality Assessment-wound module, a disease-specific instrument. *International Wound Journal, 7*(6), 493–501.

Bales, I., & Duvendack, T. (2011). Reaching for the moon: Achieving zero pressure ulcer prevalence, an update. *Journal of Wound Care, 20*(8). 374–347.

Bales, I., & Padwojski, A. (2009). Reaching for the moon: Achieving zero pressure ulcer prevalence. *Journal of Wound Care, 18*(4), 137–144.

Beeckman, D., Clays, E., Van Hecke, A., et al. (2013). A multi-faceted tailored strategy to implement an electronic clinical decision support system for pressure ulcer prevention in nursing homes: A two-armed randomized controlled trial. *International Journal of Nursing Studies, 50*(4), 475–486.

Beitz, J. M., Fey, J., & O'Brien, D. (1999). Perceived need for education vs. actual knowledge of pressure ulcer care in a hospital nursing staff. *Dermatology Nursing, 11*(2), 125.

Bolton, L., McNees, P., van Rijswijk, L., et al. (2004). Wound-healing outcomes using standardized assessment and care in clinical practice. *Journal of Wound, Ostomy, and Continence Nursing, 31*, 65–71.

Bonham, P. (2009). The role of wound, ostomy and continence (WOC) specialty nurses in managing complex cases. *Remington Report, 17*, 10.

Cary, A. H. (2001). Certified registered nurses: Results of the Study of the Certified Workforce. *The American Journal of Nursing, 101*(1), 44–52.

Chicano, S. G., & Drolshagen, C. (2009). Reducing hospital-acquired pressure ulcers. *Journal of Wound, Ostomy, and Continence Nursing, 36*(1), 45–50.

Dalhousie University Libraries. (2020). *Evaluation of health information on the Web.* https://dal.ca.libguides.com/c.php?g=257155&p=1717074. Accessed November 20, 2020.

Ehrenberg, A., Fraser, K. D., & Gunningberg, L. (2004). Can decision support improve nurses' use of knowledge? *Journal of Wound, Ostomy, and Continence Nursing, 31*(5), 256–258.

Fagervik-Morton, H., & Price, P. (2009). Chronic ulcers and everyday living: Patients' perspective in the United Kingdom. *Wounds, 21*(12), 318–323.

Fineout-Overholt, E., Berryman, D. R., Hofstetter, S., et al. (2019). Finding relevant evidence to answer clinical questions. In B. M. Melnyk, & E. Fineout-Overholt (Eds.), *Evidence-based practice in nursing & healthcare. A guide to best practice, ed 2.* Philadelphia: Lippincott Williams & Wilkins.

Fleck, C. (2008). To certify or not to certify; that is the question. *Todays Wound Clinical, 2*(3), 26.

Golinko, M. S., Clark, S., Rennert, R., et al. (2009). Wound emergencies: The importance of assessment, documentation, and early treatment using a wound electronic medical record. *Ostomy/Wound Management, 55*(5), 54–61.

Gorecki, C., Lamping, D. L., Brown, J. M., et al. (2010). Development of a conceptual framework of health-related quality of life in pressure ulcers: A patient-focused approach. *International Nursing Studies, 47*, 1525–1534.

Harris, C., & Shannon, R. (2008). An innovative enterostomal therapy nurse model of community wound care delivery: A retrospective cost-effectiveness analysis. *Journal of Wound, Ostomy, and Continence Nursing, 35*(2), 169–183.

Herber, O. R., Schnepp, W., & Rieger, M. A. (2007). A systematic review on the impact of leg ulceration on patients' quality of life. *Health and Quality of Life Outcomes, 5*, 4.

Hiser, B., Rochette, J., Philbin, S., et al. (2006). Implementing a pressure ulcer prevention program and enhancing the role of the CWOCN© impact and outcomes. *Ostomy/Wound Management, 52*(2), 48–59.

Iglesias, C. P., Birks, Y., Nelson, E. A., et al. (2005). Quality of life of people with venous leg ulcers: A comparison of the discriminative and responsive characteristics of two generic and a disease specific instruments. *Quality of Life Research, 14*(7), 1705–1718.

International best practice guidelines. (2013). *Wound management in diabetic foot ulcers.* Wound International. http://www.woundsinternational.com/pdf/content_10803.pdf. Accessed July 13, 2015.

Kelleher, A. D., Moorer, A., & Makic, M. F. (2012). Peer-to-peer nursing rounds and hospital-acquired pressure ulcer prevalence in a surgical intensive care unit: A quality improvement project. *Journal of Wound, Ostomy, and Continence Nursing, 39*(2), 152–157.

Lloyd-Vossen, J. (2009). Implementing wound care guidelines: Observations and recommendations from the bedside. *Ostomy/Wound Management, 55*(6), 50–55.

McIsaac, C. (2007). Closing the gap between evidence and action: How outcome measurement informs the implementation of evidence-based wound care practice in home care. *Wounds, 19*(11), 299–309.

Melnyk, B. M., & Fineout-Overholt, E. (2019). *Evidence-based practice in nursing & healthcare. A guide to best practice* (4th ed.). Philadelphia: Wolters Kluwer.

Milne, C. T., Trigilia, D., Houle, T. L., et al. (2009). Reducing pressure ulcer prevalence rates in the long-term acute care setting. *Ostomy/Wound Management, 55*(4), 50–59.

Moore, A., Butcher, G., Corbett, L. Q., et al. (2014). Exploring the concept of a team approach: Managing wounds as a team. *Journal of Wound Care, 23*(Suppl. 5), S1–S38.

Murad, M. H. (2017). Clinical practice guidelines: A primer on development and dissemination. *Mayo Clinic Proceedings, 92*(3), 423–433.

Orsted, H. L., Rosenthal, S., & Woodbury, M. G. (2009). Pressure ulcer awareness and prevention program: A quality improvement program through the Canadian Association of Wound Care. *Journal of Wound, Ostomy, and Continence Nursing, 36*(2), 178–183.

Padula, W. V., Mishra, M. K., Makic, M. B., et al. (2011). Improving the quality of pressure ulcer care with prevention: A cost-effectiveness analysis. *Medical Care, 49*(4), 385–392.

Pasek, T. A., Geyser, A., Sidoni, M., et al. (2008). Skin care team in the pediatric intensive care unit: A model for excellence. *Critical Care Nurse, 28*(2), 125–135.

Persoon, A., Heinen, M. M., Vleuten, C. J. M., et al. (2004). Leg ulcers: A review of their impact on daily life. *Journal of Clinical Nursing, 13*, 341–354.

Price, P., & Harding, K. (2004). Cardiff Wound Impact Schedule: The development of a condition-specific questionnaire to assess health-related quality of life in patients with chronic wounds of the lower limb. *International Wound Journal, 1*(1), 10–17.

Ribu, L., & Wahl, A. (2004). Living with diabetic foot ulcers: A life of fear, restrictions, and pain. *Ostomy/Wound Management, 50*, 57–67.

Rogers, E. M. (2003). *Diffusion of innovations* (5th ed.). New York: Free Press.

Sackett, D. L., Strauss, S. E., Richardson, W. S., et al. (2000). *Evidence-based medicine: How to practice and teach EBM.* (2nd ed.). London: Churchill Livingstone.

Thomas, M. E. (2008). The providers' coordination of care: A model for collaboration across the continuum of care. *Professional Case Management, 13*(4), 220–227.

Tippet, A. W. (2009). Reducing the incidence of pressure ulcers in nursing home residents: A prospective 6-year evaluation. *Ostomy/Wound Management, 55*(11), 52–58.

Woods, D. K. (2002). Realizing your marketing influence, Part 3: Professional certification as a marketing tool. *The Journal of Nursing Administration, 32*(7–8), 379–386.

Wound, Ostomy and Continence Nurses Society. (2011). *Position statement about the role and scope of practice for wound care providers.* Mt Laurel, NJ: Wound, Ostomy and Continence Nurses Society.

Wound, Ostomy and Continence Nurses Society. (2017). *Wound, ostomy and continence nursing: Scope & standards of practice* (2nd ed.). Mt. Laurel: Wound, Ostomy and Continence Nurses Society.

Wound, Ostomy and Continence Nurses Society™ (WOCN®). (2012). *WOC nursing salary and productivity survey.* Mount Laurel: WOCN®.

Billing, Reimbursement, and Setting Up an Outpatient Clinic

Elaine Horibe Song, Tiffany Hamm, and Jeffrey Mize

OBJECTIVES

1. Describe how wound clinics differ in their management, location, staff, and services offered.
2. List key components of a wound clinic.
3. List documentation that must be in the medical record to meet Medicare and billing requirements.
4. Distinguish among the different Medicare and insurance programs, including how they relate to billing for clinic services and supervision requirements.

Patients come to wound care clinics expecting state-of-the-art treatments. Many patients are seeking advanced technologies and evidence-based care and are anticipating improved healing by clinicians knowledgeable in wound management. Typical etiologies of an outpatient wound clinic patient include chronic and difficult-to-heal wounds, such as pressure injuries; venous, arterial, and diabetic wounds; and skin disorders and unusual wound types. The common goal of an outpatient wound clinic is to provide standardized, consistent, evidence-based wound care, which includes the comprehensive care of the patient, addressing underlying etiologies, addressing cofactors, and teaching self-care to prevent recurrence. This chapter outlines the essential components of the operation and structure of an outpatient wound clinic and the impact of various regulatory issues and reimbursement requirements.

CREATING THE BUSINESS PLAN

The first step in creating a new clinic is to establish a business plan (Box 2.1). The goal of a business plan is to provide a step-by-step guide to follow when creating a new program or project. A well-constructed business plan is an important tool when obtaining administrative support. The following are some characteristics of a well-crafted business plan:
- The business plan is formulated around the clinic's mission and vision, and related short- and long-term goals (Aviles, 2018).
- A business plan will enumerate the benefits of the service and summarize existing internal and external competitors.
- The business plan should include a pro forma or projected operating budget for the next 5 years.
- Getting started requires consideration of several topics that should be covered in the business plan: the local health care environment, referral sources, customers, competitors, regulators, and revenue sources.

- The business plan must emphasize the product or service being proposed, as well as the marketing plan. A key element of the business plan is often referred to as the unique service advantage, which is what this business will do that no other business currently does, or how this new business will do it better than the competition does.
- Completion of a business plan will reveal commitment to goals and serve as a tool to highlight focus on improved outcomes and financial advantages the new business will provide.

The benefits of a wound care clinic to a hospital or organization are numerous (Box 2.2) and should be outlined in the business plan. A completed sample business plan is available through the Wound, Ostomy and Continence Nurses Society's™ *Professional Practice Manual, 4th Edition* (The Wound Ostomy and Continence Nurses Society [WOCN], 2013).

CLINIC MANAGEMENT

Although wound clinics offer similar services, they differ in their management arrangements and structure. Management can be overseen externally by a managed contract or proprietor, or they may be self-directed (internal), similar to a provider private practice. Table 2.1 lists advantages of both types of management. Available resources are a key consideration in determining the type of management needed. Resources include guidelines for care, policies, and forms; materials for staff and patient education; and quality improvement processes. Another essential consideration is access to the staff with expertise in developing these resources. External management often has these resources ready for use. However, such an arrangement could potentially commit more than half of the wound center revenue to the management contract. Decision makers should be aware of the type and extent

---

BOX 2.1   Components of a Business Plan

I. Executive Summary
   - Summarizes the key points of the entire business plan, giving administration a "quick read": a one-page overview of the plan summarizing mission, purpose, competitive edge, evidence supporting the need, potential services provided, financial and resource requirements, and benefits including financial and patient outcomes. Keep it brief and interesting.
II. Present Situation
   - Describes factors and demographic information that support the need for this venture; includes external analysis, competitive analysis, and internal analysis. Express how the plan supports the facility's mission statement and organizational goals (consider changes to health care related to the Affordable Care Act with readmission and infection rates).
III. Goals and Objectives
   - Provides a step-by-step guide as to what has to be done and how; includes realistic timeframes.
IV. Business/Product Descriptions
   - Describes the service to be provided and the benefits of that service to the patient, the facility, and the community. Highlight increase of use in ancillary hospital services.

V. Market Analysis/Strategy
   - Identifies customers, competitors, and the service's position in the market.
VI. Critical Success Factors/Key Assumptions
   - Identifies the conditions that must be met to achieve success.
VII. Qualifications
   - Specifies the education, experience, and certification of the staff. What makes this staff or individual so well qualified to care for patients with a wound?
VIII. Financial Projections/Budgeting Process
   - Articulates a pro forma budget that projects the expected revenues and expenses for 3–5 years. A pro forma is an operating budget for the next 3–5 years and indicates a break-even point.
IX. Appendix
   - Includes all backup documents that support the data provided in the plan, curriculum vitae of the staff, and staff job descriptions.

BOX 2.2   Benefits of a Wound Clinic to an Organization

- Addresses a significant need in the community
- Provides a competitive edge through a unique offering
- Is a convenient referral source for physicians
- Keeps patient and revenue within the organization
- Creates revenue for ancillary hospital departments
- Allows continuity of care:
  - Decrease in lead time from inpatient to outpatient treatment
  - Patient, medical record, referral are already in the system
  - Patient does not have to search for a clinic

---

of support that the management company can provide before choosing that company as a partner. Some factors to consider are

- For health care systems or health care providers that lack experience and expertise in administration of wound care programs, this "turn-key" wound care model managed by an external contractor can be preferred in the initial years of operation (Kim et al., 2013).
- For clinics or providers with experience and expertise with management of wound care programs, the self-directed model may be a better fit.

Clinic Structure

Structurally, the physical space of a wound clinic can be attached to a hospital (a hospital-based clinic or hospital outpatient clinic) or freestanding (clinic or office without any physical attachment to a hospital). The hospital-based clinic is a portion of a hospital that provides diagnostic, therapeutic, and rehabilitation services to sick or injured persons who do not require hospitalization. When determining the physical location of the clinic, particularly of the hospital-based clinic, it is important to consider ease of patient access to the clinic and ease of parking. Within the clinic space itself, a variety of issues must be considered in the design of the individual treatment rooms, the floor plan, the location of stocked equipment, lighting, and the need for stretcher access or lounge chair space (Checklist 2.1). Consultation with the facility maintenance department or facility planning department early in the planning to assist with these unique clinic space issues may be beneficial.

Billing Differences

The billing of clinic services is one of the consistent differentiations between the hospital-based clinic and the freestanding clinic based on the Medicare billing system. At a hospital-based clinic (identified by Medicare by place of service codes 22 or 19), services billed to Medicare or Medicaid patients will be reimbursed at the Medicare facility rate (facility submits a facility rate for the overhead cost and physician submits a separate bill for professional services). At a freestanding clinic or office (identified by Medicare by place of service code 11), services billed to Medicare or Medicaid patients will be reimbursed at the Medicare nonfacility rate (a higher reimbursed dollar amount compared with the facility rate because the overhead cost is not billed separately) (Centers for Medicare and Medicaid Services, 2021a, 2022a).

TABLE 2.1 Advantages of External vs Internal Clinic Management	
External (Outside) Management	**Internal (Self-directed) Management**
Policy and documentation developed and available	Create policy and forms that coincide with current hospital tools
Educational tools available and outside resources identified via managed company	Establish and seek education via both national and local conferences and online wound-specific clinical decision support based on clinic focus
Able to compare productivity and internal outcome numbers with other management facilities to gauge quality outcomes	Quality care program based on internal data or nationally available data
Established evidence-based pathway provided	Create clinic pathway to fit patient population and current hospital protocols using available evidence-based resources
Decisions and goals made at the corporate level and can be implemented with corporate support	Decisions and goals made at local level with flexibility to respond based on internal assessment and preferences
Audits by oversight Chief Compliance Officer to determine compliance, alert to national changes	Verify changes to payment rate, make local coverage determinations at least quarterly, make policy/form changes as prompted from data to fit local changes
Database system to assist with reports and documentation	If database desired, may choose from many available reports and documentation; this option may offer benchmarking with other sites for outcome comparisons
Potential for faster startup/growth due to already created tool and knowledge	Potential to add services other than wound care if clinic desires (e.g., nail care, ostomy clinic, lymphedema, continence clinic)
Staffing needs determined by job descriptions	Less outgoing expense, increased clinic revenue potential
Providers are often private or independent health care providers that work one-half to two days per week in the wound center (Kim, Evans, Steinberg, Pollard, & Attinger, 2013). Providers may be able to cover each other's absence	Some providers may work full-time in the clinic, allowing for better continuity of care

CHECKLIST 2.1   Clinic Space and Supply Needs

Space-Related
- ✓ Individual treatment rooms with sinks
- ✓ Adequate front office space
- ✓ Offices
- ✓ Waiting area (include bariatric-friendly furniture)
- ✓ Clinic workspace
- ✓ Dictation area
- ✓ Storage areas
- ✓ Clean and dirty utility rooms

Hyperbaric-Related (if Applicable)
- ✓ Patient changing rooms
- ✓ Oxygen supply
- ✓ Fire safety
- ✓ Floor weight loading with consideration to wax on floor and types of lights in ceiling

Nail Care-Related (if Applicable) (See Also Chapter 18)

Debridement-Related
- ✓ Forceps (toothed and/or smooth)
- ✓ Scalpels with blade (no. 10, 11, 15)
- ✓ Clamps or hemostats
- ✓ Curettes of several sizes
- ✓ Scissors or tissue nippers (various types: bandage removal, sharp for cutting tissue or dressings)

- ✓ Rongeurs
- ✓ Punch biopsy
- ✓ Sterile drapes
- ✓ Dressings

Wound Management-Related
- ✓ Normal saline
- ✓ Dressings
- ✓ Tube stabilizers
- ✓ Ostomy and wound pouches
- ✓ Wound measuring guides
- ✓ Camera
- ✓ Monofilaments
- ✓ Doppler
- ✓ Pulsate lavage supplies/noncontact low-frequency ultrasound (if applicable)
- ✓ Durable equipment that accommodates bariatric and spinal cord-injured population
- ✓ Transfer devices (e.g., hover mat, Hoyer lift)
- ✓ Examination tables and chairs
- ✓ Offloading overlay surface
- ✓ Scales
- ✓ Full range of blood pressure cuff sizes

Lists specify items other than routine examination room-related supplies, such as gloves, gowns, masks, and drapes.

Additional Means of Financial Viability

The survival of any wound clinic will depend on more than desire and quality outcomes. No wound center can continue to provide care unless the costs of providing care are covered. Wound care conducted in the fee-for-service model is a volume business—that is, the center must see a certain number of patients in order to create a positive cash flow. The bottom-line number of patients who must be seen will depend on the center's overhead: salaries, rent, utilities, cost of supplies, and other expenses.

A hospital-based clinic can offer additional referrals to the hospital for laboratory, radiology, nuclear medicine, magnetic resonance imaging, arteriogram, and surgical procedures and even for admissions, all of which add to the clinic's financial viability. The clinic should record these referrals and communicate to administrators in regular reports to reinforce the financial contributions of the wound center (Kim et al., 2013; Treadwell, 2007). Hospital outpatient clinics have the ability to obtain the facility fee for services provided by charging the facility rate when procedures are performed; this will assist in capturing facility-operating expenses.

In contrast, the freestanding clinic may increase financial stability by performing some of the necessary supplementary procedures in the center. Vascular evaluations with Doppler, transcutaneous oxygen pressure studies, and measurements of ankle-brachial index can generate charges for the center and enhance the bottom line, as long as they meet medical necessity as defined by payers. Clinics may choose to provide outpatient intravenous antibiotic therapy, ostomy care/education, lymphedema therapy, or foot and nail services, allowing patients to come to a familiar location for multiple services. In turn, these visits provide the staff with an opportunity to keep a close eye on the patient's wound while offering one-stop convenience to the patient.

CLINIC OPERATIONS

Numerous operations-related issues must be addressed: regulatory compliance, consents, infection control, national guidelines, laboratory and radiology needs, staff education, documentation, billing guidelines, and much more. Many of these issues are common to all outpatient clinics regardless of their location.

Hours of Operation and Scheduling

Hours of operation need to accommodate the population served and be compatible with staff availability and support services, such as transportation, laboratory, and radiology departments. The schedule should include time allocated for follow-up communication, staff education, meetings, quality reviews, audits, telehealth, and emergency visits. Allowing for unscheduled emergency visits may avoid costly trips to the emergency department and unnecessary hospital admissions. The wound clinic has readily available focused resources to address wound care needs in an outpatient environment. This is significant in helping prevent unplanned readmissions, which precipitate negative financial impact as per Centers for Medicare & Medicaid Services (CMS) Hospital Readmissions Reduction Program (HRRP) (Centers for Medicare and Medicaid Services, 2022c; Graham et al., 2018).

Special scheduling considerations include a longer time slot for new patients and anticipated procedures, teaching sessions, and review of test results. As the clinic volume grows, it will be prudent to establish predetermined time slots for these types of visits. A communication process should be established so that the scheduling staff is aware of these special needs. This can be accomplished with a notation on the medical record or on the scheduling book to remind scheduling staff to consider this information before scheduling the appointment.

Another consideration for scheduling is staff and skill mix needs. For example, a plastic surgeon with many immobile individuals may require higher numbers of staff to help position and hold patients vs a podiatry clinic, where the majority of patients can self-ambulate and remove/replace their shoes.

Chart Preparation, Storage, and Electronic Medical Records

Before the appointment, the clerical staff should prepare the necessary forms and verification of insurance authorization. New patients will need to provide a history and sign consent forms, in addition to any documentation forms necessary for return visits. Locked file storage within the clinic will be necessary, with potential for offsite storage if space is limited. However, it is important to consider how accessible these records will be if a request is made to retrieve them. A master list for storage boxes should be maintained to assist with retrieval, sign-out, and replacement.

The electronic medical record (EMR) has been utilized for years in wound clinics to aid clinical documentation, financial tracking/billing, regulatory compliance, audits, and outcome tracking. A growing number of companies have focused attention on EMR use for the wound clinic; however, wound care-specific documentation templates can be created within generic EMRs as well. Privacy and security regarding the confidentiality of all patient health information is a priority, and facility policies must be implemented and followed for all patient records.

Obtaining Consents

Preprinted consent forms (treatment, photography, and surgical/biopsy) should be available and signed before the visit. Consents can be mailed, faxed, or sent electronically to the appropriate authority before the appointment to prevent delay in treatment when the patient is unable to sign independently. A policy for the frequency of renewing consents should be established. Some facility registration cycles require monthly consents with each new registration; others refer to this as a recurring series and require annual updates if the patient has continued uninterrupted visits during the course of treatment. All consents should be maintained in the legal patient's records.

Regulations and Compliance

With the numerous rules and regulations existing today that ultimately impact quality of care, reputation, and payment for services, most organizations have a compliance program to oversee both corporate and regulatory issues. The objective of a compliance program is to identify potential sources of risk and implement policy and process modifications to reduce risk (Hess, 2008). Corporate compliance addresses employee behaviors and ethical issues in an attempt to protect the corporation from criminal and civil liability. This is accomplished through corporate-sponsored training activities on topics such as code of conduct (e.g., sexual harassment, interaction with vendors, ethics, publication, and involvement with media), grievance without retribution procedures, and disciplinary processes.

Regulatory issues are dictated by whether the clinic is freestanding or hospital based. Most hospital-based clinics are included in annual hospital audits/surveys and are required to follow standard hospital policies; freestanding clinics may not have the same requirements. Several different organizations set regulatory requirements based on our geographical region. Compliance with National Patient Safety Goals (including patient identification, appropriate hand-off communication, and medication safety) and with coding and billing guidelines is essential to the financial health of a clinic. Coding experts should be used in developing the "charge master" (clinic billing charges linking codes and dollar amounts), training staff in coding visits and procedures, and ensuring accurate documentation that reflects compliance and maximizes payment (Steed, 2016).

The clinic staff should be familiar with and in compliance with the Health Insurance Portability and Accountability Act (HIPAA) of 1996 privacy rule. The HIPAA was enacted for many reasons, including improving the portability and continuity of health insurance coverage and combating waste, fraud, and abuse in health insurance and delivery of health care (U.S Department of Health & Human Services, 2009). The HIPAA privacy rule also established national standards to protect the privacy of a patient's health information from health plans, health care clearinghouses, and most health care providers. Further information and guidance on implementing the HIPAA privacy rule are available on the websites listed in Table 2.2.

Insurance Authorization

Generally, Medicare policy requires providers to update beneficiary payer information for every admission, outpatient encounter, or start of care before submitting a bill to Medicare. The provider should retain a copy of the completed questionnaire on file or online for audit purposes. It is prudent for providers to retain these records. When a provider believes Medicare may not cover his or her services as medically reasonable and necessary, the provider should give the patient an acceptable advance beneficiary notice (ABN); otherwise, the provider generally cannot hold the patient liable if Medicare denies payment. For example, hyperbaric oxygen treatment for non-CMS-approved conditions would require an ABN signed before treatment is initiated. Managed care contracts and some group health care plans may require prior authorization for care at the wound clinic. Authorizations

TABLE 2.2	Website Addresses Relevant to Clinic Function, Structure, and Operations
Information Available	**Website URL**
CMS.gov	https://www.cms.gov/
CPT® Codes	https://www.ama-assn.org/practice-management/cpt
Directory of Fiscal Intermediaries and Intermediary Carriers and Medicare Contractors	http://www.cms.gov/About-CMS/Agency-Information/Aboutwebsite/contractorwebguidlines.html
Fee schedules	https://www.cms.gov/Medicare/Medicare-Fee-for-Service-Payment/FeeScheduleGenInfo
Guidance on HIPAA privacy rules and teaching materials	http://www.hhs.gov/ocr/privacy/hipaa/understanding/index.html
Healthcare Common Procedure Coding System HCPCS	http://www.cms.gov/Medicare/Coding/MedHCPCSGenInfo/index.html
Hospital outpatient PPS	http://www.cms.gov/Medicare/Medicare-Fee-for-Service-Payment/HospitalOutpatientPPS/index.html
ICD-10 information	http://www.cms.gov/icd10
Medicare Coverage Database with current NCDs and draft and final LCDs	https://www.cms.gov/medicare-coverage-database/new-search/search.aspx
NCCI edits	http://www.cms.gov/Medicare/Coding/NationalCorrectCodInitEd/
Prior Authorization Process for Certain Durable Medical Equipment, Prosthetic, Orthotics, Supplies Items	https://www.cms.gov/Research-Statistics-Data-and-Systems/Monitoring-Programs/Medicare-FFS-Compliance-Programs/DMEPOS/Prior-Authorization-Process-for-Certain-Durable-Medical-Equipment-Prosthetic-Orthotics-Supplies-Items
Quality initiatives	http://www.cms.gov/Medicare/Quality-Initiatives-Patient-Assessment-Instruments/QualityInitiativesGenInfo/index.html

CPT, Current Procedural Terminology; *HIPAA*, Health Insurance Portability and Accountability Act of 1996; *LCD*, local coverage determination; *NCCI*, National Correct Coding Initiative; *NCD*, national coverage determination.

may come open ended or may have restricted timeframes and visit numbers. A tracking system needs to be created so that staff is alerted when reauthorization is required.

Some wound treatment orders may require authorization before implementation (e.g., cellular and/or tissue-based products—also known as skin substitutes, negative pressure wound treatments, noncontact low-frequency ultrasound); therefore, the provider and staff should be aware of these requirements to prevent loss of reimbursement. In addition, the office staff should verify that the provider is covered by the insurance plan.

Treatment Orders

In most wound clinics, a provider is present to see the patient at each visit. A physician referral or a prior physician order to treat is not required by the CMS; however, a referral may be required by the individual patient's insurance plan. The office staff should be familiar with this requirement so that they can obtain the necessary authorization. A copy of this order must remain in the patient's record.

When no physician or advanced practice provider (APP) is scheduled to see the patient, auxiliary staff (nursing, technicians, and therapist) must meet supervision criteria (as determined by state and institutional policies) before billing the incident to the physician services. In this case, the order for treatment and documentation of visit must be maintained in the medical record, including the provider's treatment plan showing his or her active involvement with prior and ongoing care. Additionally, the facility should maintain a record of the supervising physician for each visit (consider documenting in the record at the encounter); auxiliary staff must also be certain to follow the scope of practice pertaining to license and state law. "Incident to services" are further explained later in this chapter.

Documentation

Documentation alone will not guarantee reimbursement; however, to receive payment for services, appropriate and complete documentation must be provided. Clinicians are encouraged to check CMS' National Coverage Determinations (NCDs), Local Coverage Determinations (LCDs), and Articles for updated guidance. See Section "National Coverage Determinations and Local Coverage Determinations." At minimum, documentation should include the following:

- Accurate diagnoses are documented by clinic staff and the physician treating the patient.
- Exact anatomic locations of all wounds treated are denoted, including specific and consistent measurements.
- Clinic and provider documentation support each other.
- Provider documentation is present, supports the necessity of treatment, and is linked to the diagnosis code (Hess, 2018).
- Treatments, including the dressing specifics, are recorded. Many treatment modalities and dressings (e.g., cellular and/or tissue-based products, negative pressure wound therapy, debridement) are reimbursed based on the size of the affected area (Schaum, 2019).

Additional documentation needed to complete the clinic chart is listed in Table 2.3. Documentation requirements are extensive. Compliance is facilitated by building prompts within the documentation system of the medical record.

TABLE 2.3   Items in an Outpatient Clinic Chart

Comprehensive admission assessment	Patient's name, gender, race, ethnicity, primary language spoken, address, phone number, date of birth, height/weight, name and phone of any legally authorized representative, past and present diagnoses, wound history, reason for visit, barriers to care, allergies, current mediations, advanced directive, family history
Wound assessment, compliance/teaching record	Vital signs, any medicine changes, procedure or hospitalizations since last visit, reason for visit, complete wound description and photography (if applicable), compliance to treatment plan, pain, any teaching reviewed at visit and response to teaching, treatment applied before discharge, vascular assessment if lower extremity wounds, nutritional assessment, offloading
Provider progress notes	Reason for visit and relevant history, physician examination findings and prior diagnostic test results, assessment, clinical impression or diagnosis, plan of care, rationale for ordering any test, patient's progress and response to changes in treatment plan; codes reported on billing statement should be supported in the documentation; any consult advice provided or received acknowledged as reviewed
Discharge orders	Any new test or medications ordered, wound treatment orders, next follow-up appointment or consult appointment, compression or offloading instructions
Acuity	Used by hospital-based clinic if no procedure was completed to bill evaluation and management of services based on facility resources acuity score; all resources considered should be supported in the medical record (consider acuity form a permanent documentation form to prevent charges not documented; use as a documentation and scoring tool)
Billing form	Complete listing of any diagnosis codes or procedure codes used for billing; supporting documentation must be in the medical record
Consents, insurance information, HIPAA documents	Consent for treatment, consent for photography, insurance information or copy of insurance card, HIPAA notification, advance beneficiary notice as indicated

Debridement

Wound debridement is an integral part of the day-to-day care provided in wound clinics. As required by Medicare, documentation of debridement must communicate exactly what was done and the rationale. Specifically, documentation must include type of tissue removed, depth of removal, instrument used (type of instrument, dressing, medication), wound size, condition of wound/bleeding stopped, and how the wound was redressed after debridement (Cartwright, 2020). A clear picture must be presented, given the Office of the Inspector General (OIG) report revealing that 64% of claims for debridement did not meet Medicare requirements (Department of Health and Human Services, Office of Inspector General, 2007). OIG continues to review Part B payments to determine if debridement services were medically necessary (Department of Health and Human Services, Office of Inspector General, 2019). Chapter 20 provides critical information related to debridement.

Contractor or Payer Audits

Regular audits are conducted by the CMS through their Recovery Audit Contractors (RACs) program (Centers for Medicare and Medicaid Services, 2022b). Implemented in 2008, RAC's mission is to identify overpayments and underpayments to health care providers and suppliers. Contractors must comply with NCDs and LCD (see Section "National Coverage Determinations and Local Coverage Determinations").

Recent audit-related CMS initiatives include the Targeted Probe and Educate (TPE) audit program and the Supplemental Medical Review Contractor (SMRC). The goal of the TPE program is to identify errors and help providers correct them, whereas SMRC's goal is to help lower improper payment rates and protect the Medicare Trust Fund (Centers for Medicare and Medicaid Services, 2022e, 2022f). Auditors will often request specific documentation to demonstrate compliance (Checklist 2.2). Common issues reviewed by auditors include (Hamm, 2020; Hess, 2019; Weiss, 2019):

CHECKLIST 2.2 Typical Documentation Items Requested by Audit Contractor or Payer

✓ Office records (progress notes, current history and physical, treatment plan)
✓ General patient consents for treatment and procedures
✓ Documentation of identity and professional status of clinician
✓ Laboratory and radiology reports
✓ Comprehensive problem list
✓ Current list of prescribed medications
✓ Progress notes for each visit indicating patient's response to prescribed treatment
✓ Documentation supporting time spent with patient when time-based codes are used
✓ Required referrals or prescriptions (for many nonphysician services/supplies)
✓ Required Certificates of Medical Necessity

- Every service billed must be documented because the patient's record must contain clear evidence that the service, procedure, or supply actually was performed or supplied.
- The medical necessity for choosing the procedure, service, or medical supply must be substantiated.
- Every service must be coded correctly. Diagnoses must be coded to the highest level of specificity, and procedure codes must be current.
- Documentation must clearly indicate who performed the procedure or supplied the equipment.
- Legible documentation, which may be dictated and transcribed, is required. Existing documentation may not be embellished; however, additional documentation that supports a claim may be submitted.
- Voluntary disclosure of information by the provider is encouraged. When an error is discovered, any overpayment should be returned to Medicare (Centers for Medicare and Medicaid Services, 2022b).

Clinic Composition: Staffing With an Interdisciplinary Team

Much like any wound team, the outpatient wound clinic requires the coordination and contribution of a variety of individuals and professionals and an extensive referral network. Of note, a multidisciplinary approach is one of the key elements in a successful wound care program. Given the potential complexity of chronic wounds, no health care provider has the knowledge, skill, and experience to single-handedly provide comprehensive care to patients with chronic wounds (Kim et al., 2013).

Each member of the outpatient wound clinic team should have a job description and expectations that align with their educational preparation, as outlined in Chapter 1. In addition, each member will be instrumental in patient recruitment. The following describes the additional roles unique to the outpatient setting. Table 2.4 lists the examples of Wound Clinic Interdisciplinary Team Members.

Clinic Director

The clinic director can be a nurse or other qualified professional, who may or may not be certified in wound care. This position provides oversight of the clinic, including staffing, scheduling, materials management, staff preparation/education, regulatory compliance, and profitability. Routine and frequent contact of the clinic director with insurance, billing, and coding personnel will facilitate early identification of any problems in reimbursement or documentation so that corrective steps can be taken promptly. Community education programs need to be used to become acquainted with possible referral sources, such as home health care agencies, nursing homes, physician offices, urgent care centers, and emergency rooms.

Nurse Coordinator

Nurses in the clinic provide a key role in the operation of the clinic and coordination of care. Responsibilities often include

TABLE 2.4   Wound Clinic Interdisciplinary Team Members

Position	Onsite	Available as Consultant
Medical director	X	
General surgeon		X
Vascular surgeon		X
Orthopedic surgeon		X
Dermatologist		X
Reconstructive surgeon		X
Podiatry		X
Infectious disease		X
Geriatrician		X
Occupational therapist		X
Certified wound care nurse (CWCN©, CWOCN©, CWON©, CWS)	X	
Registered nurse	X	
Physical therapist (may be certified wound specialist)	X	
Medical or surgical assistant	X	
Office staff (e.g., receptionist)	X	
Diabetes educator		X
Dietitian	X	
Billing/coder	X	

checking in the patient, interviewing the patient, removing dressings, assessing the wound, and collaborating with the wound care specialist and interdisciplinary team members to evaluate and implement the plan of care. Basic competencies in physical assessment including basic wound assessment are essential to optimal functioning of the nursing staff in the wound clinic (Morrison, 2007).

Wound Care Specialist

The health care member who is wound care certified (typically a nurse or physical therapist) are key members contributing to the comprehensive treatment planning process in collaboration with the provider, who is ideally also certified in wound care. This person has insight into the range of treatment options for this patient with this particular situation and will use the response to previous treatments to guide future treatment approaches.

Insurance and Billing Coder

The value and expertise of insurance and billing coders cannot be understated. Close collaboration with the coding department will secure optimal regulatory compliance and reimbursement. In addition, insurance coordinators for the wound department may assist with preapprovals from various private insurance companies. This position may be part of the facility coding team or a person assigned to the department to obtain preapprovals and support the coders with communication to the clinic.

Ancillary Staff

Ancillary clinic staff may include schedulers, medical assistants, and surgical assistants, who may work in the clinic and assist with office duties. Expectations may include preparation of forms and consents, patient registration, placing appointment reminder calls, scheduling tests, and data entry for billing and supplies. Training ancillary staff to work in the clinical area (within their job scope and reporting significant findings to clinic nurses and physicians) and to cover the office allows for flexibility in scheduling during slow clinic times and vacation schedules.

Utilizing the ancillary staff while scrutinizing staffing ratios (nursing hours vs ancillary hours and all hours worked vs patient visits) will assist with monitoring worked hours per patient visit. Closely watching this ratio may show the need to bring on new staff as clinic visits increase, alter staff hours during slower days during the week, and shift staff hours to busier workdays.

Referral Network

Outpatient care, in large part, requires referrals to, and use of, community services: local transportation companies, durable medical equipment (DME) companies, orthotics and prosthetics suppliers, physician offices, home care agencies, laboratories, radiology, and other hospital departments. Everyone in the clinic should be familiar with how to access these resources and the requirements that must be fulfilled in order to complete a referral. This kind of detail when providing care to the clinic patient will convey a sense of calmness and confidence to the patient and facilitate the patient's ability to follow through, which ultimately will enhance outcomes.

Hospital facilities likely have access to onsite laboratory, radiology, vascular laboratory, surgical suite, and emergency rooms. The place or site to which the patient is referred must always be the patient's choice rather than a mandate that the patient be sent to a particular facility. The insurance company often drives this decision. When referral sites are freestanding, it may be beneficial to have a list of local sites where such tests can be obtained, along with their hours of business, addresses, and contact information.

DME supplies will be a common need of the wound clinic patient. Most patients are unaware of where to obtain supplies and what products may be equivalent substitutes. Therefore, the patient will need a list of local DME providers, as well as mail-order companies, to facilitate accessing supplies. The patient who has limited mobility cannot easily pick-up supplies and will need either free home delivery or mail delivery. Providing patients with written instructions detailing their wound care supplies and the wound care procedure will facilitate continuity in their care. In many situations, wound care orders can be sent directly to the DME.

Clinic Space and Equipment

Equipment needed for the wound clinic is similar to that needed in many routine outpatient clinics; however, additional equipment items unique to the care of the patient with a wound are necessary to provide the patient with efficient care (see Checklist 2.1).

Room Equipment

At a minimum, multipatient rooms should have privacy curtains separating patients. Individual rooms are preferred to facilitate privacy. From an infection control perspective, rooms in which treatments have the potential to generate aerosolization should be separated by walls rather than curtains to prevent the spread of microorganisms. Considering how the patient will arrive may be critical to determining what equipment to place in a room. Carts and large wheelchair transports may be cumbersome when turning corners and should be considered early in the planning phase.

The type of clinic room equipment may vary depending on the type of patients expected. Spinal cord injury or reconstructive surgery clinics may require space to accommodate patients arriving on stretchers, with pneumatic treatment tables and additional staff or adaptive equipment to assist with transfers. An offloading overlay surface should be added to the examination table to reduce pressure and provide comfort; it also can be used for educational purposes when teaching positioning and hand checks. Examination chairs (e.g., podiatry chairs) are preferable for the ambulatory patient with a lower extremity ulcer. The positioning made available with this type of chair will facilitate patient comfort, allow for better visualization of lower extremity wounds, promote ergonomic movements by the staff, thus reducing their risk of musculoskeletal injury, and maintain a good distance from the floor so that the risk of cross-contamination from microorganisms on the floor is minimized.

A stand for treatment supplies with wheels that can be positioned within reach of the patient and caregiver, as well as a place for documentation, will be needed for each room. Additional items needed include a stool for the clinician, a visitor chair, and good lighting. Basic equipment includes items such as thermometers, sphygmomanometers, needle boxes,

gloves boxes, dirty linen containers, trashcans, and hazardous waste receptacles.

Wound centers may want to purchase a bariatric treatment chair. Many treatment chairs have a weight limit between 275 and 400 lbs; however, a certain patient population will require a treatment chair that can hold between 500 and 800 lbs.

Another important piece of equipment for wound centers is a scale to help monitor nutrition and fluid balance, especially when diuretics are used with compression wraps. Patient safety should be considered when purchasing a scale. A scale with handrails provides a stable base for patients to step onto. A wheelchair scale may be necessary, or one with a weight limit of up to 850 lbs.

Wound Care Supplies

A formulary of wound care supplies for the wound clinic will need to be developed. The formulary should be selected with knowledge of the most common wound needs seen in the clinic and the function of the various dressings (Song et al., 2020). The range of products included in the formulary should be kept narrow to reduce the potential for confusion on utilization, ordering, or storage. Due to product expiration dates, supplies used less often or for specific procedures (e.g., biologic graft) may need to be special ordered.

Pharmaceuticals (topical anesthetics and topical creams) should be kept locked and made available for minor procedures such as debridement. Medications should not be administered without a provider's order. Patients attending a clinic where medications cannot be administered should be encouraged to take a pain medication before their visit.

Many wound care visits will require conservative sharp debridement, so appropriate tools should be available. However, no package should be opened during room setup in anticipation of debridement. Rather, package materials should be opened only after the need for the tools is confirmed. Basic sharp debridement tools can be disposable or resterilized; consider patient volumes when determining the number of tools needed and the time allotment for resterilizing equipment.

Education

Education of patients and staff is a vital component of any wound care program in any setting and is addressed throughout this textbook. In the outpatient setting, documentation of the education and handouts provided and their understanding is important, not only in providing quality wound care but also can be used to justify additional clinic visits, as well as potential referrals (e.g., psychiatrist, cognitive evaluation, and home care).

Patient education is regarded as an important element in enabling patients to be more engaged in their care. However, there is a need to consider different types of education (e.g., printed brochures, electronic media, videos, etc.), as people will respond differently to different methods (Gethin, Probst, Stryja, Christiansen, & Price, 2020). When setting up a clinic, planners should consider the variety of electronic media that can be used and made available to the patient, either on their own electronic devices (mobile, laptops, etc.)

CHECKLIST 2.3   Examples of Wound Clinic Policies and Competencies

Policies	Competencies
✓ Wound measurement	✓ Wound measurement
✓ Wound photo	✓ Wound photography
✓ Direct supervision/"incident-to" visits	✓ Wound culture
✓ Quality program	✓ Compression wraps
✓ Conservative care designation	✓ Negative pressure wound therapy
✓ Chart order	✓ Low-frequency ultrasound treatments
✓ Billing guidelines	✓ Skin inspections
✓ Form completion guidelines	✓ Room cleaning between patients
✓ Clinic scheduling	✓ Isolation/infection control
✓ Position descriptions and responsibilities	✓ Offloading techniques
✓ Insurance authorization process	✓ Ankle-brachial index
✓ HIPAA/EMR/Health information security and privacy	✓ Monofilament/sensory testing
	✓ Conservative sharp debridement
	✓ Chemical cautery with silver nitrate
	✓ Pulsate lavage

EMR, electronic medical record; *HIPAA,* Health Insurance Portability and Accountability Act.

or in a separately designated "education" room or from a library, from which the patient can access the material, review it at home, and then return it (Armstrong et al., 2008).

Staff education should be mandatory and competency based for a variety of reasons, such as patient safety, appropriate use of resources, improved patient care, standardization of care, and compliance with facility policy. The Federal Register and State Operating Manuals have requirements for policies to address education when protocols are utilized. Education time and resources are essential for staff to keep current of any new developments in their field and be informed to follow proper safety procedures (Centers for Medicare and Medicaid Services, 2020b). Checklist 2.3 provides a list of competencies to be considered for staff education in a wound clinic.

Policies, Procedures, and Guidelines

As described in Chapter 1, the wound specialist plays a pivotal role in integrating research findings into policies, procedures, and guidelines for the clinic. Evidence-based policies, procedures, and guidelines for care must be readily available to clinic personnel. Familiarity with these documents should be addressed through competency-based staff education programs as already described. See Checklist 2.3 for a list of possible wound clinic policies.

Continuous Quality Improvement Plan

Quality outcome data are necessary to evaluate compliance with evidence-based wound care and progress of the overall treatment plan. The data may be shared with the patient to encourage continued treatment, shared with insurance

companies to demonstrate medical necessity, and compared locally or nationally to display the cost benefit of treatment. Although economic factors in wound care are common measures in product evaluation, ultimately the bottom line is efficacy. An inexpensive product that makes up for its low cost with increased clinic visits due to delayed healing time quickly loses its product price advantage; additional costs will be incurred if infection develops (Fife, 2019). Healing time in relation to cost is another valuable piece of outcome data. Stratification of data by etiology, providers, and clinic days provides additional information about efficiency, effectiveness, and best practice. Further analysis includes measuring the impact of clinic-based care on the number of home care visits, use of wound care-related medications, acute care readmissions, emergency room visits, number of surgical procedures, limb salvage, and healing times. These data are useful for substantiating best practices and for marketing the clinic.

PAYMENT SYSTEMS IN THE UNITED STATES

Successful wound management is a culmination of quality wound care practices and knowledge of coverage and payment policies. Reimbursement is based on what is done and documented at the clinic visit. Knowing the type of insurance and whether authorization is required, keeping track of visits, and knowing whether the patient has Medicare/Medicaid and how this coverage affects billing are essential.

CMS is responsible for establishing the payment system for Medicare and Medicaid beneficiaries. It pays the majority of the health care dollars in the United States. Billing principles are similar for other insurance types using the billing codes established by the American Medical Association (AMA) known as Current Procedural Terminology (CPT®). The International Classification of Diseases, 10th Revision (ICD-10) codes support the disease/reason for visit. Acronyms are common in the billing process, and a directory of acronyms related to the billing process is provided in Box 2.3.

Affordable Care Act

The Affordable Care Act (ACA) is a comprehensive health care reform law enacted in March 2010. The ACA focuses on provisions to expand coverage, control health care costs, and improve the health care delivery system (Kaiser Family Foundation, 2013). Under the ACA, paying for value is a focus, as the hospital is rewarded based on the quality of care it provides to patients via the Value-Based Purchasing Program; the HRRP reduces payment to hospitals with relatively high rates of potentially preventable readmissions. Promoting better care and protecting patients are addressed via the adoption of the electronic record, as well as reporting hospital-acquired conditions, with possible payment penalties for those with high rates. Reducing health costs is addressed in the Medicare durable medical equipment, prosthetics, orthotics, and supplies (DMEPOS) competitive bidding and by fighting fraud (Centers for Medicare and Medicaid Services, 2014b).

BOX 2.3   Acronyms Related to Billing and Reimbursement Process

APC: Ambulatory Payment Classification—System used for outpatient services, attached to assigned CPT code for payment.

CPT: Current Procedural Terminology—Codes that describe the procedure performed, such as debridement.

DME: Durable Medical Equipment—Supplies ordered by physician for use in the home (item must be reusable).

DMERC: Durable Medical Equipment Regional Carrier—Contractor for CMS who provides claims processing and payment for DME.

E&M: Evaluation and Management—CPT code used to obtain the fee for the corresponding services provided.

FI: Fiscal Intermediary—Contractor for CMS who processes claims for services covered under Medicare.

HCPCS: Healthcare Common Procedure Coding System—Uniform method used by providers and suppliers to report professional services, procedures, and supplies (codes describe dressing supply) assigned and maintained by local Medicare contractors.

ICD-10: International Classification of Diseases, 10th Revision—National coding method designed to enable providers to effectively document the medical condition, symptom, or complaint that forms the basis for rendering a specific service.

LCD: Local Coverage Determination—Formal statement developed through a specifically defined process that defines the service, provides information about when the service is considered reasonable and necessary, outlines any coverage criteria and/or documentation requirements, and provides coding information.

Level II HCPCS—Method for obtaining reimbursement for products, supplies, or procedures not covered in the CPT codes.

MAC: Medicare Administrative Contractor—A single authority consisting of integrated fiscal intermediaries and carriers responsible for the receipt, processing, and payment of Medicare claims. The MAC will perform functions related to the beneficiary and provider service, appeals, provider outreach and education, financial management, program evaluation, reimbursement, payment safeguards, and information systems security.

NCCI: National Correct Coding Initiative—Developed to promote correct coding by providers and supplies (to prevent payment for noncovered and/or incorrectly coded services).

NCD: National Coverage Determination—Developed by CMS to describe the circumstances for Medicare coverage for a specific medical service procedure or device.

OPPS: Outpatient Prospective Payment System—A prospective payment system (fee schedule) that sets payments for individual services as identified by the HCPCS codes and used for hospital outpatient services, certain Part B services furnished to hospital inpatients who have no Part A coverage, and partial hospitalization services furnished by hospitals and community mental health centers.

PPS: Prospective Payment System—Method of reimbursement in which Medicare payment is made based on a predetermined, fixed amount.

The fundamentals of traditional Medicare remain with additional incentives and penalties assigned for quality outcomes, technology use, and cost containment. Being aware of key provisions and how they affect care changes and financial outcomes remain critical (i.e., reduce the number of hospital readmissions, reduce hospital-acquired conditions, bundling payments, and improved quality reporting) (Centers for Medicare and Medicaid Services, 2014b).

A hospital outpatient clinic can help prevent unnecessary readmissions via the emergency department or nonspecialist provider by conducting early assessments and preventing infections (Graham et al., 2018). In addition, clinics may provide areas of expanded value to the hospital partner by providing care of the ostomy, lymphedema, and burn patient if not already addressed.

Medicare

Title XVIII of the Social Security Act designated "Health Insurance for the Aged and Disabled," is more commonly known as Medicare. The Social Security Amendments of 1965 created a health insurance program for aged persons to complement retirement, survivor, and disability insurance benefits. When first implemented in 1966, Medicare covered most persons aged 65 years and over. In 1973, additions made to Medicare benefits included (1) persons entitled to Social Security or Railroad Retirement disability cash benefits for at least 24 months, (2) most persons with end-stage renal disease (ESRD), and (3) certain otherwise noncovered aged persons who elected to pay a premium for Medicare coverage.

Medicare traditionally has consisted of two parts: Part A and Part B (Original Medicare). A third part, Part C, or the Medicare Advantage program (also known as Medicare + Choice), is available to individuals who qualify for Original Medicare and is offered by Medicare-approved private companies that must follow rules set by Medicare. The drug coverage, known as Medicare Part D, is provided by private health plans; this coverage can be drug only or can be provided through a Medicare Advantage plan that offers comprehensive benefits.

Medicare Part A

Medicare Part A, referred to as "Hospital Insurance," helps cover services and supplies related to inpatient hospital stays. In addition, Part A covers care in a skilled nursing facility (SNF) if the care follows a Medicare Part A-covered 3-day hospital stay. Finally, Part A covers hospice and, in some situations, home health care. When the beneficiary is entitled to Part A benefits, the beneficiary's red, white, and blue Medicare identification card will indicate "Hospital (Part A)."

Medicare Part B

Medicare Part B, commonly known as "Medical Insurance," essentially helps cover doctors' services, certain medical items, and outpatient care when such services are provided under a doctor's care and are documented to be medically necessary. Specifically, clinical laboratory services, some home health care, outpatient hospital services, blood transfusions (after the first 3 pints), some preventive services, ambulance services (when other transportation would endanger health), and medical social services are provided under Part B. Physical therapy and some home health care furnished by hospitals, SNFs, and other institutional providers likewise are eligible for Part B coverage. When the beneficiary has Part B benefits, the Medicare card will stipulate "Medicare (Part B)." Part B requires payment of a monthly premium that usually is taken out of the beneficiary's Social Security, Railroad Retirement, or Office of Personnel Management Retirement payment. Otherwise, Medicare will bill for the premium every 3 months. In addition to the premium, the beneficiary must meet an annual deductible and pay all coinsurance amounts unless he or she has other supplemental insurances.

Providers who submit Part B claims should always refer to their carrier's LCDs and other billing guidance for specific coverage and payment criteria. Box 2.4 gives a list of services and supplies covered under Part B, when medically necessary.

Medicare Advantage Plan, Part C

The Medicare Advantage program was established by the Balanced Budget Act of 1997 (BBA). This program consists of a set of options created by the BBA to provide care under contract to Medicare, to possibly reduce the beneficiary's out-of-pocket expenses, and to offer more health care and contractor choices. The Medicare Advantage plan must provide the same services a beneficiary would be eligible to receive from Medicare if he or she were in Original Medicare. However, the beneficiary technically still is "on Medicare" but has selected a different contractor and is required to receive services according to that contractor's arrangements.

Providers, suppliers, and their billing personnel must be aware that Medicare Advantage plans do not operate under the same coverage and payment policy for claims processing as Original Medicare. If a beneficiary is a member of a Medicare Advantage plan, the local Part B carrier cannot process claims for that beneficiary. When claims are submitted, the local Medicare Part B carrier will deny payment (except for dialysis services). After the denial, the carrier will automatically transfer the claim to the appropriate Medicare Advantage plan. The medical managed care plan is not responsible for paying Medicare Advantage claims, except when (1) the physician or supplier is affiliated with the Medicare Advantage plan or (2) the physician or supplier furnishes emergency services, urgently needed services, or other covered services not reasonably available through the Medicare Advantage plan.

A provider may be reimbursed when filing a claim to a Medicare Advantage plan if he or she is an in-network provider. An out-of-network provider may be covered if specific criteria are met as stipulated by the Medicare Advantage plan, such as prior authorization. If the plan denies the claim, the provider has the right to appeal the claim. An out-of-plan provider may also collect the full fee directly from the patient for services provided if the patient did not receive prior authorization. Before rendering services, a provider who is an affiliate with a Medicare Advantage plan should emphasize to his or her patients what their financial liability will be if they did not receive prior authorization to see the out-of-plan provider.

BOX 2.4   Services and Supplies Covered Under Medicare Part B, When Medically Necessary

Medical Care and Other Services
- Doctor's services
- Outpatient medical and surgical services and supplies
- Diagnostic examinations and tests
- Ambulatory surgery center facility fees for approved procedures
- DME such as wheelchairs, hospital beds, oxygen, walkers
- Second surgical opinions
- Outpatient mental health care
- Outpatient physical and occupational therapy, including speech/language therapy

Clinical Laboratory Services
- Blood tests
- Urinalysis
- Other tests requested by provider

Home Health Care
- Part-time skilled nursing care
- Physical therapy
- Occupational therapy
- Speech/language therapy
- Home health aide services
- Medical social services

- DME such as wheelchairs, hospital beds, oxygen, walkers
- Medical supplies and other services

Additional Coverage Related to Wound Care
- Ambulance services when other transportation would endanger the patient's health
- Artificial limbs that are prosthetic devices and their replacement parts
- Braces (arm, leg, back, neck)
- Emergency care
- Medical nutrition therapy services for people who have diabetes or kidney disease (unless currently on dialysis), with doctor's referral
- Medical supplies, such as ostomy pouches, surgical dressings, splints, casts, some diabetic supplies
- Second surgical opinion by a doctor (in some cases)
- Services of a practitioner, such as clinical social worker, physician's assistant, nurse practitioner
- Telemedicine services in some rural areas
- Therapeutic shoes for people with diabetes (in some cases)
- X-Ray films, magnetic resonance imaging, computed tomographic scanning, electrocardiography, and some other purchased diagnostic tests

DME, durable medical equipment.

Medicaid

Title XIX of the Social Security Act is a federal/state entitlement program that pays for medical assistance for certain individuals and families with low incomes and limited resources. The program, known as Medicaid, became law in 1965 as a cooperative venture jointly funded by the federal and state governments for furnishing medical assistance to eligible needy persons. Medicaid is the largest source of funding of medical and health-related services for America's poorest individuals.

Each state (1) establishes its own eligibility standards; (2) determines the type, amount, duration, and scope of services; (3) sets the rate of payment for services; and (4) administers its own program. Medicaid eligibility and/or services within a state can change during the year. Medicare beneficiaries who have low incomes and limited resources may also receive help from the Medicaid program. For persons who are eligible for full Medicaid coverage, Medicare health care coverage is supplemented by services that are available under their state's Medicaid program, according to eligibility category. When a patient is "dual enrolled," the Medicare program pays for any services that are covered by Medicare before the Medicaid program makes any payments, as Medicaid is always the "payer of last resort."

Group Health Plans, Medicare Secondary Payer Program, and Medicare Coordination of Benefits

Until 1980, Medicare was the primary payer in all situations except those involving workers' compensation. Since 1980, changes in the Medicare law have resulted in Medicare being the secondary payer in situations. The Medicare Secondary Payer (MSP) program protects Medicare funds and ensures that Medicare does not pay for services reimbursable under private insurance plans or other government programs.

The MSP program precludes Medicare from making primary claims payment when a beneficiary has other insurance that should pay first. If a beneficiary is covered by a group health plan as a benefit of current employment, charges for medical services must first be submitted to the group health plan (Centers for Medicare and Medicaid Services, 2022d).

The Medicare Coordination of Benefits program works to identify health care coverage that beneficiaries may have that pays primarily to Medicare and to coordinate the payment process to prevent mistaken Medicare primary payments. Although the various insurance programs may set separate guidelines, they generally follow similar guidelines as established by the Medicare and/or Medicare Advantage Programs. Monthly verification for services and specific procedures may be necessary to gather payment.

Medigap (Supplemental Insurance)

A Medigap policy is a health insurance policy sold by private insurance companies to fill "gaps" in the Original Medicare plan. The Medigap policy must clearly identify it as "Medicare Supplemental Insurance." Medigap plans have variances in coverage depending on the plan you select.

FACTORS THAT INFLUENCE PROVIDER REIMBURSEMENT

When implemented in 1966, Medicare was a fee-for-service insurance plan. Part B providers were paid on a reasonable charge basis for most services. Since then, Congress has mandated several changes to the Medicare reimbursement models that vary depending on the care setting and services provided. Today most payments are based on federally established predetermined payments per procedure or item rather than randomly created clinic or hospital fees. Several factors influence the amount of payment the provider is reimbursed (e.g., the care setting, the payer or payment plan, and the type of provider).

Care Setting: Nonfacility/Freestanding Sites (Part B)

Part B providers include physicians, physician assistants, nurse practitioners, clinical nurse specialists, clinical social workers, physical therapists, occupational therapists, speech-language pathologists, clinical psychologists in private practice, and suppliers of DMEPOS. A Part B provider will always accept assignments on claims submitted on behalf of the Medicare beneficiary. When a Part B provider accepts assignment, the Part B provider agrees to bill the beneficiary only for any coinsurance or deductible that may be applicable and accepts the Medicare payment as full payment.

Physician services are paid by the carrier based on the Medicare Physician's Fee Schedule. A fee schedule is a complete listing of fees used by Medicare to pay doctors or other providers/suppliers. This comprehensive listing of "fee maximums" is used to reimburse a physician and/or other providers on a fee-for-service basis. The Centers for Medicare & Medicaid Services develops fee schedules for physicians, ambulance services, clinical laboratory services, and DMEPOS. These fee schedules provide listings for facility rates and nonfacility rates; the nonfacility rates are utilized when services are provided in a standard office setting/nonfacility site.

Care Setting: Hospital Outpatient Facility Settings (Part B)

Reimbursement is limited to a facility fee rate when services are performed in one of the following settings: (1) an inpatient or outpatient hospital setting, (2) a hospital emergency room, (3) an SNF, (4) a comprehensive inpatient or outpatient rehabilitation facility (ORF), (5) an inpatient psychiatric facility, or (6) an ambulatory surgical center. Medicare pays less for services provided in these settings because Medicare assumes the physician's overhead and other related expenses are lower than they would have been in a standard office setting. Physicians are not allowed to bill the beneficiary for the difference. The fee schedule is updated annually on January 1 and available online (see Table 2.2).

Care Setting: Hospital-Based Clinic (Part A)

Part A providers include comprehensive ORFs; ESRD facilities; home health agencies (HHAs), including hospital subunits; hospitals (including freestanding facilities or units of a medical complex, such as critical access hospitals); and ORFs.

Today, most Part A providers, including hospitals, SNFs, and HHAs, receive payments through a prospective payment system (PPS), which is designed to cover the costs of all items and services furnished to beneficiaries while they are under the care of that facility. A PPS is a method of reimbursement in which Medicare payment is made based on a predetermined, fixed amount. The payment amount for a particular service is derived based on the classification system of that service (e.g., diagnosis-related groups for inpatient hospital services and ambulatory payment classifications [APCs] for outpatient services).

Many items and services that once were billable now are covered under the "Consolidated Billing" provisions of the Part A PPS system. Under this coverage, many dressing supplies and services (e.g., physical therapy) must be billed by the facility even if the services were furnished by a Part B provider (in which the payment would generally fall within the PPS). Part B suppliers should contact their Medicare Administrative Contractor (MAC) to learn what "Consolidated Billing" provisions may apply to their provider type or services they furnish.

All services paid under the new PPS to the outpatient clinic are classified into APCs. Services in each APC are similar clinically in terms of the resources they require. A payment rate is established for each APC. Depending on the services provided, hospital clinics may be paid for more than one APC per encounter. The APC codes are attached to the assigned CPT® code as further described in Section "Procedure Codes" and in Table 2.5.

Medicare Managed Care Plan

A beneficiary can select a managed care plan to provide Medicare services. CMS will pay a fixed amount (i.e., a capitated rate) to the managed care plan selected by the beneficiary. CMS pays the plan, which then reimburses the provider for services. However, enrollment as a Part B provider does not ensure payment from a Medicare-managed care plan. Provider reimbursement in a managed care plan is based solely on the terms of the provider's agreement with the plan, regardless of the amount Medicare pays for the services.

Advance Practice Providers

Medicare allows payment for services furnished by advance practice provider (APP) providers, which includes the advanced practice registered nurse (e.g., nurse practitioner, clinical nurse specialist, nurse anesthetist, and nurse midwife) and physician assistants. The APP may provide physician services and bill as the provider with the APP's provider number. Medicare reimburses the APP at a rate of 85% of the physician rate (American Academy of Physician Associates, 2022). Medicare will pay 80% of the patient's bill for the services, and the patient will pay 20% (AAPA, 2022). A service that does not meet Medicare's definition of a "physician service" will not be reimbursed. For example, health services that are within the realm of nursing but are not "physician services" are not covered under Medicare Part B. Medicare defines physician services as diagnosis, therapy, surgery consultation, and care plan oversight AAPA (2022). Box 2.5 lists Medicare rules for APP payment.

In general, Medicare requires that practices bill services under the provider number of the individual clinician performing the service. However, Medicare rules allow "incident-to" billing (i.e., submitting bills under a physician's provider number for services provided by a supervised employee) reimbursed at a rate of 100% of the physician rate. For services billed as "incident-to," the APP must follow the incident-to rules discussed next and use the physician's provider number on the claim. In this situation, the APP provider number is not needed.

Incident-to-Physician Services and Direct Supervision

"Incident-to-physician" services may be provided by auxiliary staff (any individual acting under the supervision of a physician, regardless of whether the individual is an employee, leased, or employed independent contract) or the APP. Therapeutic services and supplies that are incident to the services of the physician in the course of diagnosis or treatment of an injury or illness are referred to as incident-to-physician's professional services. To be covered as incident-to-physician's

TABLE 2.5	Sample Types of Codes Necessary for Provider Billing		
Code	**Description**	**Caveat**	**Example**
ICD-10-CM	The first 3 digits pertaining to category, the following digits addressing etiology, anatomic sites, and severity Primary diagnosis code followed by secondary diagnosis—example showing secondary diagnosis for pressure ulcer	Identified as 3- to 7-digit numbers	L8993: Pressure Ulcer unspecified site stage 4 L89153: Pressure Ulcer sacral region stage 3 L89154: Pressure Ulcer sacral region stage 4
CPT	Describes the procedure or service provided	Identified as a 5-digit code	11041: debride skin full-thickness 97597: active wound care/20 cm or under
HCPCS	Describes dressing, supplies, drugs, or procedures that do not have a CPT code	Identified as a letter and numbers	A6234: hydrocolloid dressing 4 × 4 with adhesive A6257: transparent film, 4 × 4 size

CPT, Current Procedural Terminology; *HCPCS,* Healthcare Common Procedure Coding System; *ICD-10,* International Classification of Diseases, 10th Revision.

BOX 2.5 **Medicare Rules for Advance Practice Providers (APP) Reimbursement**

The APP meets Medicare qualification requirements.

The practice or facility accepts Medicare's payment, which is 85% of the physician fee schedule rate for bills submitted under the APP's provider number.

The services performed are "physician services" or those for which a physician can bill Medicare.

The services are performed in collaboration with a physician.

The services are within the APP's scope of practice as defined in state law.

No facility or other provider charges are paid with respect to the furnishing of the services.

---

services, the services and supplies must be furnished and represent an expense to the legal entity billing for the services or supplies (clinic, physician—in a private office) and must be an integral, although incidental, part of the physician's professional service. The services must be furnished under the order of a physician and under the direct supervision of a physician. A service or supply could be considered to be incident-to when furnished during a course of treatment where the physician performs an initial service and subsequent services of a frequency reflect the physician's active participation in the management of the course of treatment, which is documented in the medical record (Centers for Medicare and Medicaid Services, 2019a).

"Direct supervision" means the physician has performed the initial service and periodically is involved in care; the physician must be present, on the premises, and immediately available to furnish assistance and direction throughout the performance of the procedure. It does not mean that the physician must be present in the room when the procedure is performed (Vargo, 2010). In the office setting, this means the physician must be present in the office suite. In the physician-directed clinic, direct supervision may be the responsibility of several physicians as opposed to an individual attending physician; the clinic physician ordering the service need not be the physician who is supervising the service (Centers for Medicare and Medicaid Services, 2019a). A hospital service or supply would not be considered incident to a physician's service if the attending physician merely wrote an order for the services or supplies and referred the patient to the hospital without being involved in the management of that course of treatment (Centers for Medicare and Medicaid Services, 2019a). During any course of treatment rendered by the auxiliary or nonphysician provider, the physician must personally see the patient periodically and sufficiently often to assess the course of treatment and the patient's progress and, where necessary, to change the treatment regimen. Clinicians must follow scope of practice and follow state laws. CMS would expect that hospitals have credentialing procedures to ensure that services furnished are being provided by qualified practitioners in accordance with all applicable laws and regulations. In addition to the Medicare Benefit Policy Manual, supervision criteria can be verified with the local MAC.

General Supervision

Effective January 1, 2020, all hospital outpatient therapeutic services require a minimum of general supervision. However, CMS may assign certain hospital outpatient therapeutic services either direct supervision or personal supervision. Also, hospital policy and process may require a higher level of supervision. "General supervision" means the procedure or service is furnished under the physician's overall direction and control, but the physician's presence is not required during the performance of the procedure (Centers for Medicare and Medicaid Services, 2020a).

Fiscal Intermediaries, Carriers, and Medicare Administrative Contractors

Medicare Part A and Part B claims are processed by nongovernmental organizations or agencies that contract to serve as fiscal agents between providers and suppliers and the federal government. Historically these claims processors were known as fiscal intermediaries (FIs) and carriers. These contractors apply Medicare coverage rules to determine appropriateness of claims for Part A (claims for institutional services, including inpatient hospital claims, SNFs, HHAs, and hospice services) and Part B (claims submitted by institutional providers, including hospital outpatient services). Providers who submit claims should always refer to their local LCD policy and other billing guidance for specific coverage and payment criteria.

From October 2004 through October 2011, FIs and carriers were integrated into MACs. As a single authority, the MAC was responsible for the receipt, processing, and payment of Medicare claims. In addition to providing core claims processing operations for both Medicare Part A and Part B, MAC performed functions related to the beneficiary and provider service, appeals, provider outreach and education (also referred to as provider education and training), financial management, program evaluation, reimbursement, payment safeguards, and information systems security. To access the most current information on Medicare contractors, see the website reference listed in Table 2.2.

National Coverage Determinations and Local Coverage Determinations

NCDs were developed by CMS to describe the circumstances for Medicare coverage for a specific medical service procedure or device. NCDs outline the conditions for which a service is considered to be covered or not covered. Once published by the CMS, an NCD is binding on all Medicare contractors and providers or suppliers. A list of current NCDs available on the CMS website is provided in Table 2.2. Box 2.6 gives a list of Medicare NCDs pertaining to wound care.

> **BOX 2.6   Medicare National Coverage Determinations Pertaining to Wound Dressings and Modalities**
>
> - Porcine skin and gradient pressure dressings
> - Treatment of decubitus ulcers
> - Hyperbaric oxygen therapy for hypoxic wounds and diabetic wounds of the lower extremities
> - Electrical stimulation and electromagnetic therapy for treatment of wounds
> - Noncontact normothermic wound therapy
> - Nonautologous blood-derived products for chronic nonhealing wounds

The LCD is a formal statement developed through a specifically defined process that (1) defines the service, (2) provides information about when the service is considered reasonable and necessary, (3) outlines any coverage criteria and/or specific documentation requirements, (4) provides specific coding and/or modifier information, and (5) provides references upon which the policy is based. Copies of draft and final LCDs are available with the Medicare Coverage Database (see Table 2.2 for the CMS website).

Generally, the LCD is an administrative and education tool used to assist providers and suppliers in completing claims for payments correctly and to guide medical reviewers. These documents specify the clinical circumstances that qualify for select service and the correct coding. The contractor shall ensure that all LCDs are consistent with all regulations and national coverage payment and coding policies. If a contractor develops an LCD, this LCD applies only within the geographic area in which that contractor services. LCDs have related billing and coding articles or policy articles, which include billing codes related to the LCD.

Clinic personnel who are primarily responsible for ensuring fiscal success in the wound clinic should be aware of any NCD and LCD pertaining to the wound care services provided in the clinic and verify updates frequently throughout the year. A mechanism should be in place for this information to be shared with the practitioners, who are expected to read and know the information. In the event, both an NCD and an LCD address the same procedure or service, the NCD will always take precedence. In the absence of an NCD addressing a specific procedure or service, local Medicare contractors may establish an LCD that summarizes medical necessity, criteria for coverage, codes for novel procedures or supplies, and references upon which a temporary coverage policy is based.

CODING AND BILLING FOR SERVICES AND SUPPLIES

Both prospective payment billing (for the hospital outpatient department) and fee-for-services billing (for provider services) require identifying the diagnosis and services provided via the coding methods described in the following section. Table 2.5 lists the types of codes necessary for provider billing.

Medical Condition Codes (ICD-10-CM)

The national coding method designed to enable providers to effectively document the medical condition, symptom, or complaint that forms the basis for rendering a specific service is known as the International Classification of Diseases, 10th Revision, Clinical Modification (ICD-10-CM, the most recent version).

These codes have multiple parts. ICD-10 codes have 3 to 7 digits, with the first 3 digits pertaining to category and the following digits addressing etiology, anatomic sites, and severity; these codes now allow for much more specific detail to be captured from the documentation. ICD-10 codes are able to capture initial encounters or subsequent, acute or chronic, right or left, normal healing, or delayed healing (Centers for Medicare and Medicaid Services, 2014a).

To provide more detail about the diagnosis and procedures provided, ICD-10 diagnosis codes increased from ~14,500 to ~70,000. Similarly, procedure codes increased from ~4000 to ~ 72,000. The number of codes available for pressure injuries increased from 13 to 25 codes incorporating location and stage, and venous ulcer codes increased from 4 to 50. A template (crosswalk) of relevant wound-specific ICD-10 codes with CPT® codes should be created to facilitate the efficient and accurate capturing of charges.

Procedure Codes (CPT®)

Procedures provided in the clinic are billed using CPT® codes that describe the procedures performed, such as debridement, compression, biopsy, chemical cautery, application of negative pressure, and application of biologic skin substitutes. These codes are derived from a standardized numeric coding system developed and maintained by the AMA.

It is essential to match the CPT® codes to the services performed during the wound clinic visit in order to bill both CMS and private health insurance programs. A created list of all services or charge data master should be reviewed with the billing/coding department to find the most closely related code to the service provided, with frequent reviews to incorporate any changes to the frequently used codes. The physician-reported procedure codes and the facility-reported procedure codes should match and be supported via documentation in the medical record. It is vital this process is reviewed by the clinic director.

Evaluation and Management Services

When the patient receives care, yet no procedure is completed, the visit is billed using an evaluation and management (E&M) service code. There are different levels of E&M codes which are determined by the complexity of a patient visit and documentation requirements. Unlike procedure codes, the E&M code level of the physician service and the hospital outpatient department service may not always match. The facility will base the E&M level on the acuity-scoring tool.

The CMS Outpatient Prospective Payment System (OPPS) Hospital Outpatient Department Facility Evaluation and Management Code

The facility charge for a clinic visit in which the provider completes an evaluation and assessment of a patient is billed with Healthcare Common Procedure Coding System (HCPCS) code G0463, "Hospital outpatient clinic visit for assessment and management of a patient" (American Medical Coding, 2022; Centers for Medicare and Medicaid Services, 2013).

- HCPCS code G0463 was created for hospital use only, for any clinic visit under the OPPS. As such, there is no need to identify whether the patient is new or established.
- G0463 does not require an organization to use any specific criteria to determine a level of service. That is, HCPCS code G0463 is used for all facility E&M visits, regardless of the intensity of service provided.

Professional (Part B) Services

E&M codes 99211–99215 describe varying levels of complexity for an "established patient" visit. Codes 99201–99205 describe varying levels of complexity for the "new patient" visit. Taken collectively, when visit levels are graphed, the majority of visits would be expected to be in the middle level of complexity and present as a bell curve.

According to CMS, a "new patient" is a new patient who has not received any professional services from the physician/qualified health care professional or another physician/qualified health care professional of the exact same specialty and subspecialty who belongs to the same group practice within the past 3 years (Centers for Medicare and Medicaid Services, 2021c). An "established patient" is a patient who has received professional services from the physician/qualified health care professional or another physician/qualified health care professional of the exact same specialty and subspecialty who belongs to the same group practice within the past 3 years (Centers for Medicare and Medicaid Services, 2021c).

Billing for Evaluation and Management and Procedures on the Same Day

It is not appropriate to bill for an E&M service separately when billing for services that already include taking the patient's blood pressure, temperature, asking the patient how he/she feels, and getting the consent form signed (e.g., diagnostic, therapeutic procedures). However, an E&M service may be separately billed with a minor procedure as long as a new or separately identifiable problem was addressed when a minor procedure was performed by the same physician on the same day of the procedure or other service. In that case, the E&M service needs to be clearly documented and substantiated and modifier 25 needs to be properly appended to the appropriate E&M service code (Cartwright, 2020).

Supply Codes (HCPCS)

Medicare does not allow for reimbursement of routine dressing supplies provided during a clinic (hospital outpatient) visit. Under the OPPS, the cost of routine dressing supplies considered integral to the visit are bundled into the visit codes and costs of many procedures; thus, supplies are included in the payment for the service (i.e., packaged services). No separate payment is made for packaged services. Although supplies may be marked on the bill to show the cost of the visit, most insurance providers will not reimburse for wound care supplies used during an outpatient clinic visit and tend to follow the Medicare guidelines on packaged codes. For example, routine supplies, anesthesia, recovery room use, and most drugs are considered an integral part of a surgical procedure, so payment for these items is packaged into the APC payment for the surgical procedure.

Unless a facility is also a DME provider, the ability for an outpatient clinic to provide and bill supplies for use at home is cost prohibitive. The patient may qualify for home dressing supplies per Medicare guidelines if home health care is not providing the wound care. Medicaid may reimburse for supplies if home care is active, and group health plans may offer coverage at times with a possible copayment. Understanding how to assist patients in obtaining home supplies is integral to successful patient outcomes. Patients will need information about suppliers in their area, as well as those that do business by mail (electronic and postal) and by phone. The wound specialist should be aware of additional services provided by suppliers, such as billing insurance directly, offering free delivery, obtaining physician prescriptions for supplies, and making reminder phone calls for reorders. Box 2.7 lists the Medicare guidelines for DME orders.

Knowledge of coverage limits and criteria will assist with the ordering of products that are readily available in the community and reimbursed by Medicare. This valuable information on coverage can be obtained from the CMS website (see Table 2.2).

A complete list of supplies frequently used in the clinic, such as foams, hydrocolloids, alginates, or compression wraps, should be developed and matched to the corresponding HCPCS. These codes describe the dressing supply assigned and maintained by local Medicare contractors. Level II HCPCS provides a method for obtaining reimbursement for products, supplies, or procedures not covered in CPT codes.

In the OPPS, outpatient clinics are encouraged to mark on the bill all supplies used at each visit, regardless of expected reimbursement. The total cost of the visit will help ensure future reimbursement of clinic CPT and E&M services by showing the average cost of visits over time.

National Correct Coding Initiative Edits

The CMS developed the National Correct Coding Initiative (NCCI) to promote correct coding by providers and suppliers. NCCI edits apply to claims that contain more than one procedure on the same patient, on the same date, and by the same provider or supplier. Payment edits are designed and put in

---

BOX 2.7 Medicare Guidelines for DME Arrangements for the Home

1. Written orders for DME can be submitted as a photocopy, facsimile image, electronic file, or original "pen-and-ink" order.
2. For dressing supplies that will be provided on a periodic basis, the written order should include:
   - The start date of the order
   - A detailed description listing all options or additional features that will be separately billed or that will require an upgraded code
3. Medical necessity information (diagnosis code) is not considered part of the order, although it may be included within the same document.
4. Someone other than the physician may complete the detailed description of the item or service; however, the treating physician must review the detailed description and personally sign and date the order to indicate agreement.

Example: One 4 × 4 hydrocolloid dressing changed two times per week for 1 month or until the ulcer is healed.
DME, durable medical equipment.

---

place to prevent payment for noncovered and/or incorrectly coded services. The NCCI edits can be located online at the CMS website listed in Table 2.2. Wound debridement codes include the wound debridement, the dressing placed after the debridement, and the assessment and documentation of the wound; therefore, E&M would not be added to the bill along with the debridement because E&M is a necessary part of the debridement and is already captured in the debridement code.

Modifier 59: Distinct Procedural Service

Under certain circumstances, the physician may need to indicate that a procedure or service was distinct or independent from other services performed on the same day. Multiple procedures involving one wound site are almost always billed under one code. The code modifier 59, Distinct Procedural Services, applies when multiple procedures involving multiple anatomic sites or different patient encounters are performed. In this situation, it is appropriate to bill for additional procedures, adding the modifier 59 to indicate that the various procedures involved were at different wound sites even though they were performed on the same day.

Misuse of modifier 59 preceded the introduction of four HCPCS modifiers effective January 2015 that are more specific. Modifier 59 remains available; however, the most descriptive modifier should always be used.

The four HCPCS are referred to as X{EPSU} modifiers: (1) XE Separate Encounter—a service that is distinct because it occurred during a separate encounter, (2) XS

Separate Structure—a service that is distinct because it was performed on a separate organ/structure, (3) XP Separate Practitioner—a service that is distinct because it was performed by a different practitioner, and (4) XU Unusual Nonoverlapping Service—the use of a service that is distinct because it does not overlap unusual component of the main service (Centers for Medicare and Medicaid Services, 2014c; Cobuzzi, 2015). Understanding the edits for bundled services and the code modifier for multiple services is essential to comprehending expected reimbursement.

Medically Unlikely Edits

Medically Unlikely Edits (MUEs) are used by the MACs, including DME MACs, to reduce the improper payment rate for Part B claims. An MUE for a HCPCS or CPT® code is the maximum units of service that a provider would report under most circumstances for a single beneficiary on a single date of service. Not all HCPCS or CPT® codes have an MUE.

Although CMS publishes most MUE values on its website, other MUE values are confidential and are for CMS and CMS contractors use only. Confidential MUE values are not releasable. The MUEs files are updated at least quarterly.

Status Indicator

CPT codes are assigned a status indicator. A T indicates that reimbursement will be adjusted downward to a discount for multiple procedures. An S indicates that no downward adjustment will be made, that is, no discount for multiple procedures. This adjustment reflects a situation where multiple services are provided with the understanding that resources (e.g., room setup, registration) for multiple procedures will not be duplicated for each of the additional procedures. For example, if three debridements are done to three different anatomic sites on the same patient on the same day, the first debridement is paid in full and the additional debridements are paid at a discounted rate.

Waiver of Deductible and Coinsurance

Routinely waiving the collection of deductible or coinsurance from a beneficiary constitutes a violation of the law pertaining to false claims and kickbacks. Where a physician/supplier makes a reasonable collection effort for the payment of coinsurance/deductibles, failure to collect payment is not considered a reduction in the charges. To be considered reasonable collection efforts, the efforts must be similar to those made to collect from non-Medicare patients. This may include actions such as subsequent billings, collection letters, and telephone calls or personal contacts that constitute a genuine, rather than token, collection effort (Centers for Medicare and Medicaid Services, 2020b).

CLINICAL CONSULT

S: Please see attached business plan including a list of patients and interventions provided this past year by the Wound, Ostomy and Continence Nurses Society™ after readmissions within 30 days of initial hospital stays.

B: As you are aware, in addition to the financial penalty hospitals with excess Medicare readmissions receive, Medicare Hospital Readmissions Reduction Program (HRRP) provides financial incentive to lower readmission rates.

A: An outpatient wound clinic could help the hospital with the HRRP, save money, and increase patient satisfaction.

R: We respectfully request your review of the attached proposal and permission to begin meeting with key stakeholders to further explore the possibility of providing wound care services across the continuum of care.

SUMMARY

- This chapter describes the key components of a wound clinic. Staffing, supplies, consents, authorizations, and location may differ depending on type of clinic (freestanding clinic or office vs hospital outpatient department).
- Further explanation is given on the role and expectations of staff in the wound clinic. The need for consents, safekeeping of medical records, and need for intercommunication between referrals both in and out of the clinic.
- Clinics will obtain reimbursement differently depending on the clinic structure (i.e., hospital-based clinic, freestanding clinic). The freestanding clinic will mirror the physician office in utilizing the physician fee schedule for reimbursement, whereas the hospital outpatient department will utilize the hospital outpatient prospective payment system (HOPPS).
- In the hospital outpatient clinic, when a physician sees a patient while utilizing the hospital staff, a bill is submitted by the physician (at a lower reimbursement rate than if the patient were seen in his or her private office) and a bill is submitted by the facility (to capture hospital resources of room, staff, and supplies based on the HOPPS).
- Further differences between clinics consist of determining who the practitioners will be: physician, APPs (reimbursed at 85% of the physician rate when billing physician services), nurse, PT, or a combination, while also considering which multidiscipline programs will be attached to the clinic.
- Not only are the differences in reimbursement shared, we also discuss the various types of insurance coverage outpatient wound clinics may utilize for appropriate reimbursement.
- Checklist 2.4 summarizes steps to consider for establishing a successful outpatient clinic.

CHECKLIST 2.4 Establishing an Outpatient Clinic

- ✓ Determine services to be provided
- ✓ Create business plan
- ✓ Gain support and approval from administration and medical colleagues
- ✓ Decide clinic structure and staffing needs
  - Management/clinic director
  - Medical director
  - Wound specialist nationally certified as CWCN or CWS
  - Nurse
  - Physical therapist
  - Insurance and billing coders
  - Ancillary staff
- ✓ Determine clinic location and space needs
- ✓ Develop compliance program
  - HIPAA privacy rule
  - Centers for Medicare & Medicaid Services
  - The Joint Commission
  - Department of Health Certificate of Need
  - National Patient Safety Goals
  - Billing codes
  - Corporate compliance
- ✓ Meet with coders and create charge master
  - Establish policies

- Documentation
- Photography
- Frequency of visits
- Referrals for tests and consults
- Infection control
- Treatment orders
- Obtaining consents
- Debridement
- Staffing
- Staff education
- Wound care outcomes
- Insurance authorization
- ✓ Create patient and staff education and competencies
- ✓ Determine equipment needs and formulary of supplies
- ✓ Create/gather teaching documents, including list of durable medical equipment contacts
- ✓ Establish operations
  - Hours
  - Scheduling
  - Documentation forms
  - Chart storage and retrieval
  - Room cleaning
- ✓ Develop marketing plan

HIPAA, Health Insurance Portability and Accountability Act of 1996.

SELF-ASSESSMENT QUESTIONS

1. One of the key elements for a successful wound care program is:
   a. The clinic needs to be attached to a hospital
   b. The clinic needs to be managed by a contractor (i.e., external management)
   c. The clinic needs to have additional means of financial viability
   d. A multidisciplinary approach

2. Some of the items that need to be documented in an outpatient wound clinic chart include:
   a. Comprehensive admission assessment; wound assessment, compliance/teaching record
   b. Provider progress notes; modifier 79
   c. Discharge orders; modifier 82
   d. Consents, insurance information, HIPAA documents; Medically Unlikely Edits

3. True or false: Freestanding clinic or office (place of service 11) is able to bill Medicare for a facility fee.

4. The National Correct Coding Initiative (NCCI) was created by the Centers for Medicare and Medicaid Services to:
   a. Help lower improper payment rates and protect the Medicare Trust Fund
   b. Promote correct coding by providers and suppliers and prevent payment for noncovered and/or incorrectly coded services
   c. Reduce the improper payment rate for Part B claims
   d. Detection and collect overpayments made on claims of health care services provided to Medicare beneficiaries

REFERENCES

American Academy of Physician Associates. (AAPA). (2022). *The Essential Guide to PA reimbursement 2022.* American Academy of Physician Associates. Retrieved November 16, 2022, from https://www.aapa.org/shop/essential-guide-pa-reimbursement/.

American Medical Coding. (2022). G0463 HCPCS code: Coding guidelines for coders. Medical coding guide. Learn how to code. Retrieved November 16, 2022, from https://www.americanmedicalcoding.com/hcpcs-code-g0463/.

Armstrong, D. G., Ayello, E. A., Capitulo, K. L., Fowler, E., Krasner, D. L., Levine, J. M., et al. (2008). New opportunities to improve pressure ulcer prevention and treatment. *Journal of Wound, Ostomy and Continence Nursing, 35*(5), 485–492. https://doi.org/10.1097/01.WON.0000335960.68113.82.

Aviles, F. (2018). Let's be frank: How to save your wound clinic from failure. *Today's Wound Clinic, 12*(4). Retrieved 11.16.2022, from https://www.hmpgloballearningnetwork.com/site/twc/articles/lets-be-frank-how-save-your-wound-clinic-failure.

Cartwright, D. (2020). An auditor's perspective of debridement and E&M/clinic visits with modifier-25. *Today's Wound Clinic, 14*(4), 10–13. Retrieved December 15, 2020, from https://www.todayswoundclinic.com/articles/auditors-perspective-debridement-and-emclinic-visits-modifier-25.

Centers for Medicare and Medicaid Services. (2013). *Update of the hospital outpatient prospective payment system (OPPS).* Pub 100-04 Medicare Claims Processing. Transmittal 2845. CMS Manual System. Retrieved November 16, 2022 from https://www.cms.gov/Regulations-and-Guidance/Guidance/Transmittals/2013-Transmittals-Items/R2845CP.

Centers for Medicare and Medicaid Services. (2014a). *ICD-10 basics for medical practices.* Retrieved November 16, 2022, from https://www.cms.gov/medicare/coding/icd10/downloads/icd10basicsforpractices20140819.pdf.

Centers for Medicare and Medicaid Services. (2014b). *Lower costs, better care: Reforming our health care delivery system.* Retrieved December 15, 2020, from https://www.cms.gov/newsroom/factsheets/lower-costs-better-care-reforming-our-health-care-delivery-system.

Centers for Medicare and Medicaid Services. (2014c). *Specific modifiers for distinct procedural services.* Pub 100-20. One-Time Notification. CMS Manual System. Retrieved November 16, 2022 from, https://www.cms.gov/Regulations-and-Guidance/Guidance/Transmittals/2014-Transmittals-Items/R1422OTN.

Centers for Medicare and Medicaid Services. (2019a). Chapter 15. Covered medical and other health services. *Internet-Only Manuals (IOMs). Publication # 100-2.* In *Medicare benefit policy manual.* Retrieved November 17, 2022 from, https://www.cms.gov/Regulations-and-Guidance/Guidance/Manuals/Internet-Only-Manuals-IOMs-Items/CMS012673.

Centers for Medicare and Medicaid Services. (2020a). *Update of the hospital outpatient prospective payment system (OPPS).* Retrieved November 17, 2022, from https://www.cms.gov/files/document/mm11605.pdf.

Centers for Medicare and Medicaid Services. (2020b). Appendix A. Survey protocol, regulations and interpretive guidelines for hospitals. In *Internet-Only Manuals (IOMs). Publication #100-07. State operations manual.* Retrieved November 16, 2022 from https://www.cms.gov/Regulations-and-Guidance/Guidance/Manuals/Internet-Only-Manuals-IOMs.

Centers for Medicare and Medicaid Services. (2021a). *Place of service code set.* Retrieved November 16, 2022, from https://www.cms.gov/Medicare/Coding/place-of-service-codes/Place_of_Service_Code_Set.

Centers for Medicare and Medicaid Services. (2021b). Chapter 23. Fee schedule administration and coding requirements. In *Internet-Only Manuals (IOMs). Publication #100-04. Medicare claims processing manual.* Retrieved November 17, 2022, from https://www.cms.gov/Regulations-and-Guidance/Guidance/Manuals/Internet-Only-Manuals-IOMs.

Centers for Medicare and Medicaid Services. (2021c). Chapter 12. Physicians/nonphysician practitioners. In *Internet-Only Manuals (IOMs). Publication #100-04. Medicare claims processing manual.* Retrieved November 16, 2022 from, https://www.cms.gov/Regulations-and-Guidance/Guidance/Manuals/Internet-Only-Manuals-IOMs-Items/CMS012673.

Centers for Medicare and Medicaid Services. (2022a). *How to use the searchable Medicare physician fee schedule (MPFS).* Retrieved

November 16, 2022, from https://www.cms.gov/Medicare/Medicare-Fee-for-Service-Payment/PFSlookup.

Centers for Medicare and Medicaid Services. (2022b). *Medicare fee for service recovery audit program.* Retrieved November 16, 2022, from https://www.cms.gov/Research-Statistics-Data-and-Systems/Monitoring-Programs/Medicare-FFS-Compliance-Programs/Recovery-Audit-Program/.

Centers for Medicare and Medicaid Services. (2022c). *Hospital Readmissions Reduction Program (HRRP).* Retrieved November 16, 2022, from https://www.cms.gov/Medicare/Medicare-Fee-for-Service-Payment/AcuteInpatientPPS/Readmissions-Reduction-Program.

Centers for Medicare and Medicaid Services. (2022d). *Group health plan recovery.* Retrieved November 16, 2022, from https://www.cms.gov/Medicare/Coordination-of-Benefits-and-Recovery/Coordination-of-Benefits-and-Recovery-Overview/Group-Health-Plan-Recovery/Group-Health-Plan-Recovery.

Centers for Medicare and Medicaid Services. (2022e). *Supplemental medical review contractor.* Retrieved November 16, 2022, from https://www.cms.gov/Research-Statistics-Data-and-Systems/Monitoring-Programs/Medicare-FFS-Compliance-Programs/Medical-Review/SMRC.

Centers for Medicare and Medicaid Services. (2022f). *Targeted probe and educate.* Retrieved November 16, 2022, from https://www.cms.gov/research-statistics-data-and-systems/monitoring-programs/medicare-ffs-compliance-programs/medical-review/targeted-probe-and-educatetpe.

Cobuzzi, B. (2015). Knowledge Center. Specific modifiers for distinct procedural services. *AAPC.* Retrieved November 17, 2022, from https://www.aapc.com/blog/29197-specific-modifiers-for-distinct-procedural-services-from-cms/.

Department of Health and Human Services, Office of Inspector General. (2007). *Medicare payments for surgical debridement services in 2004.* Retrieved November 17, 2022 from, at http://oig.hhs.gov/oei/reports/oei-02-05-00390.pdf.

Department of Health and Human Services, Office of Inspector General. (2019). *Medicare Part B payments for podiatry and ancillary services.* Retrieved December 14, 2020, from https://oig.hhs.gov/reports-and-publications/workplan/summary/wp-summary-0000344.asp.

Fife, C. (2019). For wound care formularies, it's the infrastructure, stupid. *Today's Wound Clinic,* 13(6). Retrieved November 17, 2022 from https://www.hmpgloballearningnetwork.com/site/twc/articles/wound-care-formularies-its-infrastructure-stupid.

Gethin, G., Probst, S., Stryja, J., Christiansen, N., & Price, P. (2020). Evidence for person-centered care in chronic wound care: A systematic review and recommendations for practice. *Journal of Wound Care,* 29(Sup9b), S1–S22. https://doi.org/10.12968/jowc.2020.29.Sup9b.S1.

Graham, K. L., Auerbach, A. D., Schnipper, J. L., Flanders, S. A., Kim, C. S., Robinson, E. J., et al. (2018). Preventability of early versus late hospital readmissions in a national cohort of general medicine patients. *Annals of Internal Medicine,* 168(11), 766–774. https://doi.org/10.7326/M17-1724.

Hamm, T. (2020). Internal medical documentation auditing. In E. Song (Ed.), *WoundReference.*

Hess, C. T. (2008). Developing a wound care compliance program (part 1). *Advances in Skin & Wound Care,* 21(10), 496. https://doi.org/10.1097/01.ASW.0000323568.82755.c4.

Hess, C. T. (2018). Wound care medical record documentation. *Advances in Skin & Wound Care,* 31(10), 479–480. https://doi.org/10.1097/01.ASW.0000546121.09810.83.

Hess, C.T. (2019). Owning and auditing your documentation. *Advances in Skin & Wound Care,* 32(11), 527–528.

Kaiser Family Foundation. (2013). *Summary of the Affordable Care Act.* Retrieved December 15, 2020, from https://www.kff.org/health-reform/fact-sheet/summary-of-the-affordable-care-act/.

Kim, P. J., Evans, K. K., Steinberg, J. S., Pollard, M. E., & Attinger, C. E. (2013). Critical elements to building an effective wound care center. *Journal of Vascular Surgery,* 57(6), 1703–1709. https://doi.org/10.1016/j.jvs.2012.11.112.

Morrison, C. (2007). If you build it, they will come: Marketing your wound clinic to its fullest potential. *Today's Wound Clinic,* 1(1), 32–33.

Schaum, K. D. (2019). Fiction or fact: Reimbursement for cellular and/or tissue-based products for skin wounds. *Advances in Skin & Wound Care,* 32(2), 55–57. https://doi.org/10.1097/01.ASW.0000550738.26041.c5.

Song, E. H., Milne, C., Hamm, T., Mize, J., Harris, K., Kuplicki, S., et al. (2020). A novel point of care solution to streamline local wound formulary development and promote cost-effective wound care. *Advances in Skin & Wound Care,* 33(2), 91–97. https://doi.org/10.1097/01.ASW.0000617852.54001.46.

Steed, D. (2016). Building an effective coding compliance program in medical practices. *The Journal of Medical Practice Management,* 32(1), 28–31.

The Wound Ostomy and Continence Nurses Society (WOCN). (2013). *Professional practice manual* (4th ed.).

Treadwell, T. (2007). How are we doing? Evaluating your wound clinic operations. *Today's Wound Clinic,* 29–31.

US Department of Health & Human Services. (2009). Health Information Privacy. HITECH Act Enforcement Interim Final Rule. Retrieved 10/06/2022 from: https://www.hhs.gov/hipaa/for-professionals/special-topics/hitech-act-enforcement-interim-final-rule/index.html.

Vargo, D. M. (2010). Direct supervision requirements and incident to services. *Journal of Wound, Ostomy and Continence Nursing,* 37(2), 148–151. https://doi.org/10.1097/won.0b013e3181cf721c.

Weiss, D. G. (2019). Successfully navigating today's world of CMS audits. *Today's Wound Clinic,* 13(10), 22–25.

Postacute Care Settings

Catherine T. Milne

OBJECTIVES

1. Describe the operational and regulatory requirements for wound management in postacute settings.
2. List the requirements to receive care in a skilled nursing facility (SNF).
3. Describe the role of the Minimum Data Set (MDS) in relation to wound management and prevention.
4. List the requirements to receive home health care services.
5. Describe the role of the Outcome and Assessment Information Set (OASIS) in relation to wound management.
6. Compare and contrast differences in providing wound management in postacute settings.

Postacute settings are complex, dynamic, and diverse. Often stereotyped as a "lower level" of care, many providers are surprised at both the intensity and acuity of the patients which may not differ greatly from the acute care setting. Mechanical ventilation, intravenous medications, and dialysis are often necessary to manage the comorbidities typically present in a patient with a wound. Many postacute settings now routinely care for these complex, labor intense patient populations. With the focus on shifting from a fee-for-service to a value-based health care system, many transformational changes have been made in the delivery of health care in postacute settings. The wound management service line is affected in these transformations. The previous chapter discussed wound management in the outpatient clinic and wound center settings. This chapter will outline wound management in the other postacute settings of the skilled nursing facility (SNF) and the home health setting. While the principles of wound management do not change as the patient moves through the continuum of care, systems management of the clinical setting becomes imperative to achieve positive outcomes.

SKILLED NURSING FACILITY POSTACUTE SETTING

Operational Structure

Frequently called the long-term care (LTC) setting or an SNF nothing could be farther from reality. SNFs are varied in the services they provide. Usually a stand-alone building with its own organizational structure, they may also be situated within an acute care facility but operating separately. SNFs can be owned and operated by chains or as a part of an integrated delivery system. Others may be unaffiliated and operate as a stand-alone entity. Many SNFs are owned by investors or private individuals who pay a management fee to a corporation to provide staff and operations. Nursing home chains can be large and have a national and international presence or they can be regional with locations in just one or two states. Whether a chain or a stand-alone facility, each with a mission statement as well as structured policies and protocols, every building will have its own personality, challenges, and opportunities.

The typical organizational chart for a chain SNF includes the Chief Executive Officer (CEO), the Chief Operating Officer, and a Clinical Vice-President (CVP). The CVP may have a background in nursing, pharmacy, physical or occupational therapy, or medicine. There are standard clinical reporting lines under the CVP that include wound and management and infection prevention, as the cost of managing these specialties can be significant. Most medium- and large-size chains make purchasing decisions at the corporate level, including those for wound management. The corporate chains are either for-profit or designated nonprofit entities. As in other settings, the patient experience between different individual SNFs will differ. You et al. (2016) found that independent, nonprofits SNFs generally score higher on patient satisfaction surveys than for-profit small, medium, or large chains.

Defined by the number of buildings owned or managed, small chains (2–10 facilities), medium (11–70 facilities), and large chains (more than 70 facilities) provide services for facilities for over half of the United States. Independent organizations account for 45% of all SNFs in the United States (You et al., 2016). Independent SNFs can also have a for-profit or nonprofit status. The owner(s) may or may not be active in the on-site daily management.

The organizational structure is influenced by regulations. The skilled nursing home facility is one of the most heavily regulated industries in the United States. To participate in Medicare and Medicaid programs, nursing homes must comply with all federal requirements mandated by the Omnibus Budget Reconciliation Act (OBRA) passed by Congress in 1988. This legislation required skilled facilities to provide services and activities to attain or maintain the highest practicable physical, mental, and psychosocial well-being of each resident in accordance with a written plan of care (Kelly, 1989; Morford, 1988). The mandates of OBRA are regarded in the nursing home setting to represent minimum accepted standards of care. The failure of a nursing home to comply with the OBRA mandates while caring for a resident represents a violation of the law, which can be accompanied by a monetary fine, restriction of services, or a loss of license with the possibility of civil suits and criminal charges (Kelly, 1989; Morford, 1988).

Each SNF, regardless of its ownership or financial reporting structure, will have its own internal organizational management team. This will consist of an administrator, accountable for financial stability as well as the physical facilities as well as ensuring that regulatory requirements are met. Sitting at the helm of the clinical activities will be a Director of Nursing (DON), who is charged to oversee direct care and supporting staff. The administrator and DON must work together to oversee even the smallest of buildings as the regulatory requirements in this setting are abundant.

All SNFs will have a therapy department, usually consisting of at least one physical therapist, an occupational therapist, a physical therapy aide, and a speech therapist. Some facilities contract with companies who provide the services in the facility. If the SNF is large enough to financially support a dietician, this may be an employee. If not, a dietician is contracted to provide these required services in the facility. Also crucial to the operational structure is the facility admissions personnel. These employees are responsible for assessing potential patients for admission. They serve as a hospital and community liaison by evaluating whether the patient's needs can be met at the facility before accepting to care for them. Integral to this process is an appraisal of financial compensation for the LTC services that is expected to be provided.

Each facility decides how they operationalize their wound care program. Some have an infection preventionist nurse who is solely dedicated to providing wound care services which encompass weekly rounds, data collection, monitoring of infections, and presentation of statistics and outcomes to the medical and administrative staff. Wound care, if ordered more frequently than weekly, may be performed by the infection preventionist nurse or the shift nurse assigned to the patient. The infection preventionist nurse may oversee a "treatment" nurse or nurses who perform wound care. Other organizations structure the infection preventionist role to perform additional duties including employee health and staff development. Other key activities encompass monitoring other potential infection-related issues around the facility including surveillance activities, often working with the maintenance and kitchen staff.

Over the past several years, requirements from the Centers for Disease Control and Prevention have required the infection preventionist in LTC facilities to manage antibiotic stewardship programs. The COVID-19 pandemic added additional responsibilities to the role, often without additional manpower. The infection preventionist or the treatment nurse may or may not have formal training in wound management beyond their initial education or hold specialized wound certification. This position is often given to a Registered Nurse, though Licensed Vocational/Practical Nurses may qualify if State Scope of Practice requirements are met. Considering that 61% of all nursing homes in the United States received a citation for an infection control issue (Rau, 2020), this position is central to the success of any SNF.

The Minimum Data Set (MDS) Coordinator position requires taking documentation from the medical record from a variety of providers and entering the data into required forms that are submitted to federal and state regulatory agencies. The data are used to provide accurate reimbursement, outside oversight to determine quality, and to ensure the facility is meeting regulatory requirements. The person who holds the position of an MDS coordinator develops the plan of care based on the MDS and patient care planning meetings with the patient and their significant others. The position maybe held by a Licensed Vocational/Practical Nurse but is preferably occupied by a Registered Nurse. The accuracy of the reports and the care planning process is often in an area of intense scrutiny by state department of public health during the survey process.

Facilities may also have the staff nurse caring for the patient perform provider-ordered wound care. Patients, who are referred to as "residents" in this milieu, are admitted at various days and times. At the time of admission, a body audit is completed to identify all types of skin alterations. These may include pressure injuries, surgical wounds, venous, arterial, and diabetic-related wounds but also skin tears and rashes. It is often the staff nurse who refers to standardized institutional protocols to obtain orders for wound management at the time of admission or a change in wound characteristics. They are also responsible for patient and family education for prevention of wounds especially pressure injuries and providing teaching for wound management postdischarge.

The certified nursing aide (CNA) is integral in providing eyes and ears for the nursing staff as well as establishing rapport with the patient and their family to improve patient compliance. Monthly education for the CNA is required with at least one annual session devoted to skin care management and wound prevention.

The medical staff is expected to have basic knowledge in wound management. The Medical Director is a paid staff position though not required to be on site full time. They are expected to be available by phone 24 h/day. This position is responsible for ensuring good clinical practice is being employed at the facility. Medical Directors are held accountable by regulatory agencies and state department of public health agencies to address physician and mid-level provider practice issues as well uphold medical management standards and monitor quality measures. In this position, Medical Directors often set the tone for the medical care that is provided to residents.

Reimbursement

While general information regarding billing and reimbursement has been discussed in Chapter 2, there are specific regulations surrounding reimbursement that affect the provision of wound management services in the postacute care setting. In general, if a resident is enrolled in the Medicare Part A, they require a 3-day hospital stay prior to admission to the SNF for the stay to be covered (e.g., reimbursed) under the assistance Medicare provides. A resident must be in an SNF that has been certified by Medicare to access this benefit. Patients on Medicare that have not met a qualifying stay are financially responsible for all charges accruing at the facility for their length of stay.

The Centers for Medicare and Medicaid Services (CMS) determine the benefit rules, which may change at any time. While changes in benefit provisions are posted on the CMS website for the public to provide comment and are not made final until remarks have been received and considered, CMS did rapidly eliminate the 3-day stay requirement during the COVID-19 pandemic (Centers for Medicare and Medicaid Services, 2020a).

A skilled service is also required for an admission to be covered under the Medicare Part A benefit. A skilled service for a medical condition is defined as a hospital-related medical condition treated during a 3-day inpatient hospital stay, even if it was not the related to the reason for hospitalization. Additionally, it includes a condition that occurred in the SNF for a hospital-related medical condition (e.g., pressure injury). At least one skilled service is required daily to continue to qualify for the Medicare Part A benefit.

The first 20 days of this benefit will pay for 100% of the patient's stay. Between days 21 and 100, the patient is required to pay $176 per day of reasonable and necessary care, requiring the SNF to absorb the remaining costs (Centers for Medicare and Medicaid Services, 2020b). This includes all laboratory, diagnostics, medication, and durable medical equipment (DME) expenses in addition to room, board, nursing, and therapy services. The first 100 days of an SNF stay is known as a "Part A stay." From a wound management perspective, provision of wound care dressings and equipment such as a support surface or a negative pressure therapy device often falls to the responsibility of the SNF.

If a patient has a supplemental insurance, the costs incurred in the first 100 days of the SNF stay are usually absorbed by the insurer. Many people do not have supplemental coverage and expense anxiety about the noncovered cost of care impacts and often overrules clinical decisions. A patient without insurance may be accepted as a patient in the SNF with the expectation that Medicaid application will be initiated and payment for service will be rendered.

After 100 days, the patient is responsible for all costs associated with their stay. Many facilities recognize patients who are unlikely to be discharged before the end of their 100-day stay and actively work with the family and patient to provide information on alternative methods of meeting financial obligations to the nursing facility and other health care services prior to this. Typically, this means patients are transitioning to a state-managed Medicaid program. As each state makes its own rules and implements its programs differently, the reader is advised to contact a knowledgeable source about local requirements and terms of participation.

Not all patients coming to an SNF have traditional Medicare. Approximately 20 million people (35%) in the United States subscribed to a Medicare Advantage plan program in 2017. It is expected that this number will increase to 50 million (50%) by 2025 (Frack, Garlbaldi, & Kadar, 2017; Starc, 2014). There are a variety of Medicare Advantage programs that provide coverage for short-term stays in an SNF. These also have a variety of stipulations which are often changing in as describing each plan individually in this section is moot. The reader is advised to contact a specific patient's insurance plan for coverage details. Medicare Advantage plans must provide the same benefits as traditional Medicare, and many provide more. How these benefits are accessed by patients differ among the plans. The CMS have contracted with organizations that monitor quality and implementation of Medicare Advantage plans offered by private insurance companies. Many of these offerings will approve of up to 20 days of care in an SNF but often present the case that the patient can receive the same services at home and will not provide for payment after 20 days. There is an increasing trend for these residents in these Medicare Advantage plans to have shorter stays when compared with their traditional Medicare part A counterparts.

Evaluation and management services performed by Physician and Mid-level providers are covered under the Medicare Part B supplement, assuming the patient has enrolled in this benefit (Centers for Medicare and Medicaid Services, 2020c). Physician Assistants, Nurse Practitioners, and Clinical Nurse Specialists, also referred to as Mid-level providers, are lumped together and referred to as Nonphysician Providers (NPPs). Medicaid Services also cover provider evaluation and management services though, at a very reduced reimbursement. Some Medicaid patients may carry a Medicare Part B supplement which would provide payment for services provided by a physician or NPP. Medicare Part B pays 80% of a Physician or Physician assistant evaluation and management service regardless if the patient is in the Part A stay or not. An Advanced Practice Nurse (Nurse Practitioner of Clinical Nurse Specialist) receives 85% of 80% of the approved visit charge. Visit charges are predetermined by Medicare rate schedules and adjusted annually under the value-based payment program. A patient on a Medicare Advantage Plan may have restrictions or incentives to use an approved provider. As a result, the responsibility for the entire charge of the service for an out-of-network provider may lie solely with the patient.

Due to an often-confusing payment system, managing these patients from a financial perspective while maintaining standards of care and improving outcomes can be challenging for an SNF. The largest cost to the facility includes medication, diagnostic testing, and transportation costs associated with physician appointments outside of the SNF. This has led to the implementation of in-house interdisciplinary wound care teams with strict formulary adherence to protocols designed to maximize outcomes with the least amount of cost. During a Medicare Part A stay, bedside debridement procedures that are performed within the facility fall under consolidated billing guidelines. Under these regulations, the provider cannot bill Medicare for these services and must bill the facility for payment of the services.

Determining the Daily Rate of Care in the Skilled Nursing Facility

Prior to October 1, 2019, payment to an SNF for a Medicare Part A stay was based on resource utilization groups (RUGs). This system categorized individual patients based primarily on the rehabilitation needs (Fig. 3.1) with adjustments for geographical labor costs and case mix (MedPac, 2016). RUGs, a volume-based system, placed emphasis on the use of physical, occupational, or speech therapy utilization on the assumption that therapy was the way to obtain the highest physical well-being as mandated by OBRA was the most important.

Over time, it became a strong revenue stream for LTC facilities. As such, it led to a proliferation of therapy services, many times without corresponding gains in outcomes. Therapy services would abruptly stop at Day 100 and the patient would be placed on a "restorative" program to be provided by nursing. Patients received no therapy at all, as the incentive to tie therapy volume to payment was no longer available.

In October 2019, a new reimbursement initiative was instituted for all Medicare Part A stay patients called

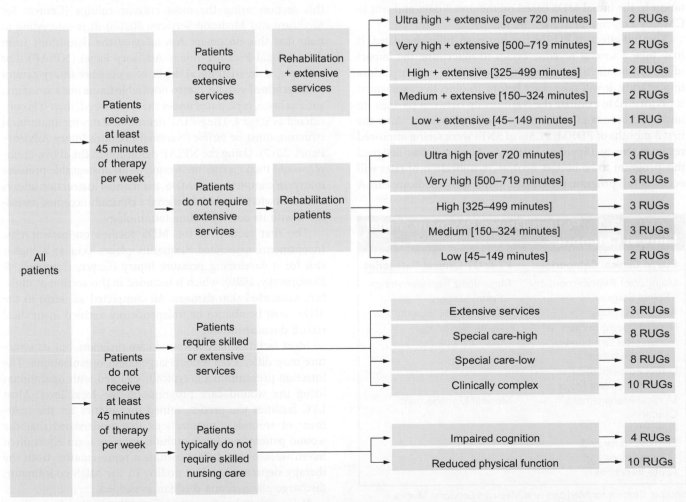

Fig. 3.1 Determinates of reimbursement using the resource utilization group (RUG) Method. Source: MedPac. (2016). *Skilled nursing facility payment system.* Retrieved 02-01-2020 from: http://medpac.gov/-documents-/payment-basics. Issue date October 11, 2019.

Patient-Driven Payment Model (PDPM). This new reimbursement system focuses on the acuity and individual needs of the patient based on the goals of care (Centers for Medicare and Medicaid Services. Medicare Learning Network, 2019a). Compensation is based on the completion of the MDS and an assignment into a case group. Patients are first grouped into a clinical classification and then scored for their nontherapy (e.g., nursing) needs as requiring extensive services, special care high services, special care low services, or clinically complex nursing categories. Functional scores that take therapy needs into consideration are also determined by clinical classification (Table 3.1). They are adjusted based on urban or rural location as well as the wage index, federal sequestration requirements, and scores received on the value-based and quality reporting measures. Service is most intense in the first few days, and payment to the facility is adjusted accordingly.

The current PDPM system pays the facility at the highest rate for the first 3 days and if there are high scores in the nontherapy ancillary group. Starting on Day 21, PT and OT groups decrease by 2% starting on Day 21 of the stay and continue to decrease by an additional 2% every 7 days thereafter. The patient must have a complete assessment and documentation in the initial MDS based on the first 3 days and sent to CMS by Day 5 of arrival at the facility.

The full effect of PDPM has not been fully elucidated. It may take a several revenue cycles to determine the impact of PDPM on the financial health on the SNF industry. More importantly, it will take years before an objective assessment is performed to evaluate the relationship between payment to improved outcomes under this value-based system. After the first 3 months of PDPM, 91.5% of SNFs were seeing improved revenue stream (Spanko, 2019). As Medicare has designed this program to be budget neutral, recalibration of rates will occur as this program progresses. While only Medicare Part A

patients are affected by PDPM, many states have modeled their Medicaid payment systems to correspond with the PDPM model.

Wound Management

Wound programs in SNFs vary in structure and implementation. When providing wound management to residents in these facilities, it is important to ask how the wound program is organized and managed (Maguire, 2014). Many facilities contract with an outside wound service who supplies a provider to visit the facility on a routine basis to assess and provide recommendations for wound management.

The LTC setting is highly regulated with emphasis on the prevention of skin conditions, particularly pressure injuries. The MDS identifies specific individualized patient characteristics to plan care. The MDS 3.0 skin condition section M (Fig. 3.2) captures skin issues including pressure injuries and their corresponding stages, venous and arterial ulcers, and other wounds such as diabetic-related foot ulcers and skin tears and attempts to capture their associated treatments (Centers for Medicare and Medicaid Services, 2019a). The MDS has a comprehensive instruction manual available for assisting the facility MDS coordinator to accurately complete this section using the most current rulings (Centers for Medicare and Medicaid Services, 2020b). It is interesting to note that this document has *adapted* the definitions from the National Pressure Injury Advisory Panel (NPIAP). For example, if an anatomical depth of a pressure injury cannot be determined visually due to nonviable tissue but a structure, such as bone, is *palpated* under the wound bed, then it is considered as Stage 4. The NPIAP definition states the anatomical structure must be *visible* (National Pressure Injury Advisory Panel, 2017). Using the NPIAP definition in the above example would then classify the wound as an unstageable pressure injury. In completing the MDS, the manual instruction always overrides what may be considered a clinically accepted assessment with its corresponding terminology.

The first section of the MDS focuses on patient risk. Incontinence-associated dermatitis places skin at a higher risk for a developing pressure injury (Coyer, Campbell, & Doubrovsky, 2020), which is included in this section as moisture associated skin damage. All completed all items in the MDS must be able to be independently verified in medical record documentation.

Most facilities have a wound care program, but its structure may differ even among large chain organizations. The infection preventionist is typically charged with operationalizing the wound care program on the local level. Most LTC facilities use predetermined formularies for the treatment of wounds. Organizations that understand that the wound patient requires a multidisciplinary team effort often haven weekly rounds that include a representative from the therapy department while pulling in the MDS coordinator, discharge planner, and dietitian as needed.

It is unclear how many SNFs in the United States have secured services of outside consultants to provide wound management services. In this model, an Advanced Practice

TABLE 3.1 Patient-Driven Payment Model Clinical Categories

PDPM Clinical Categories	PT & OT Clinical Categories
Major Joint Replacement or Spinal Surgery	Major Joint Replacement or Spinal Surgery
Acute Neurologic	Nonorthopedic Surgery and Acute Neurologic
Nonorthopedic Surgery	
Nonsurgical Orthopedic/ Musculoskeletal	Other Orthopedic
Orthopedic—Surgical Extremities Not Major Joint	
Medical Management	Medical Management
Cancer	
Pulmonary	
Cardiovascular and Coagulations	
Acute Infections	

Source: Centers for Medicare and Medicaid Services. Medicare Learning Network. (2019). *SNF PPS: Patient driven payment model training presentation.* Retrieved 7-29-20 from https://www.cms.gov/Medicare/Medicare-Fee-for-Service-Payment/SNFPPS/PDPM.

Resident	Identifier	Date

Section M — Skin Conditions

> **Report based on highest stage of existing ulcer(s) at its worst; do not "reverse" stage**

M0100. Determination of Pressure Ulcer Risk

↓ **Check all that apply**

☐ A. Resident has a stage 1 or greater, a scar over bony prominence, or a non-removable dressing/device

☐ B. Formal assessment instrument/tool (e.g., Braden, Norton, or other)

☐ C. Clinical assessment

☐ Z. None of the above

M0150. Risk of Pressure Ulcers

Enter Code ☐ Is this resident at risk of developing pressure ulcers?
- 0. No
- 1. Yes

M0210. Unhealed Pressure Ulcer(s)

Enter Code ☐ Does this resident have one or more unhealed pressure ulcer(s) at Stage 1 or higher?
- 0. No → Skip to M0900, Healed Pressure Ulcers
- 1. Yes → Continue to M0300, Current Number of Unhealed (non-epithelialized) Pressure Ulcers at Each Stage

M0300. Current Number of Unhealed (non-epithelialized) Pressure Ulcers at Each Stage

Enter Number ☐ **A. Number of Stage 1 pressure ulcers**
Stage 1: Intact skin with non-blanchable redness of a localized area usually over a bony prominence. Darkly pigmented skin may not have a visible blanching; in dark skin tones only it may appear with persistent blue or purple hues

B. Stage 2: Partial thickness loss of dermis presenting as a shallow open ulcer with a red or pink wound bed, without slough. May also present as an intact or open/ruptured blister

Enter Number ☐ 1. **Number of Stage 2 pressure ulcers** - If 0 → Skip to M0300C, Stage 3

Enter Number ☐ 2. **Number of these Stage 2 pressure ulcers that were present upon admission/reentry** - enter how many were noted at the time of admission

3. **Date of oldest Stage 2 pressure ulcer** - Enter dashes if date is unknown:

☐☐ – ☐☐ – ☐☐☐☐
Month   Day   Year

C. Stage 3: Full thickness tissue loss. Subcutaneous fat may be visible but bone, tendon or muscle is not exposed. Slough may be present but does not obscure the depth of tissue loss. May include undermining and tunneling

Enter Number ☐ 1. **Number of Stage 3 pressure ulcers** - If 0 → Skip to M0300D, Stage 4

Enter Number ☐ 2. **Number of these Stage 3 pressure ulcers that were present upon admission/reentry** - enter how many were noted at the time of admission

D. Stage 4: Full thickness tissue loss with exposed bone, tendon or muscle. Slough or eschar may be present on some parts of the wound bed. Often includes undermining and tunneling

Enter Number ☐ 1. **Number of Stage 4 pressure ulcers** - If 0 → Skip to M0300E, Unstageable: Non-removable dressing

Enter Number ☐ 2. **Number of these Stage 4 pressure ulcers that were present upon admission/reentry** - enter how many were noted at the time of admission

M0300 continued on next page

Fig. 3.2 Minimum Data Set 3.0 skin conditions. Source: Centers for Medicare and Medicaid Services. (2019b). *OASIS user manual. Outcome and assessment information set OASIS-D guidance manual.* Effective January 1, 2019. Retrieved 08-08-2020 from https://www.cms.gov/Medicare/Quality-Initiatives-Patient-Assessment-Instruments/HomeHealthQualityInits/HHQIOASISUserManual.

(Continued)

Resident _____   Identifier _____   Date _____

Section M   Skin Conditions

M0300. Current Number of Unhealed (non-epithelialized) Pressure Ulcers at Each Stage - Continued

E. Unstageable - Non-removable dressing: Known but not stageable due to non-removable dressing/device

Enter Number
☐   **1. Number of unstageable pressure ulcers due to non-removable dressing/device** - If 0 → Skip to M0300F, Unstageable: Slough and/or eschar

Enter Number
☐   **2. Number of these unstageable pressure ulcers that were present upon admission/reentry** - enter how many were noted at the time of admission

F. Unstageable - Slough and/or eschar: Known but not stageable due to coverage of wound bed by slough and/or eschar

Enter Number
☐   **1. Number of unstageable pressure ulcers due to coverage of wound bed by slough and/or eschar** - If 0 → Skip to M0300G, Unstageable: Deep tissue

Enter Number
☐   **2. Number of these unstageable pressure ulcers that were present upon admission/reentry** - enter how many were noted at the time of admission

G. Unstageable - Deep tissue: Suspected deep tissue injury in evolution

Enter Number
☐   **1. Number of unstageable pressure ulcers with suspected deep tissue injury in evolution** - If 0 → Skip to M0610, Dimension of Unhealed Stage 3 or 4 Pressure Ulcers or Eschar

Enter Number
☐   **2. Number of these unstageable pressure ulcers that were present upon admission/reentry** - enter how many were noted at the time of admission

M0610. Dimensions of Unhealed Stage 3 or 4 Pressure Ulcers or Eschar
Complete only if M0300C1, M0300D1 or M0300F1 is greater than 0

If the resident has one or more unhealed (non-epithelialized) Stage 3 or 4 pressure ulcers or an unstageable pressure ulcer due to slough or eschar, identify the pressure ulcer with the largest surface area (length x width) and record in centimeters:

☐☐.☐ cm   **A. Pressure ulcer length:** Longest length from head to toe

☐☐.☐ cm   **B. Pressure ulcer width:** Widest width of the same pressure ulcer, side-to-side perpendicular (90-degree angle) to length

☐☐.☐ cm   **C. Pressure ulcer depth:** Depth of the same pressure ulcer from the visible surface to the deepest area (if depth is unknown, enter a dash in each box)

M0700. Most Severe Tissue Type for Any Pressure Ulcer

Enter Code
☐

Select the best description of the most severe type of tissue present in any pressure ulcer bed
1. **Epithelial tissue** - new skin growing in superficial ulcer. It can be light pink and shiny, even in persons with darkly pigmented skin
2. **Granulation tissue** - pink or red tissue with shiny, moist, granular appearance
3. **Slough** - yellow or white tissue that adheres to the ulcer bed in strings or thick clumps, or is mucinous
4. **Necrotic tissue (Eschar)** - black, brown, or tan tissue that adheres firmly to the wound bed or ulcer edges, may be softer or harder than surrounding skin

M0800. Worsening in Pressure Ulcer Status Since Prior Assessment (OBRA, PPS, or Discharge)
Complete only if A0310E = 0

Indicate the number of current pressure ulcers that were **not present or were at a lesser stage** on prior assessment (OBRA, PPS, or Discharge). If no current pressure ulcer at a given stage, enter 0

Enter Number
☐   **A. Stage 2**

Enter Number
☐   **B. Stage 3**

Enter Number
☐   **C. Stage 4**

Fig. 3.2, Cont'd

(Continued)

Resident _____   Identifier _____   Date _____

Section M — Skin Conditions

M0900. Healed Pressure Ulcers
Complete only if A0310E = 0

Enter Code [ ]	**A. Were pressure ulcers present on the prior assessment (OBRA, PPS, or Discharge)?** 　0. **No** → Skip to M1030, Number of Venous and Arterial Ulcers 　1. **Yes** → Continue to M0900B, Stage 2

Indicate the number of pressure ulcers that were noted on the prior assessment (OBRA, PPS, or Discharge) that have completely closed (resurfaced with epithelium). If no healed pressure ulcer at a given stage since the prior assessment (OBRA, PPS, or Discharge), enter 0

Enter Number [ ]	**B. Stage 2**
Enter Number [ ]	**C. Stage 3**
Enter Number [ ]	**D. Stage 4**

M1030. Number of Venous and Arterial Ulcers

Enter Number [ ]	**Enter the total number of venous and arterial ulcers present**

M1040. Other Ulcers, Wounds and Skin Problems

↓ Check all that apply

Foot Problems

- [ ] **A. Infection of the foot** (e.g., cellulitis, purulent drainage)
- [ ] **B. Diabetic foot ulcer(s)**
- [ ] **C. Other open lesion(s) on the foot**

Other Problems

- [ ] **D. Open lesion(s) other than ulcers, rashes, cuts** (e.g., cancer lesion)
- [ ] **E. Surgical wound(s)**
- [ ] **F. Burn(s)** (second or third degree)

None of the Above

- [ ] **Z. None of the above** were present

M1200. Skin and Ulcer Treatments

↓ Check all that apply

- [ ] **A. Pressure reducing device for chair**
- [ ] **B. Pressure reducing device for bed**
- [ ] **C. Turning/repositioning program**
- [ ] **D. Nutrition or hydration intervention** to manage skin problems
- [ ] **E. Ulcer care**
- [ ] **F. Surgical wound care**
- [ ] **G. Application of nonsurgical dressings** (with or without topical medications) other than to feet
- [ ] **H. Applications of ointments/medications** other than to feet
- [ ] **I. Application of dressings to feet** (with or without topical medications)
- [ ] **Z. None of the above** were provided

Fig. 3.2, Cont'd

Nurse, Physician Assistant, or a Physician comes into the facility on a predetermined schedule to evaluate and manage the patient with a wound. It is imperative that the organization having a wound consultant vet the provider accordingly by asking for previous experience, continuing education documentation, if certification in wound care is held and by which certifying agency to maximize patient outcomes. The wound consultant should possess understanding of team member roles and foster collaboration.

The organization usually has predetermined documentation mechanisms and requirements for the wound consultant. Telemedicine for wound evaluation and management has increased in SNFs due to the COVID-19 pandemic as well as increased adoption of the electronic health records and other technologies in this setting. A savvy wound provider will determine if there is an ability to incorporate this into their practice.

To prevent conflicts related to treatment modalities and their associated expenses, a frank discussion between the wound consultant and the administrator should take place before attempting to initiate more expensive modalities. The wound clinician in the LTC facility should be sensitive to the financial constraints often faced in this setting whenever possible while keeping the patient outcomes at the forefront when advocating to veer from the formulary or in attempts to bring in new dressings, supplies, or pharmaceuticals.

Wound dressing supplies are provided by the facility. Some will supply scalpels, sutures, silver nitrate sticks, and suture removal sets, but the wound care provider should know if these supplies are available prior to evaluating patients. Some facilities have arrangements with outside vendors to provide dressing supplies under the Medicare Part B Surgical Dressing policy. The Medicare Part B dressing supplier will provide and bill for these supplies for eligible patients. This removes added expenses from the SNF and has been quite successful when implemented well. The staff of the organization as well as any outside wound consultant should be familiar with the requirements the Medicare Part B Surgical Dressing Policy (Centers for Medicare and Medicaid Services, 2020d) as the documentation for these supplies is facility and provider driven. The outside consultant should also be aware of other services that can be provided for wound management within the facility, such as continuous pulse up irrigation, electrical stimulation, ultrasound, or diathermy.

Scope of practice issues up affect not only the staff employees at the facility but also the outside consultant. Some states have regulations that require that the attending physician must approve all consultant orders before they are implemented. Others limit the scope of physical therapists regarding debridement or forbid wound assessments by licensed vocational/practical nurses.

SNF quality measures include avoiding return to the acute care setting within 30 days of the hospital discharge. A financial penalty is imposed when this occurs. Because the patient with the wound is at greater risk for hospital readmission than the patient without a wound (Hakkarainen, Arbabi, Willis, Davidson, & Flum, 2016), it is imperative the wound consultant actively strive to mitigate factors that could trigger readmission.

HOME HEALTH POSTACUTE SETTING

Much like the SNF, complex wounds are frequently managed in this setting. There are several similar organizational structures to the LTC setting as well as differences. Provision of formal health care services in the home setting became more structured in the early 19th century and demand has steadily grown. Demand for home health continues to grow steadily due to an aging population, shifts in healthcare delivery systems, technology use, and increased consumer engagement in the process (Landers et al., 2016). The impact of the COVID-19 pandemic increased acuity and diverted patients from admission to the SNF (Holly, 2020).

Operational Structure

Home health agencies (HHAs) may vary in the services they provide. They may be a small agency with its own organization structure, owned by and operated under the umbrella of a larger health care system or are their own health corporate entities. Some may be owned by investors or by private individuals and pay a management fee to a corporation to staff and operate them. Like SNFs, they can have local, regional, or a national presence. HHAs may be for-profit or nonprofit entities. Of the 12,000 HHAs in the United States, 80% are for-profit (Centers for Disease Control, 2016). The home health may agency have one central location or several offices throughout their defined territory.

All HHAs must meet local and state health care regulations. Only Medicare-certified HHAs can receive reimbursement for services provided to Medicare patients. Medicare is the largest single payer of home health services, with Medicaid and Managed Care providing payment for the bulk of the remaining home health patients. If accepting Medicare or Medicaid reimbursement, additional requirements from these programs must also be met as well. Clinical policies and protocols, including those for skin and wound management are required. Every HHA has unique challenges and opportunities based on the referral source, economic stability of the client base, and patient volume.

The typical organizational structure of a HHA includes a CEO or an executive administrator, a medical director, a marketing manager, an informational technology leader, a human resource executive, and a clinical administrator who is most often a nurse. Some HHAs have a director of therapy services who oversees physical therapy, occupational therapy, and speech therapy. The provision of clinical care is the predominant service given requiring intake nurses, quality assurance personnel, case managers, social work, therapy services, as well as a robust nursing staff of both registered nurses, licensed vocational/practical nurses, and home health aides. In smaller agencies, many of these roles overlap. Large agencies may have a defined wound care team, or a wound care trained nurse or therapist for each office. Midsized agencies may have a wound care trained nurse available for all staff to access. Small agencies often rely on their own expertise, local wound care centers and surgeons, or use outside wound consultants as needed.

While each organization defines how to operationalize the management of a patient with a wound, a registered nurse typically performs an assessment of the patient, including the wound, using a standardized admission process within 24–48 h after receiving the referral. Based on the patient's needs, state licensure and scope of practice requirements, a registered nurse, licensed vocational/practical nurse, or a physical therapist performs wound care following the provider's orders.

Medicare covers home health care if the patient is considered "homebound" (Centers for Medicare and Medicaid Services. Medicare Learning Network. Chronic Care Policy Group, 2014). This is defined as requiring a "considerable and taxing effort" for the patient to leave the home and some form of assistance is needed to do so. This may require help of another person or medical equipment such as crutches, a walker, or a wheelchair. If the provider believes the patient's health may suffer or current health conditions may exacerbate if the patient leaves the house, the patient can qualify for home health Medicare coverage. The ordering provider for home health services must certify homebound status, evaluate, and recertify this eligibility every 60 days. Patients may leave their home for medical treatment, religious services, and/or to attend a licensed or accredited adult day care center without the homebound status at risk. Leaving home for short periods of time or for special nonmedical events, such as a family reunion, funeral, or graduation, does affect your homebound status. The patient may take occasional trips to the barber or beauty parlor.

Additional requirements include a medical condition requiring skilled nursing services and/or skilled therapy care on an intermittent basis. Intermittent means care at a minimum of once every 60 days and a maximum of once a day for up to 3 weeks. This period can be extended if needed if more care is needed. Medicare defines skilled care as care that must be performed by a skilled professional, or under their supervision.

A provider must have a face-to-face meeting with a patient within the 90 days before starting home health care, or within 30 days after the first day you receive care. This can be an office visit, hospital visit, or in certain circumstances a face-to-face visit facilitated by technology, such as telehealth conferencing. In addition, a plan of care must also be submitted. This plan of care is also known as "the 485," referring to the government-assigned form number. Validating the patient's homebound status and recertifying the plan of care every 60 days is required, additional face-to-face meetings are not.

Until recently, only licensed physicians could order home health services and DME. Early in the COVID-19 pandemic, NPPs, including advanced practice nurses and physician assistants, were added to alleviate a long-standing provisional service gap in this setting. This ruling, as well as all administered services covered by any payor, are subject to change and the reader is advised to be aware of the current rules and regulations required by the home health setting by contacting Medicare or the primary payer.

The physician or NPP overseeing the plan of care and orders may or may not be familiar with the intricacies of wound management. Often, primary care providers rely on collaboration with the nursing staff to determine the best topical treatment for a wound. If the patient's wound is comanaged by another provider, such as a surgeon or wound center, those recommendations are often folded into and accepted by the attending home health provider.

While home health care is normally covered by Medicare Part B, Medicare Part A provides coverage in certain circumstances. Specifically, if the patient spends at least three consecutive days as a hospital inpatient or has a Medicare-covered SNF stay, Medicare Part A covers the first 100 days of home health care, assuming all other eligibility requirements are met. If the patient does not have service initiated immediately after transitioning from these settings, home health services initiated within 14 days of the discharge are also covered under Part A. After 100 days, home health benefits are covered by Part B at full cost. Regardless if care is covered by Part A or Part B, Medicare pays the full cost (Centers for Medicare and Medicaid Services, 2017).

Nursing services under the home health benefit provide for wound care, including observation and management up to 7 days a week. Generally, nursing cannot provide more than 8 h of care per day or 28 h per week, though with thorough documentation and medical necessity, up to 35 h per week is possible. In complicated wound patients, such as patients with fistulas whose loss of dressing integrity in the home health setting can be frequent and time consuming to replace, the need for increased services may be needed. The provider ordering wound services and the nurse or case manager caring for the patient may need to increase frequency of communication when high wound complexity presents.

Skilled physical therapy, speech, and occupational therapy services that are reasonable and necessary for treating gait or movement disorders, speech, and/or language skills, to improve the patient's ability to perform usual daily activities or perform self-care management of illness or disease can also be provided. The latter is particularly important for the wound provider managing the patient who needs to be able to don and doff compression garments on the lower extremity.

Home health aides fall under the purview of nursing services in this postacute space. A Medicare beneficiary can qualify for personal care services that includes bathing, toileting, and dressing if a skilled service is in place. There is full coverage under the Medicare home health program. Social services are also allowed if they are related to the illness requiring a concomitant skilled benefit.

The HHA is required to provide for most medical supplies, including primary and secondary wound dressings and catheters. Supplies for wound management are typically ordered by the agency from a third party. These are either delivered to the HHA or directly to the patient's home. There is a lag time that can be as little as 24 h but may be up to 7 days. The HHA usually keeps a supply of common wound management items in the office so that wound care can be initiated while waiting for the delivery of specific items. It is imperative for the provider to communicate necessary items and outline specific steps to the agency personnel who will provide wound care in the home setting. It is often helpful to provide the patient with the specific plan of care for wound management in case the agency staff member is unable to access this due to technology failure, as most agencies use an electronic health record.

Medicare pays 80% of its approved amount for DME to the HHA, such as a wheelchair, walker, or nondisposable negative pressure therapy devices. The patient is responsible for 20% of the charges. If a patient has a Medicare supplemental policy, this may or may not be covered, depending on the specific contract. The HHA has the option not to accept the Medicare predetermined payment. In this case, the patient will pay additional fees. For those organizations who do not accept assignment, the HHA will arrange with a DME supplier approved by Medicare to provide the ordered equipment. Disposable negative pressure therapy units have a separate distinct billing process. Wound providers can access the most current regulations (Centers for Medicare and Medicaid Services. Medicare Learning Network, 2019b). As requirements for home health services may change at any time, the wound provider can find specific information at: https://www.medicare.gov/coverage/home-health-services.

Medicare Advantage Plans must provide at least the same level of home health care coverage as traditional Medicare but may impose different rules, restrictions, or costs. Often there are preferred HHAs contracted to provide services. Many plans require a preauthorization before approving care. Copayments are often required. While time consuming for the provider, it is beneficial to determine coverage type and identify any limitations and associated patient costs for specific wound care treatment plans before initiating them when managing a patient with a Medicare Advantage Plan that includes a home health benefit (Medicare Interactive, 2020).

Determining Reimbursement in the Home Health Setting

At the time of the first in-home evaluation of the patient, the agency is required to complete a data set that helps develop the plan of care, serves as the main determinate of reportable quality measures, and assists in the establishment of reimbursement rates. The Outcome and Assessment Information Set (OASIS) form is the mechanism to achieve these three objectives. The OASIS has undergone many updates with each version having an associated updated letter attached to the OASIS name. In 2020, HHAs are using the OASIS-D. An OASIS-E version is scheduled for release in January 2021 but delayed due to the COVID-19 pandemic and is now anticipated in 2022. Current

regulations require withholding release until January 1st of the year that is at least one full calendar year after the end of the COVID-19 pandemic.

The OASIS, like the MDS in the SNF setting, walks the nurse through a variety of assessments to determine a comprehensive plan of care on the initial visit to the patient's home. OASIS, Section M (Centers for Medicare and Medicaid Services, 2019b) is specific to skin (Fig. 3.3). The upcoming OASIS-E update has been made to closely align with the MDS as the goal is to have congruency between care settings. Completion and submission of the OASIS is a requirement of participation to receive Medicare payments. The OASIS must be submitted within 5 days after the start of care, and within 5 days prior to recertification, which occurs every 60 days, within 2 days of resumption of care, and at the end-of-care (Centers for Medicare and Medicaid Services. Medicare Learning Network, 2019c).

Once submitted to Medicare, quality measurements provide opportunities for benchmarking and public reporting. The results of these measures are posted online by CMS as an initiative for consumers to compare outcomes to make informed choices in selecting the HHA when services are needed. These are available at: https://www.medicare.gov/homehealthcompare/search.html. Specific quality measures related to the patient with a wound reported during the provision as well as at the end of care include:

- Percentage of patients rehospitalized within 30 days of hospital discharge.
- Percentage of patients with a new or worsening pressure injury.
- Percentage of patients with improvement in the surgical wound.
- Need for emergent care with hospitalization or emergent care without need for hospitalization. Emergent care is defined as seeking care in a hospital emergency department.

Quality measures are important to the wound provider as 31% of all admissions to a HHA have a wound component associated with provided services (Ellenbecker, Samia, Cushman, & Alster, 2008; Quality Insights. Home Health Quality Improvement.org, 2019). It is imperative that the patient is receiving outcome-focused quality wound care as patients with a venous leg ulcer do not receive adequate compression in this setting (Harding et al., 2015; Zarchi et al., 2016). Given the frequency of cellulitis in this population seeking emergent care, regulators are seeking to improve care processes in the wound management arena. Over 76% of patients admitted to an acute care facility from the home setting were found to have pressure injuries (Corbett, Funk, Fortunato, & O'Sullivan, 2017).

The OASIS data set assesses for the presence or absence of any unhealed pressure injuries that are Stage 2 or higher as well as the number present in each stage. Stage 1 or healed pressure injuries considered by many clinicians as "red flags" that identify patients who are at higher risk for more developing severe wounds are not considered in the OASIS.

INTEGUMENTARY STATUS

(M1306)	Does this patient have at least one **Unhealed Pressure Ulcer/Injury at Stage 2 or Higher** or designated as Unstageable? (Excludes Stage 1 pressure injuries and all healed pressure ulcers/injuries)
Enter Code ☐	0 No *[Go to M1322 at SOC/ROC/FU; Go to M1324 at DC]* 1 Yes
(M1307)	The **Oldest Stage 2 Pressure Ulcer** that is present at discharge: (Excludes healed Stage 2 pressure ulcers)
Enter Code ☐	1 Was present at the most recent SOC/ROC assessment 2 Developed since the most recent SOC/ROC assessment. Record date pressure ulcer first identified: ☐☐ / ☐☐ / ☐☐☐☐ month day year NA No Stage 2 pressure ulcers are present at discharge

SOC/ROC

(M1311) Current Number of Unhealed Pressure Ulcers/Injuries at Each Stage	Enter Number
A1. Stage 2: Partial thickness loss of dermis presenting as a shallow open ulcer with a red or pink wound bed, without slough. May also present as an intact or open/ruptured blister. **Number of Stage 2 pressure ulcers**	☐
B1. Stage 3: Full thickness tissue loss. Subcutaneous fat may be visible but bone, tendon, or muscle is not exposed. Slough may be present but does not obscure the depth of tissue loss. May include undermining and tunneling. **Number of Stage 3 pressure ulcers**	☐
C1. Stage 4: Full thickness tissue loss with exposed bone, tendon, or muscle. Slough or eschar may be present on some parts of the wound bed. Often includes undermining and tunneling. **Number of Stage 4 pressure ulcers**	☐
D1. Unstageable: Non-removable dressing/device: Known but not stageable due to non-removable dressing/device **Number of unstageable pressure ulcers/injuries due to non-removable dressing/device**	☐
E1. Unstageable: Slough and/or eschar: Known but not stageable due to coverage of wound bed by slough and/or eschar **Number of unstageable pressure ulcers/injuries due to coverage of wound bed by slough and/or eschar**	☐
F1. Unstageable: Deep tissue injury **Number of unstageable pressure injuries presenting as deep tissue injury**	☐

Follow-Up

(M1311) Current Number of Unhealed Pressure Ulcers/Injuries at Each Stage	Enter Number
A1. Stage 2: Partial thickness loss of dermis presenting as a shallow open ulcer with a red or pink wound bed, without slough. May also present as an intact or open/ruptured blister. **Number of Stage 2 pressure ulcers**	☐
B1. Stage 3: Full thickness tissue loss. Subcutaneous fat may be visible but bone, tendon, or muscle is not exposed. Slough may be present but does not obscure the depth of tissue loss. May include undermining and tunneling. **Number of Stage 3 pressure ulcers**	☐
C1. Stage 4: Full thickness tissue loss with exposed bone, tendon, or muscle. Slough or eschar may be present on some parts of the wound bed. Often includes undermining and tunneling. **Number of Stage 4 pressure ulcers**	☐
D1. Unstageable: Non-removable dressing/device: Known but not stageable due to non-removable dressing/device **Number of unstageable pressure ulcers/injuries due to non-removable dressing/device**	☐
E1. Unstageable: Slough and/or eschar: Known but not stageable due to coverage of wound bed by slough and/or eschar **Number of unstageable pressure ulcers/injuries due to coverage of wound bed by slough and/or eschar**	☐
F1. Unstageable: Deep tissue injury **Number of unstageable pressure injuries presenting as deep tissue injury**	☐

Fig. 3.3 OASIS-D integumentary items. Source: Centers for Medicare & Medicaid Services. (2020d). *Surgical dressings—policy article.* Retrieved February 21, 2020 from https://www.cms.gov/medicare-coverage-database/view/article.aspx?articleid=54563Centers for Medicare and Medicaid Services, Medicare Learning Network, 2019.

(Continued)

Discharge

(M1311) Current Number of Unhealed Pressure Ulcers/Injuries at Each Stage	Enter Number
A1. Stage 2: Partial thickness loss of dermis presenting as a shallow open ulcer with a red or pink wound bed, without slough. May also present as an intact or open/ruptured blister. **Number of Stage 2 pressure ulcers** [If 0 – Go to M1311B1, Stage 3]	☐
A2. Number of <u>these</u> Stage 2 pressure ulcers that were present at most recent SOC/ROC – enter how many were noted at the time of most recent SOC/ROC	☐
B1. Stage 3: Full thickness tissue loss. Subcutaneous fat may be visible but bone, tendon, or muscle is not exposed. Slough may be present but does not obscure the depth of tissue loss. May include undermining and tunneling. **Number of Stage 3 pressure ulcers** [If 0 – Go to M1311C1, Stage 4]	☐
B2. Number of <u>these</u> Stage 3 pressure ulcers that were present at most recent SOC/ROC – enter how many were noted at the time of most recent SOC/ROC	☐
C1. Stage 4: Full thickness tissue loss with exposed bone, tendon, or muscle. Slough or eschar may be present on some parts of the wound bed. Often includes undermining and tunneling. **Number of Stage 4 pressure ulcers** [If 0 – Go to M1311D1, Unstageable: Non-removable dressing/device]	☐
C2. Number of <u>these</u> Stage 4 pressure ulcers that were present at most recent SOC/ROC – enter how many were noted at the time of most recent SOC/ROC	☐
D1. Unstageable: Non-removable dressing/device: Known but not stageable due to non-removable dressing/device **Number of unstageable pressure ulcers/injuries due to non-removable dressing/device** [If 0 – Go to M1311E1, Unstageable: Slough and/or eschar]	☐
D2. Number of <u>these</u> unstageable pressure ulcers/injuries that were present at most recent SOC/ROC – enter how many were noted at the time of most recent SOC/ROC	☐
E1. Unstageable: Slough and/or eschar: Known but not stageable due to coverage of wound bed by slough and/or eschar **Number of unstageable pressure ulcers due to coverage of wound bed by slough and/or eschar** [If 0 – Go to M1311F1, Unstageable: Deep tissue injury]	☐
E2. Number of <u>these</u> unstageable pressure ulcers that were present at most recent SOC/ROC – enter how many were noted at the time of most recent SOC/ROC	☐
F1. Unstageable: Deep tissue injury **Number of unstageable pressure injuries presenting as deep tissue injury** [If 0 – Go to M1324]	☐
F2. Number of <u>these</u> unstageable pressure ulcers that were present at most recent SOC/ROC – enter how many were noted at the time of most recent SOC/ROC	☐

Fig. 3.3, Cont'd

(Continued)

An unstageable pressure injury may meet one of two criteria in the OASIS:
- Pressure injuries that are known to be present but that are unobservable due to a dressing/device, such as a cast, that cannot be removed to assess the skin underneath. "Known" refers to when documentation is available that states a pressure injury exists under the nonremovable dressing/device.
- The most widely accepted definition from the NPIAP of an unstageable ulcer is also acceptable. This is, a pressure injury having eschar (tan, black, or brown) or slough (yellow, tan, gray, green, or brown) tissue presenting such that the anatomic depth of soft tissue damage cannot be visualized in the wound bed. Deep tissue injury injuries are coded under the unstageable category.

Pressure injuries that undergo definitive surgical treatment for closure, such as a myocutaneous flap procedure or a skin graft change the categorization from "pressure" to "surgical." Surgical sharp debridement does not fit into this definition and thus the wound remains classified as a pressure injury

(M1322)	**Current Number of Stage 1 Pressure Injuries**: Intact skin with non-blanchable redness of a localized area usually over a bony prominence. Darkly pigmented skin may not have a visible blanching; in dark skin tones only it may appear with persistent blue or purple hues.	
Enter Code	0 1 2 3 4 or more	
(M1324)	**Stage of Most Problematic Unhealed Pressure Ulcer/Injury that is Stageable**: (Excludes pressure ulcer/injury that cannot be staged due to a non-removable dressing/device, coverage of wound bed by slough and/or eschar, or deep tissue injury.)	
Enter Code	1 Stage 1 2 Stage 2 3 Stage 3 4 Stage 4 NA Patient has no pressure ulcers/injuries or no stageable pressure ulcers/injuries	
(M1330)	Does this patient have a **Stasis Ulcer?**	
Enter Code	0 No [*Go to M1340*] 1 Yes, patient has BOTH observable and unobservable stasis ulcers 2 Yes, patient has observable stasis ulcers ONLY 3 Yes, patient has unobservable stasis ulcers ONLY (known but not observable due to non-removable dressing/device) [*Go to M1340*]	
(M1332)	**Current Number of Stasis Ulcer(s) that are Observable:**	
Enter Code	1 One 2 Two 3 Three 4 Four or more	
(M1334)	**Status of Most Problematic Stasis Ulcer that is Observable:**	
Enter Code	1 Fully granulating 2 Early/partial granulation 3 Not healing	
(M1340)	Does this patient have a **Surgical Wound?**	
Enter Code	0 No [*Go to M1400*] 1 Yes, patient has at least one observable surgical wound 2 Surgical wound known but not observable due to non-removable dressing/device [*Go to M1400*]	
(M1342)	**Status of Most Problematic Surgical Wound that is Observable**	
Enter Code	0 Newly epithelialized 1 Fully granulating 2 Early/partial granulation 3 Not healing	

Fig. 3.3, Cont'd

(Centers for Medicare and Medicaid Services. Medicare Learning Network, 2019c).

In addition to staging a pressure injury or identifying the presence of a surgical wound or venous wound, the OASIS document attempts to determine where in the healing trajectory the wound (Table 3.2). These descriptions relate to pressure injuries as well as venous insufficiency ulcers and surgical wounds. Others, such a diabetic foot wounds, arterial-related ulcerations, atypical ulcerations, or skin tears/lacerations, do not need their healing status identified (Centers for Medicare and Medicaid Services. Medicare Learning Network, 2019c).

Given that staging of pressure injuries and their corresponding descriptions are inconsistent among nonwound care nurses, it is highly unlikely that accurate completion of the OASIS document would be any different. The accuracy of assigning wound bed classifications using the OASIS wound bed descriptions in the OASIS document by nonspecialists or specialists has not yet been studied.

Reimbursement

Like reimbursement change in LTC, home health has also undergone several changes. In January 2020, the home health reimbursement system changed from a prospective payment system (PPS) to a value-based system called Patient-Driven Groupings Model (PDGM). System overhaul was designed to focus payments based on patient needs for

TABLE 3.2   OASIS Wound Healing Status Descriptors

OASIS Wound Description	Defining Criteria
Fully Granulating	A wound with its bed filled with granulation tissue to the level of the surrounding skin or new epithelium; no dead space, no avascular tissue; no signs or symptoms of infection; wound edges are open
Early/Partial Granulation	A wound with $\geq$25% of the wound bed is covered with granulation tissue OR there is minimal avascular tissue (<25% of the wound bed is covered with avascular tissue) OR may have dead space with no signs OR no symptoms of infection with wound edges that are open
Not Healing	A wound having $\geq$25% avascular tissue OR signs/symptoms of infection OR clean but nongranulating wound bed OR closed/hyperkeratotic wound edges OR persistent failure to improve despite appropriate comprehensive wound management

functional improvement. Under the PPS system, it was assumed that the more visits by a physical or occupational therapist resulted in improved outcomes. Agencies who had more therapy visits reaped larger financial benefits. By changing the focus to patient clinical characteristics with matching services for those needs, payments based on therapy volume are eliminated.

PDGM uses a 30-day period as a basis for payment. These are categorized into 12 clinical categories for the purposes of adjusting payment. Payment is highest for the first 30-day reimbursement period as service intensity is greatest in this time. Subsequent 30-day reimbursement periods have lower rates. Rates for patients differ based on the referral source, with hospitalized and skilled nursing patients who transition to the home setting having higher payments rates than those referred from a provider office, clinic, or hospital outpatient departments, such as a wound service. Thirty-day periods are placed into different subgroups for each of the following broad categories based on primary diagnosis and linked with functional status and comorbidities (Fig. 3.4). A total of 432 potential rates can be determined based on the cumulation of individual patient needs (Centers for Medicare and Medicaid Services. Medicare Learning Network, 2019c).

The wound clinical grouping has its own section. Functional levels within each clinical grouping are weighted by needed intensity and placed in a low, medium, or high grouping. Each grouping has weighted point values, with the high point value corresponding to greater reimbursement. The average reimbursement for patient admitted with a primary diagnosis of a wound in 2020 is $2090.82 (Holly, 2020).

It is unclear how PDGM will impact the home health setting in terms of agency consolidation or the overall number of agencies who survive financially. Additional strategies, such as using an office-based wound expert using remote management tools to assist the agency nurse in the home providing hands on care are being trialed as are use of outside paid wound case management services and computer-aided decision support platforms.

The PDGM system is a Medicare reimbursement system. Home health services by another payor may likely reimburse the HHA by another method and may not use the PDPM system to calculate payment to the agency. These can include a per patient/per month or a flat rate for the entire episode. It is important for the wound provider to be cognizant of how the agency receives reimbursement and the associated costs of providing care.

Wound Management in the Home Health Setting

Under Medicare, the HHA must supply all necessary items to perform wound care as ordered on the plan of care, except for DME. Other payors may have different requirements, including the patient obtaining and paying for their own wound dressings. Regardless, the goal of the HHA is to have the patient care for their own wound whenever possible. Enlisting several strategies to achieve this are usually necessary, though not always successful. Comorbidities, and adherence to recommendations such as avoiding cigarette smoking, managing blood glucose and leg elevation are constant challenges in this setting.

Environmental challenges also exist in the home health setting including household pets, vermin, hoarding behaviors leading to unclean environment, significant others, relatives, and nonrelatives may undermine recovery. Access to face-to-face visits with the provider, obtaining medications and necessary supplies may be limited due to transportation barriers, expense, physical disability, or mental health reasons.

Patients must be given a choice to select the HHA they wish to receive care from. An exception to this is if their non-Medicare insurer has a preferred provider. The provider, or his/her representative, must call the agency to refer the patient and provide documentation that the face-to-face visit and homebound requirements have been met.

It is beneficial for wound providers to be familiar with the commonly selected agencies in the area and what their wound management capabilities are. Most HHAs are very accommodating in providing this information. The provider should determine the types of wounds the agency typically manages, usual outcomes, the wound formulary in use, and the ability to respond to urgent wound management issues such as loss of dressing integrity. Specifically asking about staff qualifications, including the presence of a certified wound specialist,

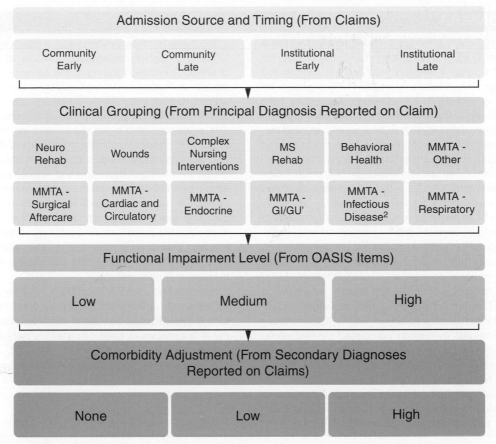

Fig. 3.4 Structure of patient-driven grouping model of reimbursement for home health agencies. Source: Centers for Medicare and Medicaid Services. Medicare Learning Network. (2019c). Overview of the patient-driven groupings model (PDGM). February 12, 2019. Retrieved 02-02-2020 from: https://www.cms.gov/Outreach-and-Education/Outreach/NPC/Downloads/2019-02-12-PDGM-Presentation.pdf.

available modalities, and equipment, can prevent communication and wound management misunderstandings prior to their occurrence.

Once a patient has initiated home health, frequent communication with staff caring for the patient in the home and the case manager at the agency responsible for the overall helps provide useful information and care coordination to assist to identify and mitigate clinical issues. The provider should know that the staff person in the home may be different from the case manager responsible for the patient. Issues that arise between scheduled visits may be handled by an on-call agency staff person, who may or may not be familiar with the patient's case.

Providers can, and do, make house calls for wound management patients. Due to regulations, the provider and the HHA nurse cannot charge for the same wound management services on the same day. Joint visits with the HHA staff and the provider are possible if the HHA staff are monitoring the patient for another condition or providing another service. House call wound management services do exist (Sterba, 2012).

Management can be particularly challenging as HHAs typically prefer to provide wound management visits three times a week or less. It is possible to order daily wound care in the home setting for a limited time with medical necessity. It is best for the provider to call the agency to discuss an intensive wound management need and agree on expected outcomes before ordering the service.

Some agencies do not have the resources to provide care for certain wounds and may refuse to accept the patient. For example, the agency may not have a vascular Doppler available to assess for peripheral pulses. Some agencies do not have certain skill sets, such as application of a multilayer compression wrap. The most challenging wounds to manage are those with high exudate such as venous leg ulcers or fistulas as both require frequent home visits, with specialized topical and systemic management interventions with someone that has considerable expertise and health care system navigational skills.

A: Ms. Jacob is an 86-year-old female is now being admitted to the skilled nursing facility from a week-long stay at the hospital for pneumonia with a Stage 4 pressure injury of her sacrum and her right trochanter. The pressure injuries have been present for more than 30 days and previously managed with orders from her primary care physician implemented by a home health agency. During hospitalization, osteomyelitis of both areas was ruled out. Additional diagnoses include: protein-calorie malnutrition, hip and knee flexion contractures, hypothyroidism, urinary and fecal incontinence, and dementia. Her primary insurance is Medicare. She has a Part B supplement. Using a systems-approach combined with patient-centered care the following was taken.

A: Physical exam of patient and wound. Evaluate for specialty pressure redistribution mattress and wheelchair pressure redistribution seating surface. OT/PT evaluation for pressure mapping of patient in specialty mattress and wheelchair cushion. PT evaluation for determination of appropriate adjunctive therapy. Nursing assessment for pressure injury risk factors, incontinence impact on wound. Wound consultant performs wound evaluation and seeks further history data from home health agency and hospital. Nutritional evaluation completed by Registered Dietician. MDS coordinator reviews medical record documentation for comprehensive completion and completes required PDPM forms for reimbursement determination.

D: Patient is on Medicare Part A stay with multiple full-thickness wounds and comorbidities impacting recovery requiring multidisciplinary team assessment and intervention.

I: Occupational therapy obtains a tilt and space chair with a static air seating cushion redistribution. A low air loss mattress is obtained. Pressure mapping of the patient in the chair and on the low air mattress in various positions are completed. Individualized turn and reposition schedules are designed. Topical wound care dressings include an absorbent primary dressing and a waterproof but moisture vapor permeable secondary dressing to prevent incontinence effluent wound contamination. The dietician recommends a ground diet based on the speech therapist's finding of dysphagia and initiates a high protein thickened nutritional supplement to promote calorie intake for wound healing. A wound consultant reevaluates the patient weekly, changing topical therapy as needed. Physical therapy determines that the patient would benefit by continuous pulse irrigation and diathermy to the wound. The MDS reviews all the documentation, completes, and submits the MDS 3.0 for reimbursement determination.

E: Wounds show weekly reductions in size and volume with no strikethrough drainage on secondary dressing. Topical wound care is altered based on wound characteristics. Dressing integrity is maintained despite persistent urinary and fecal incontinence. Patient eats 100% of diet and takes nutritional supplements. Reimbursement determination covers costs for care for facility.

SUMMARY

Postacute Care Setting:
- Regulatory requirements and the complexity of reimbursement in the postacute care setting impact wound management.
- Wound providers must be familiar with the industry regulations and reimbursement specific to prevention and management to be successful in these settings.
- Wound management in the post-acute care space is challenging but also extremely rewarding as the opportunity to manage a patient over a longer time when compared with acute care allows one to see patient progress.
- Working with a multidisciplinary team is essential in the postacute space and provides opportunities for learning and teaching for all as each member of the group provides specific expertise to the patient with a wound.
- Wound management in the post-acute setting allows the health providers to be a partner with the patient and their significant others in identifying and handling the barriers —medical, physical, social, and environmental that prevent optimal wound healing.

Home Health Setting:
- Providing wound management in the home setting is satisfying and never routine.
- Wound management in this setting allows the health provider to be a partner with the patient and their significant others in identifying and handling the barriers—medical, physical, social, and environmental that prevent optimal wound healing.
- Understanding the requirements for a patient to receive home health care and the intricacies of regulations as they apply to wound management is an important facet of providing care in this setting.

SELF-ASSESSMENT QUESTIONS

1. Which of the following would meet the requirement for Medicare coverage for a skilled nursing facility?
   a. A one-night stay in an acute care setting
   b. A two-night stay in the acute care setting
   c. A three-night stay in the acute care setting
   d. A four-night stay in the acute care setting

2. The provider in an LTC setting wants to order negative pressure therapy for a patient who has been in the facility for 88 days. Who is responsible for the costs of this therapy?
   a. Neither the patient nor the facility is responsible for the entire cost of therapy
   b. The facility is responsible for 80% of the cost and the patient is responsible for 20%
   c. The facility is responsible for 20% of the cost and the patient is responsible for 80%
   d. Medicare will cover all costs except $176.00 per day, including negative pressure therapy

3. Wound management in postacute care settings requires:
   a. Knowledge of the reimbursement systems used
   b. Ability to communicate well with others
   c. Knowledge of the formulary used in the setting
   d. All the above

4. The wound provider is referring a patient to home health for wound care. What documentation is needed for the home health agency?
   a. Written orders for management of the patient's hypertension
   b. Documentation of a face-to-face visit and homebound status
   c. A list of all medications and diagnosis obtained from the patient
   d. a and c

5. Patient-Driven Groupings Model uses which combination of characteristics to determine reimbursement in the home health setting?
   a. Patient diagnosis, functional level, and comorbidities
   b. Patient diagnosis, family history, and comorbidities
   c. Referral source, functional ability, and insurance coverage
   d. Referral source, family history, and comorbidities

REFERENCES

Centers for Disease Control. (2016). *National Center for Health Statistics*. March 11, 2016. Retrieved 8/14/2020 from https://www.cdc.gov/nchs/fastats/home-health-care.htm.

Centers for Medicare & Medicaid Services. (2017). *CMS product no. 10969 Medicare & home health care. CMS product number 10969*. Retrieved 7/15/2020 from https://www.medicare.gov/Pubs/pdf/10969-Medicare-and-Home-Health-Care.pdf.

Centers for Medicare & Medicaid Services. (2019a). *Long-term care facility resident assessment instrument 3.0 user's manual, version 1.17.1, effective 10-01-2019*. Retrieved 2-10-2020 from https://www.cms.gov/Medicare/Quality-Initiatives-Patient-Assessment-Instruments/NursingHomeQualityInits/MDS30RAIManual.

Centers for Medicare & Medicaid Services. (2019b). *OASIS user manual. Outcome and assessment information set OASIS-D guidance manual. Effective January 1,2019*. Retrieved 08-08-2020 from https://www.cms.gov/Medicare/Quality-Initiatives-Patient-Assessment-Instruments/HomeHealthQualityInits/HHQIOASISUserManual.

Centers for Medicare & Medicaid Services. (2020a). *Long term care facilities (skilled nursing facilities and/or nursing facilities): CMS flexibilities to fight COVID-19*. Retrieved 08-01-2020 from https://www.cms.gov/files/document/covid-long-term-care-facilities.pdf.

Centers for Medicare & Medicaid Services. (2020b). *Skilled nursing facility care*. Retrieved 07-22-2020 from https://www.medicare.gov/coverage/skilled-nursing-facility-snf-care.

Centers for Medicare & Medicaid Services. (2020c). *What part B covers*. Retrieved 02-12-2020 from https://www.medicare.gov/what-medicare-covers/what-part-b-covers.

Centers for Medicare & Medicaid Services. (2020d). *Surgical dressings—policy article*. Retrieved February 21, 2020 from https://www.cms.gov/medicare-coverage-database/view/article.aspx?articleid=54563Centers for Medicare and Medicaid Services, Medicare Learning Network, 2019.

Centers for Medicare & Medicaid Services. Medicare Learning Network. (2019a). *SNF PPS: Patient driven payment model training presentation*. Retrieved 7-29-20 from https://www.cms.gov/Medicare/Medicare-Fee-for-Service-Payment/SNFPPS/PDPM.

Centers for Medicare & Medicaid Services. Medicare Learning Network. (2019b). *Clarification of billing and payment policies for negative pressure wound therapy (NPWT) using a disposable device*. June 11, 2019. Retrieved 6-18-2020 from https://www.cms.gov/Outreach-andEducation/MedicareLearningNetworkMLN/MLNMattersArticles/downloads/SE17027.pdf.

Centers for Medicare & Medicaid Services. Medicare Learning Network. (2019c). *Overview of the patient-driven groupings model (PDGM)*. February 12, 2019. Retrieved 02-02-2020 from https://www.cms.gov/Outreach-and-Education/Outreach/NPC/Downloads/2019-02-12-PDGM-Presentation.pdf.

Centers for Medicare & Medicaid Services. Medicare Learning Network. Chronic Care Policy Group. (2014). *Certifying patients for the Medicare home health benefit*. Retrieved 8/14/2020 from https://www.cms.gov/Outreach-and-Education/Outreach/NPC/Downloads/2014-12-16-HHBenefit-HL.pdf.

Corbett, L. Q., Funk, M., Fortunato, G., & O'Sullivan, D. M. (2017). Pressure injury in a community population: A descriptive study. *Journal of Wound, Ostomy, and Continence Nursing, 44*(3), 221–227. https://doi.org/10.1097/WON.0000000000000320.

Coyer, F., Campbell, J., & Doubrovsky, A. (2020). Efficacy of incontinence-associated dermatitis intervention for patients in intensive care: An open-label pilot randomized controlled trial. *Advances in Skin & Wound Care, 33*(7), 375–382. https://doi.org/10.1097/01.asw.0000666904.35944.a3.

Ellenbecker, C. H., Samia, L., Cushman, M. J., & Alster, K. (2008). Patient safety and quality in home health care. In R. G. Hughes (Ed.), *Patient safety and quality: An evidence-based handbook for nurses.* Agency for Healthcare Research and Quality (US). Retrieved 7/10/2020 from https://www.ncbi.nlm.nih.gov/books/NBK2631/.

Frack, B., Garlbaldi, A., & Kadar, A. (2017). Why Medicare advantage is marching towards 70% penetration. L.E.K. *Consulting Executive Insights.*, *19*(69), 1–5. Retrieved 06-04-2020 from https://www.lek.com/sites/default/files/insights/pdf-attachments/1969_Medicare_AdvantageLEK_Executive_Insights_1.pdf.

Hakkarainen, T. W., Arbabi, S., Willis, M. M., Davidson, G. H., & Flum, D. R. (2016). Outcomes of patients discharged to skilled nursing facilities after acute care hospitalizations. *Annals of Surgery*, *263*(2), 280–285. https://doi.org/10.1097/SLA.0000000000001367.

Harding, K., Dowsett, C., Fias, L., Jelnes, R., Mosti, G., Öien, R., et al. (2015). Simplifying venous leg ulcer management. Recommendations from an expert working group (consensus recommendations). *Wounds International*, 1–25. Retrieved 05-25-2020 from https://www.woundsinternational.com/resources/details/simplifying-venous-leg-ulcer-management-consensus-recommendations.

Holly, R. (2020). Why home health agencies should gear up for PDGM's wound care opportunity. Home Health Care News. May 5, 2020. Retrieved 05-18-2020 from https://homehealthcarenews.com/2019/05/why-home-health-agenciesshould-gear-up-for-pdgms-wound-care-opportunity.

Home Health Quality Improvement.org. (2019). *Evidence-based practices for improving your wound management program. HHQI webinar.* May 16, 2019. Retrieved November 20, 2022 from https://www.youtube.com/watch?v=xchNd3qHEto.

Kelly, M. (1989). The omnibus budget reconciliation act of 1987. A policy analysis. *The Nursing Clinics of North America*, *24*(3), 791–794.

Landers, S., Madigan, E., Leff, B., Rosati, R. J., McCann, B. A., Hornbake, R., et al. (2016). The future of home health care: A strategic framework for optimizing value. *Home Health Care Management and Practice*, *28*, 262–278. https://doi.org/10.1177/1084822316666368.

Maguire, J. (2014). Wound care management. *Today's Geriatric Medicine*, *7*(2), 14–18.

Medicare Interactive. (2020). *Medicare advantage and home health.* Retrieved 06-04-2020 from https://www.medicareinteractive.org/get-answers/medicare-covered-services/home-health-services/home-health-basics.

MedPac. (2016). *Skilled nursing facility payment system.* Retrieved 02-01-2020 from http://medpac.gov/-documents-/payment-basics. Issue date October 11, 2019.

Morford, T. G. (1988 Supp.). Nursing home regulation: History and expectations. *Centers for Medicare & Medicaid Services. NTIS #PB89-188494. Health Care Financing Review.* Retrieved November 18, 2022 from, https://www.cms.gov/Research-Statistics-Data-and-Systems/Research/HealthCareFinancingReview/List-of-Past-Articles-Items/CMS1192068.

National Pressure Injury Advisory Panel. (2017). *NPUAP position statement on staging. 2017 clarifications.* Retrieved 07-15-2020 from https://npiap.com/resource/resmgr/npuap-position-statement-on-.pdf.

Rau, J. (2020). As coronavirus cases grow, so does scrutiny of nursing home infection plans. *Kaiser Health News.* Retrieved 07-20-2020 from https://khn.org/news/as-coronavirus-cases-grow-so-does-scrutiny-of-nursing-home-infection-plans/.

Spanko, A. (2019). Early PDPM claims data reveals far more winners than losers, "impossible combinations" of conditions. *Skilled Nursing News.* Retrieved 02-22-2020 from https://skillednursingnews.com/2019/11/early-pdpm-claims-data-reveals-far-more-winners-than-losers-impossible-combinations-of-conditions/.

Starc, A. (2014). Who benefits from Medicare advantage. *Wharton Public Policy Initiative Issue Briefs*, *2*(5). Scholarly Commons. PennLibraries. University of Pennsylvania. Retrieved November 18, 2022 from https://repository.upenn.edu/pennwhartonppi/26/.

Sterba, J. A. (2012). Wound care on the go. *Today's Wound Clinic*, *6*(12), 18–21.

You, K., Li, Y., Intrator, O., Stevenson, D., Hirth, R., Grabowski, D., et al. (2016). Do nursing home chain size and proprietary status affect experiences with care? *Medical Care*, *54*(3), 229–234. https://doi.org/10.1097/mlr.0000000000000479.

Zarchi, K., Theut Riis, P., Graversgaard, C., Miller, I. M., Heidenheim, M., & Jemec, G. B. E. (2016). Validation of a screening questionnaire for chronic leg ulcers. *The International Journal of Lower Extremity Wounds*, *15*(4), 320–324. https://doi.org/10.1177/1534734616671227.

FURTHER READING

Bruce, T. A., Shever, L. L., Tschannen, D., & Gombert, J. (2012). Reliability of pressure ulcer staging: A review of literature and one institution's strategy. *Critical Care Nursing Quarterly*, *35*(1), 85–101. https://doi.org/10.1097/CNQ.0b013e31823b1f22.

Centers for Medicare & Medicaid Services. (2020d). *Surgical dressings—policy article (A54563).* Retrieved 08-01-2020 from https://www.cms.gov/medicare-coverage-database/details/article-details.aspx?articleId=54563&ver=32&CoverageSelection=Local&ArticleType=All&PolicyType=Final&s=All&KeyWord=Surgical+Dressings&KeyWordLookUp=Title&KeyWordSearchType=And&bc=gAAAABAAAAAA&.

Holly, R. (2020). Predicting COVID-19's long-term impact on the home health care market. Home Healthcare News. June 10, 2020. Retrieved 07-30-2020 from https://homehealthcarenews.com/2020/06/predicting-covid-19s-long-term-impact-on-the-homehealth-care-market/.

4

Telehealth and Wound Management

Elaine Horibe Song

"Information provided in this chapter reflects the reimbursement scenario upon writing of the chapter. However, reimbursement regulations often change quickly, and thus readers are encouraged to access CMS' website for the most current information."

OBJECTIVES

1. Describe the different types of telehealth services.
2. Evaluate the effectiveness of telehealth in wound management.
3. Provide examples of use of telehealth for wound management across different care settings.
4. Describe the process of assessing the benefits telemedicine can bring to their practices.
5. Provide a pathway for implementation and reevaluation of a telehealth solution.
6. Identify barriers and facilitators to telehealth adoption.

BACKGROUND

Telehealth as a concept dates back to the 19th century (Board on Health Care Services & Institute of Medicine, 2012). The first known case of real-time video telehealth is believed to have taken place in 1959, when doctors at the University of Nebraska utilized interactive telemedicine to submit neurological examinations to colleagues (Gaydos, 2019; Rinde & Balteskard, 2002). However, the first reports on the use of telehealth for wound management were not published until the early 21st century (Gaydos, 2019). Since then, the use of telemedicine in chronic wound management has been associated with lower cost of care (Chanussot-Deprez & Contreras-Ruiz, 2013), shorter healing time (Gaydos, 2019; Sood et al., 2016; Wickström et al., 2018), fewer foot amputations (Nordheim, Haavind, & Iversen, 2014; Smith-Strøm et al., 2018), and fewer office visits (Chanussot-Deprez & Contreras-Ruiz, 2013; Gamus, Kaufman, & Chodick, 2019; Pifer, 2020; Song et al., 2020b).

Before the COVID-19 pandemic, telehealth adoption rate was relatively modest despite its promising potential, likely due to reimbursement and regulatory hurdles. The COVID-19 pandemic presented an opportunity for the rapid rise of telehealth consultations throughout the world. In the United States, the Centers for Medicare and Medicaid Services (CMS) issued temporary waivers and new rules that promoted ground-breaking flexibilities in reimbursement and privacy requirements. Those changes broadened access and payment for a wider variety of telehealth services, ultimately leading to an increase in telehealth claims by more than 11,000% in a 6-week period, starting when the public health emergency was declared (AHRQ, 2020).

During the widespread adoption of telehealth propelled by the pandemic, patients realized telehealth could be a means to solve long faced health-care challenges, such as getting faster access to care, making care more convenient, and connecting with their own providers (Advisory Board, 2020b). Telehealth visits continued to be frequent even after in-person primary care visits were allowed to be resumed during the pandemic, although not as frequent as in the beginning of this period (Advisory Board, 2020a; League & Advisory Board, 2020). From the providers' standpoint, at least two primary challenges to sustaining the hard-won momentum of telehealth adoption could be identified (League & Advisory Board, 2020):

- Streamlining telehealth workflows: many providers were forced into adopting telehealth solutions that did not integrate with their existing workflows and electronic medical records, which led to a proliferation of platforms and inefficient workflows.
- Addressing clinician lack of familiarity: many providers were not able to confidently incorporate telehealth into their practices due to lack of familiarity with the telehealth modalities and technologies.

Despite some adoption challenges, the fact that the health-care landscape has been moving from a fee-for-service to a value-based era remains unchanged. Payers have been implementing new reimbursement models that encourage providers to be cost-effective. Many clinicians still face a myriad of constraints that may pose an obstacle to better outcomes or increased access to wound care (Song et al., 2020b). A truly patient-centric approach to care delivery leverages telehealth as a tool to overcome barriers and hassles of receiving care (League & Advisory Board, 2020).

It is important to note that telehealth can be deployed in a way that benefits not only patients, but also clinicians and institutions. For providers, a well-implemented telehealth program can offer better work-balance and flexibility to continue to provide follow-up care to patients even when they cannot physically be present in their workplace (e.g., while in self-quarantine). For institutions, telehealth may help with revenue optimization, for instance, by accommodating patients who cannot travel to the clinic as virtual encounters, scheduling telehealth on evenings and weekends, and reducing overhead costs (Hostetter, 2020).

This chapter reviews definitions and types of telehealth modalities, and the evidence supporting telehealth interventions. In addition, it provides a framework for setting up a new telehealth program or evaluating an existing one.

DEFINITIONS

eHealth

The term "eHealth" is regarded as lacking a clear definition; however it generally refers to the use of electronic health records, patient administration systems, and data collection to further the health of individuals (Mahoney, 2020; Oh, Rizo, Enkin, & Jadad, 2005). eHealth encompasses telehealth and telemedicine (Fig. 4.1) (AHRQ, 2020; Song, 2019; van Dyk, 2014).

Telehealth

The Agency for Healthcare and Research Quality (AHRQ) defines telehealth as preventative, promotive, and curative health care delivered at a distance (AHRQ, 2020). Specifically, telehealth consultations are defined as the use of telehealth to facilitate collaboration between two or more providers, often involving a specialist, or among clinical team members, across

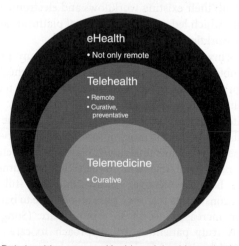

Fig. 4.1 Relationship among eHealth, telehealth, and telemedicine (AHRQ, 2020; Song, 2019; van Dyk, 2014).

time, and/or distance. While the patient may or may not be involved in the consultation, the consultation is required to be related to a specific patient or group of patients in order to differentiate this activity from training or education (Totten et al., 2019).

Telemedicine

The AHRQ defines telemedicine as the process of delivering curative care remotely. Examples include teledermatology, teleradiology, and others.

CMS-Billable Telehealth Services

CMS utilizes the term "Telehealth Services" when referring to CMS-billable remote visits with a provider using interactive audio and video telecommunications systems that permit real-time communication between the distant provider and the patient at home (CMS, 2020a). Covered health-care services include preventative and curative services (CMS, 2020b).

TYPES OF TELEHEALTH SERVICES

Telehealth modalities are generally classified as (CCHP, 2020; Song, 2019; Song et al., 2020b):
- Store-and-forward (asynchronous): e.g., digital photographs and clinical data sent over the Internet to a wound care specialist, who analyzes the data, and sends back written recommendations.
- Real-time tele-video conferencing (synchronous): e.g., live interaction/communication with a wound care specialist via a webcam.
- Remote monitoring: collection and transmission of clinical data, often from outside conventional care settings, to a provider. For instance, a provider can continually monitor vital signs, glucose, etc. of a patient who is at home or at a remote care facility.
- Mobile health (mHealth): health care and public health information provided through mobile applications on mobile devices (e.g., cell phones, tablets), to enhance health outcomes and improve health care services (Iribarren, Cato, Falzon, & Stone, 2017).

Table 4.1 summarizes virtual services covered by Medicare as of 2022 (CMS, 2020a, 2020b; Song, 2020). (Readers are encouraged to check CMS website for updates). In the United States, for reimbursement purposes by the CMS and private insurers, virtual services can be classified as:
- CMS telehealth visits,
- brief communication technology-based service (e.g., virtual check-in),
- remote evaluation of recorded video and/or images (e.g., store-and-forward),
- interprofessional Internet consultation, and
- remote monitoring.

TABLE 4.1 Virtual Services Covered by Medicare

Type of Medicare-Covered Service	Description of the Service	HCPCS
Medicare Telehealth Visits	*CMS Telehealth. A visit between a provider and a patient using telecommunication systems*	Commonly used CPT codes include 99201-5 and 99211-5 "Office or other outpatient visits" and others (check the list of telehealth services on the CMS website)
Brief communication technology-based service, e.g., virtual check-in	*CTBS. Virtual check-in by physician or other QHP, provided to an established patient*	HCPCS code G2012
Remote evaluation of recorded video and/or images (e.g., store and forward)	*CTBS. Patient submits a video/pictures to provider, who provides interpretation with follow-up with the patient within 24 business hours*	HCPCS code G2010
E-Visits: Online digital evaluation and management services or e-Visits	*CTBS. Communication between patient and provider through an online portal*	CPT 99421-99423 and G2061-G2063 or CPT 98970-98972 for some commercial players
Interprofessional Internet consultation (e.g., e-consults)	*Provider-to-provider communication involving assessment and management of a specific patient*	CPT codes 99446, 99447, 99448, 99449, 99451, 99452
Remote monitoring	*Chronic core remote physiologic monitoring (e.g., weight, blood pressure, pulse oximetry, respiratory flow rate)*	CPT codes 99453, 99454, 99457

CTBS, Communication Technology-Based Services.
Compiled from CMS (2020a, 2020b) and Song (2020).

TELEHEALTH EFFECTIVENESS ACROSS SETTINGS AND SPECIALTIES

Telehealth has been reported to have limitations such as likely overdiagnosis and dependence on functioning technology (Bolton, 2019). Nevertheless, telehealth consultations in general have been shown to produce either similar or better clinical outcomes when compared with control interventions (i.e., in-person face-to-face consultations, care without access to specialty services), with results varying by setting and condition (Totten et al., 2019). Findings of a systematic review that included 233 studies on telehealth across several specialties and care settings indicate that (Totten et al., 2019):

- Specialty telehealth consultations likely reduce patient time in the emergency department.
- Remote consultations for outpatient care likely improve access and clinical outcomes.

TELEHEALTH EFFECTIVENESS IN WOUND MANAGEMENT

In wound management, telehealth as a complement to in-person assessment has the potential to improve time to diagnosis, promote faster wound healing, and reduce likelihood of amputations (Bolton, 2019).

The clinical setting and conditions being treated are of primary importance when analyzing effectiveness of telehealth interventions (Chen et al., 2020; Totten et al., 2019). The majority of available studies involving telehealth for chronic wound management published thus far were conducted in the outpatient setting (e.g., wound clinics, community clinics) and postacute setting (e.g., long-term care facility, home health agency).

For chronic wounds treated in those settings, currently available evidence suggests that efficacy and safety of telehealth interventions are at least similar or slightly better to those of conventional standard care (Chen et al., 2020; Tchero et al., 2017).

Primary Clinical Outcomes

In general, there is moderate quality evidence that telehealth interventions promote similar or better wound healing outcomes (i.e., healing rate, healing time) and result in fewer amputations. Table 4.2 provides a summary of primary clinical outcomes reported by systematic reviews and meta-analyses described in this section.

A systematic review and meta-analysis conducted by Huang et al. (2020) included 14 studies published between 2004 and 2019 ($n = 1926$) that compared clinical outcomes in patients who received telehealth interventions with patients who received usual care. Telehealth interventions included web-based systems, teleconsultation, telemonitoring, mobile application, telephone, text messaging, and e-mail. Authors found that compared with usual care, telehealth interventions significantly improved wound healing rate and reduced adverse events. No

TABLE 4.2 Comparison of Telehealth Modalities With Wound Care Management by Primary Outcomes

Systematic Review/Meta-Analysis	Included Studies	Telehealth Modality	Outcome: Wound Healing	Outcome: Amputation
Huang, Wu, Yu, and Hu, (2020), systematic review and meta-analysis	14 Studies published between 2004 and 2019 ($n = 1926$)	Web-based systems, teleconsultation, telemonitoring, mobile application, telephone, text messaging, and e-mail	• Telehealth interventions significantly improved wound healing rate (RR 1.44, 95% CI 1.16–1.80, $P = 0.001$) • No difference in healing time (MD $= -1.20$, 95% CI -8.13 to 5.754, $P = 0.74$)	• The rate of adverse events of chronic wounds (amputation, infections, eczema, and malnutrition) was significantly lower in the telemedicine group (RR 0.52, 95% CI 0.34–0.80, $P = 0.003$)
Chen et al. (2020), systematic review and meta-analysis	12 Studies published between 2004 and 2019 ($n = 3913$)	Mobile applications, specialized interactive systems, e-mail, telephone, and videoconferencing	• No difference in wound healing at 1 year (RR 1.05, 95% CI 0.89–1.23; $P = 0.15$)	• Decreased risk in amputation for patients receiving telehealth (RR 0.45, 95% CI 0.29–0.71; $P = 0.001$)
Totten et al. (2019), systematic review	6 Studies published between 2000 and 2015	Real-time audio and video, or image and/or record review	• Telehealth interventions lead to similar or improved healing rate, healing time	• Telehealth results in fewer amputations
Tchero et al. (2017), systematic review and meta-analysis	2 Studies published between 2004 and 2015 ($n = 514$)	Real-time audio and video with patients from their homes	• No difference in wound healing time (43 vs 45 days; $P = 0.83$), and number of unhealed ulcers (3 of 20 vs 7 of 120; $P = 0.13$)	• No difference in amputation (12 of 193 vs 14 of 182; $P = 0.59$)

RR, relative risk.

significant differences were found between patients allocated to the telemedicine group or usual care group, in terms of the outcomes of healing time, change in wound size, or mortality.

A systematic review and meta-analysis by Chen et al. (2020) included 12 studies published between 2004 and 2019 ($n = 3913$) that evaluated the efficacy and safety of telehealth for chronic wound management in the community and in the wound clinic. Telehealth interventions included mobile applications, specialized interactive systems, e-mail, telephone, and videoconferencing. Data showed no statistically significant difference in wound healing rates, and mortality with a decreased risk of amputation in patients receiving telemedicine around 1 year (RR 0.45, 95% CI 0.29–0.71; $P = 0.001$).

A 2019 systematic review included six studies published between 2000 and 2015 that evaluated the effectiveness of telehealth expert consultations delivered through real-time audio and video, or image and/or record review in the treatment of patients with chronic wounds in the outpatient or postacute settings (Totten et al., 2019). Authors concluded that there is moderate certainty evidence that telehealth interventions promote similar or better wound healing outcomes (i.e., healing rate, healing time) and result in fewer amputations.

A 2017 systematic review and meta-analysis that included two studies published between 2004 and 2015 ($n = 514$) evaluated whether telehealth consultations can be effective in diabetic foot patient care, compared with usual care (Tchero et al., 2017). Interventions included teleconsultations with patients from their homes. Patients in the telehealth group, as well as in the control group had statistically similar wound healing outcomes (i.e., healing time, unhealed ulcers) and amputations. Authors concluded that care delivered via telehealth consultations is promising for the management of diabetic foot patients as the results were comparable with usual care.

As previously mentioned, the care setting where telehealth is conducted likely influences telehealth effectiveness in wound healing (Chen et al., 2020). Findings of one of the meta-analyses listed above seem to indicate that among patients living in the community or rural areas who mainly received routine wound care by general nurses, those who received expert telehealth consultations in addition to routine care had better wound healing outcomes and decreased mortality compared with those who did not. In contrast, among patients who received their care directly from wound specialists at wound centers, those who received follow-up care via telehealth showed no statistically significant difference in wound healing and mortality outcomes when compared with those who received usual care only (i.e., in-person visits) (Chen et al., 2020). These results imply that telehealth consultations are especially beneficial to patients living in the community or remote rural areas. For those patients, telehealth interventions may be able to have a substantial impact on clinical outcomes.

Intermediate Outcomes

Other outcomes of interest when analyzing effectiveness of telehealth interventions in wound management are access to specialized care, resource utilization, patient satisfaction, cost, and safety.

Access to Specialized Care

There is moderate certainty evidence that telehealth consultations improve access by reducing wait times and time to treatment, and by increasing the number of patients receiving indicated diagnostic tests or treatment (Totten et al., 2019).

Resource Utilization

Telehealth consultations may reduce resource utilization (e.g., the number of in-person visits to specialists and hospitals; number of hospitalizations and shorter lengths of stay; low certainty evidence) (Totten et al., 2019).

Patient Satisfaction

In general, patients seem to be more satisfied with telehealth consultations, especially when those consultations save time or expense compared with usual care (low certainty evidence) (Totten et al., 2019). A study showed a significant improvement of foot self-care behavior among patients with diabetic retinopathy compared with baseline ($P < 0.001$) after a 12-week educational intervention on foot self-care delivered via one-on-one training during bedside visits, leaflets, DVD or videos, telephone follow-ups, and home visits (Gethin, Probst, Stryja, Christiansen, & Price, 2020; Li, Gu, & Guo, 2019). The quality of life reported by patients with venous leg ulcers has also been shown to increase 3 months after implementation of a multidisciplinary specialist service supplemented with telehealth consultations ($P < 0.001$) (Gethin et al., 2020; Tulleners et al., 2019).

Cost

Reported cost savings derive from reductions in transfers or less transportation and from discontinuation of expensive nonevidence-based treatments in postacute care settings as a result of recommendations provided by expert telehealth consultations (low certainty evidence) (Santamaria, Carville, Ellis, & Prentice, 2004; Specht, Wakefield, & Flanagan, 2001; Stern et al., 2014; Totten et al., 2019).

Safety

There is currently insufficient evidence to determine whether telehealth interventions result in more harm compared with usual care. Existing studies report lower rates of complications with telehealth (Totten et al., 2019).

TELEHEALTH ACROSS CARE SETTINGS

Telehealth, when implemented across different care settings, ensures prompt access to specialists and facilitates transition of care. Each care setting has specific needs and requirements; thus, it is important that each program identify its priorities and adjust its telehealth workflow accordingly. For instance, wound clinics may prioritize telehealth platforms that are patient-friendly and easy to use, whereas intensive care units may require telehealth systems equipped with a myriad of sensors to enable remote monitoring of critically ill patients. This section describes how different care settings can employ models that allow them to incorporate telehealth into their practice and meet their specific needs. Boxes 4.1–4.4 provide examples of how telehealth is used in the various care settings.

Outpatient Wound Clinics

Telehealth may be used as a complement to in-person visits and greatly benefit patients. Patients with chronic wounds frequently go through difficult transfers and journeys to

---

BOX 4.1 Outpatient Wound Clinic Use Case

Use of telehealth for community-dwelling patients

- In this scenario, a new patient with a simple venous ulcer is initially evaluated at the wound clinic. Dressings and compression bandages are applied, and the patient is asked to follow-up at the clinic after 48 h. As edema shows signs of improvement, dressings and bandages are reapplied at the clinic and the patient is asked to follow-up in the clinic in a week.
- As long as edema and wound appearance continues to improve and the patient can be educated on how to perform dressing changes at home, some of the follow-up visits can be conducted via telehealth audio/video visits (for instance, one

in-person visit, followed by two real-time audio/video conferencing) (Rasmussen et al., 2015). The patient can take pictures of the ulcer upon dressing change and submit these pictures to the clinicians via a secure messaging app.
- Once the virtual visit is completed, wound care recommendations are delivered via an online patient portal, along with digital patient education materials.
- If the wound healing process stalls, the patient is brought in for a thorough evaluation and continues with in-person follow-up visits.

Based on Rasmussen, B. S. B., Froekjaer, J., Bjerregaard, M. R., Lauritsen, J., Hangaard, J., Henriksen, C. W., et al. (2015). A randomized controlled trial comparing telemedical and standard outpatient monitoring of diabetic foot ulcers. *Diabetes Care, 38*(9), 1723–1729. https://doi.org/10.2337/dc15-0332.

BOX 4.2 Home Health Agency Telehealth Use Case

Use of telehealth for patients under home health care

- In this scenario, a home care clinician visiting a patient's home can submit patient assessment and photographs to a remote home health wound care professional via a secure messaging system.
- The wound care professional performs a comprehensive analysis of the patient medical records received via secure messaging system.
- If the wound care professional has further questions, those may be clarified by the home care clinician via telephone or real-time virtual visit, during which the patient may be present as needed.

- The remote wound care professional completes a comprehensive evaluation and submits recommendations for a treatment plan, which is carried out by the home care clinician.
- Medical data and photographs sent by the home care clinician, along with assessment and recommendations sent by the wound care professional via secure messaging are easily transferred to the electronic medical record utilized by both parties. Past telehealth encounters and generated data are available for easy comparison and evaluation at subsequent visits.

Based on Mahoney, M. F. (2020). Telehealth, telemedicine, and related technologic platforms: Current practice and response to the COVID-19 pandemic. *Journal of Wound, Ostomy, and Continence Nursing, 47*(5), 439–444. https://doi.org/10.1097/WON.0000000000000694.

BOX 4.3 Telehealth in Long-Term Care and Assisted Living Facilities

Use of telehealth for patients residing in long-term care and assisted living facilities

Follow-up consultations

- A remote wound care professional is able to deliver virtual care to residents with chronic wounds via real-time audio/video visits and/or store-and-forward modalities.
- Traditional wound rounds, in which a wound care professional evaluates multiple patients/residents in a row, can be transformed into a virtual workflow. In virtual wound rounds, specialists can remotely see several patients/residents in a row and document encounters simultaneously, all on a single video visit.
- The facility-based clinician can send a list of patients to be evaluated by the wound care professional upfront.
- On the day of the televisit, the facility-based clinician facilitates the virtual encounter by first communicating vital signs

and summarizing patient and wound history, then removing wound dressings and positioning the camera so that the remote wound care professional can visualize the wounds. The wound care professional provides verbal orders for wound care, then submits a written report to the facility.
- Facility-based clinicians can also request asynchronous virtual care between the televisits, by submitting a photograph of the ulcer along with their questions via secure messaging.
- Encounters are properly documented on the electronic medical records of the facility.

Urgent consultation

- In this scenario, if a patient with chronic wounds develops an urgent condition that requires evaluation by a wound care professional (e.g., cellulitis), the facility staff can promptly arrange for a virtual visit with the specialist and prevent a visit to the emergency department.

Compiled from Mahoney (2020), Milne et al., (2020), and Ratliff, Shifflett, Howell, and Kennedy (2020).

BOX 4.4 Telehealth in Acute Care

Expediting access to wound care professionals

- In this scenario, a patient presents to the emergency department (ED) of a hospital with fever and a sacral ulcer (e.g., unstageable pressure ulcer/injury), but no wound care professional is readily available on-site.
- The provider obtains photographs of the ulcer and submits them to the remote wound care professional via secure messaging, along with reason for consultation and pertinent medical data.
- The remote wound care professional evaluates the information received and sets up a televisit with the ED provider to discuss details of the patient's condition and wound characteristics, measurements, presence of odor, exudate, erythema, warmth, and induration.

- The wound care professional submits a plan of care back to the provider, who admits the patient and requests consultation with a general surgeon for sharp wound debridement. Interventions are completed by the bedside nurses.
- A few days later, the wound care professional is able to visit the patient in-person to assess effectiveness of the plan of care.

Postoperative telemonitoring

- In this use case, a secure messaging system is used by surgical patients in their postoperative period. Patients use the system to send daily photographs of the surgical wound and to answer questions about their recovery. Clinicians evaluate the data and monitor the patient for early complications such as surgical site infections.

Compiled from Engels, Austin, Doty, Sanders, and McNichol (2020) and Haveman et al., (2019).

attend an in-person visit at the wound center. Commuting to the clinic increases risk and exposure to trauma and infectious threats. Telehealth offers patients convenience, mitigates risks, and saves resources (Bolton, 2019). Specific challenges in this model include the need to triage patients who are candidates for telehealth consultations and the need for schedulers and clinicians to teach patients and caregivers how to utilize the telehealth platform of choice. From the providers' perspective, telehealth has the potential to increase practice revenue and increase provider flexibility. Strategies include (Engels et al., 2020; Hostetter, 2020):

- offering patients the option to receive visits that typically have lower fee-for-service reimbursement as virtual visits (e.g., diabetes education, nutrition, and behavioral health);
- offering patients who cannot travel to the clinic the option to reschedule in-person visits as virtual visits;
- offering patients the option to schedule telehealth virtual visits on evenings and weekends to generate revenue while simultaneously offering providers more flexibility; and
- allowing providers who are forced to quarantine or work from home to provide virtual visits while at home.

Home Health Agencies

Wound care specialists working at home health agencies can leverage telehealth to reduce valuable time spent traveling to/from patients' homes, increase access to care, and detect and resolve complications before they require hospital admission (Bolton, 2019). One of the main advantages of this model is the efficient utilization of the wound care professional's time and expertise, as time previously allocated to traveling to patients' homes can be shifted to the provision of remote care to a greater number of patients. In addition, wound care professionals may be more available to impromptu consultation requests by home care clinicians while visiting a patient's home. Challenges in this model include lack of reliable Internet or cell phone reception at patients' homes, which poses a barrier to communication between the home health clinician and remote wound care professional. Also, the wound care professional depends on the home health clinician to provide a thorough and accurate clinical picture, such as wound measurements, wound odor, etc.

Long-Term Care and Assisted Living Facilities

As several long-term care and assisted living facilities were required to implement strict policies for external visitors during the COVID-19 pandemic, telehealth rose to become a silver-lining for residents needing specialty care (Ratliff et al., 2020). This telehealth model allows patients to receive timely access to wound care professionals. In addition, participation of facility-based clinicians in telehealth encounters with remote wound care professionals opens an opportunity for hands-on training and involvement of the facility staff in the care of the patient and wound (Mahoney, 2020). One of the challenges in this model is the need to rely on facility staff to assist with the visit, lack of adequate resources in many

facilities leading to variability in the quality of Internet connection, video and photographs, and the paucity of viable alternatives to in-person serial conservative sharp debridement when needed (Mahoney, 2020).

Inpatient Acute Care

Telehealth in the acute care setting has the potential to expedite access to specialty care, enhance continuity of care after discharge to postacute facilities and reduce hospital readmissions (Ratliff et al., 2020). It has been reported that use of telehealth to monitor patients postoperatively is associated with improved patient satisfaction and can facilitate early detection of complications (Haveman et al., 2019; Mousa et al., 2019). Challenges in this setting include the need to use generic hospital-approved telehealth platforms, which sometimes do not meet wound care professionals' specific needs (e.g., camera used for video visits is not mobile enough to be positioned in an angle that captures the wound, need to use separate platforms for photographs, video visits, etc.).

PRACTICAL FRAMEWORK FOR TELEHEALTH IMPLEMENTATION

This framework is based on the American Medical Association Digital Health Implementation Playbook (American Medical Association, 2018) and adapted to fit the needs of a wound care clinicians (Evans et al., 2019; Hess, 2020a, 2020b; Song, 2020; Song et al., 2020a, 2020b). The purpose of a framework is to

1. guide health care professionals in assessing the benefits telemedicine can bring to their practices and
2. provide a pathway for implementation of telehealth solutions.

Part 1 (Pregame): Explore Telehealth as a Solution
Step 1: Identify a Need for Telehealth Solutions
- Identify areas of opportunity.
  - Solicit feedback from wound care clinicians.
  - Develop a wound care patient triage system to identify which patients can be potential candidates for telehealth virtual services, which patients need to be evaluated in-person, or which patients can be offered a combination of services. Table 4.3 provides an example of a triage system for lower-extremity wounds.
  - Define the type of telehealth services to be provided within your practice. See Section "Types of Telehealth Services."
- Research existing telemedicine solutions/software.

Step 2: Form the Team
- Identify the key members of your implementation team: it should include clinicians, schedulers, billers, information technology (IT) specialists, and others.
- Define how the team members will work together.
- Solicit input from team members.

TABLE 4.3   Sample Triage System for Patients With Lower-Extremity Wounds and Diabetic Foot Problems

	Conditions	Care Setting	Urgency
Critical	• Severe and moderate infections (according to the Infectious Disease Society of America—IDSA classification) • Gas gangrene • Sepsis • Acute limb ischemia	Hospital	Urgent—Priority 1
Serious	• ISDA mild and some moderate infections (including osteomyelitis) • Chronic limb-threatening ischemia • Dry gangrene • Worsening foot ulcers • Active Charcot foot	Outpatient clinic Surgery center Physician's office	Priority 2
Guarded	• Improving foot ulcer • Inactive Charcot foot • Simple venous leg ulcer	Outpatient clinic Physician's office Home Telehealth	Priority 3
Stable	• Recently healed foot ulcer • Inactive Charcot foot in stable footwear • Healed amputation • Diabetic foot ulcer in remission	Home Telehealth	Priority 4

Adapted from Rogers, L. C., Lavery, L. A., Joseph, W. S., & Armstrong, D. G. (2020). All feet on deck-the role of podiatry during the COVID-19 pandemic: Preventing hospitalizations in an overburdened healthcare system, reducing amputation and death in people with diabetes. *Journal of the American Podiatric Medical Association.* https://doi.org/10.7547/20-051.

Step 3: Define Success

- Identify goals: relevant goals generally focus on health outcomes, improving patient experience, reducing cost, and/or increasing provider satisfaction.
- Identify target results: research the types of results that are feasible with the solution you are considering:
  - For clinician–patient telemedicine interactions:
    - Improve patient access to care
    - Improve patient satisfaction (as patient does not need to spend resources to be physically present for a consultation)
  - For clinician–clinician telemedicine interactions:
    - Increase clinicians' satisfaction and productivity (e.g., avoid disruptions in clinician's schedule by reducing impromptu calls, reduce clinicians' time spent on coordinating transportation to the clinic)
    - Improve clinical outcomes, decrease errors (e.g., requesting clinician can prepare a case so that consultant can better understand the case and provide more accurate assessment/recommendations, compared to impromptu calls)
    - Improve knowledge base of requesting clinician over time

Step 4: Evaluate the Vendor

- Research and compare potential vendors of telemedicine solutions
  - Select HIPAA compliant solutions that offer a business associate agreement

- Select wound care-specific solutions (e.g., with workflow integration, wound-specific decision support, documentation templates, superior quality video and photographs, etc.)
- Select user friendly solutions (e.g., that clinicians and patients can easily use)

Step 5: Make a Business Case

- Find your internal advocates
- Research implementation costs and potential reimbursement
- Review licensing requirements
- Prepare a proposal for internal approval

Step 6: Establish Contract With Telemedicine Vendor

- Negotiate terms with vendor

Part 2 (Game): Telehealth Implementation
Step 7: Design the Workflow

- Identify visit types needed. See Fig. 4.2
- Map and document your existing in-person workflow
- Identify and secure resources needed for telehealth implementation
- Establish your virtual workflow/documentation sequencing based on your visit types
- Aim for integration of the telehealth platform into the electronic medical records workflow

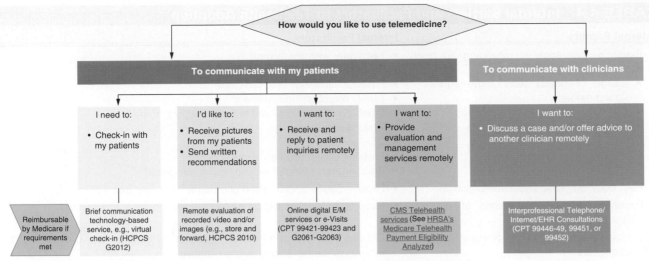

Fig. 4.2 Algorithm to identify types of telehealth services needed (Song et al., 2020a).

Step 8: Prepare the Care Team

- Talk with your vendor about available training support
- Identify staff leaders who can help develop, position, and socialize training material
- Train the care team

Step 9: Partner With the End-User/Customer

- Develop (or source from your vendor) a wide variety of training materials for patients or request clinicians to support different learning styles
- Identify and invite end-users (patient or requesting clinicians) who are more likely to try and use the telemedicine solution

Step 10: Implement the Solution

- Review the most current CMS and commercial insurers regulations and associated policies. Ensure all parts of the clinical workflow contemplate requirements imposed by these regulations and policies, from patient registration to encounter documentation and billing (Song, 2020).
- Ensure the billing department has included the billing codes in the charge master to support the telehealth services provided.
- Configure your telehealth platform: reliable Internet connection and appropriate devices, patient portal, video conferencing, consent management, secure messaging, photograph management, virtual waiting room, integration with electronic medical records workflow, etc.
- Train staff and practice the workflow internally.
- Conduct trial telehealth services with invited end-users who are more likely to try the new virtual solutions.
- Announce the new virtual services to your patients and partnering institutions (e.g., skilled nursing facilities, referring providers, etc.).

Step 11: Evaluate Success

- Gather data used to track your key success metrics and assess success
- Consult your implementation team to determine the program's future

Step 12: Scale

- Resolve any improvement opportunities identified in the initial implementation
- Select your next scaling prospect (i.e., new department, more patients, etc.)

EVALUATING YOUR TELEHEALTH PROGRAM

For wound care programs that have already implemented a telehealth program, periodical evaluation of the program is recommended, to determine if adjustments are needed. A good starting point for wound care programs to evaluate their current telehealth program is to review their initial goals and target outcomes, as described in "Step 3: Define Success" of the practical framework described above. If target outcomes are not being reached, reassessment of the initial goals, workflows, and barriers and facilitators to telehealth adoption is recommended. For workflows, refer to "Step 7: Design the Workflow" above. Barriers and facilitators, which can be internal or external, are listed in Tables 4.4 and 4.5. Webside manners, a facilitator for telehealth adoption, are summarized in Box 4.5.

- Internal factors: refer to the users' behaviors and motivations while using and interacting with the system, which are keys to patients' acceptance of the use of this technology (Almathami et al., 2020).
- External factors: refer to the environment surrounding the system's usage and the system itself that influence users' acceptance and use of telehealth services (Almathami et al., 2020).

TABLE 4.4 Internal Barriers and Facilitators to Telehealth Adoption

Internal Barriers	Internal Facilitators

• Patient's resistance to changing to new approaches:
  • Usage of digital technology requires good dexterity
  • Difficulty reading on smartphones
  • Lack of technological savviness
	• Familiarity with the system
	• Patients' past treatment experiences
	• Patients' familiarity with clinicians
	• Family members' involvement
	• Provision of emotional and technical support to patients
	• Time saved
	• Convenience
	• Enabling detection of an acute condition
	• Enabling monitoring of wound healing progress

• Poor body language and communication	• Excellent body language and communication. See Box 4.5
• Patients' negative perceptions of virtual visits privacy and security	• Patients' positive perceptions of virtual visits privacy and security
• Clinician's fear of a dehumanizing effect on patient care	• Clinician's belief that long-term relationships between the clinician and the patient can be developed over a distance

• Clinician's suboptimal clinical and technological competency:
  • Unsystematic wound care training
  • Inadequate training on the usage of digital technology
	• Competent clinicians:
	  • Adequate wound care training
	  • Adequate training on the usage of digital technology
	  • Increased wound care competency due to usage of digital technology

Almathami, Win, and Vlahu-Gjorgievska (2020), Foong, Kyaw, Upton, and Tudor Car (2020), and Gethin et al., (2020).

TABLE 4.5 External Barriers and Facilitators to Telehealth Adoption

External Barriers	External Facilitators

• Internet connectivity issues that prevent stable communication via telehealth technology:
  • Slow Internet speed
  • Poor cell phone network signal
	• Reliable Internet connectivity:
	  • High Internet speed (wired connection, strong Wi-Fi signal)
	  • Good cell phone network signal

• System difficult to use:
  • Complex installation
  • Not user friendly
  • Difficulty in taking good wound photographs
  • Lack of integration with clinician's workflow
	• System ease of use:
	  • Easy to get started, training and support for patients and clinicians
	  • User friendliness
	  • Flexible, with easy integration into clinician's workflow
	  • Allows patients to easily take pictures of their wounds

• Lack of organizational support:
  • Regulations, policies, and reimbursement hurdles
  • Lack of full support to telehealth services by health insurance companies
  • Lack of support from health-care organizations to integrate telehealth technologies with patients' health records, cross-synchronize with other system platforms, and eliminate duplicate data entry
	• Strong organizational support:
	  • Reimbursement and regulation flexibilities granted by CMS during the pandemic
	  • Access to Internet in remote and rural areas
	  • Leadership support in leveraging technology to enhance interaction with patients and clinical outcomes

• Interference during virtual visits:
  • Patients are distracted by other things happening at home and the family members around them, which affects their privacy concerns
  • Patients multitask during virtual visits
	• Training provided to patients prior to the virtual visit

Compiled from Almathami et al., (2020), Foong et al., (2020), Gethin et al., (2020).

BOX 4.5 Webside Manners for Real-Time Televisits

Before the visit
- Upon scheduling the visit, ensure patients have a compatible device, access to the telehealth technology and strong Internet. Send patients and caregivers instructions on how to use the technology upfront. If it is the first time, schedule a time to test patient's ability to initiate a video call or submit a picture
- Ensure your telehealth platform is working well
  - Ensure you have good Internet connection
  - Close extra tabs and applications to improve video quality
  - Check if your microphone and speakers are working
  - Perform weekly inspections to ensure technology is working correctly
- Set the stage
  - Dress professionally
  - Choose a quiet place or room with no distractions and a solid background with neutral color
  - Review the patient's medical history before the visit
  - Use virtual waiting room to protect patient's privacy

During the visit
- Ensure your camera is turned on and that you can hear the patient and vice versa
- Focus your eyes on the camera
- Keep your focus on the patient during the video call
- Practice patient-centered communication
  - Give body language cues like nodding your head to reassure patients you are listening to them
  - Repeat back the patient's concerns to confirm you are understanding them
  - Leave time for questions

After the visit
- Send an after-visit summary to the patient, with information on how they contact you if needed
- Ask for feedback on the patient's experience with the virtual visit

Advisory Board. (2020). Tips to improve your "webside manner." Retrieved October 8, 2020, from https://www.advisory.com/research/physician-executive-council/resources/posters/webside-manner.

SUMMARY

- Telehealth is not new; however, the COVID-19 pandemic presented an opportunity for the rapid rise of telehealth consultations throughout the world.
- Telehealth can be defined as preventative, promotive, and curative health care delivered at a distance (AHRQ, 2020). The Centers for Medicare and Medicaid Services (CMS) employs the term "Telehealth Services" when referring to CMS-billable remote visits with a provider using interactive audio and video telecommunications systems that permit real-time communication between the distant provider and the patient at home (CMS, 2020a).
- Telehealth has been reported to have limitations such as likely overdiagnosis and dependence on functioning technology (Bolton, 2019). However, in wound management, telehealth as a complement to in-person assessment has

the potential to improve time to diagnosis, promote faster wound healing, and reduce likelihood of amputations (Bolton, 2019). In addition, it can provide scheduling flexibilities to health-care professionals, and convenience, cost and time savings to patients (Santamaria et al., 2004; Specht et al., 2001; Stern et al., 2014; Totten et al., 2019).
- Telehealth implementation for wound management should be centered around patients' and providers' needs. Development of a wound care triage system and ensuring the telehealth intervention fits into existing clinical workflows can help achieve desired goals. A framework for implementation and evaluation of telehealth programs such as the one presented in this chapter facilitates implementation and adoption process.

SELF-ASSESSMENT QUESTIONS

1. What type of telehealth encounter would best describe the following virtual service? A patient submits a picture of his wound and his concerns to the wound care professional. The wound care professional evaluates and sends written wound care recommendations.
   a. Store-and-forward (asynchronous)
   b. Real-time tele-video conferencing (synchronous)
   c. Remote monitoring
   d. Mobile health (mHealth)
2. Which statement below is supported by moderate certainty evidence?
   a. Use of telehealth interventions promotes similar or better wound healing outcomes (i.e., healing rate,

healing time) and results in fewer amputations compared with usual care.
   b. Use of telehealth interventions promotes better wound healing outcomes (i.e., healing rate, healing time) and results in fewer amputations compared with usual care.
   c. Use of telehealth interventions promotes better wound healing outcomes (i.e., healing rate, healing time) but results in more lower limb amputations compared with usual care.
   d. Use of telehealth interventions results in worse wound healing outcomes (i.e., healing rate, healing time) but results in fewer lower limb amputations compared with usual care.

REFERENCES

Advisory Board. (2020a). *What you need to know about Trump's telehealth and rural health executive order, Advisory Board Daily Briefing.* Retrieved October 3, 2020, from https://www.advisory.com/daily-briefing/2020/08/04/telehealth.

Advisory Board. (2020b). *Insurers are rolling back Covid-19 telehealth benefits. (But providers should not panic.) | Advisory Board Daily Briefing.* Retrieved October 5, 2020, from https://www.advisory.com/daily-briefing/2020/10/01/insurance.

AHRQ. (2020). *The evidence base for telehealth: Reassurance in the face of rapid expansion during the COVID-19 pandemic.* Retrieved September 8, 2020, from https://effectivehealthcare.ahrq.gov/products/telehealth-expansion/white-paper.

Almathami, H. K. Y., Win, K. T., & Vlahu-Gjorgievska, E. (2020). Barriers and facilitators that influence telemedicine-based, real-time, online consultation at patients' homes: Systematic literature review. *Journal of Medical Internet Research, 22*(2), e16407. https://doi.org/10.2196/16407.

American Medical Association. (2018). *American Medical Association digital health implementation playbook.*

Board on Health Care Services, & Institute of Medicine. (2012). *The role of telehealth in an evolving health care environment: Workshop summary.* Washington (DC): National Academies Press (US). https://doi.org/10.17226/13466.

Bolton, L. (2019). Telemedicine improves chronic ulcer outcomes. *Wounds Research, 31*(4).

CCHP. (2020). *About telehealth.* Retrieved January 1, 2020, from https://www.cchpca.org/about/about-telehealth.

Chanussot-Deprez, C., & Contreras-Ruiz, J. (2013). Telemedicine in wound care: A review. *Advances in Skin & Wound Care, 26*(2), 78–82. https://doi.org/10.1097/01.ASW.0000426717.59326.5f.

Chen, L., Cheng, L., Gao, W., Chen, D., Wang, C., & Ran, X. (2020). Telemedicine in chronic wound management: Systematic review and meta-analysis. *JMIR mHealth and uHealth, 8*(6), e15574. https://doi.org/10.2196/15574.

CMS. (2020a). *Medicare telemedicine health care provider fact sheet.* Retrieved March 18, 2020 from https://www.cms.gov/newsroom/fact-sheets/medicare-telemedicine-health-care-provider-fact-sheet.

CMS. (2020b). *List of telehealth services.* CMS. Retrieved October 5, 2020b, from https://www.cms.gov/Medicare/Medicare-General-Information/Telehealth/Telehealth-Codes.

Engels, D., Austin, M., Doty, S., Sanders, K., & McNichol, L. (2020). Broadening our bandwidth: A multiple case report of expanded use of telehealth technology to perform wound consultations during the COVID-19 pandemic. *Journal of Wound, Ostomy, and Continence Nursing, 47*(5), 450–455. https://doi.org/10.1097/WON.0000000000000697.

Evans, K., Song, E., Mize, J., Hamm, T., Smith, A., Milne, C., et al. (2019). *Telemedicine/televisit implementation playbook—Part 1—Wound reference.* Retrieved January 1, 2020, from https://woundreference.com/app/topic?id=telemedicine-televisit-implementation-playbook.

Foong, H. F., Kyaw, B. M., Upton, Z., & Tudor Car, L. (2020). Facilitators and barriers of using digital technology for the management of diabetic foot ulcers: A qualitative systematic review. *International Wound Journal.* https://doi.org/10.1111/iwj.13396.

Gamus, A., Kaufman, H., & Chodick, G. (2019). Remote care of lower extremities ulcers: An observational pilot study. *The Israel Medical Association Journal, 21*(4), 265–268.

Gaydos, J. (2019). The audio-visual connection: A brief history of telemedicine. *Today's Wound Clinic, 13*(4).

Gethin, G., Probst, S., Stryja, J., Christiansen, N., & Price, P. (2020). Evidence for person-centered care in chronic wound care: A systematic review and recommendations for practice. *Journal of Wound Care, 29*(Sup9b), S1–S22. https://doi.org/10.12968/jowc.2020.29.Sup9b.S1.

Haveman, M. E., Kleiss, S. F., Ma, K. F., Vos, C. G., Ünlü, Ç., Schuurmann, R. C. L., et al. (2019). Telemedicine in patients with peripheral arterial disease: Is it worth the effort? *Expert Review of Medical Devices, 16*(9), 777–786. https://doi.org/10.1080/17434440.2019.1649595.

Hess, C. T. (2020a). Expanded telehealth services offer smart wound care workflows. *Advances in Skin & Wound Care, 33*(5), 277–278. https://doi.org/10.1097/01.ASW.0000660112.99951.f1.

Hess, C. T. (2020b). Triaging telehealth in wound care: Embracing the regulations within your workflows. *Advances in Skin & Wound Care, 33*(6), 334–335. https://doi.org/10.1097/01.ASW.0000666140.77900.62.

Hostetter, S. (2020). *6 Months into Covid-19: What's on independent physician executives' minds?.* Retrieved October 4, 2020, from https://www.advisory.com/research/physician-executive-council/prescription-for-change/2020/09/covid-19.

Huang, Z., Wu, S., Yu, T., & Hu, A. (2020). Efficacy of telemedicine for patients with chronic wounds: A meta-analysis of randomized controlled trials. *Advances in Wound Care.* https://doi.org/10.1089/wound.2020.1169.

Iribarren, S. J., Cato, K., Falzon, L., & Stone, P. W. (2017). What is the economic evidence for mHealth? A systematic review of economic evaluations of mHealth solutions. *PLoS One, 12*(2), e0170581. https://doi.org/10.1371/journal.pone.0170581.

League, J., & Advisory Board. (2020). *What should you expect from telehealth? Here are 4 perspectives from across the industry.* Retrieved October 3, 2020, from https://www.advisory.com/research/health-care-it-advisor/it-forefront/2020/09/telehealth.

Li, J., Gu, L., & Guo, Y. (2019). An educational intervention on foot self-care behaviour among diabetic retinopathy patients with visual disability and their primary caregivers. *Journal of Clinical Nursing, 28*(13–14), 2506–2516. https://doi.org/10.1111/jocn.14810.

Mahoney, M. F. (2020). Telehealth, telemedicine, and related technologic platforms: Current practice and response to the COVID-19 pandemic. *Journal of Wound, Ostomy, and Continence Nursing, 47*(5), 439–444. https://doi.org/10.1097/WON.0000000000000694.

Milne, C., Song, E., Robinson, S., Evans, K., Hamm, T., Mize, J., et al. (2020). Implementing team-based interprofessional telemedicine-based wound care management in post-acute settings leveraging a wound care-specific telemedicine software. In Wound Care Education Institute (Ed.), *Vol. 1. Wild on wounds 2020 National Wound Conference* (p. 232). Relias.

Mousa, A. Y., Broce, M., Monnett, S., Davis, E., McKee, B., & Lucas, B. D. (2019). Results of telehealth electronic monitoring for post discharge complications and surgical site infections following arterial revascularization with groin incision. *Annals of Vascular Surgery, 57*, 160–169. https://doi.org/10.1016/j.avsg.2018.09.023.

Nordheim, L. V., Haavind, M. T., & Iversen, M. M. (2014). Effect of telemedicine follow-up care of leg and foot ulcers: A systematic review. *BMC Health Services Research, 14*, 565. https://doi.org/10.1186/s12913-014-0565-6.

Oh, H., Rizo, C., Enkin, M., & Jadad, A. (2005). What is eHealth?: A systematic review of published definitions. *Journal of Medical Internet Research, 7*(1), e1. https://doi.org/10.2196/jmir.7.1.e1.

Pifer, R. (2020). *Medicare members using telehealth grew 120 times in early weeks of COVID-19 as regulations eased.* Retrieved May 28, 2020, from https://www.healthcaredive.com/news/medicare-seniors-telehealth-covid-coronavirus-cms-trump/578685/.

Rasmussen, B. S. B., Froekjaer, J., Bjerregaard, M. R., Lauritsen, J., Hangaard, J., Henriksen, C. W., et al. (2015). A randomized controlled trial comparing telemedical and standard outpatient monitoring of diabetic foot ulcers. *Diabetes Care, 38*(9), 1723–1729. https://doi.org/10.2337/dc15-0332.

Ratliff, C. R., Shifflett, R., Howell, A., & Kennedy, C. (2020). Telehealth for wound management during the COVID-19 pandemic: Case studies. *Journal of Wound, Ostomy, and Continence Nursing.* https://doi.org/10.1097/WON.0000000000000692.

Rinde, E., & Balteskard, L. (2002). Is there a future for telemedicine? *The Lancet, 359*(9322), 1957–1958. https://doi.org/10.1016/S0140-6736(02)08845-1.

Santamaria, N., Carville, K., Ellis, I., & Prentice, J. (2004). The effectiveness of digital imaging and remote expert wound consultation on healing rates in chronic lower leg ulcers in the Kimberley region of Western Australia. *Primary Intention The Australian Journal of Wound Management, 12*(2), 62–70.

Smith-Strøm, H., Igland, J., Østbye, T., Tell, G. S., Hausken, M. F., Graue, M., et al. (2018). The effect of telemedicine follow-up care on diabetes-related foot ulcers: A cluster-randomized controlled noninferiority trial. *Diabetes Care, 41*(1), 96–103. https://doi.org/10.2337/dc17-1025.

Song, E. (2019). *What is new in 2019 for telehealth and telemedicine?.* Retrieved August 8, 2019, from https://woundreference.com/blog?id=what-is-new-in-2019-for-telehealth-and-telemedicine.

Song, E. (2020). *Reimbursement for Telemedicine services in wound care.* Retrieved October 5, 2020, from https://woundreference.com/blog?find=reimbursement%20telehealth&id=reimbursement-for-telemedicine-services-in-wound-care.

Song, E., Evans, K., Mize, J., Hamm, T., Smith, A., Milne, C., et al. (2020a). *Telemedicine/televisit implementation playbook—Part 2—WoundReference.* Retrieved October 7, 2020, from https://woundreference.com/app/topic?id=1475.

Song, E., Evans, K., Robinson, S., Hamm, T., Mize, J., Milne, C., et al. (2020b). *Adopting telemedicine in wound care: Interprofessional Internet consultations.* Today's Wound Clinic.

Sood, A., Granick, M. S., Trial, C., Lano, J., Palmier, S., Ribal, E., et al. (2016). The role of telemedicine in wound care: A Review and analysis of a database of 5,795 patients from a mobile wound-healing center in Languedoc-Roussillon, France. *Plastic and Reconstructive Surgery, 138*(3 Suppl), 248S–256S. https://doi.org/10.1097/PRS.0000000000002702.

Specht, J. K., Wakefield, B., & Flanagan, J. (2001). Evaluating the cost of one telehealth application connecting an acute and long-term care setting. *Journal of Gerontological Nursing, 27*(1), 34–39. https://doi.org/10.3928/0098-9134-20010101-11.

Stern, A., Mitsakakis, N., Paulden, M., Alibhai, S., Wong, J., Tomlinson, G., et al. (2014). Pressure ulcer multidisciplinary teams via telemedicine: A pragmatic cluster randomized stepped wedge trial in long term care. *BMC Health Services Research, 14*, 83. https://doi.org/10.1186/1472-6963-14-83.

Tchero, H., Noubou, L., Becsangele, B., Mukisi-Mukaza, M., Retali, G.-R., & Rusch, E. (2017). Telemedicine in diabetic foot care: A systematic literature review of interventions and meta-analysis of controlled trials. *The International Journal of Lower Extremity Wounds, 16*(4), 274–283. https://doi.org/10.1177/1534734617739195.

Totten, A. M., Hansen, R. N., Wagner, J., Stillman, L., Ivlev, I., Davis-O'Reilly, C., et al. (2019). *Telehealth for acute and chronic care consultations.* Rockville (MD): Agency for Healthcare Research and Quality (US).

Tulleners, R., Brain, D., Lee, X., Cheng, Q., Graves, N., & Pacella, R. E. (2019). Health benefits of an innovative model of care for chronic wounds patients in Queensland. *International Wound Journal, 16*(2), 334–342. https://doi.org/10.1111/iwj.13033.

van Dyk, L. (2014). A review of telehealth service implementation frameworks. *International Journal of Environmental Research and Public Health, 11*(2), 1279–1298. https://doi.org/10.3390/ijerph110201279.

Wickström, H. L., Öien, R. F., Fagerström, C., Anderberg, P., Jakobsson, U., & Midlöv, P. J. (2018). Comparing video consultation with inperson assessment for Swedish patients with hard-to-heal ulcers: Registry-based studies of healing time and of waiting time. *BMJ Open, 8*(2), e017623. https://doi.org/10.1136/bmjopen-2017-017623.

5

Patient Engagement and Noncompliance

Denise P. Nix and Vicki Haugen

OBJECTIVES

1. Define and critique the following terms: noncompliance, nonadherence, patient engagement, and Health Belief Model (HBM).
2. Recognize the significance of nonadherence in wound management outcomes.
3. Identify interventions to support practice when patients refuse care that may put them in harm's way.
4. List the advantages of using a HBM as a framework to guide shared goal setting.
5. Summarize the Joint Commission standards related to patient education.
6. Discuss barriers and strategies to developing a sustainable plan of care.

Historically, the term *noncompliant* has been used to describe the patient who, for whatever reason, does not adopt interventions included in the plan of care. Nurses' and doctors' descriptions of behaviors from noncompliant patients have ranged from passive resistance, unintentional and intentional, to lack of motivation or overt refusal and deliberate interference with care (Iihara et al., 2014; Moffatt, Murray, Keeley, & Aubeeluck, 2017; Stacey et al., 2017; Tobiano, Marshall, Bucknall, & Chaboyer, 2015). However, patients who have been labeled noncompliant report a lack of understanding of why or what they were supposed to do or an inability to perform prescribed interventions (Aliasgharpour & Nayeri, 2012; Yan, Liu, Zhou, & Sun, 2014). This gap in perception leads to obvious questions about the billable ICD-10-CM code Z91.19 that can be used for reimbursement for "noncompliance" with treatment or medical regime (ICD 10 Data 2019) and the noncompliance label, which has been described as an arrogant term suggesting that the patient's job is to do what he or she is told to do by the health care provider (Rappl, 2004; Sandman, Granger, Ekman, & Munthe, 2012; van Rijswijk, 2004).

The term *adherence* has been used as an alternative to compliance. The World Health Organization (WHO) (Chisholm-Burns & Spivey, 2012) defines the term as "the extent to which a person's behavior (taking medication, following a diet, and/or executing lifestyle changes) corresponds with agreed recommendations from a health care provider." The critical difference between compliance and adherence requires the patient's agreement to the recommendations, recognizing patients as active partners in their own care and that good communication between patient and health professional.

Regardless of terminology, however, misperceptions remain. Discrepancies between professional and patient perspectives need to be reconciled and addressed to improve adherence to treatment regimens (Moffatt et al., 2017; Tobiano et al., 2015). The wound specialist's role should be to critique the plan of care rather than the patient. This chapter uses the Health Belief Model (HSM) and patient engagement principles to address important factors that impact the ability to achieve a sustainable plan of care.

SIGNIFICANCE

Although most health-related adherence research has focused on medication, adherence also encompasses numerous health-related behaviors that extend beyond taking prescribed pharmaceuticals. According to the WHO (Chisholm-Burns & Spivey, 2012), adherence to therapy for chronic illnesses in developed countries averages 50%. In developing countries, the rates are even lower. Poor adherence severely compromises the effectiveness of treatment making this a critical issue from the perspective of quality of life and of health economics. Interventions aimed at improving adherence would provide a significant positive return on investment through primary prevention (of risk factors) and secondary prevention of adverse health outcomes.

Wound management is reported in the literature as one of the many health-related problems associated with nonadherence (European Pressure Ulcer Advisory Panel, National Pressure Injury Advisory Panel, Pan Pacific Pressure Injury Alliance (EPUAP, NPIAP, PPPIA), 2019; Wound, Ostomy and Continence Nurses Society, 2014, 2016, 2019, 2021). It is estimated that 1%–2% of the population in developed countries will develop a chronic wound in their lifetime, similar to the prevalence rate for heart failure (Nussbaum et al., 2018). In the United States, chronic wounds affect approximately 6.5 million patients and may experience chronic pain, loss of function and mobility, increased social stress and isolation, depression and anxiety, prolonged hospitalization, increased financial burden, and increased morbidity and mortality. More than $25 billion is spent in the United States every year on treating wound-related complications (Jarbrink et al., 2016). An analysis of a large subset of older Americans (Medicare beneficiaries) conducted by Nussbaum et al. (2018) showed chronic wounds impact nearly 15% of Medicare beneficiaries (8.2 million). A conservative estimate of the annual cost is $28 billion when the wound is the primary diagnosis on the claim. When the analysis included wounds as a secondary diagnosis, the cost for wounds is conservatively estimated at $31.7 billion (Nussbaum et al., 2018). Significance and cost of care for specific types of wounds including diabetic foot ulcers, arterial ulcers, and pressure injuries and their association with nonadherence are described in the following section.

In the United States, 30.3 million people have diabetes (Centers for Disease Control and Prevention (CDC), 2017). Up to 25% of patients with diabetes will develop a foot ulcer in their lifetime; once healed, up to 30.6%–64.4% will reoccur within 3 years (Dubský, Jirkovská, Bem, et al., 2013; Hicks et al., 2020). In the year 2016, 4.9 per 1000 adults with diabetes in the United States received lower extremity amputations (US Department of Health and Human Services, 2020). According to Nussbaum et al. (2018) the cost of care for diabetic foot ulcers ranges from $6.2 to $6.9 billion. Experts describe foot offloading and blood glucose control among the most critical interventions for the prevention and treatment of diabetic foot ulcers (Armstrong, Lavery, Wu, et al., 2005; Hicks et al., 2020; Wound, Ostomy and Continence Nurses Society, 2021). Unfortunately, researchers report that nonadherence with insulin for insulin depended diabetes ranges from 20% to 38% (Doggrell & Chan, 2015) and several reports of challenges with offloading the foot (Armstrong et al., 2005; Peters, Armstrong, & Lavery, 2007; Wu, Jensen, Weber, et al., 2008). A retrospective analysis of the Medicare beneficiaries with diabetic wounds estimated annual health care costs at $6.2–6.9 billion (Nussbaum et al., 2018).

Venous leg ulcers account for 80% of lower extremity ulcerations according to a Cochrane review (O'Meara, Al-Kurdi, & Ovington, 2008). The mean direct cost of treating one VLU is estimated to be greater than $15,000, with the mean cost of surgical intervention for a VLU as high as $33,000 (Wound, Ostomy and Continence Nurses Society, 2019). Clinical practice guidelines and systemic reviews report reoccurrence rates as high as 40%–70% (Dahm, Myrhaug, Stromme, Fure, & Bruberg, 2019; O'Donnell et al., 2014; Wound, Ostomy and Continence Nurses Society, 2019). While the cornerstone of treatment for venous insufficiency is compression, "noncompliance and nonadherence" with its use is widely reported (Al Shammeri et al., 2014; Labropoulos, Wang, Lanier, et al., 2012; Mariani et al., 2011; Weller, Buchbinder, & Johnston, 2016; Wound, Ostomy and Continence Nurses Society, 2019).

According to Nussbaum et al. (2018), Medicare costs to treat pressure injuries in the United States are between $3696–$4436 billion annually. Recurrence rates range from 13% to 56% with 21% developing a new ulcer at a different anatomical location (Wound, Ostomy and Continence Nurses Society, 2016). Much is asked from patients and caregivers to prevent and treat pressure injuries (see Chapter 11). In a recent integrative review, Ledger, Worsley, Hope, and Schoonhoven (2020) identified lifestyle considerations, pain and/or discomfort, and patient engagement in the decision-making process, as key common themes for adherence to pressure injury prevention and treatment interventions.

One of the greatest costs is to the patient's health-related quality of life (HRQOL). Numerous qualitative studies reflect the lived experience of the patient living with several types of chronic wounds. Among these experiences, pain, restricted lifestyle, impaired mobility, powerlessness, and coping challenges are common (Gorecki, Brown, Nelson, et al., 2009; Jaksa & Mahoney, 2010; Price & Harding, 2004; Spilsbury et al., 2007). Patient engagement and adherence to treatment is directly related to HRQOL (CDC, 2000; Gorecki, Nixon, Madill, Firth, & Brown, 2012). The remainder of this chapter will describe strategies to address these common themes and challenges as they relate to helping every patient with a wound to achieve a sustainable plan of care.

PATIENT ENGAGEMENT

There are many definitions for patient engagement, but all share an underlying theme: the facilitation and strengthening of the role of those using services as coproducers of health, and health care policy and practice (Carman et al., 2013; Ledger et al., 2020; Tobiano et al., 2015). Patient involvement and engagement is increasingly recognized as an important management strategy (Brown, 2014; Ledger et al., 2020; Tobiano et al., 2015; WHO, 2016). *Meaningful patient involvement* is based on the premise that the patient has a specific expertise derived from being a patient and possessing experiential knowledge. *Collective patient involvement* refers to the extent to which patients, through their representative organizations, contribute to shaping the health care system through involvement in health care policymaking, organization, design and delivery (European Patient's Forum, 2017).

Best practice for optimizing patient engagement in wound management requires a whole-system approach with a need for clinicians, patients, industry, and healthcare organizations to agree on clear goals and a coherent strategy as shown in

Patients	Clinicians
• Take an active role in decisions made about treatment • Take responsibility for wound management where they can • Be prepared to learn • Provide constructive about services delivery	• Commit to involving patients in their care • Invest time in developing partnerships with patients • Provide patient education to facilitate informed decision making • Encourage and help patients to plan for future care needs

Healthcare Organizations	Industry
• Understand wound management needs • Ensure services are coordinated and patient-centered • Encourage feedback from patients and clinicians to adapt services • Ensure consistency in competency levels of wound care clinicians • Improve funding for research to allow for better risk stratification	• Respond to product feedback • Develop products that support self-management • Commit to providing evidence to support product use • Provide patient information related to product use • Make dressings available via retail outlets

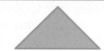

Fig. 5.1 The role of clinicians, patients, industry, and organizations in developing an empowered health service. (Adapted from International Best Practice Statement. (2016). Optimizing patient involvement in wound management. *Wounds International.*)

Fig. 5.1 (International Best Practice Statement, 2016). Box 5.1 lists factors that affect patient engagement, potential solutions, and opportunities for patient engagement (de Silva, 2013; Doherty & Stavropoulou, 2012; Domecq et al., 2014; Moffatt et al., 2017; WHO, 2016).

Shared Decision Making

"Shared Decision Making" (SDM) is a decision-making process where patients actively participate in decisions about their health, rather than delegate decision-making authority to their providers (Elwyn, Col, et al., 2012). Providers work with patients to enhance collaborative outcomes. People using health services are asking for more responsive, open, and transparent communication. They expect practitioners to engage them in the decision-making process. Patient engagement promotes mutual accountability and understanding between the patients and health care providers. Engaged patients are better able to make informed decisions about their care options and outcomes improve when patients are involved in setting goals that affect their lives (Brown, 2014; WHO, 2016). To facilitate a sustainable plan of care, health care professionals need a paradigm shift from a

directive, paternalistic style to a more collaborative interactive style in which problems, treatment goals, and management strategies are defined together (Chatterjee, 2006; Doherty & Stavropoulou, 2012; Parks, Joireman, & Van Lange, 2013).

Not surprisingly, trust and communication are central to the effectiveness of this process. A meta-analysis conducted by Zolnierek and Dimatteo (2009) attributed poor communication to a 19% higher risk of nonadherence. A provider who is willing to take the time and put in the effort to communicate effectively with the patient is perceived by the patient to be supportive. The simple perception of provider support has been shown to increase achievement of a positive outcome (International Best Practice Statement, 2016; O'Malley, Forrest, & Mandelblatt, 2002).

Patient Decision Aids

Patient decision aids are designed to support patients in this process. Patient decision aids are materials such as leaflets, interactive media, video or audio tapes that are intended to supplement rather than replace patient–clinician interaction. Patients may use them to prepare for an appointment or they may be provided at the visit to facilitate SDM. At a minimum,

---

BOX 5.1   Factors Affecting Patient Engagement and Potential Solutions

Factors Affecting Patient Engagement:
- Patient factors (e.g., demographic characteristics, health literacy)
- Health conditions (e.g., illness severity)
- Health care professional's knowledge and attitudes
- Tasks (e.g., required patient safety behavior challenges clinician's abilities)
- Health care setting (e.g., hospital or home)
- Patient perception of their role (e.g., subordinate to clinicians, fear of being labeled "difficult")

Potential Solutions:
- Patient feedback (e.g., surveys, online feedback, interviews, focus groups)
- Patient participation with advisory committees
- Patient/family engagement in resource development (e.g., patient education tool)
- Patient involvement in research (e.g., source of data)
- Patient access to their own electronic health records
- Education of health care professionals to address:
  - Importance of patient engagement
  - Barriers to communication (e.g., expert language, technical jargon)
  - Discrepancies between professional and patient perspectives need to be reconciled and addressed to improve adherence to treatment regimes

---

patient decision aids provide evidence-based information related to risks and benefits. Most strive to help the patient clarify and communicate their values to their practitioners, and to gain skills in collaborative decision making (Elwyn et al., 2006).

Evidence indicates that the use patient decision aids is superior to standard counseling and have a positive effect on patient–clinician communication and increase the likelihood of more realistic expectations, a SDM process. A Cochrane review conducted by Stacey et al. (2017) that included 105 studies and 31,043 participants, found that decision aids lead to increased knowledge of options and help the patient feel better informed, less decisional conflict and clearer about what factors matters most to them.

Although existing patient decision aids related to wound management is not yet available in the literature, the overall number of patient decision aids is growing rapidly with several available on the Internet (Syrowatka, Krömker, Meguerditchian, & Tamblyn, 2016). Regardless of form, quality varies; some do not cite their evidence sources, others contain biases. Because patient decision aids can have an important influence on the patient's choices, the International Patient Decision Aids Standards Collaboration developed quality criteria for patient decision aids (Elwyn et al., 2006). Chapter 1 provides excellent examples and resources for developing, recognizing and evaluating quality of evidence. Table 1.5 presents established criteria to assess the credibility of information on the Internet.

Family and Caregiver Involvement

In the United States, the Family Caregiver Alliance of the National Center on Care Giving data (Family Caregiver Alliance (FCA), 2015) showed 43.5 million people in the United States have cared for someone who is disabled in the past year. Therefore, to achieve a sustainable plan of care, education and goal setting must include families and caregivers. The wound specialist can help the patient and family identify their goals based on what the patient and family are able and willing to do to achieve them. This can be accomplished only if decisions are based on full disclosure and an understanding of relevant information.

Realistic Goals and Evidence-Based Interventions

The patient and care team together must monitor progress toward the goals of the plan of care to determine whether they are patient centered and realistic, identify actual or potential barriers toward achieving a sustainable plan, and modify the plan accordingly. Ideally, this process should occur while the initial plan of care is being developed so that realistic goals can be set from the onset. Identification and consideration of patient preferences and actions are central to evidence-based decision making. In many situations there may be more than one right choice for treatment. SDM works best when there is more than one option to weigh pros and cons (Atkin et al., 2019; Doherty & Stavropoulou, 2012; McCaughan, Sheard, Cullum, Dumville, & Chetter, 2018). When planned interventions are not completed and goals are not met, the best question is not, "What's wrong with the patient?" Rather, we should be asking, "What's wrong with the plan?" or "Are our goals realistic?"

The goal of wound healing as a standard for all patients is unrealistic for many patients and can lead to a lack of patient engagement and adherence to the care plan (Atkin et al., 2019; McCaugan et al., 2018). For example, a patient who is malnourished and does not care to receive enteral or elemental feedings will not achieve the goal of wound healing. Once the patient understands that wound healing is unrealistic, he or she may decide to reconsider supplemental feedings or may aim for a goal that keeps him or her at home, avoids hospital admission, controls symptoms (e.g., odor, exudate), and enhances quality of life as defined by the patient. In other cases, the treatment may produce added discomfort or risk for the patient. A patient with an overwhelming disease process, after being informed of all treatment options, may decide to decline supplemental nutrition and set a palliation goal of prevention of pain and wound extension rather than wound healing.

Wound-healing potential must be based on the most current evidence and communicated in such a way that the patient and family understand (e.g., a patient with peripheral vascular disease (PVD) with an ankle-brachial index <0.5 requires revascularization for healing to occur; venous insufficiency requires compression for wound healing to occur; pressure ulcer healing is not realistic without offloading, nutrition support, and management of urinary or fecal incontinence). When healing is no longer realistic, the plan of care should be revised to focus on goals that minimize infection and other complications and that support the patient's comfort and his or her need and desire for socialization.

In order to integrate interventions needed for optimal healing, the patient must face multiple adaptations to accommodate the wound and the underlying disease. To understand the range of adaptations facing the patient, the wound specialist must understand the effect of the wound and interventions on the patient's life. Patient beliefs and perceptions must be revealed in order to dispel any myths or misperceptions and identify teaching/learning needs.

Informed Refusal

The wound specialist must acknowledge the patient's right to decline care if the decision is based on full comprehension of the consequences. If the decision does not appear to be in the patient's best interest, refusal should be a red flag for the specialist to review all the factors that may be hindering care and seek to offer other potential options more acceptable to the patient (Keen, Thoele, Fite, & Lancaster, 2019). The current plan of care may seem too overwhelming for the patient to cope with, especially when the actions require long-term life changes. For example, the need for lifelong compression stockings may seem overwhelming or confusing if the information received is incomplete or contradictory from one care provider to another (Brown, 2014). Approaches recommended in the literature and innovation forum conducted by Keen et al. (2019) conclude that nurses need direction and institutional policies to support practice when patients refuse care that may put them in harm's way. Approaches include interdisciplinary standard and structured approach for escalation (i.e., nursing policy or pathway) and staff training to include understanding the reason behind the refusal, assessing patient care goals, engaging patients, family and caregivers in education and problem solving. Fig. 5.2 provides an example of an algorithm for patient refusal of positioning for pressure injury prevention.

PATIENT PERCEPTIONS AND THE HEALTH BELIEF MODEL

The HBM provides an appropriate framework to guide shared goal setting and development of a sustainable plan of care. Developed nearly a half-century ago by Irwin Rosenstock of the US Public Health Service, the HBM was applied to predict behavioral response to treatment of acutely or chronically ill patients. In the decades that followed, the HBM's effectiveness in predicting and explaining health-related actions with multiple medical conditions and patient population has been well documented in meta-analyses (Carpenter, 2010; Jones, Smith, & Llewellyn, 2014) and other scientific studies (Obirikorang, Obirikorang, Acheampong, et al., 2018; Tavafian, Hasani, Aghamolaei, et al., 2009). Core constructs associated with

the likelihood of adapting an intervention are listed in Table 5.1 and described in the following sections.

Perceived Threat (Perceived Severity and Susceptibility)

The combination of perceived severity and perceived susceptibility is referred to as *perceived threat*. Perceived severity and susceptibility depend on knowledge about the condition. The HBM predicts that higher perceived threat leads to higher likelihood of engagement in health-promoting interventions.

Perceived severity encompasses beliefs about the health problem itself, as well as broader effects of the disease on functioning in work and social roles (e.g., whether it is life threatening, life altering, or painful). For example, a patient may perceive that a venous wound is not medically serious. However, learning that venous ulcers lead to an estimated 2 million lost workdays in the United States annually (Morton, Bolton, Corbett, et al., 2013) may help the patient see the wound as serious or severe due to the potential financial consequences.

The HBM predicts that patients who perceive themselves at high risk for a particular health problem such as a wound are more likely to engage in activities that will decrease their risk. Patients with low perceived susceptibility may be in denial, whereas others may acknowledge the possibility but believe it is unlikely to happen to them. This potential range of perceptions underscores the importance of conducting frequent risk assessments together with the patient and family. A discussion with emphasis on each individual risk factor as it applies to the individual patient may help the patient see his or her own vulnerability and need to take action.

Perceived Benefits

Perceived benefits refer to the patient's assessment of the value or effectiveness of various interventions. If the patient believes that a particular action will reduce susceptibility to a health problem or decrease its seriousness, he or she is more likely to embrace the intervention (Obirikorang et al., 2018). For example, studies have shown that patients are significantly more likely to wear compression stockings if they believe the stockings are worthwhile, will decrease edema and prevent wounds (Jull, Mitchell, Arroll, et al., 2004; Van Hecke, Verhaeghe, Grypdonck, et al., 2011).

Perceived Barriers

Even if an individual perceives a wound as threatening and believes that a particular action will prevent or eliminate the wound, barriers may prevent implementation. Perceived benefits must outweigh the perceived barriers in order for a change to occur. Factors associated with poor adherence include lower educational level, poor socioeconomic status, cumbersome regimens, dislike of and perceived inconvenience of treatment, fear of side effects, anger about condition or its required treatment, forgetfulness or complacency (Tavafian et al., 2009; Treadwell, 2018). For instance, lack

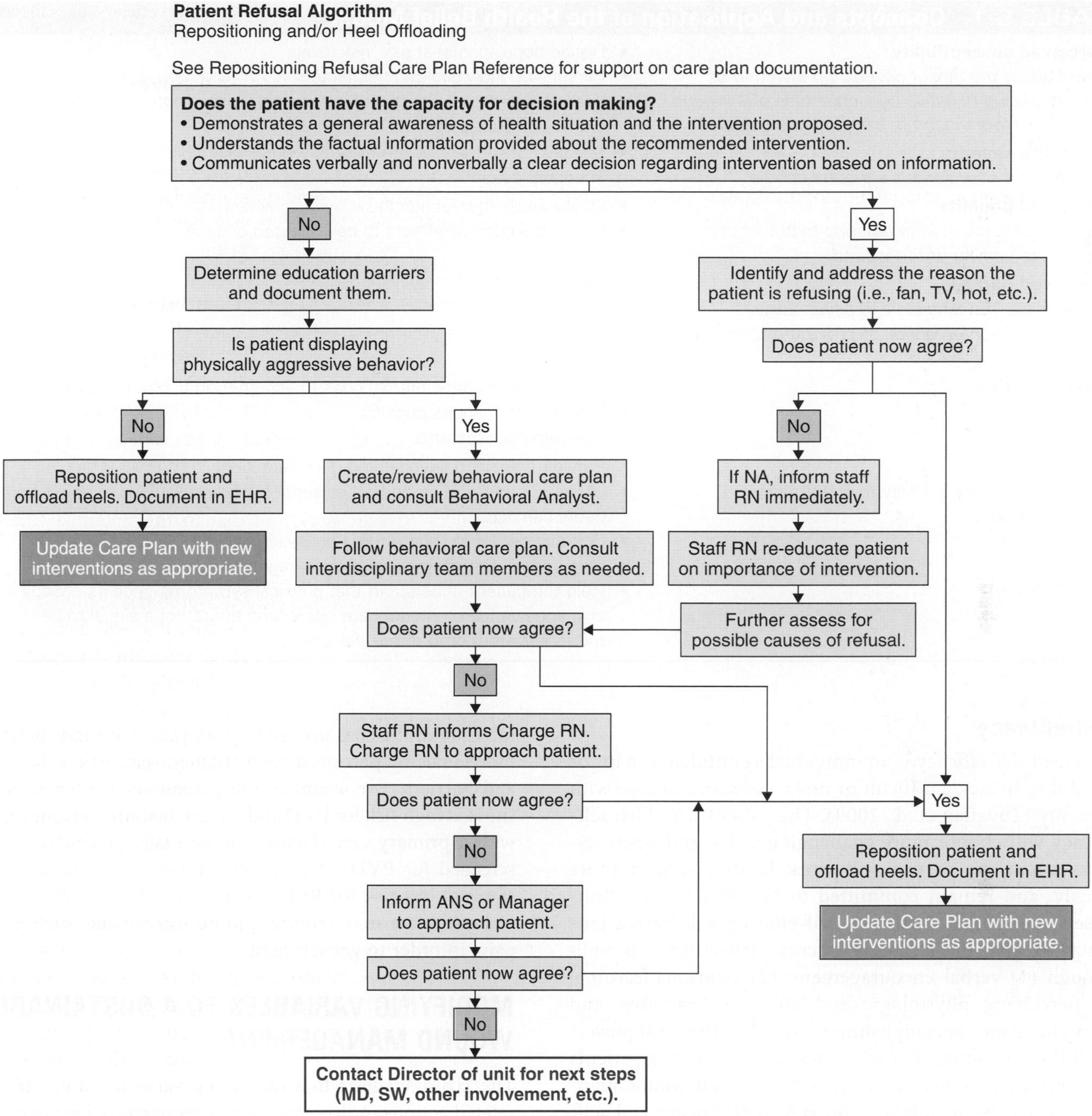

Patient Refusal Algorithm
Repositioning and/or Heel Offloading

See Repositioning Refusal Care Plan Reference for support on care plan documentation.

Does the patient have the capacity for decision making?
- Demonstrates a general awareness of health situation and the intervention proposed.
- Understands the factual information provided about the recommended intervention.
- Communicates verbally and nonverbally a clear decision regarding intervention based on information.

No

Determine education barriers and document them.

Is patient displaying physically aggressive behavior?

No

Reposition patient and offload heels. Document in EHR.

Update Care Plan with new interventions as appropriate.

Yes

Create/review behavioral care plan and consult Behavioral Analyst.

Follow behavioral care plan. Consult interdisciplinary team members as needed.

Does patient now agree?

No

Staff RN informs Charge RN. Charge RN to approach patient.

Does patient now agree?

No

Inform ANS or Manager to approach patient.

Does patient now agree?

No

Contact Director of unit for next steps (MD, SW, other involvement, etc.).

Yes

Identify and address the reason the patient is refusing (i.e., fan, TV, hot, etc.).

Does patient now agree?

No

If NA, inform staff RN immediately.

Staff RN re-educate patient on importance of intervention.

Further assess for possible causes of refusal.

Yes

Reposition patient and offload heels. Document in EHR.

Update Care Plan with new interventions as appropriate.

Fig. 5.2 Patient refusal algorithm. (From M. Health Fairview Bethesda Hospital.)

of transportation to clinic appointments and significant pain with wound debridement may act as barriers to receiving wound management follow-up.

People are less likely to adopt interventions that have unpleasant side effects (Fierheller, Anku, & Alavi, 2009; Gaude, Hattiholi, & Chaudhury, 2014; Wu et al., 2008). If patients are not informed about the side effects of treatment or don't understand the impact these side effects may have on their life, they can develop mistrust and skepticism and choose to discontinue an activity. For example, venous wound prevention and treatment studies have cited cost, appearance, discomfort, and difficulty with application among the reasons for not following recommendations for compression and offloading devices (Armstrong et al., 2005; Fierheller et al., 2009). Some manufacturers and clinicians facilitate sampling and trialing of products and interventions so the patient can learn by experience before making a full commitment to the interventions. Singh, Singh, Rohilla, et al. (2013) used a protocol for patients undergoing pressure injury surgery that involved encouraging prone positioning on a pressure redistribution support surface preoperatively in preparation for the postoperative recovery period.

TABLE 5.1	Concepts and Application of the Health Belief Model
Perceived susceptibility *Belief about the risk of developing a wound or experiencing negative consequences of a wound (e.g., lost work/income, pain, infection, death)*	• Define population(s) at risk, risk levels • Personalize individualized risk factors • Work toward making perceived susceptibility more consistent with individual's *actual* risk
Perceived severity *Belief about how serious a wound can be*	• Specify consequences of having a wound (e.g., lost work/income, pain, infection, death)
Perceived benefits *Belief in efficacy of interventions to prevent or promote healing of the wound*	• Define each intervention (how, where, when) • Clarify the positive effects to be expected of each
Perceived barriers *Belief about the tangible and psychological costs of the intervention to prevent or promote healing of the wound*	• See Table 5.2
Cues to action	• Help patient identify internal cues to act (erythema, edema, pain, etc.) • Provide information/education • Use reminder systems
Self-efficacy *Confidence in one's ability to adapt/perform intervention*	• Provide training, guidance, and demonstration • Utilize support groups and other venues where vicarious learning from peers can occur • Conduct demonstration returns or "teach backs" • Give verbal reinforcement and encouragement • Help the patient understand that physical symptoms such as change in skin appearance or integrity are not failure, but rather a signal to be more persistent or to revise the plan

Self-efficacy

Perceived self-efficacy is an individual's confidence in his or her ability to tackle difficult or novel tasks and to cope with adversity (Tavafian et al., 2009). The patient with high self-efficacy will choose more challenging tasks, and when setbacks occur, he or she will work harder, recover more quickly, and remain committed to his or her goals. Conversely, the patient with low self-efficacy will have a tendency to give up if failure occurs. Self-efficacy is built through (1) verbal encouragement; (2) vicarious learning; (3) perceiving physiologic and affective responses; and (4) performance accomplishment, which is the most powerful of the four sources of self-efficacy. Empowering patients by promoting a sense of ownership over their wound management has been shown to improve self-efficacy and self-esteem (Lindsay, 2000, 2004). Teaching foot self-care in patients with diabetes mellitus increased self-efficacy in identifying early symptoms in foot ulceration (Fan et al., 2014). Education of patients with type 2 regarding how often to observe their feet lead to earlier identification of symptoms putting them at risk for foot ulcer (Takehara et al., 2019). The wound specialist can promote self-efficacy through verbal encouragement (Brown, 2014).

Cues to Action

According to the HBM, patients with high cues to actions are more likely to adhere to their agreed plan of care (Glanz, Rimer, & Viswanath, 2008; Obirikorang et al., 2018). Cues to action can be internal (e.g., pain or wound) or external (e.g., service announcements or educational materials). The intensity of the cues needed to prompt action varies between individuals by perceived susceptibility, seriousness, benefits, and barriers. For example, the patient who believes he or she is at high risk for PVD and has an established relationship with a primary care doctor may be easily persuaded to get screened for PVD, whereas the patient who believes he or she is at low risk for PVD and does not have reliable access to health care may require a more intense cue, such as leg pain, in order to get screened.

MODIFYING VARIABLES TO A SUSTAINABLE WOUND MANAGEMENT

The HBM suggests that modifying variables affect health-related actions indirectly by affecting perceived seriousness, susceptibility, benefits, and barriers (Glanz et al., 2008). Examples of these variables include but are not limited to demographic (e.g., education, culture, economic), psychosocial (e.g., anxiety, depression, social isolation), physical (e.g., cognitive, mobility, dexterity), language skill, and structural (e.g., knowledge, experience). Not surprisingly, a number of these variables overlap with the domains of HRQOL in older adults (EPUAP, NPIAP, PPPIA, 2019). The following sections provide a discussion related to common modifying variables associated with patients with wounds and factors to consider in order to set appropriate goals, prescribe appropriate intervention, and achieve a sustainable plan of care. Possible interventions to prevent or minimize various barriers to a sustainable wound management plan are listed in Table 5.2.

TABLE 5.2 Interventions to Prevent or Minimize Barriers to a Sustainable Wound Management Plan

Barrier	Intervention
Inappropriate goals	Collaborate with patient to help him or her articulate goals; make sure goals are mutual Set goals based on best evidence Ensure goals are clearly written and understood Explain interventions needed to accomplish goals before patient commits to the goal Provide guidance by breaking goals into intermediate steps with a high likelihood of accomplishment to ensure early success Adjust goals as needed for changes in assessment parameters
Depression, pain, anxiety	Be aware that many patients with depression will not ask for help Appropriate pain assessment and management (see Chapter 28) Address aspects of wound management that trigger or exacerbate depression, pain, or anxiety Collaborate with social services and physician for appropriate referrals
Cognitive impairment, complicated regimens, impaired dexterity	Simplify procedures Divide procedures into easier intermediate steps Choose dressings that require fewer changes Choose products that are easy to use Use combination products to minimize steps Encourage use of memory aids and assistive devices when indicated Clearly label supplies Dispense appropriate number of supplies Collaborate with occupational therapy
Impaired activity and mobility	Prescribe compression that is compatible with appropriate shoe wear Prescribe offloading devices compatible with wheelchair and home environment Adapt clinical environment to accommodate patients with mobility impairment (low examination tables, closer parking) Be aware of wound management recommendations that may hinder mobility Prescribe sitting program compatible with employment and parenting needs Facilitate home care when appropriate
Financial barriers, lack of social/environmental resources	Collaborate with social services Identify payer and reimbursement sources Learn prices of products and less expensive alternatives Learn about resources and available funds available to patients with low income Financial guidance for prioritizing
Skepticism	Address concerns immediately Be honest about risk vs benefits of recommended interventions Respect and incorporate life experiences Do not minimize concerns Recommend a second opinion Provide alternative interventions (and goals as needed)
Knowledge deficit	Develop education plan that matches developmental phase, cognitive and physical abilities, and educational and cultural background (see Boxes 5.2 and 5.5) Use multiple methods of educational methods and tools (see Table 5.3)

Culture and Language

Globalization continues to expand while more people move around the world for work, educational opportunities, and escape from wars and civil conflicts. Culture refers to patterns of behavior of racial, ethnic, religious, or social groups. The National Quality Forum (NQF) says cultural competence is the ability to meet the needs of diverse patient populations so that delivered health care is safe and equitable. Culturally competent care according to the NQF (2009) tries to eliminate misunderstandings and improve patient adherence with treatments. However, evidence is clear that minorities receive a lower quality of care and suffer disproportionately from higher rates of disease and death even when factors such as access, health insurance, and income are taken into account (Anderson, Scrimshaw, Fullilove, et al., 2003; NQF, 2009).

Improving cultural competence is essential for closing the disparity gap in health care because culture and language can affect someone's beliefs about health, disease, and the behaviors that lead to both. Being respectful of—and responsive to—individuals' cultural needs ensures more effective communication so that a patient's needs can be better met (The Joint Commission (TJC), 2010).

In TJC's roadmap to advancing effective communication, cultural competence, and patient- and family-centered care (TJC, 2010), cultural competence is defined as the ability of the health care provider and health care organizations to understand and respond effectively to the cultural and language needs brought by the patient to the health care encounter. The roadmap further states that cultural competence requires organizations and their personnel to value diversity, assess themselves, manage the dynamics of difference, acquire and institutionalize cultural knowledge, and adapt to diversity and the cultural contexts of individuals and the communities served.

From the first encounter, the wound specialist must openly address the patient's individual cultural factors without stereotyping. Cultural competence is rooted in respect, validation, and openness toward someone with different social and cultural perceptions and expectations than one's own. Ensuring clear communication may require a language interpreter. Because people tend to have an "ethnocentric" view in which they see their own culture as the best, the wound specialist must be aware of his or her own cultural belief system so as not to inflict it on the patient (Jeffs, 2001). Checklist 5.1 provides examples of action steps to improve cultural competence. The best way to understand a patient's cultural needs is to simply ask, "Are there any cultural, religious, or spiritual beliefs that might influence your care?"

Use of animal-derived products in wound care (e.g., cellular or tissue based wound products (CTPs), and collagen) may interfere with the patients ability to follow a plan of care if it conflicts with their religious or ethical beliefs (Erickson, Burcharth, & Rosenberg, 2013).

Language

Language barriers are associated with longer hospital stays, and higher rates of hospital readmissions, more infections, falls, surgery delays, and pressure injuries. Approximately 25 million, 8.6 & percnt; of the US population, have limited English proficiency leaving at least 8.6% of the US population is at risk for adverse events because of barriers associated with their language ability (Betancourt, Renfrew, Green, Lopez, & Wasserman, 2012).

Access to language assistance for patients is important to the delivery of high-quality care for all populations with limited English proficiency. US law requires that healthcare organizations provide interpreter services to patients with limited English proficiency with regulations restricting use of family members and validating language skills of healthcare workers (Diamond, Wilson-Stronks, & Jacobs, 2010; Health and Human Services (HHS) Department, 2016). Ideally, every effort should be made to engage the services of a professional medical interpreter using local guidelines and greater time allowances. Professional medical interpreters are always preferable as they provide a degree of assurance around quality, accuracy, and confidentiality. That a family members and other health care worker may lack. Interpreters should be neutral and passive, which may prove difficult for family members. For example, a family member may find it hard to share difficult news or may have emotional or cultural reasons to distort your message. Family members can also be selective with translations based on their own views of the patient's condition or treatment options. There is also the possibility that the untrained translator (friend, family member, or health care worker) will not understand the language well enough to communicate complex medical information (Rimmer, 2020). Digital technologies, such as multilingual (mobile) translation apps have gained popularity especially when interpreters are not available or when time constraints do not warrant the booking of professional interpreters. Although early studies on digital translation tools report high levels of user satisfaction, there have been concerns about risks related to reduced accuracy, patient privacy, and data protection (Krystallidou, Langewitz, & van den Muijsenbergh, 2020). Regardless of method, failing to recognize how interpreters can alter the dynamic of a conversation can decrease the quality of care. Box 5.2 provides tips for working effectively with an interpreter.

Health Literacy

Full disclosure and understanding of relevant information are critical to goal setting and the decision-making process yet lack of knowledge is one of the most common barriers associated with a failed plan of care (Gaude, et al., 2014). The relationship health literacy skills and adult health outcomes is well documented. Lower health literacy has been linked to higher health care costs, misunderstanding of medical condition, delayed diagnoses, lack of adherence to treatment as well as impaired self-management skills (Meherali, Punjani, & Mevawala, 2020).

Patient-specific teaching that is structured and culturally appropriate are found to be better than ad hoc teaching or generalized teaching (Friedman, Cosby, Boyko, et al., 2011). Researchers also have found that health information that is

---

CHECKLIST 5.1   Examples of Action Steps to Improve Cultural Competence

✓ Identify what language the patient and health care decision maker prefer to discuss health care.

✓ Provide education materials that are in the patient's preferred language and have translators available.

✓ Ask the patient if there are any cultural, religious, or spiritual beliefs that might influence his or her care.

✓ Identify if the patient has cultural-based modesty issues about care provided by staff of the opposite sex.

✓ Determine whether there are certain garments or items that need to be worn.

✓ Identify any special dietary needs. Provide options that are acceptable to the patient.

✓ Collaborate with patients and families to develop solutions to requests that can't be met.

BOX 5.2   Tips for Working Effectively With an In-Person Medical Interpreter

1. Intrduce yourself and provide a brief report on the history and work needed
2. Let the patient know they can ask the interpreter anything (even if it isn't the main reason for the interpretation)[a]
3. Communicate directly with the patient. Resist the temptation to talk to or look at the interpreter (unless you need clarification of something the interpreter said)
4. Speak in shorter sentences than normal to make it easier for the interpreter to remember and improves the translation's accuracy[a]
5. If the interpreter appears confused, ask if clarification or rephrasing is needed[a]
6. Try not to interrupt the interpreter while translating the patient's reply. (Guessing what the patient is about to say may not be right, and some cultures perceive interruptions as rude behavior)[a]

7. If the interpreter seems to be taking a long time to translate for the patient, it may mean that they are trying to phrase the sentence in a way that will be best received.
8. Make sure that the interpreter interprets patients' responses completely. (Don't accept a "yes" or "no" when the patient gave a lot of information, even if you're in a hurry).
9. When the encounter finishes, ask the patient if they need anything else while the interpreter is there. (Many patients have more needs, and often the interpreter encounter makes them feel comfort able enough to express them)[a]
10. After leaving the room with the interpreter, review the encounter to ensure that both you and the interpreter ended up on the same page. The interpreter may also have some cultural insights to share that can help with care planning.

Adapted from Squires, A. (2018). Strategies for overcoming language barriers in healthcare. *Nursing Management, 49*(4), 20–27. doi:10.1097/01. NUMA.0000531166.24481.15
[a] These steps also apply to telephone or video interpretation.

CHECKLIST 5.2   Educational Assessment

✓ Age and developmental phase
✓ Cognitive abilities
✓ Physical abilities (activity, mobility, dexterity)
✓ Educational background
✓ Life experiences that may influence learning
✓ Cultural and religious practices
✓ Language skills
✓ Occupation
✓ Finances and financial implications of care choices
✓ Type of health care coverage and discharge plan
✓ Support from family and friends
✓ Pain, anxiety, and depression
✓ Learning needs and readiness to learn

BOX 5.3   Principles of Adult Learning

1. Adults want to know why they should learn.
   - Adults are motivated to put time and energy into learning if they know the benefits of learning and the costs of not learning.
2. Adults need to take responsibility.
   - Adult learners perceive themselves as being in charge of their lives and decisions and need to be seen as capable.
3. Adults bring experience to learning.
   - Adults define themselves by their experiences and need to have their experiences valued and respected. Experiences can give deeper meaning to new ideas and skills or may lead to bias.
4. Adults are ready to learn when the need arises.
   - Adults learn when they choose to learn, usually when they perceive a need to learn.
5. Adults are task oriented.
   - Education often is subject centered, and adults need education that is task centered.

Data from Knowles, M. S., Holton, E. F., III, & Swanson, R. A. (1998). *The adult learner.* Houston, TX: Gulf Publishing.

---

focused on individual needs not only increased patients' understanding of their health needs and improved their health literacy but supported self-management and promoted health outcomes (Yen & Leasure, 2019). Checklist 5.2 lists components for patient education assessment.

Cognitive impairment may be an obvious barrier toward achieving a sustainable treatment plan; however, the presence of cognitive impairment can be subtle. It is important to review past medical records and speak with family members so that cognitive deficits can be identified, and the plan of care adjusted accordingly. In many settings, occupational therapy and speech therapy can assist in identifying cognitive deficits and can assist the wound specialist in developing a plan of care that incorporates the unique learning needs of the patient. Patients tend to remember the first thing they are told. Key factors to enhance learning and retention are to use straightforward language and simple sentences. It is also important to explain why the treatment is needed, simplify the steps in the procedure, use repetition, and ask the patient to repeat back the instructions (Price, 2008).

Age-appropriate education must take into account principles of adult leaning and stages of development. Knowles principles of adult learning (Box 5.3) were introduced in the 1990 and remain widely cited today in health-related evidence-based practice (Knowles, Holton III, & Swanson, 1998; Thompson, Leach, Smith, Fereday, & May, 2020). Features of development that affect coping and learning strategies for children are described in Chapter 36.

Simplifying education and interventions are known to improve education and sustaining a successful plan of care. When large amounts of information are presented at once, less is recalled, and almost half of the recalled information is incorrect (Yen & Leasure, 2019). Complicated regimens present considerable room for error and confusion and threaten patient adherence especially in the presence of impaired cognition, mobility, or dexterity. Simple procedures and combination products may increase the likelihood of a desired action to take place (Gaude et al., 2014; Turabian, 2019; Warshaw, Nix, Kula, et al., 2002). Breaking down knowledge and steps into smaller segments and having the patient repeat back the steps will lessen the larger task (Price, 2008). Using products that combine interventions and performing procedures with routines already established (e.g., after meals) may increase the likelihood of success.

Printed materials are an economical use of time if they are well designed and match the learner's reading and literacy levels. Educational methods must be sensitive to the culture of patients who will be using them, addressing their lifestyles and using cultural language and symbols they understand (Redman, 2007). Lower educational level is associated with poor adherence (Gaude et al., 2014). Approximately half of the population in the United States struggles with basic reading skills. For many persons, the materials available are written at a higher level than they can understand—sometimes as many as five grades higher than the school level the patient has completed (Redman, 2007). Techniques that improve readership, comprehension, and memory of printed materials are summarized in Table 5.3 (Buxton, 1999).

Patients can quickly access information on the Internet; however, as mentioned previously, information on the Internet may be inaccurate or incomplete (EPUAP, NPIAP, PPPIA, 2019) and should be reviewed for credibility (Table 1.5). Online communities of patients with the same medical condition have emerged and are increasingly being used by consumers as trusted sources of information (Nielson Global Online Consumer Survey, 2009). However, some Internet sources, if followed, can sabotage the plan of care. Websites and e-learnings designed by health professionals and maintained by government and health consumer groups are more likely to contain reputable information (Brace & Schubart, 2010; EPUAP, NPIAP, PPPIA, 2019; Schubart, 2012). The wound specialist should respectfully discuss this information with the patient. Becoming defensive or dismissing the patient's concerns will leave the patient feeling alienated. Such interactions can damage trust and lead to nonadherence (Iihara et al., 2014). The patient should have his or her concerns addressed and should be encouraged to obtain a second opinion.

Research suggests that *combining educational methods* increases knowledge, reduce decisional conflict, and increases patient engagement (Friedman et al., 2011; Kim & Cho, 2017; Mattison & Nemec, 2014; Stacey et al., 2017). A systematic review conducted by Friedman et al. (2011) examined teaching strategies and methods of delivery for patient education. Strategies identified included traditional lectures, discussions, simulated games, computer technology, written material, audiovisual sources, verbal recall, demonstration, and role playing. Five teaching strategies (computer technology, audio and videotapes, written materials, demonstrations, and combination) showed an increase in knowledge and patient

TABLE 5.3 Techniques to Improve Health Education Materials

Do	Don't
Direct Readers to the Message	
• Use arrows, underlines, bold type, boxes, white space, and bullets to direct readers' eyes to the key messages.	• Use italics, all capital letters, or screens of color over text. • Require reader to look in many directions on the page to read copy and find the message.
Select an Easy-to-Read Typeface	
• Use 10- to 14-point type size. • Use a typeface with serifs in the body copy (e.g., Times Roman).	• Go below 10-point type size for good readers and 12-point for poor readers. • Mix typefaces or use more than three sizes of print on one page. • Use white letters on black background.
Create Easy-to-Read Copy	
• Use columns that are 40–50 characters wide, left justified. • Use lots of white space. Consider question-and-answer or bullets rather than paragraphs. • Use highly contrasting colors for text and background, such as black on white or cream. • Use the same dark color for headings and body copy or colors with similar intensity.	• Break margins with illustrations or other graphics. If required, break only the right margin. • Use light or unusual ink colors, such as red, green, or orange.
Create Clear Visuals	
• Convey one key message per visual. Print the message in a caption. • Make the message easy to grasp at a glance. • Show only the "desired" way to act. • Use realistic drawings, photos, or humanlike figures. • Use visuals with which the audience can identify.	• Add any visuals simply to decorate the material. • Include any details or background in the visual that are not required to communicate the message. • Use highly stylized or abstract graphics. • Portray blood cells and other body parts as cartoon characters.

Adapted from Buxton, T. (1999). Effective ways to improve health education materials, *Journal of Health Education, 30*(1), 47–50. From Redman, B.K. (2007). *The practice of patient education* (10th ed.), St. Louis, MO: Mosby.

satisfaction as well as a decrease in anxiety when compared with the other techniques.

Ample time for patient teaching has always been a challenge. With shorter hospital stays, the wound specialist must take even more care to develop a variety of strategies to ensure the patient's educational needs are identified and that progress toward meeting these needs is communicated to providers in the next care setting. In acute care, the education plan begins at admission and must be incorporated into routine care during frequent daily encounters. For example, skin inspection can be taught during the patient's bath. Protection of skin surrounding wounds and moist wound healing can be discussed during dressing changes. Each time a patient is repositioned, pressure injury prevention strategies can be taught and reinforced. Information may need to be limited to the skills and actions necessary for the patient to learn before discharge. Box 5.4 summarizes The Joint Commission International (2017) standards for patient education in hospitals.

Reinforcing or Confirming Patient Learning

Studies have shown that a majority of patients remain confused about their health care plans after being discharged from the hospital. A substantial proportion of medical information is forgotten immediately after discharge. Further, many patients do not recognize their lack of comprehension (Yen & Leasure, 2019). Findings of a systematic review support use of the teach-back method as effective in reinforcing or confirming patient education (Yen & Leasure, 2019). In the teach-back method, patients are asked to explain health information in their own words to ensure the health care provider explained the information clearly. Effective use of the teach-back method includes (Institute for Healthcare Advancement (IHA), 2020):
1. Use of appropriate materials to support learning.
2. Use of a caring tone of voice and attitude.

> ### BOX 5.4 The Joint Commission Statements for Patient and Family Education Standards
>
> - The hospital provides education that supports patient and family participation in care decisions and care processes.
> - Each patient's educational needs are assessed and recorded in his or her medical record.
> - The patient's and family's ability to learn and willingness to learn are assessed.
> - Education methods take into account the patient's and family's values and preferences and allow sufficient interaction among the patient, family, and staff for learning to occur.
> - Health care practitioners caring for the patient collaborate to provide education.
> - Patient education and follow-up instructions are given in a form and language the patient can understand.
>
> From Joint Commission International. (2017). *Accreditation standards for hospitals including standards for Academic Medical Center Hospitals.* Retrieved 12/16/2020 from: https://www.jointcommissioninternational.org/-/media/jci/jci-documents/accreditation/hospital-and-amc/jci-standards-only_6th-ed-hospital.pdf.

3. Use of open-ended questions.
4. Emphasizing that the responsibility to explain clearly is the wound specialists.
5. Explain again and recheck as needed.

Psychological Conditions

The National Institute of Mental Health estimates that tens of millions of people each year experience mental illness, and estimates suggest that only half of people with mental illnesses receive treatment. The prevalence of major depressive episode among US adults aged 18 or older in 2017 estimated 17.3 million adults in the United States had at least one major depressive episode. This number represented 7.1% of all US adults (National Institute of Mental Health (NIMH), 2018).

At least 30% of all patients in chronic wound populations suffer from *depression and/or anxiety*. This is three times more than the rate of depression diagnosed in persons without wound-healing problems in normal population (Renner, Seikowski, & Simon, 2014). Zhou and Jia (2016) described a positive correlation between depressive symptoms and wound duration >90.

Psychological conditions negatively influence patient engagement in wound management even with regular telephone and coach support (Guihan et al., 2014; Herber, Schnepp, & Rieger, 2007). Patients suffering from depression or anxiety may not ask for help, have difficulty performing activities of daily living, and may be unable to follow through with agreed-upon interventions. Anxiety and depression affect the ability to objectively assess one's own actions. The patient with anxiety and depression may interpret his or her successes negatively, underestimate his or her achievements, or simply ignore them completely.

Wound pain has been cited as an independent risk factor for the development of depression (Faria, Blanes, Hochman, Mesquita Filho, & Ferreira, 2011; Wachholz, Masuda, Nascimento, Taira, & Cleto, 2014; Zhou & Jia, 2016). It has been reported that over 70% of patients experience pain associated with their wounds. Ineffective pain management can result in delayed healing, decreased patient engagement, and an inability to follow recommended interventions (Frescos, 2011; Gaude et al., 2014; Ledger et al., 2020; McInnes, Chaboyer, Murray, Allen, & Jones, 2014). The wound specialist can help decrease pain in many ways such as with the use of nonadherent dressings to promote nontraumatic dressing removal or decrease the frequency of dressing changes by using more absorptive dressings. Adjust the wound dressing protocol and the frequency of dressing change in order to diminish pain factors. Offering pain medication before the dressing change addresses both the pain directly and the patient's apprehension about the dressing change. Chapter 28 provides detailed information related to the assessment and management of wound pain.

Whether a patient experiences depression before developing a wound or becomes depressed because of the profound challenges the wound presents (e.g., pain, embarrassing odor and exudate, interference with activities of daily living), the wound specialist is in a unique position to impact wound challenges expressed by patients with depression with use of dressings that decrease odor and exudate, provide a waterproof barrier to facilitate bathing, and increase independence and by using dressings with a longer wear time to allow for home care nurses rather than the need for long-term care for dressing changes. Beyond symptom management and wound healing, one of the most important interventions of the wound specialist, may be to ask for a psychological evaluation and recommendations further address the patient's suffering.

Physical Ability

The wound specialist must have the expertise and resources available to design a plan of care that accommodates the individual with impaired dexterity. For example, many combination dressings and products eliminate the need for cutting tape. The need for long-term use of lower extremity compression stockings requires the patient's ability to apply them. Assisting them or acquiring assistive devices will facilitate routine usage (Brown, 2014). For example, donning household rubber gloves can aid in pulling up compression stockings. Practice and return demonstrations are critical for the patient with impaired dexterity. Impaired dexterity can significantly affect procedure time; selecting dressings that require fewer changes may be more realistic and sustainable.

Impaired activity and mobility affect the patient's ability to accomplish many important activities needed for disease management and wound healing. Unfortunately, these challenges are not always understood by the health care system and lead to inaccurate assumptions about nonadherence (Box 5.5). The extent to which impaired activity and mobility affect a patient's life must be explored thoroughly before realistic goals and interventions can be put in place. For example, the wound specialist must be aware of the many interventions (e.g., sitting restrictions) and devices (e.g., bulky compression and high-profile support surfaces) that actually can create an activity or mobility deficit for the patient. Patients have reported losing their jobs or retiring early because of immobility secondary to a wound or treatment for a wound (Ashford, McGee, & Kinmond, 2000; Herber et al., 2007). Mobility issues can be addressed as a wound team, enlisting physical and occupational therapies early in the plan of care to ensure comprehensive assessment and problem solving for mobility issues. It is unreasonable to expect a patient who is homebound and wheelchair dependent to "comply" with the use of a new support surface if transfer methods from bed to chair and chair to bed were not observed and discussed before selection of the new product.

Finances and Available Resources

Lower economic status is associated with poor adherence (Gaude et al., 2014). According to a 30-year review of the literature (Eaddy, Cook, O'Day, Burch, & Cantrell, 2012), strategies designed to control the increasing cost of healthcare delivery range from trying to prevent overutilization with higher out-of-pocket expenses, copayments, and more restrictive formularies listings are associated with declines in treatment adherence and poorer outcomes. The financial impact of a wound on a patient and family ranges from lack of productivity to early retirement and job loss. For persons who are elderly, are chronically ill, or are in a low-income bracket, as much as 31% of their total income may be spent on health care.

Treatment decisions should be made, bearing in mind what is financially reasonable for the patient, as well as the less expensive alternatives. It is important to be aware of the payer source and the patient's out-of-pocket expenses for noncovered items, transportation, and loss of pay due to time missed from work. Cost is incurred from both the treatment and nontreatment of wounds—the cost of not implementing evidence-based management of wounds is likely to increase from associated complications such as infection, increased hospital admissions, higher expenditure on pharmaceuticals (analgesia, antibiotics), and surgical procedures.

The wound specialist needs to understand the logistics of obtaining equipment and other resources to ensure proper patient care. This is especially important between care settings so that the patient is discharged only after the appropriate equipment and supplies are ready at the next care setting. Resources may not be available due to a lack of funds or support from friends and family for of a variety of reasons (e.g., distance or family dynamics). Although finances are a powerful risk factor, they can be a powerful motivator as well. For example, a family member or patient who is not ready to learn how to do a dressing change may become motivated when he or she learns there will be out-of-pocket expense for another care setting or home care.

BOX 5.5 Activity/Mobility Issues That Contribute to Inaccurate Assumptions About Nonadherence

Transportation to Clinic
- Missed clinic appointments are due to unreliable transportation
- Transfer method to vehicle causes friction and shear
- Amount of time sitting in vehicle is not compatible with sitting restrictions
- Parking at the clinic is too expensive, does not accommodate vehicle, or is located too far away for patient to get to appointment on time or at all

Mobility
- Mobility deficits limit patient's ability to shop and prepare meals to meet nutrition plan

- Wound care devices prescribed for patient are too difficult to apply and remove
- Compression prescribed for patient prohibits patient from wearing an appropriate shoe for safe ambulation or exercise
- Sitting limitations threaten patient's ability to maintain employment or parental rights
- Offloading boots and cushions prescribed for patient do not fit properly in patient's wheelchair

Transfer Method
- Profile of prescribed chair cushion is not compatible with home furniture and makes transfers too difficult or unsafe
- Resources are unavailable for Hoyer lift transfers, and sliding board transfers cause friction or shear

CLINICAL CONSULT

A: Referral for management of pressure injury on coccyx of 76-year-old Caucasian gentleman discovered post op day 3. Nurses state the patient keeps refusing to turn on his side. Noted pressure redistribution visco elastic foam mattress with heels slightly floating off bed with use of pillows under the legs. Patient has head of bed at 45 degrees and is watching TV. Indwelling catheter, no reports of fecal incontinence. Discussed reason for repositioning refusal. He states it hurts too much to move, does not believe it makes sense to lie on his hip, and can't see the TV if he lies on his side. Wound 3 × 3 cm without measurable depth. Tissue smooth and pink. Periwound skin intact. No local signs of infection.

D: Stage 2 pressure injury due to pressure from immobility combined with shear from head of bed elevated above 30 degrees allowing tissue and bone to move in opposite directions.

P: Evaluate if patient is making an informed refusal to repositioning. Educate/reeducate regarding the importance of premedication to control pain, techniques for appropriate positioning for pressure injury prevention.

I: (1) Dispel the myth patient must "lie on his hip," 30-degree tilt is sufficient for offloading the coccyx. (2) Discuss the relationship between shear injury and HOB elevation and evaluate if patient can tolerate HOB at 30 degrees or less. (3) Premedicate as needed for effective repositioning. (4) Limit supine positioning as much as possible, position bed so patient can see the TV while he is positioned toward his side. (5) Keep HOB at 30 degrees or less. (6) Continue floating heels while in bed. (7) Provide moist wound healing with hydrocolloid dressing changes 2×/week. (8) Reconsult wound specialist for higher specification support surface if patient is unable to limit supine position or keep HOB at 30 degrees or less.

E: Nurse, patient, and wife understand and agree to plan of care. Will follow up in 1 week to evaluate/monitor effectiveness and adapt plan as needed. Call sooner for questions, concerns, or signs of deterioration.

SUMMARY

- The wound management team must be guided by an underlying philosophy that care providers work in partnership with the patient to develop a sustainable plan of care based upon mutually agreed-upon goals.
- Identifying and addressing realistic goals toward achieving a sustainable plan may improve the ability to achieve care plan goals, decrease recurrence rates, and, if appropriate, maximize the potential for wound healing.

- The wound specialist is in a pivotal position to avoid mislabeling patients as noncompliant. At a very minimum, a complete assessment using the HBM and documentation of interventions addressing the barriers toward achieving a sustainable plan should be completed before such a conclusion can be reached.

SELF-ASSESSMENT QUESTIONS

1. Which strategies are most effective in preventing nonadherence?
   a. Those that include cognitive, behavioral, and affective components
   b. Interactive learning with web, app, and computer-based activities
   c. Patient Education books and Brochures at a 5th Grade reading level
   d. Multiple demonstration returns
2. How does the "Health Belief Model" (HBM) help the patient adhere to the plan of care for wound management?
   a. By emphasizing the wound specialist's philosophy for wound healing
   b. By focusing on patient understanding and facilitating shared goal setting

   c. By facilitating better technology for patient education
   d. By promoting a team approach to wound management
3. The wound specialist discovers a patient with a venous ulcer is not wearing their compression garment. How should the wound specialist intervene?
   a. Emphasize the critical role compression plays in venous ulcer healing
   b. Put the patient into a different type of compression
   c. Collaborate with the patient to identify barriers to use of the compression garment
   d. Document the Z code in the patient's medical record

REFERENCES

Aliasgharpour, M., & Nayeri, N. D. (2012). The care process of diabetic foot ulcer patients: A qualitative study in Iran. *Journal of Diabetes and Metabolic Disorders, 11*(1), 27.

Al Shammeri, O., AlHamdan, N., Al-Hothaly, B., Midhet, F., Hussain, M., & Al-Mohaimeed, A. (2014). Chronic venous insufficiency: Prevalence and effect of compression stockings. *International Journal of Health Sciences, 8*(3), 231–236.

Anderson, L. M., Scrimshaw, S. C., Fullilove, M. T., et al. (2003). Culturally competent healthcare systems: A systematic review. *American Journal of Preventive Medicine, 24*(Suppl. 3), 68–79.

Armstrong, D. G., Lavery, L. A., Wu, S., et al. (2005). Evaluation of removable and irremovable cast walkers in the healing of diabetic foot wounds: A randomized controlled trial. *Diabetes Care, 28*(3), 551–554.

Ashford, R. L., McGee, P., & Kinmond, K. (2000). Perception of quality of life by patients with diabetic foot ulcers. *Diabetic Foot, 3*, 150–155.

Atkin, L., Bućko, Z., Conde Montero, E., Cutting, K., Moffatt, C., Probst, A., et al. (2019). Implementing TIMERS: The race against hard-to-heal wounds. *Journal of Wound Care, 28*(3 Suppl. 3), S1–S49.

Betancourt, J. R., Renfrew, M. R., Green, A. R., Lopez, L., & Wasserman, M. (2012). *Improving patient safety systems for patients with limited English proficiency: A guide for hospitals*. Rockville, MD: Agency for Healthcare Research and Quality.

Brace, J. A., & Schubart, J. R. (2010). A prospective evaluation of a pressure ulcer prevention and management e-learning program for adults with spinal cord injury. *Ostomy/Wound Management, 56*(8), 40–50.

Brown, A. (2014). Evaluating the reasons underlying treatment nonadherence in VLU patients: Introducing the VeLUSET part 1 of 2. *Journal of Wound Care, 23*(1), 37. 40, 42–44.

Buxton, T. (1999). Effective ways to improve health education materials. *Journal of Health Education, 30*(1), 47.

Carman, K. L., Dardess, P., Maurer, M., Sofaer, S., Adams, K., Bechtel, C., et al. (2013). Patient and family engagement: A framework for understanding the elements and developing interventions and policies. *Health Affairs, 32*(2), 223–231.

Carpenter, C. J. (2010). A meta-analysis of the effectiveness of health belief model variables in predicting behavior. *Health Communication, 25*(8), 661–669.

Centers for Disease Control and Prevention (CDC). (2000). *Measuring healthy days: Population assessment of health-related quality of life*. Atlanta, GA: Centers for Disease Control and Prevention.

Centers for Disease Control and Prevention (CDC). (2017). *National diabetes statistics report, 2017*. Available at: https://dev.diabetes.org/sites/default/files/2019-06/cdc-statistics-report-2017.pdf. Accessed 12/6/2020.

Chatterjee, J. S. (2006). From compliance to concordance in diabetes. *Journal of Medical Ethics, 32*, 507–510.

Chisholm-Burns, M. A., & Spivey, C. A. (2012). The 'cost' of medication nonadherence: Consequences we cannot afford to accept. *Journal of the American Pharmaceutical Association, 52*(6), 823–826.

Dahm, K. T., Myrhaug, H. T., Stromme, H., Fure, B., & Bruberg, K. G. (2019). Effects of preventive use of compression stockings for elderly with chronic venous insufficiency and swollen legs: A systematic review and meta-analysis. *BMC Geriatrics, 19*(76). https://doi.org/10.1186/x12877019-1087-1.

de Silva, D. (2013). *Involving patients in improving safety*. London: The Health Foundation.

Diamond, L. C., Wilson-Stronks, A., & Jacobs, E. A. (2010). Do hospitals measure up to the national culturally and linguistically appropriate services standards. *Medical Care, 48*(12), 1080–1087.

Doggrell, S. A., & Chan, V. (2015). Adherence to insulin treatment in diabetes: Can it be improved? *Journal of Diabetes, 7*(3), 315–321. https://doi.org/10.1111/1753-0407.12212. Epub 2014 Nov 10 25195971.

Doherty, C., & Stavropoulou, C. (2012). Patients' willingness and ability to participate actively in the reduction of clinical errors: A systematic literature review. *Social Science & Medicine, 75*(2), 257–263.

Domecq, J. P., Prutsky, G., Elraiyah, T., Wang, Z., Nabhan, M., Shippee, N., et al. (2014). Patient engagement in research: A systematic review. *BMC Health Services Research, 14*, 89.

Dubský, M., Jirkovská, A., Bem, R., et al. (2013). Risk factors for recurrence of diabetic foot ulcers: Prospective follow up analysis in the Eurodiale subgroup. *International Wound Journal, 10*(5), 555–561.

Eaddy, M. T., Cook, C. L., O'Day, K., Burch, S. P., & Cantrell, C. R. (2012). How patient cost-sharing trends affect adherence and outcomes: A literature review. *Pharmacy and Therapeutics, 37*(1), 45–55. 22346336. PMCID: PMC3278192.

Elwyn, G., Col, N., et al. (2012). Shared decision making a model for clinical practice. *Journal of General Internal Medicine, 27*(10).

Elwyn, G., O'Connor, A., Stacey, D., Volk, R., Edwards, A., Coulter, A., et al. (2006). Developing a quality criteria framework for patient decision aids: Online international Delphi consensus process. *British Medical Journal (Clinical Research Ed.), 333*(7565), 417. https://doi.org/10.1136/bmj.38926.629329.AE.

Eriksson, A., Burcharth, J., & Rosenberg, J. (2013). Animal derived products may conflict with religious patients' beliefs. *BMC Medical Ethics, 14*, 48. https://doi.org/10.1186/1472-6939-14-48.

European Patient's Forum. (2017). *Toolkit for patient organizations on patient empowerment*. Retrieved 12/28/2020 from: https://www.eu-patient.eu/globalassets/library/publications/patient-empowerment- - -toolkit.pdf.

European Pressure Ulcer Advisory Panel, National Pressure Injury Advisory Panel, Pan Pacific Pressure Injury Alliance (EPUAP, NPIAP, PPPIA). (2019). In E. Haesler (Ed.), *Prevention and treatment of pressure ulcers/injuries*. Osborne Park, Western Australia: Cambridge Media.

Family Caregiver Alliance (FCA). (2015). *Women and caregiving: Facts and figures. Who are the caregivers?*. Retrieved 12/18/2020 from: https://www.caregiver.org/caregiver-statistics-demographics.

Fan, L., et al. (2014). Improving foot care knowledge, self-efficacy with behaviors in patients with type 2 diabetes at low risk for foot ulceration: A pilot study. *Clinical Nursing Research, 23*(6), 627–643.

Faria, E., Blanes, L., Hochman, B., Mesquita Filho, M., & Ferreira, L. (2011). Health-related quality of life, self-esteem, and functional status of patients with leg ulcers. *Wounds, 23*(1), 4–10.

Fierheller, M., Anku, C., & Alavi, A. (2009). Encouraging patient adherence to therapeutic graduated compression therapy in venous stasis disease: A limited literature review. *Wound Care Canada, 7*(1), 10–16.

Frescos, N. (2011). What causes wound pain? *Journal of Foot and Ankle Research, 4*(Suppl. 1), P22.

Friedman, A. J., Cosby, R., Boyko, S., et al. (2011). Effective teaching strategies and methods of delivery for patient education: A systematic review and practice guideline recommendations. *Journal of Cancer Education, 26*(1), 12–21.

Gaude, G. S., Hattiholi, J., & Chaudhury, A. (2014). Role of health education and self-action plan in improving the drug compliance in bronchial asthma. *Journal of Family Medicine and Primary Care, 3*, 33–38.

Glanz, K., Rimer, B. K., & Viswanath, K. (2008). *Health behavior and health education: Theory, research, and practice* (4th ed., pp. 46–49). San Francisco, CA: Jossey-Bass.

Gorecki, C., Brown, J. M., Nelson, E. A., et al. (2009). Impact of pressure ulcers on quality of life in older patients: A systematic review. *Journal of the American Geriatrics Society, 57*, 1175.

Gorecki, C., Nixon, J., Madill, A., Firth, J., & Brown, J. M. (2012). What influences the impact of pressure ulcers on health-related quality of life? A qualitative patient-focused exploration of contributory factors. *Journal of Tissue Viability, 21*(1), 3–12.

Guihan, M., Bombardier, C. H., Ehde, D. M., Rapacki, L. M., Rogers, T. J., Bates-Jensen, B., et al. (2014). Comparing multicomponent interventions to improve skin care behaviors and prevent recurrence in veterans hospitalized for severe pressure ulcers. *Archives of Physical Medicine and Rehabilitation.*

Health and Human Services (HHS) Department. (2016). *Nondiscrimination in health programs and activities.* Retrieved 12/25/2020 from: https://www.federalregister.gov/articles/2016/05/18/2016-11458/nondiscrimination-in-health-programs-and-activities#sec-92-201%20.

Herber, O. R., Schnepp, W., & Rieger, M. A. (2007). A systematic review on the impact of leg ulceration on patients' quality of life. *Health and Quality of Life Outcomes, 5*(44), 2007.

Hicks, C. W., Canner, J. K., Mathioudakis, N., Lippincott, C., Sherman, R. L., & Abularrage, C. J. (2020). Incidence and risk factors associated with ulcer recurrence among patients with diabetic foot ulcers treated in a multidisciplinary setting. *The Journal of Surgical Research, 246*, 243–250.

Iihara, N., Nishio, T., Okura, M., Anzai, H., Kagawa, M., Houchi, H., et al. (2014). Comparing patient dissatisfaction and rational judgment in intentional medication non-adherence versus unintentional non-adherence. *Journal of Clinical Pharmacy and Therapeutics, 39*(1), 45–52.

Institute for Healthcare Advancement (IHA). (2020). *Always Use Teach-back! training toolkit.* Retrieved 12/29/2020 from: http://www.teachbacktraining.org.

International Best Practice Statement. (2016). Optimizing patient involvement in wound management. *Wounds International,* download available from: www.woundsinternational.com.

Jaksa, P. J., & Mahoney, J. L. (2010). Quality of life in patients with diabetic foot ulcers: Validation of the CWIS in a Canadian population. *International Wound Journal, 7*, 502.

Jarbrink, K., Ni, G., Sonnergren, H., Schmidtchen, A., Pang, C., Bajpai, R., et al. (2016). Prevalence and incidence of chronic wounds and related complications: A protocol for a systematic review. *Systematic Reviews, 5*(1), 152.

Jeffs, L. (2001). Teaching cultural safety the culturally safe way. *Nursing Praxis in New Zealand, 17*(3), 41–50.

Joint Commission International. (2017). *Accreditation standards for hospitals including standards for Academic Medical Center Hospitals.* Retrieved 12/16/2020 from: https://www.jointcommissioninternational.org/-/media/jci/jci-documents/accreditation/hospital-and-amc/jci-standards-only_6th-ed-hospital.pdf.

Jones, C. J., Smith, H., & Llewellyn, C. (2014). Evaluating the effectiveness of health belief model interventions in improving adherence: A systematic review. *Health Psychology Review, 8*(3), 253–269.

Jull, A., Mitchell, N., Arroll, J., et al. (2004). Factors influencing concordance with compression stockings after venous leg ulcer healing. *Journal of Wound Care, 13*, 90–92.

Keen, A., Thoele, K., Fite, L., & Lancaster, S. (2019). Competent patient refusal of nursing care: An innovative approach to a complex problem. *Journal of Wound, Ostomy, and Continence Nursing, 46*(5), 390–395. https://doi.org/10.1097/WON.0000000000000569. 31513125.

Kim, J. Y., & Cho, E. (2017). Evaluation of a self-efficacy enhancement program to prevent pressure ulcers in patients with a spinal cord injury. *Japan Journal of Nursing Science, 14*(1), 76–86. https://doi.org/10.1111/jjns.12136.

Knowles, M. S., Holton, E. F., III, & Swanson, R. A. (1998). *The adult learner.* Houston: TX, Gulf Publishing.

Krystallidou, D., Langewitz, W., & van den Muijsenbergh, M. (2020). Multilingual healthcare communication: Stumbling blocks, solutions, recommendations. *Patient Education and Counseling, S0738-3991*(20), 30513–30519. https://doi.org/10.1016/j.pec.2020.09.015.

Labropoulos, N., Wang, E. D., Lanier, S. T., et al. (2012). Factors associated with poor healing and recurrence of venous ulceration. *Plastic and Reconstructive Surgery, 129*(1), 179–186.

Ledger, L., Worsley, P., Hope, J., & Schoonhoven, L. (2020). Patient involvement in pressure ulcer prevention and adherence to prevention strategies: An integrative review. *International Journal of Nursing Studies, 101*, 103449.

Lindsay, E. (2000). Leg clubs: A new approach to patient-centred leg ulcer management. *Nursing & Health Sciences, 2*(3), 139–141.

Lindsay, E. (2004). The Lindsay Leg Club® Model: A model for evidence-based leg ulcer management. *Woundcare, 9*(Suppl. 6), S15–S20.

Mariani, F., Marone, E. M., Gasbarro, V., Bucalossi, M., Spelta, S., Amsler, F., et al. (2011). Multicenter randomized trial comparing compression with elastic stocking versus bandage after surgery for varicose veins. *Journal of Vascular Surgery, 53*(1), 115–122. https://doi.org/10.1016/j.jvs.2010.08.033.

Mattison, M. J., & Nemec, E. C. (2014). The impact of an immersive elective on learners' understanding of lifestyle medicine and its role in patients' lives. *American Journal of Pharmaceutical Education, 78*(8), 154.

McCaughan, D., Sheard, L., Cullum, N., Dumville, J., & Chetter, I. (2018). Patients' perceptions and experiences of living with a surgical wound healing by secondary intention: A qualitative study. *International Journal of Nursing Studies, 77*, 29–38. https://doi.org/10.1016/j.ijnurstu.2017.09.015.

McInnes, E., Chaboyer, W., Murray, E., Allen, T., & Jones, P. (2014). The role of patients in pressure injury prevention: A survey of acute care patients. *BMC Nursing, 13*(1), 41. https://doi.org/10.1186/s12912-014-0041-y.

Meherali, S., Punjani, N. S., & Mevawala, A. (2020). Health literacy interventions to improve health outcomes in low- and middle-income countries. *Health Literacy Research and Practice, 4*(4), e251–e266. https://doi.org/10.3928/24748307-20201118-01.

Moffatt, C., Murray, S., Keeley, V., & Aubeeluck, A. (2017). Non-adherence to treatment of chronic wounds: Patient versus professional perspectives. *International Wound Journal, 14*(6), 1305–1312. https://doi.org/10.1111/iwj.12804.

Morton, L. M., Bolton, L. L., Corbett, L. Q., et al. (2013). An evaluation of the association for the advancement of wound care venous ulcer guideline and recommendations for future research. *Advances in Skin & Wound Care, 26*(12), 553–561.

National Institute of Mental Health (NIMH). (2018). Transforming the understanding and treatment of mental illnesses. In *Depression*. Retrieved 11/11/2020 from: https://www.nimh.nih.gov/health/statistics/major-depression.shtml.

National Quality Forum (NQF). (2009). A comprehensive framework and preferred practices for measuring and reporting cultural competency: A consensus report. Washington, DC. Retrieved 9/18/2022 from https://www.qualityforum.org/projects/cultural_competency.aspx.

Nielson Global Online Consumer Survey. (2009). *Global advertising consumers trust real friends and virtual strangers the most.* Retrieved 11/11/2020 from: http://www.nielsen.com/us/en/newswire/2009/global-advertising-consumers-trust-real-friends-and-virtual-strangers-the-most.html.

Nussbaum, S. R., Carter, M. J., Fife, C. E., DaVanzo, J., Haught, R., Nusgart, M., et al. (2018). An economic evaluation of the impact, cost, and medicare policy implications of chronic nonhealing wounds. *Value in Health, 21*(1), 27–32. https://doi.org/10.1016/j.jval.2017.07.007.

Obirikorang, Y., Obirikorang, C., Acheampong, E., et al. (2018). Predictors of noncompliance to antihypertensive therapy among hypertensive patients Ghana: Application of health belief model. *International Journal of Hypertension, 2018,* 4701097. https://doi.org/10.1155/2018/4701097. 30018819. PMCID: PMC6029446.

O'Donnell, T. F., Passman, M. A., Marston, W. A., Ennis, W. J., Dalsing, M., Kistner, R. L., et al. (2014). Management of venous leg ulcers: Clinical practice guidelines of the Society for Vascular Surgery and the American Venous Forum. *Journal of Vascular Surgery, 60,* 3s–59s. https://doi.org/10.1016/j.jvs.2014.04.049.

O'Malley, A. S., Forrest, C. B., & Mandelblatt, J. (2002). Adherence of low-income women to cancer screening recommendations. *Journal of General Internal Medicine, 17,* 144–154.

O'Meara, S., Al-Kurdi, D., & Ovington, L. G. (2008). Antibiotics and antiseptics for venous leg ulcers. *Cochrane Database of Systematic Reviews,* (1), CD00355.

Parks, C. D., Joireman, J., & Van Lange, P. A. (2013). Cooperation, trust, and antagonism: How public goods are promoted. *Psychological Science in the Public Interest, 14*(3), 119–165.

Peters, E. J., Armstrong, D. G., & Lavery, L. A. (2007). Risk factors for recurrent diabetic foot ulcers: Site matters. *Diabetes Care, 30*(8), 2077–2079. https://doi.org/10.2337/dc07-0445.

Price, P., & Harding, K. (2004). Cardiff wound impact schedule: The development of a condition-specific questionnaire to assess health-related quality of life in patients with chronic wounds of the lower limb. *International Wound Journal, 1,* 10.

Price, P. E. (2008). Education, psychology and 'compliance'. *Diabetes/Metabolism Research and Reviews, 24*(Suppl. 1), S101–S105. https://doi.org/10.1002/dmrr.851.

Rappl, L. (2004). Non-compliance: Adding insult to injury. *Ostomy/Wound Management, 50*(5). 6, 8.

Redman, B. K. (2007). *The practice of patient education: A case study approach* (10th ed.). St. Louis, MO: Mosby.

Renner, R., Seikowski, K., & Simon, J. C. (2014). Association of pain level, health and wound status in patients with chronic leg ulcers. *Acta Dermato-Venereologica, 94,* 50–53.

Rimmer, A. (2020). Can patients use family members as non-professional interpreters in consultations? *British Medical Journal, 368*(2).

Sandman, L., Granger, B. B., Ekman, I., & Munthe, C. (2012). Adherence, shared decision-making and patient autonomy. *Medicine, Health Care, and Philosophy, 15*(2), 115–127. https://doi.org/10.1007/s11019-011-9336-x. 21678125.

Schubart, J. R. (2012). An e-learning program to prevent pressure ulcers in adults with spinal cord injury: A pre- and post-pilot test among rehabilitation patients following discharge to home. *Ostomy/Wound Management, 58*(10), 38–49.

Singh, R., Singh, R., Rohilla, R. K., et al. (2013). Improvisations in classic and modified techniques of flap surgery to improve the success rate for pressure ulcer healing in patients with spinal cord injury. *International Wound Journal, 10*(4), 455–460.

Spilsbury, K., Nelson, A., Cullum, N., Iglesias, C., Nixon, J., & Mason, S. (2007). Pressure ulcers and their treatment and effects on quality of life: Hospital inpatient perspectives. *Journal of Advanced Nursing, 57,* 494.

Stacey, D., Légaré, F., Lewis, K., Barry, M. J., Bennett, C. L., Eden, K. B., et al. (2017). Decision aids for people facing health treatment or screening decisions. *Cochrane Database of Systematic Reviews,* (4), CD001431. https://doi.org/10.1002/14651858.CD001431.pub5.

Syrowatka, A., Krömker, D., Meguerditchian, A. N., & Tamblyn, R. (2016). Features of computer-based decision aids: Systematic review, thematic synthesis, and meta-analyses. *Journal of Medical Internet Research, 18*(1), e20. https://doi.org/10.2196/jmir.4982.

Takehara, K., et al. (2019). Differences between patient reported versus clinician reported nonulcerative signs and symptoms of the foot in patients with diabetes mellitus. *Journal of Wound, Ostomy, and Continence Nursing, 46*(2), 133–136.

Tavafian, S. S., Hasani, L., Aghamolaei, T., et al. (2009). Prediction of breast self-examination in a sample of Iranian women: An application of the Health Belief Model. *BMC Women's Health, 9,* 37. https://doi.org/10.1186/1472-6874-9-37.

The Joint Commission (TJC). (2010). *Advancing effective communication, cultural competence, and patient- and family-centered care: A roadmap for hospitals.* Oakbrook Terrace, IL: TJC.

Thompson, D., Leach, M., Smith, C., Fereday, J., & May, E. (2020). How nurses and other health professionals use learning principles in parent education practice: A scoping review of the literature. *Heliyon, 6*(3), e03564. https://doi.org/10.1016/j.heliyon.2020.e03564.

Tobiano, G., Marshall, A., Bucknall, T., & Chaboyer, W. (2015). Patient participation in nursing care on medical wards: An integrative review. *International Journal of Nursing Studies, 52*(6), 1107–1120.

Treadwell, T. (2018). Maybe there is a reason to patient noncompliance! *Wounds, 30*(10), A8.

Turabian, J. L. (2019). Strategies to improve therapeutic compliance in general medicine. *Community Medicine and Health Education Research, 1*(1), 31–39.

US Department of Health and Human Services. (2020). *Reduce the rate of foot and leg amputations in adults with diabetes—D-08.* Retrieved 2/27/2020 from https://health.gov/healthypeople/objectives-and-data/browse-objectives/diabetes/reduce-rate-foot-and-leg-amputations-adults-diabetes-d-08.

Van Hecke, A., Verhaeghe, S., Grypdonck, M., et al. (2011). Processes underlying adherence to leg ulcer treatment: A qualitative field study. *International Journal of Nursing Studies, 48,* 145–155.

van Rijswijk, L. (2004). Non-compliance no more. *Ostomy/Wound Management*, 50(1), 6.

Wachholz, P. A., Masuda, P. Y., Nascimento, D. C., Taira, C. M. H., & Cleto, N. G. (2014). Quality of life profile and correlated factors in chronic leg ulcer patients in the mid-west of São Paulo State, Brazil. *Anais Brasileiros de Dermatologia*, 89, 73–81.

Warshaw, E., Nix, D., Kula, J., et al. (2002). Clinical and cost-effectiveness of a cleanser protectant lotion for treatment of perineal skin breakdown in low-risk patients with incontinence. *Ostomy/Wound Management*, 48(6), 44–51.

Weller, C.D., Buchbinder, R., & Johnston, R.V. (2016). Interventions for helping people adhere to compression treatments for venous leg ulceration. Cochrane Database of Systematic Reviews, Issue 3. Art.No.: CD008378. doi: https://doi.org/10.1002/14651858.CD008378.pub3.

World Health Organization (WHO). (2016). *Patient engagement: Technical series on safer primary care*. Geneva: License: CC BY-NC-SA 3.0 IGO.

Wound, Ostomy and Continence Nurses Society. (2014). Guideline for management of wounds in patients with lower-extremity arterial disease. *WOCN clinical practice guideline series 1*. Mt. Laurel: Author.

Wound, Ostomy and Continence Nurses Society. (2016). *Guideline for management of pressure ulcers, WOCN clinical practice guideline series #2*. Mt. Laurel: Author.

Wound, Ostomy and Continence Nurses Society. (2019). Guideline for management of wounds in patients with lower-extremity venous disease. *WOCN clinical practice guideline series 4*. Mt. Laurel: Author.

Wound, Ostomy and Continence Nurses Society. (2021). Guideline for management of wounds in patients with lower-extremity neuropathic disease. *WOCN clinical practice guideline series 3*. Mt. Laurel: Author.

Wu, S. C., Jensen, J. L., Weber, A. K., et al. (2008). Use of pressure offloading devices in diabetic foot ulcers. *Diabetes Care*, 31(11), 2118–2119.

Yan, J., Liu, Y., Zhou, B., & Sun, M. (2014). Pre-hospital delay in patients with diabetic foot problems: Influencing factors and subsequent quality of care. *Diabetic Medicine*, 31(5), 624–629.

Yen, P. H., & Leasure, A. R. (2019). Use and effectiveness of the teach-back method in patient education and health outcomes. *Federal Practitioner*, 36(6), 284–289.

Zhou, K., & Jia, P. (2016). Depressive symptoms in patients with wounds: A cross-sectional study. *Wound Repair and Regeneration*, 24, 1059–1065.

Zolnierek, K. B., & Dimatteo, M. R. (2009). Physician communication and patient adherence to treatment: A meta-analysis. *Medical Care*, 47(8), 826–834.

FURTHER READING

Australian Wound Management Association (AWMA) and the New Zealand Wound Care Society (NZWCS). (2011). *Australian and New Zealand clinical practice guideline for prevention and management of venous leg ulcers*. Osborne Park, WA, Australia: Cambridge Publishing.

Durso, S. (2001). Technological advances for improving medication adherence in the elderly. *Annals of Long-Term Care*, 9(4), 43.

Edwards, L. M., Moffatt, C. J., & Franks, P. J. (2002). An exploration of patients' understanding of leg ulceration. *Journal of Wound Care*, 11(1), 35–39.

Légaré, F., Ratté, S., Gravel, K., & Graham, I. D. (2008). Barriers and facilitators to implementing shared decision-making in clinical practice: Update of a systematic review of health professionals' perceptions. *Patient Education and Counseling*, 73, 526–535.

Col, N. F., & Haugen, V. (2022). Shared decision-making and short-course radiotherapy for operable rectal adenocarcinoma: A patient's right to choose. *Journal of Wound, Ostomy and Continence Nursing*, 49(2), 180–183.

Partnership to Fight Chronic Disease (PFCD). (2014). *Better care legislation a positive step in fight against the growing epidemic of chronic disease*. Accessed 11/11/2020 from: http://www.fightchronicdisease.org/media-center/releases/better-care-legislation-positive-step-fight-against-growing-epidemic-chronic-d.

6

Quality Tracking Across the Continuum

Lisa Q. Corbett

OBJECTIVES

- Describe the driving forces for quality and safety in health care including the origins of quality measures in wound care.
- Discuss the value of evaluation and quality measures for wound care.
- Summarize the role of the Wound Specialist as facilitator of Quality Improvement.

- Identify sources of external quality measures pertaining to wound care specialty practice for acute care, home care, and skilled nursing populations.
- Distinguish between prevalence and incidence and describe the clinical utility of each measure.
- Provide examples of quality metrics used for internal wound quality improvement programs.

Improving the quality of care for the acute and chronic wound population is a key competency for the wound care specialist. Measurement of outcome from the delivery of evidence-based wound care is an expectation in every practice setting. The most high-profile quality indicator for the wound specialist pertains to pressure injury. However, there are many other outcome metrics associated with wound prevention and healing that are within the scope of the wound specialist. Measures such as health care-associated infections, readmissions, end-of-life care preferences, and patient satisfaction all involve wound specialty skills. This chapter will review the driving forces behind the quality movement, sources of wound quality measures, and methods for collecting and tracking wound-related data across the care continuum.

Over the past two decades, in health systems worldwide, there has been a sharpened focus on improving health care quality. The World Health Organization (WHO) has stated:

"Even where health systems are well developed and resourced, there is clear evidence that quality remains a serious concern, with expected outcomes not predictably achieved and with wide variations in standards of health-care delivery within and between health-care systems. In every country, there is opportunity to improve the quality and performance of the health-care system, as well as growing awareness and public pressure to do so" (WHO, 2006, p. 3).

In the United States, the quality movement was spurred by a series of publications released by the Institute of Medicine (IOM) (IOM, 2001). *To Err is Human* (2000) was the first report that outlined the extent of medical errors in US hospitals, citing 44,000–98,000 preventable deaths each year

(Kohn, Corrigan, & Donaldson, 2000). A subsequent publication, *Crossing the Quality Chasm: A New Health System for the 21st Century* (2001), called for sweeping reform of the American health system and outlined six aims for improvement (Table 6.1). It also proposed the alignment of quality accountability with payment incentives. Additional publications from the IOM proposed revision of work environment for nurses, prevention of medication errors, and promotion of nursing leadership in health care (IOM, 2011a, 2011b). The IOM reports raised awareness of poor health care quality and moved transparency, service excellence and measurement to the forefront of health care goals. The evidence reported in these publications inspired changes in health care, government, insurance, education, and consumer sectors. Quality improvement concepts, tools, and methods are now part of the operating strategy for health care delivery systems around the world. Initiatives arising from the government, private and public sectors have been responsible for improvements. Driving Forces for Quality and Safety in Wound Care are described in Fig. 6.1. Organizations and websites for patient quality and safety are provided in Table 6.2.

FEDERAL POLICY DRIVES WOUND QUALITY

In the United States, collective efforts have been introduced over the past decades to drive health care quality and safety improvements through policy change. Wound care practitioners must appreciate the policy process to understand the current regulatory and reimbursement landscape. Many significant health care policies originate from federal legislation. Once passed, the intent of the legislation is interpreted by the federal agency responsible for implementing the law,

TABLE 6.1   Six Aims for Health Care Improvement

Aims	Description
Safe	• Avoid injuries to patients from the care that is intended to help them
Effective	• Provide services based on scientific knowledge to all who would benefit • Refrain from providing services to those not likely to benefit
Patient-centered	• Provide care that is respectful of and responsive to the individual patient preferences, needs, values • Ensure that patient values guide all clinical decisions
Timely	• Reduce waits and sometimes harmful delays for both those who receive and those who give care
Efficient	• Avoid waste, including waste of equipment, supplies, ideas, energy
Equitable	• Provide care that does not vary in quality because of personal characteristics such as gender, ethnicity, geographic location, and socioeconomic status

From Institute of Medicine. (2001). *Crossing the quality chasm: A new health system for the 21st century.* Washington, DC: National Academy Press.

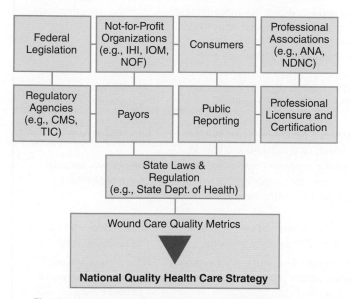

Fig. 6.1 Driving forces for quality and safety in wound care.

(LTCH), inpatient rehabilitation facilities (IRF) and home health agencies (HHA). Specific definitions, measure time windows, and coding criteria are established for each site of care as outlined by federal regulation. Nongovernmental insurance payors often follow the federal lead on quality standards.

Several significant federal laws have set standards for health care quality that impact wound care practice. The most significant public health law was the Social Security Amendments of 1965 (Public Law 89-97) which created Medicare and Medicaid, two of America's most enduring social programs. While these programs started as basic insurance programs for those in need, they have changed over the years to provide more Americans with access to quality affordable health care. Medicare has expanded to cover inpatient and outpatient care, home care, rehabilitation, dressings, prescription drug benefits, and end-stage renal disease for the elderly and disabled. Medicaid has expanded to cover medical expenses for families with low-income, pregnant women, disabled, and those who need long-term care. States tailor their Medicaid programs to best serve their constituents. A 2018 retrospective analysis identified that more than 8 million (14.5%) of Medicare beneficiaries suffer from wounds. Annual Medicare wound care expenditure is estimated at 32 billion, with the majority of costs accruing in outpatient settings (Nussbaum, Carter, Fife, et al., 2018).

The Omnibus Budget Reconciliation Act of 1987, also known as the Nursing Home Reform Act (Public Law 100-203), is another example of a law that set standards of care and established rights for elderly persons (Omnibus, 1987). The Act requires that states and federal government inspect nursing homes, conduct periodic surveys and enforce standards by using a range of sanctions. Surveyors use guidelines derived from this and other federal laws when they inspect skilled nursing facilities and evaluate resident safety related to pressure injury prevention and facility-associated infections (Wagner, Castle, Reid, & Stone, 2013).

In 1997, the Balanced Budget Act (P.L. 105-33) established the Medicare Payment Advisory Commission (MedPAC) as an independent congressional agency to advise the US Congress on issues affecting the Medicare program. MedPAC analyzes access to care, quality of care, and other issues affecting Medicare. This agency acts as a check and balance on the Medicare program to assure it continues to deliver the safety net as it was intended (https://www.medpac.gov/).

As a response to the IOM reports, Congress enacted the Healthcare Research and Quality Act of 1999 (Public Law 106-129), which established the Agency for Healthcare Research and Quality (AHRQ) within the Department of Health and Human Services (HHS). The law designated AHRQ as the lead Agency to reduce medical errors and study patient safety. Over the past 20 years, AHRQ has fostered the use of research and evidence in health care delivery and produced data to guide decisions by clinicians, system leaders, and policy makers. The AHRQ monitors adverse events, funds grants, disseminates technology assessment reports, produces patient safety tools, and creates evidence guides.

such as the Centers for Medicare and Medicaid Services (CMS) (CMS, 2015, 2020). The agency publishes proposed rules in the Federal Register with a comment period, and subsequently publishes final rules for all organizations wishing to receive Medicare and/or Medicaid funds to obey. For example, as seen in Table 6.3, CMS establishes quality metrics reporting requirements for pressure injuries for hospitals, skilled nursing facilities (SNF), long-term care hospitals

TABLE 6.2   Organizations for Patient Quality and Safety

Name	Description	Internet Site
The National Patient Safety Foundation's Lucian Leape Institute	NPSF Lucian Leape Institute members are national thought leaders in patient safety	www.npsf.org/LLI
The National Patient Safety Foundation at the Institute for Healthcare Improvement	The Institute for Healthcare Improvement (IHI) and the National Patient Safety Foundation (NPSF) joined forces to focus and energize the patient safety agenda in order to build systems of safety across the continuum of care	www.ihi.org/PatientSafety
Agency for Healthcare Research and Quality	The Agency for Healthcare Research and Quality (AHRQ) is the lead Federal agency charged with improving the safety and quality of the US healthcare system	www.ahrq.gov/
PSNet – Patient Safety Network	AHRQ Patient Safety Network (PSNet) is a national web-based resource featuring the latest news and essential resources on patient safety	https://psnet.ahrq.gov/
The Joint Commission (TJC)	TJC has established standardized core performance measure sets for hospital operations and contributes to the national strategy for improving health care quality transparency	https://www.jointcommission.org/
National Committee for Quality Assurance (NCQA)	The NCQA is one of the main certifications and accreditation organizations for patient-centric medical home initiatives, health plan accreditations, disease and case management, and other health care provider certification and recognition programs	https://www.ncqa.org/
National Quality Forum (NQF)	The National Quality Forum (NQF) is a nonprofit organization that: (1) builds consensus on national priorities and goals for performance improvement, (2) endorses national consensus standards for measuring and publicly reporting on performance, and (3) promotes the attainment of national goals through education and outreach programs	http://www.qualityforum.org
American Society for Healthcare Risk Management (ASHRM)	ASHRM promotes effective and innovative risk management strategies and professional leadership through education, recognition, advocacy, publications, networking, and interactions with leading health care organizations and government agencies	https://www.ashrm.org/
National Center for Patient Safety	The NCPS was established in 1999 to develop and nurture a culture of safety throughout the Veterans Health Administration	https://www.patientsafety.va.gov/
Partnership for Patient Safety	Partnership for Patient Safety is a patient-centered initiative to advance the reliability of health care systems worldwide	https://p4ps.net/
ECRI Institute	ECRI Institute is an independent nonprofit organization whose mission is to benefit patient care by promoting the highest standards of safety, quality, and cost-effectiveness in health care	https://www.ecri.org/solutions/patient-safety/
WHO Patient Safety World Health Organization	WHO Patient Safety, aims to coordinate, disseminate and accelerate improvements in patient safety worldwide	https://www.who.int/patientsafety/en/
Quality and Patient Safety American Hospital Association (AHA)	Delivering the right care at the right time in the right setting is the core mission of hospitals across the country	https://www.aha.org/advocacy/quality-and-patient-safety

Examples of evidence-based toolkits from the AHRQ include the "On-Time Pressure Ulcer Prevention Program" for skilled nursing facilities (AHRQ, 2016) and the "Preventing Pressure Ulcers in Hospitals" programs (Agency for Healthcare Research and Quality, 2014; Agency for Healthcare Research and Quality (AHRQ), 2014). These programs provide step-by-step instructions for implementing pressure injury programs in health care institutions. Many

publications have demonstrated the benefits of these standardized approaches to pressure injury program development (Niederhauser et al., 2012; Sullivan & Schoelles, 2013). Evidence-based tool kits for wound-related quality programs and the website links are listed in Table 6.4.

As part of its quality mission, AHRQ established the Medicare Patient Safety Monitoring System (MPSMS), a chart surveillance database to measure national rates for 21 types of

TABLE 6.3 Cross-Setting Pressure Ulcer/Injury Quality Measures* (as of July 2020)

Site of Care	Tool for Reporting Pressure Ulcers/Injury	Measure Steward/ Quality Program	Metric
Hospitals	Pressure ulcer prevalence	Joint Commission	NQF-0201: The total number of patients who have hospital-acquired stage 2 or greater pressure ulcers on the day of the prevalence measurement episode
	PSI-03	AHRQ -Hospital Acquired Conditions	Stage 3 or 4 or unstageable pressure ulcers per 1,000 discharges among surgical or medical patients ages 18 years and older
	PSI-90	AHRQ	NQF-0531: Patient Safety and Adverse Events Composite Measure
	Serious Reportable Events (SRE)	State Departments of Health (if mandatory reporting), CMS	NQF-4F: Any Stage 3, Stage 4, and unstageable pressure ulcers acquired after admission/ presentation to a healthcare setting
Skilled Nursing Facilities	Minimum Data Set (MDS)	CMS-Nursing Home Quality Initiative	NQF-0678: Percent of Residents or Patients with Pressure Ulcers Stage 2–4 That Are New or Worsened
Long-Term Care Hospitals	LTCH Continuity Assessment Record and Evaluation (LTCH CARE) Data Set	CMS-Nursing Home Quality Initiative	NQF-0678: Percent of Residents or Patients with Pressure Ulcers Stage 2–4 That Are New or Worsened
Inpatient Rehabilitation Facilities	Inpatient Rehabilitation Facility Patient Assessment Instrument (IRF-PAI)	CMS-Nursing Home Quality Initiative	NQF-0678: Percent of Residents or Patients with Pressure Ulcers Stage 2-4 That Are New or Worsened
Home Care	Outcome and Assessment Information Set (OASIS)	CMS-Home Health (HH) Quality Reporting Program	NQF-0678: Percent of Residents or Patients with Pressure Ulcers Stage 2-4 That Are New or Worsened

AHRQ, Agency for Healthcare Research & Quality; *CMS*, Centers for Medicare & Medicaid Services.
*Check with primary sources for accuracy, as policy evolves.

TABLE 6.4 Evidence-Based Tool Kits for Wound-Related Quality Programs

Tool Kit	Source
How-to Guide: Reducing Pressure Ulcers	IHI http://www.ihi.org/resources/Pages/Tools/HowtoGuidePreventPressureUlcers.aspx
Preventing Pressure Ulcers in Hospitals	AHRQ http://www.ahrq.gov/professionals/systems/hospital/pressureulcertoolkit/index.html
Preventing Hospital Acquired Pressure Ulcers	HRET http://www.hret-hiin.org/Resources/pressure-ulcers/17/hospital-acquired-pressure-ulcers-injuries-hapu-change-package
Pressure Ulcer/Injury Road Map	Minnesota Hospital Association https://www.mnhospitals.org/pressure-ulcers#/videos/list
Safety Program for Nursing Homes: On-Time Pressure Ulcer Prevention	AHRQ https://www.ahrq.gov/patient-safety/settings/long-term-care/resource/ontime/pruprev/index.html
Toolkit for Reducing CAUTI in Hospitals	AHRQ https://www.ahrq.gov/hai/tools/cauti-hospitals/index.html
Re-Engineered Discharge (RED) Toolkit	AHRQ https://www.ahrq.gov/patient-safety/settings/hospital/red/toolkit/index.html
Toolkit to Promote Safe Surgery	AHRQ https://www.ahrq.gov/hai/tools/surgery/index.html
AHRQ Safety Program for Long-Term Care: HAIs/ CAUTI	AHRQ https://www.ahrq.gov/hai/quality/tools/cauti-ltc/modules/implementation/long-term-modules/overview.html
AHRQ Tools To Reduce Hospital-Acquired Conditions	AHRQ https://www.ahrq.gov/hai/hac/tools.html

adverse events. Included are select hospital-acquired conditions (HACs), such as postsurgical complications and pressure injuries. Currently this program is transitioning to the Quality and Safety Review System (QSRS) and is developing e-measure chart-abstraction methodology to expand the array of adverse event measures captured from electronic health records. Professional wound organizations have shared public reservations about the accuracy of pressure injury data when e-measure abstraction becomes standardized.

In 2005, the US Congress passed the Patient Safety and Quality Improvement Act (Public Law 109-41) with the intention to improve patient safety by encouraging voluntary and confidential reporting of adverse events. It established a network of Patient Safety Organizations (PSOs) to collect and analyze confidential information reported by health care providers. The Act also provided legal protections to information collected by the PSOs.

The Deficit Reduction Act of 2005 (Public Law 109–171), required CMS to identify hospital-acquired conditions (HAC) that were (1) high cost or high volume or both and (2) result in the assignment of a case to a DRG that has a higher payment when present as a secondary diagnosis, and could reasonably have been prevented through the application of evidence-based guidelines. Subsequently, in 2008, CMS implemented the Hospital-Acquired Conditions (HAC) initiative which denies incremental payment to hospitals for complications of hospital care, including stage 3 and 4 pressure ulcers, catheter-associated urinary tract infections, surgical site infections, and others. Adding to the value-based programs (authorized after passage of the Patient Protection and Affordable Care Act-Public Law 111-148), CMS began adjusting payments to hospitals based on the rank performance on risk-adjusted HAC quality measures. In addition, the Hospital Readmission Reduction Program (HRRP) penalizes institutions for excess readmissions across certain diagnostic groups such as COPD, Heart Failure, and others. Poorer performers are subject to an overall 1% payment reduction. The Hospital Value-Based Purchasing Program includes rewards or penalties to incentivize high-quality care. Measures include a Patient Safety Indicators (PSI) 90 composite score, total HAC score and National Healthcare Safety Network (NHSN) hospital-associated infections (HAI) measure scores. Hospital-acquired pressure injuries (stage 3, 4, and unstageable) are configured in the score prominently. The value-based and HAC-reduction programs are rebalanced yearly determining domain weighting and penalty score levels. As of 2020, there were 14 listed HACs and CMS has reported an overall reduction in the rate of HACs of 4.5% since program inception, though pressure injury rates have not decreased (AHRQ, 2019). Checklist 6.1 provides a list of these CMS programs, initiatives, and websites.

Another significant federal law impacting health care quality is the Patient Protection and Affordable Care Act (PPACA) of 2010 (Public Law 111-148). The sweeping health reform bill was designed to make affordable health insurance available to more people through Medicaid expansion and subsidies for lower-income people. Building on existing health care reform momentum in the private and public

---

CHECKLIST 6.1 Centers for Medicare and Medicaid Services (CMS) programs, initiatives, and websites

✓ Hospital-Acquired Conditions (HAC) initiative
https://www.cms.gov/Medicare/Medicare-Fee-for-Service-Payment/HospitalAcqCond
✓ Hospital Readmission Reduction Program (HRRP)
https://www.cms.gov/Medicare/Quality-Initiatives-Patient-Assessment-Instruments/Value-Based-Programs/HRRP/Hospital-Readmission-Reduction-Program
✓ Hospital Value-Based Purchasing Program
https://www.cms.gov/Medicare/Quality-Initiatives-Patient-Assessment-Instruments/Value-Based-Programs/HVBP/Hospital-Value-Based-Purchasing
✓ Hospital Consumer Assessment of Healthcare Providers and Systems (HCAHPS)
https://www.cms.gov/Medicare/Quality-Initiatives-Patient-Assessment-Instruments/HospitalQualityInits/HospitalHCAHPS

All websites accessed 03/07/2023.

---

sectors, the law promoted change in the following three areas. First, it shifted reimbursement based on the value of care rather than volume of services provided, known as value-based purchasing. Second, the law focused on testing new models of health care delivery such as accountable care organizations (ACO) where providers are rewarded for improving quality and reducing cost. Finally, the PPACA invested in resources for systemwide improvement to provide effective, quality care.

The Act created the Patient-Centered Outcomes Research Institute to develop research priorities and fund comparative effectiveness research. Comparative effectiveness research (CER) is designed to test different health care interventions (such as drugs, devices, dressings, treatment protocols), against one or more other interventions. The goal is to understand what treatment modalities work best for different populations with different health conditions. Examples of comparative effectiveness research wound projects include work on chronic venous ulcers, skin substitutes, and pressure injury treatment strategies (AHRQ, Effective Health Program, https://effectivehealthcare.ahrq.gov/; Valle et al., 2014). To date, the PPACA has reduced the percentage of uninsured Americans to historically low levels, but its future remains uncertain due to partisan conflict. Meanwhile, states have had considerable discretion in how the ACA is implemented, creating variability in how the law has affected people across the country (Guth, Garfield, & Rudowitz, 2020).

The Improving Medicare Post-Acute Care Transformation Act of 2014 (H.R. 4994), commonly known as the Impact Act, required the standardized and interoperable reporting of patient assessment data in postacute care settings for the purpose of improving Medicare beneficiary outcomes. Specific quality measures in several domains must be submitted from home health agencies (HHAs), skilled nursing facilities

(SNFs), long-term care hospitals (LTCHs), and inpatient rehabilitation facilities (IRFs) (Table 6.3). The quality measure domains include skin integrity, functional status, cognitive function, medication reconciliation; incidence of major falls; care preferences with transfer. The data are publicly reported and provide basis for prospective payment programs in postacute settings, linking payment to quality.

States adopt health care quality and safety laws and policies consistent with the negotiated preferences of their legislatures. An example of this is the state reporting requirements for adverse events in hospitals. Only 26 states have adverse event reporting requirements authorized through state law. Reporting systems vary in terms of what events were reported, criteria used for selection, and type of information reported. Some states adopt the National Quality Forum list of Serious Reportable Events (SRE), others establish their own lists (Hanlon, Sheedy, Kniffen, & Rosenthal, 2015). The wound care specialist should be aware of all state laws and regulations related to mandatory reporting of adverse events in the state of practice.

Nonprofit Organizations Drive Wound Quality

Not-for-profit organizations have also had a strong influence on shaping health care quality. The Institute for Health Care Improvement (IHI) began in the 1980s as a demonstration project to explore quality improvement in health care. Over the decades, they have leveraged the science of improvement to develop methods for change and innovation in health care. In 2004, they launched the 100,000 Lives Campaign, engaging more than 3,000 US hospitals to improve safety and outcomes. In 2008, IHI proposed the "Triple Aim"; a transformative goal to improve the individual experience of care, the health of populations, and to reduce the per capita costs of care. The Triple Aim (Fig. 6.2) later became part of the US National Quality Strategy in the implementation of the PPACA of 2010. The IHI is a leader in the delivery of quality improvement and safety education through the web "Open School" courses. By merging with the National Patient Safety Foundation (NPSF) in 2017, the IHI has reenergized the global patient safety agenda.

The National Quality Forum (NQF) is another not-for-profit organization that exerts a major influence on quality in health care. Defined performance measures provide a method to assess health care compared with recognized standards. Measures can come from many sources, but those endorsed through the NQF process have become the US reference for high-quality appropriate care. As a consensus-based organization, the NQF uses a rigorous process appraising the evidence through scientific review with input from patients, families, clinicians, payers, and health care leaders. Today, over 300 NQF-endorsed measures are used in more than 20 federal public reporting and pay-for-performance programs as well as in private-sector and state programs. NQF has also developed and maintained the definitions of Serious Reportable Events (SRE) used for public reporting in a variety of health care settings. Previously called "never events," these are events that fit specific criteria (listed in Box 6.1) and are then adopted by other regulatory bodies for monitoring, as shown in Table 6.3. As NQF measures are continuously maintained, prioritized and improved, the reader is directed to the source sites listed in Table 6.2 for up-to-date status on measures. The NQF definitions have formed the basis for regulatory and certifying agency pressure injury benchmarks (Brown, Donaldson, Bolton, & Aydin, 2010).

Another not-for-profit organization, The Joint Commission (TJC), is the oldest accrediting body in US health care, evaluating more than 20,000 organizations and programs. The organizational mission is to continuously improve

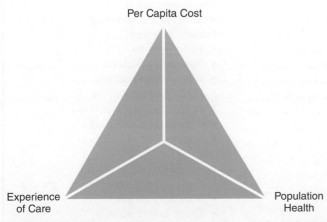

Fig. 6.2 IHI triple aim framework. Three simultaneously dimensions to optimizing health system performance.

> ## BOX 6.1 National Quality Forum (NQF): Defining Serious Reportable Events (SRE)
>
> **NQF considers a serious reportable event to be:**
> - Unambiguous
> - Largely, if not entirely, preventable
> - Serious
> - Any of the following:
>   - Adverse
>   - Indicative of a problem in a healthcare setting's safety systems
>   - Important for public credibility or public accountability
>
> **SREs are events that are:**
> - Of concern to both the public and healthcare professionals/providers
> - Clearly identifiable and measurable
> - Feasible to including in a reporting system
> - Of a nature such that the risk of occurrence is significantly influenced by the policies and procedures of the healthcare facility
>
> **NQF's list of SREs include:**
> - Injuries occurring during care management (rather than underlying disease) and
> - Errors occurring from failure to follow standard care or institutional policies and procedures.
>
> Data from National Quality Forum (NQF). (2011). *Serious Reportable Events In Health-care—2011 Update: A Consensus Report*. Washington, DC: NQF.

health care for the public and provide safe and effective care of the highest quality and value. During surveys, deficiencies are recorded based on the risk of harm and scope of occurrence, allowing organizations to prioritize high-risk deficiencies for correction. TJC develops resources for quality and safety initiatives. Examples include best practice guidance on surgical site infections and medical device-related pressure injuries. The Joint Commission recommends that hospitals report "sentinel events," defined as "an unexpected occurrence involving death or serious physiological or psychological injury, or the risk thereof" (TJC, 2020). Each year TJC designates a list of National Patient Safety goals to provide a quality focus scaffold for certifying health care organizations. Table 6.5 lists the examples of TJC's national patient safety goals across settings. Pressure injuries have been a focus of quality in TJC standards for many years. Wound specialists practicing in institutions with TJC accreditation will be familiar with the current standards, often leading their organizations in efforts to meet compliance.

Professional Organizations Drive Quality

Professional organizations also impact health care quality and safety. In 1998, the American Nurses Association (ANA) funded the development of nurse-sensitive quality indicators to provide data on acute-care outcomes that reflect the quality of nursing care delivery. These data, in the National Database of Nursing Quality Indicators (NDNQI), now managed by Press Ganey, continue to evolve as new evidence substantiates nursing-sensitive impact. Pressure injuries have been an early and enduring indicator of nursing quality. The concept of nursing-sensitive indicators, the gaps in congruence with nursing theoretical models, and implications for informing national health policy still requires clarity in nursing science (Helsop & Lu, 2014). With the evolution of interprofessional care teams, specific attribution of a clinical outcome to one profession might be questioned (Ayello, 2019). The unintended consequences of one measure impacting another may advocate for composite scores rather than singular scores on quality indicators (Boyle et al., 2016; Padula et al., 2019). For example, as patients are mobilized more to decrease pressure injury rates, an unintended consequence may be an increase in fall rates.

Standardized processes for planning and conducting pressure injury prevalence and incidence studies are an important component of a skin safety program and will be described later in this chapter. Participation in an external benchmarking program for pressure injury is required for CMS participation and Magnet designation (Ma & Park, 2015). The NDNQI is one option for institutions to report voluntary prevalence and incidence benchmarking for pressure injury and other nursing-sensitive indicators (NDNQI®, 2020). This involves a validated process with training tools and

TABLE 6.5   Examples of The Joint Commission National Patient Safety Goals Across Settings (2020)

Nursing Care Centers	Home Care	Hospitals
Identify residents correctly • 2 method identification	Identify patients correctly • 2 method identification	Identify patients correctly • 2 method identification • With medications • With blood transfusion
Use medicines safely • Anticoagulants • Medication reconciliation • Facilitate personal patient medication list	Use medicines safely • Medication reconciliation • Patient education on medications • Up-to-date list of meds with every healthcare visit	Improve staff communication • Test results on time Use Medications Safely • Label medications before procedures • Anticoagulants • Medication reconciliation
Prevent infection • Hand hygiene • Resistant infections • Central line infections • Urinary catheter infections	Prevent infection • Hand hygiene	Use Alarms safely • Settings and response Prevent Infection • Hand Hygiene • Resistant infections • Central line infections • Surgical site infections • Urinary catheter infections
Prevent residents from falling • Fall risk assessment • Medications contributing	Prevent patients from falling • Fall risk assessment • Medications contributing to falls	Identify patient safety risks • Suicide
Prevent bed sores • Risk Assessment • Prevention measures • Surveillance	Identify patient safety risks • Risks for patients on oxygen • Fire safety	Prevent mistakes in surgery • Right surgery, right patient, right site • Mark surgical site • Pause before surgery

Adapted from https://www.jointcommission.org/-/media/tjc/documents/standards/national-patient-safety-goals/2020-ncc-npsg-goals-final.pdf.

standardized summary reports. Scores are compared with peer institutions and reported as percentile rankings. The Hill-Rom-sponsored International Pressure Ulcer Prevalence (IPUP) Survey is another pressure ulcer database, with over 1000 facilities participating over a 3-day period surveying more than 100,000 patients each year. Acute care, long-term care, long-term acute care, rehabilitation, and home care organizations, globally, can participate in the data collection process (VanGilder, Cox, Edsberg, & Koloms, 2021).

The American Nurses Credentialing Center (ANCC, 2017), part of the ANA Enterprise, considers prevention of certain patient safety indicators, including pressure injuries, falls, catheter-associated urinary tract infections (CAUTI) and central line–associated bloodstream infections (CLABSI), as important indicators critical in hospitals' pathway to receive Magnet recognition. Developed in 1993, the Magnet Recognition program recognizes health care organizations that promote nursing excellence and provide superior quality patient care (ANCC, 2017). Hospitals with Magnet designation report lower rates of nursing sensitive events such as pressure injuries (Ma & Park, 2015). Improved nursing staff satisfaction, collaborative relationships, recruitment and retention, community recognition and marketing advantages are also benefitting of Magnet recognition.

In the United States, professional wound societies also contribute to quality and patient safety through the advancement of the specialty, policy advocacy and the development of scientific basis for wound practice. The Wound Ostomy Continence Nurses (WOCN) Society began in 1968 with a mission to promote educational, clinical and research opportunities to advance the practice and guide the delivery of expert health care to individuals with wound, ostomy, and continence issues (Corbett, 2012). After 50 years, it is considered the gold standard for certification, with more than 6500 board-certified nurses worldwide. The Association for the Advancement of Wound Care (AAWC) is a large interprofessional wound care organization with a mission to advance the care of patients with and at risk for wounds. The Wound Healing Society (WHS) advocates for the scientific advancement of wound healing. The National Pressure Injury Advisory Panel (NPIAP) participated in the development of international pressure injury guidelines whose language has entered the regulatory space. All of these organizations develop evidence-based clinical practice guidelines to support the specialty.

Clinical practice guidelines are "systematically developed statements to assist practitioner and patient decisions about appropriate healthcare for specific clinical circumstances" (Institute of Medicine, 2011a, 2011b) Evidence-based practice guidelines decrease unwanted variation in practice which translates to improved quality and safety. Specific examples are listed in Box 6.2. Developed through a standardized GRADE process, many wound-related CPGs can be found on professional society websites, in published literature and in guideline repositories such as ECRI. Incorporation of the patient perspective into clinical practice guideline

---

BOX 6.2 Benefits of Clinical Practice Guidelines

- Promote interventions of proven benefit
- Discourage ineffective or potentially harmful interventions
- Reduce unnecessary variation in practice
- Define disease performance measures
- Lessen disparities
- Empower consumer
- Influence public policy
- Define high-value care

Data from Murad, M. H. (2017). Clinical Practice Guidelines: A Primer on Development and Dissemination. *Mayo Clinic Proceedings, 92*(3), 423–433.

---

development is now a standard. Application of clinical practice guidelines with resulting evidence of improved outcomes has been published in many journals.

Licensure and Certification Support Wound Quality

Another safety net to support quality health care is through licensure and certification. The public relies on educational institutions and licensing bodies to ensure the competence of individual clinicians, such as nurses. Nursing professionals undergo rigorous training and pass licensing examinations to assure a basic level of skill and knowledge, but not all who have successfully passed these exams are competent. Professional competency is a fundamental concept in nursing, which has a direct relationship with quality of patient care. The American Nurses Association position statement on Professional Role Competence states:

> *"The public has a right to expect registered nurses to demonstrate professional competence throughout their careers. ANA believes the registered nurse is individually responsible and accountable for maintaining professional competence. The ANA further believes that it is the nursing profession's responsibility to shape and guide any process for assuring nurse competence. Regulatory agencies define minimal standards for regulation of practice to protect the public. The employer is responsible and accountable to provide an environment conducive to competent practice. Assurance of competence is the shared responsibility of the profession, individual nurses, professional organizations, credentialing and certification entities, regulatory agencies, employers, and other key stakeholders" (ANA, 2014).*

Institutional annual review and nursing peer review programs provide evaluation of the appropriateness and quality of care performed. State Nursing Licensing Boards respond to patient and health care professional complaints about negligence or unprofessional behavior. Individual State Boards of Nursing require specific continuing education requirements for Registered Nurses and Advanced Practice Nurses.

National nursing board certification provides another layer of protection for the public. The validation of a clinicians' specialty knowledge, such as through a nationally accredited certifying organization, signifies a level of expertise that implies quality (Summers & Bickford, 2017). The link between nursing specialty certification and quality care has been demonstrated in the literature. For example, Boyle, Bergquist-Beringer, and Cramer (2017) found a significant relationship between hospitals that employed Certified wound nurses and decreased pressure injury rates. A message to consumers from the Wound Ostomy Continence Nursing Certification Board (2020) states:

"Board certification demonstrates that your nurse has an ongoing, personal commitment to specialty education and professional growth that leads to quality patient care" (WOCNCB, 2020).

Board recertification processes require demanding levels of professional growth portfolio accomplishments and/or testing. The objectives of certification and recertification are to maintain excellence in a specialty, thereby constantly elevating the level of quality care provided to a population. Wound care specialists who maintain educational, licensure and certification requirements are contributing to the promotion of quality health care delivery for acute and chronic wound patients. There are several pathways to wound certification available to many levels of clinicians and sales professionals, Table 6.6 lists important considerations when choosing a wound certification program.

Nursing education programs at all levels now have required curriculum in quality and safety, known as the Quality and Safety Education for Nurses (QSEN)

(Cronenwett et al., 2007). Developing a health care workforce that attains quality competencies prelicensure will eventually produce a collective mindfulness of "quality-driven healthcare" (NAHQ, 2018). The six domains of competencies critical to quality and safety practice are listed in Box 6.3. Wound care practitioners from all backgrounds should consider the effective application of these six domains to improve care delivery, enhance outcomes and prevent harm.

The Role of the Consumer in Quality and Safety

The relationship between patients and health care providers has shifted from a paternalistic view toward a full partnership, characterized by more active involvement by the patient and family. "Person centered care" is a concept acknowledging the significant role that consumers play in their own health care experience. A growing body of evidence shows that improving the consumer experience and developing partnerships with patients is linked to improved

---

BOX 6.3 Quality and Safety Education for Nurses (QSEN) Competencies (QSEN)

- Patient Centered Care
- Teamwork and Collaboration
- Evidence-Based Practice
- Quality Improvement
- Safety
- Informatics

Data from Cronenwett, L., Sherwood, G., Barnsteiner J., Disch, J., Johnson, J., Mitchell, P., Sullivan, D., Warren, J. (2007). Quality and safety education for nurses. *Nursing Outlook, 55*(3), 122–131.

TABLE 6.6	Considerations for Choosing a Wound Certification Program
Accreditation	• Is the credentialing organization accredited by an independent, national certifying body? • Does the certifying organization require coursework by an accredited program?
Examination	• Is the exam created by a panel of content experts? • Is there a preparation course for the examination? • What is the passing rate? • What is the certification duration? • What is the recertification process? Frequency? Costs?
Role Specificity	• Is the certification aligned with specific wound role delineations? • What are the eligibility criteria for the certification? • Is this certification available to licensed professionals or "one size fits all"? • What is the perceived value of this certification by potential employers? Check on requirements for specific certifications based on job role.
Experience/ Preceptorship	• Have you had the minimum experience required to meet the eligibility criteria for the certification? • Does the certification require clinical preceptorship hours or experience? • For your professional development, do you need hands-on training with a preceptor to acquire the knowledge, skills, and expertise required for this specialty?
Required Course Work	• Is there required coursework or a preparation course associated with the certification? Does it offer CE/CME hours? • Is it available online or in-person? • What are the costs associated with each mode of study?
Ethical Considerations	• Once certified from this organization, can the public trust that you have attained the knowledge, skills and expertise to be called a specialist?

health outcomes. Health care leaders are systematically partnering with patient and family members in improvement efforts and research priorities. Nonprofit and governmental agencies have recruited consumer stakeholders to their advisory boards.

Health care policy has endorsed person-centered care approaches by inclusion in value-based metrics. For example, CMS uses the Hospital Consumer Assessment of Healthcare Providers and Systems (HCAHPS) survey to measure patients' perceptions of their hospital experience. Questions about nursing responsiveness to toileting needs, pain management, and patient education have direct links to wound care services delivery in the acute care setting (Checklist 6.1).

Public reporting is the practice of measuring and transparently reporting clinical outcomes. The promise of public reporting speculates that consumers will choose higher quality performing providers and market forces will drive improved patient outcomes (Romanelli, Fuchshuber, Stulberg, et al., 2019). Several organizations have undertaken complex scoring methods to produce rating systems to inform the public about safety measures; examples are provided in Table 6.7. Analysis of consumer shifts related to public reporting is still unclear, though these tools do appear to be incentivizing health care organizations to improve quality (Saghafian & Hopp, 2019).

Consumer reporting of adverse events is another mechanism for engaging the public in health care quality. State health departments, CMS and the AHRQ, have recognized that patients' reports of safety events have complemented information that is reported by institutions and providers. The consumer perspective has contributed to an improved understanding of patient safety and assisted in the detection of patterns associated with medical errors or health system failures.

The consumer perception of pressure injuries and chronic wound care has been explored in the literature. Patients living with chronic wounds express desire for shared decision making with their providers, and a goal for living a "normal independent" life while receiving appropriately skilled care for their wounds (Corbett & Ennis, 2014). Hospitalized patients may know that they need to perform certain behaviors to prevent pressure injury, though their adherence may be affected by discomfort and the partnership with their caregivers (McInnes, Chaboyer, Murray, Allen, & Jones, 2014). Patient refusal of preventive care in facilities that are financially penalized for pressure injury outcomes creates tension in the therapeutic relationship and invokes bioethics discussion (Caplan, 2012; Sharp, Schulz Moore, & McLaws, 2019).

The visually disturbing nature of pressure injuries to patients and families is compounded by the regulatory perception that all wounding is preventable. Despite significant "tort reform" efforts, litigation over pressure injuries remains common in both acute and long-term settings, resulting in frequent and costly judgments (Fife, Yankowsky, Ayello, et al., 2010). The notion of skin failure and "gap-free" adverse events pressure injuries is real in clinical practice but, currently only has a regulatory definition in the skilled nursing setting (Ayello et al., 2019). Because of these social trends, wound care practitioners need to balance sensitivity to consumer views with legal and regulatory realities and adapt practice accordingly.

National Quality Strategy and Measures Across Health Care Settings

Provisions laid out in overlapping health care law have required the alignment of federal, state, local agencies with private sector quality agencies to ensure a national strategy

TABLE 6.7 Resource Guide to Selected Public Facing Health Care Quality Metrics

Metric	Organization	Description
Hospital Compare—Quality Star Ratings Nursing Home Compare Patient Experience Star Rating https://www.medicare.gov/ hospitalcompare/search.html	Center for Medicare and Medicaid Services	Up to 60 quality measures in seven categories
Hospital Safety Grade https://www.hospitalsafetygrade.org/	Leapfrog Group	Composite safety grade A-F
Best Hospital Rankings Best Children's Hospital Rankings Best Hospitals by Specialty Rankings https://health.usnews.com/ best-hospitals/rankings	US News and World Report	Structure, process, outcome, and patient experience composite score
Top Hospitals Specialty Excellence Awards Patient Safety Ratings and Excellence Awards Provider Star Ratings https://www.healthgrades.com/	Healthgrades	Public quality measures and data bases

for quality improvements in health care. In the United States, a "cross-setting" strategy was developed as the AHRQ National Quality Strategy. The program now includes the Acute Care HAC Reduction Program, Hospital Readmission Reduction Program, Value-Based Purchasing programs, the Home Health Quality Reporting Programs, Post-Acute Care Quality Reporting Program, and provider Quality Payment Programs. All of these programs are tied to reimbursement penalty (or incentives). Private health care insurers have followed suit to require quality metrics for payment. The CMS Meaningful Measures framework (https://cms.gov, 2022) was designed to demonstrate how quality outcomes for beneficiaries are aligned with key quality indicators, CMS programs and NQF measures. Checklist 6.2 lists high priority areas for quality measurement and improvement to improve outcomes for patients, their families, and providers.

The overall CMS strategy for pressure injury reduction includes "harmonized" measures that can be implemented and collected using standardized data elements across health care settings (see Table 6.3). Pressure injuries migrate with patients across health care settings, regardless of where they begin. Therefore, "cross-setting" measures aim to facilitate implementation of best practices in each setting and reflect coordinated care (Schwartz, Nguyen, Swinson, Thaker, & Bernard, 2013). Ideally, the measures should account for the trajectory of care points where the development, worsening or healing of pressure injuries may be mitigated. In reality, there remain persistent challenges in following pressure injury occurrences by administrative claims data across sites of care (Squitieri et al., 2018). See below further discussion on the wound specialist's role in determination of present on admission pressure injuries.

In summary, regulatory policy impacting wound care has evolved from a multitude of driving forces in the government, public and professional sectors. No single law or endeavor is responsible for the focus of wound metrics in the national quality conversation. Only highlights have been discussed, though it is apparent that many decades of thoughtful policy make up the current patient protections. The prevention of

pressure injury is at the forefront of quality and safety concern. The wound care specialist must keep well-informed on shifting regulatory developments and appreciate the origins and trajectory of policy impacting practice.

Measuring for Improvement

The desire to continuously evaluate performance and adopt change is the core of improvement science. Pragmatic approaches to improvement in quality and productivity have been developed by business and industries throughout the world. Now the adoption of quality improvement practice has become standard operating procedure in health care. Government regulation and penalties have become the carrot and the stick approach to quality, though practitioners and leaders innately want health care to be safer and more effective. Quality improvement has been defined as "the use of data to monitor outcomes of care processes and use improvement methods to design and test changes to continuously improve the quality and safety of healthcare systems" (QSEN, 2017). There are numerous quality improvement approaches and philosophies based on the measurement of performance. Quality improvement is aimed at the prevention, reduction, and elimination of harm, but also the search for innovation and breakthrough improvements that contribute to better outcomes. The wound specialist aims to advance performance toward excellence with their specialty leadership and the application of improvement science.

Models of Quality Measurement

Florence Nightingale was the earliest advocate for the use of data collection to measure safe and effective health care. While serving in the Crimean War in 1858, she developed statistical graphs to summarize the causes of mortality and used data to enable health care reform in the British military. Nightingale's view that rigorous data collection yields "a uniform record of facts from which to deduce statistical results" (Nightingale, 1859) was a forerunner of the modern disease registry. Her analysis of the interaction between multiple factors and the economics of care provided early vision and leadership in quality. The wound care specialist role in every setting involves data collection on pressure injuries and wound outcomes.

A physician leader who contributed to the field of healthcare quality was Dr. Avedis Donabedian. Donabedian suggested that health care quality measures should be organized around three key points: structures, processes, and outcomes (Donabedian, 1966). The theory is that the right structure will support the right processes which, in turn, will result in desired patient outcomes. It is not enough to measure only end point outcomes. Quality measures should be developed to capture all three dimensions to fully assess the problem. Wound care specialists can consider the Donabedian dimensions of a pressure injury prevention and treatment program and plan quality measures arising from each domain (Table 6.8).

W. Edwards Deming and Walter Shewhart are known as founders of improvement science. Deming's work with

---

CHECKLIST 6.2 Meaningful Measures: High Priority Areas for Quality Measurement and Improvement

✓ Promote effective communication and coordination of care
✓ Promote effective prevention and treatment of chronic disease
✓ Work with communities to promote best practices of healthy living
✓ Make care affordable
✓ Make care safer by reducing harm, cost in the delivery of care
✓ Strengthen person and family engagement as partners in their care

https://www.cms.gov/Medicare/Quality-Initiatives-Patient-Assessment-Instruments/QualityInitiativesGenInfo/MMF/General-info-Sub-Page. Accessed 03/07/2023.

TABLE 6.8 Wound-Related Key Performance Indicators Categorized by Donabedian Framework

Dimension	Key Performance Indicators
Structures (e.g., tools, resources, organizational components)	Adequacy of wound care supplies Wound Team (access to certified specialists) Designated Unit-based Skin Champions Nursing Leadership Support Technology Supplies, Resources, Budget Specialty Beds Rehabilitation Team Advanced Dressings Orthotics Devices Compression Modalities
Processes (e.g., activities that connect patients, caregivers, providers, and staff)	Electronic Health Record/Optimized Nurse Driven Protocols Admission Skin Assessments Risk Assessment Care Planning Interprofessional Communication Internal and External Benchmarking Evidence-Based Guidelines Nutritional Supplement Protocols Consultation Processes Clinical Documentation/Coding Institutional Throughput
Outcomes (e.g., results)	Pressure Ulcer/Injury Harm Frequency (Prevalence, Incidence) Pressure Ulcer/Injury Severity (Stages, Location) Medical Devices Causing Harm (Stages, Location, Type) Discreet Populations With Pressure Ulcer/Injury Critical Care vs Noncritical Care Hospital-Acquired Infections Wound Infection Rates Readmission Rates Patient Satisfaction Regulatory Penalties Healing Rates Post-Acute Resource Utilization

Donabedian, A. (1966). Evaluating the quality of medical care. *The Milbank Memorial Fund Quarterly, 44*(Suppl. 3), 166-206. Reprinted in Milbank Q. 2005;83(4):691–729.

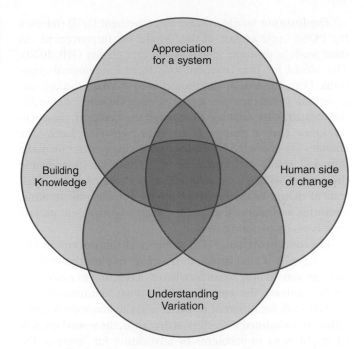

Fig. 6.3 Deming system of profound knowledge.

interrelated dimensions as a lens to view the organization. Cultivating a "systems thinking" approach will support the wound specialist in quality improvement efforts. Shewart's concepts of variation stated that one should not react to each observation, but rather plot data over time and observe patterns (Langley et al., 2009).

Quality leaders often use the Plan-Do-Study-Act (PDSA) model to guide projects. The concept of PDSA is based on the scientific method of creating a hypothesis, doing an experiment, collecting data, and evaluating the results. This model, attributed to Deming and Shewhart, provides a methodology for repeated cycles of change that produce measurement and knowledge to power the next cycle, leading to improved outcomes. An example of successive PDSA cycles to solve the problem of device-related pressure injury is included in Fig. 6.4.

Japanese industries in the 1950s helped to pioneer the Total Quality Management approach. Drawing from psychology, economics, and social theories, his "System of Profound Knowledge" detailed four key components that allow individuals to gain a clear picture of the system they are trying to improve (see Fig. 6.3). Advocating "systems thinking" as an approach for developing effective change, he promoted these

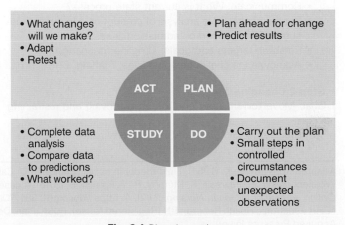

Fig. 6.4 Plan do study act.

The Institute for Healthcare Improvement (IHI) endorses the PDSA cycle as part of the "Model for Improvement" in their work to promote global health care quality (IHI, 2020). The Model for Improvement asks three fundamental questions. First, the aim of the project is established through the question, "what are we trying to accomplish?" Secondly, the measures are established through the question, "how will we know that a change is an improvement?" Lastly, the changes are predicted by asking "what changes can we make that will result in improvement?" These questions frame the project which is accomplished by rapid cycles of small tests of change using the PDSA model. Establishing the aims, measures and planned changes for an improvement project are necessary planning steps.

The concept of change is fundamental to improvement. The old adage, "If it ain't broke, don't fix it" implies that making changes should only be undertaken as a reaction to a problem. To the contrary, the wound specialist must continuously proactively look for different or better ways to accomplish goals. Often overwhelmed with clinical demands, the wound specialist might react to problems by advocating for "more of the same": more staff, equipment, and time. Using the science of improvement, we seek to develop change that fundamentally alters the system to achieve better performance. Lewin's (1951) classic theory of change posits that an assessment of forces, both driving and restraining, is necessary throughout the change process. Example of the application of change theory to a wound-related quality improvement project is illustrated in Box 6.4. Wound specialists need to be cognizant of forces in the change process that may impact the success of an improvement project. The key to quality efforts is to examine the current state, identify possible changes, design or redesign systems, implement change and eventually spread improvement (Langley et al., 2009).

Organizational Quality Structure and Collaboration

Wound care specialists collaborate with several levels of safety and quality leadership in health care settings to achieve effective change and improvement. At a clinical level, relationships with interprofessional team members, case coordinators, clinical documentation, and coding specialists are critical for the accurate accounting of wound type and attribution required for regulatory and value-based outcome measurement. Managers, Educators and Clinical Leaders coordinate with wound specialists to determine priorities for orientation and continuing education. Informatics specialists' partner with wound specialists to optimize electronic health documentation vital to accurate wound outcome measurement. Feedback of wound-related surveillance data to clinical departments and institutes provides targets for improvement projects. Validation of pressure injury severity by the wound specialists is vital for accurate internal and external quality benchmarking and regulatory compliance.

At an organizational level, wound care specialists serve as subject matter experts in wounds and pressure injury. They partner with trained Healthcare Quality Professionals (HQPs) and facilitators who possess specific competencies in quality and safety (NAHQ, 2018). Quality leaders determine the overall quality strategic plan for an organization, including ongoing requirements and focused improvements based on the internal and external stakeholders. To achieve quality capability and goals, health care organizations often ascribe a specific quality operating model, such as Lean or Six Sigma (Wojciechowski, Pearsall, Murphy, & French,

---

BOX 6.4   Implementation of Two-RN Admission Skin Assessment using Lewin's Three-Step Model for Planned Change

Step 1 Unfreezing
Goal: Increase driving forces; decrease restraining forces for change
- Convene: Stakeholders/working group
- Educate: Review latest literature and clinical practice guideline on admission skin assessment best practice
- Communicate: What is current state process?
- Set the scene: Data analysis of present-on-admission pressure injuries missed on admission assessment
- Establish targets and goals: Timeline for change
- Acknowledge challenges/obstacles: Staffing, EHR*, Time

Step 2 Changing/Moving
Goal: Move toward new equilibrium of driving and restraining forces
- Brainstorm, Simulate and Try: Review risks and benefits
- Pilot PDSA* cycle: Measure

- Role Model: Unit-based Skin Champions
- Implement: Start new process on two units; measure; spread
- Coach/Mentor: Nursing Leaders, Nurse Educators
- Show Improvement: Develop transparent dashboards

Step 3 Refreezing/Sustain
Goal: Sustain the change
- Monitor Key Performance Indicators: POA-PI, HAPI*, Care Planning
- Evaluate Process: Meet target of 100%
- Realize Benefit > Barriers: Efficiency with EHR[a] entry
- Retrain: New accountability standard for admission skin assessment
- Socialize new employees: Orientation standard
- Reward: Unit achieves lower pressure injury rates

Adapted from Lewin, K. (1951). Field theory in social science. In D. Cartwright (Ed.), Selected theoretical papers. New York: Harper & Row; Wojciechowski, E., Pearsall, T., Murphy, P., & French, E. (2016). A case review: Integrating Lewin's theory with lean system approach for change. *Online Journal of Issues in Nursing, 21*(2), 4. https://doi.org/10.3912/OJIN.Vol21Noo2Man04.
*EHR (Electronic Health Record); RN (Registered Nurse); PDSA (Plan, Do Study, Act); POA-PI (Present on Admission Pressure Injury); HAPI (Hospital Acquired Pressure Injury).

2016; Donovan, Manta, Goldsack, and Collins (2016). Knowledge of quality reporting structures and the flow of wound-related data is an important competency for the wound specialist. Alignment with the organizational strategy, mission, priorities, and methodology for wound care-related quality improvement efforts is essential.

Monitoring Pressure Injury Prevalence and Incidence

Measurement of the target phenomena is critical to understanding it and improving it. "You can't manage what you can't measure" is a quote often attributed to Peter Drucker, an international business management consultant. In any sector—business, manufacturing, health care—a clearly established metric for success is required to quantify progress and adjust the process to produce the desired outcome. Pressure injury surveillance has historically focused on intermittent measurement (quarterly prevalence) or adverse event (incident report) data, both important, but as stand-alone, incomplete measures of the problem. Similar to infectious disease monitoring, the continuous surveillance of pressure injury occurrence in a population is critical to improvement efforts. For best public health practice, the WHO encourages the "continuous, systematic collection, analysis and interpretation of health-related data needed for planning, implementation, and evaluation" (World Health Organization, 2020). The revised international guideline from the European Pressure Ulcer Advisory Panel, National Pressure Injury Advisory Panel and Pan Pacific Pressure Injury Alliance (EPUAP/NPIAP/PPPIA, 2019) states that best practice is to "use a rigorous methodological design and consistently measure variables when conducting and reporting pressure injury" (p. 35). The AHRQ Preventing Pressure Ulcers in Hospitals toolkit (2014) advocates the regular ongoing assessment of pressure injury rates and practices.

There is no uniform requirement for measuring pressure injuries in every health care setting. It is suggested that both

components of measurement should be addressed: routine surveillance and quality improvement metrics. Depending on the care setting, the minimum required data must satisfy regulatory reporting measures (see Table 6.3). For improvement efforts, the program should set up additional measures to drive improvement (Crawford, Skeath, & Whippy, 2015; Harrison, Mackey, & Friedberg, 2008; Polancich, Williamson, Poe, Armstrong, & Vander Noot, 2019; Zaratkiewicz et al., 2010). Following from Donabedian framework (see Table 6.8) for a comprehensive pressure injury program to advance, regular monitoring will minimally support an improvement effort (Agency for Healthcare Research and Quality, 2014; Agency for Healthcare Research and Quality (AHRQ), 2014). The wound care specialist relies on guidance from quality improvement science, professional societies, and regulatory policy to determine surveillance standards.

Measurement of pressure injury performance is more than just avoidance of penalty; it is the most direct measure of success in preventing harm. If the rate is low or improving, then the organization is likely doing a good job and can continue to look for opportunities to drill down to zero occurrences. If the rate is high or increasing, the data will help to support change initiatives, design alternative processes, monitor progress and sustain improvements. Checklist 6.3 list of reasons to measure pressure injuries.

Formulas to calculate prevalence and incidence data are listed in Table 6.9. Table 6.10 gives examples of how the data

CHECKLIST 6.3 Why Measure Pressure Ulcer/Injury Rates and Practices?

✓ Are there areas in which care can be improved?
✓ Are you meeting your aims?
✓ Are changes in practice improving outcomes?
✓ Are you sustaining improvements?
✓ If you don't know where you are, how do you know if you are improving?

TABLE 6.9 Formulas Used to Calculate Prevalence and Incidence

Pressure Injury Point Prevalence (%)	$\frac{\text{Number of patients with a PI at a specific point in time}}{\text{Total number of patients in the study population at a specific point in time}} \times 100$
Pressure Injury Cumulative Incidence (%)	$\frac{\text{Number of patients developing a new PI during a specific time period}}{\text{Total number of patients in the study population over a specific time period}} \times 100$
Pressure Injury Incidence Density per 1000 Patient Days	$\frac{\text{Number of patients developing a new PI}}{1000 \text{ patient days}}$
Facility Acquired Pressure Injury Rate (%)	$\frac{(\text{Number of patients with PI at a time point}) - (\text{Number of patients with PI on admission})}{(\text{Number in population at time point}) - (\text{Number with PI on admission})} \times 100$

PI, pressure injury.

Anderson, J., Langemo, D., Hanson, D., Thompson, A., & Hunter, S. M. (2013). Planning, conducting and interpreting prevalence and incidence for the wound practitioner. *Advances in Skin & Wound Care, 26*(1), 35–42; Agency for Healthcare Research and Quality. (2014). *Preventing pressure ulcers in hospitals.* Rockville: Agency for Healthcare Research and Quality. https://www.ahrq.gov/patient-safety/settings/hospital/resource/pressureulcer/tool/index.htm. Accessed July 12, 2020; Agency for Healthcare Research and Quality (AHRQ). (2014). The Patient Safety and Quality Improvement Act of 2005. Content last reviewed October 2014. Rockville, MD. https://www.ahrq.gov/policymakers/psoact.html. Accessed November 2, 2020; European Pressure Ulcer Advisory Panel, National Pressure Injury Advisory Panel and Pan Pacific Pressure Injury Alliance. Prevention and Treatment of Pressure Ulcers/Injuries. (2019). In Haesler, E. (Ed.). *Clinical Practice Guideline. The International Guideline.* EPUAP/NPIAP/PPPIA.

TABLE 6.10   Use of Prevalence and Incidence Data

Measure	Data Usage	Examples
Prevalence	Health care planning and resource utilization	• RNs needed • Specialty beds needed • Wound specialists
Incidence	Reflects risk factors and prevention efforts	• OR time • Length of stay • Repositioning

can be useful. Table 6.11 outlines steps with rationale for conducting a prevalence incidence study. Accurate prevalence and incidence measurement of pressure injury occurrence is vital to understanding the phenomena and improving patient safety. The counting of pressure injuries should be carried out in a precise way to provide robust data that truly reflects the population risk and care provided. Published reports suggest that prevalence and incidence methodology is often confused, the processes for conducting pressure injury studies are wrought with error in identification, classification, and collection, and that erroneous comparisons of

TABLE 6.11   Steps and Rationale for Conducting a Prevalence/Incidence Study

Steps	Rationale
1. Establish leadership support	• Alignment with organizational goals • Enhance project success • Plan resources, access, scheduling
2. Determine data to be collected	• Clarify purpose: Regulatory, quality, research • Plan data destination and distribution • Explore benchmarks: Internal/external • Match measures to methodology
3. Define the population	• Establish inclusion/exclusion criteria • Determine psychiatry, obstetric, outpatient, emergency population exclusions • Consistent denominator for comparisons
4. Recruit a team of data collectors	• Launch meeting schedule, membership • Determine training needs • Plan adequate size of team • Consider interprofessional group • Optimize validity of audit data • Eliminate bias • Assure clinical competency of skin examination • Strategize ongoing continuing education
5. Determine data collection method	• Explore national benchmarking organizations • Use standardized collection tool • Seek meaningful peer benchmark groupings • Consider resources for fee vs voluntary options • Paper vs electronic demographic capture • Determine definitions, data sources
6. Time frame for collection	• Plan out quarterly, monthly, weekly • Optimize time of day for best patient access • Block out schedules to prioritize • Remind and encourage team
7. Access reliable data for denominator	• Optimize EHR functionality • Establish demographic feed, patient days data
8. Analyze the data	• Plan for data review for errors • Determine data storage • Enlist statistical analyses expertise • Interpretation of data • Comparison to meaningful benchmarks • Establish confidence intervals
9. Report the data	• Determine internal and external data flow • Bring data full circle for optimal benefit • Feedback from stakeholders
10. Plan change	• Use data to formulate actionable change • Improve patient safety and quality

Adapted from Anderson, J., Langemo, D., Hanson, D., Thompson, A., & Hunter, S. M. (2013). Planning, conducting and interpreting prevalence and incidence for the wound practitioner. *Advances in Skin & Wound Care, 26*(1), 35–42.

outcome studies often result (Fletcher, Crook, & Harris, 2013; Baharestani et al., 2009; Moore, Avsar, Moore, Patton, & O'Connor, 2019). Conducting prevalence and incidence studies requires training, planning, and execution of a standardized method to achieve valid and reliable results.

Generally accepted definitions of prevalence and incidence follow from epidemiological principles (Rothman, 2012). Prevalence is a measure of a condition or disease status, as being either present or absent, in a population at a point in time. Prevalence may reflect a single point in time, called *point prevalence.* An example of pressure injury point prevalence is the measurement of the number of people with a pressure injury (numerator), in a defined population (denominator), at a single point in time, for example, the first day of the month. *Period prevalence* is a measure of the number of people with a pressure injury (numerator), in a defined population (denominator), who have a pressure injury over a particular time period, such as over a number of days or weeks. Period prevalence should be reported with the specified time period. Both prevalence measures count the number of people with the condition, not the number of pressure injuries in the population. Prevalence measures include all people with pressure injuries, including those who were admitted with pressure injury and those who developed it after admission. Prevalence can be calculated for an individual unit or an overall facility. Prevalence is expressed as a percentage.

Prevalence measurement is intended to identify the size of the problem. Prevalence does not measure disease onset, location, or duration (e.g., when the pressure injuries started, or if they are acquired inside or outside of the organization), it is a measure of disease status at a point in time. Prevalence data are useful for measuring the burden of pressure injuries and the scope of the problem in a given setting, especially if the target population requires special medical attention or services. For example, if the prevalence of pressure injuries in Noblecare Hospital is 15%, this will help to predict the need for specialty beds, wound care supplies, and wound care specialists at that institution. Attribution of cause cannot be determined with prevalence data. Prevalence provides a useful "snapshot" of the pressure injury burden but cannot determine the quality of the preventive care.

Incidence is the measurement of the new cases of a disease or condition in a given period of time (Rothman, 2012). Therefore, in the case of pressure injury incidence, it includes only new cases developed after admission. Incidence is used to describe a rate at which new cases occur and reflects direct evidence of the quality of care. Quality improvement efforts should focus on the reduction of incidence rates. There are two common measures of incidence used in pressure injury quality evaluation. *Cumulative incidence* is the proportion of a specified population that develops a new pressure injury within a specified time period (weeks or months). Cumulative incidence reflects the likelihood that a patient who is free of pressure injury will develop one (or more) over a given period of time. It is essentially a measurement of risk, and therefore reflects the effectiveness of prevention measures. *Incidence density* is another measure of pressure injury incidence, often used in post acute settings where patients reside for long periods of time, as it accounts for length of stay. Incidence density measures the number of people developing a new pressure ulcer (numerator), divided by the number of patient care days in the facility. It is also useful when comparing various units in a large facility because it controls for length of stay. When reporting incidence, the number of individuals affected is counted, not the number of pressure injuries experienced by each individual. Therefore, pressure injuries are recorded as an unduplicated count per reporting period.

Facility-acquired pressure injury rates are often determined in conjunction with point prevalence studies. After pressure injury prevalence is determined, then admission documentation is examined for each injury to determine if it was present on admission (POA). If the wound was not documented on admission, then the pressure injury is considered facility acquired. Facility-acquired pressure injury rates can reflect prevention protocol effectiveness and are less time consuming to conduct than incidence studies (European Pressure Ulcer Advisory Panel, National Pressure Injury Advisory Panel, and Pan Pacific Pressure Injury Alliance. Prevention and Treatment of Pressure Ulcers/Injuries, 2019). The accuracy of the admission skin assessment is critical to be able to determine POA status.

Timeframes for completion of admission skin assessment vary depending on regulatory and institutional policy. Clinical practice guidelines promote skin assessment "as soon as possible after admission" to a health care service (European Pressure Ulcer Advisory Panel, National Pressure Injury Advisory Panel and Pan Pacific Pressure Injury Alliance. Prevention and Treatment of Pressure Ulcers/Injuries, 2019). For the home care Oasis tool, clinicians are encouraged to complete the skin assessment "as close to the SOC/ROC as possible" (Centers for Medicare & Medicaid Services, 2023). The purpose of a prompt and accurate skin assessment is to determine risk assessment and provide appropriate care for the patient. As pressure injuries can progress rapidly, especially in the acute patient with multiple co-morbidities, determination of skin status on admission is critical. Wound specialists should become familiar with specific regulatory requirements for skin assessment completion in applicable practice settings. For example, in the acute care setting, provider documentation of pressure injury, presence as either POA or hospital acquired, is required for clinical documentation and coding.

Consistency in methodology for conducting prevalence and incidence data collection is critical to providing the most reliable and valid data. Table 6.12 describes inclusion/exclusion criteria along with important considerations for collecting valid and reliable data. If an institution participates in a standardized database nursing quality measurement program, such as the National Database of Nursing Quality Indicators (NDNQI), detailed methodology supports the integrity of the data collection. The program provides hospitals with unit-level performance comparison reports to state, national, and regional percentile distributions. Another benchmarking program, the Hill-Rom International Pressure Ulcer study, was previously described.

TABLE 6.12 Considerations for Collecting Valid and Reliable Pressure Injury Data

Inclusion/Exclusion Criteria	Considerations
Population definition	Setting Inpatient/outpatient Exclusions by diagnosis Hospice/palliative care Risk status Patient refusals
Time period	Hospital-acquired vs present on admission Define methods and time frames Prospective vs retrospective
Data sources	Clinical assessment Electronic health record capture Administrative data (i.e., ICD-10) Patient/family/caregiver self-report
Data calculation method	Method is aligned with metric Compare to benchmarks with similar methodology Statistical support
Staging	Use of standardized definitions Determination of stages and wounds included/excluded: Stage 1, mucosal, device-related Stage at point-in-time considerations (i.e., deep tissue) Medical device related Wounds covered by nonremovable device Consistent rationale for exclusion
Avoidable/unavoidable	Follow regulatory definitions Not pertinent for all settings
Accuracy	Pressure vs nonpressure wound etiology Interrater reliability Expertise of clinical evaluators
Bias	Sponsor of database/study Conflict of interest issues Influence/fear of financial penalties Retribution from manager/director Reporting structures

Data from European Pressure Ulcer Advisory Panel, National Pressure Injury Advisory Panel and Pan Pacific Pressure Injury Alliance. Prevention and Treatment of Pressure Ulcers/Injuries. (2019). In E. Haesler (Ed.), Clinical Practice Guideline. The International Guideline. EPUAP/NPIAP/PPPIA; Baharestani, M. M., Black, J. M., Carville, K., Clark, M., Cuddigan, J. E., Sanada, H., et al. (2009). Dilemmas in measuring and using pressure ulcer prevalence and incidence an international consensus. *International Wound Journal, 6*(2), 97–104. https://doi.org/10.1111/j.1742-481X.2009.00593.x; Anderson, J., Langemo, D., Hanson, D., Thompson, A., & Hunter, S. M. (2013). Planning, conducting and interpreting prevalence and incidence for the wound practitioner. *Advances in Skin & Wound Care, 26*(1), 35–42; Zaratkiewicz, S., Whitney, J., Lowe, J., Taylor, S., O'Donnell, F., & Minton-Foltz, P. (2010). Development and implementation of a hospital-acquired pressure ulcer incidence tracking system and algorithm. *The Journal for Healthcare Quality, 32*(6), 44–51. https://doi.org/10.1111/j.1945-1474.2010.00076.x; Fletcher, J., Crook, H., & Harris, C. (2013). Monitoring pressure ulcer prevalence: A precise methodology. *Wounds UK, 9*(4), 48–53; Agency for Healthcare Research and Quality. (2014). *Preventing pressure ulcers in hospitals.* Rockville: Agency for Healthcare Research and Quality. https://www.ahrq.gov/patient-safety/settings/hospital/resource/pressureulcer/tool/index.htm. Accessed July 12, 2020; Agency for Healthcare Research and Quality (AHRQ). (2014). *The Patient Safety and Quality Improvement Act of 2005.* Content last reviewed October 2014. Rockville, MD. https://www.ahrq.gov/policymakers/psoact.html. Accessed November 2, 2020.

Prevalence and incidence data provide valuable evidence to drive quality improvement at a facility level, but also provide data for national and international policy decisions and research agendas. Standardization of definitions and collection methodology and determination of a "minimum dataset" for pressure injury monitoring would facilitate scaled investigation. As pressure injury is a threat to patient safety in worldwide health care settings, the establishment of large interoperable data bases and registries has been proposed (Gaspar, Collier, Marques, Ferreira, & de Matos, 2020; Moore, Soriano, & Pokorna, 2017).

Real-time Surveillance

Several authors have described the development and implementation of pressure injury tracking systems to support health care quality and safety. Zaratkiewicz et al. (2010) reported on a surveillance algorithm implemented in a large health care system. Pressure injury occurrence was triggered by frontline nurses, verified by certified wound nurses and then followed weekly. This resulted in earlier identification of pressure injury, a reduction in the number and severity of hospital-acquired pressure injuries and facilitated quality improvement and educational efforts. Examples of tracking tools for acute care and skilled nursing settings are included in Figs. 6.5 and 6.6.

Polancich et al. (2019) described an overhaul of the pressure injury reporting process at a large southeastern academic medical center. As a response to inaccurate pressure injury reports arising from EHR, they made changes to the wound ostomy continence (WOC) nurse workflow and created a "HAPI reporting platform." WOC nurses validated every pressure injury and subsequently only validated data populated the dashboard which tracked incidence, length of stay by stage, present on admission pressure injuries and AHRQ PSI-03 data with patient specific detail. They concluded that in an acute care setting, the pressure injury workflow should support data accuracy.

The digital transformation of health care data provides increasing opportunities for real time, or continuous, wound-related data capture for concurrent quality improvement. Advances in data mining, streaming analytics and machine learning algorithms provide actionable data to predict and monitor wounds in many settings (Cramer, Seneviratne, Sharifi, Ozturk, & Hernandez-Boussard, 2019). The transparency and timeliness of performance data facilitates safety dashboards and allows for timely interventions and evaluation. Real-time EHR reports can inform clinicians of high-risk patients, monitor wound healing rates, and gather incidence and prevalence data. Using electronic alerts for clinical decision support demonstrated positive outcome in a project in skilled nursing facilities (Agency for Healthcare Research and Quality, 2014; Agency for Healthcare Research and Quality [AHRQ], 2014). The alerts provided clinical knowledge and resident-specific information to inform clinicians to deliver resident care at appropriate times. As a result of this clinical decision support, the participating facilities saw a reduction in pressure injuries.

Sample Pressure Injury Prevalence Form—Acute Care

Unit	Bed	ID	Admit Date	Risk Score	Risk Score Within 8 h? Y/N	Skin Assess Within 8 h? Y/N	Prevention Bundle Started? Y/N	Support Surface? Y/N	Nutrition Consult? Y/N	Moisture Interventions? Y/N	Protective Dressing? Y/N	PI on Admit? Y/N	Stage of PI on Admit	Location of PI on Admit	PI Acquired after admit? Y/N	Stage of Acquired PI	Location of Acquired PI	Unit of Acquired PI

Fig. 6.5 Sample pressure injury data collection tool: acute care.

Sample Weekly Pressure Injury Flow Record
Skilled Nursing

Page#					Month/Year:				Floor/Unit:				
RM#	Resident	Date of Onset	FA Faculty Acquired CA Community Acquired	Stage	Site	Week 1 L×W×D	Week 2 L×W×D	Week 3 L×W×D	Week 4 L×W×D	Week 5 L×W×D	Progress I-Improving D-Deterior U-Unchanged	Comments: Current Interventions, Equipment, Supplements

Fig. 6.6 Sample pressure injury surveillance tool: skilled nursing facility.

Validation of accurate etiology, staging and wound origin attribution remain concerns for reliance solely on electronic capture (Alvey, Hennen, & Heard, 2012; Cox, Roche, & Gandhi, 2013; Levine, Ayello, Zulkowski, & Fogel, 2012; Zrelak et al., 2015). The saying, "garbage in, garbage out" is applicable to health care electronic records. If inaccurate wound data are entered into EHR, it will produce inaccurate output reports. Most organizations recognize the challenge of accurate pressure injury staging and develop some method of validation: dual-nurse skin assessment requirement, designated skin champions, certified wound nurse team, required provider cosignatures. These challenges underscore the role of the wound specialist to assure competent clinical wound practice for all clinicians in the practice setting. In addition to clinical skills and leadership, the wound specialist may benefit from competency in informatics to promote optimization of the EHR for wound quality.

Pressure injury data are used internally for quality improvement and it also flows outside the organization to external stakeholders. External stakeholders include regulatory agencies such as CMS and AHRQ as well as private insurance programs, state quality review organizations, and consumer organizations. For each of these data exports, it is imperative to provide data consistent with the request and inclusion/exclusion criteria. For example, the CMS uses administrative codes to determine the penalties for the Hospital Acquired Conditions program. AHRQ has used direct clinical data abstraction to determine harm as part of the Medicare Patient Safety Monitoring System (see above for descriptions of these programs). Published reports have shown wide variation in the rates calculated from these two methods (Meddings, 2015; Meddings, Reichert, Hofer, & McMahon, 2013). Health care institutions would benefit from creating workflow to verify and validate all quality metrics. This strategy involves the collaboration of a wide interprofessional team including clinical documentation specialists, clinicians, providers, statisticians, informaticists, financial leaders, and quality professionals (Fig. 6.7).

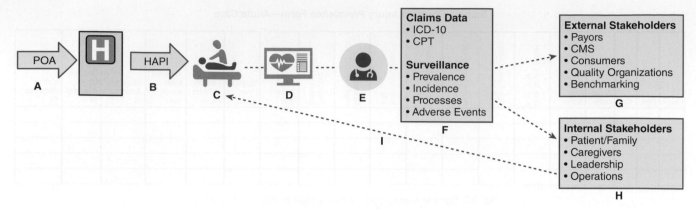

Fig. 6.7 Pressure injury data flow diagram.

Using Pressure Injury Data to Improve Patient Care

Prevalence and incidence data must be brought "full circle" and be analyzed and distributed in order to improve patient care. In addition to the targeted outcome "number" or rate obtained from the study, several other qualitative and quantitative metrics should be monitored or culled from the data as "key performance indicators." Metrics should be allocated to the work unit of pressure injury origin and displayed in graphics that are meaningful and actionable for the frontline clinician. A routine schedule of data dissemination creates the expectation for continuous improvement. These processes are essential to enable data-driven changes to improve patient outcomes (Fig. 6.8).

Dashboards are an efficient way of organizing critical quality oversight information and showing trends toward established goals. Benefits of visual dashboards include providing transparency, expectation setting, motivation, progress tracking, and engagement. Priorities and opportunities can be quickly observed. Dashboards can depict key metrics at the system, institution, service, unit, and provider level. Challenges of dashboards include ownership for maintenance, determination of audience, frequency and mode of

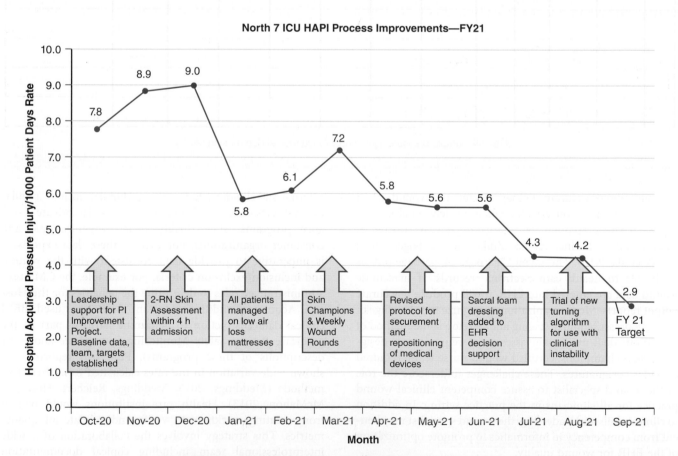

Fig. 6.8 Unit-based quality improvement efforts illustrated with rate decline.

distribution, mechanism for feedback on process changes associated with the metrics. Dashboard data should be tailored to the audience with the highest potential for benefit. For example, if the institutional dashboard is distributed monthly to the bedside clinicians but contains complex aggregate data that is not clearly actionable in their practice, data overload can occur. Various stakeholders have different levels of statistical knowledge, which impacts the type of information conveyed and level of detail necessary. Translation of dashboard metrics to maximize salience to the audience is necessary for quality impact.

Because of competing quality initiatives in health care, mangers and leaders will need to select specific quality projects or "drivers" to focus on during a time period. Nursing-sensitive indicators, such as falls and pressure injuries, tend to be monitored continuously with an eye on achieving zero occurrences. The continuous nature of these metrics can impact attention and devotion to active change projects. Identification of unit-based champions is one method for sustaining long-term quality improvement projects (Creehan, 2015). Skin champions can be local owners of wound-related quality metrics and serve to hard-wire the monitoring and sustainability of process changes as well as escalating of new issues.

The display of wound-related metrics can be simple or complex. Dashboards and graphs can be made with basic computer skills or produced with elaborate graphics by a high-level quality department. Figs. 6.9–6.14 are examples of basic dashboards. At a minimum, each work unit should know the number, severity and location of pressure injuries that occur under their care. In addition, they should be able to identify a target goal for improvement and know the

current status toward that goal. They should be able to identify the largest gaps in care related to the pressure injury events, to allow for focused improvement efforts.

Benchmarks

Wound specialists responsible for wound-related quality programs should keep abreast of the literature and clinical practice guidelines. With the rapid evolution of new evidence, this can be a daunting task. However, membership in a professional wound society and attendance at continuing education events will keep one informed of the specialty arena. Benchmarks can be found in several sources. Participation in a national database will provide institutional performance benchmarked against peer organizations (see above NDNQI, Hill-Rom IPUP). State health departments typically produce a transparent annual report of health care facility adverse events. Comparison of reportable adverse event performance against peer institutions provides one measure of benchmarking, albeit void of process learning. Statewide or regional collaborative improvement programs, often sponsored by hospital associations or PSROs, are an excellent way to compare practice and performance with area facilities. Identification and implementation of best practices are the cornerstones of the regional collaborative improvement model, which allows for a rapid assessment of relationships between process and outcomes (Share et al., 2011). Comparing institutional outcome performance in consumer facing websites such as those presented in Table 6.7 is another source of benchmarking. A literature review for studies, metanalyses or systematic reviews focused on outcomes in one type of practice site or patient population, may elucidate benchmarks by specialties such as Perioperative, Emergency Pediatrics, or

Noblecare Hospital—Quality & Safety Dashboard

		2020	2021	2021	2021					
Fiscal Year		Q4	Q1	Q2	Q3	FYTD	Threshold	Target	Stretch	Status
Quality	Pneumonia 30-day Readmission	24	32			56	140	132	126	
Safety	Serious Safety Events Rate Rolling					0.86	0.85	0.80	0.75	
Hospital Acquired Conditions	AHRQ PSI 90 Composite					0.79	0.90	0.80	0.70	
	Pressure Injury/1000 Pt Days Rate	1.25	1.56			1.41	1.50	1.20	1.00	
	AHRQ PSI -03 Pressure Injury	2	1			3	8	6	5	
	Observed/Expected Mortality									
Hospital Acquired Infections	CAUTI Number of Events									
	CLABSI Number of Events									
	Colon SSI – Number of Events									

Key
Worse Than Threshold/Target
At or Above Threshold/Below Target
At or Above Target/Below Stretch
At or Above Stretch

Fig. 6.9 Example of quality dashboard for an institution.

TABLE 6.13	Pressure Injury Data Collection in Specialty Populations and Settings
Population	**Considerations**

Peri-operative	• Benchmark: Pressure injury developing within 72 h after a surgical procedure may be attributed to periop setting (Primiano, Friend, McClure, et al., 2011).
	• Metric: Cumulative incidence rate
	• Surveillance: Cases discovered in postop settings
	• Action:
	  • Designate a Peri-op Skin Champion representative
	  • Perform a review of each occurrence
	  • Focus PDSA improvement opportunities

Emergency Departments	• Benchmark: Pressure injury develops in at-risk patients with >4 h length of stay in Emergency Departments (Dugaret et al., 2014).
	• Metric: Cumulative incidence rate
	• Surveillance: Cases discovered in inpatient areas or postacute settings
	• Action:
	  • Designate an Emergency Department Skin Champion representative
	  • Perform a review of each occurrence
	  • Focus PDSA improvement opportunities

Pediatric	• Benchmark: Pressure injury prevalence 1.4%, hospital-acquired pressure injury prevalence 1.1% (Razmus & Bergquist-Beringer, 2017)
	• Surveillance:
	  • Higher rates in critical care and rehabilitation
	  • Age-related increase in rate
	  • High use of medical devices
	• Action:
	  • Strong support for inclusion of children in routine pressure injury survey studies
	  • Advocate skin champion model in pediatric setting

Palliative Home Care	• Benchmark: Admission point prevalence 13.1%; cumulative incidence 13.0% (Artico et al., 2017) • Surveillance: High rates suggest this as a major factor in palliative care settings • Action: Focus on caregiver support for prevention

Palliative Care. Examples are provided in Table 6.13. When looking at current literature for benchmarks, it is important to carefully review the study population to determine generalizability of findings.

Culture of Safety

As stated in the introduction to this chapter, health care is in the midst of a cultural transformation. With a mission to ensure the most compassionate, complex, and technological care, this must be delivered while assuring the elimination of harm to our patients and the workforce. The development of a "culture of safety" in health care includes supporting institutions as "learning organizations," understanding the limits of human factors in error, and appreciating the need for transparent reporting mechanisms when things go wrong. Key elements in creating this culture include establishing safety as an organizational priority, fostering of teamwork, promoting patient involvement, valuing transparency and accountability (Berwick, Calkins, McCannon, & Hackbarth, 2006). Health care leaders are charged with creating the vision, engaging the board and establishing organizational behavior expectations for leaders (ACHE, 2017). Health care organizations routinely survey their workforce, using standardized tools, to take a pulse on the culture of safety climate

(Famolaro, Yount, Hare, et al., 2018). These data help to track changes and set priorities for training and education to support the attitudes and behaviors of a safe culture.

In a culture of safety, an important balance must be achieved between intolerance for unsafe behavior and avoidance of blame. The historical excessive focus on determination of blame with medical error, has led to concealing rather than reporting of error. When an error occurs, the emphasis should be on discovering what went wrong, not on who caused the problem. This is referred to as a "just culture" (Paradiso & Sweeney, 2019). Organizations typically have algorithms that determine questions to explore when a medical error occurs.

Another patient safety concept is that of high-reliability organizations (HRO). Highly reliable organizations, such as commercial aviation and nuclear power plants, operate under very stressful conditions, though manage to have few accidents. Health care has adopted the tenants of the HRO culture (Table 6.14). Pressure injury prevention is an example of a high-reliability process. An interprofessional team may focus on the reduction of harm from pressure injuries. Using evidence from the literature and clinical practice guidelines, the team constructs a pressure injury prevention bundle, a set of processes to be used consistently to prevent pressure injuries. If the processes are consistently applied by every

TABLE 6.14   Characteristics of High Reliability Organizations (HRO)

Characteristic	Elements	Example
Preoccupation With Failure	• Proactively identify high-risk activities and analyze all potential error points in processes • Be alert to "near-miss" events	• Anticoagulation therapy interactions with antibiotics
Reluctance to Simplify	• Recognize the complexity of work • Probe beyond the superficial for causes of failure	• Pressure Injury Prevention protocol has 10 components • Risk of "work arounds" • i.e., "forgot" to do dressing: what are the system factors: supply availability, unclear orders, hand-off report
Sensitivity to Operations	• Situational awareness of the environment	• Fatigue, interruptions, distractions, workload • i.e., medication administration location
Commitment to Resilience	• Ability to overcome problems, recover when something bad happens	• Perform quick situational assessment • Contain or manage the error • Then take steps to mitigate future harm
Deference to Expertise	• Collective expertise is better than any individual	• Teamwork • Deemphasize authority gradients • Speak up

Adapted from Weick, K. E. & Sutcliffe, K. (2001). *Managing the Unexpected—Assuring high performance in an age of complexity*. San Francisco: Jossey-Bass.

clinician providing care to the patient, the likelihood of harming a patient drops significantly. High reliability processes can improve quality, improve the patients experience and improve financial performance.

The Joint Commission has mandated the use of "root cause analysis" (RCA) process to examine severe health care errors, called sentinel events. An example of a sentinel event is wrong-site surgery. Root cause analysis is a systematic approach to get to the causes of problems. Tools such as fishbone diagrams, flow charts, brainstorming, or the use of the "five whys" questions help to get to the root of the problem. The National Pressure Injury Advisory Panel (NPIAP) developed an RCA format for investigating pressure injury causation (Tescher, Deppisch, Munro, Jorgensen, & Cuddigan, 2022). Wound care leaders have advocated the use of the RCA process for all full-thickness pressure injuries (Black, 2019). The process of RCA begins with examining the differential diagnosis of pressure etiology or other causation. The next step is to examine the human processes of care for any omissions that could be linked to the pressure injury. Lastly, the RCA examines the system factors for trends or patterns that could be remedies to prevent future occurrences. An example of a system factor might be the delay in start of specialty bed therapy due to delivery failure related to order or messaging error.

Avoidable/Unavoidable Pressure Injuries

The issue of whether pressure injuries are always avoidable or preventable has been the topic of debate and discussion for many years. Regulatory policy is based on the tenant that all pressure injuries are "largely preventable" (NQF, 2011) (see Box 6.1). Significant financial penalties are levied, and

resources are expended in efforts to comply with these standards. In the skilled nursing and rehabilitation environment, there is regulatory language for the unavoidable pressure injury (CMS, 42CFR 483.25.c F314). It reads, "Unavoidable means that the resident developed a pressure ulcer/injury even though the facility had evaluated the resident's clinical condition and risk factors; defined and implemented interventions that are consistent with resident needs, goals, and professional standards of practice; monitored and evaluated the impact of the interventions; and revised the approaches as appropriate." The CMS has not applied this same standard in other health care settings, leading to confusion. Professional societies have supported the notion that despite provision of best practice interventions, pressure injuries do occur and may be considered unavoidable (Schmitt et al., 2017). They recommend the development of research and dissemination of evidence that differentiates avoidable from unavoidable pressure injuries in the acute care setting. Wound care specialists are advised to keep ahead of changes in regulatory language that may impact practice.

"Data-Driven Wound Care" Improves Specialty

Although the United States spends more per capita on health care than any other country, there remain significant deficits in efficiency, quality, access, safety, and affordability in health care. Wound Care specialists have an opportunity to influence health care quality, in particular, to impact the high-profile quality indicator of pressure injury. For example, through standardized pressure injury data generation and analysis, phenomena such as skin failure and deep tissue injury may become better understood (Delmore, Cox, Rolnitsky, Chu, & Stolfi, 2015). With the consistent use of improvement science, we can reduce preventable harm and elucidate research opportunities to better understand unavoidable harm. Health economists cite the value of skilled wound specialists as a cost-effective strategy to drive down cost and improve health care quality (Padula, Nagarajan, Davidson, & Pronovost, 2019). By consistently applying quality analytics, specialists can quantify the effectiveness of wound care provision and support future resources, innovation, and funding for the specialty.

Quality Consult: Fictitious Noblecare Hospital ICU Unit North 7

North 7 has struggled with high rates and occurrences of pressure injuries (see Figs. 6.10–6.12). The Nurse Manager consults with the Quality Director, they assemble an intra-professional group and embark on a quality improvement initiative. They complete the "Organizational Readiness Checklist" from the AHRQ Pressure Ulcer Toolkit (Berlowitz, VanDeusen, Parker, et al., 2011) and determine that they have sufficient institutional support and resources for the project Padula, Valuck, Makic, & Wald, 2015) and that it is aligned with the institutional mission and vison to provide safe effective care for all patients. Using the IHI model, they determine the goal for the project is to reduce the number and severity of pressure injuries on North 7, to achieve a HAPI/1000 Patient Days rate of 3.0 by fiscal year end. They enlist the support of subject matter experts, the certified wound team, and the medical librarian to search for current evidence-based strategies for reducing pressure injury in the critical care populations. They already had baseline data from the unit-based dashboard; but they determine the frequency of data collection necessary to support the project and they adopt existing metrics.

The Quality Leader suggests a discovery technique adopted from Lean methodology, called "go to the Gemba," as a method to start their first PDSA cycle (Gallo, Doyle, Beckman, & Lizarraga, 2020). Team members observe the nursing admission process and compare findings to best practice evidence and validate a need to start their first PDSA cycle focused on admission skin assessment. Since they have a high percentage of novice nurses on the unit, they decide to adopt a best practice strategy called "2-RN Admission Skin Assessment" (EPUAP, NPIAP, PPPIA, 2019). After 2 PDSA cycles to work out the logistics of this new workflow, they achieve a 95% compliance with the new process. Coincidently, the hospital had budgeted for new replacement ICU beds and during the second month of the project, the new beds were delivered. Supported by the evidence and admission Braden risk scores, North 7 determined that a new safety standard for their population would be to care for all critically ill patients using the upgraded technology support surfaces.

Seeing demonstrable improvements in their monthly HAPI rates by January (Fig. 6.12), some of the enthusiasm for the project waned and they experienced an uptick in number and severity of pressure injuries in the spring. They decided to increase visibility for the project by starting weekly wound rounds with a team consisting of a certified wound nurse, a respiratory therapist, a nurse practitioner, a physical therapist, and the unit Clinical Nurse Leader. During weekly wound rounds, they conducted audits of expected protocol interventions and noted several opportunities. Collating data from observed gaps in the prevention protocol, they constructed a Pareto chart to identify the top opportunities for improvement (Fig. 6.14). Confirmed by surveillance data of device-related pressure injuries by location and severity (Figs. 6.11 and 6.13), they devised PDSA cycles to revise the workflow for interprofessionals to cross-cover the requirement to rotate devices and protect skin around medical devices. Hospital-wide implementation of an evidence-based sacral foam dressing nursing order was introduced that supported the unit project. The physical therapist worked with informatics department to introduce an algorithm on turning protocols for critically ill patients with hemodynamic instability, an extension to the existing mobility protocol. The weekly rounds group presented encouraging data of sustainability of best practice changes, using graphs to depict the progress (Fig. 6.12). During the last month of the fiscal year, the team achieved a pressure injury rate below 3 and they celebrated the achievement. The team presented their findings at the yearly quality improvement conference and they planned for sustainability (Creehan et al., 2016).

FY 2021 HAPI		Oct-20	Nov-20	Dec-20	Jan-21	Feb-21	Mar-21	Apr-21	May-21	Jun-21	Jul-21	Aug-21	Sep-21	Total FYTD21	Target FY21
North 7 ICU	Stage 1	0	1	1	0	1	2	1	0	1	2	2	1	12	
	Stage 2	3	2	3	1	1	1	1	2	2	1	1	1	19	
	Stage 3	0	1	0	0	0	0	0	0	0	0	0	0	2	0
	Stage 4	0	0	0	0	0	0	0	0	0	0	0	0	0	0
	DTI	2	2	1	3	1	1	2	2	1	0	0	0	15	
	Unstageable	0	0	1	0	1	0	0	0	0	0	0	0	2	0
	Total HAPI	5	6	6	4	4	5	4	4	4	3	3	2	50	35
	Total patient days	642	677	669	684	658	690	690	714	710	702	710	694	8240	
	HAPI Rate per 1000 pt days	7.79	8.86	8.97	5.85	6.08	7.25	5.80	5.60	5.63	4.27	4.23	2.88	6.07	3.0

Fig. 6.10 Unit-based pressure injury dashboard examples.

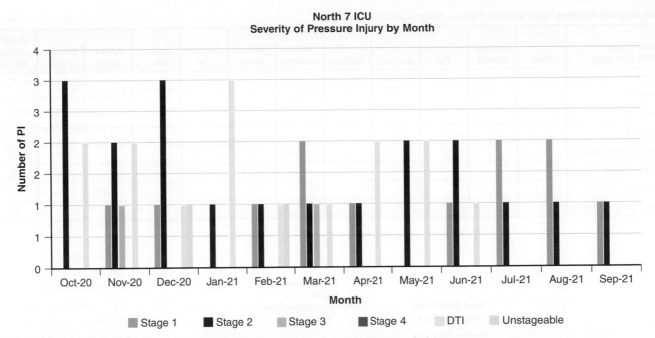

Fig. 6.11 Unit-base pressure injuries by severity/stage.

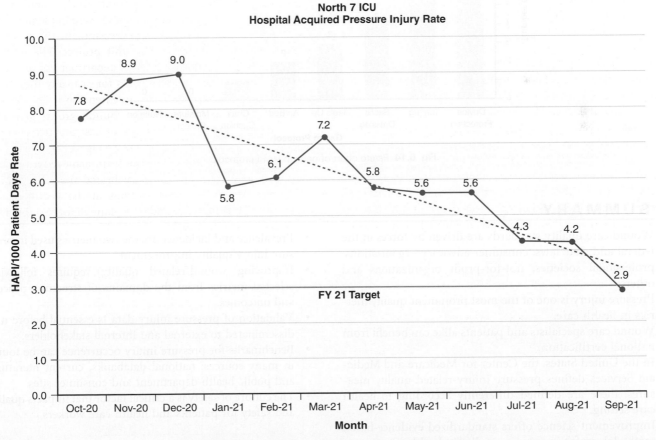

Fig. 6.12 Unit-based pressure injuries trended monthly by rate.

Unit-Acquired Pressure Injury Monthly Report – Stage – Location – Device

North 7 ICU FYTD May 2021	Heel	Coccyx/ Sacral	Hip	Ischium	Occiput	Other location	Device: Nose	Device: Lip	Device: Ear	Device: Trach	Device: Other	Stage Total FYTD
Stage 1	2	3							1			6
Stage 2	3	6		2		1 ankle	1			1		14
Stage 3		2										2
Stage 4												0
Deep Tissue Injury	2	5	1	1		2 buttock			2		1 TLSO	14
Unstageable		1			1							2
Mucosal								3				3
Location Total FYTD	7	17	1	3	1	3	1	3	3	1	1	41

Fig. 6.13 Unit-acquire pressure injury by stage, location and device.

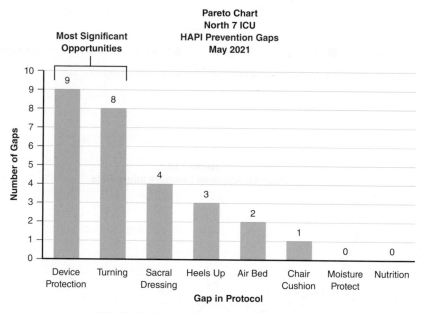

Fig. 6.14 Pareto chart of gaps in HAPI protocol.

SUMMARY

- Wound care quality standards are driven by forces in the federal and state laws, consumer advocacy organizations, professional societies, not-for-profit organizations and others.
- Pressure injury is one of the most prominent quality metrics in health care.
- Wound care specialists and patients alike can benefit from national certification.
- In the United States, the Center for Medicare and Medicaid Services defines pressure injury-related quality measures; these are defined differently according to health care setting.
- Improvement science offers standardized evidence-based methodology for improving quality in health care.

- Prevalence and incidence are the two metrics used in pressure injury quality improvement.
- Improving wound-related quality requires following selected metrics from the domains of structure, process and outcomes.
- Validation of pressure injury data is essential before it is disseminated to external and internal stakeholders.
- Benchmarks for pressure injury occurrence can be found in many sources: national databanks, current literature, and public health department and consumer sites.
- The culture of safety is a critical factor that impacts quality and safety for patients and health care workers.

SELF-ASSESSMENT QUESTIONS

1. Where do I find quality measures related to wound care?
   a. Federal regulatory agencies
   b. State laws and regulations
   c. National health care accreditation organizations
   d. Professional wound care associations
   e. All of the above

2. How do I know what I should be striving for in a PI rate?
   a. Compare your rates to nationally benchmarked data
   b. Participate in a national pressure injury prevalence survey
   c. Compare your rates to similar sized/acuity facility or setting
   d. All of the above

3. What is an example of a PDSA cycle for wound care?
   a. Plan: Can we increase resident repositioning to 90% compliance with use of musical cues?
   b. Do: On a skilled rehabilitation unit, provide overhead musical cues q 2 h; engage staff, measure repositioning documentation
   c. Study: Repositioning documentation improved to 85%; residents complained of noise on night shift
   d. Act: Revise to use musical cues 6 am to 6 pm and study again
   e. All of the above

4. Can I make up my own metrics to improve quality?
   a. Determine your aims; Define what will be an improvement (target); Plan tests of change
   b. Consider sources of data: EHR, claims, chart, interviews, observation
   c. Determine numerator, denominator, inclusion and exclusion criteria
   d. Collect data, analyze data; determine interventions to improve performance. Repeat
   e. All of the above

5. Where are the major resources for government quality metrics?
   a. Centers for Medicare and Medicaid Services (CMS)
   b. Agency for Healthcare Research and Quality (AHRQ)
   c. US Department of Health & Human Services (HHS)
   d. All of the above

6. How can I find best-practice toolkits?
   a. Search AHRQ website
   b. Search published health care literature
   c. Search professional organization sites
   d. Search clinical practice guidelines
   e. All of the above

7. Can I substitute prevalence for incidence and vice versa?
   a. Pressure injury prevalence is a measure of injuries present at a point in time
   b. Pressure injury incidence is a measure of new cases, for example, those developed since admission to a facility
   c. Prevalence and incidence are different measures of pressure injury occurrence
   d. Consistency in operational definitions of prevalence and incidence is essential for quality improvement
   e. All of the above

REFERENCES

Agency for Healthcare Research and Quality. (2014). *Preventing pressure ulcers in hospitals*. Rockville: Agency for Healthcare Research and Quality. https://www.ahrq.gov/patient-safety/settings/hospital/resource/pressureulcer/tool/index.htm. Accessed July 12, 2020.

Agency for Healthcare Research and Quality. (2016). *AHRQ's safety program for nursing homes: On-time pressure ulcer prevention*. Rockville: Agency for Healthcare Research and Quality. https://www.ahrq.gov/patient-safety/settings/long-term-care/resource/ontime/pruhealing/index.html. Accessed July 12, 2020.

Agency for Healthcare Research and Quality. (2019). *Hospital Acquired Conditions National Scorecard 2014–16*. Rockville, MD. https://www.ahrq.gov/data/infographics/hac-scorecard-2014-16.html. Accessed November 2, 2020.

Agency for Healthcare Research and Quality (AHRQ). (2014). *The Patient Safety and Quality Improvement Act of 2005. Content last reviewed October 2014. Rockville, MD*. https://www.ahrq.gov/policymakers/psoact.html. Accessed November 2, 2020.

Alvey, B., Hennen, N., & Heard, H. (2012). Improving accuracy of pressure ulcer staging and documentation using a computerized clinical decision support system. *Journal of Wound, Ostomy and Continence Nursing, 39*(6), 607–612. https://doi.org/10.1097/WON.0b013e31826a4b5c.

American College of Healthcare Executives (ACHE). (2017). *Leading a culture of safety: A blueprint for success*. ACHE. https://www.ache.org/about-ache. Accessed October 1, 2020.

American Nurses Association (ANA). (2014). *Position statement on professional role competence*. https://www.nursingworld.org/practice-policy/nursing-excellence/official-position-statements/id/professional-role-competence/.

American Nurses Credentialing Center (ANCC). (2017). *Practice Standards*. https://nursingworld.org/organizational-programs/pathway/. Accessed November 2, 2020.

Artico, M., Dante, A., D'Angelo, D., Lamarca, L., Mastroianni, C., Petitti, T., et al. (2017). Prevalence, incidence and associated factors of pressure ulcers in home palliative care patients: A retrospective chart review. *Palliative Medicine, 32*(1), 299–307.

Ayello, E. (2019). Pressure injuries: Nursing sensitive indicator or team and system-sensitive indicator? *Advances in Skin and Wound Care, 32*(5), 199–200.

Ayello, E. A., Levine, J. M., Langemo, D., Kennedy-Evans, K. L., Brennan, M. R., & Sibbald, G. R. (2019). Reexamining the literature on terminal ulcers, SCALE, skin failure, and unavoidable pressure injuries. *Advances in Skin & Wound Care, 32*(3), 109–121. https://doi.org/10.1097/01.ASW.0000553112.55505.5f. PMID: 30801349.

Baharestani, M. M., Black, J. M., Carville, K., Clark, M., Cuddigan, J. E., Dealey, C., et al. (2009). Dilemmas in measuring and using pressure ulcer prevalence and incidence: An international consensus. *International Wound Journal, 6,* 97–104. https://doi.org/10.1111/j.1742-481X.2009.00593.x.

Berlowitz, D., VanDeusen, C., Parker, V., et al. (2011). *Preventing pressure ulcers in hospitals: A toolkit for improving quality of care. (Prepared by Boston University School of Public Health under Contract No. HHSA 290200600012 TO #5 and Grant No. RRP 09-112.).* Rockville: Agency for Healthcare Research and Quality. April 2011. AHRQ. Publication No. 11-0053-EF.

Berwick, D. M., Calkins, D. R., McCannon, C. J., & Hackbarth, A. D. (2006). *The 100,000 lives campaign: Setting a goal and a deadline for improving health care quality.* Institute for Healthcare Improvement. www.ihi.org/IHI/Topics/Improvement/ImprovementMethods/Literature/100000LivesCampaign SettingaGoalandaDeadline.html. Accessed October 1, 2020.

Black, J. M. (2019). Root cause analysis for hospital-acquired pressure injury. *Journal of Wound, Ostomy, and Continence Nursing, 46*(4), 298–304.

Boyle, D. K., Bergquist-Beringer, S., & Cramer, E. (2017). Relationship of wound, ostomy and continence certified nurses and healthcare acquired conditions in acute care hospitals. *Journal of Wound, Ostomy, and Continence Nursing, 44*(3), 283–292.

Boyle, D. K., Jayawardhana, A., Burman, M. E., Dunton, N. E., Staggs, V. S., Bergquist-Beringer, S., et al. (2016). A pressure ulcer and fall rate quality composite index for acute care units: A measure development study. *International Journal of Nursing Studies, 63,* 73–81. https://doi.org/10.1016/j.ijnurstu.2016.08.020. Accessed November 2, 2020.

Brown, D. S., Donaldson, N., Bolton, L. B., & Aydin, C. (2010). Nursing-sensitive benchmarks for hospitals to gauge high-reliability performance. *The Journal for Healthcare Quality, 32* (6), 9–17. https://doi.org/10.1111/j.1945-1474.2010. 00083.x.

Caplan, A. L. (2012). Not my turn. *Lancet, 380,* 968–969.

Centers for Medicare and Medicaid Services (CMS). (2015). *Medicare and Medicaid Milestones 1937–2015.* https://www.cms.gov/About-CMS/Agency-Information/History/Downloads/Medicare-and-Medicaid-Milestones-1937-2015.pdf. Accessed November 2, 2020.

Centers for Medicare and Medicaid Services (CMS). (2020). www.cms.gov. Accessed July 24.

Centers for Medicare and Medicaid Services (CMS). (2023). *Outcome and Assessment Information Set OASIS-E-Manual.* Retrieved 3/07/2023 from: https://www.cms.gov/files/document/oasis-e-guidance-manual51622.pdf.

Corbett, L. Q. (2012). Wound care nursing: Professional issues and opportunities. *Advances in Wound Care, 1*(5), 189–193.

Corbett, L. Q., & Ennis, W. J. (2014). What do patients want? Patient preference in wound care. *Advances in Wound Care (New Rochelle), 3*(8), 537–543. https://doi.org/10.1089/wound.2013.0458.

Cox, J., Roche, S., & Gandhi, N. (2013). Critical care physicians: Attitudes, beliefs, and knowledge about pressure ulcers. *Advances in Skin & Wound Care, 26*(4), 168–176. https://doi.org/10.1097/01.ASW.0000428863.34294.9d.

Cramer, E. M., Seneviratne, M. G., Sharifi, H., Ozturk, A., & Hernandez-Boussard, T. (2019). Predicting the incidence of pressure ulcers in the intensive care unit using machine learning. *EGEMS (Washington, DC), 7*(1), 49.

Crawford, B., Skeath, M., & Whippy, A. (2015). Multifocal clinical performance improvement across 21 hospitals. *The Journal for Healthcare Quality (JHQ), 37*(2), 117–125. https://doi.org/10.1111/jhq.12039.

Creehan, S. (2015). Building nursing unit staff champion programs to improve clinical outcomes. *Nurse Leader, 13*(4), 31–35. https://doi.org/10.1016/j.mnl.2015.06.001.

Creehan, S., Cuddigan, J., Gonzales, D., et al. (2016). The VCU pressure ulcer summit—Developing centers of pressure ulcer prevention excellence. *Journal of Wound, Ostomy and Continence Nursing, 43*(2), 121–128. https://doi.org/10.1097/WON.0000000000000203.

Cronenwett, L., Sherwood, G., Barnsteiner, J., Disch, J., Johnson, J., Mitchell, P., et al. (2007). Quality and safety education for nurses. *Nursing Outlook, 55*(3), 122–131.

Delmore, B., Cox, J., Rolnitsky, L., Chu, A., & Stolfi, A. (2015). Differentiating a pressure ulcer from acute skin failure in the adult critical care patient. *Advances in Skin & Wound Care, 28*(11), 514–524.

Donabedian, A. (1966). Evaluating the quality of medical care. *The Milbank Memorial Fund Quarterly, 44*(Suppl. 3), 166–206. Reprinted in Milbank Q. 2005;83(4):691–729.

Donovan, E. A., Manta, C. J., Goldsack, J. C., & Collins, M. L. (2016). Using a lean six sigma approach to yield sustained pressure ulcer prevention for complex critical care patients. *The Journal of Nursing Administration, 46*(1), 43–48. https://doi.org/10.1097/NNA.0000000000000291. PMID: 26641470.

Dugaret, E., Videau, M.-. N., Faure, I., Gabinski, C., Bourdel-Marchasson, I., & Salles, N. (2014). Prevalence and incidence rates of pressure ulcers in an emergency department. *International Wound Journal, 11,* 386–391. https://doi.org/10.1111/j.1742-481X.2012.01103.x ECRI. Accessed July 2, 2020. From https://www.ecri.org/about/.

European Pressure Ulcer Advisory Panel, National Pressure Injury Advisory Panel and Pan Pacific Pressure Injury Alliance. Prevention and Treatment of Pressure Ulcers/Injuries. (2019). In E. Haesler (Ed.), *Clinical Practice Guideline. The International Guideline.* EPUAP/NPIAP/PPPIA.

Famolaro, T., Yount, N., Hare, R., et al. (2018). *Hospital Survey on Patient Safety Culture: 2018 User Database Report.* Rockville: Agency for Healthcare Research and Quality.

Fife, C. E., Yankowsky, K. W., Ayello, E. A., et al. (2010). Legal issues in the care of pressure ulcer patients: key concepts for healthcare providers—A consensus paper from the International Expert Wound Care Advisory Panel© [published correction appears in Adv Skin Wound Care. 2010 Dec; 23(12):540]. *Advances in Skin & Wound Care, 23*(11), 493–507. https://doi.org/10.1097/01.ASW.0000390494. 20964.a5.

Fletcher, J., Crook, H., & Harris, C. (2013). Monitoring pressure ulcer prevalence: A precise methodology. *Wounds UK, 9*(4), 48–53.

Gallo, A. M., Doyle, R. A. C., Beckman, J., & Lizarraga, C. (2020). Blending evidence-based practice and Lean Six Sigma methodology to reduce hospital-acquired pressure injuries in a progressive care unit. *Journal of Nursing Care Quality, 35*(4), 295–300. https://doi.org/10.1097/NCQ.0000000000000455.

Gaspar, S., Collier, M., Marques, A., Ferreira, C., & de Matos, M. G. (2020). Pressure ulcers: The challenge of monitoring in hospital context. *Applied Nursing Research, 53*(151266), 1–5.

Guth, M., Garfield, R., & Rudowitz, R. (2020). The Effects of Medicaid Expansion under the ACA: Updated Findings from a Literature Review. *Kaiser Family Foundation,* 2002.

Hanlon, C., Sheedy, K., Kniffen, T., & Rosenthal, J. (2015). *National Academy for State Health Policy, Guide to State Adverse Event Reporting Systems.* Retrieved 11/2/2020 From: https://www.nashp.org/wp-content/uploads/2015/02/2014_Guide_to_State_Adverse_Event_Reporting_Systems.pdf.

Harrison, M. B., Mackey, M., & Friedberg, E. (2008). Pressure ulcer monitoring: A process of evidence-based practice, quality and research. *The Joint Commission Journal on Quality and Patient Safety, 34*(6), 355–359.

Helsop, L., & Lu, S. (2014). Nursing sensitive indicators: A concept analysis. *Journal of Advanced Nursing, 70,* 2469–2482. https://doi.org/10.1111/jan.12503 (PubMed: 25113388).

Institute for Healthcare Improvement (IHI). (2020). *Model for improvement.* www.ihi.org. Accessed October 2.

Institute of Medicine. (2001). *Crossing the quality chasm: A new health system for the 21st century.* Washington, DC: National Academy Press.

Institute of Medicine. (2011a). *Clinical practice guidelines we can trust.* Washington, DC: The National Academies Press. https://doi.org/10.17226/13058.

Institute of Medicine. (2011b). *The future of nursing: Leading change, advancing health.* Washington, DC: The National Academies Press. https://doi.org/10.17226/12956.

Kohn, L. T., Corrigan, J., & Donaldson, M. S. (2000). *To err is human: Building a safer health system.* Washington, DC: National Academy Press.

Langley, G. J., Moen, R. D., Nolan, K. M., Nolan, T. W., Norman, C. L., & Provost, L. P. (2009). *The improvement guide.* San Francisco: Jossey-Bass.

Levine, J. M., Ayello, E. A., Zulkowski, K. M., & Fogel, J. (2012). Pressure ulcer knowledge in medical residents: An opportunity for improvement. *Advances in Skin & Wound Care, 25,* 115–117 (PMID: 22343598).

Lewin, K. (1951). Field theory in social science. In D. Cartwright (Ed.), *Selected theoretical papers.* New York: Harper & Row.

Ma, C., & Park, S. H. (2015). Hospital magnet status, unit work environment, and pressure ulcers. *Journal Nursing Scholarship, 47*(6), 565–573. https://doi.org/10.1111/jnu.121732.

McInnes, E., Chaboyer, W., Murray, E., Allen, T., & Jones, P. (2014). The role of patients in pressure injury prevention: A survey of acute care patients. *BMC Nursing, 13*(1), 41. https://doi.org/10.1186/s12912-014-0041-y.

Meddings, J. (2015). Using administrative discharge diagnoses to track hospital-acquired pressure ulcer incidence—Limitations, links, and leaps. *The Joint Commission Journal on Quality and Patient Safety, 41*(6), 243.

Meddings, J. A., Reichert, H., Hofer, T., & McMahon, L. F. (2013). Hospital report cards for hospital-acquired pressure ulcers: How good are the grades? *Annals of Internal Medicine, 159*(8), 505–513.

Moore, Z., Avsar, C. L., Moore, D. H., Patton, D., & O'Connor, T. (2019). The prevalence of pressure ulcers in Europe, what does the European data tell us: A systematic review. *Journal of Wound Care, 28*(11), 710–719.

Moore, Z., Soriano, J. V., & Pokorna, A. (2017). The joint EPIAP & EWMA pressure ulcer prevention & patient safety advocacy project. *Wounds UK, 13*(3), 16–20.

National Association for Healthcare Quality (NAHQ). (2018). *The road to healthcare value is driven by quality workforce integration.* https://www.qualitydrivenhealthcare.org/. Accessed September 20, 2020.

National Database of Nursing Quality Indicators™ (NDNQI®). 2020. http://www.health-links.me/web/ndnqi.html Accessed June 2020.

National Quality Forum (NQF). (2011). *Serious reportable events in healthcare—2011 Update: A consensus report.* Washington, DC: NQF.

Niederhauser, A., VanDeusen, L. C., Parker, V., Ayello, E. A., Zulkowski, K., & Berlowitz, D. (2012). Comprehensive programs for preventing pressure ulcers: A review of the literature. *Advances in Skin & Wound Care, 25,* 167–188; quiz 189–190. https://doi.org/10.1097/01.ASW.0000413598.97566.d7.

Nightingale, F. (1859). *Notes on nursing.* Philadelphia: Lippincott.

Nussbaum, S. R., Carter, M. J., Fife, C. E., et al. (2018). An economic evaluation of the impact, cost, and Medicare policy implications of chronic nonhealing wounds. *Value Health, 21,* 27–32.

Omnibus Budget Reconciliation Act of 1987. (1987). *H.R. 3545, Public Law 100-203.*

Padula, W. V., Nagarajan, M., Davidson, P. M., & Pronovost, P. J. (2019). Investing in skilled specialists to grow hospital infrastructure for quality improvement. *Journal of Patient Safety, Publish Ahead of Print.* https://doi.org/10.1097/PTS.0000000000000623.

Padula, W. V., Pronovost, P. J., Makic, M. B. F., Wald, H. L., Moran, D., Mishra, M. K., et al. (2019). Value of hospital resources for effective pressure injury prevention: A cost-effectiveness analysis. *BMJ Quality & Safety, 28*(2), 132–141.

Padula, W. V., Valuck, R. J., Makic, M. B. F., & Wald, H. L. (2015). Factors influencing adoption of hospital acquired pressure ulcer prevention programs in US academic medical centers. *Journal of Wound, Ostomy, and Continence Nursing, 42*(4), 327–330.

Paradiso, L., & Sweeney, N. (2019). Just culture. *Nursing Management, 50*(6), 38–45. https://doi.org/10.1097/01.NUMA.0000558482. 07815.ae.

Polancich, S., Williamson, J., Poe, T., Armstrong, A., & Vander Noot, R. M. (2019). Innovations in pressure injury reporting: Creating actionable data for improvement. *Journal for Healthcare Quality, 41*(3), 180–187. https://doi.org/10.1097/JHQ.0000000000000196.

Preventing Pressure Ulcers in Hospitals. (2014). *Content last reviewed October 2014.* Rockville: Agency for Healthcare Research and Quality. https://www.ahrq.gov/patient-safety/settings/hospital/resource/pressureulcer/tool/index.htm. Accessed July 12, 2020.

Primiano, M., Friend, M., McClure, C., et al. (2011). Pressure ulcer prevalence and risk factors during prolonged surgical procedures. *AORN Journal, 94*(6), 555–566. https://doi.org/10.1016/j.aorn.2011.03.014.

QSEN Institute. (2017). *Pre-licensure KSs: Quality Improvement.* http://qsen.org.

Razmus, I., & Bergquist-Beringer, S. (2017). Pressure injury prevalence and the rate of hospital acquired pressure injury among pediatric patients in acute care. *JWOCN, 44*(2), 110–117.

Romanelli, J. R., Fuchshuber, P. R., Stulberg, J. J., et al. (2019). Public reporting and transparency: A primer on public outcomes reporting. *Surgical Endoscopy, 33*(7), 2043–2049. https://doi.org/10.1007/s00464-019-06756-4.

Rothman, K. J. (2012). *Epidemiology: An introduction.* New York: Oxford University Press.

Saghafian, S., & Hopp, W. J. (2019). *The role of quality transparency in health care: Challenges and potential solutions. NAM Perspectives.* Washington, DC: Commentary, National Academy of Medicine. https://doi.org/10.31478/201911a.

Schmitt, S., Andries, M. K., Ashmore, P. M., Brunette, G., Judge, K., & Bonham, P. A. (2017). WOCN society position paper: Avoidable versus unavoidable pressure ulcers/injuries. *Journal of Wound, Ostomy and Continence Nursing, 44*(5), 458–468.

Schwartz, M., Nguyen, K., Swinson, T., Thaker, S., & Bernard, S. (2013). *Development of a cross-setting quality measure for pressure ulcers, OY2: Information gathering. Final report prepared for the Centers for Medicare & Medicaid Services.* Research Triangle Park: RTI International.

Share, D. A., Campbell, D. A., Birkmeyer, N., Prager, R. L., Hitinder, S. G., Moscucci, M., et al. (2011). How a regional collaborative of hospitals and physicians in michigan cut costs and improved the quality of care. *Health Affairs, 30*(4), 636–645.

Sharp, C. A., Schulz Moore, J. S., & McLaws, M. L. (2019). Two-hourly repositioning for prevention of pressure ulcers in the elderly: Patient safety or elder abuse? *Journal of Bioethical Inquiry, 16*(1), 17–34. https://doi.org/10.1007/s11673-018-9892-3.

Squitieri, L., Waxman, D. A., Mangione, C. M., Saliba, D., Ko, C. Y., Needleman, J., et al. (2018). Evaluation of the present on admission indicator among hospitalized fee-for-service medicare patients with a pressure ulcer diagnosis: Coding patterns and impact on hospital-acquired pressure ulcer rates. *Health Services Research, 53*, 2970–2987. https://doi.org/10.1111/1475-6773.12822.

Sullivan, N., & Schoelles, K. M. (2013). Preventing in-facility pressure ulcers as a patient safety strategy: A systematic review. *Annals of Internal Medicine, 158*(5 Pt. 2), 410–416.

Summers, L., & Bickford, C. J. (2017). *Nursing's Leading Edges: Specialization, credentialing and certification of RNs and APRNs.* Silver Spring: American Nurses Association.

Tescher, A., Deppisch, M., Munro, C., Jorgensen, V., & Cuddigan, J. (2022). Perioperative pressure injury prevention: National Pressure Injury Advisory Panel root cause analysis toolkit 3.0. *Journal Wound Care, 31*(Suppl. 12), S4–S9. https://doi.org/10.12968/jowc.2022.31.Sup12.S4. PMID: 36475846.

The Joint Commission, National Patient Safety Goals. (2020). https://www.jointcommission.org/en/standards/national-patient-safety-goals/. Accessed July 1, 2020.

Valle, M. F., Maruthur, N. M., Wilson, L. M., Malas, M., Qazi, U., Haberl, E., et al. (2014). Comparative effectiveness of advanced wound dressings for patients with chronic venous leg ulcers: A systematic review. *Wound Repair and Regeneration, 22*(2), 193–204. https://doi.org/10.1111/wrr.12151. PMID: 24635169.

VanGilder, C. A., Cox, J., Edsberg, L. E., & Koloms, K. (2021). Pressure injury prevalence in acute care hospitals with unit-specific analysis: Results from the International Pressure Ulcer Prevalence (IPUP) Survey database. *Journal of Wound, Ostomy and Continence Nursing, 48*(6), 492–503.

Wagner, L. M., Castle, N. G., Reid, K. C., & Stone, R. (2013). U.S. Department of health adverse event reporting policies for nursing homes. *Journal for Healthcare Quality, 35*, 9–14. https://doi.org/10.1111/j.1945-1474.2011.00177.x.

Wojciechowski, E., Pearsall, T., Murphy, P., & French, E. (2016). A case review: Integrating Lewin's theory with lean system approach for change. *Online Journal of Issues in Nursing, 21*(2), 4. https://doi.org/10.3912/OJIN.Vol21No2Man04.

World Health Organization. (2006). Quality of care: A process for making strategic choices in health systems. *World Health Organization.* https://apps.who.int/iris/handle/10665/43470. Accessed November 2, 2020.

World Health Organization. (2020). https://www.who.int/. Accessed July 25, 2020.

Wound Ostomy Continence Nursing Certification Board. (2020). *Consumers.* WOCNCB. http://www.wocncb.org/consumers.

Zaratkiewicz, S., Whitney, J., Lowe, J., Taylor, S., O'Donnell, F., & Minton-Foltz, P. (2010). Development and implementation of a hospital-acquired pressure ulcer incidence tracking system and algorithm. *The Journal for Healthcare Quality, 32*(6), 44–51. https://doi.org/10.1111/j.1945-1474.2010. 00076.x.

Zrelak, P., Utter, G. H., Tancredi, D. J., Mayer, L. G., Cerese, J., Cuny, J., et al. (2015). How accurate is the AHRQ patient safety indicator for hospital-acquired pressure ulcer in a national sample of records? *The Journal for Healthcare Quality, 37*(5), 287–297. https://doi.org/10.1111/jhq.12052.

FURTHER READING

Agency for Healthcare Research and Quality. (2011). *Patient safety and quality improvement act of 2005.* http://www.ahrq.gov/qual/psoact.htm. Accessed June 21, 2020.

Al-Mansour, L. A., Dudley-Brown, S., & Al-Shaikhi, A. (2020). Development of an interdisciplinary healthcare team for pressure injury management: A quality improvement project. *Journal of Wound, Ostomy, & Continence Nursing, 47*, 349–352. https://doi.org/10.1097/WON.0000000000000652.

Bouyer-Ferullo, S., O'Connor, C., Kinnealey, E., Wrigley, P., & Osgood, P. M. (2021). Adding a visual communication tool to the electronic health record to prevent pressure injuries. *AORN Journal, 113*, 253–262. https://doi.org/10.1002/aorn.13323.

Fleming, S. L., McFarlane, K. H., Thapa, I., Johnson, A. K., Kruger, J. F., Shin, A. Y., et al. (2022). Performance of a commonly used pressure injury risk model under changing incidence. *Joint Commission Journal on Quality & Patient Safety, 48*, 131–138. https://doi.org/10.1016/j.jcjq.2021.10.008.

Maguire, J., Hastings, D., Adams, M., Phillips, D., McKenna, J., Lin, J. R., et al. (2021). Development and implementation of an individualized turning program for pressure injury prevention using sensor technology in nursing homes: A quality improvement program. *Wound Management & Prevention, 67* (11), 12–25. Retrieved from http://ovidsp.ovid.com/ovidweb.cgi?T=JS&PAGE=reference&D=med20&NEWS=N&AN=35030094.

Padula, W. V., Nagarajan, M., Davidson, P. M., & Pronovost, P. J. (2021). Investing in skilled specialists to grow hospital infrastructure for quality improvement. *Journal of Patient Safety, 17*, 51–55. https://doi.org/10.1097/PTS.0000000000000623.

Pittman, J., Horvath, D., Beeson, T., Bailey, K., Mills, A., Kaiser, L., et al. (2021). Pressure injury prevention for complex cardiovascular patients in the operating room and intensive care unit: A quality improvement project. *Journal of Wound, Ostomy, & Continence Nursing, 48*, 510–515. https://doi.org/10.1097/WON.0000000000000815.

Polancich, S., Coiner, S., Barber, R., Poe, T., Roussel, L., Williams, K., et al. (2017). Applying the PDSA framework to examine the use of the clinical nurse leader to evaluate pressure ulcer reporting. *Journal of Nursing Care Quality, 32*(4), 293–300. https://doi.org/10.1097/NCQ.0000000000000251.

Seton, J. M., Hovan, H. M., Bogie, K. M., Murray, M. M., Wasil, B., Banks, P. G., et al. (2022). Interactive evidence-based pressure injury education program for hospice nursing: A quality improvement approach. *Journal of Wound, Ostomy, & Continence Nursing, 49*, 428–435. https://doi.org/10.1097/WON.0000000000000911.

Shirey, M. R. (2013). Lewin's theory of planned change as a strategic resource. *Journal of Nursing Administration, 43*(2), 69–72. https://doi.org/10.1097/NNA.ob013e31827f20a9.

Tayyiba, N., Coyer, F., & Lewis, P. A. (2016). Implementing a pressure ulcer prevention bundle in an adult intensive care. *Intensive and Critical Care Nursing, 37*, 27–36. https://doi.org/10.1016/j.iccn.2016.04.005.

Zubkoff, L., Neily, J., McCoy-Jones, S., Soncrant, C., Young-Xu, Y., Boar, S., et al. (2021). Implementing evidence-based pressure injury prevention interventions: Veterans health administration quality improvement collaborative. *Journal of Nursing Care Quality, 36*, 249–256. https://doi.org/10.1097/NCQ.0000000000000512.

Anatomy and Physiology of Skin and Soft Tissue

Annette B. Wysocki

OBJECTIVES

1. Describe the mechanisms by which the skin is able to provide its six major functions.
2. Describe the structures, function, and cellular composition of the skin layers, including layers within the dermis and epidermis.
3. Explain the relationship between skin pigmentation and protection against ultraviolet radiation.
4. Compare and contrast the structural and cellular development of the skin in the fetus, premature infant (23–32 weeks' gestation), full-term neonate, adolescent, and adult.
5. Describe at least two effects on the skin of the following: hydration, sun, nutrition, soaps, and medications.
6. Compare and contrast the structure and function of dark and lightly pigmented skin.

The skin is the one organ of the body that is constantly exposed to a changing environment. Maintaining its integrity is a complex process, and without appropriate treatment, assaults from surgical incisions, injuries, or burns can lead to life-threatening consequences.

The skin of the average adult covers approximately 3000 in^2, or an area almost equivalent to 2 m^2. From birth to maturity the skin covering will undergo a sevenfold expansion. It weighs about 6 lbs (or up to 15% of total adult body weight), is the largest organ of the body, and receives one third of the body's circulating blood volume. The skin forms a protective barrier against the external environment while maintaining a homeostatic internal environment. Epidermal appendages (nails, hair follicles, sweat, or sebaceous glands) that are lined with epidermal cells are also present in the skin. During healing of partial-thickness wounds, these epidermal cells migrate to resurface the wound. This organ is capable of self-regeneration and can withstand limited mechanical and chemical assaults. The skin varies in thickness from 0.5 mm in the tympanic membrane to 6 mm in the soles of the feet and the palms of the hands. Variations are attributable to differences in the thickness of the skin layers covering underlying organs, bones, muscle, and cartilage. Diseases of the skin can result from genetic causes, so-called genodermatoses, infection, immune dysfunction, and trauma. Skin diseases can involve some or all skin layers and, in the case of various skin cancers, metastasize to other organs and/or tissues.

Population projections indicate that changing demographics will occur over the next decades and that by 2043, a majority of the US population will be composed of people with skin of color, a "majority–minority" population. By 2060 the population is expected to be 31% Hispanic, 14.7% African American, 8.2% Asian, 1.5% American Indian and Native Alaskan, and 0.3% Native Hawaiian and other Pacific Islanders (US Census Bureau, 2014). Unique characteristics of darker vs lighter pigmented skin (Box 7.1) are described throughout the chapter.

SKIN LAYERS

Human skin is divided into two primary layers: epidermis (outermost layer) and dermis (innermost layer) (Fig. 7.1). These two layers are separated by a structure called the basement membrane. Beneath the dermis is a layer of loose connective tissue called the hypodermis, or subcutis.

Epidermis

The epidermis, the outermost skin layer, is avascular and derived from embryonic ectoderm. This layer is relatively uniform in thickness over the body, between 75 and 150 μm, except on the soles and palms, where thickness is between 0.4 and 0.6 mm. The epidermal layer is constantly being renewed, with turnover time ranging from 26 to

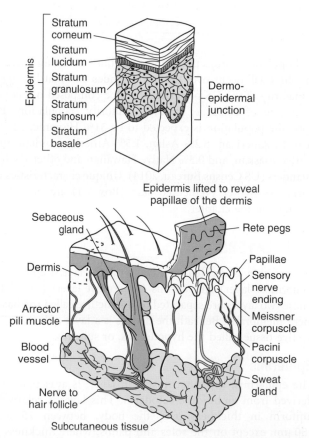

Fig. 7.1 Schematic diagram of anatomy of skin and subcutaneous tissue. (From Hooper, B. J., & Goldman, M. P. (1999). *Primary dermatologic care*. St. Louis, MO: Mosby.)

42 days. Complete epidermal renewal occurs over a period lasting between 45 and 75 days, or about every 2 months (Odland, 1991). The epidermal layer is composed of stratified squamous epithelial cells, or keratinocytes, and is divided into five layers (see Fig. 7.1). These layers, beginning from the outermost to the innermost, are the stratum corneum, stratum lucidum, stratum granulosum, stratum spinosum, and stratum basale (stratum germinativum or, simply, the basal layer).

Stratum Corneum

The stratum corneum, or horny layer, is the top layer and is composed of dead keratinized cells. These squames, or corneocytes, are the cells that are abraded by the daily mechanical and chemical trauma of hand washing, scratching, bathing, exercising, and changing of clothes. The stratum corneum is composed of layers of thin, stacked, pancake-appearing, anucleate cells. Approximately 80% of these cells are filled with keratin, a tough, fibrous, insoluble protein; hence, they are called keratinocytes. The α-keratin subclass that is found in mammalian skin can be acidic or basic. Keratins are critical to the maintenance of cell shape and polarity and in addition to protect the skin from assaults propagated from mechanical forces. Keratinocytes are initially formed in the basal layer and undergo the process of differentiation. The normal stratum corneum is composed of completely differentiated keratinocytes. Keratin is resistant to changes in temperature and pH and to chemical digestion by trypsin and pepsin. This same protein is found in hair and nails; in these structures, keratin is referred to as "hard" keratin compared with the "soft" keratin of the skin (Jacob, Francone, & Lossow, 1982; Solomons, 1983). Stratum corneum thickness varies with age, gender, and disease. In the deeper layer of the stratum corneum, the stratum compactum, the keratin is more densely packed, and the cells have a diminished capacity to bind water (Haake, Scott, & Holbrook, 2001). In the upper layer, the stratum dysjunctum, cells are partly shed as a result of proteolytic degradation of the desmosomes.

The stratum corneum is enriched with a lipid matrix that enhances the barrier properties of the skin. This lipid-rich matrix is composed of about 50% ceramides, 25% cholesterol, and 15% free fatty acids and has a unique lamellar organization (the mortar) seen between corneocytes (the bricks) that is first detected in the upper layer of the stratum spinosum where their assembly begins (Feingold & Elias, 2014). The composition of the lipid-rich matrix changes with aging. Although not universally agreed upon, across the skin color spectrum, the differences in the stratum corneum exist as summarized by Taylor (2002). At least two studies (La Ruche & Cesarini, 1992; Rienertson & Wheatley, 1959) report that black stratum corneum has a higher lipid content and this may in part contribute to the conflicting results regarding stratum corneum thickness. The stratum corneum in darkly pigmented skin has been reported to have increased junctional integrity as evidenced by the increased number of tape strippings required to remove the stratum corneum. Whether the stratum corneum is thicker in darkly pigmented skin is unclear (Taylor, 2002).

Stratum Lucidum

The stratum lucidum is directly below the stratum corneum. This layer is found in areas where the epidermis is thicker, such as the palms of the hands and the soles of the feet, but it is absent from thinner skin, such as the eyelids. This layer can be one to five cells thick and is transparent. Cell boundaries often are difficult to identify in histologic sections under a light microscope. The stratum lucidum is a transitional layer where active lysosomal enzymes degrade the nucleus and cellular organelles before they are moved into the stratum corneum (Jacob et al., 1982; Wysocki, 1995).

Stratum Granulosum

The stratum granulosum, or granular layer, is beneath the stratum lucidum when the stratum lucidum is present; otherwise, the stratum granulosum lies beneath the stratum corneum. This layer is one to five cells thick and is so named because of the granules present in the keratinocytes of this layer. The cells of the stratum granulosum have not yet been compressed into a flattened layer and are diamond shaped. The structures contained in these cells are keratohyalin granules, which become intensely stained with the appropriate acid and basic dyes. The proteins contained in these granules (profilaggrin, intermediate keratin filaments, and loricrin) help to organize the keratin filaments in the intracellular space. Profilaggrin is cleaved to form filaggrin, which is further degraded to form urocanic acid and pyrrolidone carboxylic acid. Both urocanic acid and pyrrolidone carboxylic acid provide additional hydration to the stratum corneum and limited filtering against ultraviolet radiation (UVR). The major component of the cornified envelope is loricrin, which is cross-linked to other protein components (involucrin, cystatin A, small proline-rich proteins [SPRR1, SPRR2], elafin, envoplakin) that together form up to 70% of the molecular mass of the cells in this layer. Cells in this layer still have active nuclei (Millington & Wilkinson, 1983; Wheater & Burkitt, 1987).

Stratum Spinosum

The stratum spinosum is below the stratum granulosum. This layer often is described as the prickly layer because cytoplasmic structures in these cells take on this morphology. Generally, the cells of this layer are polyhedral. A prominent feature of the prickle layer is the desmosome, a type of cell–cell junction. The desmosomes provide adhesion between cells and resistance to mechanical forces. Cells in this layer begin to synthesize involucrin, a soluble precursor of the cornified envelopes (Millington & Wilkinson, 1983). The spinous cells contain large bundles of newly synthesized keratin filaments (K1/K10) in addition to K5/K14 still present from the basal layer (Haake et al., 2001). The identification of various classes of desmosomal proteins (plakoglobin, desmoplakin, plakophilins) and transmembrane glycoproteins (desmogleins, desmocollins) has led to the identification of their roles in various epidermal pathologies, such as bullous impetigo, pemphigus vulgaris, and other genodermatoses.

Stratum Basale or Stratum Germinativum

The stratum basale, or stratum germinativum, is the innermost epidermal layer. It often is referred to simply as the basal layer (see Fig. 7.1). It is a single layer of mitotically active cells called basal keratinocytes, or basal cells. These active cells respond to several factors, such as extracellular matrix, growth factors, hormones, and vitamins. Skin metabolism is mediated by glucose. Glucose utilization in the skin is comparable to that in muscle. Glucose leaving the circulation crosses the basement membrane and forms a concentration gradient that decreases as the glucose moves to the upper layers of the epidermis.

Once cells leave the basal layer, they begin an upward migration, which can take 2–3 weeks. A cell takes approximately 14 days to move to the stratum corneum and another 14 days to move through the stratum corneum and desquamate (Haake et al., 2001). After leaving the basal layer, the cells begin the process of differentiation. All layers of the epidermis consist of peaks and valleys, but this arrangement is more dramatic in the basal layer such that these protrusions are partly responsible for anchoring the epidermis, thus providing structural integrity. These epidermal protrusions of the basal layer point downward into the dermis and are called rete ridges, or rete pegs. The basal layer is the primary location of mitotically active cells of the epidermis and has been noted to have increased proliferative capacity compared with cells at the top of the ridges (Briggaman, 1982).

Epidermal stem cells compose about 10% of the basal cell population. These stem cells have a slow cell cycle. When labeled with a radiolabeled DNA precursor, epidermal stem cells retain the label for long periods; thus, they are identified as label-retaining cells (Bickenbach, 1981). Once cell division occurs, daughter cells that will undergo differentiation as they move toward the stratum corneum are called transient amplifying cells. These transient amplifying cells make up approximately 50% of the basal keratinocyte population (Lavker & Sun, 2000). Transient amplifying cells progress to become postmitotic cells that then terminally differentiate. A portion of the stem cell population is found in the epidermal crypts of the rete pegs and in the bulge region of hair follicles. Dividing cells go through the cell cycle, and the G_1 phase is shortened in states such as wound healing. The normal keratinocyte cell cycle time is 300 h but may be as short as 36 h when psoriasis is present. These stem cell compartments and the transient amplifying cells both are capable of limited or continuing cell division and thus are the cells most likely to reside long enough in the skin to undergo genetic modifications that lead to the development of skin cancers. The use of stem cells alone and in combination with tissue-engineering approaches is an area of active research and development in wound care (Griffith & Naughton, 2002).

Tissue oxygenation data have shown that the oxygen pressure in the epidermis is low compared with other tissue, at around 0.2%–8%, compared with 10% in the dermis. These low partial pressures result in a mildly hypoxic microenvironment with a resulting expression of hypoxia inducible factor-1α (HIF-1α). HIF-1α targets a number of genes important for skin homeostasis and repair, including genes that encode proteins for cell growth and apoptosis, cell adhesion and migration, angiogenesis, melanogenesis, DNA repair, and extracellular matrix synthesis and repair and mediates glucose uptake for cell metabolism (Rezvani, Ali, Nissen, et al., 2011).

Melanocytes, the cells responsible for skin pigmentation as a result of melanin synthesis, also are distributed in the basal layer. Melanocytes are dendritic cells that arise from melanoblasts, which derive from the neural crest. During development, they migrate to other locations, including the bulge region of hair follicles, the choroid of the eye, the heart, and the brain (Goding, 2007). Melanocytes are also required for hearing; genetic mutations resulting in a loss of melanocytes are a major cause of deafness (Steel & Barkway, 1989). Benign accumulations of melanocytes in the epidermis and/or dermis are commonly referred to as "moles" or naevi. Melanin is packaged inside the cell into melanosomes, which are transported via the cytoskeletal network of microfilaments and microtubules to the dendritic processes of the melanocyte, where they are then transferred to keratinocytes. Incorporation into the keratinocytes is thought to occur via one or more of the following processes: release and endocytosis, engulfment, active transport, or passage through channels or pores between the melanocyte and neighboring keratinocytes (Boissy, 2003). Melanocytes can be detected by 50 days' gestation in fetal development (Holbrook, Vogel, Underwood, et al., 1998). Under normal conditions, melanocytes rarely divide. In normal skin, the number of melanocytes present is nearly the same, regardless of skin color. There is approximately 1 melanocyte for every 36 basal cells. Dendritic melanocyte structures are responsible for the transfer of pigment to a large number of keratinocytes. The primary difference between light- and dark-skinned individuals is the size, number, and distribution of melanosomes, the structures containing the melanin pigment, and the activity of the melanocytes. Carotene or carotenoids are responsible for imparting the yellow hue to the skin of some individuals (Jacob et al., 1982; Sams, 1990; Solomons, 1983).

Melanin pigment is a complex polymer that is synthesized from tyrosine by activity of the tyrosinase gene pathway. Melanin is difficult to study because it is relatively insoluble (Boissy, 2003). The two primary types of melanin are brown/black eumelanin and red/yellow pheomelanin (Lin & Fisher, 2007). Pheomelanin is more photolabile, and damage leads to release of oxygen radicals such as hydrogen peroxide, superoxide, and hydroxyl radicals, resulting in oxidative stress and DNA damage (Lin & Fisher, 2007). Constitutive synthesis, or the synthesis that occurs at basal levels, results primarily from genetic regulation. Facultative synthesis is the additional up- or downregulation of melanin synthesis in response to UVR, hormones, cytokines, immune regulation, chemical exposure, or other agents (Boissy, 2003). Interestingly, once delivered to the keratinocytes, melanosomes are preferentially, although not exclusively, clustered around the apical side of the nucleus, where they can more effectively provide protection from UVR to prevent DNA damage leading to mutations (Boissy, 2003). In addition to its photoprotective effect, melanin is thought to act as a sink for highly reactive oxygen species

that can also lead to DNA damage (Goding, 2007). Pathologies associated with melanocytes or pigmentation are melanoma, dyschromias such as vitiligo and melasma, xeroderma pigmentosa, and albinism.

As a result of genetics, genetic recombination, and selective environmental pressures (e.g., UVR intensity and exposure, age, hormonal influences), skin pigmentation demonstrates considerable variation across the human population. Presently more than 150 genes have been identified that either directly or indirectly affect skin color (Yamaguchi & Hearing, 2009). Key proteins and receptors identified with the synthesis and transport of melanin or melanosomes include melanocyte-stimulating hormone, melanocortin-1 receptor (MC1R), keratinocyte growth factor, and protease-activated receptor-2. The red hair/light skin phenotype is associated with mutations found in the residues of MC1R, which lead to increased risk for skin cancer (Miyamura, Coelho, Wolber, et al., 2006). Thus, the skin color spectrum ranges from dense black, with the highest level and distribution of melanosomes, to various shades of brown to white and finally to albino, or the complete absence of pigment (but not an absence of melanocytes). In general, Caucasian and Asian skin has smaller melanosomes that form small clusters or aggregates, whereas dense African skin has larger melanosomes that are distributed primarily as single units (Montagna, Prota, & Kenney, 1993; Szabo, Gerald, Pathak, et al., 1969; Szabo, Gerald, Pathak, Fitzpatrick, et al., 1972). In darkly pigmented skin, despite the hydrolytic degradation that occurs with keratinocyte differentiation, some melanosomes can still be seen in the stratum corneum, whereas in light skin no melanosomes are seen in the stratum corneum (Boissy, 2003). Various shades of brown skin occur across African, African American, Hispanic, Asian, Caucasian, and Native American peoples; these shades are influenced by the number, size, and distribution of melanosomes. The range of variation can even occur in the same individual, depending on skin location and sun exposure (Szabo, 1954). In general, the density of melanocytes is slightly higher in skin covering the upper dorsal surfaces compared with skin on the lower dorsal surfaces, and the amount of melanin present in the skin correlates well with visible skin pigmentation seen on physical examination (Miyamura et al., 2006).

Intensely pigmented skin can mask the detection of skin inflammatory reactions, which is seen as reddened areas in light-skinned individuals that may appear in response to conditions such as contact dermatitis, pressure, or folliculitis. Inflammation may appear as darker areas in black skin, violet-black in intensely black skin, or black in brown skin. Other signs of inflammation may include the detection of heat or warmth to touch or induration detected as skin tightening or hardening over areas where there is skin damage. Dermatologic disorders accompanied by inflammation can result in postinflammatory hypopigmentation or hyperpigmentation that can be especially distressing to individuals with more darkly pigmented skin in which the color contrast can be dramatically evident. Other dermatologic disorders more commonly associated with darkly pigmented skin include vitiligo and keloids. Keloids occur 3–18 times more frequently in darkly pigmented skin, and the incidence has been reported as between 4.5% and 16% in Chinese, Hispanic, and African American individuals (Oluwasanmi, 1974; Robles & Berg, 2007; Taylor, 2002, 2003).

Universal agreement concerning comparative differences, if any, across the skin color spectrum for transepidermal water loss (TEWL), stratum corneum structure, epidermal thickness, and sweat and sebaceous gland number or distribution is fraught with numerous points of criticism that include low numbers of subjects, variation in age, gender, circadian rhythms, use of emollients, relative temperature and humidity, geographic location, location of skin sample, sun-exposed vs sun-protected areas, nutrition, validity and reliability of instrumentation, and accurate indexing to skin color (McDonald, 1988; Taylor, 2002). It has been noted that there are 31 climate zones around the globe subject to the adaptation, lifestyle, and conditions of people with various customs and resources, and climate can influence birth weight, body shape, and cranial morphology (Lambert, Mann, & Dugas, 2008). Thus, definitive studies of skin biology across the range of the skin color spectrum relative to age and gender await more exhaustive and comprehensive research studies and may require more precise instrumentation for some measures.

Basement Membrane Zone

The basement membrane zone (BMZ), or dermal–epidermal junction, is the area that separates the epidermis from the dermis. Closer examination of the BMZ in the past decade has revealed the BMZ to be more complex than previously believed. Basal keratinocytes use hemidesmosomes to structurally and functionally attach to the BMZ. The BMZ is subdivided into three distinct zones: the lamina lucida, the lamina densa, and the lamina fibroreticularis. The lamina lucida is so named because it is an electron-translucent zone compared with the electron-dense zone of the lamina densa. The major proteins found in the BMZ are fibronectin, an adhesive glycoprotein; laminin, a glycoprotein; type IV collagen, a nonfiber-forming collagen; and heparin sulfate proteoglycan, a glycosaminoglycan. A lesser amount of type VII collagen has also been detected that forms anchoring fibrils linking the extracellular matrix of the dermis to the basement membrane. The BMZ anchors the epidermis to the dermis and is the layer that is affected in blister formation associated with dermatologic diseases, second-degree burns, full-thickness wounds, and mechanical trauma. During wound healing the BMZ is disrupted and must be reformed (Sams, 1990). The BMZ also acts to as a nutrient flow for metabolites and other molecules into the epithelium since no blood vessels occur in the epidermis.

Dermis

The dermis, or corium, is the thickest tissue layer of the skin. Compared with the cellular epidermal layer, the dermis is sparsely populated (primarily by fibroblast cells) and is vascularized and innervated. The dermal layer is derived from the middle embryonic germ layer, the mesoderm.

Dermal thickness ranges from 2 to 4 mm, but on average is 2 mm. Variations in dermal thickness account for differences in total skin thickness that have been measured throughout the body. The dermis of the back is thicker than the dermis covering the scalp, forehead, abdomen, thigh, wrist, and palm.

The dermal vasculature consists of a network of papillary loops, supported by a deep horizontal plexus. The vasculature functions to provide nutritional support, immune surveillance, wound healing, thermal regulation, hemostasis, and the inflammatory response. Formation of the vascular system involves vasculogenesis and angiogenesis. Vasculogenesis is the process that occurs de novo during embryonic development and is mediated by angioblasts derived from the mesoderm. Angiogenesis is the process whereby new vessels are formed from preexisting vessels. It is involved in wound healing, tumor growth and metastasis, hemangiomas, telangiectasia, psoriasis, and scleroderma. Vascular endothelial growth factor (VEGF), or vascular permeability factor, is secreted by keratinocytes in response to hypoxia. It is increased in wound healing and is responsible for stimulating angiogenesis. Other factors that stimulate angiogenesis include acidic and basic fibroblast growth factor, interleukin-8, platelet-derived endothelial growth factor, placental growth factor, transforming growth factor-α and transforming growth factor-β, oncostatin M, angiogenin, and heparin-binding epidermal growth factor. Inhibitors of angiogenesis include angiostatin, thrombospondin, endostatin, interferon-γ, interleukin-12, and platelet factor-4.

The major proteins found in the dermis are collagen and elastin. The other category of proteins found occupying the space between collagen and elastin fibers is referred to as the ground substance. The ground substance in black skin is distinctly more abundant in both the papillary and reticular layers than in white skin (Montagna & Carlisle, 1991). This category of proteins is largely composed of proteoglycans and glycosaminoglycans. Included in this category of proteins are chondroitin sulfates and dermatan sulfate (also called mucopolysaccharide), versican, aggrecan, a class of small leucine rich proteoglycans (decorin, asporin, biglycan, lumican, fibromodulin), hyaluronate or hyaluronic acid, keratan sulfate, heparan and heparan sulfate proteoglycans (syndecan, perlecan), aggrecan, decorin, and chondroitin-6 sulfate proteoglycans. Although these proteins account for only approximately 0.2% of the dry weight of the dermis, these large molecules are capable of binding up to 1000 times their volume. Thus, proteoglycans and glycosaminoglycans play a role in regulating the water-binding capacity of the dermis, which can determine dermal volume and compressibility. Hyaluronan is also found in the dermis and in higher abundance in fetal skin, where it forms a watery, less stable matrix that allows greater cell movement; it also is a critical factor in scarless healing (Longaker, Adzick, Hall, et al., 1990). Hyaluronan can bind growth factors and provide cellular linkages with other matrix materials that together function to regulate cell migration, adhesion, proliferation, differentiation, morphogenesis, and tissue repair (Haake & Holbrook, 1999). Other glycoproteins found in the dermis include fibronectin, thrombospondin, laminin, vitronectin, and tenascin. These glycoproteins are synthesized and secreted by fibroblasts in the dermis.

Data indicate that skin fibroblasts from different anatomic locations contain different transcriptional patterns that can indicate position and can be differentiated from fibroblasts in other locations using microarray analysis (Chang, Chi, Dudoit, et al., 2002). Fibroblasts present in the dermis range in size and number. It has been reported that fibroblasts in black facial skin were larger, occurred in greater numbers, and were more likely to be binucleated or multinucleated compared with white skin. Overall, the dermis in black skin was thick and compact compared with thinner and less compact in white skin (Montagna & Carlisle, 1991). In this same study, collagen fiber bundles were observed to be smaller, more tightly packed and were oriented parallel to the epidermis in black skin and had more fiber fragments. Somewhat in contrast, white skin was noted to have larger collagen fiber bundles with some degraded collagen fragments, which may have resulted from sun exposure, but had greater variability in the number of fibroblasts. No differences in mast cells were observed. However, black skin did have more binucleated and multinucleated macrophages in the papillary dermis, and the accompanying melanophages in black skin contained melanosomes both singly and in complexes, whereas in white skin the melanophages were almost exclusively in complexes (Montagna & Carlisle, 1991). Again, these findings should be viewed with caution given the lack of comprehensive studies across the skin color spectrum. The dermis is a matrix that supports the epidermis. It can be divided into two areas: papillary dermis and reticular dermis (see Fig. 7.1). The papillary and reticular layers appear more distinct in white skin and less distinct in black skin (Montagna & Carlisle, 1991).

Papillary Dermis

The papillary dermis lies immediately below the BMZ and forms interdigitating structures with the rete ridges of the epidermis called dermal papillae. The dermal papillae contain papillary loops (Fig. 7.2), which supply the necessary oxygen and nutrients to the overlying epidermis via the BMZ. The collagen fibers contained in the papillary dermis are much smaller in diameter and form smaller, wavy, cable-like structures compared with the reticular dermis. This portion of the dermis also contains small elastic fibers and has a greater proportion of ground substance than the reticular dermis. The superficial subepidermis in darkly pigmented skin contains more numerous blood vessels, along with many more dilated lymph channels (Montagna & Carlisle, 1991). The papillary dermis also contains lymphatic vessels that play a role in controlling interstitial fluid pressure by resorption of fluid and assist in clearing the tissues of cells, lipids, bacteria, proteins, and other degraded substances. The papillary lymph vessels drain into the horizontal plexus of larger lymph vessels located in the deep subpapillary venous plexus. This system is further connected to the lymph system in the reticular dermis. Fluid flow through this system is partially controlled through arterial pulsations, muscle contractions, and body movement. Renewed interest in the skin lymphatic system has resulted from the identification of markers such as VEGF-C, VEGFR-3, and lymphatic vessel endothelial receptor-1 and the findings of the role of these lymphatic vessels in tumor promotion (Chu, 2008).

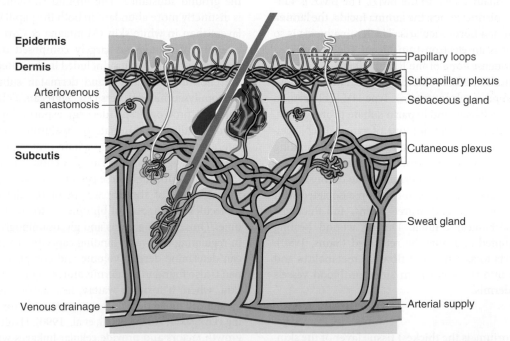

Fig. 7.2 Blood circulation in the skin with papillary loops, which supply oxygen and nutrients to the epidermis, and dermal cutaneous plexuses, which arise from the deeper blood supply located in the hypodermis. (From Young, B., O'Dowd, G., & Woodford, P. (2006). *Wheater's functional histology: A text and colour atlas* (5th ed.). Edinburgh: Churchill Livingstone.)

Reticular Dermis

The reticular dermis (the area below the papillary dermis) forms the base of the dermis. The collagen fibers in the reticular dermis are thicker in diameter and form larger cable-like structures than in the papillary dermis. There is no clear separation of papillary and reticular dermis because the collagen fibers change in size gradually between the two layers. Thicker elastic fibers are found in the reticular dermis, but substantially less ground substance is present. A complex of cutaneous blood vessels is found in this part of the dermis.

Dermal Proteins

Collagen, the protein that gives the skin its tensile strength, is the major structural protein found in the dermis and accounts for 25% of the skin's total weight (Stryer, 1995). The primary constituents of collagen are proline, glycine, hydroxyproline, and hydroxylysine. Collagen is secreted by dermal fibroblasts as tropocollagen, which undergoes additional extracellular processing so that mature collagen fibers are formed. Normal human dermis is primarily composed of type I collagen, a fiber-forming collagen. Type I collagen represents 77%–85% of the collagen present; type III collagen, also a fiber-forming collagen, represents the remaining 15%–23% (Gay & Miller, 1978; Wysocki et al., 2005). Very small amounts of type V collagen (less than 5%) and type VI collagen also are present. Type XII collagen has been detected that decorates the surface of type I, III, and V collagen to maintain skin matrix structure and modulates growth factor availability and regulates cell composition and function (Schonborn, Willenborg, Schulz, et al., 2020).

Elastin, another protein found in the dermis, provides the skin's elastic recoil, a feature that prevents the skin from being permanently reshaped. It is a fiber-forming protein, like collagen. Elastin has a high amount of proline and glycine. However, unlike collagen, elastin lacks large amounts of hydroxyproline. Elastin fibers form structures, similar to coils, that allow this protein to be stretched and, when released, to return to its inherent configuration. Elastin accounts for less than 2% of the skin's dry weight (Millington & Wilkinson, 1983; Sams, 1990; Wysocki, 1995). Elastin is distributed with collagen but in smaller amounts and can also be found in association with two other fibers, oxytalan and elaunin as part of the system of elastic forming fibers. Large concentrations of elastin are found in blood vessels (especially the aortic arch near the heart) and lymphatic vessels. The distribution of elastic fibers ranges from less abundant in darkly pigmented skin to more abundant in light skin. Upon exposure to sunlight, elastic fibers in darkly pigmented skin show no obvious signs of damage, whereas elastic fibers in light skin show obvious signs of elastosis (Montagna et al., 1993). The lower distribution of elastic fibers in darkly pigmented skin also extends to the anchorage of hair follicles, leading to an increase in hair breakage and a higher prevalence of traumatic alopecia in both men and women (Taylor, 2002). Furthermore, the curvature of hair follicles and the spiral configuration seen in Africans and African Americans lead to pseudofolliculitis, especially in men who shave.

Other cells found in the dermis are mast cells, macrophages, and lymphocytes. All of these cells are involved with immune surveillance of the skin, often referred to as the skin immune system. The dermis also contains dermal appendages that include hair follicles, sebaceous glands, and eccrine and apocrine sweat glands. Glomus bodies that can act as arteriovenous shunts are also found in the dermis of the fingertips, hands, and feet that can control skin blood flow at these sites that are prone to the effects of cold temperatures. This body is composed of muscular vessel forming tissue in combination with dense collagenous tissue that are under nerve control.

Hypodermis

Hypodermis, or superficial fascia, forms a subcutaneous layer below the dermis. It is an adipose rich layer containing a subdermal plexus of blood vessels giving rise to the cutaneous plexus in the dermis, which in turn gives rise to the papillary plexus and loops of the papillary dermis (see Fig. 7.2). The hypodermis attaches the dermis to underlying structures. This layer provides insulation for the body, a ready reserve of energy, and additional cushioning; it also adds to the mobility of the skin over underlying structures (Haake & Holbrook, 1999). Growing hair follicles and apocrine and eccrine sweat glands can extend into this layer. The hypodermis is largely absent in certain pathologic disease states, such as Werner syndrome and scleroderma. Adipocytes form the primary cells in this tissue layer, and their activity is regulated by leptin. This layer also contains a reservoir of adipose derived stem cells that are of mesodermal origin and modulate skin repair and in concert with other cells exert paracrine and endocrine effects (Zuk, Zhu, Ashjian, et al., 2002). With aging this reservoir of stem cells is decreased and the ability of these cells to respond is diminished.

Mucous Membranes

Mucous membranes are specialized soft tissue structures that are distributed across a variety of visible external and unseen internal surfaces that interface with the external environment. Mucous membranes are typically composed of a layer of epithelial tissue attached to a basement membrane over an underlying layer of connective tissue or lamina propria that is further supported by a thin layer of smooth muscle tissue. Mucous membranes are found in the respiratory (nose, trachea, and lungs), gastrointestinal (GI) (lips, mouth stomach, lining the digestive tract and anus), urogenital tracts (urethra, urinary bladder, ureters, and vagina) and in the eye. It is estimated that mucous membranes cover 400 m^2 compared with the 2 m^2 of the skin. Typically, these mucous membranes are formed by a layer(s) of unkeratinized stratified squamous epithelium or simple columnar epithelium. These layers can be traversed by blood vessels, nerves, fibrous tissue structures, and lymphatic channels. These layers are able to withstand abrasions and wear encountered in the daily interface with their exposure to air, wind, urine, and food. Mucous membranes have specialized cells or associated glands (lacrimal gland in the eye) that can secrete and/or absorb substances that can provide lubrication and control or kill bacteria.

Mucous membranes are colonized with bacteria, most notably in the GI tract and form part of the immune system. Embryologically, a majority of mucous membranes are of endodermal origin. However, the palate, cheeks, floor of the mouth, gums, lips, and a portion of the anal canal below the pectinate line are of ectodermal origin.

These membranes are referred to with various names, for example, the conjunctiva in the eye lines the eyelids and covers the sclera. In the eye, mucous membranes also contain melanocytes and T and B cell lymphocytes. In the uterus, the endometrium is a specialized mucous membrane.

Mucus in the primary substance secreted by these specialized membranes along with a host of other substances such as water, lipids, lysozyme, lipocalin, lactoferrin, lacritin, immunoglobulins, urea, sodium, glucose, and potassium. Mucin is the principal component of mucus that is a mucopolysaccharide. This slippery watery substance provides protection, moisture and lubrication across these surfaces.

Injury to these tissues is often visible to wound care providers as a consequence of catheter tubing such as feeding tubes, nasal cannula, and urinary catheters that can visibly be seen to erode these thin epithelial layers on the surface of these mucous membranes and/or the underlying supporting structures.

SKIN FUNCTIONS

The skin provides several functions: protection, immunity, thermoregulation, sensation, metabolism, and communication (Jacob et al., 1982; Millington & Wilkinson, 1983; Woodburne & Burkel, 1988).

Protection

The skin protects the body against aqueous, chemical, and mechanical assaults; bacterial and viral pathogens; and UVR. It also prevents excessive loss of fluids and electrolytes in order to maintain the homeostatic environment. The effectiveness of the skin in preventing excessive fluid loss can be seen in patients with burns. Patients with burns involving 30% of their body can lose up to 4.1 L of fluid compared with 710 mL for normal adults (Rudowski, 1976). The skin maintains the internal milieu, and a progressive decrease in water content across the epidermal layers helps to prevent excessive TEWL under basal conditions. Water constitutes 65%–70% of the basal layer and decreases to 40% in the granular layer and 15% in the stratum corneum (Warner, Myers, & Taylor, 1988). The skin's barrier function is so effective that percutaneous drug delivery is limited except in premature babies and in newborns. In general, compounds are restricted to those with a molecular mass of 500 Da or less with a daily dose of 10 mg or less. Protection against mechanical assaults is mainly provided by the tough fibroelastic tissue of the dermis, collagen, and elastin.

Protection Against Pathogens

Protection against aqueous, chemical, bacterial, and viral pathogens is provided by the stratum corneum, secretions from the sebaceous glands, and the skin immune system. Epithelial cells have pattern recognition receptors as part of the skin immune system that are capable of recognizing microbes via their cell wall components, nucleic acids, and flagella and have the ability to recruit immune cells. The primary line of defense against all of these agents is an intact stratum corneum (Roth & James, 1988). The insoluble protein keratin, found in the horny layer, provides good resistance. In addition, the constant shedding of squames from the stratum corneum prevents the entrenchment of microorganisms.

Sebum, a lipid-rich, oily substance secreted by the sebaceous glands onto the skin surface, usually via hair follicles and shafts, provides an acidic coating with a pH ranging from 4 to 6.8 (Spince & Mason, 1987) and a mean pH of 5.5 (Roth & James, 1988; Wysocki et al., 2005). Salt and electrolytes from eccrine sweat provide additional acidification. This acidity, together with natural antibacterial substances found in sebum, retards the growth of microorganisms. These glands are stimulated by sex hormones (androgens) and become very active during adolescence. Sebum, along with keratin, provides resistance to aqueous and chemical solutions. When sebaceous glands occur in association with hair follicles, they are called a pilosebaceous unit. Sebaceous glands are not found on palms or soles; they occur in areas that lack hair, such as lips. These glands are largest when they are located on the face and when associated with hair follicles. Sebaceous glands may increase in size by 100–150 times as sebum accumulates. Maximum secretion occurs in persons in their late teens to early twenties. Rates of secretion are higher in men and decline 32% per decade in females compared with 23% per decade in males.

Resistance to pathogenic microorganisms is also provided by normal skin flora through bacterial interference (Noble, 2004; Weinberg & Swartz, 1987). Conceptually, the two categories of skin flora are (1) resident (bacteria normally found on a person) and (2) transient (bacteria not normally found on a person and usually shed by daily hygienic practices, such as bathing and hand washing). Resident bacteria are found on exposed skin; moist areas such as the axillae, perineum, and toe webs; and covered skin. Bacterial microcolonies are found in hair follicles and at the edges of squames as halos in the upper loose surface layers. It has been estimated that in healthy skin a $1\text{-}cm^2$ area is covered with 1 million or more bacteria, including those in appendages such as the hair follicle and sebaceous glands (Grice, Kong, Renaud, et al., 2008). The skin microbiome has been examined using 16S rRNA, a highly conserved gene across different species of bacteria, in combination with polymerase chain reaction to provide a more comprehensive topographic map that demonstrates the regional diversity across air-exposed and covered skin surfaces where creases and moisture can shift the bacterial populations (Grice, Kong, Conlan, et al., 2009) and varies depending on epidermal vs dermal compartment. The epidermal microbiota compartment has higher variability due to environmental exposure, whereas the dermal compartment is more stable. It is estimated that only 1% of bacterial species are identified using standard laboratory methods using bacterial culture media.

The most predominant phyla represented are Actinobacteria (51.8%), represented by the genera and *Propionibacteria*; Firmicutes (24.4%), represented by the genera *Staphylococci*; Proteobacteria (16.5%); and Bacteroidetes (6.3%) (Grice et al., 2009). A noteworthy finding is that gram-negative bacteria are abundant on dry surfaces, having previously thought to be rare skin colonizers. Furthermore, sequence data using the 16S approach indicate that swab, scrape, or punch biopsy are each sufficient to obtain a representative sample of the community membership of the bacteria present (Grice et al., 2008). Generally, the following species of bacteria are routinely found on human skin: Staphylococcus, Micrococcus, Peptococcus, Corynebacterium, Brevibacterium, Propionibacterium, Streptococcus, Neisseria, and Acinetobacter. The yeast Pityrosporum, the fungi Malassezia, and the mite Demodex are also found. Not all species are found on any one individual, but most individuals have at least five of these genera. Normal viral florae are not known to exist (Noble, 2004). However, viruses have been detected in compromised skin and in individuals who are not immunocompetent.

An association exists between skin pH and bacteria. For example, *Propionibacterium acnes* grow well at pH values of 6 and 6.5, but its growth is markedly decreased at pH 5.5 (Korting & Braun-Falco, 1996). However, this association can vary depending on the specific bacterial species involved and the body location. The formation of bacterial biofilms has been scrutinized (Wysocki, 2002), and the role of normal skin flora in the formation of these biofilms is an area of active investigation. Biofilms are essentially an extracellular polysaccharide matrix, or glycocalyx, in which microorganisms are embedded. Biofilms are composed of mixed bacterial species living in their own microniche in a complex, metabolically cooperative microbial community that maintains its own form of homeostasis and rudimentary circulatory system (Costerton, Lewandowski, Caldwell, et al., 1995). Biofilms are resistant to host immune responses and are markedly more resistant to antibiotic and topical bactericidals (Xu, McFeters, & Stewart, 2000). Reports indicate that biofilm cells can be at least 500 times more resistant to antibacterial agents (Costerton et al., 1995). Biofilm formation is familiar to clinicians and can be identified on endotracheal tubes, Hickman catheters, central venous catheters, contact lenses, and orthopedic devices. *Pseudomonas aeruginosa* forms biofilms in conjunction with other bacterial species. Quorum sensing by bacteria is a feature in biofilm formation. These biofilms complicate the eradication of infections because they give rise to sessile and planktonic bacteria. Planktonic bacteria can be cleared by phagocytosis, antibodies, and antibiotics (Costerton, Stewart, & Greenberg, 1999). Sessile bacteria in biofilms can evade antibiotics by giving rise to planktonic bacteria, which respond to antibiotics and host immune responses, but the sessile bacteria remain. Cycles of antibiotic treatment often are administered without success, and the symptoms of infection recur. In these situations, biofilm formation should be suspected, and surgical removal of the sessile population most likely will be required to eliminate the pathogenic bacteria. Moist skin areas, such as the axillae,

perineum, toe webs, hair follicles, nail beds, and sweat glands, are especially prone to an increased presence of bacteria. Protection from bacterial invasion is mediated in part by antimicrobial peptides (AMPs), proteins called defensins (Hoffmann, Kafatos, Janeway, et al., 1999), cathelicidins, and protegrins and RNases (Simanski, Köten, Schröder, et al., 2012). More than 1200 AMPs have been identified, and in the skin, they are found in keratinocytes, mast cells, neutrophils, sebocytes, and eccrine epithelial cells (Nakatsuji & Gallo, 2012). Findings show that β-defensin is abundant in skin and may be important for wound healing. Defensins act in conjunction with phagocytosing neutrophils and the membrane attack complex of complement. Thus, optimal skin and wound care is a cornerstone of clinical practice in preventing the progression from bacterial colonization to infection (Wysocki, 2002).

Protection Against Ultraviolet Radiation

Protection against UVR is provided by skin pigmentation, which results from synthesis of the pigment melanin. Harmful effects are primarily attributable to UVA, the long wave form of UVR, which ranges spectrally from 320 to 400 nm, and UVB, the short-wave ultraviolet form, which ranges from 290 to 320 nm (Council on Scientific Affairs, 1989). Approximately 90%–99% of UVA reaches the planet's surface compared with only 1%–10% of UVB. The shorter the waves, the more dangerous they are. UVC is effectively blocked by an intact ozone layer. Holes appearing in the ozone layer have raised concern over the effects of UVR in causing skin diseases. Because darker-skinned individuals have increased synthesis, amount, and distribution of melanin, they are better protected against skin cancer. More melanin is distributed in all layers of the epidermis in dark skin than in light skin (Spince & Mason, 1987).

Darkly pigmented black skin provides more efficient protection from both UVB and UVA. The mean transmission of UVB is approximately 7.4% and that of UVA is 17.5% in darkly pigmented skin compared with 29.4% and 55.5%, respectively, in white skin. The mechanism for the more efficient absorption and scattering of UVB and UVA in darkly pigmented skin is attributed to the larger size and number of melanosomes in black skin. The superior UVB/UVA efficiency in black skin can provide a skin protection factor of approximately 13.4 compared with 3.4 for white skin (Montagna et al., 1993), with a range from 10- to 15-fold that is seen in the absence of melanin when the minimal erythematous dose is used as a measure (Lin & Fisher, 2007). However, in terms of protection against various types of skin cancer, highly pigmented skin affords a 500–1000 times reduction in risk (Lin & Fisher, 2007). An inverse relationship exists between melanin levels and DNA damage, with darker skin having less DNA damage. Higher melanin levels also decrease damage to basal stem cells and melanocytes in the deep epidermis. Thus, DNA damage in darkly pigmented skin is largely restricted to the upper layers of the epidermis, whereas DNA damage in lightly pigmented skin occurs throughout all layers of the epidermis (Miyamura et al.,

2006). Melanocytes in darkly pigmented skin are more efficient than melanocytes in lighter skin in their response to the same UVR challenge (Miyamura et al., 2006). The immediate response in darkly pigmented skin leads to a more efficient distribution and trafficking of melanosomes to the upper epidermis. An actual increase in melanin synthesis is largely a delayed response (Tadokoro, Yamaguchi, Batzer, et al., 2005). Finally, UV-induced apoptosis leading to removal of damaged cells is higher in darkly pigmented skin, resulting in an overall lower incidence of skin carcinogenesis (Yamaguchi, Beer, & Hearing, 2008). However, even individuals with darkly pigmented skin can develop skin cancers, and the increased melanin content often can mask precancerous and cancerous lesions, leading to poorer outcomes when the lesions eventually are detected and treated.

Clinically, the skin phototype (SPT) system was developed as a valid and practical tool to characterize the reactivity of human skin to UVR based on the minimal erythematous dose and the ability to tan upon sun exposure (Fitzpatrick, 1988; Pathak, Nghiem, & Fitzpatrick, 1999). It is one of the most widely used systems to classify skin pigmentation by dermatologists and the Food and Drug Administration (Fitzpatrick, 1988; Taylor, 2002). Originally this system was developed to guide the exposure of individuals receiving psoralen ultraviolet A for psoriasis when it was found that hair and eye color were not sufficient to determine the level of exposure (Fitzpatrick, 1988). Over time the system was expanded from primarily one that defined various light-skinned individuals to include darkly pigmented skin. The SPT system ranges from I (ivory, white) to VI (dark brown or black) and is now defined based on (1) constitutive or unexposed skin color, (2) minimal erythematous dose and minimal melanogenic dose for UVB and UVA, (3) reactivity to ultraviolet light, (4) sunburn and tanning history, (5) immediate pigment darkening, (6) delayed tanning, (7) extent of photoaging, and (8) susceptibility to skin cancer (Pathak, Fitzpatrick, Nghiem, et al., 1999).

Exposure to UVR can lead to skin cancer, sunburn (first- or second-degree burns), compromised immunity, and long-term skin damage. Sun-exposed epidermal skin is thicker and rougher than unexposed skin, is more prone to benign and malignant growths, and tends to have a greater decrease in Langerhans cells (which seems to occur independent of skin color) (Scheibner, Hollis, McCarthy, et al., 1986). And the increase in skin pigmentation that occurs in sun-exposed skin also leads to an increase in pigmentation in sun-protected skin (Stierner, Rosdahl, Augustsson, et al., 1989). Infrequent sun exposure may be more harmful than regular exposure (Miyamura et al., 2006). Sun-exposed dermis has increased elastogenesis and a greater decrease in mature collagen with fragmented collagen fibrils compared with unexposed dermis.

Skin Immune System

The skin immune system also provides protection against invading microorganisms and antigens. The cells of the skin that provide immune protection are the Langerhans cells, which are antigen-presenting cells found in the epidermis; interstitial dendritic cells in the dermis; tissue macrophages,

which ingest and digest bacteria and other substances; mast cells, which contain histamine (released in inflammatory reactions); and dendrocytes. Immune cells (dendritic cells, monocytes, macrophages, B cells, T cells) and some nonimmune cells (fibroblasts, epithelial cells, and endothelial cells) found in the skin have pattern recognition receptors, most notably toll-like receptors that can initiate an immune response especially against microbial molecules. Both skin resident B and T cell populations modulate skin homeostasis where B cell populations can secrete IgM and IgA to control commensal and invading microorganisms, enhance efferocytosis by macrophages, limit inflammation with secretion of IL-10, and produce cytokines and growth factors that support wound healing (Debes & McGettigan, 2019). Both macrophages and mast cells are found in the dermis (Auger, 1986; Benyon, 1989; Wolff & Stingl, 1983). Using a standard panel of 41 allergens, allergic contact dermatitis and irritant contact dermatitis overall do not appear to be different in white compared with black individuals, although their response to specific allergens is different (DeLeo, Taylor, Belsito, et al., 2002).

Langerhans cells are responsible for the recognition, uptake, processing, and presentation of soluble antigens and haptens to sensitized T lymphocytes. This occurs through binding of T cells to Langerhans cells. Exposure to UVB light decreases the functional capability of Langerhans cells (Bergstresser, Toews, & Streilein, 1980). Dermal dendritic cells are now recognized as having a more prominent role in antigen presentation, with Langerhans cells remaining important for activation of regulatory cells.

Tissue macrophages are derived from monocytes, which arise from bone marrow precursor cells. Macrophages are among the most important cells of the skin's immune system because they are versatile. Once monocytes migrate into the tissue, they differentiate and become macrophages. Cells in the dermis that are not completely differentiated are difficult to distinguish, and much effort has been made in the past decade to recognize the various cells in the dermis. Macrophages, in addition to their antibacterial activity, can process and present antigens to immunocompetent lymphoid cells; are tumoricidal; and can secrete growth factors, cytokines, and other immunomodulatory molecules. Macrophages are involved in coagulation, atherogenesis, wound healing, and tissue remodeling (Haake & Holbrook, 1999).

Mast cells are usually distributed in the papillary dermis, around epidermal appendages, blood vessels and nerves in the subpapillary plexus, and in subcutaneous fat. These cells are distributed in connective tissue throughout the body in places where organs interface with the environment. Mast cells contain or secrete a host of proteins on demand. Thus, mast cells are the primary effector cells in allergic reactions. They also are involved in conditions of subacute and chronic inflammatory disease. Increased numbers of mast cells have been detected in tissues affected by chronic eczema, psoriasis, scleroderma, porphyria cutanea tarda, lichen simplex chronicus, lichen planus, and in healing wounds. As a part of the skin immune system, mast cells play a role in protecting against parasites, stimulating chemotaxis, and promoting phagocytosis; are involved in the activation and proliferation of eosinophils; are capable of altering vasotension and vascular permeability; and can promote connective tissue repair and angiogenesis (Haake & Holbrook, 1999).

Dermal dendrocytes are highly phagocytic cells found in the papillary and upper reticular dermis. They also are distributed near vessels in the subpapillary plexus, reticular dermis, and subcutaneous fat. These immunologically competent cells are highly phagocytic and can be recognized as melanophages. Their numbers are increased in fetal, infant, and photoaged skin and in pathologic skin conditions such as psoriasis and eczema (Headington, 1989). Their numbers are decreased in malignant fibrotic tumors and fibroproliferative lesions, such as keloids, scars, and scleroderma (Headington & Cerio, 1990).

Thermoregulation

Thermoregulation of the body is provided by the skin forming a barrier between the outside and inside environments, thus maintaining the body's temperature. The two primary thermoregulatory mechanisms are circulation and sweating. Blood vessels can either dilate to dissipate heat or constrict to shunt heat to underlying body organs. When dilated, these vessels have increased blood flow and release heat by conduction, convection, radiation, and evaporation. Vasoconstriction is often accompanied by the action of arrector pili muscle attached to hair follicles. This action results in the hair standing vertically. In mammals that depend on hair for warmth, this action fluffs up the fur to increase thermal capacity. The resulting visible bulge around hair shafts is commonly referred to as goose bumps. In humans, shivering is more important than the vertical orientation of hair for maintaining body temperature when the outside environment is cold (Jacob et al., 1982; Sams, 1990). In cold weather the "core" body temperature encompasses a smaller zone, whereas in warm weather the "core" is expanded. Sensations of cold and warm are generally detected below 30°C and above 37°C, respectively. Clinically it has been estimated that for each 1°C (1.8°F) increase in fever, a patient's fluid and calorie needs increase by 13%. At rest, the trunk, viscera, and brain account for 70% of heat production but compose only 36% of body mass. However, during exercise, muscle and skin account for 90% of heat production but represent 56% of body mass (Wenger, 1999).

Unlike other skin structures, hair follicles have a repeated cycle of growth and regression. Follicle development begins in month 4 of gestation. The hair growth cycle consists of anagen (growth phase), catagen (follicle involution), and telogen (dormant or resting phase) phases. In addition, a population of epidermal stem cells in the bulge region of the hair follicle contributes to reepithelialization in partial-thickness wounds. Hair shape varies depending on ethnicity and location. Asians have the largest diameter scalp hair and Caucasians the smallest. In the scalp, approximately 85% of hair is in anagen phase and 15% in telogen phase. The anagen phase lasts from 2 to 5 years. On the extremities, anagen lasts from 22 to 28 days (Freinkel, 2001).

Sweating occurs when the activity of the sweat glands is increased. It has been estimated that the human body has from 2 to 5 million sweat glands ranging in size from 0.05 to 0.1 mm. Sweat glands are of two types—eccrine and apocrine. Eccrine glands arise from epidermal invagination and are found abundantly on the palms of the hands and the soles of the feet. These glands are largely under the control of the nervous system, responding to temperature differences and emotional stimulation. Their secretory activity also is influenced by muscular activity. These sweat glands, located in the dermis as a coil, secrete fluid that is 99%–99.5% water; the remainder consists of sodium chloride, urea, sulfates, and phosphates (Solomons, 1983; Spince & Mason, 1987). The pH is slightly acidic. Thermoregulatory control occurs as a result of cooling when fluid evaporates from the skin surface, since evaporation requires heat. The odor associated with sweat is largely a result of bacterial action. Eccrine sweat glands are capable of producing 1–4 L of sweat per hour, resulting in a 75%–90% reduction in body heat. Man is capable of losing heat more rapidly and for longer periods than is any other animal (Quinton, 1983).

Apocrine sweat glands usually are found in association with hair follicles; they do not play a significant role in thermoregulation. These coiled, tubular glands are present in the axillae and in the anogenital area; modifications of these glands are found in the ear and secrete ear wax, or cerumen (Spince & Mason, 1987). There are approximately 100,000 apocrine glands, each 2–3 mm in diameter. Apocrine glands produce secretions in small amounts. The secretions are turbid, and they contain iron, carbohydrates, and lipids.

In general, no differences in the quantity, structure, or function of eccrine or apocrine sweat glands between individuals have been identified (Badreshia-Bansal & Taylor, 2009). However, scant data on functional activity indicate that white individuals have a higher degree of sweating with physical labor than do black Africans or Asian Indians and that eccrine gland activity for Hispanic individuals falls between that of white and black individuals (Badreshia-Bansal & Taylor, 2009). Other data indicate that the sodium content in sweat is lower in Africans, indicating the existence of a more efficient electrolyte conservation system in Africans (Badreshia-Bansal & Taylor, 2009). It has been reported that apocrine glands, sweat glands that are a combination of exocrine and eccrine glands, are more abundant in the facial skin of blacks compared with whites (Montagna & Carlisle, 1991). The significance of these findings, if any, awaits more comprehensive study.

Sensation

Nerve receptors located in the skin are sensitive to pain, touch, temperature, and pressure. Nerve fibers are located in the dermis and throughout the epidermis. Nerve structures in the skin originate from the neural crest and are detectable in the developing embryo at approximately 5 weeks' gestation. When stimulated, these receptors transmit impulses to the cerebral cortex, where they are interpreted. Combinations of the four basic types of sensations result in burning, tickling, and itching (Jacob et al., 1982). These sensations are propagated by unmyelinated free nerve endings, Merkel cells, Meissner corpuscles, Krause end bulbs, Ruffini terminals, and pacinian corpuscles. Identification of particular responses with specific nerve structures has not been successful, in part because some receptors seem to respond to a variety of stimuli. However, Meissner corpuscles are involved in touch reception and are positioned at the top of the dermal papillae; pacinian corpuscles (see Fig. 7.1) respond to pressure, coarse touch, vibration, and tension and are found deep in the skin; free nerve endings respond to touch, pain, and temperature (Wheater & Burkitt, 1987) and nociceptive Schwann cells that are found along the upper dermal border and project into the epidermis in association with nociceptive fibers can propagate pain signals (Abdo, Calvo-Enrique, Lopez, et al., 2019). Merkel cells are instrumental in propagating light sensory touch in the skin (Maricich, Wellnitz, Nelson, et al., 2009) and are distributed in the rete ridges among basal keratinocytes. They can be identified in association with hair follicles, digits, lips, and regions of the oral cavity.

Skin sensation is a part of the body's integrative response to protect itself from the surrounding environment. Sensation assists with the skin's regulatory function and can signal sweating, shivering, weight shifts (Parish, Lowthian, & Witkowski, 2007), laughter, and scratching.

Merkel cells function as mechanoreceptors. In the epidermis these cells produce nerve growth factor, whereas in the dermis, Merkel cells express receptors for nerve growth factor (Narasawa, Hashimoto, Nihei, et al., 1992). Merkel cells are found around the arrector pili muscle in the bulge region of hair follicles and contribute to the development of eccrine sweat glands, nails, and nerves of the skin (Boulais & Misery, 2008; Kim & Holbrook, 1995; Narasawa, Hashimoto, & Kohda, 1996).

Sensation also moderates the psychobiologic phenomena made famous by Harlow (Harlow & Zimmermann, 1959; van der Horst, Leroy, & van der Veer, 2008), who demonstrated the preference of young animals for objects that were warm and those that provided better tactile sensitivity. In addition, early studies by Spitz (1947) point to the importance of touch in mediating social interactions with children and infants. Deprivation of touch can lead to psychomotor retardation and increased risk of death (Ottenbacher, Muller, Brandt, et al., 1987). Stroking, handling, talking, and playing resulted in a 60% decrease in aortic atherosclerotic lesions (Nerem, Levesque, & Cornhill, 1980), even though study groups had the same cholesterol-containing diet, blood pressures, heart rates, and serum cholesterol levels.

In healing wounds, sensory nerves sprout abundantly for about the first 3 weeks, then return to their normal density. The role of neuropeptides in stimulating growth of connective tissue is increasingly being recognized. This includes a role for these neuropeptides in modulating matrix production by fibroblasts and in acting as growth factors for keratinocytes (Baraniuk, 1997; Kiss, Wlaschek, Brenneisen, et al., 1995; Metze & Luger, 2001).

Metabolism

Synthesis of vitamin D in the skin occurs in the presence of sunlight. UVR converts a sterol (7-dehydrocholesterol) to cholecalciferol (vitamin D). Vitamin D participates in calcium and phosphate metabolism and is important in the mineralization of bone. Because vitamin D is synthesized in the skin but then transmitted to other parts of the body, it is considered an active hormone when converted to calcitriol (1,25-dihydroxycholecalciferol) (Lehninger, 1982; Stryer, 1995). Synthesis of vitamin D is higher in lightly pigmented skin and lower in darkly pigmented skin (Badreshia-Bansal & Taylor, 2009; Wilkins, Birge, Sheline, et al., 2009), a condition that may have implications for mood and cognitive status (Wilkins et al., 2009) and for protection against cardiovascular disease, diabetes, and some cancers (Harris, 2006). On the other hand, the reduced level of vitamin D in darkly pigmented skin does not seem to be associated with a higher level of osteoporotic fractures (Harris, 2006). Consequently, clinicians are being encouraged to promote an increased level of vitamin D intake, especially among individuals with darkly pigmented skin (Harris, 2006; Wilkins et al., 2009).

Communication

In addition to its biologic, structural, functional, and physiologic functions, human skin functions as an organ of communication and identification. The skin over the face is especially important for identification of a person and plays a role in internal and external assessments of beauty. Injury to the skin can result not only in functional and physiologic consequences, but also in changes in body image. Scarring from trauma, surgery, or incisions can lead to changes in clothing choices, avoidance of public exposure, and decreased self-esteem. Research (Koblenzer, 2005; Shuster, Fisher, Harris, et al., 1978) indicates that self-image is progressively reduced with increased scarring from facial acne. Adolescents are especially sensitive to physical appearance (Bernstein, 1976a, 1976b, 1976c; Van Loey & Van Son, 2003). As an organ of communication, facial skin, along with underlying muscles, is capable of expressions such as smiling, frowning, and pouting. The sensation of touching can convey feelings of comfort, concern, friendship, and love.

FACTORS ALTERING SKIN CHARACTERISTICS

Many factors alter the normal characteristics of the skin. Predominate factors include age, sun, hydration, soaps, nutrition, smoking, obesity, medications, and allergens and irritants. Although normal age-related changes in the skin cannot yet be changed, the effects of the other variables that affect the skin can be modified or prevented.

Age

The aging process is associated with numerous morphologic and functional changes in the skin (Tables 7.1 and 7.2). Distinctive differences exist in fetuses, premature infants (23–32 weeks' gestation), full-term newborns, adults, and

TABLE 7.1   Morphologic Differences in Skin at Various Ages

	Premature Newborn	Term Newborn	Adult	Aged
Skin thickness (total)	Approximately 50% of adult Higher surface-to-weight ratio Approximately 13% of body weight	Approximately 70% of adult Higher surface-to-weight ratio	Full thickness Approximately 3% of body weight	Approximately 65%–70% of adult
Periderm	Present up to approximately 120 days	Absent	Absent	Absent
Epidermis	Thinner (2–3 cells thick) Stratum corneum absent until 2–4 weeks after air exposure Melanin production absent/low Immature junctional integrity Fewer desmosomes Immature keratin filament bundles	Equivalent to smaller adult, more uniform cell size Reduced melanin production Vernix caseosa present Immature melanin granule formation	Mature stratum corneum Junctional integrity Immune cells and melanin production relative to skin phototype	Epidermal thinning is minimal (10%–50%) Increased corneocyte surface area Decreased number of active melanocytes by 10%–20% each decade Increased time for epidermal turnover Loss of epidermal stem cell population Progressive reduction in moles from 15–40 in the 30s to 4 at 60–80 years Increase in apoptosis below granular layer
Dermal–epidermal junction	Flat Absent to few rete pegs/dermal papillae before 34 weeks with immature hemidesmosomes	Rete ridges only weakly developed at birth	Mature with full junctional integrity	Flat with loss of rete pegs/dermal papillae
Dermis	Thin Higher type I-to-type III collagen ratio Approximately 24% soluble collagen compared with 1% in the adult Smaller, more uniform collagen fibers/fiber bundles in both papillary and reticular dermis High amount of hyaluronic acid Higher water content More immature elastin fiber bundles Fibroblasts more abundant in reticular dermis	Thinner (approximately 60% of adult) Much higher cellular component compared with mature adult skin Higher type I-to-type III collagen ratio persists Collagen development continues up to 3–6 months postnatally Smaller, finer collagen fiber bundles Some immature elastin fiber bundles become mature at approximately 3 years Fibroblasts more abundant in reticular dermis	Mature array of collagen and elastin fibers Larger, denser collagen fiber bundles in reticular dermis 1% of collagen is soluble Elastin fibers mature in size, distribution Fibroblasts more abundant in papillary dermis Level of advanced glycation end-products begins to increase around age 35 years	Approximately 20% loss of dermal thickness (1% reduction each year) Increase in size, number, diameter of elastic fibers Decrease in elastin synthesis Decrease in number of fibroblasts Decrease in synthesis and turnover of collagen types I and III Increase in collagen cross-linking Slight decrease in levels of hyaluronic acid, glycosaminoglycans, proteoglycans Increased matrix metalloproteinase expression Increase in advanced glycation end-products

Continued

TABLE 7.1	**Morphologic Differences in Skin at Various Ages—cont'd**			
	Premature Newborn	**Term Newborn**	**Adult**	**Aged**
Subcutaneous	No/little subcutaneous tissue	Thinner subcutaneous tissue	Mature subcutaneous tissue	Contraction of septae in subcutaneous fat Loss of subcutaneous fat Changes more dramatic in papillary than reticular dermis
Vasculature	Capillary beds not organized Poor/reduced vasoconstriction/ vasodilation of cutaneous vessels	Capillary beds not completely organized, continues up to 14–17 weeks postnatally	Mature organization of cutaneous vessels in papillary and reticular dermis	Approximately 30% reduction in venular cross-sections Approximately 60% reduction in peak cutaneous blood circulation Reduced vascular response Up to 50% reduction in vascular wall thickness at age 80 years Decreased vasoconstriction/ vasodilation arteriole response Decrease in vascular endothelial growth factor Decreased endothelial cell permeability response
Innervation/ sensation	Meissner corpuscles not fully developed Nervous network not as organized Axon flare response attenuated	Meissner corpuscles not fully developed Axon reflex muted	Mature complement of Meissner and pacinian corpuscles	Reduced number of pacinian and Meissner corpuscles to one third that in adult Pain threshold increases up to 20%
Apocrine glands	Present	Present	Present and active	Reduction in gland size, function
Immune cells	Decreased immune function	Reduced immune function	Mature immune function	Langerhans cells reduced by 20%–50% Up to 50% reduction in mast cells Increase in autoantibodies (bullous pemphigoid, antinuclear antibodies, antithyroglobulin, rheumatoid factor)
Eccrine glands	Structure present by 24–29 weeks but not responsive until 36 weeks, with cells more undifferentiated	Structure present but not responsive for one to several days after birth, with complete neural control by age 2–3 years		15% Reduction in number of glands, with 70% reduction in sweating
Sebaceous glands	Large and active	Large and active but decreased in size, activity Sebum composition different from adult	Increased estrogen and androgens at puberty Increase activity of pilosebaceous glands	Decreased sebum production by approximately 65%, but number and size remain similar to adult

TABLE 7.1 Morphologic Differences in Skin at Various Ages—cont'd

	Premature Newborn	Term Newborn	Adult	Aged
Hair	Lanugo hair may be present	Vellus and terminal hair present	Axillary and pubic hair appear at puberty	Reduced hair follicle density Reduced/absent hair follicle melanocyte activity Increased time for hair growth Up to approximately 50% gray/white hair by age 50 years 20% Decrease in number of hair follicles by 60 years Reduction in hair diameter Bitemporal hair line recession in both genders Increased baldness in at-risk individuals

Data for this table compiled from the following resources: complete references provided at end of chapter.
Braverman (1986); Bullard, Longaker, and Lorenz (2003); Chang and Orlow (2008); Evans and Rutter (1989); Gilchrest (1989, 1991); Gilchrest, Murphy, and Soter (1982); Harpin and Rutter (1983); Holbrook (1991); Kalia, Nonato, Lund, et al. (1998); Lavker, Zheng, and Dong (1986); Lin and Carter (1986); Longaker, Adzick, et al., 1990; Metze and Luger (2001); Nordlund (1986); Rutter (1998); Sauder (1986); Silverberg and Silverberg (1989); Varani, Dame, Rittie, et al. (2006); Yaar and Gilchrest (2007); Yanagishita (1994).

TABLE 7.2 Functional Differences in Skin Among Premature Newborn, Term Newborn, Adult, and Aged

	Premature Newborn	Newborn	Adult	Aged
Protection	Highly permeable TEWL 10 times higher at 24 weeks of prematurity TEWL up to 100 g/m^2/h Skin maturation may require up to 5–7 weeks Higher surface-to-body weight ratio leading to greater absorption and toxicity from topical agents Excessive fluid loss and risk of hypernatremia Low melanin production leading to increased sunburn risk Increased risk of bacterial invasion Increased risk of trauma up to 15% or more of body surface area from monitor probes, rubbing, tape stripping Higher pH becomes more acidic over time (up to 8 days or more) Stratum corneum hydration higher than newborn or adult	Somewhat permeable leading to increased risk of toxicity from topical agents TEWL 6–8 g/m^2/h More readily sunburns Active sebaceous glands due to maternal hormone exposure Sebum secretion higher at birth than at 6 months Slightly higher pH compared with adult that stabilizes over 2 days Reduced stratum corneum hydration initially	Mature barrier function with good resistance to penetration Protection from UV radiation related to skin phototype	Decreased barrier function Delayed barrier recovery of stratum corneum Dry, flaky stratum corneum Higher pH (<5.0 vs 4.5) at 80+ years (increased risk of infection) Decline in lipid content Decline in sebum production Loss of UV protection due to decrease in melanocyte activity Delayed wound healing Increased risk of mechanical injury (i.e., skin tears) Decrease in skin turgor Higher risk of premalignant and malignant lesions

Continued

TABLE 7.2   Functional Differences in Skin Among Premature Newborn, Term Newborn, Adult, and Aged—cont'd

	Premature Newborn	Newborn	Adult	Aged
Immune	Antimicrobial peptides (dermcidin, LL-37) in sweat absent Decreased IgG, IgM Reduced neutrophil chemotaxis and neutrophil phagocytosis Decreased T lymphocytes			Muted allergic and contact reactions Decreased inflammatory reaction Sun-protected skin more reactive than sun-exposed skin Impaired humoral/cell-mediated immunity Decreased DNA repair capacity Increased oncogene activation
Sensation	Sensory nerve endings present and functioning			Decreased/delayed sensory perception Increased risk of burn injury 20% Increase in radiant pain threshold
Metabolism	Immature metabolism Oxygen absorption and carbon dioxide excretion 6–11 times higher before 30 weeks but upon air exposure for 2–3 weeks approaches that of adult		Vitamin D production peaks with decreased synthesis depending on skin phototype	Decreased metabolism Reduced vitamin D production contributing to osteoporosis, diabetes, hypertension, tumor formation Decreased clearance of transepidermal substances Increased UV-induced reactive oxygen species damage
Thermoregulation	High risk of hypothermia Reduced/no sweating for up to 24 days Compromised ability to regulate body temperature requires humidified thermal incubator Evaporative heat loss can exceed resting heat production	Reduced sweating for up to 5 days	Full sweating capability	Loss of ability to control/maintain body temperature when exposed to cold or excessive heat by vasoconstriction, vasodilation, shunting

IgG, immunoglobulin G; *IgM*, immunoglobulin M; *TEWL*, transepidermal water loss; *UV*, ultraviolet.

older adults. By 2040, approximately one in five Americans will be 65 years or older (AARP, n.d.); therefore, understanding age-related changes in the skin is important for all health care providers in any health care setting so that complications can be averted.

A key feature of fetal tissue that has come under more intense investigation is its ability for scarless healing (Longaker, Whitby, Adzick, et al., 1990; Siebert, Burd, McCarthy, et al., 1990). Until 120 days' gestation, wounds in the fetal lamb heal without scarring. Differences in chemical composition and growth factor concentrations of fetal skin contribute to its capacity for scarless healing and are summarized in Box 7.2 (Bullard et al., 2003; Longaker, Adzick, et al., 1990). An understanding of the factors that

contribute to the phenomenon may lead to the achievement of scarless healing in adults. For example, in the laboratory setting, topical application of hyaluronic acid has been associated with a reduction in scar formation in postnatal wounds and can bind growth factors and cytokines.

At birth, the skin and nails are thinner than those in an adult, but with aging they will gradually increase in thickness. Formation of the epidermal and dermal layers occurs within the first 2 weeks of embryonic development. Epidermal development is complete by the end of the second trimester, and at birth, epidermal thickness is almost that of adult skin, although newborn skin is not as effective as adult skin in providing a barrier to transcutaneous water loss. On the other hand, development of the dermis lags behind and does not

BOX 7.2   Unique Characteristics of Fetal Skin

- Collagen deposition occurs more rapidly (Longaker, Adzick, et al., 1990)
- Collagen deposition follows normal dermal pattern (Longaker, Adzick, et al., 1990)
- Approximately 30%–60% of collagen is type III (10%–15% in adult skin) (Bullard et al., 2003)
- Higher concentrations of hyaluronic acid than in adult (Siebert et al., 1990)
- Less TGF-β1 in fetal wounds (Roberts & Sporn, 1996)
- Differential patterns of expression of various isoforms of TGF-β in fetal wounds
- Difference in cell responses
  - Decrease in inflammatory cells, particularly polymorphonuclear leukocytes and macrophage
  - Platelets do not aggregate in response to collagen
  - Platelets do not release same amount of TGF-β1 and platelet-derived endothelial growth factor-AB as adult cells
  - Fibroblasts can migrate at faster rate
  - Fibroblasts synthesize more total collagen
- Differences in protease and inhibitor activity, level of growth factors, and expression of homeobox genes detected (Bullard et al., 2003)

TGF, transforming growth factor.

take on the characteristics of adult dermis until after birth. Until about 6 months of age, the ratio of type I to type III collagen is similar to that in the fetus; soluble collagen is approximately 24%, compared with 1% in the adult.

Immature skin, or skin from premature infants between 23 and 24 weeks' and up to 32 weeks' gestation, requires special attention compared with that of infants beyond 32 weeks' gestation. In particular, before 28 weeks' gestation the skin is thin and poorly keratinized and functions weakly as a barrier. An article appearing in *Lancet* (Immature skin, 1989) has characterized the skin of infants born at the limits of viability as more suitable to an "aquatic environment" than to atmospheric conditions. TEWL is high, and application of adhesives to the outer immature epidermal layer can leave behind raw, damaged skin prone to infection and occasional scarring. At 24 weeks' gestation, TEWL can be 10 times greater per unit area compared with an infant born at term (Rutter, 1996). Infants born between 22 and 25 weeks' gestation may require up to 4 weeks to develop a functional stratum corneum (Evans & Rutter, 1989; Harpin & Rutter, 1983; Kalia et al., 1998; Rutter, 1996). In addition, premature infants have high evaporative heat losses that result in increased risk for hypothermia.

Because premature infants have a greater surface-area-to-volume ratio compared with full-term infants, they are at an increased risk for skin complications and systemic toxicity from topically applied agents. These infants may also have alterations in metabolism, excretion, distribution, and protein binding of chemical agents, placing them at increased risk for local or systemic toxicity from soaps, lotions, or other topical

agents (Weston & Lane, 1999). Other dangers are percutaneous absorption of topical agents, including antiseptics. Hemorrhagic necrosis of the dermis from alcohol absorption has been reported if the alcohol does not quickly evaporate and is sometimes mistaken for bruising. The use of topical antibiotic sprays containing neomycin should be avoided, since it is an ototoxic aminoglycoside. Thus water-based topical antiseptics are preferred but should be used sparingly. Cleaning should be done with care, using normal saline or water. Chlorhexidine, a commonly used antiseptic, is not known to have any adverse effects, but it is probably absorbed from the skin and should be used judiciously. Likewise, iodine has been reported to be absorbed, leading to goiter and hypothyroidism (Rutter, 1998). If required, moisturizing creams or ointments may be applied to dry, flaking, or fissured skin, and the best agents appear to be those with few or no preservatives, since these offer the greatest benefit with decreased risk (Weston & Lane, 1999). Other topical agents that can place the premature or neonate at risk are aniline dyes (methemoglobinemia), hexachlorophene (neurotoxicity), corticosteroids (adrenal suppression), lidocaine–prilocaine cream or EMLA (methemoglobinemia, seizures, petechiae), *N,N*-dimethyl-*meta*-toluamide or DEET (neurotoxicity), salicylates (salicylism, metabolic acidosis, encephalopathy), and silver sulfadiazine (kernicterus, agranulocytosis) (Mancini, 2004).

The next period of change occurs in adolescence, when hormonal stimulation results in increased activity of sebaceous glands and hair follicles. Sebaceous glands increase their secretory rate, and hair follicles become activated, giving rise to secondary sexual characteristics. From adolescence to adulthood there is a gradual change in skin characteristics. By the time the skin reaches mature adulthood, several changes become apparent. The dermis decreases in thickness by about 20% and collagen fibrils become thicker and more fragmented, whereas the epidermis remains relatively unchanged. Epidermal turnover time is increased; this means that wound healing may take longer. For instance, in young adults, epidermal turnover takes about 21 days, but by 35 years of age this turnover time is doubled. Barrier function is reduced, and such reduction may increase the risk of irritation. The number of active melanocytes per unit body surface area decreases with aging, which means that protection against UVR is diminished. However, across the lifespan, darker skin offers greater protection against photoaging or dermatoheliosis (Miyamura et al., 2006). Skin dryness is also associated with aging and an increase in wrinkles. Sensory receptors are diminished in capacity, meaning that the skin is more likely to be burned or traumatized without perception. Vitamin D production is decreased and may be a factor in osteomalacia.

With aging there is a decrease in the number of Langerhans cells, which affects the immunocompetence of the skin and can lead to an increased risk of skin cancer and infection by invading microorganisms. The density of Langerhans cells changes from 10 per 3 mm cross-section of unexposed skin in 22–26-year-old persons to 5.8 per 3 mm cross-section in 62–68-year-old persons (Gilchrest et al., 1982). There is also a decrease in the number of mast cells and melanocytes. The inflammatory response is decreased, and such a decrease may alter allergic reactions and healing. A decrease in the number of sweat glands, diminished vascularity, and a reduction in the amount of subcutaneous fat compromise the thermoregulatory capacity of the skin. Epidermal–dermal junction changes, such as the flattening of the prominent dermal papillae and of the rete ridges, alter junctional integrity. Consequently, the skin is more easily torn in response to mechanical trauma, especially shearing forces. Because the epidermal rete pegs flatten, the unique microenvironment of the basal keratinocytes changes; it is thought that this explains the decrease in epidermal proliferative capacity that occurs with aging (Lavker et al., 1986).

Skin elasticity decreases with age and is related to a combination of aging and solar damage. Microscopic analysis of collagen and elastin fibers reveals that these are more compact, with a loss of ground substance from the spaces between these cable-like structures. Collagen fibers appear to be unwinding, whereas elastin fibers appear to be lysing. The degradation of elastin can be detected at about 30 years of age but becomes marked at 70 years of age (Braverman, 1986). Changes in dermal proteoglycans usually occur after 40 years of age (Yanagishita, 1994). By 70 years of age, most of the elastin network is affected. Changes in collagen content and structure are mediated by an under expression of procollagen; an overexpression of collagenase (MMP-1), stromelysin (MMP-3), and gelatinase A (MMP-2); and a decreased expression of tissue inhibitors of matrix metalloproteinase-1. Fibroblasts in aged skin have a reduced ability to synthesize collagen type I and type III, and collagen fragments further reduce the ability of fibroblasts to synthesize new collagen. In addition, fibroblasts in young adult skin have a higher amount of their cell surface in contact with collagen and exhibit more extensive cell spreading compared with fibroblasts in old skin (Varani et al., 2006). There is also a marked reduction in vascular beds in the vertical capillary loops in the dermal papillae. There is an approximately 35% decrease in the cross-sectional area of these loops in aged skin. It is thought that this leads to atrophy of the hair bulbs, the sweat glands, and the sebaceous glands. Because the hypodermis also becomes thinner, mature individuals are more prone to pressure necrosis (Gilchrest, 1989). With aging, a progressive loss of mechanoreceptors to one third of their average density occurs from the second to the ninth decades (Metze & Luger, 2001).

The density of skin melanocytes is relatively constant until about 40 years of age. By about 45 years of age, skin melanocytes have decreased in density to approximately half that seen between 30 and 39 years of age (Nordlund, 1986). Melanocytes decrease 6%–8% each decade after age 30. It is thought that the loss of skin melanocytes contributes to an increase in the formation of skin cancers. Other overt changes are wrinkling and sagging, which occur as a result of the loss of underlying tissue, in addition to changes seen in collagen and elastin.

Changes in hair color and hair follicles also accompany aging. Age-related changes in active melanocytes result in gray hair. About 50% of the body's hair will be gray by the age of 50 in about 50% of the population. This change is accompanied by a reduction in the number of hair follicles and a decrease in the diameter of the hair. The rate of hair growth is also decreased (Silverberg & Silverberg, 1989). Nail growth rates also decrease by 40%–50%.

Changes in thermoregulatory capacity occur with age, and older individuals are more prone to hypothermia and heat stroke. This has been attributed to changes in blood capillaries and eccrine sweat glands. In healthy older individuals, sweating may be decreased by up to 70% (Gilchrest, 1991). Sebum secretion also declines with age. Barrier function decreases with aging due to the decreased level of all the major lipid species, especially ceramides. In addition, corneocytes are larger and less cohesive. In addition to these changes, pain perception is dulled, and there is reduced skin reactivity upon exposure to irritants. Cutaneous immune function also changes with aging, as seen by a reduction in Langerhans cell density. Skin damaged by sun exposure, or actinically damaged skin, has been found to have a 50% reduction of Langerhans cell density compared with sun-protected skin (Sauder, 1986). Reduced immunocompetence of the skin is thought to contribute in part to skin cancer in the elderly.

Other factors that may contribute to the development of skin cancer in aged individuals are cumulative exposure to carcinogens, diminished DNA repair capacity, decreased melanocyte density, and alterations in dermal matrix (Lin & Carter, 1986). Not surprisingly, wound healing in older individuals is delayed compared with that of younger individuals.

Additional factors than can accelerate skin changes include nicotine use, exposure to pollution, repetitive movements, diet or exposure to radiation treatment. Radiation treatment can exhaust the regenerative capacity of the skin by triggering cellular senescence in response to DNA damage. The most adverse consequence of radiation treatment can result in depletion of the stem cell pool leading to impaired skin regeneration in the epidermal layers resulting in moist desquamation and less-frequently radiation induced ulcerations (Strnadova, Sandera, et al., 2019).

Menopausal changes appear to somewhat accelerate skin changes in women where the decrease in circulating levels of estrogen result in a reduction in dermal collagen and elasticity. Other changes include a reduction in dermal hydration, increased dryness, dermal thinning, reduced vascularity, an altered response to oxidative stress, and wrinkling. Surface lipids are also reduced due to changes in sebaceous gland function. Changes in estrogen and progesterone affect inflammatory response, keratinocyte proliferation, collagen and hyaluronic acid synthesis, and matrix metalloproteinase (MMP) activity (Yaar & Gilchrest, 2007).

Together many of these changes associated with aging and menopause are now being referred to as dermatoporosis and described as the general cutaneous changes that are often visible such as solar or senile purpura, capillary hematomas following skin injury and the whitish stellate scar like spider formations that accompany skin atrophy or thinner skin (Kaya & Saurat, 2007; Strnadova et al., 2019). Dermatoporosis is especially notable by age 70 and upward where skin atrophy due to the loss of extracellular matrix, flattening of the epidermal/dermal interface and associated skin aging changes leads to loss of mechanical and structural support.

Biomechanical Skin Tension

Skin tension lines or cleavage lines have been identified dating from the seminal work of Karl Langer in 1861 (reviewed by Paul, 2017a) and these lines are defined by the biomechanical load that is propagated by the distribution of collagen and elastin in the dermal layers that when disrupted can result in how well or how poorly skin edges can be reapproximated depending on whether incisional vs excisional wounds are created. Skin as an organ tissue is anchored over the surface of the body by a series of underlying connective tissue attachments: anchoring fibrils in the epidermis/basement membrane, that interface with the dermis, and that are then attached and supported by the hypodermis overlying muscle. Thus, it is an organ that is under tension similar to that of a drumhead that is stretched over a drum shell under tension to make a percussive sound. Depending on the level of tension, and depth of injury, the elastic recoil when wounded can vary across areas of the body. For example, the eyelids have loose skin and underlying connective tissue with minimal elastic recoil whereas other areas of the body and the ear drum have varying but higher levels of tension and elastic recoil that can lead to large gaps depending on the size of the incision. If wounds occur that are perpendicular to the long axis of the collagen fibers these can result in a gaping wound that cannot be well approximated. As expected, the higher the tension and recoil, the greater the tension required to close the wound upon suturing with often multiple layers of sutures being needed to obtain satisfactory closure when disturbed with surgical procedures. In the case of surgical excisions or debridements, the ability to reapproximate edges can range from possible to not possible depending on the size, depth, orientation and extent of the excision and age of the individual. In general, incisional wounds have lower biomechanical loading and are primarily under the influence of elastin, whereas excisional wounds have higher biomechanical loading and are primarily under the influence of collagen (Paul, 2017b). More recently tensiometry has been used to define biodynamic excisional skin tension (BEST) lines to guide the creation of excisional wounds (Paul, 2018). It should be noted that wrinkle lines do not always align with skin tension lines and that skin tension can vary among individuals who have a range of variation in underlying bone, cartilage, and muscle. Many of these same principles are operating when performing circumcisions where the loss of the specialized mucosa of the ridged band of the prepuce leads to loss of Meissner's corpuscles (Taylor, Lockwood, & Taylor, 1996). Of further note is that in the case of chronic wounds that occur due to injury, erosion and degradation of skin layers, the extent of scar formation and contraction is likely beyond the direct control of clinicians. Thus, an understanding of skin tension lines, relaxed skin tension lines, BEST lines, and wrinkle lines by clinicians can lead to minimizing scar formation and wound contraction when more directly under surgically controlled conditions.

Sun

Excessive exposure to UVR can have harmful effects that accelerate aging of the skin. For this reason, the condition associated with UVR-damaged skin is referred to as photoaging. Dermatologically, the condition is called dermatoheliosis. Across the lifespan, darker skin offers greater protection against photoaging and dermatoheliosis (Miyamura et al., 2006). Obvious clinical signs of photodamaged skin are dryness, tough and leathery texture, wrinkling as a result of collagen and elastin degeneration, and irregular pigmentation from changes in melanin distribution (Box 7.3) (Silverberg & Silverberg, 1989; Young & Walker, 2008). Excessive exposure to UVR increases the risk of developing skin cancers such as basal or squamous cell carcinoma and malignant melanoma, especially in white or lightly pigmented skin. Damage to the DNA of skin cells leads to transformation of cells and cancer (Council on Scientific Affairs, 1989). Changes also occur in epidermal and dermal cells. Epidermal cells become thickened (Varani et al., 2006) and more numerous, and dermal vessels become dilated and tortuous. Langerhans cells are reduced in number by approximately 50%, thereby diminishing the immunocompetence of the skin (Lober & Fenske, 1990).

BOX 7.3 Photoaging Effects on Skin Characteristics

- Hyperkeratosis
- Atrophy
- Leathery appearance, especially in lighter skin phototypes
- Melanosomes may be increased with increase in dopa-positive melanocytes up to twofold
- Telangiectasia
- Further elastogenesis/degeneration accompanied by mass accumulations
- Increased lysozyme deposition on elastic fibers
- Decreased amounts of mature collagen
- Further increased matrix metalloproteinase activity
- Presence of hyperplastic fibroblasts
- Perivascular infiltrate of lymphocytes, histiocytes, mononuclear cells, mast cells
- Prominent grenz zone (a zone of normal-appearing dermis just below the epidermis, but below this normal-appearing zone is abnormal dermis)
- Glycosaminoglycans and proteoglycans increase
- Reduction in vascular circulation
- Venule wall thickening
- Further reduction in number of Langerhans cells
- More infiltrating mononuclear cells present
- Increased CD4[+] T cells

Exposure to excessive UVR results in the production of reactive oxygen species that lead to activation of several cell surface receptors such as interleukin-1, epidermal growth factor, and keratinocyte growth factor, which signal the induction of the nuclear transcription complex AP-1. The AP-1 complex blocks synthesis of collagen types I and III by suppressing expression of transforming growth factor-β. These same reactive oxygen species lead to damage of the lipid cell membrane, which results in release of prostaglandins that are responsible for mediating inflammatory reactions (Yaar & Gilchrest, 2007). Together these processes can create a pattern of heightened inflammation that is responsible for the net degradation of collagen tissue by the activation and overexpression of MMPs, particularly MMP-1, MMP-3, MMP-8, and MMP-9. Other cell-mediated damage results from damage to mitochondrial DNA, protein oxidation (especially in the upper dermis), and telomere shortening (Yaar & Gilchrest, 2007).

The effects of reactive oxygen species in aged skin are not effectively countered by the presence of the naturally occurring antioxidant enzymes, such as catalase, superoxide dismutase, and glutathione peroxidase, and nonenzymatic molecules, such as coenzyme Q10, ascorbate or vitamin C, tocopherol or vitamin E, and carotenoids, which are present at higher levels in young adult skin. Over the past decade, the study of the reactive oxygen species system and its role in skin damage has resulted in the use of various antioxidants in topical sunscreens and cosmetics. Among the antioxidants used are tocopherol acetate, stable forms of vitamin C, vitamin E, polyphenolic molecules such as procyanidin and flavonoids, curcumin, genistein (found in soybeans), and resveratrol (found in red wine, nuts, and grapefruit) (Yaar & Gilchrest, 2007). Other agents that have been investigated or are being used to reverse the effects of photodamaged skin include dietary lipids such as omega-3 fatty acids and eicosapentaenoic acid, osmolytes, and α-hydroxy acids derived from fruit, sugarcane, and dairy products. Retinoids have been used since the 1980s to abrogate the effects of sun damage that can be seen visually and histologically. More recently, retinoids have been used as a pretreatment approach (Yaar & Gilchrest, 2007).

Exposure to UVR can lead to sunburn. Sunburn is partly the result of a vasodilatory response that increases blood volume. Whether an individual will become sunburned depends on the extent of skin pigmentation. Naturally, those with the least pigmentation are more prone to sunburn and the harmful, long-term effects of UVR. Severe short-term exposure of unprotected, lightly pigmented skin can lead to blistering (a second-degree burn).

There is an association between melanoma and sunburn. An individual who has sustained more than six serious sunburns is at increased risk for melanoma (Green, Siskind, Bain, et al., 1985). Exposure to UVR and the rise of malignant melanomas have led to the development of more effective sun-blocking agents. Over time the lifetime risk of malignant melanoma has increased from 1:1500 people in 1930 to 1:250 in 1980 to 1:62 in 2005, and as of 2015, it is expected to be 1:50

(Potts, 1990; Rigel, Russak, & Friedman, 2010). It is estimated that 65%–90% of all melanomas result from UVR exposure. While melanomas account for 3% of all skin cancers, they are responsible for 75% of all deaths from skin cancer, with basal cell carcinoma accounting for 80%–85% and the remaining 15%–20% accounted for by squamous cell carcinoma. Sunscreens should be used on a regular basis, applied at least 30 min before sun exposure, and have a sun protection factor ranging from 15 to 30 (Pathak, Fitzpatrick, et al., 1999). Individuals with moderately pigmented skin require about three to five times more exposure to UVR to induce sunburn inflammation compared with Caucasians; individuals with darker skin require 10 times more exposure (McGregor & Hawk, 1999; Young & Walker, 2008). The age-adjusted incidence rates for melanoma have been reported as 1.0 per 100,000 for blacks vs 4.5 for Hispanics and 21.6 for white non-Hispanics (Rouhani, Hu, & Kirsner, 2008).

Hydration

Adequate skin hydration is normally provided by sebum secretion and an intact stratum corneum with its keratinized cells. Several factors can affect skin hydration, including relative humidity, removal of sebum, and age. Each of these factors increases water loss from the skin, leading to dryness and scaling. Application of emollients to the skin replaces the barrier function of lost sebum or decreased evaporative water loss when the relative humidity is low. Retention of water in the epidermal layers after application of a lotion leads to swelling of the skin, which is perceived as smoothness and softness.

Various products often are promoted with claims of superiority over other products without adequate in vitro, in vivo, or clinical data. The superiority of oil baths over water baths was found to be only marginal (Stender, Blichmann, & Serup, 1990). Twenty minutes after both kinds of baths, skin hydration was increased when measured by water evaporation and electrical conductance and capacitance. A small but significantly greater amount of water was bound in the skin after the oil bath, but no change was seen in evaporation, conductance, or capacitance. Thus, increases in water-holding capacity of the skin after an oil bath may not be of importance. However, a difference in skin-surface lipids was found, and the difference lasted at least 3 h. This effect is comparable to that seen with application of a traditional moisturizing lotion. The authors of the study concluded that because daily use of bath oil is not practical, application of moisturizing lotions may be more advantageous, and the beneficial effects of bath oils are related to lipidization of the skin surface (Stender et al., 1990).

Soaps

Washing or bathing with an alkaline soap reduces the thickness and number of cell layers in the stratum corneum (White, Jenkinson, & Lloyd, 1987). Generally, soap emulsifies the lipid coating of the skin and removes it, along with resident and transient bacteria. Excessive use of soap or detergents can interfere with the water-holding capacity of the skin and may impair bacterial resistance. Use of alkaline soaps increases skin pH, which may change bacterial resistance. The time for recovery to normal skin pH of 5.5 depends on the length of exposure. Ordinary washing requires 45 min to restore skin pH, whereas prolonged exposure can require 19 h (Bettley, 1960). Other agents that can lead to delipidization or dehydration of skin are alcohol and acetone. Currently, acidic skin cleansers appear to be less irritating than neutral or alkaline cleansers, and some evidence suggests that acidic cleansers decrease the number of acne lesions on the face (Korting & Braun-Falco, 1996).

Nutrition

Normal, healthy skin integrity can be maintained by adequate dietary intake of protein, carbohydrate, fats, vitamins, and minerals. Under normal conditions in healthy persons, supplementary nutrition is not beneficial if dietary intake is adequate. If the skin is damaged, increased dietary intake of some substances, such as vitamin C for collagen formation, may be beneficial. A healthy diet of protein supplies the necessary amino acids for protein synthesis. Fats are broken down into essential fatty acids, which cells can use to form their lipid bilayer. Carbohydrates are digested to supply energy for cell metabolism. Maintenance of normal, healthy skin requires ingestion of the following: vitamins C, D, and A; the B vitamins pyridoxine and riboflavin; the mineral elements iron, zinc, and copper; and many others. Adequate dietary intake can be ensured by ingestion of amounts consistent with the recommended daily allowances (Boelsma, Hendriks, & Roza, 2001; Roe, 1986).

Smoking

Smoking decreases capillary blood flow and changes the oxygen gradient in skin via its vasoconstrictive effects. Data indicate that the dermis in smokers has a reduced level of collagen and elastin fibers, leading to tissue that is less elastic and hardened as a result of an increase in reactive oxygen species and MMPs. Epidermal effects include keratinocyte dysplasia, telangiectasias, roughness, and excessive wrinkling (Kennedy, Bastiaens, Bajdik, et al., 2003; Leow & Maibach, 1998). Furthermore, a dose–response effect of smoking and wrinkle formation has been identified, leading to premature skin aging (Kennedy et al., 2003). Yellow discolored nails and mustaches are frequently seen in heavy users of tobacco products, including cigarettes and pipes. Tobacco smoke contains a number of mutagens and carcinogens, including polycyclic aromatic hydrocarbons, heterocyclic amines, and nitrosamines. Premature graying of hair can be seen in both men and women, and frequently accelerated hair loss can be seen in men (Ortiz & Grando, 2012).

Obesity

Obesity (body mass index >30 kg/m^2) is now a recognized risk factor for a number of skin diseases. These include an increased risk of melanoma and nonmelanoma skin cancers (Tobin, Ahern, Rogers, et al., 2013). High circulating levels of leptin, detected in obesity, have been found to confer a 1.56-times increase in risk for melanoma. Obese individuals exhibit changes in immune capacity as measured by lower levels of cytotoxic T lymphocytes and natural killer cells. Both of these cell populations are important to defend the body against cancer (Tobin et al., 2013). Obesity is also associated with increased inflammation and the presence of psoriasis, an inflammatory dermatosis. Other skin conditions associated with obesity are lymphedema and cellulitis, hidradenitis suppurativa, intertrigo with candida infection, observation of acanthosis nigricans, and various cutaneous infections. Obese individuals are more likely to become diabetic, and uninjured diabetic skin has been found to be mechanically compromised (Bermudez et al., 2011).

Medications

Various medications affect the skin, and the prevalence rate of skin reactions to medications in hospitalized individuals is 2%–3% (Gerson, Sriganeshan, & Alexis, 2008; Ramdial & Naidoo, 2009). Some of the best-studied medications are the corticosteroids, which interfere with epidermal regeneration and collagen synthesis (Ehrlich & Hunt, 1968; Pollack, 1982; Ramdial & Naidoo, 2009; Wicke, Halliday, Allen, et al., 2000). Medications also cause photosensitive and phototoxic reactions. Some categories of medications that can affect the skin are antibacterials, antihypertensives, analgesics, tricyclic antidepressants, antihistamines, antineoplastic agents, antipsychotic drugs, diuretics, hypoglycemic agents, sunscreens, and oral contraceptives (Potts, 1990; Ramdial & Naidoo, 2009). Skin eruptions have been more frequently reported for antibiotics, antiepileptics, antiarrhythmic, and anticoagulants (Gerson et al., 2008). Skin flora can be changed by the use of antibacterials, orally administered steroids, and hormones. Analgesics, antihistamines, and nonsteroidal anti-inflammatory drugs can alter inflammatory reactions. Thus, whenever drugs are prescribed and skin reactions occur, medications should always be checked to determine whether they are responsible.

Allergens and Irritants

Additionally, metals such as nickel, cobalt, gold, and chromate; plants such as poison ivy and poison oak; and foods such as chamomile, tomatoes, mango, citrus, garlic, and shiitake mushrooms can lead to inflammatory skin changes resulting in contact dermatitis with exposure. Nickel is recognized as one of the most common allergens, with an increasing prevalence as high as 28% in females and 5% in males (Schram, Warshaw, & Laumann, 2010). Other sources of skin reactions are associated with cosmetics, including personal care products that contain fragrances, preservatives, antioxidants, botanicals, and cosmetic vehicles. Reactions to these personal care products have been reported in up to 23% of women and 17.8% in men (Alani, Davis, & Yiannias, 2013).

CLINICAL CONSULT

A: Referral received from primary provider for an 88-year-old woman with persistent diffuse fine macular–papular rash over lower back, buttocks, and both legs. Rash has become bothersome and increasingly pruritic. Significant macular–papular rash with satellite lesions under both breasts; slight erythema. Pruritus more intense under both breasts. Patient well dressed, independent, and physically active. Describes self as 30 lbs overweight. Recently developed UTI and is finishing 10-day course of antibiotic. Patient describes hands as very sore. Denies any medication allergies. Acknowledges she recently changed both laundry detergent and bath soap. Reports daughter recently bought her new bath soap and laundry detergent that had a fragrant smell. Lower extremities thin, no discoloration in skin tone, no edema, dry flaking skin apparent. Macular–papular rash present under pendulous breasts; skin intact. Hands very dry with cracks apparent in fingertips. Applies lotion occasionally to her hands.

D: Dry skin and candidiasis under pendulous breasts.

P: Treat candidiasis, moisturize skin, reduce exposure to possible irritants.

I: (1) Antifungal powder to apply under breasts twice daily. (2) Apply an over-the-counter, high-grade moisturizing cream daily to her dry skin on legs and hands. (3) Increase water intake to 8 glasses daily. (4) Provided with education about loss of emollients, elasticity, and moisture with aging skin. (5) Discontinue new bath soap and evaluate for improvement in overall skin condition, especially on back. Discontinue laundry detergent if condition has not improved.

E: Return to wound clinic in 4 weeks; if condition worsens, call wound clinic for referral to dermatologist.

SUMMARY

- As the body's largest organ, the skin serves several complex functions: protection, thermoregulation, sensation, metabolism, and communication.
- Numerous factors influence the skin's integrity and ability to adequately provide these protective functions such as age, UVR exposure, hydration, medications, nutrition, obesity, irritants, and soaps.

- Wound management and skin care must be grounded in a comprehensive knowledge base of the structure and function of the skin.
- After reviewing this chapter, the care provider should closely scrutinize many of the skin care practices and bathing routines that are subconsciously engrained in day-to-day patient care activities and that may compromise the function and integrity of the skin.

SELF-ASSESSMENT QUESTIONS

1. Which are the primary functions of the skin?
   a. protection, communication, beauty, identification, metabolism, thermoregulation
   b. protection, immunity, thermoregulation, sensation, metabolism, communication
   c. filtration, protection, identification, strength, identification, warmth
   d. protection, beauty, nutrition, strength, thermoregulation, filtration, detoxification
2. Which of the following is true about darkly pigmented skin compared to lighter skin?
   a. Darker skin has less functional integrity.
   b. Darkly pigmented skin can mask erythema or redness seen with pressure injuries or dermatitis.
   c. Light skin has a higher prevalence of keloids.
   d. All of the above.
3. Which of the following is true about the dermis?
   a. The dermis is the thickest tissue layer of the skin
   b. The dermis is vascular
   c. Dermal thickness ranges from 2 to 4 mm
   d. All of the above
4. Which statement best describes the effects of smoking on the epidermis
   a. Roughness, and excessive wrinkling
   b. Decrease in capillary blood flow
   c. Increase in collagen
   d. Depletion of melanin

REFERENCES

AARP, n.d. https://www.aarp.org/politics-society/history/info-2018/older-population-increase-new-report.html#:~:text=Looking%20ahead%2C%20the%20report%20predicts%20that%20the%20number,%E2%80%94%20increasing%20from%206.4%20million%20to%2014.6%20million. Accessed 9.16.22.

Abdo, H., Calvo-Enrique, L., Lopez, J. M., et al. (2019). Specialized cutaneous Schwann cells initiate pain sensation. *Science, 365,* 695–699.

Alani, J. I., Davis, M. D. P., & Yiannias, J. A. (2013). Allergy to cosmetics: A literature review. *Dermatitis, 24,* 283–290.

Auger, M. J. (1986). Mononuclear phagocytes. *British Medical Journal, 298,* 546–548.

Badreshia-Bansal, S., & Taylor, S. C. (2009). The structure and function of skin of color. In A. P. Kelly, & S. C. Taylor (Eds.), *Dermatology for skin of color.* New York: McGraw-Hill.

Baraniuk, J. N. (1997). Neuropeptides in the skin. In J. D. Bos (Ed.), *Cutaneous immunology and clinical immunodermatology* (2nd ed., pp. 311–323). Boca Raton: CRC Press.

Benyon, R. C. (1989). The human skin mast cell. *Clinical and Experimental Allergy*, 19(4), 375–387.

Bergstresser, P. R., Toews, G. B., & Streilein, J. W. (1980). Natural and perturbed distributions of Langerhans cells: Responses to ultraviolet light, heterotopic skin grafting, and dinitrofluorobenzene sensitization. *The Journal of Investigative Dermatology*, 75, 73–77.

Bermudez, D. M., Herdrich, B. J., Xu, J., Lind, R., Beason, D. P., Mitchell, M. E., et al. (2011). Impaired biomechanical properties of diabetic skin implications in pathogenesis of diabetic wound complications. *The American Journal of Pathology*, 178(5), 2215–2223. https://doi.org/10.1016/j.ajpath.2011.01.015.

Bernstein, N. R. (1976a). Appearance: Concepts of perception and disfigurement. In *Emotional care of the facially burned and disfigured* (pp. 13–22). Boston: Little, Brown & Co. Chapter 1.

Bernstein, N. R. (1976b). Body and face images: Personality and self-representation. In *Emotional care of the facially burned and disfigured* (pp. 23–40). Boston: Little, Brown & Co. Chapter 2.

Bernstein, N. R. (1976c). Disfigurement and personality development. In *Emotional care of the facially burned and disfigured* (pp. 41–75). Boston: Little, Brown & Co. Chapter 3.

Bettley, F. R. (1960). Some effects of soap on the skin. *British Medical Journal*, 1, 1675–1679.

Bickenbach, J. R. (1981). Identification and behavior of label-retaining cells in oral mucosa and skin. *Journal of Dental Research*, 60, 1611–1620.

Boelsma, E., Hendriks, H. F., & Roza, L. (2001). Nutritional skin care: Health effects of micronutrients and fatty acids. *The American Journal of Clinical Nutrition*, 73(5), 853–864.

Boissy, R. E. (2003). Melanosome transfer to and translocation in the keratinocyte. *Experimental Dermatology*, 12(Suppl. 2), 5–12.

Boulais, N., & Misery, L. (2008). The epidermis: A sensory tissue. *European Journal of Dermatology*, 18, 119–127.

Braverman, I. M. (1986). Elastic fiber and microvascular abnormalities in aging skin. *Dermatologic Clinics*, 4, 391–405.

Briggaman, R. A. (1982). Epidermal-dermal interactions in adult skin. *The Journal of Investigative Dermatology*, 79(Suppl. 1), 21–24.

Bullard, K. M., Longaker, M. T., & Lorenz, H. P. (2003). Fetal wound healing: Current biology. *World Journal of Surgery*, 27, 54–61.

Chang, H. Y., Chi, J. T., Dudoit, S., et al. (2002). Diversity, topographic differentiation, and positional memory in human fibroblasts. *Proceedings of the National Academy of Sciences of the United States of America*, 99(20), 12877–12882.

Chang, M. W., & Orlow, S. J. (2008). Neonatal, pediatric and adolescent dermatology. In K. Wolff, B. Gilchrest, S. Katz, et al. (Eds.), *Fitzpatrick's dermatology in general medicine* (7th ed.). New York: McGraw-Hill.

Chu, D. H. (2008). Development and structure of skin. In K. Wolff, B. Gilchrest, S. Katz, et al. (Eds.), *Fitzpatrick's dermatology in general medicine* (7th ed., pp. 57–73). New York: McGraw-Hill.

Costerton, J. W., Lewandowski, Z., Caldwell, D. E., et al. (1995). Microbial biofilms. *Annual Review of Microbiology*, 49, 711–745.

Costerton, J. W., Stewart, P. S., & Greenberg, E. P. (1999). Bacterial biofilms: A common cause of persistent infections. *Science*, 284, 1318–1322.

Council on Scientific Affairs. (1989). Harmful effects of ultraviolet radiation. *Journal of the American Medical Association*, 262, 380–384.

Debes, G. F., & McGettigan, S. E. (2019). Skin-associated B cells in health and inflammation. *Journal of Immunology*, 202, 1659–1666.

DeLeo, V. A., Taylor, S. C., Belsito, D. V., et al. (2002). The effect of race and ethnicity on patch test results. *Journal of the American Academy of Dermatology*, 46, S107–S112.

Ehrlich, H. P., & Hunt, T. K. (1968). Effects of cortisone and vitamin A on wound healing. *Annals of Surgery*, 167, 324–328.

Evans, N. J., & Rutter, N. (1989). Development of the epidermis in the newborn. *Biology of the Neonate*, 49, 74–80.

Feingold, K. R., & Elias, P. M. (2014). Role of lipids in the formation and maintenance of the cutaneous permeability barrier. *Biochimica et Biophysica Acta*, 1841, 280–294.

Fitzpatrick, T. B. (1988). The validity and practicality of sun-reactive skin types I through IV. *Archives of Dermatology*, 124, 869–871.

Freinkel, R. K. (2001). Hair. In R. K. Freinkel, & D. T. Woodley (Eds.), *The biology of the skin* (pp. 77–86). New York: Parthenon.

Gay, S., & Miller, S. (1978). *Collagen in the physiology and pathology of connective tissue*. Stuttgart, Germany: Gustav Fischer Verlag.

Gerson, D., Sriganeshan, V., & Alexis, J. B. (2008). Cutaneous drug eruptions: A 5-year experience. *Journal of the American Academy of Dermatology*, 59, 995–999.

Gilchrest, B. A. (1989). Skin aging and photoaging: An overview. *Journal of the American Academy of Dermatology*, 21, 610–613.

Gilchrest, B. A. (1991). Physiology and pathophysiology of aging skin. In L. A. Goldsmith (Ed.), *Physiology, biochemistry, and molecular biology of the skin* (2nd ed., pp. 1425–1444). New York: Oxford University Press.

Gilchrest, B. A., Murphy, G. F., & Soter, N. A. (1982). Effect of chronologic aging and the ultraviolet irradiation on Langerhans cells in human epidermis. *The Journal of Investigative Dermatology*, 79, 85–88.

Goding, C. R. (2007). Melanocytes: The new black. *The International Journal of Biochemistry & Cell Biology*, 39(2), 275–279.

Green, A., Siskind, V., Bain, C., et al. (1985). Sunburn and malignant melanoma. *British Journal of Cancer*, 51, 393–397.

Grice, E. A., Kong, H. H., Conlan, S., et al. (2009). Topographical and temporal diversity of the human skin microbiome. *Science*, 324, 1190–1192.

Grice, E. A., Kong, H. H., Renaud, G., et al. (2008). A diversity profile of the human skin microbiota. *Genome Research*, 18, 1043–1050.

Griffith, L. G., & Naughton, G. (2002). Tissue engineering—Current challenges and expanding opportunities. *Science*, 295, 1009–1014.

Haake, A. R., & Holbrook, K. (1999). The structure and development of skin. In I. M. Freedberg, et al. (Eds.), *Fitzpatrick's dermatology in general medicine* (5th ed., pp. 70–114). New York: McGraw-Hill.

Haake, A., Scott, G. A., & Holbrook, K. A. (2001). Structure and function of the skin: Overview of the epidermis and dermis. In R. K. Freinkel, & D. T. Woodley (Eds.), *The biology of the skin* (pp. 19–46). New York: Parthenon.

Harlow, H. F., & Zimmermann, R. R. (1959). Affectional responses in the infant monkey. *Science*, 130, 421–432.

Harpin, V. A., & Rutter, N. (1983). Barrier properties of the newborn infant's skin. *The Journal of Pediatrics*, 102, 419–425.

Harris, S. S. (2006). Vitamin D and African Americans. *The Journal of Nutrition*, 136(4), 1126–1129.

Headington, J. T. (1989). The dermal dendrocyte. *Advances in Dermatology*, 1, 159–171.

Headington, J. T., & Cerio, R. (1990). Dendritic cells and the dermis. *The American Journal of Dermatopathology*, 12, 217–220.

Hoffmann, J. A., Kafatos, F. C., Janeway, C. A., et al. (1999). Phylogenetic perspectives in innate immunity. *Science*, 284, 1313–1318.

Holbrook, K. A. (1991). Structure and function of the developing human skin. In L. A. Goldsmith (Ed.), *Physiology, biochemistry, and molecular biology of the skin* (2nd ed., pp. 64–101). New York: Oxford University Press.

Holbrook, K. A., Vogel, A. M., Underwood, R. A., et al. (1998). Melanocytes in human embryonic and fetal skin: A review and new findings. *Pigment Cell Research, 1*(Suppl), 6–17.

Immature skin. (1989). *Lancet, 334*(8672), 1138. https://doi.org/10.1016/S0140-6736(89)91497-9.

Jacob, S. W., Francone, C. A., & Lossow, W. J. (1982). *Structure and function in man* (5th ed.). Philadelphia: Saunders.

Kalia, V. N., Nonato, L. B., Lund, C. H., et al. (1998). Development of skin barrier function in premature infants. *The Journal of Investigative Dermatology, 111*, 320–326.

Kaya, G., & Saurat, J.-H. (2007). Dermatoporosis: A chronic cutaneous insufficiency/fragility syndrome—Clinicopathological features, mechanisms, prevention and potential treatments. *Dermatology, 215*, 284–294.

Kennedy, C., Bastiaens, M. T., Bajdik, C. D., et al. (2003). Effect of smoking and sun on aging skin. *The Journal of Investigative Dermatology, 120*, 548–554.

Kim, D. K., & Holbrook, K. A. (1995). The appearance, density and distribution of Merkel cells in human embryonic and fetal skin: Their relation to sweat glands, and hair follicle development. *The Journal of Investigative Dermatology, 104*, 411–416.

Kiss, M., Wlaschek, M., Brenneisen, P., et al. (1995). Alpha-melanocyte stimulating hormone induces collagenase/matrix metalloproteinase-1 in human dermal fibroblasts. *Biological Chemistry Hoppe-Seyler, 376*, 425–430.

Koblenzer, C. S. (2005). The emotional impact of chronic and disabling skin disease: A psychoanalytic perspective. *Dermatologic Clinics, 23*(4), 619–627.

Korting, H. C., & Braun-Falco, O. (1996). The effect of detergents on skin pH and its consequences. *Clinics in Dermatology, 14*(1), 23–27.

Lambert, M. I., Mann, T., & Dugas, J. P. (2008). Ethnicity and temperature regulation. *Medicine and Sport Science, 53*, 104–120.

La Ruche, G., & Cesarini, J. P. (1992). Histology and physiology of black skin. *Annales de Dermatologie et de Vénéréologie, 119*(8), 567–574.

Lavker, R. M., & Sun, T. T. (2000). Epidermal stem cells: Properties, markers, and location. *Proceedings of the National Academy of Sciences of the United States of America, 97*(25), 13473–13475.

Lavker, R. M., Zheng, P. S., & Dong, G. (1986). Morphology of aged skin. *Dermatologic Clinics, 4*, 379–389.

Lehninger, A. L. (1982). *Principles of biochemistry*. New York: Worth.

Leow, Y. H., & Maibach, H. I. (1998). Cigarette smoking, cutaneous vasculature, and tissue oxygen. *Clinics in Dermatology, 16*, 579–584.

Lin, A. N., & Carter, D. M. (1986). Skin cancer in the elderly. *Dermatologic Clinics, 4*(3), 467–471.

Lin, J. Y., & Fisher, D. E. (2007). Melanocyte biology and skin pigmentation. *Nature, 445*, 843–850.

Lober, C. W., & Fenske, N. A. (1990). Photoaging and the skin: Differentiation and clinical response. *Geriatrics, 45*(36–40), 42.

Longaker, M. T., Adzick, N. S., Hall, J. L., et al. (1990). Studies in fetal wound healing, VII. Fetal wound healing may be modulated by hyaluronic acid and stimulating activity in amniotic fluid. *Journal of Pediatric Surgery, 25*, 430–433.

Longaker, M. T., Whitby, D. J., Adzick, N. S., et al. (1990). Studies in fetal wound healing, VI. Second and early third trimester fetal wounds demonstrate rapid collagen deposition without scar formation. *Journal of Pediatric Surgery, 25*, 63–68.

Mancini, A. J. (2004). Skin. *Pediatrics, 113*, 1114–1119.

Maricich, S. M., Wellnitz, S. A., Nelson, A. M., et al. (2009). Merkel cells are essential for light-touch responses. *Science, 324*, 1580–1582.

McDonald, C. J. (1988). Structure and function of the skin. Are there differences between black and white skin? *Dermatologic Clinics, 6*(3), 343–347.

McGregor, J. M., & Hawk, J. L. M. (1999). Acute effects of ultraviolet radiation on the skin. In I. M. Freedberg, et al. (Eds.), *Fitzpatrick's dermatology in general medicine* (5th ed., pp. 1555–1561). New York: McGraw-Hill.

Metze, D., & Luger, T. (2001). Nervous system in the skin. In R. K. Freinkel, & D. T. Woodley (Eds.), *The biology of the skin* (pp. 153–176). New York: Parthenon.

Millington, P. F., & Wilkinson, R. (1983). *Skin*. Cambridge: Cambridge University Press.

Miyamura, Y., Coelho, S. G., Wolber, R., et al. (2006). Regulation of human skin pigmentation and responses to ultraviolet radiation. *Pigment Cell Research, 20*(1), 2–13.

Montagna, W., & Carlisle, K. (1991). The architecture of black and white facial skin. *Journal of the American Academy of Dermatology, 24*, 929–937.

Montagna, W., Prota, G., & Kenney, J. A. (1993). *Black skin: Structure and function*. San Diego, CA: Academic Press.

Nakatsuji, T., & Gallo, R. L. (2012). Antimicrobial peptides: Old molecules with new ideas. *The Journal of Investigative Dermatology, 132*, 887–895.

Narasawa, Y., Hashimoto, K., & Kohda, H. (1996). Merkel cells participate in the induction and alignment of epidermal ends of arrector pili muscles of human fetal skin. *The British Journal of Dermatology, 134*, 494–498.

Narasawa, Y., Hashimoto, K., Nihei, Y., et al. (1992). Biological significance of dermal Merkel cells in development of cutaneous nevus in human fetal skin. *The Journal of Histochemistry and Cytochemistry, 40*, 65–71.

Nerem, R. M., Levesque, M. J., & Cornhill, J. F. (1980). Social environment as a factor in diet-induced atherosclerosis. *Science, 208*, 1475–1476.

Noble, W. C. (Ed.). (2004). *The skin microflora and microbial skin disease*. Cambridge: Cambridge University Press.

Nordlund, J. J. (1986). The lives of pigment cells. *Dermatologic Clinics, 4*, 407–418.

Odland, G. F. (1991). Structure of the skin. In L. A. Goldsmith (Ed.), *Physiology, biochemistry, and molecular biology of the skin* (2nd ed.). New York: Oxford University Press.

Oluwasanmi, J. O. (1974). Keloids in the African. *Clinics in Plastic Surgery, 1*, 179–195.

Ortiz, A., & Grando, S. A. (2012). Smoking and the skin. *International Journal of Dermatology, 51*, 250–262.

Ottenbacher, K. J., Muller, L., Brandt, D., et al. (1987). The effectiveness of tactile stimulation as a form of early intervention: A quantitative evaluation. *Journal of Developmental and Behavioral Pediatrics, 8*, 68–76.

Parish, L. C., Lowthian, P., & Witkowski, J. A. (2007). The decubitus ulcer: Many questions but few definitive answers. *Clinics in Dermatology, 25*(1), 101–108.

Pathak, M. A., Fitzpatrick, T. B., Nghiem, P., et al. (1999). Sun-protective agents: Formulations, effects, and side effects. In I. M. Freedberg, et al. (Eds.), *Fitzpatrick's dermatology in general medicine* (5th ed.). New York: McGraw-Hill.

Pathak, M. A., Nghiem, P., & Fitzpatrick, T. B. (1999). Acute and chronic effects of the sun. In I. M. Freedberg, et al. (Eds.), *Fitzpatrick's dermatology in general medicine* (5th ed., pp. 1598–1607). New York: McGraw-Hill.

Paul, S. P. (2017a). Biodynamic excisional skin tension (BEST) lines: Revisiting Langer's lines, skin biomechanics, current concepts in cutaneous surgery, and the (lack of) science behind skin lines used for surgical excisions. *Journal of Dermatological Research, 2,* 77–87.

Paul, S. P. (2017b). Are incisional and excisional skin tension lines biomechanically different? Understanding the inter play between elastin and collagen during surgical procedures. *International Journal of Biomedicine, 7,* 111–114.

Paul, S. P. (2018). Biodynamic excisional skin tension lines for surgical excisions: Untangling the science. *Annals of the Royal College of Surgeons of England, 100,* 330–337.

Pollack, S. V. (1982). Systemic medications and wound healing. *International Journal of Dermatology, 21,* 489–496.

Potts, J. F. (1990). Sunlight, sunburn, and sunscreens. *Postgraduate Medicine, 87.* 52–55, 59–60, 63.

Quinton, P. M. (1983). Sweating and its disorders. *Annual Review of Medicine, 34,* 429–452.

Ramdial, P. K., & Naidoo, D. K. (2009). Drug-induced cutaneous pathology. *Journal of Clinical Pathology, 62*(6), 493–504.

Rezvani, H. R., Ali, N., Nissen, L. J., et al. (2011). HIF-1α in epidermis: Oxygen sensing, cutaneous angiogenesis, cancer, and non-cancer disorders. *The Journal of Investigative Dermatology, 131,* 1793–1805.

Rienertson, R. P., & Wheatley, V. R. (1959). Studies on the chemical composition of human epidermal lipids. *The Journal of Investigative Dermatology, 32,* 49–59.

Rigel, D. S., Russak, J., & Friedman, R. (2010). The evolution of melanoma diagnosis: 25 years beyond the ABCDs. *CA: A Cancer Journal for Clinicians, 60,* 301–316.

Roberts, A. B., & Sporn, M. B. (1996). Transforming growth factor-B. In R. A. F. Clark (Ed.), *The molecular and cellular biology of wound repair* (2nd ed., pp. 275–308). New York: Plenum Press.

Robles, D. T., & Berg, D. (2007). Abnormal wound healing: Keloids. *Clinics in Dermatology, 25*(1), 26–32.

Roe, D. A. (1986). *Nutrition and the skin.* New York: Liss.

Roth, R. R., & James, W. D. (1988). Microbial ecology of the skin. *Annual Review of Microbiology, 42,* 441–464.

Rouhani, P., Hu, S., & Kirsner, R. S. (2008). Melanoma in Hispanic and black Americans. *Cancer Control, 15,* 248–253.

Rudowski, W. (1976). *Burn therapy and research.* Baltimore: Johns Hopkins University Press.

Rutter, N. (1996). The immature skin. *European Journal of Pediatrics, 155,* S18–S20.

Rutter, N. (1998). The immature skin. *British Medical Bulletin, 44,* 957–970.

Sams, W. M. (1990). Structure and function of the skin. In W. M. Sams, & P. J. Lynch (Eds.), *Principles and practice of dermatology.* New York: Churchill Livingstone.

Sauder, D. N. (1986). Effect of age on epidermal immune function. *Dermatologic Clinics, 4,* 447–454.

Scheibner, A., Hollis, D. E., McCarthy, W. H., et al. (1986). Effects of sunlight exposure on Langerhans cells and melanocytes in human epidermis. *Photodermatology, 3,* 15–25.

Schonborn, K., Willenborg, S., Schulz, J.-N., et al. (2020). Role of collagen XII in skin homeostasis and repair. *Matrix Biology, 94,* 57–76.

Schram, S. E., Warshaw, E. M., & Laumann, A. (2010). Nickel hypersensitivity: A clinical review and call to action. *International Journal of Dermatology, 49,* 115–125.

Shuster, S., Fisher, G. H., Harris, E., et al. (1978). The effect of skin disease on self-image. *The British Journal of Dermatology, 90* (Suppl. 16), 18–19.

Siebert, J. W., Burd, A. R., McCarthy, J. G., et al. (1990). Fetal wound healing: A biochemical study of scarless healing. *Plastic and Reconstructive Surgery, 85,* 495–502.

Silverberg, N., & Silverberg, L. (1989). Aging and the skin. *Postgraduate Medicine, 86,* 131–136.

Simanski, M., Köten, B., Schröder, J. M., et al. (2012). Antimicrobial RNases in cutaneous defense. *Journal of Innate Immunity, 4,* 241–247.

Solomons, B. (1983). *Lecture notes on dermatology* (5th ed.). Oxford: Blackwell Scientific.

Spince, A. P., & Mason, E. B. (1987). *Human anatomy and physiology.* Menlo Park, CA: Benjamin/Cummings.

Spitz, R. (1947). An inquiry into the genesis of psychiatric conditions in early childhood. In H. Nagera (Ed.), *Vol. 2. Psychoanalytical studies of the child.* London: International.

Steel, K. P., & Barkway, C. (1989). Another role for melanocytes: Their importance for stria vascularis development in the mammalian inner ear. *Development, 107,* 453–463.

Stender, I. M., Blichmann, C., & Serup, J. (1990). Effects of oil and water baths on the hydration state of the epidermis. *Clinical and Experimental Dermatology, 15,* 206–209.

Stierner, U., Rosdahl, I., Augustsson, A., et al. (1989). UVB irradiation induces melanocyte increase in both exposed and shielded human skin. *The Journal of Investigative Dermatology, 92,* 561–564.

Strnadova, K., Sandera, V., et al. (2019). Skin aging: The dermal perspective. *Clinics in Dermatology, 37,* 326–335.

Stryer, L. (1995). *Biochemistry* (4th ed.). New York: Freeman.

Szabo, G. (1954). The number of melanocytes in human epidermis. *British Medical Journal, 1,* 1016–1017.

Szabo, G., Gerald, A. B., Pathak, M. A., Fitzpatrick, T. B., et al. (1972). The ultrastructure of racial color differences in man. In V. Riley (Ed.), *Pigmentation: Its genesis and biological control* (pp. 23–41). New York: Appleton-Century-Crofts.

Szabo, G., Gerald, A. B., Pathak, M. A., et al. (1969). Racial differences in the fate of melanosomes in human epidermis. *Nature, 222,* 1081–1082.

Tadokoro, T., Yamaguchi, Y., Batzer, J., et al. (2005). Mechanisms of skin tanning in different racial/ethnic groups in response to ultraviolet radiation. *The Journal of Investigative Dermatology, 124,* 1326–1331.

Taylor, S. C. (2002). Skin of color: Biology, structure, function, and implications for dermatologic disease. *Journal of the American Academy of Dermatology, 46*(2 Suppl. Understanding), S41–S62.

Taylor, S. C. (2003). Epidemiology of skin diseases in people of color. *Cutis, 71,* 271–272.

Taylor, J. R., Lockwood, A. P., & Taylor, A. J. (1996). The prepuce: Specialized mucosa of the penis and its loss to circumcision. *British Journal of Urology, 77,* 291–295.

Tobin, A.-M., Ahern, T., Rogers, S., et al. (2013). The dermatological consequences of obesity. *International Journal of Dermatology, 52,* 927–932.

US Census Bureau. (2014). *An older and more diverse nation by midcentury.* The Free Library.

van der Horst, F. C. P., Leroy, H. A., & van der Veer, R. (2008). "When strangers meet": John Bowlby and Harry Harlow on attachment behavior. *Integrative Psychological and Behavioral Science, 42,* 370–388.

Van Loey, N. E., & Van Son, M. J. (2003). Psychopathology and psychological problems in patients with burn scars: Epidemiology and management. *American Journal of Clinical Dermatology, 4*(4), 245–272.

Varani, J., Dame, M. K., Rittie, L., et al. (2006). Decreased collagen production in chronologically aged skin: Roles of age-dependent alteration in fibroblast function and defective mechanical stimulation. *The American Journal of Pathology, 168,* 1861–1868.

Warner, R. R., Myers, M. C., & Taylor, D. A. (1988). Electron probe analysis of human skin: Determination of the water concentration profile. *The Journal of Investigative Dermatology, 90*(2), 218–224.

Weinberg, A. N., & Swartz, M. N. (1987). General considerations of bacterial diseases. In T. B. Fitzpatrick (Ed.), *Dermatology in general medicine: Textbook and atlas.* New York: McGraw-Hill.

Wenger, C. B. (1999). Thermoregulation. In I. M. Freedberg, et al. (Eds.), *Fitzpatrick's dermatology in general medicine* (5th ed.). New York: McGraw-Hill.

Weston, W. L., & Lane, A. T. (1999). Neonatal dermatology. In I. M. Freedberg, et al. (Eds.), *Fitzpatrick's dermatology in general medicine* (5th ed.). New York: McGraw-Hill.

Wheater, P. R., & Burkitt, H. G. (1987). *Functional histology: A text and colour atlas* (2nd ed.). Edinburgh: Churchill Livingstone.

White, M. I., Jenkinson, D. M., & Lloyd, D. H. (1987). The effect of washing on the thickness of the stratum corneum in normal and atopic individuals. *The British Journal of Dermatology, 116,* 525–530.

Wicke, C., Halliday, B., Allen, D., et al. (2000). Effects of steroids and retinoids on wound healing. *Archives of Surgery, 135*(11), 1265–1270.

Wilkins, C. H., Birge, S. J., Sheline, Y. I., et al. (2009). Vitamin D deficiency is associated with worse cognitive performance and lower bone density in older African Americans. *Journal of the National Medical Association, 101*(4), 349–354.

Wolff, K., & Stingl, G. (1983). The Langerhans cell. *The Journal of Investigative Dermatology, 80,* 17S–21S.

Woodburne, R. T., & Burkel, W. E. (1988). *Essentials of human anatomy.* New York: Oxford University Press.

Wysocki, A. B. (1995). A review of the skin and its appendages. *Advances in Wound Care, 8*(2 Pt. 1). 53–54, 56–62.

Wysocki, A. B. (2002). Evaluating and managing open skin wounds: Colonization versus infection. *AACN Clinical Issues, 13*(3), 382–397.

Wysocki, A. B., et al. (2005). Skin, molecular cell biology of. In R. A. Meyers (Ed.), *Vol. 13. Encyclopedia of molecular cell biology and molecular medicine* (2nd ed., pp. 217–250). Weinheim, Germany: Wiley-VCH Verlag GmbH & Co. KgaA.

Xu, K. D., McFeters, G. A., & Stewart, P. S. (2000). Biofilm resistance to antimicrobial agents. *Microbiology (Reading), 146,* 547–549.

Yaar, M., & Gilchrest, F. A. (2007). Photoaging: Mechanism, prevention and therapy. *The British Journal of Dermatology, 157,* 874–887.

Yamaguchi, Y., Beer, J. Z., & Hearing, V. J. (2008). Melanin mediated apoptosis of epidermal cells damaged by ultraviolet radiation: Factors influencing the incidence of skin cancer. *Archives of Dermatological Research, 300*(Suppl. 1), S43–S50.

Yamaguchi, Y., & Hearing, V. J. (2009). Physiological factors that regulate skin pigmentation. *BioFactors, 35*(2), 193–199.

Yanagishita, M. (1994). A brief history of proteoglycans. *Experientia Supplementum, 70,* 3–7.

Young, A. R., & Walker, S. L. (2008). Acute and chronic effects of ultraviolet radiation on the skin. In K. Wolff, et al. (Eds.), *Fitzpatrick's dermatology in general medicine* (7th ed.). New York: McGraw-Hill.

Zuk, P. A., Zhu, M., Ashjian, P., et al. (2002). Human adipose tissue is a source of multipotent stem cells. *Molecular Biology of the Cell, 13,* 4279–4295.

8

Wound-Healing Physiology and Factors That Affect the Repair Process

Greg Bohn and Ruth A. Bryant

OBJECTIVES

1. Compare and contrast wound-healing processes for each type of closure: primary intention, secondary intention, and tertiary intention.
2. Distinguish between partial-thickness wound repair and full-thickness wound repair, addressing the key components, phases, usual timeframes, and wound appearance.
3. Describe features distinguishing an acute wound from a chronic wound.
4. Describe the role of the following cells in the wound repair process: platelets, polymorphonuclear leukocytes, macrophages, fibroblasts, endothelial cells, and keratinocytes.
5. Explain the role of bioactive agents (e.g., growth factors and cytokines) and extracellular matrix proteins in regulating wound repair.
6. Describe features and characteristics of scarless healing.
7. Distinguish the manifestations and treatment of keloid and hypertrophic scars.
8. Identify conditions and comorbidities that affect the wound-healing process.

For centuries, wound healing was regarded as a mysterious process, with wound management based on practitioner preference as opposed to scientific principles. Research over the past 3 decades has contributed much information regarding the wound-healing process and the factors that facilitate it. We now know that repair is an extremely complex process involving hundreds, possibly thousands, of overlapping and "linked" processes (Goldman, 2004). It is critical for all wound care clinicians to base their interventions and recommendations on current evidence and to remain abreast of new findings and their implications for care. This chapter reviews the process of wound healing and discusses the implications for wound management.

MECHANISM OF WOUND HEALING

The ability to repair tissue damage is an important survival tool for any living organism. Regardless of the type or severity of injury, repair occurs by only two mechanisms—regeneration, or replacement of the damaged or lost tissue with more of the same, and scar formation, replacement of damaged or lost tissue with connective tissue that lacks some of the functions of the original tissue. Regeneration is the preferred mechanism of repair because normal function and appearance are maintained. Scar formation is a less satisfactory alternative and occurs when the tissues involved are incapable of regeneration. Many invertebrate and amphibian species have the ability to regenerate entire limbs. Humans have only limited capacity for regeneration, and most wounds heal by scar formation (Calvin, 1998; Mast & Schultz, 1996; Wilgus, 2007).

In humans, the mechanism of repair for any specific wound is determined by the tissue layers involved and their capacity for regeneration. Wounds that are confined to the epidermal and superficial dermal layers heal by regeneration because epithelial, endothelial, and connective tissue can be reproduced. In contrast, deep dermal structures (e.g., hair follicles, sebaceous glands, and sweat glands), subcutaneous tissue, muscle, tendons, ligaments, and bone lack the capacity to regenerate; therefore, loss of these structures is permanent, and wounds involving these structures must heal by scar formation (Martin, 1997; Mast & Schultz, 1996).

The standard repair mechanism for human soft tissue wounds is connective tissue (scar) formation; however, an exception to this rule is the early-gestation fetus. Intrauterine surgical procedures performed during the second trimester result in scarless healing, a phenomenon that has been consistently reproduced in laboratory studies. Interestingly, the fetus loses the ability to heal without scarring at approximately 22–24 weeks' gestation. Repair during the third trimester and the postnatal period follows the "usual" rules for repair and results in scar formation. A number of differences in the molecular environment for repair in the early-gestation fetus are thought to contribute to scarless repair and are discussed throughout this chapter (Bullard, Longaker, & Lorenz, 2002; Dang, Ting, Soo, et al., 2003; Wilgus, 2007; Yang, Lim, Phan, et al., 2003).

The mechanism of healing for a specific wound depends on the tissue layers involved (partial thickness vs full thickness), onset and duration (acute vs chronic), and type of wound closure (primary, secondary, or tertiary intention).

Partial Thickness/Full Thickness

Partial-thickness wounds involve only partial loss of the skin layers; that is, they are confined to the epidermal and superficial dermal layers. Full-thickness wounds involve total loss of the skin layers (epidermis and dermis) and frequently involve loss of the deeper tissue layers as well (subcutaneous tissue, muscle, and bone) (see Fig. 7.1). The timeframe for repair and the repair process itself differs significantly for partial-thickness and full-thickness wounds.

Acute/Chronic

Acute wounds typically are traumatic or surgical in origin. Acute wounds occur suddenly, and in most individuals, move rapidly and predictably through the repair process and result in durable closure. In contrast, chronic wounds fail to proceed normally through the repair process. Chronic wounds frequently are caused by vascular compromise, chronic inflammation, or repetitive insults to the tissue, and they either fail to close in a timely manner or fail to result in durable closure (Brissett & Hom, 2003; Pradhan, Nabzdyk, Andersen, et al., 2009). Acute wounds can become chronic if complicated by infection, vascular compromise, or closure failure occur.

Primary, Secondary, and Tertiary

Classification of repair as primary-, secondary-, or tertiary-intention healing is based on the ideal of primary surgical closure for all wounds. Primary closure minimizes the volume of connective tissue deposition required for wound repair and restores the epithelial barrier to infection (Fig. 8.1A). Approximated surgical incisions are said to heal by primary intention; they usually heal quickly, with minimal scar formation, as long as infection and secondary breakdown are prevented. Wounds that are left open and allowed to heal by scar formation are classified as healing by secondary intention (Fig. 8.1B). These wounds heal more slowly because of the volume of connective tissue required to fill the defect. They are vulnerable to infection because they lack the epidermal barrier to microorganisms until late in the repair process. These wounds are characterized by prolongation of the inflammatory and proliferative phases of healing. Chronic wounds such as pressure ulcers and dehisced incisions typically heal by secondary intention. Wounds managed with delayed closure are classified as healing by tertiary intention, or delayed primary closure (Fig. 8.1C). This approach is sometimes required for abdominal incisions complicated by significant infection (Gabriel, Mussman, Rosenberg, et al., 2018). Closure and/or approximation of the wound is delayed until the risk of infection is resolved and the wound is free of debris.

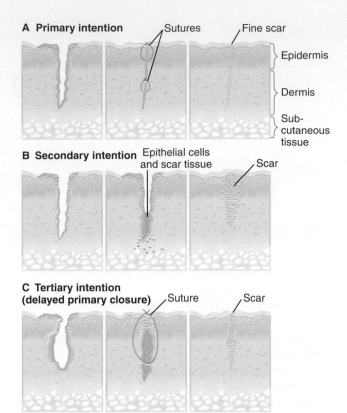

Fig. 8.1 (A) Wound healing by primary intention, such as with a surgical incision. Wound edges are approximated and secured with sutures, staples, or adhesive tapes, and healing occurs by epithelialization and connective tissue deposition. (B) Wound healing by secondary intention. Wound edges are not approximated, and healing occurs by granulation tissue formation, contraction of the wound edges, and epithelialization. (C) Wound healing by tertiary (delayed primary) intention. Wound is kept open for several days. The superficial wound edges then are approximated, and the center of the wound heals by granulation tissue formation. (From Black, J. M., & Hawks, J. H. (2005). *Medical surgical nursing, clinical management for positive outcomes* (7th ed.). St. Louis, MO: Saunders.)

WOUND-HEALING PROCESS

Wound healing is best understood as a cascade of events. Injury sets into motion a series of physiologic responses that are coordinated and sequenced and that, under normal circumstances, result in durable repair. Critical factors in the repair process include the cells that establish a clean wound bed and generate the tissue to fill the defect, the bioactive molecules that control cellular activity (growth factors and cytokines), and the wound-healing environment (extracellular matrix [ECM]). The wound-healing environment (matrix) provides a scaffold that promotes cell migration, and it contains a number of substances that regulate the activity of growth factors and cytokines and promote cell migration (e.g., matrix metalloproteinases) (Cheresh & Stupack, 2008; Gill & Parks, 2008; Macri & Clark, 2009).

Upon injury, exposure of endothelial collagen activates platelet aggregation and clot formation. Platelets degranulate releasing chemokines and cytokines initiating next step functions. The release of these factors initiates the Inflammatory

Phase attracting macrophages to the wound site. Their role is to remove devitalized tissues and stimulate cells to prepare for proliferation. Wound fibroblasts are attracted to the wound and via signaling for next step functions, lay down collagen and matrix which stimulates proliferation of granulation tissues. As the proliferation phase develops the supportive base, epithelialization occurs from the wound edges. Remodeling follows until the closure is healed and matured.

Our current understanding of wound repair is based primarily on acute wound-healing models. Therefore, the processes for partial-thickness wound healing and full-thickness wound healing by primary intention are presented first, followed by a discussion of the repair process for wounds that heal by secondary intention.

Partial-Thickness Wound Repair

Partial-thickness wounds are shallow wounds involving epidermal loss and possibly partial loss of the dermal layer (see Plate 1). Partial-thickness wounds typically are less than 0.2 cm in depth. These wounds are moist and painful because of the loss of the epidermal covering and the resultant exposure of nerve endings. When the wound involves loss of the epidermis with exposure of the basement membrane, the wound base appears bright pink or red. In the presence of partial dermal loss, the wound base usually appears pale pink with distinct red "islets." These "islets" represent the basement membrane of the epidermis, which projects deep into the dermis to line the epidermal appendages. These islands of epidermal basement membrane are important in partial-thickness wound healing because all epidermal cells are capable of regeneration, and each islet will serve as a source of new epithelium (Hunt & Van Winkle, 1997; Winter, 1979).

The major components of partial-thickness repair include an initial inflammatory response to injury, epithelial proliferation and migration (resurfacing), and reestablishment and differentiation of the epidermal layers to restore the barrier function of the skin (Monaco & Lawrence, 2003; Winter, 1979). If the wound involves dermal loss, connective tissue repair (granulation tissue formation) will proceed concurrently with epithelial repair (Table 8.1) (Jahoda & Reynolds, 2001).

Epidermal Repair

Tissue trauma triggers the processes that result in epidermal repair: an acute inflammatory response followed by epidermal mitosis and migration (Harrison, Heaton, Layton, et al., 2006). The inflammatory response produces erythema, edema, and a serious exudate containing leukocytes. When this exudate is allowed to dry on the wound surface, a dry crust, commonly referred to as a "scab," is formed. In partial-thickness wounds, the inflammatory response is limited, typically subsiding in less than 24 h (Winter, 1979).

Epidermal resurfacing begins as the inflammatory phase subsides and is dependent on two processes: proliferation of epidermal cells throughout the wound bed and lateral migration of the epidermal cells at the leading edge. In order to migrate laterally, the keratinocytes at the wound edge must

Level of Injury (Tissue Layers Involved)	Primary Phases of Repair	Outcomes
Epidermal loss	Inflammation (brief) Epithelial resurfacing Restoration of normal epithelial thickness/ repigmentation	No loss of function No scar No change in skin appearance or color
Possible partial dermal loss	Dermal repair (if dermal loss involved)	Restoration of rete ridges/dermal papillae when dermis involved

TABLE 8.1 Partial-Thickness Repair

undergo several changes. First they must acquire a migratory phenotype. This involves breakdown of their attachments to adjacent cells, the basement membrane, and the underlying dermis. These attachments normally prevent lateral migration and provide epithelial stability. The keratinocytes then must undergo cytoskeletal alterations that support lateral movement. These alterations include flattening of the cells at the advancing edge of the epithelium and formation of protrusions known as lamellipodia, which attach to binding sites in the wound bed. The migratory keratinocytes then move across the wound bed by alternately attaching to the ECM and then detaching and reattaching at a more distal point (Harrison et al., 2006; Monaco & Lawrence, 2003).

The epithelial cells within the wound bed continue this pattern of lateral migration until they contact epithelial cells migrating from the opposite direction. Once the epithelial cells meet, lateral migration ceases; this phenomenon is known as contact inhibition (Hunt & Van Winkle, 1997; Monaco & Lawrence, 2003).

Epithelial resurfacing is supported by increased production of basal cells just behind the advancing edge and throughout the wound bed. The process typically peaks between 24 and 72 h after injury. The rate of reepithelialization is affected by a number of factors of clinical significance. For example, resurfacing is promoted by maintenance of a moist wound surface. Winter (1979) found that partial-thickness wounds left open to air required 6–7 days to resurface, whereas moist wounds reepithelialized in 4 days. This is because cells can migrate much more rapidly in a moist environment (Fig. 8.2). In contrast, when the surface of the wound is covered with a scab, migration is delayed while the epithelial cells secrete enzymes known as matrix metalloproteinases (MMPs). The MMPs lift the scab by cleaving the bonds that attach it to the wound bed, creating a moist pathway that supports keratinocyte migration (Harrison et al., 2006; Monaco & Lawrence, 2003; Winter, 1979). Interestingly, hypoxic conditions in the wound bed also serve to stimulate keratinocyte migration, probably through increased production of the

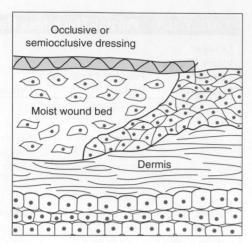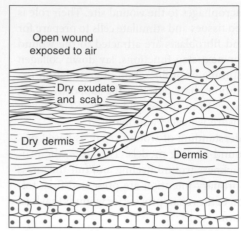

Fig. 8.2 Migration of epidermal cells in moist environment and dry environment.

MMPs that promote lateral migration. This positive response to wound bed hypoxia is lost in the elderly, which may be one factor contributing to slower rates of reepithelialization in the aged (O'Toole, van Koningsveld, Chen, et al., 2008). In contrast, high bacteria levels may serve as an impediment to reepithelialization. Data indicate that keratinocyte migration is inhibited by bacterial byproducts such as lipopolysaccharide (Loryman & Mansbridge, 2008). In vivo evidence strongly suggests that elevated glucose levels are another major impediment to epidermal proliferation and migration. This may be one factor contributing to delayed healing of superficial wounds in diabetic patients with poorly controlled glucose levels (Lan, Liu, Fang, et al., 2008).

The newly resurfaced epithelium appears pale, pink, and dry in people of all races (see Plate 1B). Because it is only a few cell layers thick, the new epithelium is very fragile and requires protection against mechanical forces such as superficial shear and friction.

Once epithelial resurfacing is complete, the epithelial cells resume vertical migration and epidermal differentiation so that normal epidermal thickness and function are restored. The normal anchors to adjacent epidermal cells and to the basement membrane are reestablished (Harrison et al., 2006). The "new" epidermis gradually repigments, matching the individual's normal skin tone. It should be noted that repigmentation in darkly pigmented skin will take longer than lighter skin. It is important as partial-thickness wounds heal to avoid interpreting the absence of pigmentation in the darkly pigmented skin as scar tissue (see Plate 1B).

Regulatory factors. The processes of epithelial proliferation and migration are regulated by a complex interplay between various MMPs and selected growth factors. Specifically, lateral migration is dependent on normal levels and function of multiple MMPs, which serve to break the attachments that bind the edge keratinocytes to adjacent cells and the underlying wound bed. In addition to playing a key role in establishment of a migratory phenotype, MMPs facilitate continued resurfacing by assisting the migrating keratinocytes to detach from the wound bed. Repetitive detachment and distal reattachment are critical to the resurfacing process

(Gill & Parks, 2008). Epithelial proliferation is dependent in part on keratinocyte attachment to the ECM and in part on exposure to growth factors. Keratinocyte attachment is required for the cell to exit from the G_0 phase of mitosis, and growth factors are required to stimulate cellular reproduction. A number of growth factors promote keratinocyte proliferation including transforming growth factor-α (TGF-α), keratinocyte growth factor, platelet-derived growth factor (PDGF), and epidermal growth factor (EGF). See Chapter 23 for a detailed discussion of the molecular factors regulating wound repair.

Dermal Repair

In wounds involving both dermal and epidermal loss, dermal repair proceeds concurrently with reepithelialization. By the fifth day after injury, a layer of fluid separates the epidermis from the dermal tissue. New blood vessels begin to sprout, and fibroblasts become plentiful by about the seventh day. Collagen fibers are visible in the wound bed by the ninth day. Collagen synthesis continues to produce new connective tissue until about 10–15 days after injury. This new connective tissue grows upward into the fluid layer. At the same time, the flat epidermis falls down around the new vessels and collagen fibers, recreating ridges at the dermal–epidermal junction. As the new connective tissue gradually contracts, the epidermis is drawn close to the dermis (Winter, 1979). Insulin and insulin-like growth factor may contribute to reformation of the dermal–epidermal junction.

Full-Thickness Wound Repair: Wounds Healing by Primary Intention

Full-thickness wounds, by definition, extend at least to the subcutaneous tissue layer and possibly as deep as the fascia–muscle layer or bone. Full-thickness wounds may be either acute or chronic (see Plates 2–5). This section addresses acute wound healing by primary intention, such as a surgical incision.

Many steps are involved in full-thickness repair, but they are commonly conceptualized as four major phases: hemostasis, inflammation, proliferation, and remodeling. Considerable

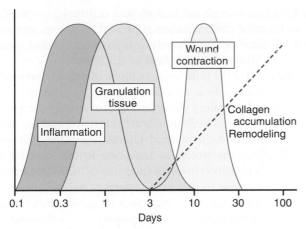

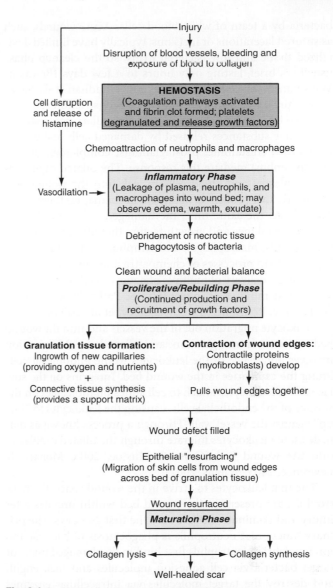

Fig. 8.3 Orderly phases of healing. Time line (in days) reflects healing trajectory of acute wound-healing model. (Modified from Clark, R. A. (1991). Cutaneous wound repair. In L. A. Goldsmith (Ed.), *Physiology, biochemistry and molecular biology of the skin* (2nd ed., Vol. 1). New York: Oxford University Press. Found in Kumar, V., Cotran, R. S., & Robbins, S. T. (2003). *Robbins basic pathology* (7th ed.). Philadelphia: Saunders.)

overlap exists among the phases, and the cells involved in one phase produce the chemical stimuli and substances that serve to move the wound into the next phase. Thus, normal repair is a complex and well-orchestrated series of events (Fig. 8.3) and is affected by a number of systemic and local factors, including the wound environment.

Hemostasis

Any acute injury extending beyond the epidermis causes bleeding, which activates a series of overlapping events designed to control blood loss, establish bacterial control, and seal the defect. Immediately upon injury, disruption of blood vessels exposes the subendothelial collagen to platelets, which trigger platelet activation and aggregation. Simultaneously, injured cells in the wound area release clotting factors that activate both the intrinsic and extrinsic coagulation pathways. As part of the coagulation pathway, circulating prothrombin is converted to thrombin, which is used to convert fibrinogen to fibrin. The end result is formation of a clot composed of fibrin, aggregated platelets, and blood cells. Hemostasis is further accomplished by a brief period of vasoconstriction mediated by thromboxane A_2 and prostaglandin 2-α, substances released by the damaged cells and activated platelets. Clot formation seals the disrupted vessels so that blood loss is controlled. The clot also provides a temporary bacterial barrier, a reservoir of growth factors, and an interim matrix that serves as scaffolding for migrating cells (Brissett & Hom, 2003; Monaco & Lawrence, 2003; Phillips, 2000).

Clot formation, followed by fibrinolysis (clot breakdown), is a critical event in the sequence of wound healing (Fig. 8.4). The activation and degranulation of platelets cause the α-granules and dense bodies of the platelets to rupture, releasing a potent "cocktail" of energy-producing compounds and cytokines/growth factors (including complement factor C5a). These substances attract the cells needed to begin the

Fig. 8.4 Cascade of events in wound repair process.

repair process. They also provide fuel for the energy-intensive process of wound healing. The platelet-derived substances thought to be most critical to repair include PDGF, TGF-β, and fibroblast growth factor-2. Thus hemostasis, which is the body's normal response to tissue injury, actually initiates the entire wound-healing cascade. The importance of hemostasis to wound healing is underscored by the finding that inadequate clot formation is associated with impaired wound healing and that the extrinsic coagulation pathway is critical to repair (Brissett & Hom, 2003; Monaco & Lawrence, 2003).

Inflammation

Once the bleeding is controlled, the focus becomes control of infection and establishment of a clean wound bed. This process can be compared with the repair of a damaged home or building. Before rebuilding can begin, the damaged components must be removed. Wound "cleanup" involves breakdown of any devitalized tissue and elimination of excess bacteria by a team of white blood cells. Acute wounds, such as sutured lacerations or incisions, typically have limited devitalized tissue and low bacterial loads, so the cleanup phase usually is brief, lasting only hours to a few days (Braiman-Wiksman, Solomonik, Spira, et al., 2007; Pradhan et al., 2009).

Within 10–15 min after injury, vasoconstriction subsides, followed by vasodilation and increased capillary permeability. Vasoactive substances released by damaged cells and by clot breakdown (histamine, prostaglandins, complement factor, and thrombin) mediate this response. The dilated capillaries permit plasma and blood cells to leak into the wound bed. Clinically, this process is observed as edema, erythema, and exudate. At the same time, the damaged cells and platelets produce cytokines and growth factors that attract leukocytes (neutrophils, macrophages, and lymphocytes) to the wound bed. The twin processes of chemoattraction and vasodilation result in the delivery of multiple phagocytic cells to the wound site within minutes of injury (Gill & Parks, 2008; Pradhan et al., 2009; Rodriguez, Felix, Woodley, et al., 2008).

Leukocyte migration out of the vessels and into the wound bed occurs via margination and diapedesis. Margination involves adherence of the leukocytes to the endothelial cells lining the capillaries in the wound bed. Integrins on the surface of the leukocytes attach to cell adhesion molecules on the surface of the endothelial cells, causing the leukocytes to "line up" against the vessel wall. Through a process known as diapedesis, the leukocytes migrate through the dilated capillaries into the wound bed (Cross & Mustoe, 2003; Monaco & Lawrence, 2003; Wilgus, 2007).

The first leukocytes to arrive in the wound space, the neutrophils, are present in the wound bed within minutes after injury and dominate the scene for the first 2–3 days. The primary function of neutrophils is phagocytosis of bacteria and foreign debris. Neutrophils first bind to the damaged tissue or target bacteria via cell adhesion molecules and then engulf and destroy the target molecules via intracellular enzymes and free oxygen radicals. In addition, growth factors released by the neutrophils attract additional leukocytes to the area (Cross & Mustoe, 2003).

By days 3–4 after injury, the neutrophils begin to spontaneously disappear as a result of apoptosis and are replaced by macrophages (activated monocytes). The macrophages continue to phagocytize bacteria and break down damaged tissues as already described. In addition, the macrophages release a large number of potent growth factors that stimulate angiogenesis, fibroblast migration and proliferation, and connective tissue synthesis.

T lymphocytes are present in the wound tissue in peak quantities between days 5 and 7 after injury. T lymphocytes contribute to the inflammatory phase of wound healing by secreting additional wound-healing cytokines and by destroying viral organisms and foreign cells. Thus significant deficiencies of T lymphocytes can delay or compromise the repair process (Monaco & Lawrence, 2003).

Although all leukocytes contribute to elimination of bacteria and establishment of a clean wound bed, macrophages contribute the most significantly to the repair process. Studies indicate that wounds can heal without neutrophils, especially if no bacterial contamination is present. However, elimination of macrophages severely compromises wound repair (Cross & Mustoe, 2003; Gabriel et al., 2018).

The result of the inflammatory phase of wound healing is a clean wound bed. In acute wounds healing by primary intention, the inflammatory phase lasts approximately 3 days. At this point, bacterial levels usually are controlled, and any devitalized tissue has been removed. Elimination of these noxious stimuli allows the wound to transition to the "rebuilding" phase. This transition involves apoptosis of the inflammatory cells, possibly due in part to the effects of antiinflammatory cytokines and increased production of growth factors that promote proliferation as opposed to inflammation (Demidova-Rice, Hamblin, & Herman, 2012; Goldman, 2004). However, in wounds complicated by necrosis and/or infection, the inflammatory phase is prolonged and wound healing is delayed (Burns, Mancoll, & Phillips, 2003). A prolonged inflammatory phase increases the risk for wound dehiscence because approximation of the incision is totally dependent on the closure material (sutures, staples, and fibrin glue) until sufficient connective tissue has been synthesized to provide tensile strength to the incision. (Tensile strength during the inflammatory phase is 0%.)

Factors affecting the duration and intensity of inflammation. The intensity and duration of the inflammatory phase appear to be critical factors in the amount of scar tissue produced. Numerous studies support a strong link between prolonged inflammation and hyperproliferative scarring (Dubay & Franz, 2003; Pradhan et al., 2009; Rahban & Garner, 2003; Robson, 2003). Thus the clinician needs to have a clear understanding of both proinflammatory and antiinflammatory factors and the implications for wound management. As noted, local factors such as bacterial load and presence of devitalized tissue are major proinflammatory factors that should be aggressively managed through debridement and appropriate use of topical dressings and antimicrobial agents (Demidova-Rice et al., 2012). Necrotic tissue and infection trigger production of cytokines that attract excessive numbers of inflammatory cells to the wound bed; these inflammatory cells produce reactive oxygen species (ROS) that, in conjunction with proinflammatory cytokines, cause degradation of the growth factors needed for normal function of proliferative cells such as fibroblasts. Thus, necrosis and infection are major impediments to wound healing.

The ECM is another important determinant; it can either promote or inhibit inflammation, depending on the types of MMPs produced and their functions. Some MMPs promote inflammation by releasing proinflammatory cytokines from the cells in the wound bed; proinflammatory cytokines attract inflammatory cells to the wound bed (Pradhan et al., 2009). Other MMPs inhibit inflammation by degrading proinflammatory cytokines or inhibiting their release. For example, tumor necrosis factor-α (TNF-α) is a proinflammatory cytokine that normally is present at high levels during the early inflammatory phase, and levels of TNF-α are controlled by two ECM proteins. One protein, a disintegrin and metallo-proteinase (ADAM-17), promotes release of TNF-α. Another protein, a tissue inhibitor of metalloproteinase-3 (TIMP-3), controls ADAM-17, thereby reducing production of TNF-α. Research is ongoing into factors that determine the combination and concentration of ECM proteins and into strategies for measuring and controlling levels of various MMPs to achieve therapeutic outcomes (Gill & Parks, 2008; Macri & Clark, 2009).

Diabetes is a clinical condition associated with prolonged inflammation. Some data suggest that leukocyte migration may be impaired in people with this condition; in addition, the leukocytes that do migrate to the wound bed frequently are dysfunctional, especially in the presence of hyperglycemia. The end result of diminished leukocyte migration and impaired leukocyte function is failure to effectively control bacterial loads. This situation results in a persistent stimulus for proinflammatory cytokines, chronic inflammation, and delayed healing (Pradhan et al., 2009). Conditions resulting in ischemia/hypoxia also produce prolonged inflammation, because oxygen and ROS are required for oxidative killing of bacteria. The inability to control bacteria that accompanies hypoxia results in chronic inflammation and failure to heal. Hyperbaric oxygen therapy can improve tissue oxygen levels, contribute to bacterial control, and reduce the production of proinflammatory cytokines, thus promoting the repair process (Rodriguez et al., 2008; Thom, 2009).

Conditions and medications that affect the function of autonomic and sensory nerves and their receptors may also affect inflammation. For example, diabetes is associated with diminished production of substance P, a neuropeptide that normally contributes to a healthy inflammatory response by supporting vasodilation and leukocyte migration. Diminished production of substance P may be one factor leading to compromised inflammation and impaired healing in the diabetic population (Pradhan et al., 2009). Preliminary research suggests β-adrenergic agents may reduce inflammation by reducing neutrophil recruitment and production of inflammatory cytokines (Pullar, Manabat-Hidalgo, Bolaji, et al., 2008).

Proliferation

The third phase of acute full-thickness wound healing is the proliferative phase. During this phase, the wound surface is covered with new epithelium that restores the bacterial barrier, vascular integrity is restored, and the incisional defect is mended with new connective tissue. The key components of the proliferative phase are epithelialization, neoangiogenesis, and matrix deposition/collagen synthesis. Limited contraction of the newly formed ECM also may occur.

Epithelialization. Epithelialization of a full-thickness wound healing by primary intention begins within hours after injury and typically is complete within 24–48 h. This "neoepithelium" is only a few cells thick but is sufficient to provide a closed wound surface and a bacterial barrier. This process is the basis for the Centers for Disease Control and Prevention's recommendation that new surgical incisions be covered with

a sterile dressing for the first 24–48 h postoperatively. Until reepithelialization is complete, the potential for bacterial invasion exists, and the wound should be managed with sterile wound care and a cover dressing that provides a bacterial barrier (Mangram, Horan, Pearson, et al., 1999; Yamamoto & Kiyosawa, 2014). As with partial-thickness wound repair, the processes of lateral migration, vertical migration, and differentiation continue throughout the proliferative phase and gradually reestablish epidermal thickness and function (Braiman-Wiksman et al., 2007; Myers, Leigh, & Navsaria, 2007). In full-thickness wounds, the new epidermis is slightly thinner than the original epidermis. Because the neoepidermis is covering scar tissue rather than normal dermis, the rete pegs that normally dip into the dermis are lacking (Monaco & Lawrence, 2003).

Granulation tissue formation. A hallmark outcome of the proliferative phase is the formation of granulation tissue, which begins as the inflammatory phase subsides, at 3–4 days postinjury (Braiman-Wiksman et al., 2007). Granulation tissue is composed primarily of capillary loops and newly synthesized connective tissue proteins and is often referred to as the ECM. Fibroblasts and inflammatory cells also are present in this new matrix. Neoangiogenesis and connective tissue synthesis occur simultaneously in a codependent fashion to form the new ECM that will fill the wound defect. Through angiogenesis, new capillaries are formed and joined with existing severed capillaries, thus restoring the delivery of oxygen and nutrients to the wound bed. At the same time, a new "provisional" ECM is formed through the synthesis of connective tissue proteins such as type III collagen (Fig. 8.5) (Pradhan et al., 2009).

Neoangiogenesis

Endothelial cells typically are quiescent. Neoangiogenesis requires stimulation by growth factors, which convert the quiescent cells to actively proliferating cells. Molecules in the ECM also play a critical role by influencing the response of endothelial cells to angiogenic growth factors (Cheresh & Stupack, 2008). Neoangiogenesis occurs by two mechanisms: production of new vessels by local endothelial cells and recruitment of circulating stem progenitor cells to form new vessels de novo (Thom, 2009).

The growth factors that stimulate production of new vessels are produced by the cells in the wound bed (injured endothelial cells, macrophages, fibroblasts, and keratinocytes) and include vascular endothelial growth factor (VEGF), basic fibroblast growth factor, and possibly PDGF. The most important angiogenic growth factor is VEGF; in addition to stimulating local endothelial cells to proliferate and migrate, VEGF attracts stem progenitor cells to the wound bed and stimulates them to differentiate into endothelial cells (Braiman-Wiksman et al., 2007; Gill & Parks, 2008; Thom, 2009). A number of ECM factors also affect neoangiogenesis. One is the provisional matrix itself, which affects the migration of endothelial cells (Gill & Parks, 2008). Another is the level of TIMP-3, which has a very negative effect on

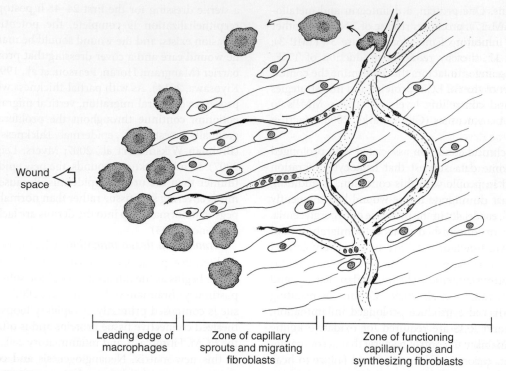

Wound space ◁

Leading edge of macrophages | Zone of capillary sprouts and migrating fibroblasts | Zone of functioning capillary loops and synthesizing fibroblasts

Fig. 8.5 Advancing module of reparative tissue during proliferative and remodeling phases. (From Whalen, G. F., & Zetter, B. R. (1992). Angiogenesis. In I. K. Cohen, R. F. Dieglemann, & W. J. Lindbald (Eds.), *Wound healing: Biochemical and clinical aspects.* Philadelphia: Saunders.)

angiogenesis. TIMP-3 binds to the receptor sites for VEGF and blocks its angiogenic effects (Gill & Parks, 2008). A third factor is the level of nitric oxide, which promotes angiogenesis by activating MMP-13 (Lizarbe, García-Rama, Tarín, et al., 2008).

Clinical factors affecting neoangiogenesis include oxygen levels within the wound bed, patient age, gender, diabetes, coronary artery disease, radiation therapy, and chemotherapy. Hypoxia acts as an initial stimulus to angiogenesis, but persistent hypoxia interferes with endothelial cell proliferation and new vessel formation. Hyperglycemia and glycolysis are associated with production of substances that are toxic to endothelial cells. Diabetes, aging, female gender, coronary artery disease, radiation therapy, and chemotherapy all interfere with angiogenesis by reducing mobilization of stem progenitor cells, thus compromising the potential for de novo development of new vessels. Aging is also associated with dysfunction and impaired mobilization of local endothelial cells, partly due to impaired expression of VEGF and other angiogenic stimuli. Of interest, some data suggest that exercise can partially reverse these age-related changes (Hoenig, Bianchi, Rosenzweig, et al., 2008; Rodriguez et al., 2008; Thom, 2009). Therapeutic modalities that may promote angiogenesis include exogenous application of basic fibroblast growth factor and topical or systemic administration of erythropoietin (EPO). Animal studies and limited human case reports indicate potent stimulation of angiogenesis and granulation tissue formation with each of these therapies; EPO has also been associated with inhibition of excessive inflammation (Hamed, Bennett, Demiot, et al., 2014; O'Goshi & Tagami, 2007).

Matrix Deposition/Collagen Synthesis

Fibroblasts are responsible for synthesis of the connective tissue proteins that compose the provisional ECM; therefore, fibroblasts are critical to the repair process. Fibroblasts migrate into the wound bed from the surrounding tissues in response to growth factors and interleukins released by degranulating platelets, activated leukocytes (neutrophils and macrophages), and keratinocytes. Migration requires upregulation of binding sites (integrin receptors) on the cell wall, which is mediated by PDGF and TGF-β. This upregulation of binding sites is essential because fibroblasts migrate by maintaining attachment to one binding site while extending lamellipodia in search of another site. Once the fibroblast is able to bind to a new site, it releases the original attachment and "moves" in the direction of the wound bed (Monaco & Lawrence, 2003; Myers et al., 2007).

Fibroblasts begin to appear in the wound bed toward the end of the inflammatory phase, 2–3 days after injury. By day 4, fibroblasts are the predominant cells in the wound matrix (Dubay & Franz, 2003). Once fibroblasts arrive at the wound site, growth factors bind to fibroblast receptor sites and trigger intracellular processes that move the fibroblasts into the reproductive phase of the cell cycle, thus stimulating proliferation of the fibroblast. Finally, the fibroblasts are converted into "wound fibroblasts" by TGF-β, a growth factor secreted by macrophages. These wound fibroblasts differ from typical dermal fibroblasts in that they exhibit decreased proliferative behavior but increased synthesis of connective tissue proteins such as collagen (Frank, Kämpfer, Wetzler, et al., 2002).

Collagen synthesis follows the established process for synthesis of any protein. The collagen molecule is characterized by a glycine-X-Y repeating sequence. The collagen molecule must undergo a series of intracellular modifications before the molecule is secreted into the extracellular environment and becomes part of the ECM. One of the most critical modifications is "cross-linking" of the proline and lysine molecules, a process known as hydroxylation. These cross-links are essential for the development of tensile strength. A number of factors are required for normal hydroxylation, including oxygen, ascorbic acid, iron, copper, and selected enzymes. Thus hypoxia, vitamin C deficiency, copper deficiency, and iron deficiency all can compromise hydroxylation and the development of tensile strength. High-dose corticosteroids also can impair tensile strength because corticosteroids suppress the enzymes needed for hydroxylation. Following intracellular modifications, the collagen molecule is secreted into the extracellular environment as the triple helix procollagen. It then undergoes additional steps that culminate in the formation of cross-linked fibrils. The enzyme lysyl oxidase is essential to these processes and to the development of stable collagen fibers (Monaco & Lawrence, 2003).

The early granulation tissue is a provisional matrix characterized by unstructured collagen and high levels of fibronectin. This provisional matrix also includes fibronectin, laminin, and proteoglycans such as hyaluronic acid (Braiman-Wiksman et al., 2007; Gill & Parks, 2008; Schneider, Garlick, & Egles, 2008). As the ECM matures, collagen becomes the predominant protein, representing a little over 50% of the new ECM. Proteoglycans such as hyaluronic acid are present in small amounts but serve critical functions. For example, hyaluronic acid facilitates cell migration, protects cells against free-radical and proteolytic damage, and contributes viscoelastic properties to the new matrix (Chen & Abatangelo, 1999; Monaco & Lawrence, 2003).

The provisional matrix is remodeled by wound fibroblasts throughout this proliferative phase. In this process, matrix is formed, modified, degraded and replaced. The process releases essential factors critical to healing (Bohn, 2020a, 2020b; Bohn, Liden, Schultz, Yang, & Gibson, 2016; Dempsey, Miller, Schueler, et al., 2020). A factor know to attract stem cells has been identified from this process. Provisional Matrix not only provides structure and sites for attachment triggering cellular next step functions, but recent research has also identified stem cell attractant factors that recruit native stem cells to the wound site. The May-Day factor is one such protein. May-Day factor is created by the macrophage cleavage of N-terminal end of decorin found in the matrix by MMP-12. The release of this is a potent signaling factor highlights one more key function of matrix processing in healing wounds (Dempsey et al., 2020). The failure of wounds to develop a provisional matrix would then lack these essential signaling proteins. Wounds would then stall and fail to progress. The recruitment of native stem cells is well known to influence healing. Chemotactic isolates such as May-Day factor may serve therapeutic roles in conditions such as arthritis, muscle repair, and others (Dempsey et al., 2020).

Wounds healing by primary intention, such as sutured incisions, require a limited amount of connective tissue to mend the defect. In these wounds, ECM production is essentially complete within 14–21 days (Hunt & Van Winkle, 1997; Monaco & Lawrence, 2003). Although the granulation tissue is not visible in these wounds, a "healing ridge" can be palpated just under the intact suture line by days 5–9. The healing ridge is produced by the newly formed connective tissue proteins. Absence of this healing ridge indicates impaired healing and increased risk for dehiscence (Hunt & Van Winkle, 1997).

Factors Affecting Granulation Tissue Formation

Factors affecting granulation tissue formation include perfusion status, oxygen levels, nutritional status, and glucose levels/diabetes. Granulation tissue formation is very much an oxygen-dependent process. Hypoxia can act as a stimulus to fibroblast proliferation and initial collagen synthesis, but adequate levels of oxygen (30–40 mm Hg) are absolutely essential for the latter steps in collagen synthesis and for the cross-linking that provides tensile strength. Adequate oxygen levels are also required for prevention of infection. Infection rates in surgical wounds are inversely proportional to oxygen levels (Rodriguez et al., 2008). Tissue oxygenation of acute wounds is discussed in more detail in Chapter 31. Nutritional status affects granulation because granulation tissue formation requires adequate levels of protein and micronutrients such as ascorbic acid, iron, and copper. Diabetes is associated with delayed deposition of granulation tissue and insufficient production of collagen to establish a mature matrix (Braiman-Wiksman et al., 2007).

Contraction

Contraction occurs when specialized fibroblasts known as myofibroblasts exert tractional forces on the ECM, reducing the size of the wound. Wounds healing by primary intention have limited or no contraction because the wound edges have been surgically approximated (Monaco & Lawrence, 2003).

Maturation/Remodeling

The final phase in full-thickness wound healing is the maturation, or remodeling, phase, which begins around day 21 after wounding and continues beyond 1 year. The early collagen is characterized by poorly organized fibers having limited tensile strength. At 3 weeks after injury, the healing wound exhibits only 20% of the strength of intact dermis. The provisional matrix is gradually converted to a mature and relatively acellular scar, a process that involves replacement of the type III collagen in the provisional matrix with type I collagen, the type normally found in dermal tissue. However, even the final form of collagen does not exhibit the normal basket-weave pattern of the collagen in unwounded dermis. Rather, the fibers of "repair collagen" are aligned parallel to the stress lines of the wound. The new ECM also lacks elastin, which provides the uninjured skin with elasticity; thus scar tissue is "stiff" compared with normal tissue (Monaco & Lawrence, 2003; Rodriguez et al., 2008).

Remodeling involves the dual processes of synthesis and degradation of the ECM and is regulated by fibroblasts and

ECM proteins (MMPs). The new collagen that is formed is more orderly and provides more tensile strength to the wound; tensile strength improves steadily during the 2–3 months following initial injury and repair. However, the tensile strength of the remodeled ECM (scar tissue) is never more than 80% of the tensile strength in nonwounded tissue (Hunt & Van Winkle, 1997).

An imbalance between the dual processes of matrix synthesis and matrix breakdown can complicate wound healing. For example, hypertrophic scarring and keloid formation are believed to be caused in part by an excess of matrix synthesis compared with matrix degradation (Rahban & Garner, 2003; Wilgus, 2007). In contrast, hypoxia, malnutrition, or excess levels of MMPs can interfere with synthesis and deposition of new matrix proteins, resulting in wound breakdown (Monaco & Lawrence, 2003).

Full-Thickness Wound Repair: Wounds Healing by Secondary Intention

Although full-thickness wounds healing by secondary intention (e.g., pressure ulcers) proceed through the same phases as full-thickness wounds healing by primary intention, key differences do exist within each phase. These differences are summarized in Table 8.2 and discussed here.

Absence of Hemostasis

The absence of hemostasis has a tremendous impact on the healing trajectory of wounds. Bleeding and hemostasis do not occur in wounds healing by secondary intention. Failure to bleed and clot compromises the repair process because the wound-healing sequence of events is normally initiated by clot breakdown and the subsequent release of growth factors. One theorized benefit of surgical debridement of chronic wounds is to trigger clot formation and the release of growth factors so that the repair process is reactivated.

Prolonged Inflammatory Phase

The inflammatory phase frequently is prolonged. Because the goal of this phase is to establish a clean wound bed and to obtain bacterial balance, the wound will remain in this phase until necrotic tissue has been eliminated and bacterial loads have been controlled. Wounds healing by secondary intention frequently are characterized by large amounts of devitalized tissue and heavy bacterial loads. Thus the inflammatory phase generally lasts considerably longer than the 3 days that are typical in the approximated incision.

Prolonged Proliferative Phase

The proliferative phase is prolonged, and the sequence of events is different. In wounds healing by primary intention, epithelialization occurs first, followed by angiogenesis and formation of a limited volume of connective tissue proteins (ECM); contraction does not occur or is very limited. These processes usually are complete within 14–21 days. In secondary intention wound healing, the proliferative phase begins with granulation tissue formation (to fill in the soft tissue defect), followed by contraction (to minimize the defect); epithelialization is the final phase.

The volume of granulation tissue required to fill the defect (and the time required for this phase of repair) is determined by the size of the wound and the degree to which contraction is able to reduce the size of the defect. Because the wound bed

TABLE 8.2	Full-Thickness Repair Process	
	Primary Intention	**Secondary Intention**
Examples	Laceration Surgical incision	Chronic wound (e.g., pressure ulcer, venous ulcer) Wound dehiscence
Hemostasis	Bleeding Platelets rupture and release growth factors Coagulation pathways (intrinsic and extrinsic) activated	No bleeding No coagulation Hemostasis absent
Inflammatory phase	Any necrotic tissue removed Bacterial balance restored Duration usually limited to 1–3 days unless complicated by infection	Necrotic tissue removed Bacterial balance restored Duration prolonged until nonviable tissue eliminated, and bacteria controlled; also prolonged by presence of excess proinflammatory cells
Proliferative phase	Epithelialization (first event in proliferative phase) Synthesis of connective tissue Duration typically 14–21 days	Granulation tissue formation • Neoangiogenesis • Synthesis of connective tissue proteins • Contraction of wound edges Epithelialization (last event in proliferative phase) Duration is dependent on size and depth of wound and host's ability to synthesize new extracellular matrix
Maturation (remodeling phase)	Collagen synthesis and lysis Tensile strength partially reestablished	Collagen synthesis and lysis Tensile strength partially reestablished

is visible, the clinician is able to assess progress in healing. Healthy granulation tissue presents as a red, vascular, granular wound bed as a result of the numerous capillary loops in combination with the newly synthesized ECM proteins (see Plates 3 and 5B).

Increased Amount of Contraction

Contraction is much more important in secondary intention wound healing than in closed wounds because contraction reduces the size of the soft tissue defect and thus reduces the amount of granulation tissue required. The rate of contraction for open wounds averages 0.6–0.7 mm/day (Gabbiani, 2003; Monaco & Lawrence, 2003). The degree to which a specific wound will contract is determined partly by the mobility of the surrounding tissue. For example, the tissue surrounding sacral and abdominal wounds is quite mobile and can contract easily. In contrast, the tissue surrounding a wound on the extremity or overlying a bony prominence has limited potential for contraction. Contraction is considered undesirable in some wounds because it can cause cosmetic deformities or flexion contractures of joints.

Contraction is mediated by myofibroblasts, modified fibroblasts that contain actin and myosin monofilaments and smooth muscle proteins. Differentiation of fibroblasts into myofibroblasts is stimulated by growth factors such as TGF-β1 and PDGF. Substances within the ECM itself are also thought to contribute to the development of myofibroblasts. Intracellular actin filaments and extracellular fibronectin work jointly to establish a contractile force that compresses and "shrinks" the ECM, thus pulling the wound edges toward each other (Demidova-Rice et al., 2012; Gabbiani, 2003).

Delayed Epithelialization

Because full-thickness wounds involve loss of the deep dermis and epidermal appendages (along with their epithelial lining), epithelialization in these wounds proceeds from the periphery of the wound inward in a centripetal fashion. Epithelial migration requires an open, proliferative wound edge. Closed, nonproliferative wound edges, also known as epibole, are sometimes seen in open wounds healing by secondary intention, probably due to premature keratinization of the wound edges (Fig. 8.6 and Plate 4). In these wounds, an open edge must be reestablished, by either surgical excision or chemical cauterization, before epithelial migration can occur (Schultz, Sibbald, Falanga, et al., 2003).

Prolonged Remodeling

The remodeling process for wounds healing by secondary intention is essentially the same as that for wounds healing by primary intention. Clinicians and caregivers must remain acutely aware that newly "healed" wounds initially lack tensile strength, and measures should be initiated to minimize stress on the remodeling wound until tensile strength has developed, which occurs 2–3 months after closure. For example, the patient with a newly healed pressure injury should remain on a therapeutic support surface and should minimize time spent lying on the involved surface.

WHAT MAKES A CHRONIC WOUND CHRONIC?

An acute wound in a relatively healthy host will heal fairly quickly because of a cascade of growth factors, cytokines, and matrix proteins that tend to keep the acute wound on the "healing track." In clinical practice, however, chronic wounds such as pressure ulcers, vascular ulcers, and neuropathic wounds behave much differently and may be extremely slow to heal. In order to intervene effectively, the clinician must be knowledgeable regarding the various factors contributing to delayed healing.

Over the past decade, extensive research analyzing the cellular, biochemical, and molecular components of acute and chronic wounds has significantly expanded the understanding of the detailed complexities of normal wound healing and the pathophysiologic mechanisms of chronic wounds. Box 8.1 summarizes the characteristics of a chronic wound.

Underlying Pathology

The nature of the injury differs between acute and chronic wounds. Acute wounds usually begin with a sudden, solitary insult and proceed to heal in an orderly manner. In contrast, chronic wounds are commonly caused by an underlying pathologic process, such as vascular insufficiency, that produces repeated and prolonged insults to the tissues. Failure to correct or control the underlying pathology can result in a persistent cycle of injury that causes repetitive tissue damage. In

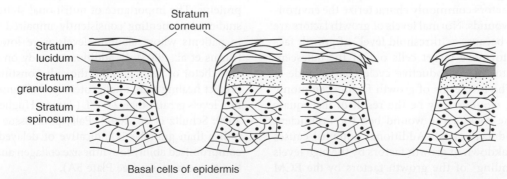

Stratum corneum
Stratum lucidum
Stratum granulosum
Stratum spinosum

Basal cells of epidermis

Fig. 8.6 *Left,* closed wound edges in which epidermis of wound edges has rolled under so that epithelial cells cannot migrate (also known as epibole). *Right,* open wound edges from which epithelial cells can migrate.

contrast, correction of the underlying pathology frequently can shift the wound to a healing pathway (Goldman, 2004).

Increased Levels of Inflammatory Substances

Chronic wounds frequently are complicated by impediments to healing, such as ischemia, necrotic tissue, heavy bacterial loads, and high levels of proinflammatory MMPs. These factors prolong the inflammatory phase of wound healing by continuing to recruit macrophages and neutrophils into the wound bed. In particular, the recognition of biofilm development in and on the wound bed helps explain high MMP levels. The innate immune response to biofilm recruits inflammatory cells which leads to higher MMP levels. Biofilm protects the bacteria contained within it and inflammatory cells fail to be able to remove or eliminate the biofilm. High levels of proinflammatory MMPs are associated with ongoing destruction of the ECM (Bohn et al., 2016; Demidova-Rice et al., 2012; Gill & Parks, 2008; Goldman, 2004). Studies indicate that the levels of inflammatory substances in chronic wounds are 100 times higher than the levels in acute wounds (Berg Vande & Robson, 2003). Debridement of necrotic tissue and control of the bacterial burden has been shown to be helpful (Goldman, 2004).

The high levels of protease can be modulated by application of effective collagen. Layering of collagen will also allow for the adjustment of effective dosing for wounds and one can infer from the consumption of the collagen whether MMPs are effectively treated (Bohn, 2020a, 2020b; Bohn et al., 2016). Wound healing can be observed when MMP levels are buffered sufficiently (Bohn et al., 2016).

Low Levels of Growth Factors

In addition to high levels of inflammatory proteases, low levels of growth factors commonly characterize the environment of chronic wounds. Normal levels of growth factors are critical to repair, because a "threshold level" of growth factors is required to move target cells out of the quiescent G_0 phase and into the reproductive cycle (Berg Vande & Robson, 2003). The low levels of growth factors commonly found in chronic wounds may be the result of inadequate production by the cells of the wound bed (or insufficient numbers of "producer" cells). Additional potential causes include rapid breakdown of growth factors by the high levels of MMPs or "binding" of the growth factors by the ECM

(Berg Vande & Robson, 2003; Steed, 2003). Although this imbalance between inflammatory and proliferative stimuli usually is thought to be the cause of impaired healing, some investigators suggest that the imbalance instead may be a result of chronicity. When the wound begins to heal, the ratio of inflammatory to proliferative stimuli normalizes (Goldman, 2004; Henry & Garner, 2003).

Cellular and ECM Abnormalities

Current evidence suggests distinct phenotypic differences in the fibroblasts and keratinocytes found in chronic wounds compared with those found in acute wounds. Specifically, both fibroblasts and keratinocytes exhibit reduced proliferative behavior and reduced motility, possibly due in part to abnormalities in the ECM (Demidova-Rice et al., 2012). Additional differences noted in the fibroblasts and keratinocytes of chronic wounds include reduced numbers of growth factor receptor sites and increased cellular senescence (that is, decreased ability to proliferate) (Telgenhoff & Shroot, 2005). Because all phases of wound healing are controlled primarily by growth factors, reduced binding sites or reduced responsiveness would significantly alter the cells' ability to contribute to wound healing. Cellular senescence may occur in the elderly as a normal component of aging and may contribute to the delayed healing commonly seen in this population. In addition, the high levels of ROS common to the chronic wound environment can cause DNA damage and loss of the cells' ability to replicate normally, regardless of age. The accumulation of senescent cells in chronic wounds creates an environment of prolonged inflammation. Increasing evidence demonstrates cellular senescence can be prevented or senescent cells removed, to mitigate chronic wounds (Wang & Shi, 2020). Optimal wound management is also a key tactic to manage and reverse cellular senescence (Berg Vande & Robson, 2003; Pittman, 2007; Telgenhoff & Shroot, 2005).

Miscellaneous Host Conditions

Additional "host factors" that trigger chronicity in a wound include ischemia, malnutrition, and comorbidities such as diabetes (Steed, 2003). Malnutrition is a particularly common contributor to wound chronicity. Fibroblasts that lack the requisite raw ingredients cannot synthesize connective tissue proteins. The importance of nutritional status is reflected in studies documenting consistently impaired wound healing in patients whose albumin levels were lower than 2.0 g/L (Burns et al., 2003). In addition, a study on wound fluid as a predictor of healing found the only constituents to reliably predict healing were total protein and albumin, that is, albumin levels greater than 2.0 g/L (James, Hughes, Cherry, et al., 2000; Schultz et al., 2003). Pale, pink tissue that is smooth rather than granular is indicative of delayed healing and a compromised ability to synthesize collagen and other connective tissue proteins (see Plate 5A).

Denervation

Denervation is another potential cause of failure to heal. Sensory nerves secrete neuropeptides (e.g., substance P) that are highly chemotactic for inflammatory cells. Therefore, denervated wounds are subject to impaired inflammation and compromised healing. Denervation may be one of the factors contributing to chronicity of pressure ulcers in patients with spinal cord injury and neuropathic ulcers in diabetic patients (Macri & Clark, 2009; Richards, Mitsou, Floyd, et al., 1997).

In summary, differences in the healing trajectory for acute and chronic wounds stem from the nature of the injury, the cellular events that follow injury, and miscellaneous host factors. In general, healing wounds are characterized by high mitotic activity, therapeutic levels of inflammatory cytokines, low levels of proteases, and mitotically competent cells. In contrast, chronic wounds exhibit low mitotic activity, excessive levels of inflammatory cytokines, high levels of proteases, and senescent or mitotically incompetent cells.

MEDIATORS OF WOUND HEALING

In order for healing to occur normally, the critical cells must be recruited to the wound bed (at the appropriate time), stimulated to reproduce, and then directed to carry out essential functions, such as neoangiogenesis, connective tissue synthesis, and reepithelialization. This complex process is controlled and coordinated by an equally complex array of regulatory substances; key elements include bioactive molecules, matrix proteins, and the matrix itself. The effect of these regulatory factors is further influenced by "host" factors, such as cell receptor sites, cellular senescence, availability of nutrients, and cofactors required for phagocytosis and collagen synthesis, and comorbid conditions, such as hypoxia and diabetes. This section provides a brief overview of regulatory factors, which are discussed further in Chapter 23.

Bioactive Molecules

Bioactive molecules include growth factors and cytokines. They are produced by the cells in the wound bed (e.g., platelets, neutrophils, macrophages, and fibroblasts) and act as "directors" of cell function and thus of the repair process. They do so by attracting the needed cells to the wound bed, stimulating them to proliferate, and then directing the cells to carry out specific aspects of repair. For example, TNF-α is a proinflammatory cytokine that attracts neutrophils and macrophages to the wound bed and is present in high concentrations during the inflammatory phase, whereas VEGF is a growth factor that supports proliferation and migration of endothelial cells and therefore is important during angiogenesis (Gill & Parks, 2008; Macri & Clark, 2009; Thom, 2009).

Matrix Proteins

Growth factors and cytokines act as "controllers" for the cells critical to the repair process. However, it is increasingly apparent that proteins within the ECM control the levels and function of growth factors and cytokines. Key categories of matrix proteins include MMPs, ADAMs, and tissue inhibitors of metalloproteinase (TIMPs). MMPs and ADAMs can "upregulate" the levels of growth factors and cytokines by cleaving them from the cell and thus activating them; however, they also can "downregulate" the levels of growth factors and cytokines by degrading them or by inhibiting their release. TIMPs control the activity of MMPs by binding to them, thus blocking their effects (Gill & Parks, 2008).

ECM remodeling releases protein factors that recruit and attract mesenchymal stem cells. May-Day factor attracts and recruits mesenchymal stem cells have been identified as a result of MMP-12 activity. N-terminal Pecorin is cleaved by MMP-12 releasing May-Day protein that attracts stem cells to the wound site. (Dempsey et al., 2020).

Extracellular Matrix

The ECM serves as a scaffold for migrating cells and as a repository for growth factors. It also influences the response of the cells to growth factors. For example, keratinocyte proliferation requires both attachment to the ECM and stimulation by growth factors. Cell migration is another aspect of repair that is dependent on both matrix proteins and integrins within the matrix itself. Matrix proteins promote migration by degrading the bonds between the migrating cells and the underlying wound bed, and the matrix promotes reattachment through the expression of binding sites (integrins) within the matrix. The matrix also supports cell-to-cell communication. The ECM needs to be porous and pliable in order to support the movement of cells, nutrients, and growth factors through the wound environment (Cheresh & Stupack, 2008; Schultz & Wysocki, 2009). Cellular based tissue products that contain a dermal matrix dressing (see Chapter 22) are often used to support cell migration and granulation tissue formation, in select wounds (Nataraj, Ritter, Dumas, et al., 2007).

Host Factors

A number of host factors influence cells' response to growth factors, cytokines, and matrix proteins. One of these factors is the type of receptors on the cell wall. This is an important factor because all cells within the wound bed are exposed to the same mix of regulatory substances, but only select cells respond. In addition, different cells may exhibit different responses to the same regulatory substance because regulatory substances exert their effects primarily through binding with cell receptors. Therefore, only cells with the specific receptor sites respond to the regulatory substance, and the effects of receptor binding vary based on cell type. For example, PDGF stimulates migration of some cells and mitosis in others, but it has no effect on other cells (Martin, 1997; Witte & Barbul, 1997). Furthermore, fibroblasts and keratinocytes in elderly individuals have a decreased number of receptor sites, which may explain why elderly patients tend to exhibit a diminished response to some regulatory substances (Ashcroft, Mills, & Ashworth, 2002).

Other factors that impact an individual's ability to heal normally are systemic factors such as nutritional status, perfusion, oxygenation, and comorbidities such as diabetes. These factors are addressed briefly in this chapter and in greater depth in other chapters in this text.

EXTREMES OF REPAIR: SCARLESS HEALING VS EXCESSIVE SCARRING

Not all full-thickness wounds heal in an ideal fashion. Hypertrophic and keloid scars (see Plate 7 C and D) are examples of abnormal repair or excessive scarring. As we learn more about the factors that lead to "normal" and excessive scarring, we hope to be able to optimize repair and minimize scarring for all patients.

Scarless Healing

As mentioned earlier in this chapter, the early-gestation fetus typically heals without scarring, an ability that is lost at 22–24 weeks of gestation (Samuels & Tan, 1999). Features and characteristics of early-gestation healing are listed in Box 8.2. One significant difference is a markedly diminished inflammatory response. Multiple studies using various models have demonstrated that inflammation is minimal or essentially absent in early-gestation (scarless) healing. This finding is consistent with other studies showing a strong link between the intensity and duration of the inflammatory response and the subsequent development of scar tissue (Wilgus, 2007). The specific factors thought to contribute to this very minimal inflammatory response include the following: (1) Fetal platelets release much lower levels of proinflammatory growth factors and cytokines, most specifically the profibrotic isoforms of TGF-β. TGF-β is responsible for attracting inflammatory cells to the wound bed, for promoting angiogenesis and fibroblast activity, and for remodeling of the ECM; (2) Marked reduction in migration of inflammatory cells (neutrophils, macrophages, and T cells); this is partially due to the lower levels of proinflammatory growth factors and partially due

to the fact that the fetal immune system is poorly developed; (3) Marked reduction in angiogenic stimuli linked to scar formation (VEGF, TGF-β1, PDGF, and prostaglandin E2) (Walraven, Gouverneur, Middelkoop, et al., 2014; Wilgus, 2007).

Another difference in early-gestation healing is the rate at which epithelial resurfacing occurs. Rapid upregulation of the adhesion molecules within the ECM allows cells to move laterally, which promotes early keratinocyte migration (Wilgus, 2007).

Most importantly, a number of differences in fetal healing contribute to production of a new ECM that retains the characteristics of unwounded tissue. One contributing factor may be the high levels of hyaluronic acid and hyaluronic-acid-stimulating activity factor. This factor is significant because hyaluronic acid supports rapid cell migration. In addition, high levels of MMPs compared with TIMPs favor degradation of the ECM, which is thought to help prevent overproduction of collagen. Finally, fetal fibroblasts retain the ability to produce new matrix proteins that retain the basket-weave configuration characteristic of normal dermis (Wilgus, 2007).

In summary, early-gestation fetal repair is characterized by a significantly reduced inflammatory response and a rapid and balanced proliferative phase that restores the dermal architecture without scarring (see Box 8.2).

Excessive Scarring

Excessive or hyperproliferative scarring is a complication of acute full-thickness wound healing that presently is not well understood. The two types of hyperproliferative scarring are keloid scars (Plate 7C) and hypertrophic scars (Plate 7D). Both types appear raised, are red or pink, and are pruritic. Hypertrophic scars are confined to the original incisional or scar area, whereas keloids expand beyond the incision into the surrounding tissue. This expansion, sometimes described as a mushroom effect, is the result of continued proliferation of connective tissue proteins that may continue indefinitely (Atiyeh, 2005; Slemp & Kirschner, 2006).

Hypertrophic scars are characterized by increased vasculature, increased numbers of white blood cells and fibroblasts, and a thickened epidermal layer (Atiyeh, 2005). The collagen fibers in hypertrophic scars are organized and oriented parallel to the epidermal layer; however, they contain an abundance of myofibroblasts, which leads to contracture formation. One positive feature of hypertrophic scars (compared with keloids) is their potential to eventually regress during the remodeling phase (Slemp & Kirschner, 2006).

Keloids are a much more serious problem than hypertrophic scars. Keloids may continue to expand, creating both functional and cosmetic deficits. In addition, scars that initially appear to be "normal" may deviate into a pattern of keloid growth over time. Biochemical analysis of keloid scars reveals increased numbers of receptor sites for growth factors and major abnormalities in the behavior of fibroblasts and keratinocytes, which may partially explain the excessive production of ECM. Most importantly, the balance between

---

BOX 8.2   Characteristics of Scarless Healing

Decreased amount of platelet-derived growth factor
Decreased amount of proinflammatory proteases and growth factors
Increased levels of fibronectin and hyaluronic acid
Balance of TIMP and MMP
New collagen structure and function indistinguishable from native collagen

MMP, matrix metalloprotease; *TIMP*, tissue inhibitor of matrix metalloprotease.

synthesis and degradation of connective tissue proteins is lost. This loss of balance is theorized to result from abnormalities in cell-to-cell communication and immune function, failure of apoptosis (spontaneous cell death), and the effects of hypoxia and oxygen free radicals. Keloid scars are characterized by disorganized collagen bundles; however, these scars do not contain myofibroblasts and are not associated with contracture formation (Atiyeh, 2005; Hahn, Glaser, McFarland, et al., 2013; Slemp & Kirschner, 2006).

Risk factors for hyperproliferative scarring include a strong family history (particularly important with keloid formation), age 10–30 years, and darkly pigmented skin. In the United States, individuals of African American descent have a 5%–15% increased risk compared with Caucasians (Atiyeh, 2005; Slemp & Kirschner, 2006). Exposure to mechanical stretch may be a trigger for keloid production (Ogawa, Okai, Tokumura, et al., 2012).

Strategies designed to prevent or correct hyperproliferative scarring have provided inconsistent and often suboptimal results. Surgical excision, intralesional steroids (either single or combination steroids), and topical silicone sheeting are the most commonly prescribed therapies. Table 8.3 lists current treatment options. Research is ongoing, with the goals of accurately identifying the cellular and biochemical abnormalities that produce these scars and designing therapies to prevent and correct them (Kieran, Knock, Bush, et al., 2013; Syed & Bayat, 2013; Yamamoto & Kiyosawa, 2014). The use of a provisional matrix may have a beneficial effect on keloid formation. New reports of surgical treatment of keloid implementing the use of a provisional matrix may result in less scar formation and more orderly healing (Mancuso et al., 2018). Signaling and stem cell recruitment may also play a role (Bohn, 2020a, 2020b; Dempsey et al., 2020).

TABLE 8.3 Therapy Options for Hyperproliferative Scarring

Treatment	Indications	Considerations
Surgical excision	Hypertrophic scars Keloid scars	Recurrence rare with hypertrophic Recurrence common (45%–100%) with keloid if surgical excision is done without adjunctive therapies
Radiation (as adjunct to surgical excision)	Hypertrophic scars Keloid scars	Promotion of fibroblast apoptosis (death) Low recurrence rates (1%–35%) Theoretical risk of radiation-induced malignancy (no data)
Corticosteroid therapy (systemic), intralesional injections (single or combined agents)	Hypertrophic scars Keloid scars	Reduces scar overgrowth, pruritus, contractures Pain of repeated injections may limit patient adherence Adverse effects: skin atrophy, depigmentation, telangiectasias
Silicone gel, sheeting	Hypertrophic scars Keloid scars	Increases wound hydration Decreases fibroblast activity Down-regulates fibrogenic isoforms of TGF-β Worn 12–24 h/day for at least 2–3 months Risk of maceration and skin breakdown with gel (gel use limited to areas where sheeting will not conform)
Laser (CDL, PDL)	Hypertrophic scars Keloid scars	Stimulates regression of keloid Reduces pruritus with hypertrophic (PDL) Variable results if used independently; best if used in conjunction with steroids or silicone gel CDL: recurrence rate as high as 50% PDL: Works best with steroids + silicone No comparative studies of laser, surgery, and adjunctive therapy
Retinoids (topical)	Hypertrophic scars Keloid scars	Suppresses collagen synthesis Increases epithelial cell turnover May be applied topically both preoperatively/postoperatively 80% of lesions have favorable short-term outcomes

Continued

TABLE 8.3 Therapy Options for Hyperproliferative Scarring—cont'd

Treatment	Indications	Considerations
Intralesional cryotherapy	Hypertrophic scars Keloid scars	Scar regression through reduction of hyperproliferative response
Compression garments	Hypertrophic scars (primary indication) Keloid scars	Hypoxic and thermal effects in compressed areas reduce fibroblast activity Must be worn 8–24 h/day for first 6 months Must fit correctly
Antiproliferative agents (5-fluorouracil, bleomycin)	Hypertrophic scars Keloid scars	Induce scar regression 5-Fluorouracil more effective with hypertrophic Provide short-term suppression of small keloids Few small studies support use of bleomycin topically Side effects: pulmonary fibrosis, fever, rash, and hyperpigmentation
Intralesional injections of verapamil	Keloid scars	Inhibit inflammation Stimulate production of collagenase and other enzymes to degrade excess extracellular matrix Used for both prevention and treatment
Immunotherapy (immunomodulators, immunosuppressants, antibody therapy [e.g., imiquimod, tacrolimus, sirolimus, tumor necrosis factor-α, interferons, interleukins])	Keloid scars	Suppress fibroblast activity Promote fibroblast apoptosis Help reduce inflammation and regulate cellular activity Significant side effects depending on agent and dose
Suture ligature	Keloid scars	Deprives tissue of nutrients and oxygen, thus promoting tissue death Keloid must be amenable to suture ligature Requires weekly office visits and daily maintenance of local wounds

CDL, carbon dioxide laser; *PDL*, pulsed dye laser; *TGF*, transforming growth factor. Data from Al-Attar, A., Mess, S., Thomassen, J. M., et al. (2006). Keloid pathogenesis and treatment. *Plastic and Reconstructive Surgery, 117*, 286–300; Berman, B. (2007). A review of the biologic effects, clinical efficacy, and safety of silicone elastomer sheeting for hypertrophic and keloid scar treatment and management. *Dermatologic Surgery, 33*(11), 1291–1302; D'Andrea, F. (2002). Prevention and treatment of keloids with intralesional verapamil. *Dermatology, 204*(1), 60–62; Franz, M., Steed, D. L., & Robson, M. C. (2007). Optimizing healing of the acute wound by minimizing complications. *Current Problems in Surgery, 44*(11), 691–763; Funayama, E., Chodon, T., Oyama, A., et al. (2003). Keratinocytes promote proliferation and inhibit apoptosis of the underlying fibroblasts: An important role in the pathogenesis of keloid. *The Journal of Investigative Dermatology, 121*(6), 1326–1331; Gupta, S., & Kumar, B. (2001). Intralesional cryosurgery using lumbar puncture and/or hypodermic needles for large, bulky, recalcitrant keloids. *International Journal of Dermatology, 40*(5), 349–353; Har-Shai, Y. (2003). Intralesional cryotherapy for enhancing the involution of hypertrophic scars and keloids. *Plastic and Reconstructive Surgery, 111*(6), 1841–1852; Kieran, I., Knock, A., Bush, J., et al. (2013). Interleukin-10 reduces scar formation in both animal and cutaneous wounds: Results of two preclinical and phase II randomized controlled trials. *Wound Repair and Regeneration, 21*(3), 428–436; Parikh, D. (2008). Keloid banding using suture ligature: A novel technique and review of literature. *Laryngoscope, 118*(11), 1960–1965; Stashower, M. (2006). Successful treatment of earlobe keloids with imiquimod after tangential shave excision. *Dermatologic Surgery, 32*(3), 380–386; Syed, F., & Bayat, A. (2013). Superior effect of combination vs single steroid therapy in keloid disease: A comparative in vitro analysis of glucocorticoids. *Wound Repair and Regeneration, 21*(1), 88–102; Xia, W., Phan, T. T., Lim, I. J., et al. (2004). Complex epithelial-mesenchymal interactions modulate transforming growth factor-beta expression in keloid-derived cells. *Wound Repair and Regeneration, 12*(5), 546–556.

FACTORS AFFECTING THE REPAIR PROCESS

By observing a number of similar wounds and tracking their time to healing, it is possible to construct a curve that represents the healing "trajectory" for that type of wound. For example, epithelialization of a surgical wound healing by primary intention typically is complete by 48 h, although difficult to palpate; a healing ridge develops by days 5–9; and initial collagen deposition should be complete by postoperative day 21. Interestingly, it also is possible to plot a "healing trajectory" for neuropathic ulcers, venous ulcers, and pressure ulcers. As described in Chapter 6, studies indicate that the usual "time to healing" is similar for all patients with a particular type of wound (Steed, 2003). Multiple factors affect the time to healing for a specific wound; it is critical for the clinician to identify and correct factors that are known to delay healing. Factors that can delay the healing process and shift the trajectory to the right are outlined in Table 8.4.

TABLE 8.4 Factors Affecting Wound Healing

Factor	Effects on Repair Process	Clinical Implications
Perfusion/ oxygenation Hypoxia Adequate oxygen levels	Initiates new vessel development, promoting fibroblast proliferation Critical for cellular production of ATP, bacterial killing, collagen synthesis, development of tensile strength Critical oxygen levels ≥30–40 mm Hg (higher for bacterial killing)	Hypovolemia, hypotension, vasoconstriction, vascular impairment, edema, hypoxia all deleterious to repair Intervene to promote perfusion and oxygenation: warmth, hydration, pain control, management of edema, maintenance or restoration of blood flow Supplemental oxygen may be beneficial See Chapter 31
Excessive bioburden	Causes direct tissue damage and breakdown of growth factors; inhibits keratinocyte migration, collagen synthesis, and development of tensile strength Bacteria compete with fibroblasts for oxygen and nutrients, thus delaying repair Inflammatory response to high bacterial loads keeps wound "stuck" in inflammatory phase and prevents progression to proliferative phase of repair	Debride necrotic tissue to eliminate environment favorable to bacterial growth Monitor wound for signs and symptoms of invasive infection (cellulitis or osteomyelitis); treat any invasive infection with systemic antibiotics Monitor for signs of biofilm Mechanically debride biofilm Use appropriate antimicrobial after debridement to prevent regrowth of biofilm Chapter 18
Smoking/tobacco use	Byproducts (nicotine, carbon monoxide, hydrogen cyanide) reduce oxygenation, impair immune response, reduce fibroblast activity, increase platelet adhesion and thrombus formation Smoking associated with significantly higher infection rates	Counsel patients on negative effects of tobacco use Offer comprehensive program for smoking cessation: support groups, nicotine replacement, medications (No increase in wound infection with nicotine patch) See Chapter 31
Nutritional status	Adequate nutritional status critical for collagen synthesis, tensile strength, immune function Critical nutrients include micronutrients (vitamins, minerals), key amino acids (glutamine, L-arginine), adequate protein	Nutritional assessment and support are critical aspects of effective wound care program and must include attention to micronutrients and calorie and protein intake See Chapter 29
Diabetes mellitus	Associated with • Abnormal and prolonged inflammation • Reduced collagen synthesis • Decreased tensile strength • Impaired epithelial migration • Compromised vasculature • Hyperglycemia associated with compromised neutrophil function, impaired epithelial migration	Tight Glycemic control (glucose levels <150 mg/dL) associated with a reduced incidence of postoperative wound infections See Chapter 17
Obesity	Adipose tissue poorly vascularized Large volumes of adipose tissue put additional stress on incisional lines, increasing risk of dehiscence Associated with higher incidence of infection, seroma formation, wound dehiscence	Monitor intake to ensure adequate intake of protein and micronutrients and appropriate caloric intake Incisional support (binders) beneficial in reducing risk of dehiscence See Chapter 36
Medications	Chemotherapeutic agents impair production of white blood cells and fibroblasts, interfering with both inflammatory and proliferative phases of repair and increasing risk of infection Corticosteroids suppress inflammation and reduce proliferation of keratinocytes and fibroblasts, thereby impairing both granulation and epithelial resurfacing; impact is time and dose dependent, with impairment limited primarily to patients receiving steroids in doses >40 mg/day and for at least 30 days before wounding High doses of NSAIDs may impair healing	Delay chemotherapy when possible to permit healing (delay in healing most significant when chemotherapy given within first weeks following surgery/injury) Limited data suggest that topical vitamin A may partially reverse negative effects of corticosteroids (applied to clean wound bed before dressing application). Systemic administration is not recommended at present due to concerns that this could block the intended effects of the steroids Recommended dose range is 25,000–100,000 international units per day (note this recommendation based on limited and anecdotal data)

Continued

TABLE 8.4   Factors Affecting Wound Healing—cont'd

Factor	Effects on Repair Process	Clinical Implications
		For patient with impaired healing taking high-dose NSAIDs, collaborate with prescribing provider to reduce dose if possible Chapter 30
Advanced age	Diminished proliferation of cells critical to repair Hormonal changes Increased number of senescent cells iminished production of growth factors and possible reduction in receptor sites for growth factors Multiple existing comorbidities	Correct any reversible comorbidities Optimize nutritional status Provide evidence-based wound care
Immunosuppression	Increased susceptibility to infection Compromises body's ability to manifest signs of infection	Provide meticulous wound care to minimize risk of infection Monitor wound closely for muted signs of infection (faint erythema, mild increase in exudate, pain) and treat appropriately
Stress	Increased production of corticosteroids	Implement strategies to minimize stress: pain control, environmental management, patient education and counseling
Cellular senescence	Impairs healing due to reduced ability of cells involved in repair to replicate normally Associated with aging and with chronic wound environment, specifically high levels of ROS	Control bioburden and inflammation/levels of ROS to avoid damage to cellular DNA and "induced senescence"
Other	Malignancy Multisystem failure Failure to maintain clean, moist wound bed	Provide holistic wound management that addresses comorbidities Implement topical therapy to eliminate necrotic tissue and heavy bacterial loads Keep wound surface clean and moist

ATP, adenosine triphosphate; *NSAID*, nonsteroidal antiinflammatory drug; *ROS*, reactive oxygen species.Data from Anstead, G. (1998). Steroids, retinoids, and wound healing. *Advances in Wound Care, 11*, 277–285; Burns, J. L., Mancoll, J. S., & Phillips, L. G. (2003). Impairments to wound healing. *Clinics in Plastic Surgery, 30*, 47–56; Ehrlich, P., & Hunt, T. (1968). Effects of cortisone and vitamin A on wound healing. *Annals of Surgery, 167*(3), 324–328; Ehrlich, P., & Hunt, T. (1969). The effects of cortisone and anabolic steroids on the tensile strength of healing wounds. *Annals of Surgery, 170*(2), 203–206; Greenhalgh, D. G. (2003). Wound healing and diabetes mellitus. *Clinics in Plastic Surgery, 30*, 37–45; Hardman, M., & Ashcroft, G. (2008). Estrogen, not intrinsic aging, is the major regulator of delayed human wound healing in the elderly. *Genome Biology, 9*(5), R80; Howard, M., Asmi, R., Evans, K., et al. (2013). Oxygen and wound care: A review of current therapeutic modalities and future direction. *Wound Repair and Regeneration, 21*(4), 503–511; Manassa, E. H., Hertl, C. H., & Olbrisch, R. R. (2003). Wound healing problems in smokers and nonsmokers after 132 abdominoplasties. *Plastic and Reconstructive Surgery, 111*(6), 2082–2087; Pittman, J. (2007). Effect of aging on wound healing: Current concepts. *Journal of Wound, Ostomy, and Continence Nursing, 34*(4), 412–417; Sorensen, L. T., Karlsmark, T., & Gottrup, F. (2003). Abstinence from smoking reduces incisional wound infection: A randomized controlled trial. *Annals of Surgery, 238*(1), 1–5; Telgenhoff, D., & Shroot, B. (2005). Cellular senescence mechanisms in chronic wound healing. *Cell Death and Differentiation, 12*, 695–698; Wang, A., Armstrong, E., & Armstrong, A. (2013). Corticosteroids and wound healing: Clinical considerations in the perioperative period. *American Journal of Surgery, 206*(3), 410–417; Whitney, J. D. (2003). Supplemental perioperative oxygen and fluids to improve surgical wound outcomes: Translating evidence into practice. *Wound Repair and Regeneration, 11*(6), 462–467; Wicke, C., Bachinger, A., Coerper, S., et al. (2009). Aging influences wound healing in patients with chronic lower extremity wounds treated in a specialized wound care center. *Wound Repair and Regeneration, 17*(1), 25–33; Wientjes, K. A. (2002). Mind-body techniques in wound healing. *Ostomy/Wound Management, 48*(11), 62–67; Williams, J. Z., Barbul, A. (2003). Nutrition and wound healing. *The Surgical Clinics of North America, 83*, 571–596; Wilson, J. A., & Clark, J. J. (2003). Obesity: Impediment to wound healing. *Critical Care Nursing Quarterly, 26*(2), 119–132.

CLINICAL CONSULT

A: Referral received to assess for interventions to promote wound healing. Patient is 62-year-old African American female who underwent abdominal hysterectomy and bilateral salpingo-oophorectomy 10 days ago for endometrial cancer and now has dehisced surgical incision. She was discharged form hospital 3 days postop and lives at home with her husband; daughter has been active in helping her at home. Medical history includes type 2 diabetes mellitus (last HbA1c 8.2), obesity (height 5′5″; weight 250 lbs), gastroesophageal reflux disease (GERD), cigarette smoking (one pack per day for 42 years; stopped smoking 3 months ago), hypertension, and chronic obstructive lung disease. Upon assessment, patient is alert, oriented × 3, and very engaged in optimizing her healing potential. She is coughing at intervals and states that she has moderately severe pain with coughing. Dehisced incisional wound measures 12 cm (L) × 6 cm (W) × 3 cm (D). The wound base is

CLINICAL CONSULT—cont'd

60% red and smooth; 40% of the wound bed is covered with mixed yellow-tan adherent nonviable tissue. There is a moderate amount of serosanguineous drainage. The periwound skin is intact with mild erythema extending 2 cm from wound edge and slight induration. Currently on day 3 of antibiotic therapy for a surgical site infection (SSI). Daughter is helping with wound care and they recently began NPWT with instillation.

D: Dehisced abdominal incision in inflammatory phase of repair. Mild erythema and slight induration indicative of resolving surgical site infection. Obesity, diabetes, and lung disease contributed to risk for SSI.

P: Optimize systemic factors to enhance wound repair; provide external support to reduce strain on wound with decreased tensile strength.

I: (1) Nutritional consult to ensure macronutrients and micronutrients sufficient for repair (e.g., protein, vitamin C, zinc, and magnesium). (2) Consult with provider to monitor blood sugars with goal of <180. (3) Abdominal binder to support incision since patient is obese and is coughing. (4) Instruct patient on characteristics of healthy granulating wound bed, transition from nonviable tissue to granulation tissue, anticipated decrease in wound exudate. (5) Provide encouragement to continue nonsmoking; offer additional smoking cessation tools as needed. (6) Check pO_2 and provide supplemental oxygen to maintain >95% particularly with exercise.

E: Will follow to evaluate/monitor effectiveness and will adapt plan as indicated.

SUMMARY

- Wound healing is a complex series of events.
- Normally wound healing is
  - initiated by an injury that leads to clot formation and platelet degranulation
  - controlled by a myriad of cytokines and growth factors
  - is affected significantly by systemic factors such as perfusion, nutritional status, and steroid levels.

- Effective management of any wound requires an understanding of the normal repair process and the factors that may interfere with normal repair. This understanding provides the foundation for comprehensive assessment of the wound and of the patient and for selection of interventions designed to optimize healing.

SELF-ASSESSMENT QUESTIONS

1. Which of the following cells are responsible for collagen synthesis?
   a. Neutrophils
   b. Fibroblasts
   c. Platelets
   d. Macrophages

2. The process of contraction is important to achieve closure in the wound healing of which of the following?
   a. Superficial abrasions
   b. Partial-thickness wounds
   c. Full-thickness wounds
   d. Primarily closed wounds

3. Which of the following explains why obesity is a risk factor for poor healing?
   a. Obesity is associated with diabetes

   b. Adipose tissue if less vascular than lean tissue.
   c. Obesity is associated with hypertension.
   d. The obese patient has low levels of neutrophils.

4. Which of the following statements about wound-healing differences between patients with light and dark pigmented skin is TRUE?
   a. Lighter skin has a higher prevalence of keloid formation.
   b. Darker skin has a slower response to recruitment of inflammatory cells to the wound site.
   c. Repigmentation of full-thickness wounds in people with darker skin occurs is delayed.
   d. Lighter skin has high levels of proteases present.

REFERENCES

Ashcroft, G. S., Mills, S. J., & Ashworth, J. J. (2002). Aging and wound healing. *Biogerontology*, 3(6), 337–345.

Atiyeh, B. (2005). Keloid or hypertrophic scar: The controversy. Review of the literature. *Annals of Plastic Surgery*, 54(6), 676–680.

Berg Vande, J. S., & Robson, M. C. (2003). Arresting cell cycles and the effect on wound healing. *The Surgical Clinics of North America*, 83, 509–520.

Bohn, G. A. (2020a). Using ovine extracellular matrix in difficult to close excisions of common skin Cancer: An evolving new technique. *Surgical Technology International*, 28(37), 49–53 (PMID: 33276415).

Bohn, G. A. (2020b). Complex problem, simple solution: Using Endoform to provide a functional extracellular matrix in chronic wounds. *Ostomy/Wound Management*, 65(10), 8–10.

Bohn, G., Liden, B., Schultz, G., Yang, Q., & Gibson, D. J. (2016). Ovine-based collagen matrix dressing: Next-generation collagen dressing for wound care. *Advances in Wound Care (New*

Rochelle)., 5(1), 1–10. https://doi.org/10.1089/wound.2015.0660. PMID: 26858910; PMCID: PMC4717509.

Braiman-Wiksman, L., Solomonik, I., Spira, R., et al. (2007). Novel insights into wound healing sequence of events. *Toxicologic Pathology, 35*, 767–779.

Brissett, A. E., & Hom, D. B. (2003). The effects of tissue sealants, platelet gels, and growth factors on wound healing. *Current Opinion in Otolaryngology & Head and Neck Surgery, 11*(4), 245–250.

Bullard, K. M., Longaker, M. T., & Lorenz, H. P. (2002). Fetal wound healing: Current biology. *World Journal of Surgery, 27*, 54–61.

Burns, J. L., Mancoll, J. S., & Phillips, L. G. (2003). Impairments to wound healing. *Clinics in Plastic Surgery, 30*, 47–56.

Calvin, M. (1998). Cutaneous wound repair. *Wounds, 10*(1), 12–32.

Chen, W. Y. J., & Abatangelo, G. (1999). Functions of hyaluronan in wound repair. *Wound Repair and Regeneration, 7*, 79–89.

Cheresh, D., & Stupack, D. (2008). Regulation of angiogenesis: Apoptotic cues from the ECM. *Oncogene, 27*, 6285–6298.

Cross, K. J., & Mustoe, T. A. (2003). Growth factors in wound healing. *The Surgical Clinics of North America, 83*, 531–545.

Dang, C., Ting, K., Soo, C., et al. (2003). Fetal wound healing: Current perspectives. *Clinics in Plastic Surgery, 30*, 13–23.

Demidova-Rice, T., Hamblin, M., & Herman, I. (2012). Acute and impaired wound healing: Pathophysiology and current methods for drug delivery, part 1: Normal and chronic wounds: Biology, causes, and approaches to care. *Advances in Skin & Wound Care, 25*(7), 304–314.

Dempsey, S. G., Miller, C. H., Schueler, J., et al. (2020). A novel chemotactic factor derived from the extracellular matrix protein decorin recruits mesenchymal stromal cells in vitro and in vivo. *PLoS One, 15*(7), e0235784.

Dubay, K. A., & Franz, M. G. (2003). Acute wound healing: The biology of acute wound failure. *The Surgical Clinics of North America, 83*, 463–481.

Frank, S., Kämpfer, H., Wetzler, C., et al. (2002). Nitric oxide drives skin repair: Novel functions of an established mediator. *Kidney International, 61*, 882–888.

Gabbiani, G. (2003). The myofibroblast in wound healing and fibrocontractive diseases. *The Journal of Pathology, 200*, 500–503.

Gabriel A., Mussman J., Rosenberg L.Z., et al (2018). Wound healing, growth factors. *Medscape* Retrieved 1/16/2021 from: https://emedicine.medscape.com/article/1298196-overview.

Gill, S., & Parks, W. (2008). Metalloproteinases and their inhibitors: Regulators of wound healing. *The International Journal of Biochemistry & Cell Biology, 40*, 1334–1347.

Goldman, R. (2004). Growth factors and chronic wound healing: Past, present, and future. *Advances in Skin & Wound Care, 17*(1), 24–35.

Hahn, J., Glaser, K., McFarland, K., et al. (2013). Keloid derived keratinocytes exhibit an abnormal gene expression profile consistent with a distinct causal mechanism in keloid pathology. *Wound Repair and Regeneration, 21*(4), 530–544.

Hamed, S., Bennett, C., Demiot, C., et al. (2014). Erythropoietin, a novel repurposed drug: An innovative treatment for wound healing in patients with diabetes mellitus. *Wound Repair and Regeneration, 22*(1), 23–33.

Harrison C., Heaton M.J., Layton C.M. and Neil SM: et al (2006). Use of an in vitro model of tissue-engineered human skin to study keratinocyte attachment and migration in the process of reepithelialization, *Wound Repair and Regeneration* 14:203–209.

Henry, G., & Garner, W. L. (2003). Inflammatory mediators in wound healing. *The Surgical Clinics of North America, 83*, 483–507.

Hoenig M., Bianchi C., Rosenzweig A., and Sellke FW: et al (2008). Decreased vascular repair and neovascularization with ageing: Mechanisms and clinical relevance with an emphasis on hypoxia-inducible factor, *Current Molecular Medicine* 8(8):754–767.

Hunt T.K., Van Winkle W. Jr (1997). Normal repair. In Hunt T.K., Dunphy J.E., editors: *Fundamentals of wound management*, New York, Appleton-Century-Crofts.

Jahoda, C. A. B., & Reynolds, A. J. (2001). Hair follicle dermal sheath cells: Unsung participants in wound healing. *Lancet, 358*(9291), 1445–1448.

James, T. J., Hughes, M. A., Cherry, G. W., et al. (2000). Simple biochemical markers to assess chronic wounds. *Wound Repair and Regeneration, 8*, 264–269.

Kieran, I., Knock, A., Bush, J., et al. (2013). Interleukin-10 reduces scar formation in both animal and cutaneous wounds: Results of two preclinical and phase II randomized controlled trials. *Wound Repair and Regeneration, 21*(3), 428–436.

Lan, C. C., Liu, I. H., Fang, A. H., et al. (2008). Hyperglycaemic conditions decrease cultured keratinocyte mobility: Implications for impaired wound healing in patients with diabetes. *The British Journal of Dermatology, 159*, 1103–1115.

Lizarbe, T., García-Rama, C., Tarín, C., et al. (2008). Nitric oxide elicits functional MMP-13 protein-tyrosine nitration during wound repair. *The FASEB Journal, 22*, 3207–3215.

Loryman, C., & Mansbridge, J. (2008). Inhibition of keratinocyte migration by lipopolysaccharide. *Wound Repair and Regeneration, 16*, 45–51.

Macri, L., & Clark, R. (2009). Tissue engineering for cutaneous wounds: Selecting the proper time and space for growth factors, cells, and extracellular matrix. *Skin Pharmacology and Physiology, 22*(2), 83–93.

Mancuso, C., et al. (2018). Utilization of ovine collagen extracellular matrix in surgical excision of recurrent keloids. *Journal of the American Osteopathic College of Dermatology, 41*, 53–54.

Mangram, A. J., Horan, T. C., Pearson, M. L., et al. (1999). Guideline for prevention of surgical site infection. *Infection Control and Hospital Epidemiology, 20*(1), 250–278.

Martin, P. (1997). Wound healing: Aiming for perfect skin regeneration. *Science, 276*, 75–81.

Mast, B. A., & Schultz, G. (1996). Interactions of cytokines, growth factors, and proteases in acute and chronic wounds. *Wound Repair and Regeneration, 4*, 411–420.

Monaco, J. L., & Lawrence, W. T. (2003). Acute wound healing: An overview. *Clinics in Plastic Surgery, 30*, 1–12.

Myers, S., Leigh, I. M., & Navsaria, H. (2007). Epidermal repair results from activation of follicular and epidermal progenitor keratinocytes mediated by a growth factor cascade. *Wound Repair and Regeneration, 15*, 693–701.

Nataraj, C., Ritter, G., Dumas, S., et al. (2007). Extracellular wound matrices: Novel stabilization and sterilization method for collagen-based biologic wound dressings. *Wounds, 19*(6), 148–156.

Ogawa, R., Okai, K., Tokumura, F., et al. (2012). The relationship between skin stretching/contraction and pathologic scarring: The important role of mechanical forces in keloid generation. *Wound Repair and Regeneration, 20*(2), 149–157.

O'Goshi, K.-I., & Tagami, H. (2007). Basic fibroblast growth factor treatment for various types of recalcitrant skin ulcers: Reports of nine cases. *Journal of Dermatological Treatment, 18*, 375–381.

O'Toole, E., van Koningsveld, R., Chen, M., et al. (2008). Hypoxia induces epidermal keratinocyte matrix metalloproteinase-9 secretion via the protein kinase C pathway. *Journal of Cellular Physiology, 214,* 47–55.

Phillips, S. J. (2000). Physiology of wound healing and surgical wound care. *ASAIO Journal, 46*(6), S2–S5.

Pittman, J. (2007). Effect of aging on wound healing: Current concepts. *Journal of Wound, Ostomy, and Continence Nursing, 34*(4), 412–417.

Pradhan, L., Nabzdyk, C., Andersen, N. D., et al. (2009). Inflammation and neuropeptides: The connection in diabetic wound healing. *Expert Reviews in Molecular Medicine, 11,* e2.

Pullar, C., Manabat-Hidalgo, C. G., Bolaji, R. S., et al. (2008). β-Adrenergic receptor modulation of repair. *Pharmacological Research, 58*(2), 158–164.

Rahban, S. R., & Garner, W. L. (2003). Fibroproliferative scars. *Clinics in Plastic Surgery, 30,* 77–89.

Richards, A. M., Mitsou, J., Floyd, D. C., et al. (1997). Neural innervation and healing. *Lancet, 350*(9074), 339–340.

Robson, M. C. (2003). Proliferative scarring. *Surgical Clinics of North America, 33,* 557–569.

Rodriguez, P., Felix, F. N., Woodley, D. T., et al. (2008). The role of oxygen in wound healing: A review of the literature. *Dermatologic Surgery, 34,* 1159–1169.

Samuels, P., & Tan, A. K. W. (1999). Fetal scarless wound healing. *The Journal of Otolaryngology, 28*(5), 296–302.

Schneider, A., Garlick, A. J., & Egles, C. (2008). Self-assembling peptide nanofiber scaffolds accelerate wound healing. *PLoS One, 3*(1), e1410.

Schultz, G. S., Sibbald, R. G., Falanga, V., et al. (2003). Wound bed preparation: A systematic approach to wound management. *Wound Repair and Regeneration, 11*(Suppl. 1), S1–S28.

Schultz, G., & Wysocki, A. (2009). Interactions between extracellular matrix and growth factors in wound healing. *Wound Repair and Regeneration, 17*(2), 153–162.

Slemp, A., & Kirschner, R. (2006). Keloids and scars: A review of keloids and scars, their pathogenesis, risk factors, and management. *Current Opinion in Pediatrics, 18*(4), 396–402.

Steed, D. L. (2003). Wound-healing trajectories. *The Surgical Clinics of North America, 83,* 547–555.

Syed, F., & Bayat, A. (2013). Superior effect of combination vs single steroid therapy in keloid disease: A comparative in vitro analysis of glucocorticoids. *Wound Repair and Regeneration, 21*(1), 88–102.

Telgenhoff, D., & Shroot, B. (2005). Cellular senescence mechanisms in chronic wound healing. *Cell Death and Differentiation, 12,* 695–698.

Thom, S. (2009). Oxidative stress is fundamental to hyperbaric oxygen therapy. *Journal of Applied Physiology, 106,* 988–995.

Walraven, M., Gouverneur, M., Middelkoop, E., et al. (2014). Altered TGF-β signaling in fetal fibroblasts: What is known about the underlying mechanism? *Wound Repair and Regeneration, 22*(1), 3–13.

Wang, Z., & Shi, C. (2020). Cellular senescence is a promising target for chronic wounds: A comprehensive review. *Burns & Trauma.* https://doi.org/10.1093/burnst/tkaa021.

Wilgus, T. (2007). Regenerative healing in fetal skin: A review of the literature. *Ostomy/Wound Management, 53*(6), 16–31.

Winter, G. (1979). Epidermal regeneration studied in the domestic pig. In T. Hunt, & J. Dunphy (Eds.), *Fundamentals of wound management.* New York: Appleton-Century-Crofts.

Witte, M., & Barbul, A. (1997). General principles of wound healing. *The Surgical Clinics of North America, 77*(3), 509–528.

Yamamoto, N., & Kiyosawa, T. (2014). Histological effects of occlusive dressings on healing of incisional skin wounds. *International Wound Journal, 11*(6), 616–621.

Yang, G. P., Lim, I. J., Phan, T. T., et al. (2003). From scarless fetal wounds to keloids: Molecular studies in wound healing. *Wound Repair and Regeneration, 11*(6), 411–418.

FURTHER READING

Barendse-Hofmann, M. G., Steenvoorde, P., van Doorn, L., et al. (2007). Extracellular wound matrix (OASIS): Exploring the contraindications and results of 32 consecutive outpatient clinic cases. *Wounds, 19*(10), 258–263.

9

Skin Damage: Types and Treatment

Ruth A. Bryant

OBJECTIVES

1. Describe the process of at least five factors that contribute to skin damage.
2. Distinguish among the following terms: macule, papule, plaque, nodule, wheal, pustule, vesicle, and bulla.
3. Describe the extent of tissue damage and skin manifestations associated with the following four types of skin injury: mechanical trauma, moisture-associated skin damage (MASD), medical adhesive-related skin injury (MARSI), and skin irradiation.
4. Discuss at least three interventions for the prevention and treatment of each type of mechanical trauma, MASD, MARSI, candidiasis, and radiation skin damage.
5. Distinguish between an irritant contact dermatitis and an allergic contact dermatitis.
6. Identify factors that predispose a patient to candidiasis.
7. Describe the types of lesions and distribution common to candidiasis, folliculitis, impetigo, and herpes.
8. Discriminate among incontinence-associated dermatitis (IAD), candidiasis intertrigo, Stage 1 or Stage 2 pressure injury, suspected deep tissue injury (sDTI), perianal herpes, tinea cruris, and inverse psoriasis.

Skin integrity can be jeopardized or compromised by a multitude of factors: mechanical, moisture, chemical, vascular, infectious, allergy, inflammatory, intrinsic disease, burn, radiation, and miscellaneous assaults. Each type of injury creates a complex set of skin responses, such as erythema, macules, papules, pustules, vesicles/bullae, erosion, and ulcers. Primary lesions of the skin are the first recognizable lesions in the skin. Plate 6 shows the definition and appearance of common primary lesions. Secondary skin lesions evolve from primary lesions due to the natural history of the disease or as a result of scratching/infection. Common secondary lesions are depicted and defined in Plate 7. Because periwound skin can develop skin complications and because many of these conditions provide clues to the etiology of the skin alteration, the health care provider for patients in acute care, home care, outpatient, and long-term care facilities must be familiar with these terms.

ASSESSMENT

A systematic skin assessment and an accurate description of any lesions are essential to obtain a reasonable list of differential diagnoses. Additional assessments and diagnostic tests then can be used to derive the most likely diagnosis. Lesions should be described by five morphologic parameters: distribution, shape or arrangement, border and margins, associated changes within the lesion(s), and pigmentation. These parameters, including options for descriptive terminology, are listed in Table 9.1.

Before a treatment plan for any skin lesion or wound can be initiated, the underlying cause of that condition must be determined. Clues to the underlying cause are derived from the patient's history and physical assessment and specifically by an assessment of the following parameters: location, characteristics, and distribution. These clues can be used to direct subsequent tests that may be necessary to develop a definitive diagnosis. Once the cause of the wound or skin lesion is identified, realistic goals for care can be established and a comprehensive, interdisciplinary treatment plan devised. This chapter introduces a classification system for types of skin damage, briefly describes the pathophysiologic process, and discusses the prevention and treatment of the most common types of skin damage (Box 9.1). The more uncommon skin lesions, particularly those associated with intrinsic disease, are addressed in Chapter 32.

MECHANICAL FORCES

The forces that are applied externally to the skin, such as pressure, shear, friction, and skin stripping (skin tears), create mechanical skin damage. Each may occur in isolation or in combination with other mechanical insults, such as pressure and shear. This chapter presents shear, friction, and skin stripping. Pressure damage and preventive interventions are discussed in Chapter 11.

TABLE 9.1 Morphologic Characteristics of Skin Lesions

Characteristic	Description	Examples
Distribution		
Localized	Lesion appears in one small area	Impetigo, herpes simplex (e.g., labialis), tinea corporis ("ringworm")
Regional	Lesions involve a specific region of the body	Acne vulgaris (pilosebaceous gland distribution), herpes zoster (nerve dermatomal distribution), psoriasis (flexural surfaces and skin folds)
Generalized	Lesions appear widely distributed or in numerous areas simultaneously	Urticaria, disseminated drug eruptions
Shape/Arrangement		
Round/discoid	Coin or fine shaped (no central clearing)	Nummular eczema
Oval	Ovoid shape	Pityriasis rosea
Annular	Round, active margins with central clearing	Tinea corporis, sarcoidosis
Zosteriform (dermatomal)	Following a nerve or segment of the body	Herpes zoster
Polycyclic	Interlocking or coalesced circles (formed by enlargement of annular lesions)	Psoriasis, urticaria
Linear	In a line	Contact dermatitis
Iris/target lesion	Pink macules with purple central papules	Erythema multiforme
Stellate	Star shaped	Meningococcal septicemia
Serpiginous	Snake-like or wavy line track	Cutanea larva migrans
Reticulate	Net like or lacy	Polyarteritis nodosa, lichen planus lesions of erythema infectiosum
Morbilliform	Measles like: maculopapular lesions that become confluent on the face and body	Measles, roseola
Border/Margin		
Discrete	Well demarcated or defined, able to draw a line around it with confidence	Psoriasis
Indistinct	Poorly defined, have borders that merge into normal skin or outlying ill-defined papules	Nummular eczema
Active	Margin of lesion shows greater activity than center	*Tinea* spp. eruptions
Irregular	Nonsmooth or notched margin	Malignant melanoma
Border raised above center	Center of lesion is depressed compared with the edge	Basal cell carcinoma
Advancing	Expanding at margins	Cellulitis
Associated Changes Within Lesions		
Central clearing	An erythematous border surrounds lighter skin	Tinea eruptions
Desquamation	Peeling or sloughing of skin	Rash of toxic shock syndrome
Keratotic	Hypertrophic stratum corneum	Calluses, warts
Punctation	Central umbilication or dimpling	Basal cell carcinoma
Telangiectasias	Dilated blood vessels within lesion blanch completely, may be markers of systematic disease	Basal cell carcinoma, actinic keratosis
Pigmentation		
Flesh	Same tone as the surrounding skin	Neurofibroma, some nevi
Pink	Light red undertones	Eczema, pityriasis rosea
Erythematous	Dark pink to red	Tinea eruptions, psoriasis
Salmon	Orange-pink	Psoriasis
Tan-brown	Light to dark brown	Most nevi, pityriasis versicolor
Black	Black or blue-black	Malignant melanoma
Pearly	Shiny white, almost iridescent	Basal cell carcinoma
Purple	Dark red-blue-violet	Purpura, Kaposi sarcoma
Violaceous	Light violet	Erysipelas
Yellow	Waxy	Lipoma
White	Absent of color	Lichen planus

From Ball, W., Dains, J. E., Flynn, J. A., Solomon, B. S., & Stewart, R. W. (2019). *Seidel's guide to physical examination. An interprofessional approach* (9th ed.). St. Louis: Elsevier.

BOX 9.1   Classification of Skin Damage Based on Source and Irritant*

Mechanical
Pressure
Shear
Friction
Skin stripping
- Skin tears
- Medical adhesives

Moisture
Moisture-donating wound dressing
  Urinary incontinence
  Perspiration
  Medical adhesives

Chemical
Feces
Gastrointestinal contents
Drainage from percutaneous tubes
Povidone-iodine complex (Betadine)
Alkaline soaps
Alcohol

Vascular/Neuropathic
Venous
Arterial
Neuropathic

Infectious
Fungal
Candidiasis
Dermatophyte (tinea)

Bacterial
Cellulitis
Erysipelas
Erythrasma
Folliculitis
Impetigo
Bullous impetigo
Nonbullous impetigo

Viral
Herpes simplex
Varicella-zoster virus

Allergic
Medical adhesive

Radiation

*See Chapter 32 for atypical types of skin damage.

Shear

Shear is a mechanical load to the skin that is applied parallel to the skin surface. Shear injury is caused by tissue layers sliding against each other and results in disruption, stretching, or angulation of cells and blood vessels. Shear force can be created by the sliding or stretching of the top superficial skin layers over a support surface and/or the sliding movement of subcutaneous soft tissue over muscle layers as well as the sliding movement of the muscle layers over a bony prominence while the underlying muscle and bone are stationary (Gefen, 2007). Skin damage is created by the interaction of tangential shear forces on the internal tissue and frictional forces (resistance) against the surface of the skin. Thus, friction is always present when shear force is present. Shear occurs when transferring a patient laterally onto the operating room table or onto a stretcher. The classic example of a shear injury occurs when the patient is in a semi-Fowler position. Because of the pull of gravity, anytime the head is higher than the foot, even when the head of bed is elevated as little as 30 degrees, shear can still occur (Gefen, Farid, & Shaywitz, 2013) (Fig. 9.1). Ultimately, the skin is held in place while the skeletal structures pull the body (by gravity) toward the foot of the bed. Consequently, blood vessels in the area are stretched and angulated, the vasculature is disrupted, and small-vessel thrombosis and tissue death may develop.

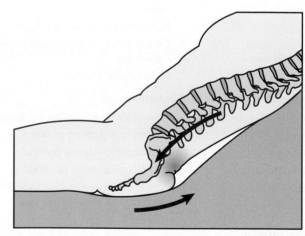

Fig. 9.1 Shearing force. (Adapted from Loeper, J. M. (1986). *Therapeutic positioning and skin care*. Minneapolis: Sister Kenny Institute.)

Shear may cause shallow or deep ulcerations and extends the tissue damage of pressure injuries. This extension is manifested in the pressure injury by the presence of undermining (dissection or separation of tissue parallel to the skin surface; see Figs. 9.1, 10.5). Shear injury is predominantly localized at the sacrum or coccyx and is commonly a consequence of elevating the head of the bed or improper transfer technique. However, it may also occur in other locations such as under contact casts. Prevention requires an awareness of those situations in which the skin is subjected to shear. For example, the patient with pulmonary distress requires the head of the bed to be elevated to facilitate adequate ventilation; however, the patient is at great risk for shear injury. Likewise, the patient with a cerebrovascular accident may experience shear injury when being transferred from the bed to the wheelchair. In the operating room, shear may be present with lateral transfers of the patient from the stretcher to the operating table (Association of periOperative Registered Nurses [AORN], 2021).

Most strategies for prevention of shear have derived from expert opinion and have been incorporated into safe patient handling guidelines by the Centers for Disease Control and Prevention (CDC), American Nurses Association, and National Institute for Occupational Safety and Health (Centers for Disease Control and Prevention, 2014; Waters & Rockefeller, 2010; Waters, Short, Lloyd, et al., 2011). Because shear is an important contributing factor to pressure injuries, strategies to simultaneously prevent shear and pressure are warranted (see Chapter 11). The primary intervention for reducing shear is the use of lifts when repositioning the patient; this eliminates drag on the sacral skin. The head of the bed should be maintained at less than 30 degrees; elevations higher than 30 degrees may be needed for meals but should be limited to short periods of time. Also, the knee gatch can be used to interrupt gravity's pull on the body toward the foot of the bed. Many support surfaces have a slick fabric covering, which anecdotally and intuitively seems to reduce shear. A standardized method to objectively measure the ability of a support surface to reduce shear is not currently available.

Friction

The National Pressure Injury Advisory Panel defines friction as the resistance to motion in a parallel direction relative to the common boundary between two surfaces (National Pressure Ulcer Advisory Panel [NPUAP], 2018). Skin injury by friction initially appears as erythema and progresses to an abrasion. As stated previously, shear is created by the interaction of tangential forces and friction (resistance) against the surface of the skin. Friction is frequently seen on elbows or heels because the patient easily abrades these surfaces against sheets when repositioning. Injury is characteristically very shallow and limited to the epidermis. Friction primarily affects superficial layers and thus does not result in tissue necrosis, whereas shear forces commonly affect deeper tissue layers (Wound, Ostomy and Continence Nurses Society™ [WOCN], 2016).

Interventions to prevent friction and superficial shear involve the use of protective padding over the elbows or heels and moisturizers applied to vulnerable areas to maintain proper hydration of the epidermis. Both maneuvers decrease friction and thereby decrease shear. Transparent adhesive dressings, thin hydrocolloids, low-adhesion foam dressings, and liquid skin protectants are effective at reducing friction. Adhesive dressings are contraindicated if the shear is sufficient to loosen the dressing. Braces, splints, prosthetic devices,

and shoes should be assessed frequently for evidence of shear, and modifications (e.g., reshaping, molding, and extra padding) implemented as needed.

Skin Stripping

Skin stripping is the inadvertent removal of the epidermis, with or without the dermis, by mechanical means. The International Skin Tear Advisory Panel (ISTAP) defines a skin tear as "a traumatic wound caused by mechanical forces (such as shear or friction), including removal of adhesives. Severity may vary by depth (not extending through the subcutaneous layer)" (LeBlanc et al., 2018). A skin tear results from a separation in skin layers and can create a partial- or full-thickness wound (LeBlanc, Baranoski, Christensen, et al., 2013). For most patients, skin tears do not extend hospital stay, but they are painful and distressing in appearance and can be interpreted as being the result of poor care (Ratliff & Fletcher, 2007). In the neonate or premature infant, however, skin tears are a significant portal of entry that can lead to septicemia (Irving, Bethell, & Burtin, 2006). Unique considerations concerning skin tears in the neonate or premature infant are addressed in Chapter 37. Uncomplicated skin tears (i.e., those that are not on the lower extremities or in patients with multiple coexisting conditions) are reported to heal within approximately 4 weeks (LeBlanc et al., 2018).

The ISTAP classification system for skin tears is a simple classification tool developed through consensus by LeBlanc et al. (2013) (Table 9.2). Type I skin tears are distinguished by a resulting skin flap or avulsed skin that can cover the exposed wound (see Plate 8). Type II skin tears (see Plates 9–11) are distinguished by partial flap loss that cannot be repositioned to cover the wound bed. Type III skin tears (see Plate 12) are defined by total flap loss. The frequency of various locations of skin-stripping injuries is more common on the upper extremities (73%–80%) first then legs and feet (20%), head (3%–4%), and torso (3%) (Malone Rozario, Gavinski, et al., 1991; McGough-Csarny & Kopac, 1998; Payne & Martin, 1990). The most frequent site of injury on the upper extremity is the forearm, followed by the arm, hand, and lower extremities (PA Patient Safety Authority, 2006).

Risk factors for a skin tear include advanced age, impaired mobility, sensory loss, dehydration and malnutrition, history

TABLE 9.2 Skin Tears: ISTAP Skin Tear Classification System	
Type	**Description**
I: No skin loss	Linear or flap tear that can be repositioned to cover the wound bed (see Plate 8)
II: Partial flap loss	Partial flap loss that cannot be repositioned to cover the wound bed (see Plates 9–11)
III: Total flap	Total flap loss exposing entire wound bed (see Plate 12)

LeBlanc et al. (2013).

of previous skin tears, cognitive impairment, dependency, poor locomotion, and presence of ecchymosis (LeBlanc et al., 2018; Strazzieri-Pulido, Peres, Campanilli, & Santos, 2017). Skin tears have been reported to be associated with blunt trauma, a fall, performing activities of daily living, getting dressed, performing treatments, patient transfers, and the presence of equipment (e.g., side rails, wheelchair); however, as many as 50% of skin tears may not have an apparent cause identified (LeBlanc et al., 2013).

Elderly skin and immature skin both are vulnerable to skin tears because the dermal–epidermal junction is not optimally functional. The interlocking dermal papillae and epidermal rete pegs at the dermal–epidermal junction are critical to providing resiliency and the ability to withstand mechanical forces. In the premature infant's skin, the dermal–epidermal junction is undeveloped and weak. As the skin ages, the epidermis thins, the dermal–epidermal junction flattens, and cohesion is diminished. In addition, the amounts of collagen and elastin present in the aging skin decrease so that the skin becomes wrinkled, thin, and less compliant. Furthermore, similar connective tissue changes around blood vessels increase the fragility of capillaries. Therefore, mechanical stresses can trigger a subcutaneous hemorrhage (e.g., senile purpura) between the skin layers, which results in further separation of the dermis and epidermis. Disease management regimens also can alter the skin's vitality. For example, corticosteroids reduce tissue collagen strength and elasticity and thereby increase the patient's risk of skin tears. Long-term consequences of radiation therapy are epidermal atrophy, microvascular occlusions, reduced fibroblast proliferation, and tissue fibrosis.

Skin tears cannot be prevented by one individual. Because the typical individual at risk for skin tears is dependent on caregivers for many aspects of care, preventive interventions must be embraced by all staff members. Therefore, staff education is a critical component of a skin tear prevention and treatment program (LeBlanc et al., 2018).

A standardized care plan for patients at high risk for skin tears consists of strategies that address risk factors pertinent to the skin, mobility, and general health (Box 9.2) (LeBlanc et al., 2018). Recognizing "at-risk" individuals and implementing key preventive strategies has been shown to decrease the incidence of skin tears. Extreme care and a gentle touch are critical when touching the patient or performing patient care because most skin tears occur during the course of providing routine patient care activities (e.g., bathing, dressing, and transferring). Because harsh soaps and frequent bathing can reduce the skin's natural lubrication and lead to dry skin, gentle skin cleansers and frequent moisturizing are important components of skin tear prevention (LeBlanc et al., 2018). It may be necessary to decrease bathing schedules and use humidifiers to increase environmental moisture (LeBlanc & Baranoski, 2009; LeBlanc, Christensen, Orstead, et al., 2008). Rooms should be adequately lit to reduce the risk of bumping into furniture and equipment. Beyond these measures, the current focus of prevention is on the application of products and garments that serve as barriers between the skin and potential trauma; such products include commercially available skin sleeves, roll gauze, pants, and long-sleeve shirts (Bank & Nix, 2006).

If adhesives must be used, liquid skin protectants can be placed on the skin before the tape is applied to provide

---

BOX 9.2 Standardized Care Plan for Patients at High Risk for Skin Tears

1. Provide a safe environment.
   - Free room of obstacles that obstruct pathway around bed and bathroom.
   - Provide adequate lighting in resident's room.
   - Leave on nightlight in bathroom and leave door open.
   - Leave side rails down at night.
   - Make hourly rounds.
   - Provide safe area for wandering.
   - Implement bed alarm.
   - Provide well-fitting supportive shoes with skid-free soles.
   - Use protective garments for arms, legs, areas of purpura (e.g., fleece-lined jogging suits, knee-length athletic socks, stockinette doubled, skin sleeves).
   - Pad rough edges of furniture.
   - Relocate or loosen ID band when determined to be cause of skin tears.
2. Maintain nutrition, hydration, and skin health.
   - Optimize nutrition and hydration.
   - Obtain dietary consult.
   - Offer fluids between meals twice every shift.
   - Encourage fluids at every meal.
   - Inspect and moisturize arms and legs twice daily.
   - Use emollient to rehydrate skin.
   - Implement skin-friendly cleanser and warm water
   - Be aware of increased risk due to extremes of age.
   - Be aware of medications that may directly affect skin (i.e., topical and systematic steroids).
3. Protect from self-inflicted injury or injury incurred during routine cares.
   - Keep nails clipped.
   - Use wheelchair for transport only.
   - Use sling around chair legs to prevent feet from falling off footrests.
   - Use padding for equipment and furniture to protect skin.
   - Use palm of hands and lift sheet instead of fingers to position patient.
   - Use mechanical lift for transfers.
   - Obtain occupational or physical therapy consultation if needed for safe positioning.
   - Avoid adhesives when possible.
   - Use appropriate methods to avoid medical adhesive-related skin injury (MARSI) (see Box 9.3).

Modified from LeBlanc, K., et al. (2018). Best practice recommendations for the prevention and management of skin tears in aged skin. *Wounds International*. Available to download from www.woundsinternational.com and White, M. W., Karam, S., & Cowell, B. (1994). Skin tears in frail elders: A practical approach to prevention. *Geriatric Nursing, 15*(2), 95–99.

BOX 9.3 Prevention of Medical Adhesive-Related Skin Injury (MARSI)*

1. Secure dressings with roll gauze, tubular stockinette, or self-adhering tape (avoids unnecessary tape on skin).
2. Apply tape without tension (prevents blistering of skin under tape).
3. Use porous tapes (allows moisture to evaporate).
4. Use skin sealants, thin hydrocolloids, or solid-wafer skin barriers under adhesives (provides protective layer over skin for adhering tapes).
5. Secure dressings with Montgomery straps (prevents repeated tape applications).
6. Remove tape slowly, peel away from anchored skin, or pull one corner of tape at an angle parallel with skin. Solvents

can be used to break bond with skin, although solvents have drying effect on skin. Plain tap water can often serve this purpose effectively (decreases trauma to epidermis and dermal–epidermal junction).

Neonates (See Also Chapter 37)
- Solvents and adhesive removers should not be used with the neonate due to reports of skin toxicity.
- Skin sealants should not be used with neonates less than 30 days old. Alcohol-free skin sealants may be used for the neonate greater than 30 days old.

*Rationale for intervention is given in parentheses.

---

protection from skin tears. Only alcohol-free skin protectants should be used when the skin is denuded or when contact with wound edges is likely to avoid discomfort and stinging. It is important to allow the skin sealant to dry completely before applying tape. Many central-line dressing kits are prepackaged with a liquid skin protectant.

When frequent tape removal is needed for dressing changes, application of an adhesive barrier (e.g., solid-wafer skin barrier or thin hydrocolloid) can be used on intact periwound skin to anchor tape and prevent skin stripping. The protocol should clearly indicate that the barrier is not changed routinely. The barrier should be left undisturbed and allowed to fall off. Loose edges should be clipped rather than removing the old barrier and applying a new one. Used in this way, the skin barrier or hydrocolloid dressing can remain in place for several days while caregivers easily apply and reapply the tape without traumatizing the epidermis. Box 9.3 summarizes interventions for preventing skin tears in conjunction with the use of medical adhesives.

Goals for topical care of skin tears include maintaining an approximated residual skin flap if applicable (gently reposition the flap over the wound surface) and maintaining a physiologic wound environment; atraumatic dressing removal is critical (LeBlanc et al., 2018). Hydrocolloids, transparent films, and closure strips are contraindicated. Silicones, foams, alginates, hydrofibers, and hydrogel dressings are recommended, and selection is based on moisture management and control of exudate (LeBlanc et al., 2013). Approximated edges also may be secured with careful use of 2-octylcyanoacrylate (also referred to as topical skin bandage or skin glue) (Baranoski, 2003; LeBlanc et al., 2018, 2013, 2008; Roberts, 2007).

MOISTURE-ASSOCIATED SKIN DAMAGE

When the skin is exposed to moisture, such as body fluids, perspiration, or cleansers, for extended periods of time or repeatedly (i.e., frequent cleansing), the normal barrier function of the stratum corneum is diminished (Voegeli, 2016). As a result, skin pH rises and the risk of bacterial colonization increases, predisposing the patient to development of

cutaneous infections. The two most common organisms are *Candida albicans* (from the gastrointestinal tract) and *Staphylococcus* (from the perineal skin).

The nomenclature used to describe and classify skin damage caused by these conditions is extensive and confusing. For example, dermatitis caused by chemical irritants has been referred to as irritant contact dermatitis. The term *diaper dermatitis*, familiar to most health care providers, specifically refers to inflammation of the skin in the diaper area (perineal or perigenital areas) of the infant (Zulkowski, 2008). However, when the same condition develops in the perineal area in the adult, it is often called *perineal dermatitis*. The dilemma with both terms is that they do not adequately address the irritant, and the terms exclude locations outside of the diaper or perineum, such as the inner thighs or buttocks.

Recognizing the multiplicity of terms and their limitations, the term *moisture-associated skin damage* (MASD) has been adopted to capture the "inflammation and erosion of the skin caused by prolonged exposure to various sources of moisture, including urine or stool, perspiration, wound exudate, mucus or saliva" (Gray, Black, Baharestani, et al., 2011). Sources of moisture that contain chemicals or enzymes (e.g., gastrointestinal secretions, stool, harsh cleansing solutions and solvents) are harmful to the skin due to their acidic pH, or high volume of enzymes, and will erode the top layers of the epidermis. In addition, when the presence of moisture is accompanied by mechanical factors such as friction and/or the presence of potentially pathogenic microorganisms, skin damage is accentuated. Coexisting infections that occur with MASD most often include candidiasis. Additional infections that can arise include herpes zoster or herpes simplex virus (HSV), tinea cruris (a dermatophyte infection of the squamous cells and trapped in a skin fold), and inverse psoriasis (Visscher, 2009).

There are four common conditions captured by the category of MASD: incontinence-associated dermatitis (IAD), periwound dermatitis, peristomal dermatitis, and intertrigo dermatitis (ITD). IAD is defined as a reactive response of the skin to chronic exposure to urine and fecal material, which could be observed as inflammation and erythema, with or without erosion or denudation (Gray, Bliss, Doughty, et al., 2007) (see Plate 13).

Pathophysiologic Process

The prolonged presence of moisture (more than 2 h) on the skin places the skin at risk for overhydration and maceration of the epidermis. Although maceration is a seemingly innocent and common experience for anyone who soaks in the hot tub or washes dishes by hand, the corresponding weakening of the collagen fibers can reduce the skin's resiliency or ability to remain intact in the presence of mechanical action (e.g., friction, tape removal, and pressure) or chemical exposure (e.g., gastrointestinal contents). In addition to urine, wound exudate, and perspiration, moisture-donating wound dressings such as hydrogel and saline-saturated gauze can be a source of moisture. Moisture can be trapped against the skin by clothing, diapers, gauze, wound dressings, and skin folds.

Maceration compromises protective skin mechanisms such as pH and normal flora. Increased skin pH can be triggered by exposure to ammonia in urine and to alkaline soaps; it has also been reported in the skin of persons with diabetes. As moisture penetrates the epidermis, it interacts with keratinocytes and fibroblasts, stimulating the release of cytokines, which act on the vasculature of the dermis to trigger inflammation. Consequently, the lipid bilayer structure of the stratum corneum is damaged, which may allow microorganisms to enter the epidermis (Visscher, 2009). Prolonged moisture also reduces the ability of the skin to resist additional stresses, such as shear, friction, and pressure, because of a higher frictional coefficient (Visscher, 2009), leading to secondary skin breakdown. The increased permeability of the skin and decreased barrier function contributes to bacterial overgrowth on the skin and cutaneous infection (Beeckman, Woodward, & Gray, 2011). Thus, clinical manifestations of skin macerated by the presence of excess or prolonged moisture include pale skin color and a wrinkling, swollen appearance of the exposed skin surface (see Plate 14). As the length of exposure continues, the skin may become erythematous. Fissures may eventually develop from exposure to friction and shear. For example, linear shallow fissures may develop in the cleft between the buttocks, in skin folds, and between the toes.

Chemical Irritants and Moisture-Associated Skin Damage

MASD precipitated by exposure to harsh solutions or effluent can occur in the perineum, periwound, peritube, and peristomal area. When the epidermis is exposed to moisture that contains caustic or enzymatic contents, the skin will be further damaged by the chemical exposure. Fluids containing chemicals include, but are not limited to, povidone–iodine complex (Betadine), alkaline soaps, alcohol, gastrointestinal contents, and drainage from percutaneous tubes. Exposure to fecal incontinence (especially liquid to loose consistency) results in MASD because of the chemical composition of the fecal material (e.g., enzymes) combined with moisture and mechanical factors of shear and friction. Skin damage may be evident within only a few hours in the presence of a strong irritant (e.g., small bowel discharge). In fact, infants may develop a chemical-related skin injury as soon as they pass a loose stool into the diaper. In other situations, skin breakdown may occur only after repeated or prolonged exposure over several days, such as with soft or formed stool.

MASD triggered by chemical irritants can be distinguished from maceration by examining the exposure sites. Initially, irritants extract water-binding chemicals and lipids from the stratum corneum, and the skin decompensates so that it becomes dry and erythematous or develops an erythematous macular rash (Habif, Dinulos, Chapan, & Zug, 2018) (see Plate 13). With continued exposure to chemical irritants, the protective layer of the stratum corneum becomes damaged, resulting in a loss of epidermis in the area of exposure, which is described as superficial erosion or moist denudement. MASD resulting from exposure to chemicals is uncomfortable for the patient because the chemicals stimulate neurocutaneous pain receptors. In differentiating IAD from the various possible skin conditions in the perineal, perianal, or buttocks region, it is also important to recognize that chemical-induced IAD will only appear in the area that is directly in contact with the irritant. To facilitate further distinctions, Table 9.3 lists the typical assessment features of a variety of perineal–perianal skin conditions, including IAD, candidiasis, HSV, herpes zoster, and pressure injuries.

Conditions Associated With IAD

Acute fecal incontinence is a common instigator of IAD. The etiology of acute fecal incontinence can be the result of a number of factors: nutritional (hyperosmolar enteric solutions, rapid rate of administration of enteric solutions, hypoalbuminemia), medications (antibiotics, cathartics), gastrointestinal function (short bowel syndrome, fat malabsorption, antibiotic-associated diarrhea, incomplete bowel obstruction, fecal impaction), and gastrointestinal disease (inflammatory bowel disease (IBD), infection, radiation enteritis). The patient's medical history is helpful in identifying the most likely etiology; additional laboratory tests or radiologic examinations may be indicated for confirmation. A digital rectal examination should be conducted to rule out a fecal impaction causing an incomplete bowel obstruction. When a fecal impaction is present, the stool will be dry and hard, and the patient will not be able to pass the stool unassisted; diarrheal stool will be passed around the impaction (Niederhuber, Armitage, Doroshow, Kastan, & Tepper, 2014). When an impaction is present, a sodium phosphate enema (i.e., Fleet enema) and oral cathartics may be indicated. A colonoscopy may be indicated to rule out other potential etiologies for diarrhea, including cytomegalovirus in immunocompromised patients, graft vs host disease, IBD, and ischemic colitis.

Antibiotic-associated diarrhea is an increasingly frequent cause of fecal incontinence. Broad-spectrum antibiotics, such as fluoroquinolones, ampicillin, amoxicillin, clindamycin, and cephalosporins, are the most common culprits (Higa & Kelly, 2013; Imhoff & Karpa, 2009; Leffler et al., 2015). Antibiotics alter the gastrointestinal microflora, thus increasing the concentration of pathogenic organisms within the bowel.

Clostridium difficile was first identified to be related to antibiotic-associated diarrhea in the late 1970s (Martin et

TABLE 9.3 Differential Diagnosis of Perineal/Perianal Skin Conditions

	Incontinence-Associated Dermatitis	Candidiasis	Herpes Zoster	Pressure
Location	Perineum Buttocks Inner thighs Groin Low abdominal skin folds	Perineum Buttocks Inner thighs Groin Low abdominal skin folds	Perianal Buttocks Genitals	Near bony prominences Coccyx, sacrum, ischium Under device/tube
Confirmed risk factors	Urinary and/or fecal incontinence	Moisture Antibiotics Immunosuppression	Immunosuppression Elderly Stress	Limited mobility or activity Dependent on others for repositioning, transferring, etc.
Blisters	Yes	No	Initially vesicles then pustules	Sometimes (Stage 2)
Distribution pattern	Confluent or patchy Irregular edges with erythema Shallow denudement, and/or maceration Fleshy part of buttocks	Confluent or patchy rash Small round pustules, plaques, and/or satellite lesions	Grouped unilateral distribution of rash or ulcerations along dermatome Pustules erode into ulcerations Clusters or isolated individual shallow lesions or blisters	Isolated individual lesions on or near bony prominence or pressure-causing device Damage ranges from intact discoloration to partial- or full-thickness wounds
Color	Pink/red	Pink/red	Initial: Pink/red Ulcer may have yellow slough Later: Crust Severe cases: Necrosis	Pink, red, yellow, tan, gray, brown, black
Discomfort	Pain may be mild to severe	Itching, burning	Tingling sometimes noted initially Often very painful	Pain may be absent to severe
Diagnostic tests	None	Potassium hydroxide preparation scraping (KOH)	DNA polymerase chain reaction assay and direct immunofluorescent stain of skin scraping for VZV antigen Tzanck preparation Tissue culture	None

al., 2016). When this anaerobic spore-forming Gram-positive bacillus is ingested, particularly following changes in the colonic flora such as with antibiotics, it will colonize and proliferate in the gut. Although other pathogens may be responsible for diarrhea, *C. difficile* is the most common pathogen and more severe than *Escherichia coli* and *Salmonella*. *C. difficile*, spores remain on surfaces for extended periods of time. Only bleach is effective at killing *C. difficile* on surfaces. *C. difficile* infection (CDI) has become the most common nosocomial diarrheal pathogen in hospitalized patients, identified as the culprit for 15%–25% of cases (Higa & Kelly, 2013; Stanley, Bartlett, Dart, & Ashcraft, 2013; Leffler & Lamont, 2015).

CDI ranges from being an asymptomatic carrier, to mild or moderate diarrhea, to fulminant pseudomembranous colitis. Diarrhea usually begins within 1–3 days after colonization; colonization can occur anywhere from 14 days to 3 months after antibiotic exposure (Higa & Kelly, 2013). Symptoms include foul-smelling, nonbloody, watery diarrhea (defined as the passage of three or more unformed stools in 24 or fewer consecutive hours), a stool test positive for toxigenic *C. difficile* or its toxins, or colonoscopic or histopathology findings demonstrating pseudomembranous colitis. Half of the patients will experience abdominal cramping and tenderness, abdominal distention, fever, leukocytosis, nausea, and dehydration (Stanley et al., 2013; Martin et al., 2016; Leffler & Lamont, 2015).

Three primary risk factors for CDI are hospitalization, recent history of antibiotic use, and over the age of 65 (Stanley et al., 2013; Leffler & Lamont, 2015). Modifiable secondary risk factors include postpyloric tube feedings, gastric-acid-reducing therapy, and double-occupancy rooms. Significant inflammation of the colonic mucosa develops when *C. difficile* strains adhere to colonic cells and produce toxins. Both secretory diarrhea and osmotic diarrhea occur with *C. difficile*-associated diarrhea (CDAD) (Eddins & Gray, 2008). As the mucosal surface is damaged, liquid accumulates in the bowel lumen, resulting in secretory diarrhea. Toxins attract proinflammatory cytokines, binding to the colonic epithelium, which further damage the bowel wall and impair its ability to absorb water, electrolytes, and nutrients, thus precipitating osmotic diarrhea (Eddins & Gray, 2008).

CDI is confirmed by clinical presentation of symptoms (usually diarrhea), exclusion of other causes of diarrhea, and a stool culture or positive toxin assay (Martin et al., 2016; Leffler & Lamont, 2015). An anaerobic stool culture for *C. difficile* is the most sensitive test, but is not widely available (Leffler & Lamont, 2015; Stanley et al., 2013). The 2017 Clinical Practice Guidelines for *Clostridium difficile* recommends two-step approach when the institution does not regulate stool specimens (i.e., patient not receiving laxatives and unexplained onset new onset and three or more unformed stools in 24 h) (McDonald et al., 2018). This requires a stool toxin test plus glutamate dehydrogenase (GDH), which may be arbitrated by nucleic acid amplification tests (NAAT), or NAAT plus toxin. NAAT alone may be used when the institution regulates stool specimen submissions. Before *C. difficile* toxin assays were available, colonoscopic examinations were common; a colonic biopsy positive for pseudomembranes in the presence of diarrhea is diagnostic of CDAD (Bartlett, 2015).

Standard treatment of CDAD is (1) prompt discontinuation of the antibiotic, (2) stool toxin assay, (3) oral metronidazole for initial episode of mild to moderate CDI (500 mg three times per day for 10–14 days), (4) correction of fluid and electrolyte imbalance, and (5) discontinuation of antiperistalsis medications. Metronidazole should be started even before the stool culture results are available when the systemic symptoms present create a high level of suspicion of CDAD. Oral vancomycin is the drug of choice for initial episodes of severe CDI (125 mg four times per day for 10–14 days) (Cohen et al., 2010). This can also be given rectally when an ileus is present (500 mg in approximately 100 mL normal saline every 6 h as retention enema). After initial antibiotic therapy, almost one-fourth of patients with CDAD relapse within 2 months because spores can prevent peristalsis and delay exposure to antibiotics by "hiding" in the mucosal folds. A more virulent strain has been discovered and is associated with increased disease severity and death (Stanley et al., 2013). CDI prevention measures emphasize infection control (gowns, gloves, isolation), hand hygiene with soap and water by all people in contact with the patient (including family and visitors), environmental disinfection (chlorine-containing compounds or vaporized hydrogen peroxide on areas of potential contamination), and antibiotic stewardship (minimal use of antibiotics for the shortest duration possible and narrow-spectrum antibiotics) (Stanley et al., 2013).

Intertrigo Dermatitis

ITD is defined as inflammation resulting from moisture trapped in skin folds subjected to friction (Sibbald, Kelley, Kennedy-Evans, et al., 2013). Risk factors for ITD are hyperhidrosis, obesity, pendulous breasts, deep skin folds, immobility, and diabetes. ITD is diagnosed based on clinical findings and supplemented with laboratory tests when a secondary infection is suspected. The distribution of ITD is a mirror image with erythema, inflammation, and/or erosion (often linear) in the skin fold. Symptoms may include pruritus, pain, and odor.

Moisture-Associated Skin Damage Prevention and Treatment

The plan of care to prevent and treat MASD begins with identification of the moisture source (Zulkowski, 2012). At that point, one can implement steps to reduce the presence of moisture. For example, when the source of moisture is urine, steps should be implemented to facilitate bladder control, such as with behavioral interventions, diet, and fluids.

In a systematic review of the literature, a structured skin care protocol was demonstrated to reduce the incidence of IAD (Beeckman, et al., 2009). A structured skin care protocol is a three-step process: gentle skin cleansing, moisturization, and the application of a skin protectant; the type of fluid on the skin and frequency of exposure will dictate the type of skin protectant used. Box 9.4 lists interventions and products that can be used to prevent and treat MASD. Table 9.4 lists a formulary of products used to prevent and manage MASD. Unique considerations concerning the prevention and management of MASD, and specifically IAD in the neonate or premature infant, are addressed in Chapter 37.

Skin cleansers with a pH near the skin's pH are more effective than soap and water at preventing IAD (Beeckman et al., 2009). Moisturizers are an important second step in the perineal skin care regimen and often are incorporated into commercially prepared skin cleansers. The three categories of skin protectants are skin sealant, moisture barrier ointment, and moisture barrier paste. Skin sealants provide a polymer film to protect the skin from maceration but may have limited effectiveness at protecting the skin from enzymes. Moisture barrier ointments protect the skin from effluent with enzymes but may be inadequate with high-volume output or excessively frequent effluent production or diarrhea. In these situations, a moisture barrier paste should be used. Proper use of an ointment or paste consists of applying the product and, when the surface becomes soiled, using a soft pad to gently wipe off the stained surface of the product. The skin should not be scrubbed in an attempt to completely remove the product. When the product must be completely removed, mineral oil can be used to facilitate removal. Commercially available incontinence cleansers also can be used to remove a barrier paste.

Containment devices include external pouches and indwelling catheters. Containment devices may be indicated for containment of contaminated stool for infection control purposes and/or when the frequency or volume of stool overwhelms the moisture barrier ointment or paste. Rectal pouches are adhesive ostomy pouches specifically designed to fit the perianal contours and contain the incontinent stool. By protecting the skin from chemicals and moisture buildup, these products can be extremely cost-effective by reducing linen changes and freeing up nursing time for other types of care. Rectal pouches also preserve the patient's dignity by containing odor and feces. Acceptable wear time for the

BOX 9.4 MASD: Types and Interventions*

Periwound
- Routine hygiene to keep skin clean and dry using skin cleanser and moisturizer.
- Use skin sealant, skin barrier ointment, skin barrier paste, or solid-wafer skin barrier to protect periwound skin.
- Use dressing with adequate absorptive capacity (see also Chapter 21).
- Change dressings before saturation occurs.
- Use low air loss support surface for moisture control of large surface areas that cannot be adequately protected with dressings, absorptive pads, or skin barrier.

Peritube or Drain (See Also Chapter 39)
- Collaborate with appropriate service (i.e., intervention radiology) to determine cause of leakage, confirm proper placement, and optimal stabilization.
- Routine mild cleansing with skin cleanser and moisturizer.
- Use skin sealant, skin barrier ointment, skin barrier paste, or solid-wafer skin barrier to protect peritube skin.
- Use dressing with adequate absorptive capacity.
- Change dressings before saturation occurs.

Between Skin Folds (ITD)
- Routine hygiene to keep skin clean and dry.
- Dust intertriginous skin surfaces with absorbent skin barrier powder.

- Separate intertriginous skin surfaces with skin sealant, barrier, and/or soft cotton material (i.e., t-shirt).
- Place commercially available textile in skin fold (do not use emollients with this product).

Incontinence
- Determine and treat etiology.
- Identify patients at risk for skin damage.
- Use absorptive padding (without plastic back) as needed; change after incontinent episodes.
- Cleanse with mild incontinence skin cleanser; repeat after each incontinent episode.
- Apply moisturizer to skin.
- Apply appropriate skin barrier to keep urine and feces off epidermis.
- Apply condom catheter or external pouch.
- Use indwelling catheters *only* with clear indication, assessment of contraindications, and order; change per manufacturer's instructions.
- *Low risk* of skin breakdown (urine and/or formed, soft stools): Apply skin sealant or moisture barrier ointment; reapply skin sealant per manufacturer's instructions; reapply moisture barrier ointment with each incontinent episode.
- *High risk* of skin breakdown (impaired skin integrity apparent, actual or anticipated loose stools): Apply skin barrier *paste* and repeat per manufacturer's instructions.

*See Table 9.4 for product examples.

TABLE 9.4 Formulary of Products* Used to Prevent and Manage MASD**

Product	Purpose	Examples*	Additional Information
Perineal cleanser	Perineal skin cleansing	Coloplast CarraFoam or CarraWash, Medline Soothe & Cool, Smith & Nephew Secura	Liquid, foam, or impregnated cloth products available in rinse or no rinse
Perineal cleanser and protectant	Combination product for cleansing and protecting perineal skin	Coloplast Baza Cleanse and Protect, Sage Comfort Shield, Medline Remedy	Skin cleanser that does not have to be rinsed off and simultaneously applies a skin protectant. Available in liquid, foam, or impregnated cloth products
Moisture barrier ointment	Perineal skin protection	Calmoseptine ointment, Lantiseptic skin protectant, Proshield Plus skin protectant, Critic-Aide clear hydrophilic ointment	May impair adhesion if used in combination with perianal pouches
Moisture barrier paste	Periwound, perifistula, peritube, high-risk perineal skin protection	Critic-Aide skin paste, Ilex skin protectant paste, Remedy Calazime protectant paste	More durable than moisture barrier ointment. Appropriate for open, denuded skin. Only need to remove top soiled layer of ointment before reapplication. Do not use force to remove. Mineral oil and selected perineal cleansers. May impair adhesion if used in combination with adhesive dressings and pouches. Some wound care treatments cannot be used with zinc-based pastes
Solid skin barrier	Peristomal, perifistula, peritube, periwound skin protection	Stomahesive, Eakin, premium skin barrier	More durable than moisture barrier ointments and pastes. Available in multiple sizes and shapes (e.g., wafer, rings, strips). Waterproof; can be worn for several days

Continued

TABLE 9.4   Formulary of Products Used to Prevent and Manage MASD—cont'd

Product	Purpose	Examples	Additional Information
Liquid skin protectant	Perineal, peristomal, perifistula, peritube, periwound skin protection	No Sting Skin Prep protective dressing, Cavilon No Sting barrier film, skin gel wipe Butyl and octyl cyanoacrylate blend (e.g., Marathon)	Liquid transparent cyanoacrylate delivered by a wipe, wand, or spray. Provides a copolymer film. Some products contain isopropyl alcohol. Nonalcohol-based products should be used when skin is compromised Butyl and octyl cyanoacrylates are wound closure adhesives intended for closure of full-thickness wounds
Skin barrier powder	Absorbs and dries weepy denuded skin to improve adherence of ointments, pastes, adhesive barriers	Stomahesive protective powder, Karaya powder, premium powder	Will impair adhesion if used on intact skin or if used in excess. Discontinue when the skin is no longer denuded
External perianal pouch	Perianal, peristomal skin protection, containment of stool	Hollister fecal incontinence collector, ConvaTec fecal collector	Combines pouch with solid skin barrier for nonambulatory patients. Attached spout can be connected to bedside bag; spout can be cut off and replaced with provided tail closure. Odorproof and waterproof with gas filter option
External urinary catheter	Perineal skin protection, containment of urine	Mentor-Coloplast Freedom Hollister extended wear, Hollister retracted penis pouch, Kendall Uri-Drain	Products made in variety of sizes and must be properly fit. Available in latex and nonlatex. Application involves self-adhesives or added adhesive strips
Indwelling fecal management device	Perianal skin protection, containment of loose stool	Hollister ActiFlo indwelling bowel catheter, ConvaTec Flexi-Seal fecal management system, Bard DigniCare stool management system, ConSure Medical Qora Stool Management Kit	Do not use without provider's order. Critical to read manufacturer's instruction for contraindications and safe use. May need additional perianal protection with moisture barrier paste
Textile	Skin fold protection	InterDry Ag textile with antimicrobial silver complex	Wicks away moisture from skin-to-skin contact areas to manage moisture, odor, and inflammation. Comes in rolls; cut amount needed

*Examples of product names are not inclusive or intended as an endorsement.
**Some of these products may not be appropriate for neonates; please see Chapter 37 and Table 37.2 specifically for important considerations in selecting skin care products for neonates.

rectal pouch is 24 h. Extra care should be used when repositioning the patient to prevent excess shear on the pouch and the surrounding skin. Step-by-step directions for application are provided by the manufacturer and should be followed closely.

Historically, large indwelling urinary catheters or devices called rectal or colon tubes designed for enema and medication administration have been inserted into the rectum and left in place. This practice is not safe because it has the potential to damage the anal sphincter and/or perforate the bowel. Only indwelling bowel and fecal management systems approved by the FDA are designed to safely divert, collect, and contain potentially harmful and contaminated gastrointestinal waste without damaging the anal sphincter. It is important to review the manufacturer's instructions for each product to understand differences in features, indications, and contraindications. Researchers have reported

efficient evacuation with minimal leakage or anorectal mucosal injury, reduction of perineal skin breakdown and pressure injuries, and no anorectal mucosal injury (Kim, Shim, Choi, et al., 2001; Kowal-Vern, Poulakidas, Barnett, et al., 2009). Reduction of perineal skin injury and pressure injuries, as well as decreased rates of urinary tract, soft tissue, skin, and bloodstream infections, also have been reported (Benoit & Watts, 2007; Kowal-Vern et al., 2009). These studies highlight the potential of these devices beyond the scope of skin protection and into the realm of managing infection and cross-contamination.

Drainage around catheters and tubes should be managed such that the drainage is eliminated, when possible, or the skin is not directly exposed to the drainage. For example, when leakage occurs around a gastrostomy tube, the first step is to ascertain proper placement and stabilization of the tube. If drainage persists once this is accomplished, appropriate use of skin barriers (particularly moisture barrier ointments, solid-wafer skin barriers, thin hydrocolloids, or foam dressings) is indicated. A solid-wafer skin barrier, hydrocolloid, or foam dressing can be trimmed to fit around a tube site; it can remain in place for several days and changed only when it loosens at the tube site. When ointment is the selected treatment, it should be reapplied periodically throughout the day to ensure adequate skin protection. However, ointments can never be used under an adhesive dressing. Regardless of the type of skin protection selected, gauze dressings are applied over the barrier to absorb drainage and are changed when damp.

Improper use of skin care products, particularly solvents, adhesives, and skin sealants, can contribute to chemical skin damage. Only pH-neutral skin cleansers should be used. Adhesive solvents must be thoroughly rinsed from the skin to prevent buildup of harmful substances. Soaps should be avoided to prevent disruption of the skin's normal acid pH. Skin sealants and adhesives, such as cements, must be allowed to dry adequately so that solvents evaporate before other products are applied.

The prevention and treatment of ITD are based on minimizing skin-to-skin contact and friction, removing irritants and moisture from the skin fold, and wicking moisture away from the vulnerable area (Sibbald et al., 2013). Prevention measures include (1) skin cleansing with pH-balanced product; (2) gentle cleansing, no scrubbing; (3) soft cloth, no washcloths; and (4) pat dry. Talc, cornstarch, antiperspirants in the skin fold, and placing bed or bath linens in the skin fold are contraindicated. Many people with obesity will offer that they routinely use a natural fiber type of material such as a cotton "t-shirt" in their skin fold to prevent moisture entrapment. A moisture-wicking textile with silver is recommended; if a secondary infection is present, appropriate systemic or topical antimicrobials will be needed.

Medical Adhesive-Related Skin Injury

Medical adhesives precipitate several forms of skin damage and are broadly labeled medical adhesive-related skin injury, or MARSI. These are extremely common complications that are often erroneously dismissed as unavoidable. Damage to the skin from medical adhesives is also a significant source of pain and discomfort for the patient. The definition of MARSI is "an occurrence in which erythema and/or other manifestation of cutaneous abnormality (including, but not limited to, vesicle, bulla, erosion, or tear) persists 30 minutes of more after removal of the adhesive" (McNichol, Lund, Rosen, et al., 2013). Types of MARSI include epidermal stripping, skin tears, tension blisters, maceration, folliculitis, irritant contact dermatitis, and allergic contact dermatitis. Factors that contribute to tape trauma include product-related factors (peel force, tape occlusiveness, rigidity of backing, rheology of adhesive), user technique (process of application and removal), and patient factors (age, general health, application of solvents, preps, cleansers, and anatomic site). Of these factors, the least familiar issues to most health care providers pertain to tape-related factors.

Medical adhesives contain several layers. The two key layers that affect the adhesive's properties and performance are the adhesive layer and the backing. The adhesive layer contacts with the skin and may be an acrylate, silicone, hydrogel, hydrocolloid, polyurethane, or latex. The backing of the adhesive is the more commonly used descriptor: paper, plastic, silk, cloth, foam, and elastic. This backing provides the properties of stretch, conformability, occlusion, and rigidity, which are important criteria to consider in selecting an adhesive product.

Medical adhesives are both pressure sensitive and time sensitive. When the adhesive contacts the skin, firm pressure activates the adhesive to conform to the microscopic uneven surfaces of the epidermis. Over time the adhesive also warms and begins to flow to fill in the gaps in the irregular skin surface, further increasing the strength of the bond. Acrylate adhesives fill the skin gaps slowly, thus taking more time to adhere. In contrast, silicone adhesives are considered a "softer adhesive" that fills the skin gaps more quickly and provides a constant level of adherence rather than becoming more adherent over time. Box 9.5 provides a list of consensus statements for the assessment, prevention, and treatment of MARSI.

VASCULAR DAMAGE

Ulcerations, particularly on the legs or feet, can occur as a result of venous hypertension, arterial insufficiency, neuropathy, or a combination of these factors. Although these types of lesions commonly develop incidental to benign trauma (i.e., by bumping against the leg of a chair), each ulcer has distinct distinguishing features, pathologic processes, and treatment regimens. Arterial ulcers, venous ulcers, and lymphedema wounds are discussed in detail in Chapters 13–16. Neuropathic ulcers, such as diabetic ulcers, are discussed in Chapter 17.

INFECTIOUS AGENTS

Many skin rashes or ulcers are indicative of an infectious process and can occur around wounds or be misinterpreted as a pressure, shear, or chemical injury. Infections can be categorized according to infecting organism: fungus, bacteria, virus, or arthropod. The wound care specialist may be the first person to observe some of these infections. In many cases, the wound specialist will be responsible for identifying and managing the infections. The common skin infections are discussed here; the more unusual skin infections are addressed in Chapter 32.

Fungal
Candidiasis
Candidiasis is the most common opportunistic fungal infection (Kauffman, 2008). *Candida* spp., which are yeast-like organisms that reproduce by budding, normally colonize the skin, gastrointestinal tract, genitourinary tract, and vagina. When immunologic defenses are compromised or the normal flora is altered, *Candida* spp. become opportunistic pathogens.

BOX 9.5   MARSI: Consensus Statement for Assessment, Prevention, Treatment

Assessment

1. During the use of adhesive-containing products, the skin should be assessed for evidence of damage on a daily basis or with adhesive device changes; this is especially important for those patients deemed to be at high risk for adhesive-related injury.
2. For all medical adhesive-related skin injuries, a comprehensive assessment should be performed to determine severity and guide management.
3. Obtain a history of patient's known or suspected allergies and sensitivities to minimize the risk of medical adhesive-related skin injury.
4. The incidence of true allergic contact dermatitis related to adhesives is not known; suspected allergic contact dermatitis should be considered for referral and/or appropriate investigation (such as patch or scratch tests).

Prevention
General

1. Identification of patients at high risk for medical adhesive-related skin injury is a key component of prevention.
2. Care of the skin, including prevention of adhesive-related injury, should be a standard of care for all health care providers.
3. Prevention of medical adhesive-related skin injuries is facilitated by good nutrition and hydration.

Selection, Application, and Removal

1. Select the most appropriate adhesive product based on its intended purpose, the anatomic location the adhesive will be applied to, and the ambient conditions present at application site.
2. Appropriate product selection entails consideration of properties of adhesive-containing products such as adhesive gentleness, breathability, stretch, conformability, and flexibility.
3. Consider the potential adverse consequences of insufficient adhesion and/or adhesive failure when selecting medical adhesive products for use in securing a critical device.
4. Exercise caution when using silicone adhesives to secure some devices, as this may result in suboptimal adherence or adhesion failure.

Selection and Application

1. Anticipate changes in skin and/or joint movement following surgery and operative or other procedures when selecting and applying medical adhesive products.
2. Anticipate skin movement with edema when selecting and applying medical adhesives.

Application

1. Consider the role of skin tension (Langer's lines) and the effects of medical adhesive products when applied with the lines or against/across the lines.
2. Consider application of a skin barrier before applying an adhesive product.
3. Limit or avoid substances that increase the stickiness of adhesives, such as compound tincture of benzoin.

Application and Removal

1. Use proper application and removal techniques for adhesive-containing products.
2. Consider use of medical adhesive removers to minimize discomfort and skin damage associated with removal of adhesive products.

Electrodes

1. To prevent electrochemical burns under adhesive electrodes, powered (battery and line voltage) equipment should be maintained and monitored for dangerous leakage currents.

Infection Prevention

1. Adhesives may promote overgrowth of microorganisms. Monitor sites exposed to adhesive materials for manifestations of infection.
2. Store and use adhesive-containing products in a manner that prevents contamination.
3. Single-patient-use adhesive products are preferred.

Treatment

1. Apply evidence-based wound care principles when treating medical adhesive-related skin injuries.
2. Consult an appropriate skin or wound care specialist if a medical adhesive-related skin injury does not respond to conservative management within 7 days or if the wound deteriorates despite conservative care.

Future Research

1. Further research is needed to expand the scientific knowledge of adhesive performance and use, including mechanisms of medical adhesive-related skin injury, prediction, prevention, assessment and documentation, and treatment.

Cutaneous candidiasis is an epidermal infection with *Candida* spp. Although more than 150 species of *Candida* exist, the most common is *C. albicans* (see Plates 15 and 16). The primary lesion of candidiasis is a pustule or erythematous papules or plaques that may have associated scaling or crusting or a cheesy white exudate. Maceration is common. Lesions typically are beefy red, with satellite erythematous papules and pustules. Satellite lesions (outside the advancing edge of candidiasis) are an important diagnostic feature of candidiasis (Habif et al., 2018). Intact pustules are not always visible because opposing skin and clothing will unroof the pustule so that the lesion appears to be a macule or papule. Pruritus is the key indicator of candidiasis and may be severe.

A common location for development of candidiasis is in skin folds; *intertrigo* is the term used for an inflammatory condition of skin folds (see Plate 17). Intertrigo can be induced by heat, moisture, maceration, and friction. In addition to *Candida* spp., intertrigo can be complicated by other fungal infections (tinea) and by bacterial infection (erythrasma). *Candida* intertrigo is located in the skin folds (intertriginous areas) and is characterized by an intensely red, macerated, glistening, confluent macular papular rash. The half-moon-shaped edge of the rash or plaque often extends just beyond the limits of the opposing skin folds. Satellite lesions usually are present (Brannon, 2021).

Predisposing factors to candidiasis include the presence of a moist environment, a hot and humid environment, tight underclothing, diabetes, and antibiotic therapy. Skin under damp surgical dressings, the perineum, the perineal area, and intertriginous areas (beneath pendulous breasts, overhanging abdominal folds, and inguinal skin folds) are typical moist areas that provide an excellent medium for yeast growth. Diabetes predisposes the patient to development of candidiasis because the associated increase in the amount of glucose in the saliva, sweat, and urine in patients with diabetes prevents bacteria from inhibiting yeast growth (Carpenter, 2015). Antibiotics predispose the patient to development of candidiasis by removing the competing organisms. An altered skin pH also increases susceptibility to yeast infection. Immunosuppressed patients and patients with irritant contact dermatitis are vulnerable to candidiasis.

Folliculitis and contact dermatitis can be confused with candidiasis. Furthermore, candidiasis can be disguised by being superimposed on irritant contact dermatitis. The distribution and types of lesions are important to identifying the underlying problem. Folliculitis, the inflammation of a hair follicle, is characterized by the presence of pustules pierced in the center by a hair (see Plate 18), whereas candidiasis causes nonfollicular pustules. Manifestations of contact dermatitis include erythema with papules, whereas pustules are unusual and warrant culture to rule out superimposed infection. Distribution can help distinguish contact dermatitis from candidiasis because a contact dermatitis conforms to the specific shape of the irritant and therefore has well-defined borders, does not have satellite lesions, and does not have pruritus.

Intertrigo candidiasis is also easily confused with tinea cruris, erythrasma (both discussed later), and inverse psoriasis. Psoriasis is a chronic inflammatory papular skin disease characterized by scaly plaques that may affect skin, nails, and joints. It is attributed to abnormal T-lymphocyte function rather than an infection (Habif et al., 2018). One of the many unique clinical forms is intertriginous psoriasis (also known as inverse psoriasis). It is uncommon but can occur in the groin or under the breasts. The skin appears macerated with smooth, red, sharply defined plaques. Satellite lesions will not be present unless a candidal infection is superimposed on the psoriasis. The application of a topical steroid is associated with contributing to the added complication of candidiasis.

Candidiasis is most often determined clinically by signs, symptoms, and predisposing factors. Pruritus and burning at the site are common. The most relevant laboratory test for confirming candidiasis is a potassium hydroxide preparation scraping. Scrapings from an intact pustule and the contents are needed to yield the best results. Budding spores and elongated pseudohyphae are observed. Because the skin can be colonized with *C. albicans* but not infected, swab cultures for *Candida* are not informative, as such cultures cannot distinguish between infection and colonization (Carpenter, 2015).

Nonpharmacologic treatment includes reduction of predisposing factors, such as humidity, moisture, antibiotics, hyperglycemia, and tight-fitting clothes. Body powders (e.g., Zeasorb-AF) or wide-mesh gauze can be placed in intertriginous areas to absorb moisture. Prevention of moisture buildup is the most important intervention to prevent candidiasis. Box 9.4 lists additional strategies to protect the skin from moisture-related complication. Table 9.4 lists a formulary of products used to prevent moisture- or chemical-related skin damage.

Burow's solution soaks followed by air drying are soothing when maceration or severe pruritus is present. Topical antifungal creams can be applied twice daily for limited involvement, and antifungal powders can be used in less severe cases. When creams are used, they should be applied sparingly to reduce moisture entrapment. Recalcitrant or severe fungal infections require orally administered therapy.

Dermatophyte (Tinea)

The dermatophyte is a type of fungus that is responsible for the majority of fungal infections on the skin, nails, and hair (Dinulos, 2021). Known as *tinea*, a dermatophyte infection infects only dead keratin, so the stratum corneum on the skin is vulnerable. A tinea infection cannot survive in the mouth or vagina because these sites do not have a keratin layer. As a pruritic superficial fungal infection, tinea can be challenging to diagnose and treat (Wiederkehr & Schwartz, 2011). The manifestations of tinea infections vary according to body site. Box 9.6 lists the types of tinea based on body location. Tinea pedis occurs on the feet and is more familiar as *athlete's foot*. Tinea cruris occurs in the groin skin folds and is more commonly known as *jock itch*. Tinea corporis is present on the body and is also known as *ringworm*, although no worm is involved with this infection.

Fungi live on damp surfaces, and most tinea infections develop on moist surfaces (e.g., skin folds, web between toes, soles of the feet). Dermatophytes can be picked up from the floor of public showers or lockers, from a pet that is infected, or from loaning or borrowing clothing items from other individuals. Some individuals may be genetically predisposed to tinea infections (Dinulos, 2021). The active border of tinea will be scaly, red, and slightly elevated. When inflammation is significant, vesicles may be present along this active border.

BOX 9.6 Tinea Patterns

- Tinea pedis (foot)
- Tinea cruris (jock itch) (groin)
- Tinea corporis (ringworm) (body)
- Tinea faciei (face)
- Tinea manuum (hand)
- Tinea capitis (scalp)
- Tinea of barbae (beard)
- Tinea of onychomycosis (nails)

Tinea can be diagnosed by directly visualizing the branches of keratinized strands under the microscope. This is done with a potassium hydroxide wet mount preparation where a scale is removed from the active edge of the infection with a no. 15 surgical blade, placed on the microscope slide, and prepared for viewing (Dinulos, 2021). Dermatophytes will appear as translucent, branching, rod-shaped strands (hyphae) with uniform width. A Wood's light examination of hair will fluoresce blue to green when infected with *Microsporum* spp. of the dermatophyte fungi. Fungal infections of the skin do not fluoresce.

Box 9.7 lists the interventions for prevention of tinea infections. Treatment varies slightly by body site but primarily consists of topical antifungal medications such as butenafine (Lotrimin Ultra), terbinafine (Lamisil), or sertaconazole (Ertaczo) applied twice daily for 2–4 weeks. When interdigital web spaces are severely macerated, the antifungal medication econazole nitrate (Spectazole) also provides an antibacterial effect that addresses common secondary bacterial infections (Dinulos, 2021; Weller, Hamish, & Mann, 2015; Wiederkehr & Schwartz, 2011). Moist lesions also can be treated with a Burow's solution dressing for 20–30 min two to six times daily until the skin is dry.

Topical corticosteroid creams are commonly prescribed for inflammatory skin lesions, particularly in the groin; however, corticosteroids must be avoided when a dermatophyte infection is suspected. Use of these products can alter the clinical presentation of a dermatophyte infection, creating a condition called *tinea incognito*. When topical steroids are applied, they decrease the inflammation, which is interpreted as improvement. However, the dermatophyte fungus will flourish in the localized steroid-induced immunosuppression. When the corticosteroid is discontinued because the inflammation is resolving, the rash will return, but then the appearance will be different (absent scaling at the margins, diffuse

erythema, scattered pustules or papules, and brown hyperpigmentation) and the area of involvement greatly expanded. Treatment remains topical antifungal agents; oral antifungal medications may be needed for extensive lesions (red papules and pustules).

Bacterial

Folliculitis, impetigo, and erysipelas are bacterial skin infections caused by coagulase-positive *Staphylococcus (aureus)*, coagulase-negative *Staphylococcus (epidermidis)*, or β-hemolytic streptococcus (Bradley, 2015; Dinulos, 2021; Stevens, Mebane, & Madaras-Kelly, 2015). Although *Staphylococcus aureus* can be recovered from normal intact skin, especially in the nares, axillae, and groin, it is rarely a true member of resident bacterial flora and is considered a highly invasive pathogen. Staphylococci are able to quickly develop resistance to antibiotics; all staphylococci should be considered resistant to penicillins. Methicillin-resistant *S. aureus* (MRSA) and methicillin-resistant *Staphylococcus epidermidis* account for up to 50% of *S. aureus*-identified nosocomial infections in some medical centers (Bradley, 2015). Community-associated methicillin-resistant *S. aureus* (CA-MRSA) strains also have been reported. Vancomycin-resistant *S. aureus* has developed as a consequence of prolonged use of vancomycin as the primary treatment of serious MRSA infections. First-generation cephalosporins and penicillinase-resistant penicillins are the most effective drugs for treating mild to moderate infections.

Cellulitis

Cellulitis is an infection of the dermis and subcutaneous tissue that is most commonly caused by *S. aureus, Staphylococcus pyogenes*, and group A streptococcus (Vij & Tomecki, 2015). Cellulitis is preceded by some type of break in the skin, such as an ulcer, laceration, surgical incision, bite, burn, or body piercing, which becomes the portal of entry for the infecting organism (Dinulos, 2021). The most frequent sites on the body for occurrence of cellulitis are the posterior legs and hands. The head, abdomen, back, neck, buttocks, perigenital and perineal areas, and inner thighs are uncommon to rare sites for cellulitis (Dinulos, 2021).

Cellulitis should be differentiated from the erythema associated with venous dermatitis (see Table 15.X) or contact allergic dermatitis (distribution has very precise edges and shape is consistent with outline of offending agent). In the perineal and perigenital areas, cellulitis can be distinguished from the erythema associated with a Stage 1 pressure injury based on the location of the lesion (a Stage 1 pressure injury is most often limited to skin overlying a bony prominence). Relative to IAD, cellulitis should be distinguished from intertrigo, erythrasma, chemical denudation, and psoriasis.

Assessment findings characteristic of cellulitis include localized erythema with diffuse borders, tenderness upon palpation, warmth, and edema. Crepitus (palpation of gas in the subcutaneous tissue), however, is pathologic for aerobic infections, such as *Clostridia*, most often *Clostridia perfringens*. An elevated white blood cell count and erythrocyte

---

BOX 9.7   Preventing Tinea Infections

- Expose feet to air whenever home.
- Change socks and underwear daily, especially in warm weather.
- Dry feet carefully (especially between toes) after using locker room or public shower.
- Avoid walking barefoot in public areas; wear flip-flops, sandals, or water shoes.
- Do not wear thick clothing for long periods of time in warm weather; heavy clothes will cause increased sweating, which can encourage growth of fungal infections.
- Discard worn exercise shoes. Never borrow other people's shoes.
- Do not borrow or lend personal towels or clothing to other people.
- Check pets for areas of hair loss and ask veterinarian to check pets as well. Determine whether pets are causing patient's fungal infection; otherwise, patient may become infected again, even after treatment.
- Make sure shared exercise equipment (e.g., treadmill at gym) is clean before using it.

sedimentation rate may be present. Recurrent cellulitis will impair lymphatic drainage and lead to lymphedema, dermal fibrosis, and epidermal thickening. A culture is required to discern the invading organism and the appropriate antibiotic initiated. Empiric treatment may begin before the culture results are obtained, but should be effective for both staphylococcal and streptococcal organisms (Dinulos, 2021). Most patients respond to oral antibiotic therapy; reevaluation and consideration of intravenous antibiotics should be considered if the patient does not respond. Clostridial infections will require high-dose intravenous penicillin in addition to prompt debridement and surgical exploration of the cellulitis site (Vij & Tomecki, 2015).

Erysipelas

Erysipelas is an acute inflammatory form of cellulitis that occurs as a complication of a break in skin integrity, which occurs with abrasions or dry skin. Erysipelas differs from other types of cellulitis because it involves the cutaneous lymphatics, in the form of "streaking." Group A streptococci are the most common causative organism (Dinulos, 2021).

Erysipelas most commonly occurs in infants, young children, and older adults. Additional risk factors include malnutrition, alcoholism, recent infections, stasis dermatitis, lymphedema, nephrotic syndrome, and diabetes mellitus. Small, seemingly insignificant breaks in the skin can serve as a portal of entry for infection; in most cases, a portal of entry cannot be found. The extremities and the face are the most common sites (Vij & Tomecki, 2015).

Erysipelas means "red skin," and the involved body part is characterized by well-defined erythema. (In contrast, cellulitis is less demarcated.) The classic primary lesion is a plaque. Prodromal symptoms, such as malaise, myalgias, chills, and high fever, may occur within 4–48 h of infection. The surrounding skin rapidly progresses to become erythematous, edematous, and intensely painful. Secondary lesions are vesicles, bullae, and cutaneous hemorrhage. Within 5–10 days of onset, desquamation of the affected area occurs. Associated lymphangitis is demonstrated by the presence of erythematous streaking over lymphatics draining the area of infection.

Erysipelas usually is diagnosed by clinical findings of sharply defined erythema, edema, and/or streaking. Accompanying systemic complaints of fever, chills, malaise, and localized pain also raise suspicion for the presence of the condition. Although cultures (via needle aspiration) of any drainage from the advancing edge and skin biopsies are appropriate, the organism is difficult to culture, leaving the test uninformative. When septicemia is suspected, a white blood cell count and blood cultures are warranted.

Nonpharmacologic interventions include bed rest, elevation of the affected extremity, and hot packs. Uncomplicated cases of erysipelas can be treated with oral antibiotics. Toxic, debilitated, and elderly patients or children with extensive facial involvement or any patients with rapidly evolving erythema, pain, and swelling require intravenous antibiotics; penicillin, a cephalosporin, or nafcillin is warranted.

Symptoms should diminish within 24 h of treatment. Pain control measures are essential.

Erythrasma

A bacterial infection (corynebacterium) can develop in skin folds (e.g., axilla, groin), resulting in the condition known as *erythrasma*. This chronic condition is mildly pruritic, with a reddish-brown pigmentation, well-defined borders, and little scaling. Overweight patients, those with diabetes, and people living in warmer climates are at increased risk for developing erythrasma. This infection can be diagnosed by microscopy or culture. Erythrasma is often confused with candidiasis intertrigo based on clinical presentation but is easily distinguished because the erythrasma rash, when exposed to long-wave ultraviolet radiation, will fluoresce to a coral pink color due to the action of the corynebacterium. The absence of satellite lesions should also help distinguish erythrasma from candidiasis. Treatment of erythrasma consists of washing the area vigorously with antibacterial soap and either applying clotrimazole lotion three times per day for 7 days, administering erythromycin tablets (500 mg) four times per day for 7–10 days, or applying erythromycin gel to the affected area. As with tinea infections, erythrasma can be prevented by keeping the skin dry, wearing absorbent clean clothing, and practicing good hygiene (Dinulos, 2021).

Folliculitis

Folliculitis is an inflammation of the hair follicle (see Plate 18). It can be mechanical, bacterial, or fungal in origin. Mechanical folliculitis is the result of tight clothing or persistent trauma. Bacterial folliculitis is most commonly caused by *S. aureus*. Fungal folliculitis is associated with tinea (dermatophyte infection) of the skin where hair is present (e.g., beard, head). Fungal folliculitis also can develop in the presence of untreated tinea corporis (Dinulos, 2021). Occlusion of the skin from occlusive ointment or the prolonged presence of oil or grease on the skin also will cause development of folliculitis (occlusion folliculitis). Improperly cleaned hot tubs are also responsible for causing *Pseudomonas folliculitis*. Steroids will trigger steroid folliculitis characterized by multiple small pustules and papules, resulting in a neutrophilic inflammation of the hair follicle.

The primary lesions in folliculitis are dome-shaped, 2- to 5-mm erythematous papules that surround the hair follicle and may manifest central pustules; secondary lesions are crusts and erythema (Dinulos, 2021). Folliculitis may be limited to the superficial area of the hair follicle or progress deeper into the follicle. Although most common on the scalp or the extremities, folliculitis may develop on any hairy body location, particularly under adhesive wound dressings. Folliculitis also may develop as a secondary infection in the presence of excoriations from scratching that accompanies scabies and insect bites.

Risk factors for developing folliculitis are diabetes mellitus, obesity, malnutrition, immunodeficiency, and chronic staphylococcal infections. When treating folliculitis, avoid or reduce heat, friction, and occlusion. Antibacterial soaps should be used and hygiene improved. Potassium hydroxide examination of the hair and surrounding skin is warranted to exclude a dermatophyte infection (i.e., tinea) so that the appropriate oral antifungal medications, such as Lamisil, can be used. When folliculitis is limited and superficial, topical mupirocin is effective (Dinulos, 2021).

Impetigo

Impetigo, most commonly seen in children, is a highly contagious, superficial, vesiculopustular skin infection that is caused primarily by the gram-positive bacterium *S. aureus*. *Streptococcus pyogenes* occasionally may be the offending pathogen, causing a more significant infection. Poor hygiene or malnutrition is typical of patients with impetigo. Lesions develop within 10–14 days (Stevens et al., 2016). The initial onset is a vesicle involving the superficial layer of the stratum corneum. The patient may experience itching and mild soreness; systemic symptoms are uncommon. Impetigo most often develops on seemingly intact skin, although it also may develop with minor breaks in the skin, such as insect bites and minor abrasions.

It is important to distinguish impetigo from HSV. HSV can be distinguished from impetigo by culture and by early manifestations. HSV begins with grouped, clear vesicles that are uniform in size, and it recurs at the same site.

Impetigo is often self-limited and resolves spontaneously, although it may also become chronic and/or recurrent. The treatment of choice for impetigo is topically administered 2% mupirocin cream (Bactroban). It has been shown to be as effective as oral erythromycin without the side effects (Dinulos, 2021). The cream should be applied three times daily until the lesions clear. Oral penicillin is indicated when streptococci are present. Impetigo may present clinically as bullous or nonbullous.

Bullous Impetigo. Bullous impetigo is a primarily staphylococcal disease that develops when certain strains of *S. aureus* produce a specific epidermolytic toxin (Dinulos, 2021). They may occur anywhere on the body, but the most common location is the face. One or more vesicles enlarge, creating a superficial, fragile, clear fluid-filled bulla that gradually becomes filled with cloudy fluid. When the center of the bulla collapses, a rim of the bulla roof often remains, encircling the lesion. The center of the lesion then develops a thin, honey-colored crust. When this is removed, a red, inflamed, moist base is revealed that is exudative with serous fluid. Eventually the outer edges of the bulla become dry and flaky, and a crust forms. Bullous impetigo lesions have little, if any, surrounding erythema; they can range in size from 2 to 8 cm and remain for several months. Infants must be monitored for signs and symptoms of serious secondary infections, such as septic arthritis and pneumonia (Dinulos, 2021).

Nonbullous Impetigo. The lesions associated with nonbullous impetigo are asymptomatic, with minimal surrounding erythema. Lesions begin as small vesicles or pustules but soon rupture, exposing a moist, red base that becomes crusted over. The most common sites affected are around the mouth, the nose, and the extremities. In the usual sequence of events, the infectious agent is present on intact skin and, after minor trauma such as scratching, the skin is broken and an infection develops (Dinulos, 2021). During the early development of the lesions, group A β-hemolytic streptococci may be isolated; however, the lesions quickly become contaminated with staphylococci. Predisposing factors for streptococcal impetigo are warm, moist climates and poor hygiene.

Viral

Viral infections, particularly HSV and varicella-zoster virus (VZV), are commonly triggered by stress and illness. It is important to recognize these highly contagious infections to facilitate prompt appropriate treatment and prevent spread to other individuals.

Herpes Simplex Virus

HSV infections of the epidermis are highly contagious and can be spread when a susceptible, noninfected person comes into direct contact (via mucous membrane or broken skin) with a person shedding the virus. Viral shedding occurs even in the absence of symptoms. Most transmission of HSV occurs during periods of asymptomatic shedding (Kimberlin & Whitley, 2008). Consequently, HSV infection should be considered a chronic process rather than an intermittent process, and all HSV-infected people should be treated as potentially contagious. Furthermore, because the primary infection often is subclinical, a negative history of vesicles or blisters does not rule out previous HSV infection.

HSV has been divided into two types: HSV-1 (oral herpes) and HSV-2 (genital herpes). HSV-1 is associated with cold sores (fever blisters); HSV-2 causes genital and perianal herpes. However, genital lesions from HSV-1 and oral lesions from HSV-2 are becoming more common, a trend that may be a consequence of sexual freedom and the ease of transmission. Ultimately, HSV lesions are not limited to the lips and genital area and may occur anywhere on the skin.

HSV infections have two phases: primary infection and secondary phase. During the primary infection, the virus becomes established in a nerve ganglion. HSV-1 most often occurs during childhood, whereas HSV-2 commonly occurs after sexual contact in sexually active individuals. Symptoms of the primary infection range from being undetectable to localized pain, headache, generalized aching, malaise, and tender regional adenopathy. A significant inflammatory response develops that extends from the base of the lesions down into the dermis, which results in the classic presentation of uniform, grouped vesicles on an erythematous base; the vesicles contain large numbers of infective viral particles. As more inflammatory cells are recruited to the site, vesicles become pustules that erode, drain, and crust (see Plates 19 and 20). Primary lesions last for 2–6 weeks and heal without scarring. As the lesion heals, the virus enters the skin nerve endings and ascends through peripheral nerves to the dorsal root ganglia, where it remains in a latent stage.

Reactivation of the virus can occur in response to local trauma (abrasion, ultraviolet light) or systemic changes (e.g., stress, illness, fatigue, fever, compromised immune system). The virus then travels back down the peripheral nerve to the site, or in the vicinity, of the initial infection to trigger a recurrence. Prodromal symptoms of burning at the site may precede the recurrence. The reactivated virus presents as vesicles on an erythematous base, or ulcers. Crusts cover the eruptions within 24–48 h and are shed in approximately 12 days, exposing a reepithelialized surface (Weller et al., 2015).

Clinical presentation of grouped vesicles on an erythematous base is a key indicator of HSV and can be confirmed with a Tzanck smear. However, the Tzanck smear is most reliable when the lesion sampled is a vesicle; the smear becomes less reliable with pustules, crusts, and ulcers.

Primary HSV-1 infections are generally asymptomatic. When symptoms are present, the lesions include painful vesicles or shallow ulcers on the lips or lower face or in the oral cavity, and they last for 2–3 weeks. Recurrent HSV-1 infections are foreshadowed by pain and tingling or a burning sensation 2–24 h before the eruption of vesicles (Kimberlin & Whitley, 2008). Recurrent HSV-1 lasts about 2 days as vesicles, which progress to pustules, ulcers, and eventually crusts. Complete healing occurs in 8–10 days.

Primary genital herpes (typically HSV-2 infection) lesions initially are macules and papules, followed by vesicles, pustules, and ulcerations. Lesions may occur on the genitalia, the perineum, and the buttocks. The lesions are extremely painful and persist for 2–3 weeks. Spontaneous resolution of the primary infection is common. Recurrent genital herpes is less pronounced and lasts for 8–10 days. Ulcers are shallow and may or may not be painful.

Herpes lesions may occur on the buttocks and are commonly misinterpreted as pressure, chemical IAD, or scabies (see Plate 20). Therefore, the differential diagnosis for ulcers located in the perianal area or on the buttocks must include HSV. HSV lesions in this location will be extremely painful and have a "punched out" appearance with a pale pink wound bed and surrounding erythema. Herpes lesions can be distinguished from pressure injuries in that the lesions are not limited to a bony prominence and are more typical over the fleshy part of the buttocks. These can also be distinguished from chemical irritation (such as occurs with diarrhea) by the presence of several isolated ulcers rather than the confluence of superficial denudement or erythema that impinges on the anal opening.

The clinical presentation of grouped vesicles on an erythematous base is highly suggestive of HSV, regardless of body site. The most definitive method for confirming the infection is to unroof the intact vesicle so that the vesicular fluid can be cultured. Rapid testing (within a few hours) also can be done with direct fluorescent antibody examination. Commercially available kits can distinguish among HSV-1, HSV-2, and VZV.

Antiviral medications are effective in treating HSV infection and are available for topical, oral, and intravenous administration. Early initiation of oral acyclovir for genital herpes decreases healing time, viral shedding, and duration of pain.

Nursing care should be directed at absorbing excess moisture, avoiding trauma, and providing comfort. Alginate dressings with a secondary dressing, such as a transparent dressing or foam, can be used to absorb exudate (Chacon & Ferreira, 2009). When the lesions are relatively dry yet painful, Burrow's solution (aluminum acetate) soaks and refrigerated hydrogel dressings can relieve the topical pain. When shedding HSV lesions are present, skin cleansing should be done cautiously to prevent spreading of the virus, particularly when the lesions are present on the buttocks.

Varicella-Zoster Virus

VZV causes varicella (chickenpox) and herpes zoster (shingles). VZV is highly contagious and is transmitted by direct contact with either vesicular fluid or airborne droplets from the infected host's respiratory tract. Airborne transmission as a mode for spreading VZV is very serious. Spread of varicella with no direct contact has been reported; the sole exposure was to air that flowed from the room of the infected individual to another room. Herpes zoster is contagious to patients who have never had VZV (they will get VZV not HSV) but not to individuals who have already had VZV.

Herpes zoster is an infection within the epidermis that is characteristically unilateral and occurs along one or two adjacent dermatome distributions (Fig. 9.2). Eruptions result from the reactivation of VZV in cranial or spinal nerve ganglia that then spread to cutaneous nerves. Reactivation, which can occur as a result of immunosuppression, fatigue, radiation therapy, and emotional trauma, occurs in 15% of people (American Academy of Dermatology, 2008; Habif et al., 2018). The elderly may be predisposed to herpes zoster as a consequence of a potential decline in immunologic function. Individuals who are immunocompromised are at risk for developing VZV and experience more severe infections. These patients are more likely to develop disseminated disease with extensive skin lesions, pneumonia, hepatitis, or encephalitis (Zaia, 2008). Diagnosis is most often based on history and clinical appearance. The DNA polymerase chain reaction assay and direct immunofluorescent stain of a skin scraping for VZV antigen are accurate and rapid diagnostic tests for chickenpox and zoster and are preferred over the Tzanck preparation or tissue culture (Zaia, 2015).

Herpes zoster has characteristic manifestations that begin with a burning pain, followed by erythema and red, swollen plaques of various sizes and across part or all of a dermatome (Dinulos, 2021). Variously sized vesicles erupt in clusters and become purulent. This is in contrast to the uniformly sized vesicles typical of herpes simplex. These pustules then rupture and crust over. In some debilitated patients, the eruptions become more extensive and inflammatory, with blisters, necrosis, or secondary infections developing. VZV in the immunocompromised patient may last from weeks to months, and the resulting ulcer may develop a black, adherent eschar (see Plate 21). Postherpetic neuralgia (pain that

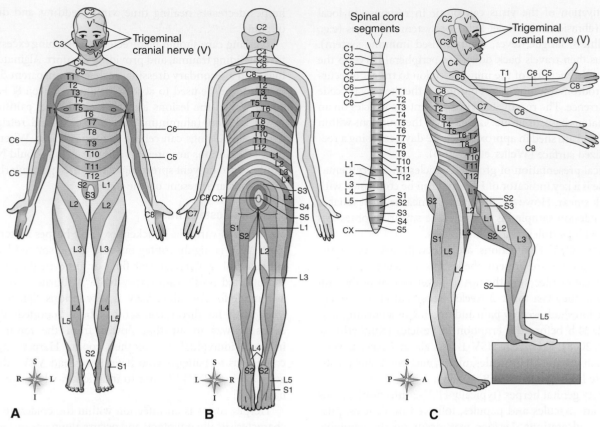

Fig. 9.2 Segmental dermatome distribution of spinal nerves to the front, back, and side of the body. Dermatomes are specific skin surface areas innervated by a single spinal nerve or group of spinal nerves. *C,* cervical segments; *CX,* coccygeal segment; *L,* lumbar segments; *S,* sacral segments; *T,* thoracic segments. (From Patton, K. T., & Thibodeau, G. A. (2015). *Anatomy and physiology* (9th ed.). St. Louis: Mosby.)

persists beyond 1 month after healing) is a major complication of shingles; thus aggressive analgesia is an essential component of treatment.

Treatment of herpes zoster requires acyclovir (Zovirax) 800 mg five times daily for 7–10 days, valacyclovir (Valtrex) 1000 mg three times per day, or famciclovir (Famvir) 500 mg three times per day (Dinulos, 2021). Early intervention with systemic antiviral medications lessens postherpetic neuralgia and decreases healing time and viral shedding. Topical antivirals are not recommended in the management of herpes zoster. Burrow's solution can be applied to act as an astringent on the lesions. Daily soaks with salt solutions may minimize bacterial infection (Zaia, 2015). Anecdotally, dressings that reduce moisture in the zoster lesion, such as foam, can be used to protect the lesion from trauma and friction and reduce pain at the site. Moisture-donating dressings such as hydrocolloids or transparent dressings, however, should be avoided.

ALLERGIC FACTORS

Numerous allergic responses, both local and systemic, can be manifested on the skin. Because the wound specialist is in a likely position to observe such reactions, it is important to be able to describe the manifestations accurately and to report the assessment to the provider in a timely fashion. This section focuses on those allergic responses that are localized reactions to items such as adhesives, wound care products, and solutions. These types of skin damage are commonly referred to as *allergic contact dermatitis.*

Allergic contact dermatitis is an immunologic response to an allergen. Contact dermatitis occurs more readily in the presence of a preexisting skin disorder in which the cutaneous barrier is disrupted.

A true allergic dermatitis requires exposure to an allergen and has two phases:

1. The sensitization phase (the skin of a nonsensitized individual is exposed to a substance or chemical) transpires over a 7- to 10-day period. Small molecules from the allergen pass through the epidermis and attach to an epidermal protein found on the surface of the Langerhans cell. From here, these cells migrate through the dermis to the lymph nodes, where they present the allergen to T lymphocytes. Subsequently, effector and memory T lymphocytes proliferate in the lymph node, are released to circulate in the blood, and ultimately return to the skin. Here the body develops the ability to recognize the antigen when it reappears on the skin, and the T lymphocytes are now "primed" (Weller et al., 2015).

2. When the individual is reexposed to the allergen, the elicitation phase occurs within 48–72 h. Once the Langerhans cell delivers the antigen to memory T cells in the skin, effector T cells begin to produce lymphokines. Inflammatory cells are summoned by the lymphokines, and allergic manifestations can be observed. Suppressor T cells are believed to end the inflammatory reaction.

An acute inflammatory response occurs within 48 h of reexposure to an allergen. Clinical manifestations begin with erythema, followed by pruritus. Primary lesions are vesicles, bullae, papules, plaques, and wheals (Plate 6). Secondary lesions include moist desquamation (see Plate 23), edema, fissure, excoriation, and crust (Plate 7). An acute reaction usually resolves in days to weeks, after the allergen has been removed.

The cause or source of the allergen may be obvious, or it may be obscured by other concurrent processes. A careful, detailed assessment and interview are imperative to identify the skin reaction as an allergic response. Common allergic sensitizers include poison ivy, nickel (used in jewelry), rosins, rubber compounds (used in elastic, gloves), benzocaine (used in antipruritic creams), paraphenylenediamine (dye used to color hair), and preservatives. Topical preparations with one of the following ingredients are other common allergic offenders: aloe vera, fragrances, parabens, quaternium 15, diphenhydramine (Benadryl spray or Caladryl lotion), neomycin (Neosporin), and *para*-aminobenzoic acid (PABA) (Dinulos, 2021). Overuse of soaps, cleansers, moisturizers, and cosmetics can produce reactions. Many chemicals with similar structures cross-react, so a person who is sensitive to one product may be sensitive to several other products.

The location and distribution of the skin inflammation are important clues in identifying the causative agent. Allergic contact dermatitis is localized to the skin where the product is applied, and involved areas typically have sharp margins (Plate 23B). For example, an allergic reaction to an adhesive will be in the shape of the adhesive and will have well-defined borders. Allergic contact dermatitis can spread from the original site of application through inadvertent transfer of the allergen by the hands or, as the disease progresses, by the circulating T lymphocytes. However, the skin reaction begins and remains most severe in the area in which contact with the antigen occurred (Weller et al., 2015).

Patch tests can be conducted to confirm the suspected agent that is causing the allergic reaction; however, these tests must be properly conducted and interpreted. Suspected allergens are applied to the skin and secured with tape. The patient's back usually is the preferred site for patch testing. After 48 h, the patches are removed and the test site assessed for skin damage, which is graded using a standard scale as listed in Box 9.8. Although the patch test seems simple to apply and read, it is a complicated procedure that requires training and experience to obtain valid results (Fowler & Zirwas, 2019).

Simply avoiding contact with allergens can prevent allergic contact dermatitis. However, recognizing or identifying

BOX 9.8 Scale for Interpretation of Patch Test Results

Score	Signifies
+	Weak (nonvesicular) positive reaction: erythema, infiltration, possibly papules
++	Strong (edematous or vesicular) positive reaction
+++	Extreme (spreading, bullous, ulcerative) positive reaction
–	Negative reaction
IR	Irritant reactions of different types
NT	Not tested
Macular erythema only is a doubtful reaction.	

Adapted from Dinulos, J. G. H. (2021). *Habif's clinical dermatology: A color guide to diagnosis and therapy* (7th ed.). St. Louis: Elsevier.

potential allergens is the key to prevention and may not be an easy task.

When an allergic response is suspected, use of the offending product or chemical should be discontinued. Often a substitute can be used. Use of antiinflammatory medications may be warranted topically or systemically and usually is determined based on the severity of the allergic reaction.

RADIATION

Radiation therapy is an established, essential treatment of most types of cancer. It is estimated that as many as half of all patients with cancer will receive radiation therapy as a primary, adjunctive, or palliative intervention (Leventhal & Young, 2017). Although the techniques and technologies for radiotherapy have improved, radiation-induced skin damage, or radiation dermatitis, will affect up to 95% of people receiving radiation (Singh, Alavi, Wong, & Akita, 2016). The evidence for the optimal treatments for prevention and management remains lacking and inconsistent; without a gold standard for care, decisions for prevention and management are based on professional opinion and anecdotal evidence rather than clinical evidence (Chan et al., 2014; Haruna, Lipsett, & Marignol, 2017).

Mechanisms of Injury

Ionizing radiation exerts direct tissue injury to curtail the growth of neoplastic cells; however, it also generates free radicals and reactive oxygen intermediates that further damage cellular components, including DNA, proteins, and cellular membranes. In response to the free radicals, the damaged keratinocytes recruit inflammatory cytokines, specifically interleukin-1 and interleukin-6, tumor necrosis factor-α, and transforming growth factor-β (Kole, Kole, & Moran, 2017; Singh et al., 2016; Yang, Ren, Guo, Hu, & Fu, 2020). Unfortunately, the effects of radiation therapy are not restricted to malignant cells. Rapidly proliferating tissues, such as intestinal mucosa, bone marrow, and skin, are more susceptible to radiation. In addition, radiosensitization techniques and breast-preserving procedures are often used to enhance the effect of radiation on tumor cells that also impact healthy tissues (Leventhal & Young, 2017; Singh et al., 2016; Yang et al., 2020).

The skin is particularly vulnerable to the effects of radiation because it is in a continuous state of cellular renewal. Damage is incurred by rapidly dividing cells, such as keratinocytes, hair follicles, sebaceous glands, epidermal basal cells, endothelial cells, and vascular components. A reduction of Langerhans cells also occurs. Because radiation damages the mitotic ability of stem cells in the basal layer, regrowth of new cells is slowed and skin integrity becomes impaired (Leventhal & Young, 2017; Singh et al., 2016; Yang et al., 2020).

Pathophysiologic Characteristics

The onset of radiation dermatitis depends on dose intensity and the individual's normal tissue sensitivity. The spectrum of skin reactions that can occur with radiation therapy (radiation dermatitis) as categorized by the National Cancer Institute is listed in Table 9.5. Treatment effects will be confined to the treatment area. Early effects will generally manifest within 2–3 weeks after beginning therapy. Because acute radiation effects are cumulative, the greatest reactions occur toward the end of therapy. However, side effects usually are self-limiting, and most subside 2–4 weeks after therapy has ended (Kole et al., 2017; Leventhal & Young, 2017).

Table 9.6 describes clinical symptoms and time of onset of acute radiation dermatitis. Initially the skin in the treatment field will develop faint, transient erythema, which may become increasingly brisk and persistent. Erythema will appear as a red, macular rash on warm-appearing skin that may feel sensitive and tight. It is an inflammatory response thought to be caused by dilation of the capillaries and increased vascular permeability; therefore, edema may accompany erythema.

Dry desquamation may occur 3–6 weeks into the regimen with cumulative doses above 20 Gy and will appear as red or tan pigmented skin that is dry, itchy, and peeling or flaky (Leventhal & Young, 2017). This reaction is a result of the decreased ability of the basal cells of the epidermis to replace the surface layer cells and the decreased ability of the sweat and sebaceous glands to produce sweat. As the cumulative dose of radiation increases (above 30–40 Gy), the erythema and dry desquamation may evolve into moist desquamation, which is characterized by exposure of the dermis as a result of blisters, peeling, and sloughing. Moist desquamation is characterized by tender red skin with serous exudate, and the potential for bullae. This break in the skin barrier poses a risk of infection, discomfort from friction, and pain, possibly requiring interruption of the treatment plan to allow for healing (Kole et al., 2017; Leventhal & Young, 2017). A combination of erythema and dry and moist desquamation may be seen within a single treatment field.

Eventually irradiated skin will develop epidermal atrophy; the epidermis is thin, dry, and translucent. Sweat and sebaceous glands and hair follicles usually are absent. Telangiectasias and blood vessels are easily visible. Subendothelial connective tissue in small arteries proliferate, causing narrowing and thrombosis of the microvasculature (i.e., progressive obliterative endarteritis), and loss of elasticity due to damage to the elastic fibers in the dermis causes fibrosis (Kole et al., 2017; Yang et al., 2020). As many as 23% of women with breast cancer treated with excisional biopsy and primary radiation therapy will experience

TABLE 9.6   Clinical Symptoms and Time of Onset of Acute Radiation Dermatitis

Skin Condition	Time of Onset	Radiation Dose at Onset (Gy)
Hyperpigmentation/erythema	1–2 weeks after RT	10–40
Dry desquamation	3–4 weeks after RT	20–30
Moist desquamation	≥4 weeks after RT	30–40

From Leventhal, J., & Young, M. R. (2017). Radiation dermatitis: Recognition, prevention, and management. *Cancer Network.* https://www.cancernetwork.com/view/radiation-dermatitis-recognition-prevention-and-management.

TABLE 9.5   Grading Systems for Radiation Dermatitis

	Grade 1	Grade 2	Grade 3	Grade 4
CTCAE 4.0	Faint erythema or dry desquamation	Moderate to brisk erythema; patchy moist desquamation, mostly confined to skin folds and creases; moderate edema	Moist desquamation other than skin folds and creases; bleeding induced by minor trauma or abrasion	Life threatening skin necrosis or ulceration of full-thickness dermis, spontaneous bleeding and a need for skin grafts
RTOG	Faint erythema Dry desquamation Epilation Decreased sweating	Tender or bright erythema Moderate edema Patchy moist desquamation	Moist desquamation in areas other than skin folds Pitting edema	Ulceration Hemorrhage Necrosis

CTCAE, Common Terminology Criteria for Adverse Events; *RTOG,* Radiation Therapy Oncology Group.
Adapted from Leventhal, J., & Young, M. R. (2017). Radiation dermatitis: Recognition, prevention, and management. *Cancer Network.* https://www.cancernetwork.com/view/radiation-dermatitis-recognition-prevention-and-management.

radiation-induced fibrosis; a complication that typically develops within the first 3 months following radiation therapy (Ramseier, Ferreira, & Levanthal, 2020). These effects develop gradually over several months or years and are a function of the daily dose, total dose, high volume of the area irradiated, energy and particles used, interval between fractions, and concomitant chemotherapy or biologic modifier. Late effects are more likely to be significant when acute reactions are significant. Late radiation damage can be further complicated by several conditions: secondary ulceration, impaired joint mobility, shedding or deformity of the nails, malignancies (basal and squamous cell), and lymphedema (caused by fibrosis of the lymph glands). When ulceration and necrosis occur years after radiation therapy, they usually occur in conjunction with trauma or infection. These lesions can become very painful and difficult to manage.

Another reaction to radiation is termed *radiation recall*, which is defined as the "recalling" of an inflammatory reaction of the skin that occurred in a previous irradiated area following the administration of certain chemotherapeutic agents and occurs greater than 1 week after completion of radiation therapy (Bray, Simmons, Wolfson, & Nouri, 2016; Camidge & Price, 2001). The estimated incidence of this poorly understood phenomenon is 1%–10% in patients who receive a systemic agent after radiation therapy. The extent of damage can range from erythema to erosion and ulceration. Although radiation recall reaction has been observed from most classes of chemotherapeutic medications, those most commonly associated with radiation recall are docetaxel, doxorubicin, gemcitabine, and paclitaxel (Burris & Hurtig, 2010). Additional medications associated with radiation recall include antimicrobial/antibacterial agents (cefotetan, cefaxoline, trimetrexate, and levofloxacin), nimesulide (nonsteroidal antiinflammatory agent), simvastatin, anti-TB medications, phentermine (an anorexiant), and hypericin (St. John's wort) (Burris & Hurtig, 2010). Once recall dermatitis is detected, the precipitating medication may be withheld until the dermatitis resolves or continued based on the severity or extent of the reaction. Treatment with corticosteroids is often indicated. Skin reactions can develop from 8 months to 3 years following radiation therapy and may be sporadic in that they may not occur each time that medication is received (Burris & Hurtig, 2010).

Risk Factors

Substantial variations in the degree of acute and late normal tissue reactions exist even in patients who have received identical treatments. Thus identifying patients at risk for severe radiation-induced skin reactions is difficult. Treatment schedule and total dose in radiation therapy are based on the tumoricidal doses and the tolerance dose of the perifocal normal tissue.

The quality of the irradiation and its modalities, including total dose, fractionation, and interfractional interval, appear to affect functional and cosmetic outcome the most. Risk factors that appear to influence the severity, onset, and duration of radiation skin reaction include age, general skin condition, and nutritional status. At risk for the highest stages of reaction are body areas within the treatment field, including bony prominences and moist areas on the body, such as skin folds, under the breast, the axillae, neck, perineum, and groin (Singh et al., 2016; Yang et al., 2020). Patients who are receiving combination therapy also are at risk because concomitant use of chemotherapy may sensitize the basal cells to radiation (Leventhal & Young, 2017).

Care of Irradiated Skin

Radiation triggers inflammatory processes in the skin and cytokine overproduction. Skin care before, during, and after radiation is aimed at minimizing these effects and preventing dessication or dry desquamation (Haruna et al., 2017). Topical skin care should be based on best evidence of effectiveness, the ability to soothe the skin and promote patient comfort, and compatibility with ionizing radiation.

Patient education on skin care is critical when preparing the patient for radiation and during therapy. Patients should be instructed on the typical effects of radiation on the skin (dry desquamation), measures to promote moisture retention in the treatment area, the potential for radiation recall (when applicable), to protect the area from trauma and potential irritants (i.e., alcohol, perfumes, products containing α-hydroxy acid), and to only use products in the treatment field that have been approved by the health care team.

Many studies have been conducted exploring the use of topical products to both prevent and treat radiation dermatitis. In general, results are mixed or insignificant findings often owing to methodological issues (small sample size, lack of controls, absence of randomization, etc.). Table 9.7 provides a summary of evidence for topical skin care products. It is common to recommend an emollient or moisturizer throughout the radiation therapy course to prevent dermatitis and reduce dry desquamation (Haruna et al., 2017; Leventhal & Young, 2017). Once radiation dermatitis develops, topical corticosteroids can be applied to reduce inflammation and cytokine production and significantly reduce the severity of radiation dermatitis. The incidence of wet desquamation has been reported as 2.5–5 times less likely with the use of a steroid (Haruna et al., 2017; Salvo et al., 2010). A practice guideline for skin care and prevention of acute skin reactions based on these reports is given in Checklist 9.1.

Dressings

Numerous topical dressings have been used to treat acute radiation dermatitis, including film dressings, hydrogels, foams, alginates, slow-released silver hydrofiber dressing, silver sulfadiazine cream, and hydrocolloid dressings (Kole et al., 2017; Leventhal & Young, 2017; Ramseier et al., 2020; Yang et al., 2020). When a topical dressing is needed to manage a radiation skin injury, the type of dressing selected must be compatible with the priority needs of the skin condition. For example, transparent film dressings absorb little exudate and would be inappropriate for moist desquamation. In contrast, hydrocolloids or foam dressings can be used with

TABLE 9.7 Skin Care Products and Radiation Therapy: Summary of Evidence

Product	Description	Findings
Evidence for Use or FDA Approved		
Hydrophilic lotions and creams	Moisturizers: Lubriderm, Glaxal base, Eucerin, Keri lotion, Aquaphor	• May be helpful in preventing radiation skin reactions • Product should be unscented, lanolin free • Gently apply (do not rub) twice per day
Calendula ointment	Pot marigold believed to have antiviral and antiinflammatory effects Has been used to treat acne, control bleeding, soothe irritated tissue	• May decrease occurrence of radiation dermatitis (limited evidence) • Compared with Biafine, reported to provide statistically significant reduction in skin reaction, pain, and need for treatment interruption
Hyaluronic acid cream	Lubricating agent found in the body	• May be radioprotective (limited evidence) • Used to treat very dry, scaly skin
Aloe vera gel	Extracted from pulp of aloe vera leaves	• May be used to soothe, cool radiated skin for comfort • Lack of evidence supporting or refuting use for prevention or treatment of radiation dermatitis • Product does not moisturize and should be discontinued if skin becomes dry
Miaderm cream (Aiden Industries)	Formulated with aloe vera, calendula, hyaluronic acid	• FDA approved for prevention or treatment of radiation dermatitis of skin (limited evidence)
Biafine emulsion (Valeant Pharmaceuticals, Int.)	Water-based emulsion with paraffin wax, trolamine, triethanolamine and avocado oil among the many ingredients	• FDA approved for treatment of radiation dermatitis, burns, other superficial wounds (limited evidence) • Do not interrupt use during course of therapy; use until skin has fully recovered • Temporary tingling sensation may occur 10–15 min after application • Apply three times per day, massage until completely absorbed; do not apply 4 h prior to radiation treatment
Topical corticosteroid creams	Used to decrease proinflammatory mediators, histamine and pruritus	• Radioprotective effect may be present with use of mometasone furoate (MMF) • Inhibits upregulation of IL-6 expression in epithelial cells • Preventive and sustained use of 0.1% betamethasone delays onset of acute radiation dermatitis during breast cancer chest wall radiation therapy
Contraindicated, Off Label, or Lack of Evidence for Use		
α-Hydroxy acid (AHA) cream	Glycolic acid and lactic acid most common AHAs Exfoliates and soothes dry, scaly skin (xerosis)	• Can increase radiation skin reaction • Stinging, burning may occur when applied to irritated skin
Skin sealant wipes, wands, sprays	Protective transparent film containing plasticizing agents such as copolymer Some products contain isopropyl alcohol	• Lack of evidence supporting or refuting use for prevention or treatment of radiation dermatitis • See Table 9.4 for examples of skin sealants • Do not use products with alcohol on radiated skin
Chamomile cream	Extracted from chamomile plant	• Lack of evidence supporting or refuting use for prevention or treatment of radiation dermatitis
Almond ointment	Made with almond oil	• Lack of evidence supporting or refuting use for prevention or treatment of radiation dermatitis
Petrolatum jelly-based products	Hydrophobic/water repelling	• Do not use for prevention or treatment of radiation dermatitis
Aqueous cream	Paraffin-based emulsion containing petroleum jelly, phenoxy ethanol, and purified water	• No evidence supporting use for prevention of radiation skin reactions • Contains petroleum, which is not recommended for prevention or treatment of radiation dermatitis of skin
Sucralfate/ sucralfate derivatives	Antiulcer drug for many years Protects mucous membranes during radiotherapy and chemotherapy Recently demonstrated in animal model to stimulate regeneration of the skin and accelerate wound healing	• Not FDA approved for topical use for prevention or treatment of radiation dermatitis of skin • Small studies in radiation therapy reported that cream significantly prevented acute skin reactions and damaged skin healed significantly faster (findings not consistent in subsequent studies)

FDA, Food and Drug Administration.

Information compiled from the following sources: Leventhal & Young, 2017; Ramseier et al., 2020; Yang et al., 2020; Singh et al., 2016; Del Rosso & Bikowski, 2008; Pozoulakis, Cheng, Han, & Quon, 2021; Haruna et al., 2017; Kole et al., 2017; Wei et al., 2018.

CHECKLIST 9.1   Prevention and Management of Radiation Skin Reactions

Promote (Do Not Limit) Personal Hygiene Practices
✓ Continue showers and baths.
✓ Wear loose-fitting clothing to minimize friction and unnecessary trauma to the skin in the treatment field.
✓ Avoid exposing skin to sun, or extremes of heat or cold.
✓ Use lukewarm water and mild pH-neutral and nonalkaline soaps (e.g., baby soap, Dove, Ivory, Basis).
✓ Use mild nonmedicated shampoo (i.e., baby shampoo) for scalp in patients receiving radiation therapy to the head.
✓ Use electric razor for shaving; avoid preshave or aftershave agents.
✓ Apply deodorant as usual to intact skin throughout treatment.

Promote Comfort
✓ Gently apply (do not rub) unscented, lanolin-free hydrophilic moisturizer twice per day (see Table 9.7 for product examples).
✓ Do not use petrolatum-based products; products with irritants such as alcohol, perfumes, or additives; or products containing α-hydroxy acids.
✓ May use aloe vera to soothe and cool the skin (does not moisturize, so discontinue if skin becomes dry).

✓ For burning and itching, apply normal saline compresses as needed or hydrocortisone cream (if ordered).
✓ Wear loose, soft, breathable, nonbinding clothing that protects skin from sun and wind.
✓ Use cool-mist humidifier if humidity is needed.

Prevent Trauma
✓ Avoid swimming in chlorinated pools, hot tubs, and lakes to minimize exposure to chemicals and bacteria.
✓ Avoid heating pads and ice packs to prevent thermal injury.
✓ Avoid adhesives and tapes to prevent skin tears.

Manage Radiation Dermatitis
✓ Normal saline soaks to provide cooling sensation and loosen crusting in treatment field.
✓ Plain, nonscented, lanolin-free hydrophilic cream for dry desquamation, but discontinue when skin breakdown occurs.
✓ Nonadherent dressings may be used for moist desquamation when it occurs during the course of radiation therapy, but should be removed during the treatment.
✓ Dressings may be used based on the wound/skin care needs (i.e., absorb moisture) once radiation therapy has concluded.

---

minimal to moderate amounts of exudate, such as what occurs with moist desquamation. Given that irradiated skin is characterized by a loss of elasticity, atrophy, and fibrosis, nonadhesive wound dressings are generally preferred to minimize trauma to irradiated skin, avoid skin tears, and prevent pain upon dressing removal (see Chapter 21 for further information about wound care dressings).

Adjunctive Interventions

Hyperbaric oxygen, growth factors, biologic skin substitutes, pentoxifylline, proinflammatory cytokines, and surgery have been used for treatment of radiation-induced necrotic wounds (Ramseier et al., 2020; Yang et al., 2020). Hyperbaric oxygen improves collagen formation, neovascularization, epithelialization, and leukocyte bactericidal activity to improve acute radiation injury by reducing tissue hypoxia and edema (see Chapter 25 for further discussion of hyperbaric oxygen therapy).

Growth factors can be used to manipulate the wound environment to stimulate healing of radiation ulcers.

Platelet-derived growth factor, epidermal growth factor, granulocyte macrophage-colony stimulating factor, plasma-rich protein and interleukins have been reported to stimulate tissue regeneration, remodeling, and proliferation of capillary endothelial cells, chemoattract neutrophils, monocytes, and fibroblasts to the wound site and inhibit inflammation (see Chapter 23 for a discussion of growth factors).

Pentoxifylline, used to treat peripheral vascular disease and improve peripheral microcirculation by increasing the flexibility of red blood cells, provides an antiinflammatory effect by targeting inflammatory cytokines and inhibiting transforming growth factor-β expression (Yang et al., 2020). Additional studies using comparison groups and larger samples are needed to replicate these findings.

Surgical interventions may be used for treatment of some radiation-induced wounds. These procedures involve extensive surgical debridement and removal of all poor-quality tissue and timely reconstruction with well-vascularized soft tissue flaps (see Chapter 35 for further discussion of surgical interventions for wound closure).

CLINICAL CONSULT

A: Referral received for a home-visit consult with a 55-year-old female with diabetes type 2, lupus, and a BMI of 42. She was recently discharged from acute care and is receiving home care for glucose monitoring and IV antibiotics following a dehisced surgical incision. She admits that she does not have an appetite and is struggling to maintain adequate intake. Recently she has developed a rash under her breasts and around her surgical incision. She also reports she has a painful blister over her "tail bone." Following a skin inspection under her breasts and around her incision you find a mixed macular–pustular rash with satellite lesions and surrounding erythema. The integrity and condition of her skin in her abdominal folds is intact with moisture and erythema; no macular pustular lesions and no pruritis. When you examine her sacral and fleshy buttocks area you note four distinct 1 cm round ulcerations with surrounding erythema; grouping of vesicles also present with erythematous base. Lesions are

CLINICAL CONSULT—CONT'D

aligned with the perirectal dermatome. The rim of each ulcer is inflamed and the wound bed is pale pink with a thin layer of tan-white debris. As you obtain your measurements and palpate around the ulcers, she volunteers these are very painful and seemed to develop overnight.

D: MASD under the breasts and surrounding the surgical site with candidiasis present likely associated with moisture entrapment in skin folds and under surgical dressing and change in normal skin flora due to antibiotics. Lesions present on sacrum and fleshy part of buttocks are consistent with herpes which could be precipitated by stress of her illness, steroid medications for lupus, and decreased nutritional intake.

P: Reevaluation type of dressings for surgical incision and frequency of change to better absorb and contain wound exudate. Light dusting of antifungal powder under breasts and surrounding surgical incision to manage candidiasis. Antimicrobial textile

under breasts to absorb moisture. Culture fluid from vesicle. Apply occlusive adherent foam dressing over ulcerations on buttocks to contain drainage and reduce pain. Consider implementing antiviral medication orally. Encourage protein and vitamins to meet wound healing needs.

I: (1) Consult with dietary for recommendations on nutritional supplements. (2) Instruct patient on indications of resolution or worsening of candidiasis. (3) Reassure patient that this type of herpes is not a reflection on hygiene or sexual behavior. (4) Monitor for resolution of candidiasis and erythema; convert to antifungal cream with mild steroid if macular–pustular rash or erythema persists.

E: Follow-up home visit in 1 week to evaluate effectiveness of interventions, dietary intake, and wound healing of surgical incision.

SUMMARY

- Intact skin provides the first line of defense against microbial invasion and trauma. Different factors can jeopardize the skin's integrity.
- It is important to be able to recognize the skin-related signs of these factors so that the factors can be eliminated, or their intensity reduced substantially.
- Most often, the type of skin damage that the wound specialist will encounter is mechanical or vascular.
- Only with an in-depth skin assessment and history of the skin eruption can the etiology of the skin damage be identified, and the negative sequelae arrested through appropriate prevention and treatment interventions.

- Because the rarer inflammatory, infectious, or disease-related skin lesions often require prompt treatment to be effective, the wound specialist should also be familiar with these types of lesions.
- Although the underlying disease is the critical determinant for wound healing in these situations, the wound specialist is an important partner and interdisciplinary team member because he or she can provide valuable recommendations for wound management that will best address the requirements of the wound and the needs of the patient.

SELF-ASSESSMENT QUESTIONS

1. List six factors known to damage the skin.
2. Which of the following is described as a lesion that is raised, solid, and less than 1 cm in diameter?
   a. Macule
   b. Papule
   c. Pustule
   d. Nodule
3. A blister that measures 1.5 cm in diameter may also be called which of the following?
   a. Bulla
   b. Pustule
   c. Vesicle
   d. Wheal
4. Which of the following statements about erosion is *true*?
   a. Erosion involves the loss of epidermis and dermis.
   b. Erosion heals by scar formation.
   c. Erosion involves partial loss of epidermis.
   d. Erosion extends into subcutaneous tissue.

5. Which of the following accurately characterizes chemical skin irritation?
   a. Erythema with satellite lesions
   b. Erythema and erosion of skin
   c. Ulcerations with necrotic tissue in wound bed
   d. Ulcerations with pustules
6. Which of the following characterizes varicella-zoster virus?
   a. It requires prior exposure to genital herpes.
   b. It is reactivated by mechanical trauma.
   c. It consists of a bilateral vesicular rash.
   d. It develops along one or two dermatomes.
7. State the two phases of an allergic contact dermatitis.
8. Candidiasis can be described as which of the following?
   a. Pustular or macular papular rash with erythema
   b. Papular rash within the hair follicle
   c. Pustular rash in clusters
   d. Vesicular rash with plaque formation

9. Which of the following statements about herpes simplex virus is *true*?
   a. It initially develops as papules.
   b. Secondary lesions consist of necrotic plaques.
   c. Erythema signifies a secondary infection.
   d. Vesicles are uniformly shaped and grouped.

REFERENCES

Association of periOperative Registered Nurses (AORN). (2021). AORN recommended practices for positioning the patient in the perioperative practice setting. In *AORN standards, recommended practices, and guidelines.* Denver: AORN.

Bank, D., & Nix, D. (2006). Preventing skin tears in a nursing and rehabilitation center: An interdisciplinary effort. *Ostomy/Wound Management, 52*(9), 38–46.

Baranoski, S. (2003). How to prevent and manage skin tears. *Advances in Skin & Wound Care, 16*(5), 268–270.

Bartlett, J. G. (2015). Antibiotic-associated diarrhea. In D. Schlossberg (Ed.), *Clinical infectious disease.* New York: Cambridge University Press.

Beeckman, D., Schoonhoven, L., Verhaerghe, S., et al. (2009). Prevention and treatment of incontinence-associated dermatitis: Literature review. *Journal of Advanced Nursing, 65*(6), 1141–1154.

Beeckman, D., Woodward, S., & Gray, M. (2011). Incontinence-associated dermatitis: Step-by-step prevention and treatment. *British Journal of Community Nursing, 16*(8), 382–389.

Benoit, R. A., Jr., & Watts, C. (2007). The effect of a pressure ulcer prevention program and the bowel management system in reducing pressure ulcer prevalence in an ICU setting. *Journal of Wound, Ostomy, and Continence Nursing, 34*(2), 163–175.

Bradley, S. F. (2015). Staphylococcus. In D. Schlossberg (Ed.), *Clinical infectious disease.* New York: Cambridge University Press.

Brannon, J. (2021). Intertrigo. In *Yeast infection in skin folds.* About.com: dermatology, updated June 16, 2021 http://dermatology.about.com/od/fungalinfections/a/intertrigo.htm. Accessed August 18, 2021.

Bray, F. N., Simmons, B. J., Wolfson, A. H., & Nouri, K. (2016). Acute and chronic cutaneous reactions to ionizing radiation therapy. *Dermatology and Therapy, 6*(2), 185–206.

Burris, H. A., & Hurtig, J. (2010). Radiation recall with anticancer agents. *The Oncologist, 15,* 1227–1237.

Camidge, R., & Price, A. (2001). Characterizing the phenomenon of radiation recall dermatitis. *Radiotherapy and Oncology, 59,* 237–245.

Carpenter, C. F. (2015). Candidiasis. In D. Schlossberg (Ed.), *Clinical infectious disease.* New York: Cambridge University Press.

Centers for Disease Control and Prevention. (2014). *Workplace safety and health topics: Safe patient handling.* http://www.cdc.gov/niosh/topics/safepatient/. Accessed August 25, 2021.

Chacon, J., & Ferreira, L. (2009). Hemicellulose dressing for skin lesions caused by herpes zoster in a patient with leukemia—An alternative dressing. *Wounds, 21*(1), 10–14.

Chan, R. J., Webster, J., Chung, B., Marquart, L., Ahmed, M., & Garantzoitis, S. (2014). Prevention and treatment of acute radiation-induced skin reactions: A systematic review and meta-analysis of randomized controlled trials. *BMC Cancer, 14,* 53. http://www.biomedcentral.com/1471-2407/14/53.

Del Rosso, J. Q., & Bikowski, J. (2008). Trolamine-containing topical emulsion: Clinical applications in dermatology. *Cutis, 81*(3), 209–214. PMID: 18441842.

Dinulos, J. G. H. (2021). *Habif's clinical dermatology: A color guide to diagnosis and therapy* (7th ed.). St. Louis: Elsevier.

Eddins, C., & Gray, M. (2008). Are probiotic or symbiotic preparations effective for the management of clostridium difficile-associated or radiation-induced diarrhea? *Journal of Wound, Ostomy, and Continence Nursing, 35*(1), 50–58.

Fowler, J. F., & Zirwas, M. H. (2019). *Fisher's contact dermatitis* (7th ed.). Phoenix: Contact Dermatitis Institute.

Gefen, A. (2007). Risk factors for pressure-related deep tissue injury: A theoretical model. *Medical & Biological Engineering & Computing, 45*(6), 563–573.

Gefen, A., Farid, K. J., & Shaywitz, I. (2013). A review of deep tissue injury development, detection, and prevention: Shear savvy. *Ostomy/Wound Management, 59*(2), 26–35.

Gray, M., Black, J. M., Baharestani, M. M., et al. (2011). Moisture-associated skin damage: Overview and pathophysiology. *Journal of Wound, Ostomy, and Continence Nursing, 38*(3), 233–241.

Gray, M., Bliss, D. Z., Doughty, D. B., et al. (2007). Incontinence associated dermatitis: A consensus. *Journal of Wound, Ostomy, and Continence Nursing, 34*(1), 45–54.

Habif, T. P., Dinulos, J. G. H., Chapan, M. S., & Zug, K. A. (2018). *Skin disease: Diagnosis and treatment* (4th ed.). St. Louis, MO: Elsevier.

Haruna, F., Lipsett, A., & Marignol, L. (2017). Topical management of acute radiation dermatitis in great cancer patients: A systematic review and meta-analysis. *Anticancer Research, 37,* 5343–5353.

Higa, J. T., & Kelly, C. P. (2013). New drugs and strategies for management of *Clostridium difficile* colitis. *Journal of Intensive Care Medicine, 29,* 190–199.

Imhoff, A., & Karpa, K. (2009). Is there a future for probiotics in preventing Clostridium difficile-associated disease and treatment of recurrent episodes? *Nutrition in Clinical Practice, 4*(1), 15–32.

Irving, V., Bethell, E., & Burtin, F. (2006). Neonatal wound care: Minimizing trauma and pain. *Wounds UK, 2,* 33–41.

Kauffman, C. A. (2008). Candidiasis. In J. S. Tan, M. J. Tan, R. A. Salata, T. M. File Jr., et al. (Eds.), *Expert guide to infectious diseases* (2nd ed., pp. 527–540). Philadelphia: ACP Press.

Kim, J., Shim, M. C., Choi, B. Y., et al. (2001). Clinical application of continent anal plug in bedridden patients with intractable diarrhea. *Diseases of the Colon and Rectum, 44,* 1162–1167.

Kimberlin, D. W., & Whitley, R. J. (2008). Herpes simplex viruses 1 and 2. In D. Schlossberg (Ed.), *Clinical infectious disease.* New York: Cambridge University Press.

Kole, A. J., Kole, L., & Moran, M. S. (2017). Acute radiation dermatitis in breast cancer patients: Challenges and solutions. *Breast Cancer: Targets and Therapy, 9,* 313–323.

Kowal-Vern, A., Poulakidas, S., Barnett, B., et al. (2009). Fecal containment in bedridden patients: Economic impact of 2 commercial bowel catheter systems. *American Journal of Critical Care, 18,* 2–14.

LeBlanc, K., & Baranoski, S. (2009). Prevention and management of skin tears. *Advances in Skin & Wound Care, 22,* 325–332.

LeBlanc, K., Baranoski, S., Christensen, D., et al. (2013). International Skin Tear Advisory Panel: A tool kit to aid in the prevention, assessment, and treatment of skin tears using a Simplified Classification System ©. *Advances in Skin & Wound Care, 26*(10), 459–476.

LeBlanc, K., Christensen, D., Orstead, H. L., et al. (2008). Best practice recommendations for the prevention and treatment of skin tears. *Wound Care Canada, 6*(1), 14–32.

LeBlanc, K., et al. (2018). Best practice recommendations for the prevention and management of skin tears in aged skin. *Wounds International.* Available to download from www.woundsinternational.com

Leventhal, J., & Young, M. R. (2017). Radiation dermatitis: Recognition, prevention, and management. *Cancer Network.* https://www.cancernetwork.com/view/radiation-dermatitis-recognition-prevention-and-management.

Malone, M. L., Rozario, N., Gavinski, M., et al. (1991). The epidemiology of skin tears in the institutionalized elderly. *Journal of American Geriatric Society, 39*(6), 591–595.

Martin, J. S., Monaghan, T. M., & Wilcox, M. H. (2016). Clostridium difficile infection: Advances in Epidemiology, Diagnosis and Transmission. *Nature Reviews Gastroenterology and Hepatology, 13*(4), 206–216. ISSN 1759-5045.

McDonald, L. C., Gerding, D. N., Johnson, S., Bakken, J. S., Carroll, K. C., Coffin, S. E., et al. (2018). Clinical practice guidelines for *clostridium difficile* infection in adults and children: 2017 update by the Infectious Diseases Society of America (ISDA) and Society for Healthcare Epidemiology of America (SHEA). *Clinical Infectious Diseases, 66*(7), e1–e48.

McGough-Csarny, J., & Kopac, C. A. (1998). Skin tears in institutionalized elderly: An epidemiological study. *Ostomy Wound Management, 44*(Suppl. 3A), 14S–24S.

McNichol, L., Lund, C., Rosen, T., et al. (2013). Medical adhesives and patient safety: State of the science: Consensus statements for the assessment, prevention, and treatment of adhesive-related skin injuries. *Journal of Wound, Ostomy, and Continence Nursing, 40*(4), 365–380.

National Pressure Ulcer Advisory Panel (NPUAP). (2018). *Terms and definitions related to support surfaces.* https://cdn.ymaws.com/npiap.com/resource/resmgr/s3i_terms-and-defs-feb-5-201.pdf. Accessed August 18, 2021.

Niederhuber, J., Armitage, J. O., Doroshow, J., Kastan, M., & Tepper, J. (2014). *Abeloff's clinical oncology* (5th ed.). Philadelphia: Elsevier.

PA Patient Safety Authority. (2006). Skin tears: The clinical challenge. *PA PSRS Patient Safety Advisory, 3*(3),1, 5–10. Accessed February 4, 2023 from http://patientsafety.pa.gov/ADVISORIES/Pages/200609_01b.aspx.

Payne, R. L., & Martin, M. L. (1990). The epidemiology and management of skin tears in older adults. *Ostomy/Wound Management, 26*, 26–37.

Pozoulakis, E. C., Cheng, Z., Han, P., & Quon, H. (2021). Radiation-induced skin dermatitis. *Clinical Journal of Oncology Nursing, 25*(4), E44–E49.

Ramseier, J. Y., Ferreira, M. N., & Levanthal, J. S. (2020). Dermatologic toxicities associated with radiation therapy in women with breast cancer. *International Journal of Women's Dermatology, 6*, 349–356.

Ratliff, C. R., & Fletcher, K. R. (2007). Skin tears: A review of the evidence to support prevention and treatment. *Ostomy Wound Management, 53*(3), 32–34.

Roberts, M. J. (2007). Preventing and managing skin tears: A review. *Journal of Wound Ostomy and Continence Nursing, 34*(3), 256–259.

Salvo, N., Barnes, E., van Draanen, J., Stacey, E., Mitera, G., Breen, D., et al. (2010). Prophylaxis and management of acute radiation induced skin reactions: A systematic review of the literature. *Current Oncology, 17*(4), 94–112.

Schutze, G. E., Willougby, R. E., Committee on Infectious Diseases, et al. (2013). *Clostridium difficile* infections in infants and children (policy statement). *Pediatrics, 131*(1), 196–200.

Sibbald, R. G., Kelley, J., Kennedy-Evans, K. L., et al. (2013). A practical approach to the prevention and management of intertrigo, or moisture-associated skin damage, due to perspiration: Expert consensus on best practice. *Wound Care Canada, 11*(Suppl. 2), 4–21.

Singh, M., Alavi, A., Wong, R., & Akita, S. (2016). Radiodermatitis: A review of our current understanding. *American Journal of Clinical Dermatology, 17*, 277–293.

Stanley, J. D., Bartlett, J. G., Dart, B. W., 4th, & Ashcraft, J. H. (2013). Clostridium difficile infection. *Current Problems in Surgery, 50*(7), 302–337.

Stevens, D. L., Mebane, J. A., & Madaras-Kelly, K. (2015). Streptococcus groups A, B, C, D, G. In D. Schlossberg (Ed.), *Clinical infectious disease* (2nd ed.). New York: Cambridge University Press.

Strazzieri-Pulido, K. C., Peres, G. R. P., Campanilli, T. C. G. F., & Santos, V. L. C. G. (2017). Incidence of skin tears and risk factors. A systematic literature review. *Journal of Wound, Ostomy, and Continence Nursing, 44*(1), 29–33.

Vij, A., & Tomecki, K. J. (2015). Cellulitis and erysipelas. In D. Schlossberg (Ed.), *Clinical infectious disease* (2nd ed.). New York: Cambridge University Press.

Visscher, M. L. (2009). Recent advances in diaper dermatitis: Etiology and treatment. *Pediatric Health, 3*(1), 81–89.

Voegeli, D. (2016). Incontinence-associated dermatitis: New insights into an old problem. *British Journal of Nursing, 325*(5), 256–262.

Waters, T. R., & Rockefeller, K. (2010). Safe patient handling for rehabilitation professionals. *Rehabilitation Nursing, 35*(5), 216–222.

Waters, T. R., Short, M., Lloyd, J., et al. (2011). AORN ergonomic tool 2: Positioning and repositioning the supine patient in the OR bed. *AORN Journal, 93*(4), 445–449.

Wei, J., Meng, L., Hou, X., Qu, C., Wang, B., Xin, Y., & Jiang, X. (2018). Radiation-induced skin reactions: Mechanism and treatment. *Cancer Management Research, 11*, 167–177. https://doi.org/10.2147/CMAR.S188655.

Weller, R. B., Hamish, J. A. H., & Mann, M. W. (2015). *Clinical dermatology* (5th ed.). Oxford: Wiley Blackwell.

Wiederkehr, M., & Schwartz, R. A. (2011). *Tinea cruris: Treatment and medication.* http://emedicine.medscape.com/article/1091806-overview. Accessed August 25, 2021.

Wound, Ostomy and Continence Nurses Society™ (WOCN). (2016). *Guideline for management of pressure ulcers (WOCN® clinical practice guideline series no. 2).* Mt Laurel: Author.

Yang, X., Ren, H., Guo, X., Hu, C., & Fu, J. (2020). Radiation-induced skin injury: Pathogenesis, treatment, and management. *Aging, 12*(22), 23379–23393.

Zaia, J. A. (2015). Varicella-zoster virus. In D. Schlossberg (Ed.), *Clinical infectious disease.* New York: Cambridge University Press.

Zulkowski, K. (2008). Perineal dermatitis versus pressure ulcer: Distinguishing characteristics. *Advances in Skin & Wound Care, 21*(8), 382–388.

Zulkowski, K. (2012). Diagnosing and treating moisture-associated skin damage. *Advances in Skin & Wound Care, 25*(5), 231–236.

FURTHER READING

LeBlanc, K., & Baranowski, S. (2011). Skin tears: State of the science: Consensus statements for the prevention, prediction, assessment, and treatment of skin tears. *Advances in Skin & Wound Care, 24*(9 Suppl), 2–15.

National Cancer Institute. (2010). *Common terminology criteria for adverse events version 4.0 (CTCAE).* http://ctep.cancer.gov/protocolDevelopment/electronic_applications/ctc.htm. Accessed December 18, 2020.

Yan, J., Yuan, L., Wang, J., Li, S., Yao, M., Wang, K., et al. (2020). Mepitel film is superior to Biafine cream in managing acute radiation-induced skin reactions in head and neck cancer patients: A randomized intra-patient controlled clinical trial. *Journal of Medical Radiation Sciences, 678*, 208–216.

10

Skin and Wound Inspection and Assessment

Denise P. Nix

OBJECTIVES

1. Differentiate between skin inspection and skin assessment.
2. List six factors to consider when assessing darkly pigmented skin.
3. Distinguish between wound assessment and evaluation of healing.
4. Define partial-thickness and full-thickness tissue loss.
5. Compare and contrast normal and abnormal findings for each wound assessment parameter.
6. Describe how to measure the length, width, depth, tunneling, and undermining of a wound.

An initial skin and wound assessment provides a baseline and foundation for developing a patient's plan of care. Ongoing skin and wound assessments are crucial because they provide the mechanism for monitoring the effectiveness of that plan, thus allowing determination of progress or deterioration of the wound. Documentation of assessment findings facilitates communication among caregivers. Because of the myriad of etiologic, systemic, and local factors commonly involved in the pathogenesis of a wound, a comprehensive patient assessment is vital to the identification of cofactors that may impair wound healing and jeopardize skin integrity. Although all patients, with or without a wound, require a skin assessment on admission, the patient with a wound requires additional assessments, including underlying causes for the wound and healing impediments.

SIGNIFICANCE

To adequately convey the condition of a wound or a skin lesion, wound and skin assessment requires access to a unique vocabulary. As with monitoring blood pressure, temperature, and pulse rate, those attending to a wound need to use specific parameters to reflect its present status. The state of the science is such that both subjective and objective measures are required to adequately capture the condition of the wound. Because subjective measures can vary in interpretation from one user to another, it is essential that accurate use of wound assessment terminology be emphasized in staff education and that competencies for wound and skin assessment be used (Williams & Deering, 2016; Young, Rohwer, Volmink, et al., 2014). Appendix A contains examples of competencies related to skin and wound management.

The economics of health care impose additional motivation for conducting and documenting a systematic measurement of wound healing. Without objective criteria of the status or progress of repair, it is difficult to justify treatments or assign appropriate reimbursement for services. The standard of care is to provide accurate and routine skin and wound assessments. Failure to assess the patient systematically also carries a great legal liability risk (Halpern & Ravitz, 2017; Painter, Dudjak, Kidwell, Simmons, & Kidwell, 2011). Without accurate, consistent, and retrievable documentation, it is difficult to retrospectively create a clear picture of the patient's condition and of the care that was provided.

ASSESSMENT

Assessment is a two-step process that requires inspection and collection of data and then interpretation of that data so that a plan of care can be derived. During the initial encounter, an assessment provides the baseline data to which comparisons can be made to determine the changes; this is the process of *monitoring*.

The word *assessment* alone as it relates to the prevention and management of wounds can be confusing because several assessments are required: risk assessment (see Chapter 11), skin assessment, wound assessment, and physical assessment. For clarity and safety, findings from each type of assessment must be documented using appropriate terms to describe the patient's skin or wound condition. Staff education and competencies should include how to conduct the assessments and how to link appropriate interventions to the findings (Institute for Healthcare Improvement [IHI] & National Pressure Injury Advisory Panel [NPIAP], 2021).

Skin Inspection and Monitoring

Skin *inspection* involves data collection related to skin changes based on visual and palpable observation, along with the patient's reports of changes in sensation/discomfort. A complete skin inspection must be completed by trained staff on admission (for baseline data). For patients at risk for pressure injuries, it is important to inspect all the skin from head to toe on admission and at least daily (including under and around medical devices, between skin folds and buttocks and under prophylactic dressings) (European Pressure Ulcer Advisory Panel, National Pressure Injury Advisory Panel, & Pan Pacific Pressure Injury Alliance [EPUAP, NPIAP, & PPPIA], 2019; Wound, Ostomy and Continence Nurses Society, 2016). Skin inspection under and around medical devices may need to be performed more frequently (more than twice daily) because most medical devises are in anatomical locations that lack subcutaneous tissue and can therefore develop full-thickness pressure injuries quickly. Examples include skin behind the ears under oxygen tubing or the bridge of the nose under an oxygen mask. International pressure injury guidelines recommend inspection under and around devices greater than twice daily at anatomical locations vulnerable to fluid shifts and edema formation (EPUAP, NPIAP, & PPPIA, 2019). Clinical examples include skin under a new tracheostomy, lower extremity splints in the presence of congestive heart failure or venous insufficiency, or an indwelling urinary catheter securement that fails to stretch as skin expands with edema such as when fluid moves from the intravascular space (blood vessels) into the interstitial tissue (third spacing). Additional device-related skin inspections can be conducted while other routine cares are provided (Table 10.1). See Chapter 11 for further discussion of device-related skin injury.

An adequate skin inspection requires the removal of garments (including shoes and stockings) and effective positioning for optimal visualization (EPUAP, NPIAP, & PPPIA, 2019;

WOCN, 2016). Staff conducting the inspection will need to gently spread skin folds (including the buttocks), check between the toes, and remove or reposition medical devices to inspect for pressure-related skin damage from devices such as oxygen tubing, nasogastric tubes, urinary tubing, drainage tubing, therapeutic stockings, and splints (EPUAP, NPIAP, & PPPIA, 2019; WOCN, 2016). Staff performing the skin inspection should be expected to report the overall skin condition, such as change in skin condition (e.g., intact, broken, denuded), skin color (e.g., red, dusky), texture (e.g., pinpoint macular–papular rash, dry skin), and wounds. These findings then are communicated to a registered nurse or a provider for interpretation, and additional information is collected as needed to further describe and understand the present condition.

The skin and wound condition should be monitored on a routine and regular basis as defined by the facility policy and the severity of the condition. *Monitoring* allows the staff to keep track or "watch" for changes that deviate from the baseline data. For example, 3 days after admission, a reddened area is identified through routine monitoring, whereas the baseline assessment and documentation indicated no redness on admission. The new finding should prompt further assessment to identify etiology so that modifications to the plan of care can be implemented. Part of the plan of care will include continued monitoring and perhaps more frequent repositioning.

Frequency of wound assessment is discussed later in this chapter. However, when dressings over wounds are intact and do not require changing, the dressing should be left in place to allow the wound to proceed through the phases of wound healing without interruption (Brindle & Farmer, 2019). The dressing should be monitored for intactness and the surrounding skin inspected for the presence or absence of discoloration (erythema, bruising), change in texture (induration, edema, boggy) rash, break in skin integrity, and pain. If the dressing is loose or leaking or new observations are made (swelling, pain, erythema), the dressing should be removed, and a thorough wound assessment be obtained.

Skin Assessment

The standard of care is to conduct a routine and systematic skin assessment on all patients on admission. Subsequent skin assessments should be performed routinely. Frequency of reassessment is based on baseline data, care setting, and risk for skin breakdown. For example, patients require daily skin assessments when they (1) are at increased risk for skin breakdown, (2) have impaired skin integrity, or (3) are in an acute care or long-term acute care setting.

Skin with deviations from normal (e.g., firm to touch, boggy, warmth, coolness) should be compared with the adjacent skin or contralateral body part and documented. Techniques for accurate assessment of edema are described and illustrated in Chapter 13, Fig. 13.1 and Box 13.1. Since there has been some indication that localized skin pain is a precursor to skin breakdown, pain should be evaluated with each skin assessment (EPUAP, NPIAP, & PPPIA, 2019). Skin assessment parameters and deviations from normal are listed in Table 10.2. Examples and descriptions of lesions are presented in Chapter 9, Table 9.1, and Plates 6 and 7.

TABLE 10.1 Routine Activities Coordinated With Skin Inspection	
Routine Activity	**Skin Inspection Site**
Oral care and medications	Back of ears, bridge of nose, nares, and lips
Listening to lung sounds	Occiput, spinous process, neck, scapula, coccyx, and sacrum
Perineal skin care/bath	Between and under skin folds of pannus and groin
Application or removal of antiembolism stockings or splints	Feet, heels, toes
Transferring in or out of chair	Coccyx, sacrum, and ischial
Repositioning side to side	Feet, heels, toes, coccyx, sacrum, occiput, scapula, spinous process, trochanter

TABLE 10.2   Skin Assessment Parameters

Findings and Interpretation

Parameter	Technique and Tips	Findings	Interpretation
Color	Conduct inspection in good light; artificial light often distorts colors and masks jaundice Ask patients/family if they have noticed any skin color changes	Pallor	Anemia, decreased blood flow, or arterial insufficiency Advanced lung disease Congestive heart failure Anemia
		Central cyanosis (lips, oral mucosa, or tongue)	Venous obstruction
		Yellow	Jaundice in sclera and skin with liver disease or excessive hemolysis of red blood cells
		Brown discoloration in lower extremities	Hemosiderin staining from venous insufficiency
		Redness	Erythema, an inflammatory response, stage 1 pressure injury
		Dark red/maroon	See Chapter 11, Box 11.3
Moisture	Visual inspection in good light Palpate using the back of fingers	Dry skin	Xerosis Hypothyroidism
		Dermatitis or macular–papular rash in skin folds, perineum, thighs, groin	Intertrigo, tinea, or psoriasis
Turgor	Pinch fold of skin and note speed with which it returns (normally, skin returns quickly to baseline state)	Decreased turgor	Dehydration
Temperature	Palpate using the back of fingers Infrared thermography	Generalized increased warmth	Fever Hyperthyroidism
		Local increased warmth	Inflammation, pressure injury
		Generalized cool	Hypothyroidism or poor vascularization
		Local increased coolness	Pressure injury, necrosis
Texture	Palpate using back of fingers	Roughness	Hypothyroidism
		Edema	See Chapter 13, Fig. 13.1 and Box 13.1
Olfaction	Note odor	Present	Bacteria, metabolic acidosis, hygiene issues
Lesions	Observe any lesions of the skin, noting characteristics such as type, location, color, distribution, arrangement	Primary or secondary skin lesions (macule, papule, pustule)	See Chapter 9, Table 9.1 and Plates 5, 6, 7 and 32
Skin injury	Skin should be intact If skin is open, assess for type of injury	Denuded	Chemical damage, fecal incontinence
		Ulcerated	Unrelieved pressure
		Excoriated	Pruritus, xerosis
Nails (see Chapter 18 for nail abnormalities)	Inspect and palpate fingernails and toenails Note color, shape, and presence of lesions	Clubbing of the fingers	Lung problems
		Onycholysis	Painless separation of nails from nail bed beginning distally
Hair	Inspect and palpate Note quantity, distribution, texture	Alopecia	Hair loss (diffuse)
		Hirsutism	Excessive body hair (may be patchy or total)

Skin assessments require *optimal lighting* for accurate visualization. Alterations including edema, dry skin or xerosis, and color changes such as erythema and dark discoloration should be noted. *Gentle touch and palpation* must be used to assess skin temperature, edema, and tissue consistency and texture in all patients and is of particular importance when assessing darkly pigmented skin since signs of erythema difficult to identify (Baumgarten, Margolis, van Doorn, et al., 2004, 2009; EPUAP, NPIAP, & PPPIA, 2019; WOCN, 2016).

Assessment of Darker Skin Tones

Unfortunately, detection and accurate identification of erythema and stage 1 pressure injuries with standard visual inspection are unreliable in persons with darkly pigmented skin (Bates-Jensen, McCreath, & Pongquan, 2009; EPUAP, NPIAP, & PPPIA, 2019; WOCN, 2016). Unique characteristics of darker versus lighter pigmented skin are summarized in Box 7.1. Teaching points and unique considerations when assessing darkly pigmented skin are provided in Checklist 10.1 (Bennett, 1995). Research has been conducted on enhanced methods for detecting erythema and soft tissue edema through increased levels of subdermal moisture (SEM) as possible methods of predicting early inflammatory signs of pressure injury development. SEM research will be discussed later in this section and in Chapter 11.

CHECKLIST 10.1 Detecting Pressure Injuries on Darkly Pigmented Skin

Color
✓ Tangential light and slight moisturization may aide in detection
✓ Skin color may not change or blanch when pressure is applied to the affected area
✓ Color changes that do occur will differ from the patient's usual skin tone
✓ Localized area of skin injury may be darker than their usual skin tone, or purple/blue or violet (eggplant) instead of red
✓ Skin may be lighter than its original color at the site of a previously closed or healed pressure injury
✓ A color chart can be used to aide in objective assessment of color

Temperature
✓ When compared to adjacent skin, an intact pressure injury may be warm; as the tissue changes color, it will likely be cool (a sign of tissue devitalization)
✓ Gloves may diminish sensitivity to changes in skin temperature
✓ Consider the use of a subepidermal moisture (SEM)/edema measurement device

Texture
• Edema (nonpitting swelling) may occur with induration and may appear taut and shiny

Pain
• Patient may complain of discomfort at a site that is predisposed to pressure injury development

---

Color

Erythema (from the Greek *erythros*, meaning red) is redness or inflammation of the skin or mucous membranes, caused by dilation and congestion of superficial capillaries (O'Toole, 2017). Erythema occurs with many skin injuries, infection, or inflammation, therefore differential diagnosis is critical for an appropriate plan of care. If erythema is identified, it is important to determine whether it is blanchable or nonblanchable. *Blanchable erythema* (Plate 24) turns white when brief pressure is applied, then red when pressure is relieved (capillary refill), indicating reactive hyperemia or inflammatory erythema with an intact capillary bed. *Nonblanchable erythema* is redness that persists after pressure is applied and released, indicating lack of capillary refill (capillary damage). Nonblanchable erythema is known as an independent predictor of skin damage such as with a pressure injury, purpura or petechia (EPUAP, NPIAP, & PPPIA, 2019; Sterner, Lindholm, Berg, et al., 2011). More recently, systemic review and meta-analysis conducted by Shi, Bonnett, Dumville, and Cullum (2020) has shown that people with nonblanchable erythema are more likely to develop stage 2–4 pressure injuries within 28 days than people without nonblanchable erythema, regardless of their age, baseline pressure ulcer risk or received support surfaces.

Two methods of applying pressure to assess for nonblanchable versus blanchable erythema have been reported in the literature and are described in Box 10.1. Both methods have been investigated for reliability with mixed results; however, education, training, and experience appear to improve reliability of both methods (EPUAP, NPIAP, & PPPIA, 2019; Kottner, Dassen, & Lahmann, 2009; Sterner et al., 2011; Vanderwee, Grypdonck, De Bacquer, et al., 2006).

Temperature

Core body temperature and skin temperature plays an important role in wound and skin assessment. A rise *core temperature* is not only indicative of infection, but it's also considered a risk factor for pressure injury risk assessment (EPUAP, NPIAP, & PPPIA, 2019). A rise in *localized skin temperature* (compared with adjacent skin) is also one of the indicators for infection. The use of *infrared thermography* continues to play a role in pressure injury research showing temperatures of deep tissue pressure injury can be normal, elevated, or decreased when compared with adjacent tissue (see Chapter 11).

BOX 10.1 Methods to Assess for Nonblanchable vs Blanchable Erythema

1. Press a finger on the erythema for 3 s and then assessing for blanching immediately upon removal
2. Apply pressure with a transparent disk, watching for blanching underneath the disk

Results
Blanchable erythema—turns white when pressure is applied
Nonblanchable erythema—redness persists when pressure is applied

Physiologically, nonviable tissue is not perfused with a cooler temperature due to lack of blood flow. With reperfusion and severe inflammation, the temperature could increase in an ischemic area (Bhargava, Chanmugam, & Herman, 2015; Cox, Kaes, Martinez, & Moles, 2016; EPUAP, NPIAP, & PPPIA, 2019). Although pressure injury guidelines recommend assessing the temperature of skin and soft tissue, feasibility of integrating thermography into clinical practice has yet to be determined (Bhargava et al., 2015; Cox et al., 2016; EPUAP, NPIAP, & PPPIA, 2019).

Moisture/Dryness

Assessing ski turgor, edema, and third spacing of fluid are well known assessments for suspicion of dehydration or fluid overload (Asim, Alkadi, Asim, & Ghaffar, 2019). Localized dry or moist skin (e.g., maceration, incontinence-associated dermatitis, wound exudate, or perspiration) can render the skin vulnerable to further skin injury. As discussed in Chapter 9, interventions to hydrate as well as protect the skin for excess moisture are important components of any skin safety program. Studies have indicated that devices such as ultrasound and subepidermal moisture (SEM)/edema are promising for the detection of underlying fluid/edema as signs of inflammation and early tissue damage (Bates-Jensen et al., 2009; Clendenin, Jaradeh, Shamirian, & Rhodes, 2015; Guihan, Bates-Jenson, Chun, et al., 2012; Harrow & Mayrovitz, 2014; O'Brien, Moore, Patton, & O'Connor, 2018; Olivieri et al., 2018; Sprigle, Zhang, & Duckworth, 2009). International pressure injury guidelines suggest that SEM/edema devices should be considered as an adjunct to routine skin assessment to detect early inflammatory signs of pressure injury (EPUAP, NPIAP, & PPPIA, 2019). In contrast, the National Institute for Health and Care Excellence (2020) states it shows promise but there is not enough good-quality evidence to support the case for routine adoption. Details about this technology will be discussed in Chapter 11.

Focused Physical Assessment

A focused physical assessment is essential to (1) identify contributing factors precipitating a wound, (2) determine the etiology of the wound, (3) identify existing factors that require attention to reduce the likelihood of wound exacerbation, and (4) identify factors that are needed to facilitate wound repair/healing. Healing is a phenomenon composed of multiple processes (see Chapter 8), each of which must function properly and sequentially. Although all patients require a physical assessment, the patient with a wound requires particular attention to systemic, psychosocial, and local factors that uniquely impact wound healing. A wound specialist is specifically educated to conduct this type of focused physical assessment and to interpret the results (Wound, Ostomy and Continence Nurses Society™, 2017). The focused physical assessment should be obtained on admission and with a change in condition. Components of a wound-focused physical assessment are listed in Checklist 10.2.

CHECKLIST 10.2   Wound-Focused Physical Assessment Parameters

✓ Wound etiology and differential diagnosis
✓ Duration of wound
✓ Cofactors that impede healing:
  • Comorbid conditions (malignancy, diabetes, cardiac, respiratory, renal issues)
  • Medications (corticosteroids, cancer medications, immunosuppressants)
  • Host infection
  • Pressure injury risk factors
  • Decreased oxygenation and tissue perfusion
  • Alteration in nutrition and hydration
  • Psychosocial barriers, family support, impaired access to appropriate resources, financial limitations
  • Past therapies (e.g., radiation near the site of the wound)

Etiology and Differential Diagnosis

The data obtained from the wound-focused physical assessment will contribute to formulating a differential diagnosis and the likely etiology of the wound. This information will drive intervention choices and treatment strategies. It is important to note, however, that determining the etiology of many wounds is a subjective process requiring integration of several sources of data, expertise, and attention to detail. The etiology of many skin injuries or wounds will not be readily apparent or could be mixed etiologies. It is critical to understand this and to engage discussions with other team members such as dermatology, infectious disease, cardiology, intensivists, etc. The completed physical assessment often helps exclude possible wound etiologies and will also exclude treatment options. For example, compression is a key intervention for successful management of the patient with venous insufficiency; however, compression may be contraindicated for many patients with arterial disease (see Chapter 14). Off-loading is needed for management of the pressure injuries (see Chapters 11), and glucose must be managed when the patient has diabetes (see Chapter 17). Wound etiology will also provide clues regarding the type of healing to anticipate. For example, a venous ulcer generally has little depth, so it often heals by epithelialization rather than wound contraction, which is in contrast to the deeper stage 3 or 4 pressure injury, which requires contraction for healing to occur. Wound depth measurement in a full-thickness (stage 3 or 4) pressure injury is an important piece of information but may be of little relevance in a venous ulcer. Various types of skin damage are discussed in Chapter 9 and throughout this text. Interpretation of the data gathered through the focused physical assessment will guide the plan of care so that wound etiology and existing cofactors can be addressed.

Duration of Wound and Critical Cofactors That Impair Healing

Factors that impede healing are described in chapters throughout the text and listed in Checklist 10.2. Approaches used to assess systemic cofactors that affect wound healing,

TABLE 10.3 Assessment of Cofactors That Impact Wound Healing

Cofactor	Diagnostic Test
Tissue oxygenation	Transcutaneous oxygen (TCO_2)
	Hemoglobin (Hgb)
Bacterial load/ inflammation	Culture
	Biopsy
	White blood count (WBC)
	C-reactive protein (CRP)
	Sedimentation rate (ESR)
Circulation	Ankle-brachial index (ABI)
	Toe-brachial index (TBI)
Nutrition	Weight
	Body mass index (BMI)
	Albumin
	Total lymphocyte count
Glycemic control	Blood glucose
	Hemoglobin A1c (HbA1c)

CHECKLIST 10.3 Wound Assessment Parameters

✓ Anatomic and directional location of wound (Fig. 10.1, Table 10.4)
✓ Extent of tissue loss (e.g., stage, category, full thickness, partial thickness)
✓ Percentage of wound containing each type of tissue/structure observed (see Table 10.5)
✓ Dimensions of wound in centimeters (length, width, depth, tunneling, undermining)
✓ Wound edges
✓ Exudate (amount, type)
✓ Odor
✓ Periwound skin
✓ Presence or absence of local signs of infection (Chapter 19)
✓ Wound pain (Chapter 28)

along with the chapters that describe them in detail, are listed in Table 10.3. A 2-week-old pressure injury that has not improved suggests the presence of cofactors that have not been adequately addressed (EPUAP, NPIAP, & PPPIA, 2019; WOCN, 2016). Guidelines for pressure injuries and arterial wounds recommend consideration of referral and biopsy for wounds that are unresponsive following 2–4 weeks of appropriate topical therapies (Wound, Ostomy and Continence Nurses Society, 2014, 2019).

Any clinical cause for suspicion, such as raised borders, unusual wound base, unexplained pain, changes in shape or color, previous history, or family history of skin cancer, requires referral for biopsy (Alavi, Niakosari, & Sibbald, 2010; Panuncialman, Hammerman, Carson, & Falanga, 2010) to rule out less common conditions such as pyoderma gangrenosum or the conversion of the wound to a malignancy such as squamous cell carcinoma or Marjolin ulcer as discussed in Chapters 32.

Wound Assessment

Wound assessment is the collection of subjective data that characterize the status of the wound and periwound skin (see Plate 25). Parameters that compose a wound assessment are listed in Checklist 10.3 and described in this section. Conducting a wound assessment is a skill and requires precision and appropriate use of unique terms; use of appropriate terms is critically important. Therefore, competency-based education for wound assessment is an important component of any nursing program (IHI & NPIAP, 2021). Before assessment, the wound must be cleansed of loose debris, particulate matter, and dressing residue so that the normal architecture and color of the wound bed and surrounding skin can be fully appreciated.

Anatomic Location

The anatomic location of the wound is important to record using proper terminology that will also provide clues about the etiology. Anatomic locations such as the sacrum and the coccyx must be clearly delineated (Fig. 10.1). Directional anatomic directional terms (Table 10.4) provide additional detail that may be as important especially in the context of multiple wounds (O'Toole, 2017). Anatomic location will also convey plan-of-care needs. For example, a wound on the ischial tuberosity should prompt caregivers to explore the patient's sitting surface. A typical venous ulcer commonly appears on the medial aspect of the lower leg and will require compression. A patient with diabetes and a plantar surface foot ulcer typically has neuropathy and will need adequate blood glucose control and offloading.

Extent of Tissue Involvement

The extent of tissue damage guides the selection of appropriate interventions to restore tissue integrity; it also provides some information about the length of time required for the healing process. Extent of tissue involvement can be described as partial thickness or full thickness, or "staged" if indicated. Numerous staging and classification systems exist that are primarily based on wound etiology and therefore are precise and descriptive for that type of wound.

Partial thickness and full thickness. A partial-thickness wound is confined to the skin layers; damage does not penetrate below the dermis and may be limited to the epidermal layers only. These wounds heal primarily by reepithelialization (see Table 8.1 and Plate 1). A full-thickness wound indicates that the epidermis and dermis have been damaged into the subcutaneous tissue or beyond; tissue loss extends below the dermis (see Table 8.2 and Plates 2–5). Wound repair will occur by neovascularization, fibroplasia, contraction, and then epithelial migration from the wound edges. Partial thickness and full thickness can be used to describe most wounds but are not precise terms for

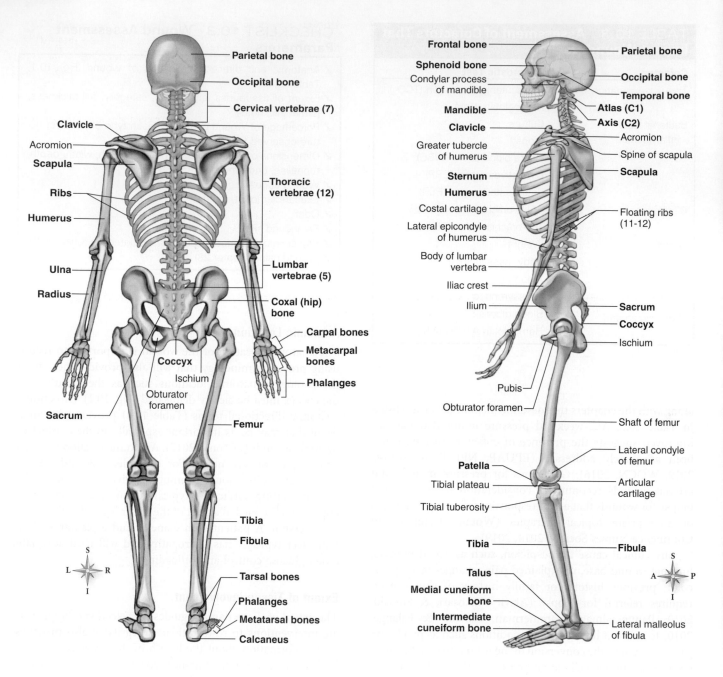

Fig. 10.1 Bony structures of human body; note delineation of sacrum and coccyx. (From Patton, K. T., & Thibodeau, G. A. (2010). *Anatomy and physiology* (7th ed.). St Louis: Mosby.)

specific types of tissue loss and depths of the wound. For example, a full-thickness wound can expose subcutaneous tissue, or it may extend to bone.

Classification systems. Accurate classification requires knowledge of the anatomy of skin and deeper tissue layers, the ability to recognize these tissues as well as structures such as ligaments or tendon, and the ability to differentiate among these. Careful evaluation of the wound bed facilitates accurate classification, a complex skill that can take time to develop. Classification systems exist for various types of wounds and may or may not indicate wound severity. For example, classification systems for vascular and diabetic wounds assign a "grade" to the wound based on levels of tissue involvement,

history of previous ulceration, presence of bony deformity, presence and severity of ischemia, and presence and severity of infection (Wound, Ostomy and Continence Nurses Society, 2014). Pressure injury classification or pressure injury staging (Chapter 11) however, was not designed for and should not be used to evaluate severity of a pressure injury. As with all classification systems, they tell only a small part of the story and therefore should be used in conjunction with wound descriptors and assessment components. Additional classification systems are provided throughout the text and include skin tears (Chapter 9), vascular wounds (Chapters 14–16), diabetic wounds (Chapter 17), and burns (Chapter 34).

TABLE 10.4	Directional Location Descriptors
Proximal	Near proximity to
Distal	Away distant from
Lateral	Outside edge/aspect
Medial	Inside edge/aspect
Posterior	Behind
Anterior	In front
Plantar	Sole of foot
Dorsal	Upper aspect/front of foot
Palmar	Surface/palm of hand
Superior	Above/over
Inferior	Below/under

Wound Tissue

The amount (percent) and type of tissue in the wound bed provide insight into the severity and duration of the wound, the extent to which the wound is progressing toward healing, and the effectiveness of current interventions. Healing wounds are characterized by increasing amounts of viable tissue (e.g., granulation tissue) and decreasing amounts of nonviable tissue (e.g., eschar or slough). When the wound bed contains a combination of tissue types, each should be described in percentages—for example, "50% of the wound bed contains eschar and 50% contains granulation tissue." Terms used to describe tissue and the wound bed, as well as other descriptions used for wound assessment, are listed in Table 10.5 (Black et al., 2010; Edsberg et al., 2016).

Viable tissue. Viable tissue is healthy tissue, such as granulation, epithelialization, or subcutaneous tissue. Healthy

TABLE 10.5 Wound Bed Descriptors

TISSUE TYPES

Term	Description	Appearance
Epithelium	Epithelialization is regeneration of epidermis across a wound surface	Flat, thin, and lighter than unusual pigmentation (often pink)
Granulation tissue	Comprised of new capillary tufts, matrix, fibroblasts, and collagen. Does not mature into epithelium. As healing occurs, a layer of epidermis will cover the granulation tissue	Healthy granulation tissue is red, shiny, bumpy (cobblestone) granulation tissue without adequate blood flow becomes pale
Hypergranulation tissue	Overproduction of granulation tissue generally caused by excess moisture or friction	Red friable, shiny granulation above the level of the surrounding skin
Slough	Inflammatory byproduct (not a physical tissue). Mixture of serum proteins (e.g., fibrin, albumin, immunoglobulin) and denatured matrix proteins (e.g., collagen)	Appears attached stringy, loosely or adherent in a range of colors (white, yellow, green, or brown) depending on its bacterial composition
Necrotic, nonviable, devitalized	Tissue that has died and therefore has lost its physical properties and biologic activities	Yellow, brown, black. Consistency may vary from soft to hard (e.g., eschar). It may be attached, adherent, loose, stringy
Eschar	Necrotic (desiccated) nonviable tissue	Black or brown. Stable eschar is dry, hard, and leathery. Unstable eschar is boggy, spongy, and slimy, with purulent drainage, periulcer edema, erythema, warmth, tenderness, and/or pain
Scab	Crust or hardened blood and serum over wound. (Not a physical tissue)	Brown hard crust
Epibole	Rolled (also called closed) wound edges that prevent *epithelial migration*	Raised, rolled paler, or pinker than surrounding tissue
Epidermis	Outermost layer of the skin. Avascular composed of keratinocytes, melanocytes, Langerhans cells, Merkel cells (see Chapter 7)	Various skin pigmentations. Thickness varies by location from 0.07 mm (eyelids) to 0.12 mm (soles of feet)
Dermis	Beneath the epidermis. Highly vascular consists of two major layers (upper and papillary). Contains collagen, elastin, hair follicles, sweat, sebaceous, and apocrine glands (see Chapter 7)	Pink, smooth. Thickness varies by location from 0.3 mm (eyelids) to 3.0 mm (back)
Superficial fascia	Beneath the dermis. The tissue network that surrounds subcutaneous fat	In healthy skin, it looks like a thin, glistening web
Subcutaneous fat	Beneath the skin. Stores energy, aids in thermal regulation	Pale yellow, waxy, globular and oily, and glistens when enmeshed in superficial fascia. When dry, it congeals (crystallizes) and turns to tan or yellow-brown

Continued

TABLE 10.5 Wound Bed Descriptors—cont'd

TISSUE TYPES

Term	Description	Appearance
Muscle	Highly vascular, contracts to move skeletal bones	Shiny red with visible striations, spring back when touched (not to be confused with red bumpy, cobblestone granulation tissue). *Ischemic avascular muscle* becomes dull red, cyanotic or pale, and mushy. *Necrotic muscle* eventually liquefies and produces dark brown, odorous drainage
Deep fascia	Essentially avascular, connective tissue surrounding muscles, bones, nerves, and blood vessels. High density of collagen and elastin fibers	Dense fibrous with glistening surface on top of muscle
Tendon	Tough band of fibrous connective tissue that connects muscle to bone	Shiny white with fibrous striations, tendon springs back when touched. Intact tendon moves when joint is moved and will dry and not survive once exposed to the environment
Ligament	Short band of connective tissue holding bones together	Ribbon-like, striated, and pearly white. Broader, flatter, and more loosely woven than tendons
Bursa	Provides cushion between bones, tendons, and/or muscles around joints	Small fluid-filled sac of white fibrous tissue lined with synovial membrane filled with synovial fluid. If bursae open, they leak a sticky, mucous-like fluid

granulation tissue is characteristically described as beefy, red, moist, and cobblestone-like or berry-like in appearance (see Plate 3). New epithelial tissue is light pink and dry (see Plate 1). Deviations from an optimal state should be described carefully and correlated with conditions that may account for the abnormality, such as the patient's fluid status, serum hemoglobin level, nutrition, or bioburden.

Nonviable (devitalized) tissue. Color, texture, moisture, and adherence of nonviable tissue to the wound bed should be noted. As with viable tissue, nonviable tissue can provide information related to wound status. Nonviable tissue in the wound is generally associated with altered tissue oxygenation, wound desiccation, increased bacterial burden, and/or a prolonged inflammation.

Slough (cellular byproduct) vs necrotic (nonviable) tissue. Necrotic tissue, which is caused by a loss of blood supply is brown, black, or tan dead tissue. Eschar is characterized by a black and/or dark brown leathery appearance. However, necrotic tissue can also be moist and boggy. In contrast, slough is the accumulation of the cellular byproducts from the inflammatory process and the continuous normal cycle of tissue breaking down and remodeling. During this inflammatory phase, matrix metalloproteinase levels increase and degrade the used growth factors and proteins resulting in the accumulation of slough (Angel, 2019). Slough is described as yellow, tan, gray, green, or brown. It can be stringy and loose or thick and adherent to the wound bed. However, both slough and necrotic tissue provide an environment for bacterial proliferation, increasing inflammation, and wound chronicity (Angel, 2019; Black et al., 2010; Percival & Suleman, 2015).

A wound initially described as nonviable dry adherent eschar (see Plate 26) may become moist, softening, brown, necrotic tissue that is lifting, loosening, or demarcating from the wound base due to a through the body's natural debridement process called autolysis (see Plate 27). The process of autolysis is facilitated by appropriate topical care and a moist wound environment. Chapters 20 and 21 provide details of the significance and process for debridement and moist wound healing.

Tissue color. A myriad of colors is often found in the wound bed (e.g., red, pink, yellow, tan, black, green). It is helpful to record the color of the tissue in the wound bed because the color gives a general indication of healing status. For example, if the wound bed is red and granulation tissue is present, these are considered a positive sign that conditions for healing are right. Eschar is black (see Plate 26); as it softens (thus moving closer to being debrided through autolysis), the color will transition to yellow (see Plate 27) or yellow tan; then small red islets of granulation tissue develop and emerge within the nonviable tissue. More granulation tissue is revealed as the wound progresses with continued autolysis and/or desloughing and debridement (see Plates 28A and 28B).

Color can be used to differentiate normal structures from the wound bed. However, as shown in Table 10.5, color alone does not sufficiently describe viable or nonviable tissue and trivializes the complexities of the healing process. For example, nonviable tissue and slough could be various shades of yellow; however, viable tendon and adipose are also yellow. The distinction for viable tendon, however, is that it will contain striations to strands; adipose tissue will be globular in appearance. A wound base may be red but with an unhealthy smooth surface (lacking the cobblestone or berry-like appearance) in which case the wound should be described as "clean, nongranulating" (see Plate 5A). In contrast, healthy granulation tissue will have a red color with a cobblestone appearance (as shown in Plate 5B). A pale red color can be indicative of anemia or hypoxia. Hypergranulation tissue is also red or pink in color but is not considered healthy. Hypergranulation tissue is the overproduction of granulation tissue generally caused by excess moisture or friction (see Plate 29).

Wound Size

Wound measurements aide in determining wound progress, deterioration, and time to heal (Bull et al., 2022). For massive tissue loss, calculation of the percentage of body surface area wounded using the Lund–Browder chart is the most common and realistic measure (see Chapter 34, Fig. 34.1).

Surface area is a two-dimensional measure (length and width), while volume is a three-dimensional measure (length, width, and depth). Two figures can have the same volume but different surface areas. Three-dimensional measurements are required with full-thickness wounds because, by definition, full-thickness wounds are below the dermis and therefore should have depth; however, shallow full-thickness wound depth may not be measurable (<1 mm). Measurements should be recorded in centimeters or millimeters and include the extent and location of undermining and tunneling when present. From these dimensions, the area of the wound can be estimated by multiplying length by width by depth. To strengthen the accuracy of wound measurement, a uniform approach among staff should be used. This can be facilitated by consistent patient positioning and identifying specific wound landmarks from which to align the measuring instrument (EPUAP, NPIAP, & PPPIA, 2019). Documentation requirements for consistency should be described in policies, procedures, and flow sheets (examples in Appendix A).

As with each wound assessment parameter, wound measurements should be interpreted within the context of the other parameters enumerated in Checklist 10.3. For example, as an eschar-covered ulcer undergoes autolysis, the percentage of eschar will decrease, and consequently wound depth will predictably increase. Looking only at wound dimensions as an assessment parameter may lead to misinterpretation of the increase as an indication of delayed or absent wound healing. However, because wound dimensions are changing while the type and volume of tissue in the wound bed are evolving from eschar to slough to granulation tissue, the increase in size that accompanies the removal of nonviable tissue is considered desirable and indicative of a positive trend in the wound-healing process.

Traditional ruler technique. The ruler technique involves manually *measuring length, width, and depth using* a head-to-toe orientation, the longest *length* head to toe and the widest *width* perpendicular to length. Researchers have found that if the width is not measured perpendicular to the longest length, the wound area can be overestimated by 70% on some wound shapes (EPUAP, NPIAP, & PPPIA, 2019; Langemo, Anderson, Hanson, et al., 2008) (Fig. 10.2).

The most common method of obtaining wound depth is by inserting a moist cotton-tipped applicator into the wound bed at the greatest depth and placing a mark on the applicator at the level of the skin (Fig. 10.3). This mark may simply be the

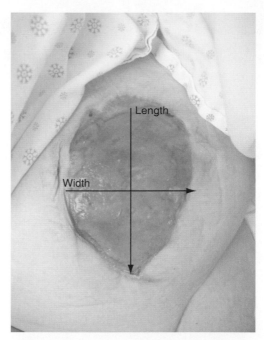

Fig. 10.2 Measuring wound length and width.

examiner's thumb and index finger, but an ink mark applied to the applicator at skin level should provide more accuracy in the measurement. The cotton-tipped applicator then is held against a metric ruler to determine the depth of the wound (Doughty, 2004; EPUAP, NPIAP, & PPPIA, 2019). This procedure can be made simpler by using a commercially available measuring guide integrated into a cotton-tipped applicator.

Measuring tunneling and undermining. The terms *tunnel* and *sinus tract* are often used interchangeably. A *tunnel* is a channel that extends from any part of the wound through subcutaneous tissue or muscle (Fig. 10.4). *Undermining* is tissue destruction that occurs under intact skin around the wound perimeter. Pressure injuries that have been subjected to shear often are accompanied with undermining. Undermining and tunneling can be documented by measuring depth and noting the location using the face of the clock as a model. The superior aspect of the wound (12 o'clock position) points toward the patient's head, whereas the inferior aspect of the wound (6 o'clock position) points toward the patient's feet. Examples are shown in Figs. 10.4 and 10.5.

Limitations to the ruler technique. Unfortunately, numerous potential reliability problems exist with hand wound measurements. Because the perimeter of open wounds often is irregular, it can be difficult to determine the best position on the wound surface from which to obtain the measurements.

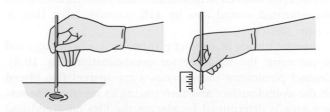

Fig. 10.3 Measuring wound depth.

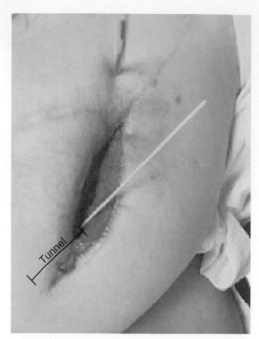

Fig. 10.4 Wound tunneling. Tunneling is present in this abdominal wound at the 7 o'clock position and measures 2 cm in length. Tunnel and sinus tract are often used interchangeably.

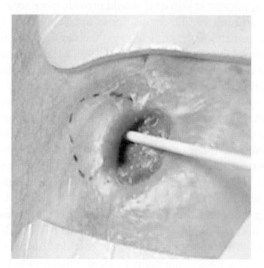

Fig. 10.5 Undermining extends 2 cm from 7 to 11 o'clock.

Even defining the edge of the wound from which measurements should be taken will vary among providers and will introduce inconsistencies in dimensions. All of these methods overestimate wound area because they assume that wounds are a perfect square or rectangle (Langemo et al., 2008). A retrospective analysis of 2768 wounds demonstrated that hand measurements overestimated wound area by 44% (Darwin, Jaller, Hirt, & Kirsner, 2019).

Acetate tracing or contact planimetry has been suggested to overcome the tendency for overestimation (Fig. 10.X). Contact planimetry incorporates a transparent film placed on the wound surface and then tracing its margins. The surface area is determined by placing the film on a grid and counting the number of squares (Khoo & Jansen, 2016).

Regardless of limitations, ruler measurements are still commonly used and can at least reveal a trend in the presence or absence of size of the wound and consequently healing. However, as discussed later in the chapter, smart devices, digital photography, and other technologies to assist with more accurate wound assessment and monitoring are relied on more and more in clinical settings (Foltynski, 2018; Nair, 2018).

Wound Shape

Terms used to describe the shape of the wound include adjectives such as round, oval, triangular, irregular, and butterfly shaped. Documenting the shape of the wound provides not only a more accurate clinical description but also clues to wound etiology. For example, device-related pressure injuries may be apparent because they will replicate the shape of the device, such as tubing, telemetry cable, or needle cap. Similarly, acute onset of a butterfly-shaped area of erythema over the upper buttocks and coccyx is consistent with unrelieved pressure while the patient is in the supine position.

Wound Exudate

The *Type* of exudate can range from clear, serosanguineous [thin, watery or blood tinged, sanguineous (bloody) or purulent]. Subjective indicators used to quantify the *volume* of wound exudate include frequency of dressing change and persistent presence of periwound maceration. Volume of wound exudate can be described as none, minimal, moderate (e.g., dressing wet), or heavy (e.g., dressing soaked) (Grey, Enoch, & Harding, 2006). However, as described in Chapter 21, the type of dressing used will also provide an indication of the volume of exudate, as hydrofiber and alginate dressings are much more absorbent than hydrocolloid dressings. Sodium-impregnated gauze also can be expected to contain more exudate than plain gauze. Exudate volume generally varies with the type of wound. For example, a venous ulcer is more exudative than an arterial ulcer. An increase in wound exudate often coincides with hyperplasia, biofilm, edema, or wound infection and can therefore be used as an indicator for those conditions (Haesler, Swanson, Ousey, & Carville, 2019). Objective measurement of the volume of wound exudate can be obtained by using a wound containment system, such as a wound pouch or closed suction.

Odor

Odor can be described as absent, faint, moderate, or strong and often varies according to wound moisture, the type and density of microorganism's present, and the amount of nonviable tissue present. Odorous, purulent exudate is suggestive of an infection (Haesler et al., 2019).

Wound Edge

The rim of the wound or wound edge provides information regarding epithelialization, chronicity, and even etiology. Ideally, the wound edges should be attached, moist, and flush with the wound base so that epithelial cells can migrate from the wound edges across the surface of the wound bed.

Unattached wound edges are those in which undermining is present between the dermis and subcutaneous tissue. Closed wound edges are characterized as dry with a loss of the intervening moist, red reproductive epithelium. In some situations, closed wound edges are also thickened and "rolled." This premature closure of the wound edge is a common complication of chronic wounds and is referred to as *epibole* (Doughty, 2004). Epibole results when squamous cells from the epidermis migrate along the wall and edge of the wound, thus preventing migration of epithelial cells across the wound bed and wound closure (see Plate 4). Cautery or sharp debridement of epibole is needed to "open" the wound edges.

Periwound Skin

The periwound skin should be described in terms of color (erythema, pale, white, blue, darkly pigmented, maroon), texture (moist, dry, indurated, boggy, macerated), skin temperature (warm, cool), integrity (denudement, maceration, excoriation, stripping, erosion, papules, pustules), and presence or absence of lesions. It is particularly beneficial to assess the periwound skin using the contralateral surface away from the wound as a comparison. This can be most notably valuable when assessing dark or non-Caucasian skin tones.

The periwound assessment can give clues to the effectiveness of the treatment plan and the technique used for dressing application or removal. For example, maceration (see Plate 14), dermatitis, or denudement of periwound skin occurs when exudate pools on intact skin for prolonged periods or when a moist dressing is inappropriately applied, is left on too long, and/or overlaps onto intact skin. Periwound skin stripping may indicate inappropriate adhesive removal.

Venous/arterial insufficiency, infection, pressure damage, peripheral neuropathy, pyoderma gangrenosum, vasculitis, and calciphylaxis may be present with distinct periwound features. Table 10.6 lists some pathologies that may be revealed through a careful periwound skin inspection.

Bacterial Burden

All wounds have some degree of bioburden. The extent and significance of that bioburden are conveyed with terms such as *contamination*, *colonization*, *biofilm*, and *infection*. The presence or absence of local signs of infection should be documented as part of the assessment. However, it's important to remember that many chronic wounds with significant bioburden may not exhibit the classic signs of infection due to factors such as immunosuppression or the presence of biofilm. Indicators of a subclinical infection or overwhelming bioburden include delayed healing despite optimal care, discolored or friable granulation tissue, pocketing or breakdown at the wound base, and/or foul odor. A "stagnant" wound despite optimal care may indicate biofilm. Chapter 19 presents a thorough discussion of the assessment and management of bacterial burden (including biofilm) and infection.

TABLE 10.6 Common Periwound Features by Wound Pathology

Pathology	Periwound Feature
Venous insufficiency (Chapter 15)	Edema, brawny discoloration, hemosiderin-staining lipodermatosclerosis, dermatitis, scaling, weeping, scarring, varicose veins, maceration
Arterial (Chapter 14)	Elevation pallor, cool, dependent rubor, absent hair, xerosis, atrophy
Infection (Chapter 19)	Erythema, pain, heat, swelling, induration
Pressure (Chapter 11)	Hyperemia, edema, induration, discoloration
Peripheral neuropathy (Chapter 17)	Insensate, edema, cellulitis, erythema, induration, xerosis, fissures, callus
Pyoderma gangrenosum (Chapter 32)	Ragged borders, elevated borders, dusky red or purple, halo
Vasculitis (Chapter 32)	Palpable, nonblanchable purpura; may be associated with petechiae; nodules and vesicles may be present
Calciphylaxis (Chapter 32)	Dusky, purple, and palpable nodules progress to necrosis and ulceration; associated with renal disease; may include mottled, reticulated patches, plaques with focal central necrosis
Candidiasis (Chapter 9)	Pustular or macular–papular rash; erythematous satellite lesions

Wound Pain

As the fifth vital sign, pain has gained a much-deserved focus in today's health care environment. Yet wound pain is infrequently assessed and inadequately managed. Wound pain can indicate infection or deterioration and inappropriate or inadequate treatment choices. Pain can be directly related to patient satisfaction and has been shown to have a negative impact on wound-healing progress. Pain should be measured regularly and frequently. Chapter 28 provides detailed discussions related to the assessment and management of wound pain.

Wound Photography

Wound photos supplement the written record but should never replace it. Advantages to wound photography are listed in Box 10.2 (Ervin, 2005; Goh & Zhu, 2017; King, 2014; Kinsella, 2002; Santamaria, Glance, Prentice, & Fielder, 2010; Sood et al., 2016; Stern et al., 2014; Wang, Anderson, Jones, & Evans, 2016). Insufficient imaging can lead to problematic encounters in the legal setting (Onuh et al., 2022). A blurred photograph or photography that does not follow facility policy can give the impression of poor work quality, supporting negative outcomes in a courtroom rather than the intended purpose of conveying progression of healing. If a photograph of the wound is not available, the jury could be

---

BOX 10.2 Advantages to Wound Photography

- Records monitoring and evaluation of healing
- Facilitates consultation with multiple disciplines for challenging differential diagnosis
- Prevents overexposure of wound by multiple health care providers
- Provides clarity for complex step-by-step procedures
- Enhances teaching, clinical coaching and mentoring
- Aids with research and publications
- Assists with communication to payers to provide rationale and justification of treatment
- Helps patients and families to make informed choices
- Increases access through telemedicine to remote and rural settings (see Chapter 4)

BOX 10.3 Wound Photography Tips

- Prep the room
  - Use natural lighting when possible
  - Remove clutter to make the wound the only focus
  - Avoid black or gray solid colors, or brightly patterned backgrounds
- Prep the patient
  - Position and drape to promote comfort and preserve dignity
  - Clean and measure wound
  - Use marker to illustrate the extent of undermining, cellulitis, dermatitis, etc.
  - Place paper ruler near wound
- Take photo
  - Prevent contamination of camera
  - Position camera parallel to patient
  - Include a close-up of the wound and periwound skin
  - Include a longer-view for an anatomical reference
  - Capture relevant clinical features when possible (e.g., contractures, pitting edema)

---

shown a photograph of a different wound as an example of how bad it could be. States differ regarding their stance on the admissibility of photographs in court cases.

When photography is used, the facility should have specific protocols or policies in place that facilitate a standardized approach, compliance with The Joint Commission, the American Health Information Management Association (AHIMA) and Health Insurance Portability and Accountability Act (HIPAA) guidelines. Checklist 10.4 provides issues to be addressed in a wound photography protocol or policy.

Tips for wound photography are provided in Box 10.3. Educational programs and competencies for wound photography should include patient confidentiality (including transmission and storage of electronic patient information), camera technique, infection control, and the accompanying nursing assessment (Buckley, Adelson, & Hess, 2005). Photos should be obtained in a serial fashion, for example, at baseline

---

CHECKLIST 10.4 Issues to Address in Policy or Protocol for Wound Photography

✓ Informed consent (who can obtain the consent and what is included)
✓ Timing of photographs (when or under what circumstances photographs are to be taken and repeated)
✓ Criteria about who can take the photographs
✓ Method of validating competency to photograph wounds (include frequency of competency revalidations)
✓ Type of camera being used
✓ Techniques used to ensure consistency in photographing and methods used to ensure photographs are not enhanced or altered (e.g., image size, distance from the wound, sample measure in frame, such as measuring guide)
✓ Appropriate patient identification (initials, medical record number, date and time markings)
✓ Maintenance and storage of photographs effectively (where they will be stored and who will have access to them)
✓ Method for releasing copies to patients upon request (authorization form)

---

with the initial assessment and then weekly. In this way, the progression of the wound is documented and can accompany the descriptive terms used to convey the wound condition.

REASSESSMENT AND EVALUATION OF HEALING

Evaluation of healing involves wound assessment documented over time to reveal patterns and trends that indicate improvement or deterioration in the wound. In this way, assessment is linked to outcomes so that an evaluation of the plan of care can follow objective criteria.

Frequency of Reassessment

In general, the patient's overall condition, wound severity, health care setting, type of dressings used, and goals determine the appropriate frequency of wound assessment. Because frequency of reassessment is dependent on so many variables, the frequency interval commonly changes over time and across care settings. For example, a patient who is immunosuppressed and in acute care has greater risk for developing a wound infection and may warrant more frequent monitoring. Once the patient is stable in long-term care, the "at-risk" patient's skin should be monitored daily but may require a full wound assessment only on admission and weekly. Once the patient is home, assessments are generally dependent on the frequency of home health worker or clinic visits. Family members should be instructed to make assessments between clinic visits and may be able and willing to monitor for trends.

National and international pressure injury guidelines (EPUAP, NPIAP, & PPPIA, 2019; WOCN, 2016) make specific recommendations on the frequency of monitoring, assessment, and evaluation of pressure injury healing, as summarized in Box 10.4. When topical wound therapy is being selected, the frequency with which the wound should be

BOX 10.4 **Guidelines for Frequency of Monitoring, Assessment, and Evaluation of Pressure Injury Healing**

1. Patients at risk for skin breakdown should have at least daily skin inspections.
2. At least twice-daily skin assessments are recommended under and around medical devices (more often than twice daily in individuals experiencing or vulnerable to developing fluid shifts and edema).
3. Pressure injuries should be assessed and monitored at each dressing change, or sooner if the wound or the patient's condition deteriorates.
4. Evaluation of pressure injury healing should occur within 2 weeks, or sooner if the patient or wound condition deteriorates.

assessed must be considered. For example, a hydrocolloid on a stable wound should not be removed daily simply to conduct a wound assessment. Rather, the assessment should be obtained at the time the dressing is scheduled to be changed (i.e., every 4 days). Chapter 21 discusses the principles of wound management and the various features of local wound care options.

Experts encourage the use of the word closed rather than healed with regard to full-thickness pressure injuries. These wounds may close, meaning the integrity of the skin is repaired but not healed. Wound collagen never achieves the normal structure of dermal collagen and therefore the scar remains vulnerable to breakdown (Black et al., 2010).

Predicting Wound Healing

It is generally agreed that the percentage of reduction in wound surface area during the initial weeks of treatment is the most reliable indicator for complete healing, and the initial size of the wound is a significant predictor of time to heal. van Rijswijk and the Multicenter Leg Ulcer Study Group (van Rijswijk, 2003) monitored the healing of 61 patients with 72 full-thickness venous leg ulcers. They found that a greater than 30% reduction in ulcer area after 2 weeks of treatment was a significant ($P < 0.004$) predictor of the time required for healing. Kantor and Margolis (2000) conducted a cohort multicenter study of 104 patients and found that the percentage change in ulcer area during the first 4 weeks of treatment was the best prognostic indicator that the ulcers would eventually heal within 24 weeks. Similarly, Phillips, Machado, Trout, et al. (2000) found baseline ulcer area and duration of leg ulcer were important predictors of healing in a multicenter retrospective review of 165 patients with venous ulcers. Falanga and Sabolinski (2000) reported data based on randomized, controlled, clinical trials and presented reliable and specific findings for predicting complete healing. Initial healing time of 0.11 cm/week or greater predicts healing, whereas rates of 0.06 cm/week or less predict nonhealing. A prospective multicenter study of 203 patients with diabetic foot ulcers (DFUs) found that 4-week healing rates correlated

significantly with healing at 12 weeks ($P < 0.01$) (Sheehan, Jones, Caselli, et al., 2003). Snyder, Cardinal, Dauphinée, et al. (2010) conducted a post hoc analysis of DFU treatment outcomes from two published, randomized, controlled studies ($n = 133$ and 117) to assess the relationship between percentage area reduction (PAR) during early standard wound care and ulcer closure by week 12. Findings confirmed that PAR in wound size is an early predictor of treatment outcome ($P \leq 0.001$). The author suggested that protocols for care should be reevaluated if greater than 50% PAR is not achieved by week 4.

Studies of neuropathic and ischemic ulcers suggest a linear relationship between initial wound radius or size and healing time (Robson, Hill, Woodske, et al., 2000; Zimny, Schatz, & Pfohl, 2002). During a controlled prospective trial examining 338 serial tracings of venous ulcers, Cardinal, Eisenbud, and Armstrong (2009) noted faster healing rates with wounds that maintained a linear relationship between margin size and wound surface size ($P < 0.001$).

Jones, Fennie, and Lenihan (2007) conducted a multisite retrospective review of medical records of patients from various care settings to determine the factors that influence wound healing within 3 months and nonhealing after 5 months. Researchers evaluated at least 3 months of data from 400 patients with pressure, venous, and diabetic wounds who received routine wound care by typical staff. Results showed a difference in wound healing by size, location, and socioeconomic status. Large and deep wounds were less likely to heal than small and shallow wounds. Lower extremity wounds were more likely to heal than wounds located on the iliac crest or trochanter. Patients who were not Caucasian and patients on Medicare had poor healing outcomes. Not surprisingly, nonhealing wounds were also associated with infection, heavy exudate, necrosis, and inappropriate use of wound care dressings. Edsberg, Wyffels, and Ha (2011) had similar findings related to initial size as a significant predictor of time to heal ($P < 0.023$), with smaller stage 3 and 4 pressure injuries healing faster than larger stage 3 and 4 pressure injuries.

Tools for Documentation and Evaluation of Healing

Several tools that enable the clinician to assess wounds are available, presented throughout the text and in Box 10.5, and described in this section. These instruments attempt to enhance communication among clinicians, define a common language, and standardize assessment. Clinicians should be familiar with the strengths and limitations of the several methods currently available for assessing wound status. Staging and assessment tools are not designed to replace a comprehensive ongoing assessment. Ideally, tools should be reliable, valid, clinically useful, and theoretically based (Arndt & Kelechi, 2014).

Pillen, Miller, Thomas, et al. (2009) conducted a systematic literature review to examine available wound-healing instruments in terms of validity, reliability, and sensitivity measures of wound healing. Their review identified substantial gaps in

> ## BOX 10.5   Assessment of Wound-Healing Instruments
>
> - Pressure Ulcer Scale for Healing (PUSH)
> - Bates-Jensen Wound Assessment Tool (BWAT)
> - Sessing Scale (SS)
> - Sussman Wound Healing Tool (SWHT)
> - Wound Healing Scale (WHS)
> - DESIGN (Depth, Exudate, Size, Inflammation/infection, Granulation tissue, Necrotic tissue)
> - Leg Ulcer Measurement Tool (LUMT)
> - ASEPSIS
> - Barber Measuring Tool (BMT)
> - Granulometer

Data obtained from Pillen, H., Miller, M., Thomas, J., et al. (2009). Assessment of wound healing: Validity, reliability and sensitivity of available instruments. *Wound Practice and Research, 17*(4), 208–217.

the literature with regard to validation of the 10 wound-healing evaluation instruments (see Box 10.5) found in their search. Authors reported the Pressure Ulcer Scale for Healing (PUSH) and Pressure Sore Status Tool (PSST) had been validated to the greatest extent, whereas those describing healing in leg ulcers and general or surgical wounds tended to lack comprehensive and quality evaluation. International guidelines advocate the combined use of clinical judgment and a valid and reliable pressure injury assessment scale to assess progress toward healing (EPUAP, NPIAP, & PPPIA, 2019).

Pressure Ulcer Scale for Healing

The PUSH was developed by the NPIAP to monitor pressure injury healing over time. The PUSH tool is designed to monitor three parameters that are considered the most indicative of healing: size (length and width), exudate amount, and tissue type. Each parameter has at least four sublevels. The subscore for each parameter is totaled, and the overall total score is calculated ranging from 0 to 17 (0 = closed or healed). A comparison of total scores measured over time provides an indication of wound improvement or deterioration (Günes, 2009; WOCN, 2016). Numerous validation studies have been conducted using the PUSH tool. George-Saintilus, Tommasulo, Cal, et al. (2009) questioned the reliability of the PUSH tool when they discovered little agreement between traditional nursing observations and PUSH scores of patients with a wound residing in an extended care facility. However, subsequent studies found the PUSH tool to be valid and responsive for assessing healing for pressure, venous, and diabetic lower extremity ulcers (Hon, Lagden, McLaren, et al., 2010).

Bates-Jensen Wound Assessment Tool

The Bates-Jensen Wound Assessment Tool (BWAT) was originally known as the PSST. The tool addresses 13 wound characteristics (Bates-Jensen, McCreath, Harputlu, & Patlan, 2019; Harris, Bates-Jensen, Parslow, et al., 2010). Specific definitions are provided for each characteristic.

Individual items are scored on a modified Likert scale (ranging from 1 for best for that characteristic to 5 for worst). Individual items are summed, and the total provides a measure of overall wound status. Total scores range from 13, which indicates tissue health, to 65, which indicates wound degeneration.

The BWAT has been used in various health care settings with various chronic wounds (Bolton, McNees, van Rijswijk, et al., 2004; Carlson, Vigen, Rubayi, et al., 2017; de Laat, Scholte, Reimer, et al., 2005; de Leon, Barnes, Nagel, et al., 2009; Ebid, El-Kafy, & Alayat, 2013). Bates-Jensen et al. (2019) reported high reliability for all subjects all participants and anatomic locations with use of the BWAT ($r = 0.90$; $P < 0.0001$; $n = 1161$ observations) during assessment of 305 pressure injuries among 142 ethnically and racially diverse nursing home residents. BWAT scores showed strongest agreement coefficients for stage 4 pressure injury ($r = 0.69$), pressure injuries among Asian and White ethnicity/racial groups ($r = 0.89$ and 0.91, respectively), and sacrum anatomic location ($r = 0.92$) indicating scores are better correlated to fair skin tones. Lower agreement coefficients were demonstrated for stage 2 pressure injury ($r = 0.38$) and pressure injuries among African American and Hispanic ethnicity/racial groups ($r = 0.88$ and 0.87, respectively). BWAT scores were significantly different by pressure injury stage ($F = 496.7$, df = 6, $P < 0.001$) and anatomic location ($F = 33.76$, df = 8, $P < 0.001$). BWAT scores correlated with pressure injury progress or deterioration (ulcer closed 18.4 ± 7.4, ulcer persisted 24.9 ± 10.0; $F = 70.11$, df = 2, $P < 0.001$), but not with comorbidities. The BWAT provides reliable, objective data for assessing pressure injury healing progress.

DESIGN and DESIGN-R Tools

Developed in Japan, the DESIGN and the revised DESIGN-R tools classify pressure injury severity and monitor progression toward healing. DESIGN interrater reliability results showed a high correlation with photos and real-life pressure injuries ($r = 0.98$ with $r = 0.91$, respectively). For validity, a high correlation was found between DESIGN-R and PSST scores. A positive change in at least one DESIGN-R score significantly correlated with total healing within 30 days with good interrater reliability with BWAT scores (Lizaka, Sanada, Matsui, et al., 2012; Sanada, Moriguchi, Miyachi, et al., 2004).

A Chinese version of DESIGN-R was developed and tested for validity and reliability (Zhong et al., 2013). Using a purposive sampling method, 44 registered nurses (RNs) and 11 physicians (MDs) were recruited from 52 departments in a hospital in China. They used the Chinese version of DESIGN-R to assess eight photographs of pressure injuries and descriptors. In addition, eight experienced medical staff used the BWAT to assess the same wounds. Interrater reliability was high (tICC score = 0.960). ICC inflammation/infection scores were 0.530 and 0.759 and ICC Granulation scores were 0.532 and 0.794 for general (less experienced) medical staff and experienced medical staff, respectively. The correlation coefficients between the BWAT and DESIGN-R tool were >0.80 for all eight raters. The results suggest the Chinese version of DESIGN-R is valid and reliable and may be a useful scoring tool for RNs and MDs to monitor pressure injury status in daily clinical practice.

Regulatory Documents

Medicare's Outcome and Assessment Information Set (OASIS-D) and Continuous Assessment Record and Evaluation (CARE) are postacute care patient assessment data sets that contain information about wounds and wound management. These documents do not contain comprehensive wound assessments and should not replace comprehensive and focused assessments for patients with wounds. Because payment is directly affected by how several wound-related questions are answered, the Wound, Ostomy and Continence Nurses Society™ (WOCN®) developed an OASIS Guidance Document for clarification of how these questions could best be answered (Wound, Ostomy and Continence Nurses Society, 2019).

The Photographic Wound Assessment Tool (PWAT) was developed from the PSST to examine the validity and reliability of wound photography. The intraclass correlation coefficient (ICC) for interrater reliability was excellent, varying from 0.86 to 0.96. Interrater reliability was dependent on the clinicians having experience in wound care. Clinicians with more than 5 years of experience had an ICC of 0.75, but only 0.34 for inexperienced students. Based on these findings, Houghton, Kincaid, Campbell, et al. (2000) concluded that when used by experienced wound clinicians, the PWAT suffices when a full bedside assessment is not possible. However, assessment methods such as wound palpation and measurement of tunneling and undermining and variables such as pain and odor, cannot be obtained through photography (Jesada et al., 2013), therefore experts agree that photography should be complementary to a bedside assessment (EPUAP, NPIAP, & PPPIA, 2019; Jesada et al., 2013).

Thompson, Gordey, Bowles, Parslow, and Houghton (2013) conducted a multicenter trial to examine the validity and reliability of the revised Photographic Wound Assessment Tool (revPWAT) on 206 digital images taken of various types of chronic wounds. Photographs assessed by the same rater on different occasions and by different raters showed moderate to excellent intrarater ICCs (ICC = 0.52–0.93), as well as test–retest (ICC = 0.86–0.90) and interrater (ICC = 0.71) reliability. There was excellent agreement between bedside assessments and assessments using photographs (ICC = 0.89).

State of the Art Wound Assessment and Evaluation of Healing

With all its limitations, visual evaluation of wounds alone, is not the future of wound care. Newer strategies involve laser to determine the topography of the wound area and imaging

with use of digital camera for planimetry and a specialized software for analysis. These methods can determine the margins of the wound and the size of the wound without contact with the wound. Some of the imaging devices can also determine the tissue type as well as the topography of the wound area and volume. Thermal imaging devices for wound assessment can assist with monitoring inflammation, infection, or ischemia (Kekonen & Viik, 2021). Features vary by device and are described in Boxes 10.6 and 10.7 (Kekonen & Viik, 2021).

If used correctly, these devices can increase precision and accuracy of wound measurement (Foltynski, 2018; Nair, 2018) while saving significant time and inconvenience for the clinician and patient. It must be emphasized that these modalities measure undermining or tunneling again

---

BOX 10.6 Features of Digital Wound Assessment and Monitoring Systems

- 3D Measurement
- Automated Alert Notifications on Wound Status
- Data Export
- Diagnostic Capabilities
- Digital Imaging
- EMR-Compatible
- HIPAA Compliant
- Mobile Capability
- Noncontact
- Progress Tracking
- Reference/Resource Availability
- Reporting Capabilities
- Smart Device Enables
- Software Integrated
- System Hardware Components

BOX 10.7 Wound Assessment Technology

Standard noncontact planimetry (or digital planimetry) uses a digital camera and a known sized object for scaling (e.g., ruler). Image is uploaded to a computer, tablet, or phone. Software is used to outline wound for calculation of surface area

Structured light or laser-assisted medical wound measurement (LAWM) uses digital camera images and laser beams that distort according to topography of the wound. Image is uploaded to a computer. Software is used to outline wound for calculation of surface area and volume

3D wound measurement (3DWM) uses an application on a cell phone. Digital images with 3D structure sensor or similar uses infrared to obtain surface area, volume and % tissue color in read time

Autofluorescence or endogenous fluorescence is used in a device to identify quantity of pathogenic bacteria in wounds without need for using exogenous contrast agents. The device is portable, noncontact, real-time and provides a digital planimetry feature (Fig. 19.1)

CLINICAL CONSULT

A: Consulted for "DTPI pressure injury under leg brace, see photo in chart." Mr. Johnson is A&O × 3, 53-year-old gentleman, admitted yesterday for increased weakness and atrial fibrillation. Photo in chart shows defined purple round lesion. No documentation noted on wound flow sheet. PMH shows multiple sclerosis. Patient states he was up ad lib until yesterday, when he became extremely tired and weak. Nurse applied heel-offloading boots after use of pillows was ineffective due to leg spasms. Patient verbalized good understanding of pressure injury prevention and demonstrates ability to reposition effectively when asked. Left posterior leg lesion 3 × 3 cm, intact, round and slightly edematous, periwound skin intact, no local sign of infection. PT and pedal pulses palpable, no history or signs of venous insufficiency. Patient denies pain, states he didn't know it was there.

D: Complete wound assessment and differential diagnosis is not consistent with a deep tissue pressure injury as it is not located over a bony prominence nor under the heel-offloading device. Suspect bruise from bumping into furniture. (Patient is on anticoagulants and states he commonly bumps into furniture at home).
P: Discussed importance for protecting himself from skin injury while on anticoagulants. Patient states he has just purchased new leather furniture to replace mission style wood furniture at home.
I: Recommendations: (1) Protect bruise from further injury especially during transfers and ambulation. (2) Continue interventions for pressure injury prevention.
E: Monitor bruise daily with skin inspection and call provider if it increases in dimensions, becomes painful, or deteriorates. No further plans for follow up. Please reconsult as needed.

underscoring their use is an adjunct rather than replacement for a comprehensive bedside assessment (EPUAP, NPIAP, & PPPIA, 2019; Jesada et al., 2013). Medical imaging (e.g., CT, SPECT/CT, MRI, ultrasound), techniques for detecting specific wound biomarkers (e.g., fluorescence, NIR, luminescence imaging) and their potential implications in wound monitoring (Li, Mohamedi, Senkowsky, Nair, & Tang, 2020) are beyond the scope of this chapter.

SUMMARY

- Few pathologic conditions are evaluated with a single instrument or parameter.
- The more intricate the process (e.g., congestive heart failure), the more clinicians rely on several measures (e.g., radiologic examination, physical examination, pulse characteristics, treadmill tests, hematocrit) to accurately capture a full description of the extent of the condition.
- Similarly, several parameters are required to best capture the condition of the wound.

- Recognizing the difference between simply measuring the dimensions of a wound and the more complex process of assessing the status of the wound's multiple components and healing status is essential to successful wound management and holistic patient care.
- Evaluating wounds as if they exist separately from the patient not only is inadequate but also is inconsistent with evidence-based practice.

SELF-ASSESSMENT QUESTIONS

1. Gently pinching a fold of skin on a patient's arm is a test for:
   a. Skin turgor
   b. Edema
   c. Capillary refill
   d. Erythema
2. Nonblanchable erythema over a bony prominence of a patient with a spinal cord injury is indicative of:
   a. Moisture-associated skin damage
   b. Stage 1 pressure injury
   c. A yeast infection
   d. Healthy skin
3. Epibole indicates:
   a. Attached wound edges
   b. Dry wound edges
   c. Rolled wound edge
   d. Infection

4. Slough is:
   a. Not a true tissue rather a byproduct of wound healing
   b. Necrotic tissue
   c. Biofilm
   d. Fibrin
5. How would you document 1 cm of undermining from the top of the wound to the bottom of the wound
   a. 1 cm of undermining from 12 to 6 o'clock
   b. 1 cm of undermining from the top of the wound to the bottom of the wound
   c. 1 cm shelf at the wound edges of half of the wound
   d. Any of the above

6. Advantages to wound photography include:
   a. Facilitates consultation with multiple disciplines for challenging differential diagnosis
   b. Prevents over exposure of wound by multiple health care providers
   c. Provides clarity for complex step-by-step procedures
   d. All of the above

7. Hypergranulation tissue is:
   a. An overproduction of granulation tissue generally caused by excess moisture or friction
   b. Red friable, shiny granulation above the level of the surrounding skin
   c. Treated with silver nitrate
   d. All of the above

REFERENCES

Alavi, A., Niakosari, F., & Sibbald, R. G. (2010). When and how to perform a biopsy on a chronic wound. *Advances in Skin & Wound Care, 23*(3), 132–140.

Angel, D. (2019). Slough what does it mean and how can it be managed. *Wound Practice and Research, 27*(4), 164–167. https://doi.org/10.33235/wpr.27.4.164-167.

Arndt, J. V., & Kelechi, T. J. (2014). An overview of instruments for wound and skin assessment and healing. *Journal of Wound, Ostomy, and Continence Nursing, 41*(1), 17–23.

Asim, M., Alkadi, M. M., Asim, H., & Ghaffar, A. (2019). Dehydration and volume depletion: How to handle the misconceptions. *World Journal of Nephrology, 8*(1), 23–32.

Bates-Jensen, B. M., McCreath, H. E., Harputlu, D., & Patlan, A. (2019). Reliability of the Bates-Jensen wound assessment tool for pressure injury assessment: The pressure ulcer detection study. *Wound Repair and Regeneration, 27*(4), 386–395.

Bates-Jensen, B. M., McCreath, H. E., & Pongquan, V. (2009). Subepidermal moisture is associated with early pressure ulcer damage in nursing home residents with dark skin tones: Pilot findings. *Journal of Wound, Ostomy, and Continence Nursing, 36*(3), 277–284.

Baumgarten, M., Margolis, D. J., Selekof, J. L., Moye, N., Jones, P. S., & Shardell, M. (2009). Validity of pressure ulcer diagnosis using digital photography. Wound Repair and Regeneration, *17*(2), 287–290. https://doi.org/10.1111/j.1524-475X.2009.00462.x.

Baumgarten, M., Margolis, D., van Doorn, C., et al. (2004). Black/white differences in pressure ulcer incidence in nursing home residents. *Journal of the American Geriatrics Society, 52*(8), 1293–1298.

Bennett, A. M. (1995). Report of the task force on the implications for darkly pigmented intact skin in the prediction and prevention of pressure ulcers. *Advances in Wound Care, 8*(6), 34–35.

Bhargava, A., Chanmugam, A., & Herman, C. (2015). Heat transfer model for deep tissue injury: A step towards early thermography diagnostic capability. *Diagnostic Pathology.* Retrieved 1/12/2021 from www.diagnosticpathology.org/content/9/1/36.

Black, J., Baharestani, M., Black, S., Cavazos, J., Conner-Kerr, T., Edsberg, L., et al. (2010). An overview of tissue types in pressure ulcers: A consensus panel recommendation. *Ostomy/Wound Management, 56*(4), 28–44.

Bolton, L., McNees, P., van Rijswijk, L., et al. (2004). Wound-healing outcomes using standardized assessment and care in clinical practice. *Journal of Wound, Ostomy, and Continence Nursing, 31*(2), 65–71.

Brindle, T., & Farmer, P. (2019). Undisturbed wound healing: A narrative review of the literature and clinical considerations. *Wounds International, 10*(2).

Buckley, K. M., Adelson, L. K., & Hess, C. T. (2005). Get the picture! Developing a wound photography competency for home care nurses. *Journal of Wound, Ostomy, and Continence Nursing, 32*(3), 171–177.

Bull, R. H., Staines, K. L., Collarte, A. J., Bain, D. S., Ivins, N. M., & Harding, K. G. (2022). Measuring progress to healing: A challenge and an opportunity. International Wound Journal, *19*(4), 734–740. https://doi.org/10.1111/iwj.13669.

Cardinal, M., Eisenbud, D. E., & Armstrong, D. G. (2009). Wound shape geometry measurements correlate to eventual wound healing. *Wound Repair and Regeneration, 17*(2), 173–178.

Carlson, M., Vigen, C. L., Rubayi, S., et al. (2017). Lifestyle intervention for adults with spinal cord injury: Results of the USC-RLANRC pressure ulcer prevention study. *The Journal of Spinal Cord Medicine, 17*, 1–18.

Clendenin, M., Jaradeh, K., Shamirian, A., & Rhodes, S. L. (2015). Inter-operator and inter-device agreement and reliability of the SEM Scanner. *Journal of Tissue Viability, 24*(1), 17–23. https://doi.org/10.1016/j.jtv.2015.01.003. Epub 2015 Feb 3 PMID:25682271. Retrieved 1/15/2021 from https://www.sciencedirect.com/science/article/pii/S0965206X15000042?via%3Dihub.

Cox, J., Kaes, L., Martinez, M., & Moles, D. (2016). A prospective, observational study to assess the use of thermography to predict progression of discolored intact skin to necrosis among patients in skilled nursing facilities. *Ostomy/Wound Management, 62*(10), 14–33. PMID:27768578. Retrieved 1/16/2021 from https://www.o-wm.com/article/prospective-observational-study-assess-use-thermography-predict-progression-discolored.

Darwin, E. S., Jaller, J. A., Hirt, P. A., & Kirsner, R. S. (2019). Comparison of 3-dimensional wound measurement with laser-assisted and hand measurements: A retrospective chart review. *Wound Management & Prevention, 65(1),* 36–41.

de Laat, E. H., Scholte, O. P., Reimer, W. H., et al. (2005). Pressure ulcers: Diagnostics and interventions aimed at wound-related complaints: A review of the literature. *Journal of Clinical Nursing, 14*(4), 464–472.

de Leon, J. M., Barnes, S., Nagel, M., et al. (2009). Cost-effectiveness of negative pressure wound therapy for postsurgical patients in long-term acute care. *Advances in Skin & Wound Care, 22*(3), 122–127.

Doughty, D. B. (2004). Wound assessment: Tips and techniques. *Advances in Skin & Wound Care, 17*, 369–372.

Ebid, A. A., El-Kafy, E. M., & Alayat, M. S. (2013). Effect of pulsed Nd:YAG laser in the treatment of neuropathic foot ulcers in children with spina bifida: A randomized controlled study. *Photomedicine and Laser Surgery, 31*(12), 565–570.

Edsberg, L. E., Black, J. M., Goldberg, M., McNichol, L., Moore, L., & Sieggreen, M. (2016). Revised national pressure ulcer advisory panel pressure injury staging system: Revised pressure injury staging system. Journal of Wound, Ostomy, And Continence Nursing, *43*(6), 585–597. https://doi.org/10.1097/WON.0000000000000281.

Edsberg, L. E., Wyffels, J. T., & Ha, D. S. (2011). Longitudinal study of stage III and stage IV pressure ulcer area and perimeter as healing parameters to predict wound closure. *Ostomy/Wound Management*, 57(10), 50–62.

Ervin, N. E. (2005). Clinical coaching: A strategy for enhancing evidence-based nursing practice. *Clinical Nurse Specialist*, 19(6), 296–301.

European Pressure Ulcer Advisory Panel, National Pressure Injury Advisory Panel, & Pan Pacific Pressure Injury Alliance (EPUAP, NPIAP, & PPPIA). (2019). In E. Haesler (Ed.), *Prevention and treatment of pressure ulcers/injuries*. Osborne Park, Western Australia: Cambridge Media.

Falanga, V., & Sabolinski, M. L. (2000). Prognostic factors for healing of venous ulcers. *Wounds*, 12(Suppl. 5A), 42A–46A.

Foltynski, P. (2018). Ways to increase precision and accuracy of wound area measurement using smart devices: *Advanced app Planimator. PLoS One*, 13(3), e0192485. https://doi.org/10.1371/journal.pone.0192485.

George-Saintilus, E., Tommasulo, B., Cal, C. E., et al. (2009). Pressure ulcer PUSH score and traditional nursing assessment in nursing home residents: Do they correlate? *Journal of the American Medical Directors Association*, 10(2), 141–144.

Goh, L. J., & Zhu, X. (2017). Effectiveness of telemedicine for distant wound care advice towards patient outcomes: Systematic review and meta-analysis. *International Archives of Nursing and Health Care*, 3, 070.

Grey, J. E., Enoch, S., & Harding, K. G. (2006). Wound assessment. *BMJ (Clinical Research Ed.)*, 332(7536), 285–288. https://doi.org/10.1136/bmj.332.7536.285.

Guihan, M., Bates-Jenson, B. M., Chun, S., et al. (2012). Assessing the feasibility of subepidermal moisture to predict erythema and stage 1 pressure ulcers in persons with spinal cord injury: A pilot study. *The Journal of Spinal Cord Medicine*, 35(1), 46–52.

Günes, U. Y. (2009). A prospective study evaluating the Pressure Ulcer Scale for Healing (PUSH Tool) to assess stage II, stage III, and stage IV pressure ulcers. *Ostomy/Wound Management*, 55(5), 48–52.

Haesler, E., Swanson, T., Ousey, K., & Carville, K. (2019). Clinical indicators of wound infection and biofilm: Reaching international consensus. *Journal of Wound Care*, 28(Suppl. 3b), s4–s12.

Halpern, N. J., & Ravitz, J. R. (2017). Malpractice liability considerations for wound clinics. *Today's Wound Clinic*, 11(9). Retrieved 1/14/2021 from https://www.todayswoundclinic.com/articles/malpractice-liability-considerations-wound-clinics.

Harris, C., Bates-Jensen, B., Parslow, N., et al. (2010). Wound assessment tool. *Journal of Wound, Ostomy, and Continence Nursing*, 37(3), 253–259.

Harrow, J. J., & Mayrovitz, H. N. (2014). Subepidermal moisture surrounding pressure ulcers in persons with a spinal cord injury: A pilot study. *The Journal of Spinal Cord Medicine*, 37(6), 719–728. https://doi.org/10.1179/2045772313Y.0000000193. Retrieved 1/15/2021 from https://www.ncbi.nlm.nih.gov/pmc/articles/PMC4231959/.

Hon, J., Lagden, K., McLaren, A. M., et al. (2010). Prospective, multicenter study to validate use of the PUSH in patients with diabetic, venous, and pressure ulcers. *Ostomy/Wound Management*, 56(2), 26–36.

Houghton, P., Kincaid, C., Campbell, K., et al. (2000). Photographic assessment of the appearance of chronic pressure and leg ulcers. *Ostomy/Wound Management*, 46(4), 20–30.

Institute for Healthcare Improvement (IHI), & National Pressure Injury Advisory Panel (NPIAP). (2021). *Pressure ulcer prevention: A nursing competency-based curriculum*. Retrieved from http://www.ihi.org/resources/Pages/Tools/PressureUlcerPreventionAnNursingCompetencybasedCurriculum.aspx.

Jesada, E. C., Warren, J. I., Goodman, D., Iliuta, R. W., Thurkauf, G., McLaughlin, M. K., et al. (2013). Staging and defining characteristics of pressure ulcers using photographs by staff nurses in acute care settings. *Journal of Wound, Ostomy, and Continence Nursing*, 40(2), 150–156. https://doi.org/10.1097/WON.0b013e31828093a4.

Jones, K. R., Fennie, K., & Lenihan, A. (2007). Chronic wounds: Factors influencing healing within 3 months and nonhealing after 5-6 months of care. *Wounds*, 19(3), 51–63.

Kantor, J., & Margolis, D. J. (2000). A multicentre study of percentage change in venous leg ulcer area as a prognostic index of healing at 24 weeks. *The British Journal of Dermatology*, 142(5), 960–964.

Kekonen, A., & Viik, J. (2021). Monitoring wound healing. In P. Annus, & M. Min (Eds.), *Bioimpedance and spectroscopy* Academic Press, Elsevier Inc.

Khoo, R., & Jansen, S. (2016). The evolving field of wound measurement techniques: A literature review. *Wounds*, 28(6), 175–181.

King, B. (2014). Influencing dressing choice and supporting wound management using remote "tele-wound care". *British Journal of Community Nursing*, 19(Suppl. 6), S24–S31.

Kinsella, A. (2002). Advanced telecare for wound care delivery. *Home Healthcare Nurse*, 20(7), 457–461.

Kottner, J., Dassen, T., & Lahmann, N. (2009). Comparison of two skin examination methods for grade 1 pressure ulcers. *Journal of Clinical Nursing*, 18(17), 2464–2469.

Langemo, D. K., Anderson, J., Hanson, D., et al. (2008). Measuring wound length, width, and area: Which technique? *Advances in Skin & Wound Care*, 21, 42–45.

Li, S., Mohamedi, A. H., Senkowsky, J., Nair, A., & Tang, L. (2020). Imaging in chronic wound diagnostics. *Advances in Wound Care*, 9(5), 245–263.

Lizaka, S., Sanada, H., Matsui, Y., et al. (2012). Predictive validity of weekly monitoring of wound status using DESIGN-R score change for pressure ulcer healing: A multicenter prospective cohort study. *Wound Repair and Regeneration*, 20(4), 473–481.

Nair, H. K. R. (2018). Increasing productivity with smartphone digital imagery wound measurements and analysis. *Journal of Wound Care*, 27(Suppl. 9a), S12–S19.

National Institute for Health and Care Excellence. (2020). SEM Scanner 200 for preventing pressure ulcers. In *Medical technologies guidance*. NICE guideline no. 51. Retrieved 1/15/2021 from https://www.nice.org.uk/guidance/mtg51.

O'Brien, G., Moore, Z., Patton, D., & O'Connor, T. (2018). The relationship between nurses' assessment of early pressure ulcer damage and subepidermal moisture measurement: A prospective explorative study. *Journal of Tissue Viability*, 27(4), 232–237.

Olivieri, B., Yates, T. E., Vianna, S., Adenikinju, O., Beasley, R. E., & Houseworth, J. (2018). On the cutting edge: Wound care for the endovascular specialist. *Seminars in Interventional Radiology*, 35(5), 406–426.

Onuh, O. C., Brydges, H. T., Nasr, H., Savage, E., Gorenstein, S., & Chiu, E. (2022). Capturing essentials in wound photography past, present, and future: A proposed algorithm for standardization. *Nursing Management*, 53(9), 12–23. https://doi.org/10.1097/01.NUMA.0000855948.88672.7a.

O'Toole, M. T. (2017). *Mosby's medical dictionary* (10th ed.). St. Louis: Mosby Elsevier.

Painter, L. M., Dudjak, L. A., Kidwell, K. M., Simmons, R. L., & Kidwell, R. P. (2011). The nurse's role in the causation of compensable injury. *Journal of Nursing Care Quality, 26*(4), 311–319. https://doi.org/10.1097/NCQ.0b013e31820f9576. 21386717.

Panuncialman, J., Hammerman, S., Carson, P., & Falanga, V. (2010). Wound edge biopsy sites in chronic wounds heal rapidly and do not result in delayed overall healing of the wounds. *Wound Repair and Regeneration, 18*(1), 21–25. https://doi.org/10.1111/j.1524-475X.2009.00559.x.

Percival, S., & Suleman, N. (2015). Slough and biofilm: Removal of barriers to wound healing by desloughing. *Journal of Wound Care, 24*(11). 498, 500–3, 6–10.

Phillips, T. J., Machado, F., Trout, R., et al. (2000). Prognostic indicators in venous ulcers. *Journal of the American Academy of Dermatology, 43*(4), 627–630.

Pillen, H., Miller, M., Thomas, J., et al. (2009). Assessment of wound healing: Validity, reliability and sensitivity of available instruments. *Wound Practice and Research, 17*(4), 208–217.

Robson, M. C., Hill, D. P., Woodske, M. E., et al. (2000). Wound healing trajectories as predictors of effectiveness of therapeutic agents. *Archives of Surgery, 135*(7), 773–777.

Sanada, H., Moriguchi, T., Miyachi, Y., et al. (2004). Reliability and validity of DESIGN, a tool that classifies pressure ulcer severity and monitors healing. *Journal of Wound Care, 13*, 13–18.

Santamaria, N., Glance, D. G., Prentice, J., & Fielder, K. (2010). The development of an electronic wound management system for Western Australia. *Wound Practice and Research, 18*(4), 174–179.

Sheehan, P., Jones, P., Caselli, A., et al. (2003). Percent change in wound area of diabetic foot ulcers over a 4-week period is a robust predictor of complete healing in a 12-week prospective trial. *Diabetes Care, 26*, 1879–1882.

Shi, C., Bonnett, L. J., Dumville, J. C., & Cullum, N. (2020). Nonblanchable erythema for predicting pressure ulcer development: A systematic review with an individual participant data meta-analysis. *The British Journal of Dermatology, 182*(2), 278–286. https://doi.org/10.1111/bjd.18154. Epub 2019 Aug 25 PMID:31120145.

Snyder, R. J., Cardinal, M., Dauphinée, D. M., et al. (2010). A post hoc analysis of reduction in diabetic foot ulcer size at 4 weeks as a predictor of healing by 12 weeks. *Ostomy/Wound Management, 56*(3), 44–50.

Sood, A., Granick, M. S., Trial, C., Lano, J., Palmier, S., Ribal, E., et al. (2016). The role of telemedicine in wound care: A review and analysis of a database of 5,795 patients from a mobile wound-healing center in Languedoc-Roussillon, France. *Plastic and Reconstructive Surgery, 138*(3 Suppl), 248S–256S.

Sprigle, S., Zhang, L., & Duckworth, M. (2009). Detection of skin erythema in darkly pigmented skin using multispectral images. *Advances in Skin & Wound Care, 22*(4), 172–179.

Stern, A., Mitsakakis, N., Paulden, M., Alibhai, S., Wong, J., Tomlinson, G., et al. (2014). Pressure ulcer multidisciplinary teams via telemedicine: A pragmatic cluster randomized stepped wedge trial in long term care. *BMC Health Services Research, 14*, 83.

Sterner, E., Lindholm, C., Berg, E., et al. (2011). Category I pressure ulcers: How reliable is clinical assessment? *Orthopaedic Nursing, 30*(3), 194–205.

Thompson, N., Gordey, L., Bowles, H., Parslow, N., & Houghton, P. (2013). Reliability and validity of the revised photographic wound assessment tool on digital images taken of various types of chronic wounds. *Advances in Skin & Wound Care, 26*(8), 360–373.

Vanderwee, K., Grypdonck, M. H. F., De Bacquer, D., et al. (2006). The reliability of two observation methods of nonblanchable erythema, grade 1 pressure ulcer. *Applied Nursing Research, 19*(3), 156–162.

van Rijswijk, L. (2003). Full-thickness leg ulcers: Patient demographics and predictors of healing. *The Journal of Family Practice, 36*(6), 625–632.

Wang, S. C., Anderson, J. A., Jones, D. V., & Evans, R. (2016). Patient perception of wound photography. *International Wound Journal, 13*(3), 326–330.

Williams, E. M., & Deering, S. (2016). Achieving competency in wound care: An innovative training module using the long-term care setting. *International Wound Journal, 13*(5), 829–832.

Wound, Ostomy and Continence Nurses Society. (2014). Guideline for management of wounds in patients with lower-extremity arterial disease. In *WOCN clinical practice guideline series 1*. Mt. Laurel: Author.

Wound, Ostomy and Continence Nurses Society. (2016). Guideline for patients with pressure ulcers injuries. In *WOCN clinical practice guideline series #2*. Mt. Laurel: Author.

Wound, Ostomy and Continence Nurses Society™. (2017). *Position statement about the role and scope of practice for wound care providers*. Mt. Laurel, NJ: WOCN®.

Wound, Ostomy and Continence Nurses Society. (2019). *Wound, Ostomy and Continence Nurses Society's guidance on OASIS-D integumentary items: Best practice for clinicians*. Mt. Laurel: Author. Retrieved 1/9/2023 from https://cdn.ymaws.com/member.wocn.org/resource/resmgr/document_library/oasis-d_best_practice_docume.pdf.

Young, T., Rohwer, A., Volmink, J., et al. (2014). What are the effects of teaching evidence-based health care (EBHC)? Overview of systematic reviews. *PLoS One, 9*(1), e86706.

Zhong, X., Nagase, T., Huang, L., Kaitani, T., Iizaka, S., Yamamoto, Y., et al. (2013). Reliability and validity of the Chinese version of DESIGN-R, an assessment instrument for pressure ulcers. *Ostomy/Wound Management, 59*(2), 36–43. 23388396.

Zimny, S., Schatz, H., & Pfohl, M. (2002). Determinants and estimation of healing times in diabetic foot ulcers. *Journal of Diabetes and Its Complications, 16*, 327–332.

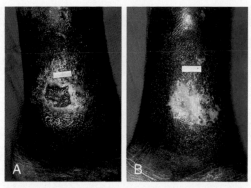

Plate 1 **A,** Partial thickness (typically less than 0.2 cm in depth) venous ulcer healing by epithelialization from the wound edges. **B,** Resurfaced venous ulcer lacks normal dark pigmentation because of depth of damage (below basement membrane). Repigmentation occurs over time and should not be confused with scar tissue.

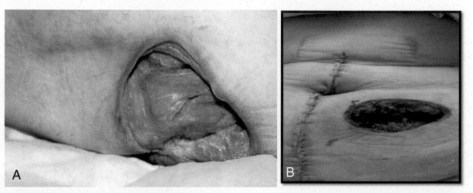

Plate 2 Full-thickness wounds. **A,** Chronic full-thickness wound: Stage 4 pressure injury/ulcer with exposed muscle. **B,** Acute full-thickness wound.

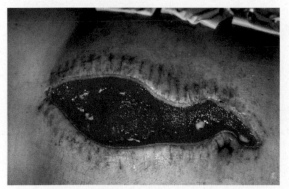

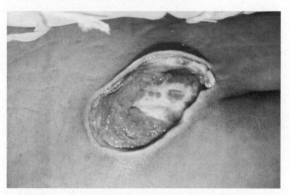

Plate 3 Full-thickness abdominal wound healing by secondary intention with healthy (*red*, cobblestone) granulation tissue and attached wound edges.

Plate 4 Stage 4 sacral pressure injury/ulcer wound edges are rolled (epibole), which is an impediment to wound healing.

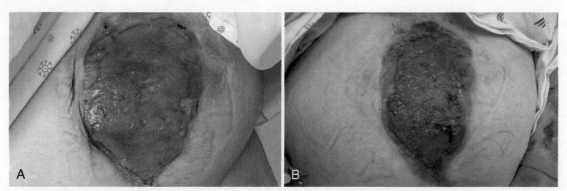

Plate 5 **A,** Pale, pink smooth tissue. Absence of granulation tissue suggesting heavy bacterial load, biofilm, or other impediments to wound healing. **B,** Same wound with granulation tissue after 1 week of topical antiseptic dressing use (note red cobblestone appearance).

PLATE 6 Primary Skin Lesions

Description

Examples

A. Macule

Flat, circumscribed area that is a change in the color of the skin less than 1 cm in diameter

Freckle, flat mole (nevus), petechia, measles, scarlet fever

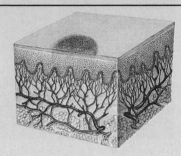

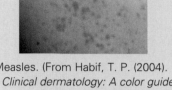

Measles. (From Habif, T. P. (2004). *Clinical dermatology: A color guide to diagnosis and therapy* (5th ed.), St. Louis: Mosby.)

B. Papule

Elevated, firm, circumscribed area less than 1 cm in diameter

Wart (verruca), elevated mole, lichen planus

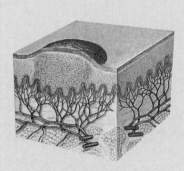

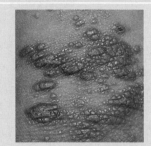

Lichen planus. (From Weston, W., et al. (1996). *Color textbook of pediatric dermatology* (4th ed.). Edinburgh: Mosby.)

C. Patch

Flat, nonpalpable, irregular-shaped macule greater than 1 cm in diameter

Vitiligo, port-wine stain, Mongolian spot, café au lait spot

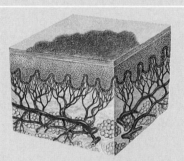

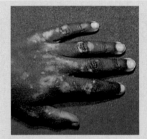

Vitiligo. (From Weston, W., et al. (1991). *Color textbook of pediatric dermatology* (4th ed.). Edinburgh: Mosby.)

D. Plaque

Elevated, firm, rough lesion with flat top surface greater than 1 cm in diameter

Psoriasis, seborrheic keratosis, actinic keratosis

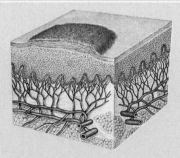

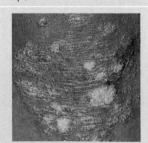

Plaque. (From Habif, T. P. (2004). *Clinical dermatology: A color guide to diagnosis and therapy* (5th ed.), St. Louis: Mosby.)

PLATE 6   **Primary Skin Lesions—cont'd**

Description	Examples		

E. Wheal
Elevated, irregular-shaped area of cutaneous edema; solid, transient, variable diameter

Insect bite, urticaria, allergic reaction

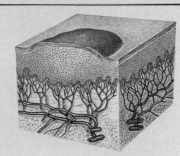 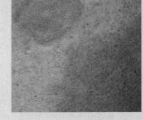

Wheal. (From Farrar, W. E., et al. (1992). *Slide atlas of infectious diseases.* St. Louis: Mosby.)

F. Nodule
Elevated, firm, circumscribed lesion; deeper in dermis than a papule; 1–2 cm in diameter

Erythema nodosum, lipoma

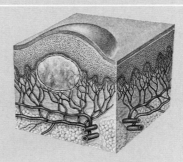 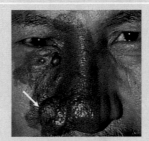

Hypertrophic nodule. (From Goldman, M. P. (1994). *Cutaneous and cosmetic laser surgery.* Edinburgh: Mosby.)

G. Tumor
Elevated and solid lesion; may or may not be clearly demarcated; deeper in dermis; greater than 2 cm in diameter

Neoplasm, benign tumor, lipoma, hemangioma

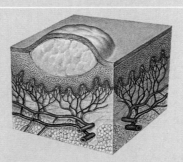 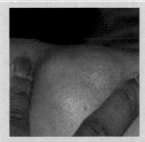

Lipoma. (From Lemmi, F. O., & Lemmi, C. A. E. (2000). *Physical assessment findings CD-ROM.* St. Louis: Saunders.)

H. Vesicle
Elevated, circumscribed, superficial, not into dermis; filled with serous fluid; less than 1 cm in diameter

Varicella (chicken pox), herpes zoster (shingles)

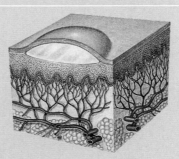 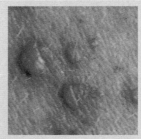

Vesicles caused by varicella. (From Farrar, W. E., et al. (1992). *Slide atlas of infectious diseases.* St. Louis: Mosby.)

Continued

PLATE 6   Primary Skin Lesions—cont'd

Description	Examples		
I. Bulla Vesicle greater than 1 cm in diameter	Blister, pemphigus vulgaris	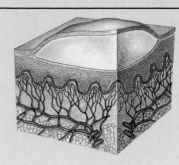	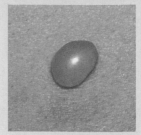 Blister. (From White, D. E., & Fenner, F. J. (1994). *Medical virology* (4th ed.). San Diego, CA: Academic Press.)
J. Pustule Elevated, superficial lesion; similar to vesicle but filled with purulent fluid	Impetigo, acne	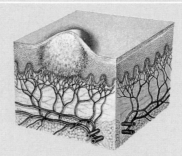	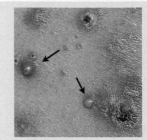 Acne. (From Weston, W., et al. (1996). *Color textbook of pediatric dermatology* (4th ed.). Edinburgh: Mosby.)
K. Cyst Elevated, circumscribed, encapsulated lesion; in dermis or subcutaneous layer; filled with liquid or semisolid material	Sebaceous cyst, cystic acne	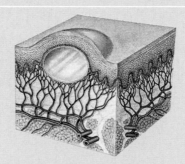	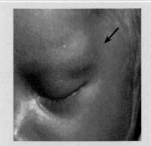 Sebaceous cyst. (From Weston, W., et al. (1996). *Color textbook of pediatric dermatology* (4th ed.). Edinburgh: Mosby.)
L. Telangiectasia Fine, irregular red lines produced by capillary dilation	Telangiectasia in rosacea	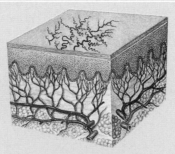	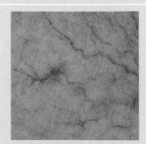 Telangiectasia. (From Lemmi, F. O., & Lemmi, C. A. E. (2000). *Physical assessment findings CD-ROM*. St. Louis: Saunders.)

PLATE 7 **Secondary Skin Lesions**

Description	Examples		

A. Scale
Heaped-up, keratinized cells; flaky skin; irregular; thick or thin; dry or oily; varies in size

Flaking of skin with seborrheic dermatitis following scarlet fever or flaking of skin following drug reaction, dry skin

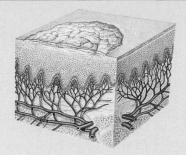

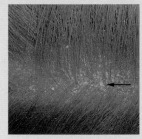

Fine scaling. (From Baran, R., et al. (1991). *Color atlas of the hair, scalp, and nails.* St. Louis: Mosby.)

B. Lichenification
Rough, thickened epidermis secondary to persistent rubbing; itching, or skin irritation; often involves flexor surface of extremity

Chronic dermatitis

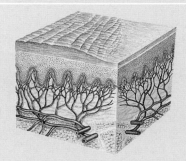

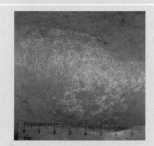

Lichenification. (From Lemmi, F. O., & Lemmi, C. A. E. (2000). *Physical assessment findings CD-ROM.* St. Louis: Saunders.)

C. Keloid
Irregular-shaped, elevated progressively enlarging scar; grows beyond boundaries of wound; caused by excessive collagen formation during healing

Keloid formation following surgery

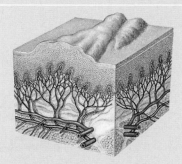

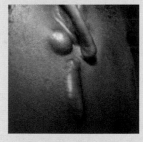

Keloid. (From Weston, W., et al. (1996). *Color textbook of pediatric dermatology* (4th ed.). Edinburgh: Mosby.)

D. Hypertrophic scar
Overproduction of collagen, causing the scar to be raised above skin level but not outside the boundaries of the wound

Healed wound or surgical incision

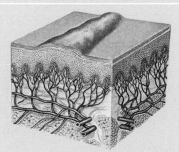

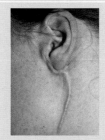

Hypertrophic scar. (From Eisele, D., & Smith, R. (2009). *Complications in head and neck surgery* (2nd ed.). Philadelphia: Mosby/Elsevier.)

Continued

PLATE 7   Secondary Skin Lesions—cont'd

Description	Examples		
E. Excoriation Loss of epidermis; linear hollowed-out, crusted area	Abrasion or scratch	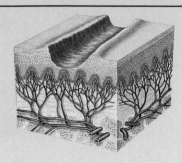	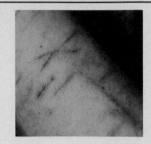 Excoriation from a tree branch. (From Lemmi, F. O., & Lemmi, C. A. E. (2000). *Physical assessment findings CD-ROM.* St. Louis: Saunders.)
F. Fissure Linear crack of break from epidermis; may be moist or dry	Athlete's foot, crack at corner of mouth	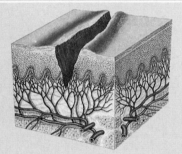	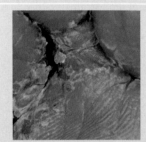 Scaling and fissures of tinea pedis. (From Lemmi, F. O., & Lemmi, C. A. E. (2000). *Physical assessment findings CD-ROM.* St. Louis: Saunders.)
G. Erosion Loss of part of epidermis; depressed, moist, glistening; follows rupture of vesicle or bulla	Varicella, variola after rupture	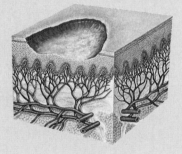	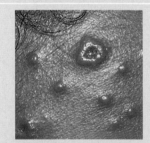 Erosion. (From Cohen, I. K., et al. (1993). *Wound healing.* Philadelphia: Saunders.)
H. Ulcer Loss of epidermis and dermis; concave; varies in size	Neuropathic wound ulcer	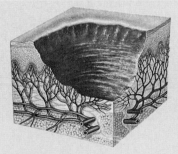	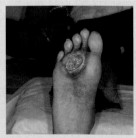 Neuropathic foot ulcer. (Courtesy of J. Lebretton and V. Driver.)

PLATE 7   Secondary Skin Lesions—cont'd

Description	Examples	
I. Crust Dried serum, blood, or purulent exudates; slightly elevated; varies in size; brown, red, black, tan, or straw color	Scab on abrasion, eczema	Scab.
J. Atrophy Thinning of skin surface and loss of skin markings; skin translucent and paper-like	Striae, aged skin	Striae. (Courtesy of Antoinette Hood, MD, Department of Dermatology, School of Medicine, University of Indiana, Indianapolis, IN.)

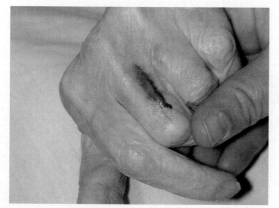

Plate 8 Type I skin tear without tissue loss: linear type (full thickness). (From LeBlanc, K., Christensen, D., Orsted, H. L., et al. (2008). Best practice recommendations for the prevention and treatment of skin tears. *Wound Care Canada, 6*(1), 22. Image courtesy of K. LeBlanc.)

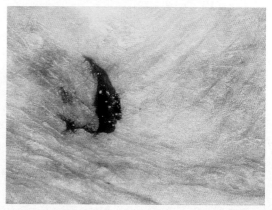

Plate 9 Type I skin tear without tissue loss: flap type (full thickness). (From LeBlanc, K., Christensen, D., Orsted, H. L., et al. (2008). Best practice recommendations for the prevention and treatment of skin tears. *Wound Care Canada, 6*(1), 22. Image courtesy of K. LeBlanc.)

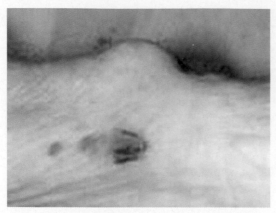

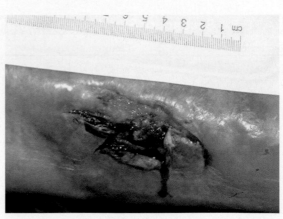

Plate 10 Type II skin tear with less than 25% partial tissue loss. (From LeBlanc, K., Christensen, D., Orsted, H. L., et al. (2008). Best practice recommendations for the prevention and treatment of skin tears. *Wound Care Canada, 6*(1), 22. Image courtesy of K. LeBlanc.)

Plate 11 Type II skin tear with greater than 25% partial tissue loss. (From LeBlanc, K., Christensen, D., Orsted, H. L., et al. (2008). Best practice recommendations for the prevention and treatment of skin tears. *Wound Care Canada, 6*(1), 22. Image courtesy of K. LeBlanc.)

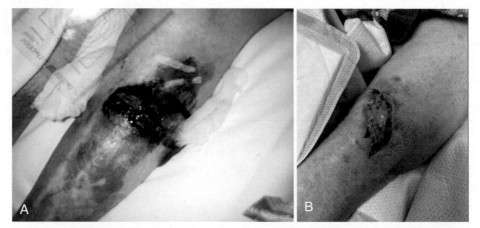

Plate 12 A, Type III skin tear with complete tissue loss. (From LeBlanc, K., Christensen, D., Orsted, H. L., et al. (2008). Best practice recommendations for the prevention and treatment of skin tears. *Wound Care Canada, 6* (1), 22. Image courtesy of K. LeBlanc.) **B,** Type 3 skin tear after fall. Complete skin loss exposing adipose tissue.

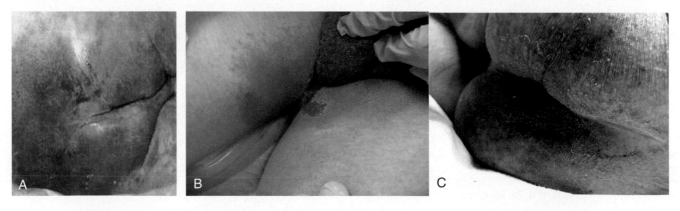

Plate 13 Incontinence-associated dermatitis (IAD). A type of MASD. **A,** Perianal skin, sacral area, and buttocks. **B,** Superficial epidermal erosion involving the scrotum and inner thighs. **C,** Manifestations in person with darkly pigmented skin complicated by candidiasis apparent in the periphery with open linear erosion on the upper aspect of the gluteal cleft not to be confused with pressure related etiology.

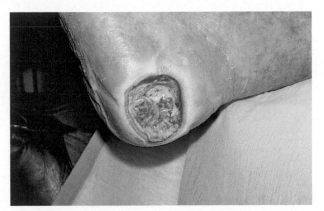

Plate 14 Unstageable right heel pressure injury/ulcer with periwound maceration (a type of MASD).

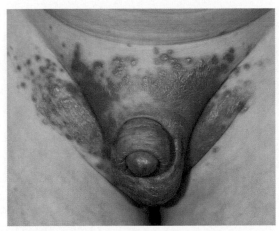

Plate 15 Candidiasis in moist diaper area with characteristic satellite lesions. (From Habif, T. P. (2009). *Clinical dermatology* (5th ed.). London: Mosby/Elsevier.)

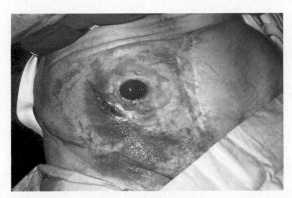

Plate 16 Peristomal dermatitis; a type of MASD. Patient with an ileostomy developed peristomal abscess that was incised. Dermatitis present due to inadequate protection of skin from stool (chemical irritant). Candidiasis also presents as papular satellite lesions and solid plaque-like rash advancing into groin and over suprapubic area.

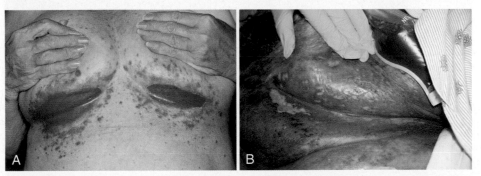

Plate 17 Intertrigo or intertriginous dermatitis (ITD); a type of MASD that develops in skin folds. **A,** ITD under breasts with visible satellite lesions. **B,** ITD in abdominal skin folds of patient with darkly pigmented skin. (**A**, From Habif, T. P. (2009). *Clinical dermatology* (5th ed.). London: Mosby/Elsevier.)

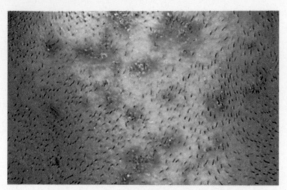

Plate 18 Folliculitis, an infection of hair follicles resulting from inappropriate hair removal technique. (From Jarvis, C. (2004). *Physical examination & health assessment* (4th ed.). St Louis: Saunders.)

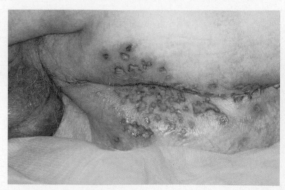

Plate 19 Herpes simplex virus (HSV) infection. Vesicles become pustules that erode, drain, and crust.

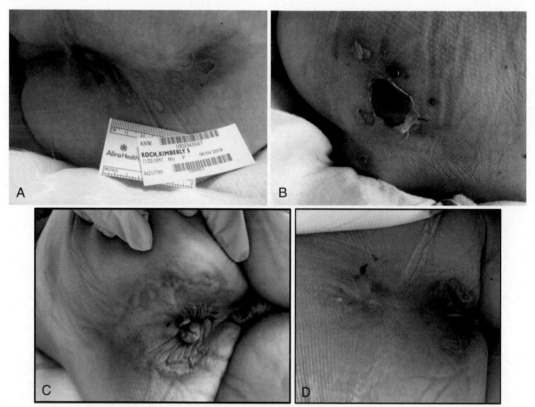

Plate 20 Laboratory confirmed HSV lesions originally mistaken and treated for IAD and/or pressure ulcers/injuries. Note variation in the extent of erythema present. **A,** Scattered shallow ulcerations along right perianal dermatome. **B,** Ulcerations predominantly located on dermatome encompassing left upper lateral buttocks. Dark discoloration within ruptured bulla may be indicative of dual etiology. **C and D,** Middle-aged female with multiple medical history including cancer and COVID-19 related pneumonia. Lesions initially managed as dermatitis/irritant (**A**) and later as a pressure injury (**B**). Identification of labial ulceration triggered further testing and confirmation of HSV-1 positive.

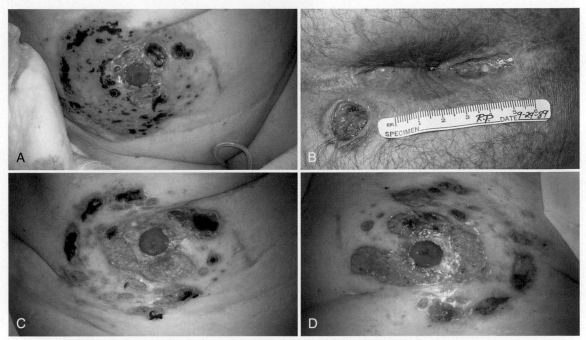

Plate 21 A, Peristomal HSV lesions initially suspected to be pyoderma gangrenosum. Islands of thick, soft adherent black, and tan necrosis with moist denudation; abdominal skin extremely painful. **B,** Same patient with perianal HSV lesions initially misclassified as pressure ulcers. Note proliferative edges and "punched-out" appearance that is characteristic of herpes lesions. **C,** Peristomal HSV lesions after initiation of antiviral medication. Note decreased erythema and fewer islands of necrosis; also experienced less pain in abdominal skin. **D,** Same patient after 1 week of antiviral medication. Necrosis has resolved. Epithelization and granulation have occurred. Pain significantly diminished.

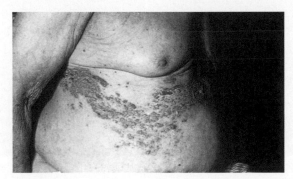

Plate 22 Herpes zoster viral (HSV) lesions involving simple thoracic dermatome. Vesicles are clustered and erythematous.

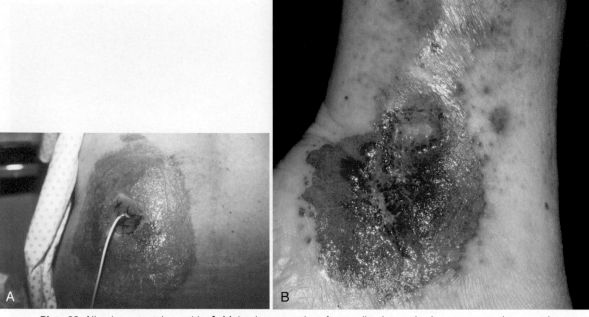

Plate 23 Allergic contact dermatitis. **A,** Moist desquamation after an allergic reaction in response to the second application of benzoin to a percutaneous nephrostomy site. **B,** Patients routinely apply neomycin ointment to leg ulcers. An allergic contact dermatitis occurred suddenly. The patient had previously used neomycin for years without any ill effects. (From Dinulos, J. G. H. (2021). *Habif's clinical dermatology: A color guide to diagnosis and therapy* (7th ed.). Philadelphia: Elsevier.)

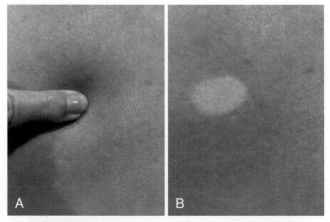

Plate 24 Blanchable erythema. **A,** Light compression applied with finger. **B,** Compressed area blanches white briefly.

Wound Assessment: Anatomy of a Wound

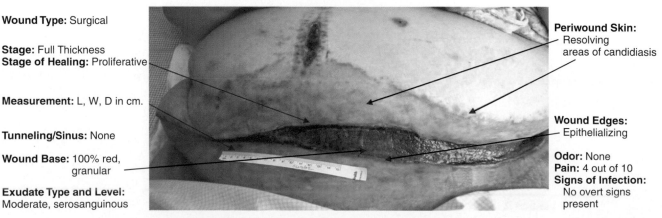

Wound Type: Surgical

Stage: Full Thickness
Stage of Healing: Proliferative

Measurement: L, W, D in cm.

Tunneling/Sinus: None

Wound Base: 100% red, granular

Exudate Type and Level: Moderate, serosanguinous

Periwound Skin: Resolving areas of candidiasis

Wound Edges: Epithelializing

Odor: None
Pain: 4 out of 10
Signs of Infection: No overt signs present

Plate 25 Anatomy of a wound. (Courtesy of BS Rolstad.)

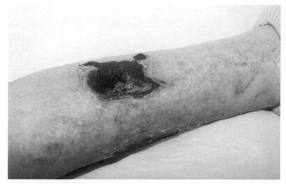

PLATE 26 Arterial ulcer with dry, stable eschar covering. Note dry condition of leg.

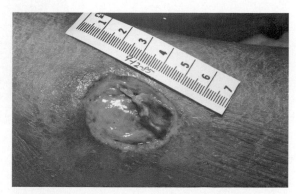

Plate 27 Arterial ulcer with loose and adherent yellow nonviable tissue present in wound bed. Mild erythema present along left lateral edge.

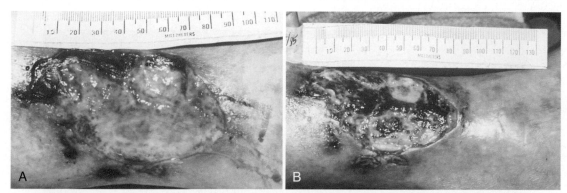

Plate 28 A, Moderately exudative venous ulcer with slough and nonviable tissue present in the wound bed and eschar present along superior aspect. **B,** After 1 week of hydrocolloids and compression therapy, autolysis has occurred, and venous ulcer has presence of granulation tissue. Amount of slough, nonviable tissue, and eschar is reduced; remaining eschar is softened.

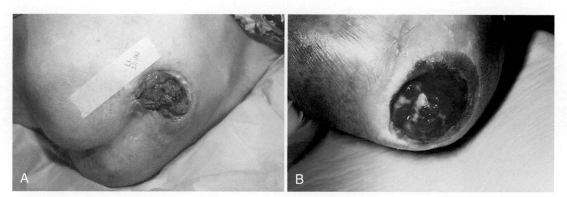

Plate 29 A, Stage 3 sacral pressure ulcer/injury with excess granulation tissue (hypergranulation tissue) due to overhydration from wound exudate. **B,** Stage 3 pressure injury/ulcer of the heel. (**B,** From Cain, J. E. (2009). *Mosby's PDQ for wound care.* St. Louis: Mosby/Elsevier.)

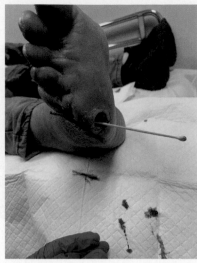

Plate 30 Diabetic foot ulcer with extensive tunneling from lateral planter surface through dorsal surface of foot. (Courtesy of Karen Bauer.)

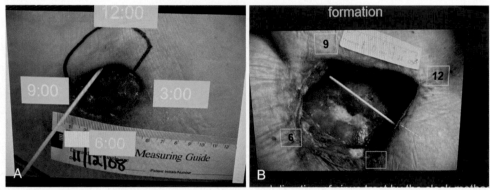

Plate 31 A, Stage 4 pressure injury/ulcer with undermining present between 9 and 2 o'clock. Cotton tip applicator and *black line* indicates dimensions of undermining. **B,** Stage 4 pressure injury/ulcer with undermining present from 9 to 3 o'clock. The *blue arrow* serves to identify extent of undermining. (Courtesy of Cara Couch.)

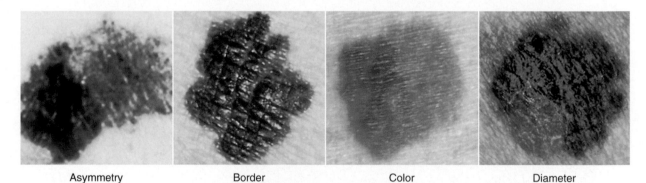

| Asymmetry | Border | Color | Diameter |

Plate 32 ABCDE Changes in Malignant Skin Moles. **A, A**symmetry-one half does not match the other. **B, B**order-ragged, notched, uneven, or blurred. **C, C**olor-uneven shades black, brown, tan, white, gray, red, and/or blue. **D, D**iameter-larger than 6 (mm). **E** (not pictured), **E**volving in size, shape, color, appearance, or texture.

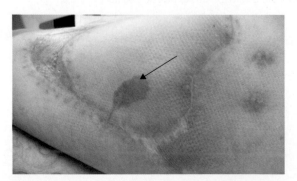

Plate 33 Right trochanter Stage 1 pressure ulcer at surgical flap site.

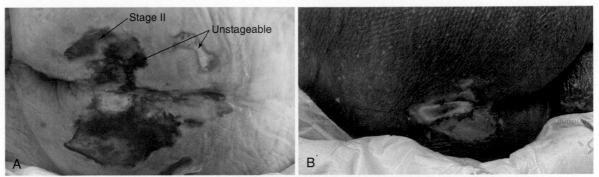

Plate 34 A, Sacral, coccygeal, buttocks ulcers. Mixed etiologies: pressure, friction, and IAD (fecal incontinence). Multiple degrees of tissue loss and stages with surrounding erythema. **B,** Coccyx pressure injury/ulcer with mixed stages. Initial DTI was not identified due to darkly pigmented skin until it began to evolve revealing multiple levels of tissue loss including Stage 2 (partial thickness) and unstageable (full thickness).

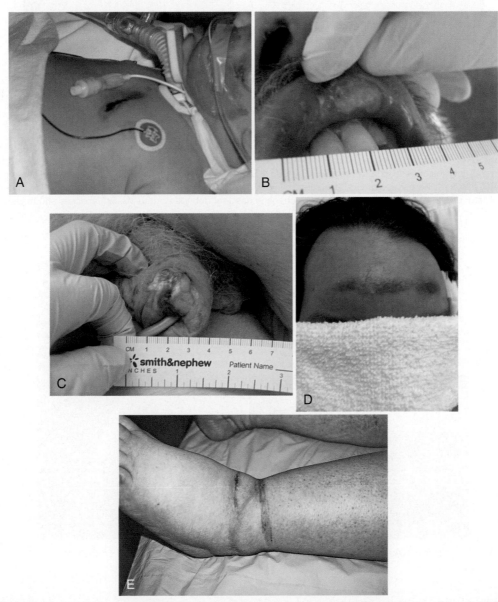

Plate 35 Medical Device Reacted Pressure Injuries (MDRPI) in a variety of stages. **A,** Shallow Stage 3 MDRPI on the right upper chest from respiratory equipment. **B,** Mucosal MDRPI from ET tube on the inner surface of the upper lip. **C,** Mucosal MDRPI on the glans penis from an indwelling urinary catheter. **D,** MDRPI on the forehead immediately following surgery in prone position. Injury resolved without tissue loss within 48 hours. **E,** Stage 2 (partial thickness) device related pressure injury/ulcer from a poorly fitting compression stocking. (**E,** From Morison, M., et al. (2004). *Chronic wound care: A problem-based learning approach.* London: Mosby.)

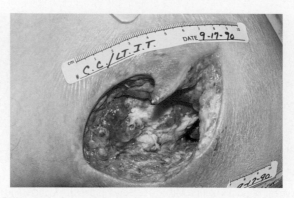

Plate 36 Left ischial tuberosity, Stage 4 pressure injury/ulcer.

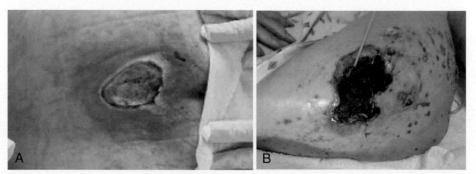

Plate 37 **A,** Unstageable sacral pressure injury/ulcer with yellow, adherent, nonviable wound base. Periwound skin shows signs of deep tissue pressure injury (DTPI). **B,** Right trochanter unstageable eschar covered pressure injury/ulcer with herpes lesions on the surrounding skin secondary to significant malnutrition. Cotton-tipped applicator demonstrates dead space under eschar and need for debridement to prevent abscess and massive infection.

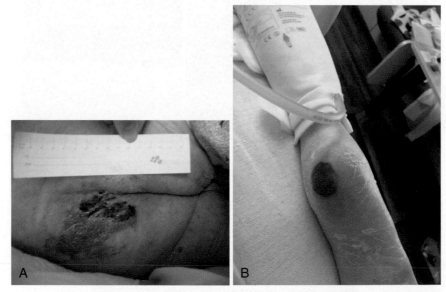

Plate 38 **A,** DTPI on left buttock following surgical procedure. **B,** DTPI on the heel.

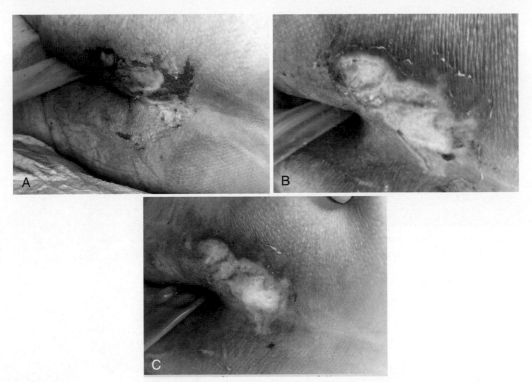

Plate 39 Evolution of a deep tissue pressure injury/ulcer (DTPI). **A,** DTPI over sacral/coccygeal area with varying levels of tissue damage. Eschar over upper lateral wound edges mixed with superficial loss of tissue. **B,** Evolution of DTPI after 2 weeks revealing unstageable (full thickness) tissue loss. **C,** Continued evolution with more consolidation of nonviable (unstageable) tissue over lateral sacrum.

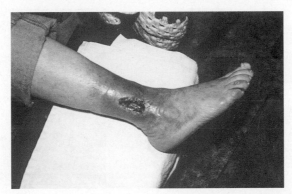

Plate 40 Typical appearance and location of venous ulcer. Surrounding skin has been moisturized to eliminate dry skin. Note hemosiderin staining of surrounding skin and ruddy red color of wound bed.

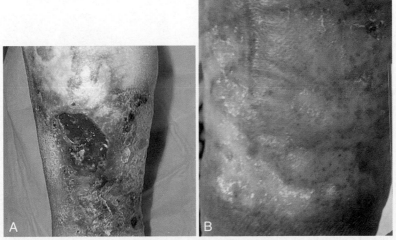

Plate 41 **A** and **B,** Atrophie blanche dermal sclerosis with dilated abnormal vasculature and ivory white plaques on the lower extremity and hemosiderin borders. (**B,** Courtesy of JoAnn Ermer-Seltun at Mercy Medical Center-North Iowa.)

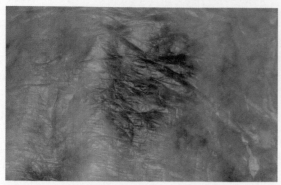

Plate 42 Senile purpura. Red-purple discoloration greater than 0.5 cm in diameter. Note these are not caused by pressure and may be confused with DTPI.

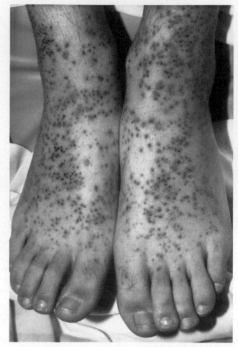

Plate 43 Petechiae on dorsal surface of feet and ankles. (Ball, J. W., et al. (Eds.), (2015). *Seidel's guide to physical examination* (8th ed.). Philadelphia: Mosby/Elsevier.)

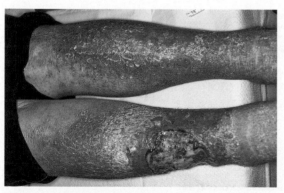

Plate 44 Venous dermatitis bilateral lower legs. Note extensive hemosiderin staining and lipodermatosclerosis. Venous ulceration present with densely adherent yellow slough. White residue from zinc compression wraps.

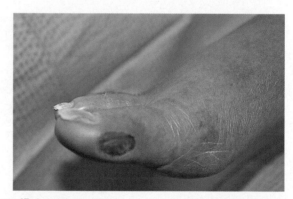

Plate 45 Arterial ulcer with necrotic base and halo of periwound erythema.

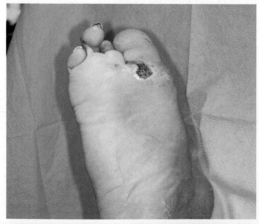

Plate 46 Diabetic foot ulcer. Charcot foot with neuropathic plantar ulcer on the first metatarsal head. Note callus and foot and toe deformities. (Courtesy of J. Lebretton and V. Driver.)

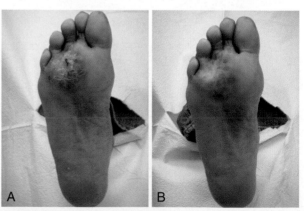

Plate 47 Callus removal. **A,** Hyperkeratotic callus causing increased plantar pressure. **B,** After rotary debridement, the surface is smooth and conducive to pressure redistribution. (Courtesy of J. Lebretton and V. Driver.)

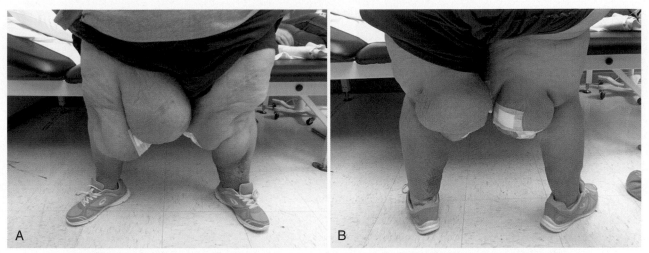

Plate 48 Lymphedema. **A** and **B,** Pattern of edema associated with lymphedema does not resolve with leg elevation and usually encompasses the entire leg. (Courtesy of JoAnn Ermer-Seltun at Mercy Medical Center-North Iowa.)

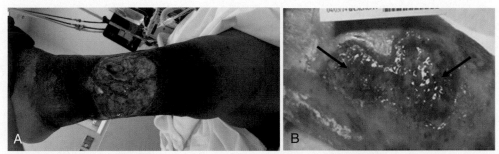

Plate 49 A, Signs of inflammation consistent with the presence of biofilm: friable granulation, odor, serous exudate, and/or pocketing in granulation tissue leading to delayed healing. **B,** Inflamed lateral calf wound covered with thick, adherent, opaque film. *Arrows* depict inconsistent wound topography (e.g., irregular surface and variation in color).

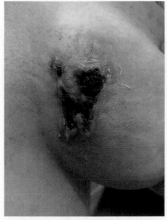

Plate 50 Overt or Classic signs of acute infection: periulcer erythema, local warmth, edema, induration, increasing pain.

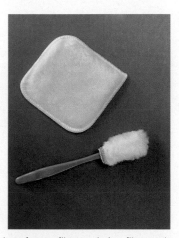

Plate 51 Examples of monofilament/microfiber pads used for bedside mechanical debridement.

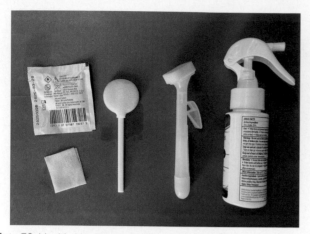

Plate 52 Liquid skin protectants formulated as wipes, sprays, wands (often referred to as skin sealants).

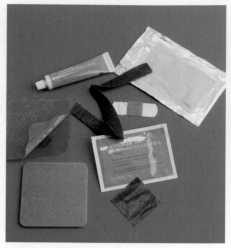

Plate 53 Antimicrobial dressings are available in a variety of formulations. (Courtesy of Bonnie Sue Rolstad.)

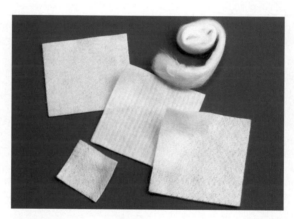

Plate 54 Variety of calcium alginate dressings. (Courtesy of Bonnie Sue Rolstad.)

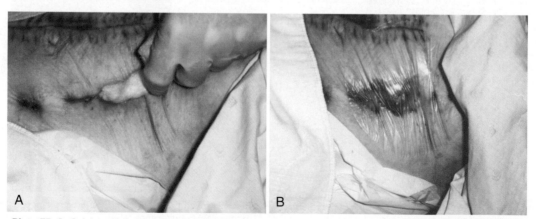

Plate 55 A, Calcium Alginate dressing applied to fill dead space and absorb exudate in a full-thickness abdominal wound. **B,** Alginate dressing secured with a secondary transparent dressing. Note that 2 days later at the scheduled dressing change, the alginate had formed an expected gel-like appearance as the wound fluid was absorbed. The periwound skin has been protected with a liquid skin barrier.

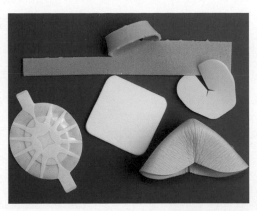

Plate 56 Variety of foam dressings. (Courtesy of Bonnie Sue Rolstad.)

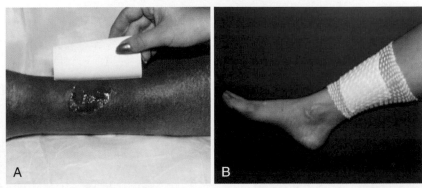

A

B

Plate 57 **A,** Application of nonadhesive foam dressing to venous ulcer by family member. **B,** Nonadhesive foam dressing secured with stretch-net secondary dressing.

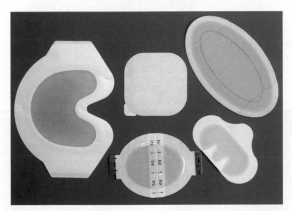

Plate 58 Variety of sizes and shapes of hydrocolloid dressings. (Courtesy of Bonnie Sue Rolstad.)

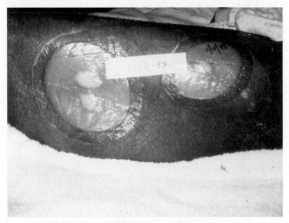

Plate 59 Hydrocolloid dressing prior to removal. Note the gel developing under the dressing, which is expected as the wound exudate is absorbed by the hydrocolloid.

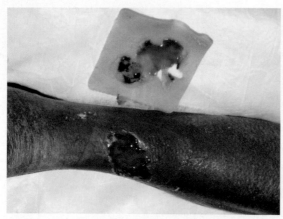

Plate 60 Hydrocolloid dressing after removal from a venous ulcer. Purulent-appearing exudate is present on the dressing and wound. This is expected with autolysis under a hydrocolloid dressing and should not be misinterpreted as evidence of infection. Upon cleansing, the wound bed is clean and granular.

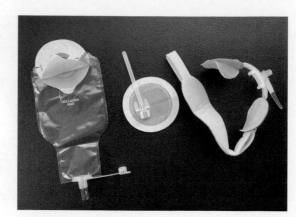

Plate 61 Hydrocolloid technology incorporated into medical device securement products.

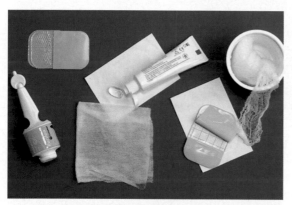

Plate 62 Variety of hydrogel dressings. (Courtesy of Bonnie Sue Rolstad.)

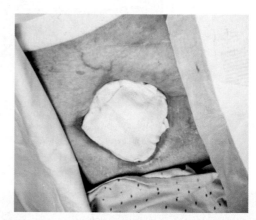

Plate 63 Hydrogel-impregnated gauze used to maintain a moist wound bed and fill dead space in this deep abdominal wound with undermining present.

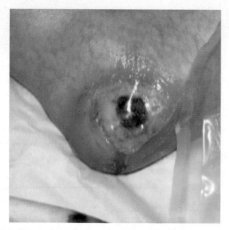

Plate 64 This illustrates inappropriate use of a hydrogel sheet dressing because (1) it overlaps onto intact periwound skin and (2) hydrogel will facilitate autolysis, which is not recommended on a stable eschar covered heel ulcer.

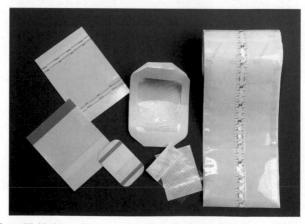

Plate 65 Variety of transparent film dressings. (Courtesy of Bonnie Sue Rolstad.)

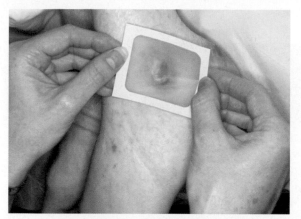

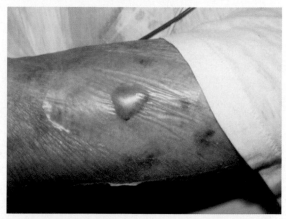

Plate 66 Application of a transparent dressing by a family member in the home setting.

Plate 67 Transparent dressing prior to removal. Note collection of fluid under the dressing, which is to be expected as autolysis occurs.

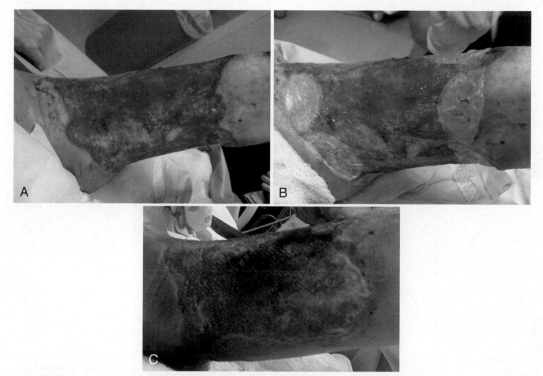

Plate 68 A, Circumferential left upper thigh debrided wound with dermal wound bed on 75-pound, middle-aged adult female. **B,** Epidermal CPT (Apligraf) applied along perimeter of wound to stimulate epidermal resurfacing. Note this is an off-label use of this product and is untested in this type of wound due to rarity of the condition. **C,** One week post application with epithelial advancement along wound edges apparent.

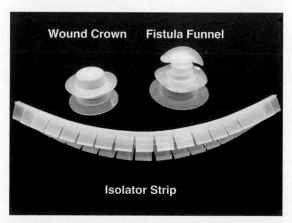

Plate 69 Example of commercially available devices for isolating a fistula, stoma, or drain to diverting effluent away from wounds. One-piece devices are compressible and customizable for different sizes and number of fistulas. (Photo courtesy of Mary Anne Obst.)

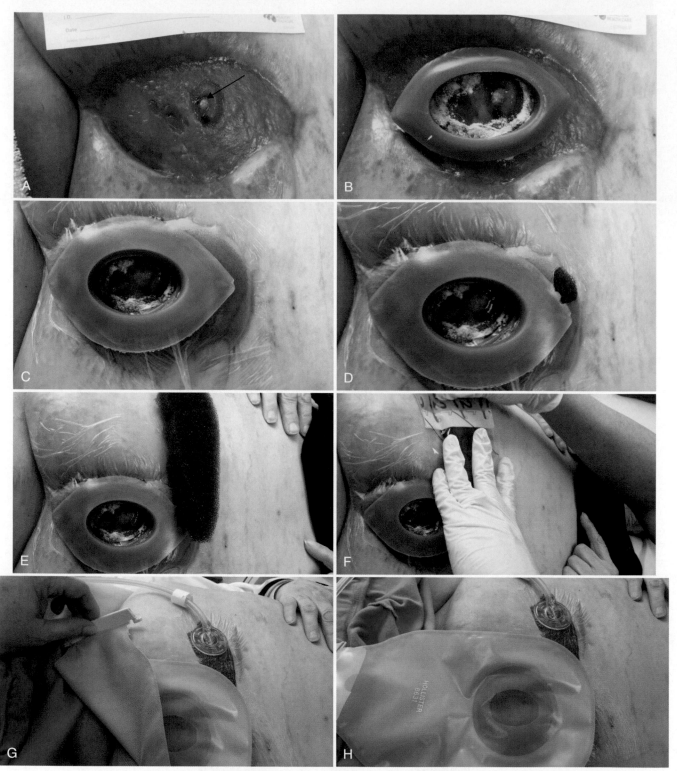

Plate 70 A, EAF within granular wound bed. **B,** Skin barrier powder dusted over wound bed where skin barrier ring will contact. Convex oval skin barrier ring applied with flat side down to wound bed, encircling fistula orifice. **C,** Black NPWT foam trimmed to fit remaining exposed wound bed contacting with skin barrier ring. Drape applied over inverted skin barrier ring and foam and sealed to skin barrier with stoma opening cut out. Second oval convex skin barrier ring inverted and applied (creating flat surface). **D,** Create slit in foam/drape all allow for track pad. **E,** Foam applied to lead away from wound area. **F,** Drape applied over foam (only) and track pad applied. Attached to negative pressure to confirm seal. **G,** Pouch opening created to size of skin barrier ring over EAF and attached. **H,** Separation of wound bed via NPWT from EAF and pouch apparent because pouch does not tract or suck down into fistula orifice.

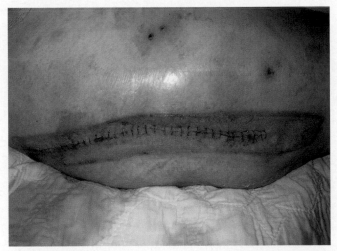

Plate 71 Damage to periwound approximated surgical incision managed with negative pressure wound therapy without appropriate protection between black foam and periwound skin.

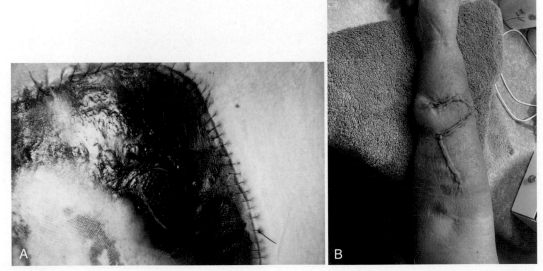

Plate 72 A, Edges of approximated incision with sutures and evidence of compromised profusion. Significant pooling of subcutaneous bleeding that evolved into eschar. This photograph illustrates the importance of assessing and documenting not only the condition of the incision but also the condition of the periwound skin. **B,** Skin flap following melanoma incision insufficient perfusion contributed to ischemia followed by necrosis and need for debridement.

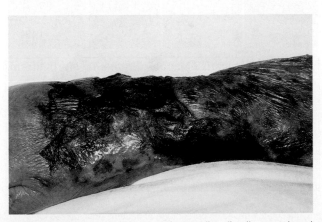

Plate 73 Necrotizing fasciitis affecting left lower arm and extending distally onto dorsal surface of hand. Note significant amount of eschar distributed over entire surface of lower arm and edema in dorsal surface of hand. (From Bolognia, J. L., et al. (2008). *Dermatology* (2nd ed.). Edinburgh: Mosby/Elsevier.)

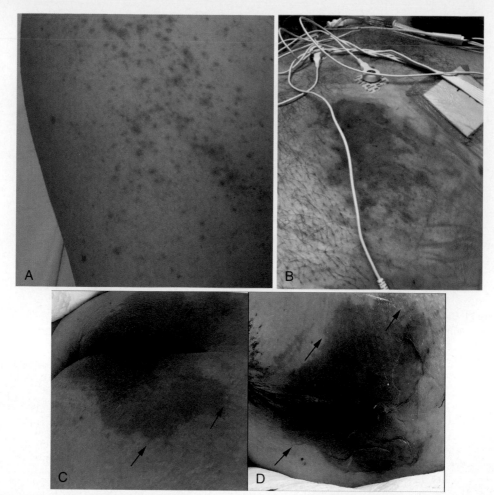

Plate 74 Cutaneous manifestations of COVID-19. **A,** Defuse macular papular and vesicular rash. **B,** Retiform purpura over the chest initially thought to be pressure injury after proning. **C,** Retiform purpura over sacral/buttocks region confirmed by biopsy initially mistaken for pressure injury. **D,** Retiform purpura over sacral/buttocks beginning to reveal extent of underlying tissue damage as it begins to slough nonviable tissue. (**A,** From Carrascosa, J. M., et al. (2020). Cutaneous manifestations in the context of SARS-CoV-2 infection (COVID-19). *Actas Dermo-Sifiliografics (English Edition), 111*(9), 734–742. **C** and **D,** From McBride, J. D., et al. (2021). Development of sacral/buttock retiform purpura as an ominous presenting sign of COVID-19 and clinical and histopathologic evolution during severe disease course. *Journal of Cutaneous Pathology, 48*(9), 1166–1172.)

Severity of COVID-19*

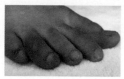 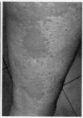 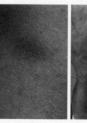 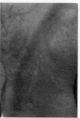 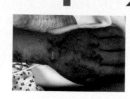

Pernio

- Feet (84%) and hands (32%)
- Pain/burning (71%) and pruritus (36%)
- After other COVID-19 symptoms (49%)
- Fever (35%), cough (35%);19% asymptomatic
- 16% hospitalized

Vesicular/ Urticarial/ Macular Erythema/ Morbilliform

- Trunk and extremities
- Pruritus in 61%–74%
- Typically after other COVID-19 symptoms (19%)
- Fever (65%–74%), cough (52%–66%), sore throat (39%–50%), shortness of breath (28%–45%)
- 22%–45% hospitalized across groups

Retiform purpura

- Extremities and buttocks
- Often asymptomatic (73%)
- After other COVID-19 symptoms (91%)
- Fever (64%), cough (73%), and shortness of breath (73%)
- 100% hospitalized
- 82% with ARDS

*Severity calculated based on percentage of patients hospitalized for COVID-19

Plate 75 Spectrum of COVID-19 dermatologic manifestation by severity of disease. (From Freeman, E. E., et al. (2020). The spectrum of COVID-19-associated dermatologic manifestations: An international registry of 716 patients from 31 countries. *Journal of the American Academy of Dermatology, 83*(4), 1118–1129.)

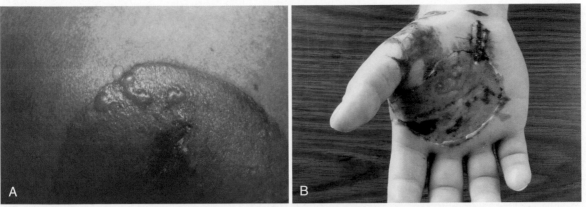

Plate 76 A, Brown recluse spider bite. Note central necrosis surrounded by purplish area and blisters. **B,** Another example of brown recluse spider bite following debridement 7 days after the bite initially presented with ischemia that progressed to eschar. Note persistent edema in the entire hand and fingertips. (**A,** From Hockenberry, M., & Wilson, D. (2009). *Wong's essentials of pediatric nursing* (8th ed.). St. Louis: Mosby/Elsevier.)

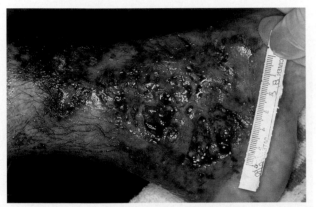

Plate 77 Classical ulceration form of pyoderma gangrenosum. Note violaceous (*purple*) color of skin surrounding ulceration.

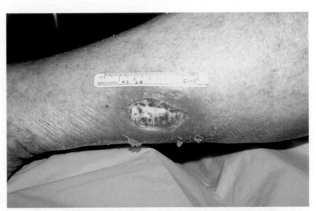

Plate 78 Vasculitis-related ulcer that developed in patient with rheumatoid arthritis. Wound bed has attached dry, yellow slough present, and surrounding skin is slightly erythematous.

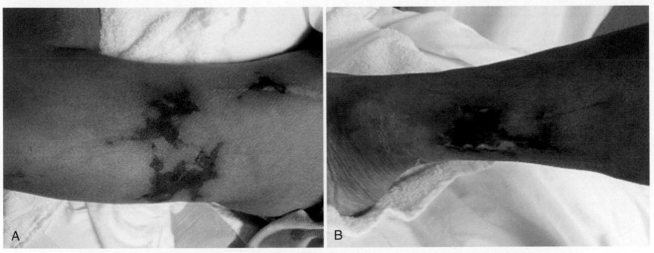

Plate 79 A, Calciphylaxis (CUA) in young patient with end-stage renal disease. Initial appearance can be similar to bruising or sDTI but accompanied by severe pain and erythematous margins. **B,** Calciphylaxis (CUA) has a range of manifestations in this patient and is eschar covered in this wound with continued periwound erythema and extreme pain.

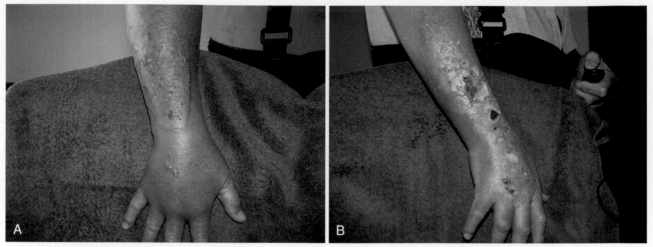

Plate 80 Untreated doxorubicin (Adriamycin) extravasation of the dorsum of the hand, with tissue damage extending throughout his forearm. **A,** Swelling, redness, and blistering apparent 3 days after the extravasation occurred. **B,** Early stages of tissue necrosis appearing 1 month later. (Copyright © 2008 by Lisa Schulmeister. Reprinted with permission.)

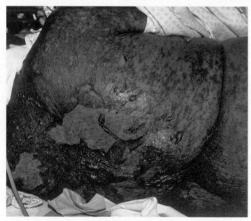

Plate 81 Clinical features of toxic epidermal necrosis (TEN) with detachment of large sheets of epidermis (more than 30% of body surface area), leading to extensive areas of denudement. A few intact bullae are still present. Wrinkling and lateral sliding of skin near blisters (positive Nikolsky sign) are apparent. (From Bolognia, J. L., et al. (2008). *Dermatology* (2nd ed.). Edinburgh: Mosby/Elsevier.)

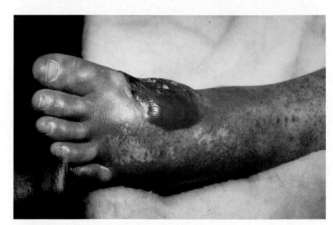

Plate 82 Graft-vs-host disease (GVHD) in a patient after allogenic bone marrow transplantation. Note macular–papular rash is barely distinguishable and has become confluent. Edema, erythema, and bulla formation are present.

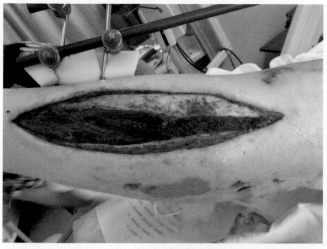

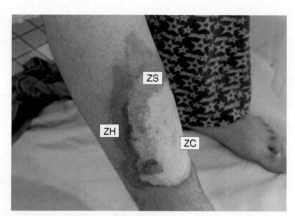

Plate 84 Burn zones. *ZC*, zone of coagulation; *ZH*, zone of hyperemia; *ZS*, zone of stasis.

Plate 83 Fasciotomy incision performed to address compartment syndrome following numerous fractures and placement of a fixation device in the lower left leg. Note viable exposed muscle and ligaments apparent in the wound bed.

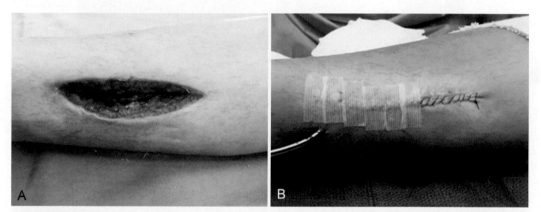

Plate 85 A, Surgically created wound on right medial leg wound. **B,** Surgical wound closed at a later date (delayed primary closure) by approximating wound edges; drain placed to reduce fluid accumulation.

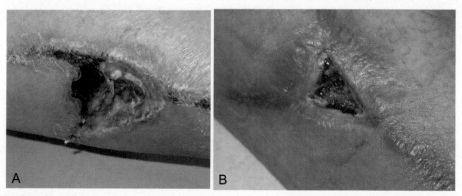

Plate 86 A, Left medial leg traumatic wound with nonviable tissue. **B,** Healing by secondary intention following surgical debridement.

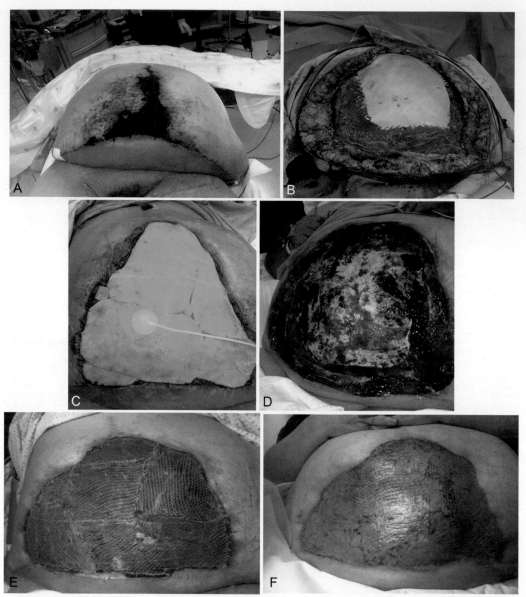

Plate 87 STSG following post panniculectomy and hernia repair on patient with obesity. **A,** Extensive necrosis post panniculectomy and ventral hernia repair. **B,** Status post debridement. **C,** Negative pressure wound therapy placed. **D,** Increase granulation tissue in wound bed. **E,** Status post meshed split-thickness skin graft (early presentation). **F,** Healed skin graft.

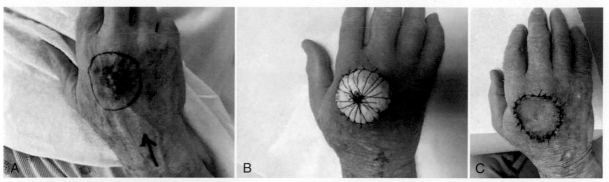

Plate 88 A, Right dorsal hand squamous cell carcinoma. **B,** Bolster dressing applied over full-thickness skin graft following excision of cancer. **C,** 1 week post graft application.

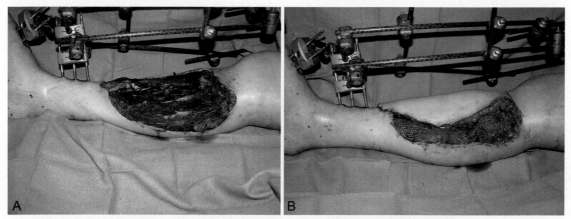

Plate 89 A, Traumatic wound, right leg with soft tissue loss and bone fracture. **B,** Defect covered with free-flap and skin graft.

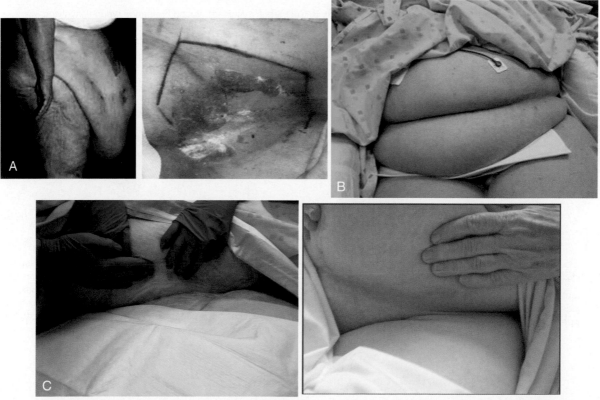

Plate 90 A, Abdomen of obese patient with skin breakdown under pannus due to pressure and moisture. **B,** Skin folds in patient with obesity; textile garment in place to protect from moisture entrapment. **C,** Linear ITD fissure present in skin folds. (**A,** Courtesy of Judith L. Gates.) **D,** Dermatitis present within a lower abdominal skin fold indicative of ITD.

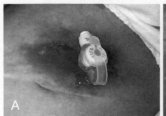
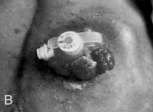

Plate 91 Complications at the site of the gastrostomy button. **A,** Cellulitis. (Courtesy of Teri Crawley Coha.) **B,** Hyperplasia/hypergranulation.

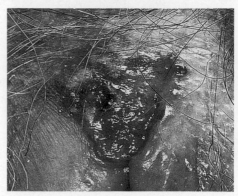

Plate 92 Basal cell carcinoma may be a primary lesion anywhere on the body. Existing chronic wounds of various etiologies may convert to malignant cutaneous wounds also known as *Marjolin's ulcer*. (From Habif, T., Campbell, M., Chapman, S., et al. (2011). *Skin disease: Diagnosis and treatment* (3rd ed.). London: Mosby.)

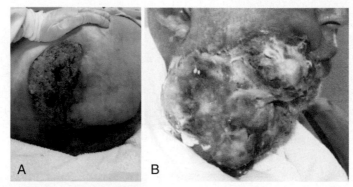

Plate 93 A, Squamous cell carcinoma on buttock. **B,** Cutaneous malignant wound (fungating wound) involving the right side of the face and neck. (**B,** From Morison, M., et al. (2004). *Chronic wound care: A problem-based learning approach.* London: Mosby.)

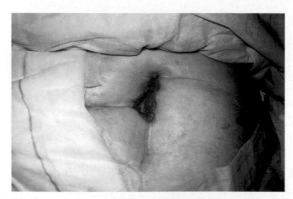

Plate 94 Patient with enterocutaneous fistula with irregular surrounding skin surfaces and depression along fistula–skin junction at interior aspect and upper left aspect.

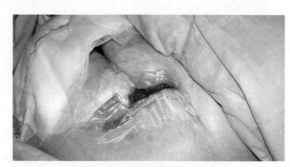

Plate 95 Tapered layers of solid–wafer skin barrier used to help level skin depression at inferior aspect. Skin barrier paste has been applied to surrounding wound margins and in all three depressions (over skin barrier wafer wedges) to level and protect the skin from effluent. Cement has been painted onto adhesive field (over paste and wedges) to increase adhesion.

11

Pressure Ulcers/Injuries

Denise P. Nix and Ruth A. Bryant

OBJECTIVES

1. Describe the pathophysiologic processes involved in the mechanics of a pressure injury.
2. Describe the incidence and prevalence of pressure injuries.
3. Summarize the features of current staging criteria for pressure injuries.
4. Distinguish between an avoidable and an unavoidable pressure injury.
5. List components of a best-practice bundle of a pressure injury prevention program.
6. Distinguish between a pressure injury risk assessment and a skin assessment.
7. Identify the risk factor subscales in the Braden Scale for predicting risk of pressure injury.
8. Describe the components of a successful pressure injury prevention program.
9. Provide examples of how an organization demonstrates skin safety as an organizational priority.

A pressure injury is a localized injury to the skin and/or underlying tissue, usually over a bony prominence, as a result of pressure or pressure in combination with shear (EPUAP, NPIAP, & PPPIA, 2019). Pressure injuries present a significant health care threat to patients of all ages who experience restricted mobility or an acute or chronic disease. Because of this threat, many professional organizations have published guidelines addressing prevention and management of pressure injuries (Box 11.1). Clearly pressure injuries remain a serious threat to patient safety and comprise a key focus of the drive to zero harm.

SCOPE OF THE PROBLEM

The scope of the pressure injury problem in the United States extends across the lifespan (e.g., geriatrics, pediatrics), in all patient care settings (long-term care, home care, acute care) and in select patient populations (e.g., spinal cord injured, surgical population, intensive care). To adequately grasp the significance of the problem, it is important to understand the magnitude of the pressure injury problem in terms of prevalence and incidence. The concepts of prevalence and incidence and the methods for calculation are discussed in Chapter 6.

Prevalence and Incidence

Prevalence and incidence (or facility acquired) will differ by health care setting and patient population (Table 11.1). In general, prevalence is not used as a metric to reflect quality of care as it will be higher in those settings where caring for the patient with a wound care is a program of focus or a surgical specialty. For example, it would be expected that prevalence in long-term care (LTC) would be greater than in an acute care setting since patients are often discharged to an LTC for strength training, recovery, and wound healing. Prevalence is typically used as a measure of burden of care for staffing-related decision making. However, a steady trend of decreasing prevalence over time could be interpreted as an indication of improved prevention. For example, the prevalence of pressure injuries in acute care has gradually declined between 2007 (13.4) and 2019 (9.14) (Van Gilder, Cox, Edsberg, & Koloms, 2021). As a measure of new onset of any condition such as pressure injuries, incidence is considered more reflective of the quality of care. As with prevalence, incidence will vary by clinical setting. Hospital- or facility-acquired pressure injuries are synonymous with incident pressure injuries.

BOX 11.1   Professional Organizations With Pressure Injury Guidelines

- *Prevention and Treatment of Pressure Ulcers/Injuries. Clinical Practice Guideline* (EPUAP, NPIAP, PPPIA, 2019)
- Wound, Ostomy and Continence Nurses Society's (WOCN) *Guideline for management of patients with pressure ulcers (injuries)* (WOCN®, 2016)
- *Association for the Advancement of Wound Care's (AAWC) Venous and Pressure Ulcer Guidelines* (Bolton, Girolami, Corbett, et al., 2014)
- American College of Physicians' *Risk Assessment and Prevention of Pressure Injuries: A Clinical Practice Guideline from the American College of Physicians* (Qaseem, Mir, Starkey, et al., 2015)
- *Treatment of Pressure Injuries: A Clinical Practice Guideline from the American College of Physicians* (Qaseem, Humphrey, et al., 2015)
- *Assessment and Management of Pressure Injuries* for the Interprofessional Team, Third Edition (Registered Nurses' Association of Ontario, 2016)
- *Guidelines for Pressure Ulcers* by the Wound Healing Society (Gould et al., 2016)
- Canadian Association of Wound Care's *Best Practice Recommendations for the Prevention and Treatment of Pressure Injuries: Update 2006* (Keast, Parslow, Houghton, et al., 2007)

TABLE 11.1   Incidence and Prevalence of Pressure Injuries by Care Setting and Patient Population

Patient Population	Prevalence	Incidence
Acute care	8.75–9.14[a]	2.61[a]
Critical care	14%[a]	9.4%–27.5%[b]
Medical surgical	7.7%[a]	1.9%[a]
US long-term care	8.2%–32.2%[c]	3.6%–59%[c]
Spinal cord injured	1.48%[d]–12%[e]	N/A
Pediatrics	1.4%[f]	2.2%[f]

[a]Data from Van Gilder et al. (2021).
[b]Data from Chaboyer et al. (2019).
[c]Data from Pieper (2012).
[d]Data from Hoh, Rahman, Fargen, Neal, and Hoh (2016).
[e]Data from Ploumis et al. (2011).
[f]Data from Razmus & Berquist-Beringer (2017).

Economic Impact

Pressure injuries are a resource intense complication requiring additional dressings, adjuvant therapy, nursing care, physical therapy, medications, nutrition support, and provider services. Facility-associated pressure injuries extend length of stay, delay recuperation, and increase the patient's risk for developing complications. In addition, patients with a pressure injury often require rehospitalization because of sepsis, complications, or the need for debridement or surgical repair.

Approximately 60,000 patients die each year from pressure injury complications (AHRQ, 2011). Mortality rates in Blacks with a pressure injury are four times greater than pressure injury related mortality rates in whites (adjRR = 4.22; 95% CI, 4.16–4.27) (Redelings, Lee, & Sorvillo, 2005). Additional notable differences between patients classified as "Black" compared to patients classified as "White" include severity at time of diagnosis and time to heal. Pressure injury stage is higher (more severe) at the time of diagnosis in the "Black" patient as compared to the "White" patient (Bates-Jensen et al., 2021; Harms, Bliss, Garrand, et al., 2014). Furthermore, an older adult admitted to the LTC setting with a pressure injury is less likely to heal in 90 days when the patient is classified as "Black" (Bliss et al., 2017). Diabetes, chronic renal failure, congestive heart failure, metastatic cancer, and low serum albumin increase the risk for 90-day and 180-day mortality in hospitalized patients with pressure injuries (Flattau & Blank, 2014).

Approximately 2.5 million patients are treated each year in US acute care facilities for pressure injuries, and the cost of treating pressure injuries is estimated to range from $9.1 to $11.6 billion annually (AHRQ, 2011) to as much as $15 billion (USD) per year (Markova & Mostow, 2012). The additional cost for a hospital-acquired pressure injury among adult inpatients is estimated between $10,708 and $12,712 (AHRQ, 2017; Padula & Delarmente, 2019). Mean hospital costs in the management of a pressure injury increase as the severity of the pressure injury increases; prevention is less costly than treatment (Ocampo et al., 2017).

TERMINOLOGY

Over the years, several terms have been used to describe pressure injuries: bedsore, decubitus ulcer, decubiti, pressure sore and pressure ulcer. *Pressure injury* is currently the preferred term because it incorporates both the pressure-related tissue damage in intact skin (e.g., DTI) and skin with tissue loss (Gefen, Brienza, Cuddigan, Haesler, & Kottner, 2021). However, pressure ulcer is the preferred term in many countries; therefore, pressure ulcer and pressure injury are often used interchangeably. *Decubitus*, a Latin word referring to the reclining position (Fox & Bradley, 1803), is commonly used in clinical settings. This term however is inaccurate because it ignores the damage that can be incurred in positions other than the reclining position.

A *pressure injury* is defined as localized injury to the skin and/or underlying tissue, usually over a bony prominence, as a result of pressure, including pressure in combination with shear (EPUAP, NPIAP, & PPPIA, 2019). They occur most commonly over a bony prominence with the majority of pressure injuries located on the pelvis (i.e., sacrum, ischial tuberosity, trochanter), heels, or occiput. Because a pressure injury can develop under a medical device or other object, a pressure injury can develop anywhere on the body, for example, under a cast, splint, nasal tube, or cervical collar. Fig. 11.1 shows the common sites for pressure injuries and frequency of ulceration per site.

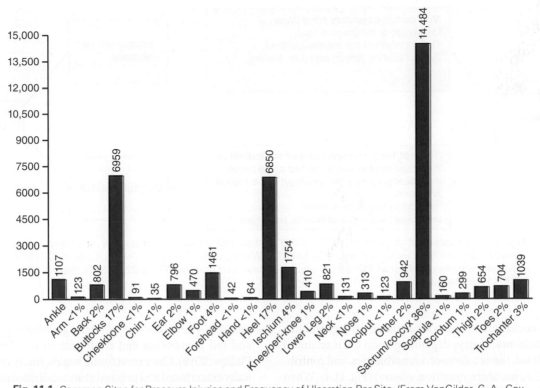

Fig. 11.1 Common Sites for Pressure Injuries and Frequency of Ulceration Per Site. (From VanGilder, C. A., Cox, J., Edsberg, L. E., & Koloms, K. (2021). Pressure injury prevalence in acute care hospitals with unit-specific analysis. Results from the International Pressure Ulcer Prevalence (IPUP) Survey database. *Journal of Wound, Ostomy, and Continence Nursing, 48*(6), 492–503.)

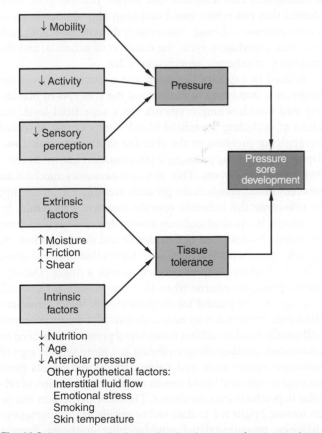

Fig. 11.2 Factors contributing to the development of pressure ulcers. (From Braden, B., & Bergstrom, N. (1987). A conceptual schema for the study of the etiology of pressure sores. *Rehabilitation Nursing, 12*(1), 8–12.)

ETIOLOGICAL PATHWAYS

While pressure and occlusion of blood vessels has long been accepted as the cause of a pressure injury, the primary cause is now understood to be mechanical load in the form of pressure and shear (EPUAP, NPIAP, & PPPIA, 2019). Several models for pressure ulcer/injury formation have been proposed over the years. Braden and Bergstrom (1987) presented a model of the factors that contribute to the intensity and duration of pressure injuries (Fig. 11.2), in combination with intrinsic and extrinsic factors that affect tissue tolerance. This model guided the development of the Braden Scale for Predicting Pressure Ulcer Risk that has been widely adopted into clinical practice. Defloor introduced a pressure injury conceptual scheme in 1999 arguing that the known causative factors are pressure (compressive force) and shear (shearing force) and that tissue tolerance is a modifying factor rather than causative (Defloor, 1999). In DeFloor's model, factors affecting intensity of compression and intensity of shearing force were identified as well as factors that affect tissue tolerance for pressure and tissue tolerance for oxygen. A new pressure ulcer conceptual framework further integrating new findings pertinent to pressure injury formation was proposed in 2015 by an international expert group. This model emphasizes the role of mechanical load (when compared with pressure and vascular occlusion) and expands tissue tolerance to include susceptibility and tolerance of the *individual*. The model depicts the interaction of these two factors and their role in pressure injury formation (Coleman et al., 2014) (Fig. 11.3).

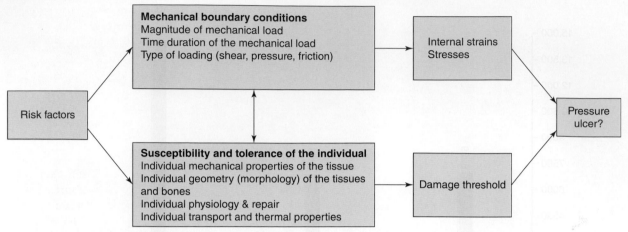

Fig. 11.3 Enhancement of NPUAP/EPUAP (2009) Factors that influence susceptibility of pressure ulcer development. (From Coleman, S., Nixon, J., Keen, J., Wilson, L., McGinnis, E., Dealey, C., et al. (2014). A new pressure ulcer conceptual framework. *Journal of Advanced Nursing, 70*(10), 2222–2234. https://doi.org/10.1111/jan.12405.)

Sustained mechanical load can cause tissue damage within a few minutes, to hours, or days depending upon the mechanical load, type of tissue, tissue tolerance, comorbidities, and contributing factors (i.e., moisture, nutrition, edema) (Fig. 11.4). When loaded, skin and soft tissue respond to the load by distorting and deforming. At the cellular level, sustained mechanical load and the subsequent stretching and deforming of cells damages the cytoskeleton thus compromising cellular integrity. It is this sustained deformation that will result in the initial cell death. Subsequent additional tissue damage occurs due to the effects of (1) inflammatory damage, (2) impaired lymphatic function that results in accumulation of metabolic waste products, proteins, and enzymes, and (3) ischemic damage (Berlowitz & Brienza, 2007; Gefen et al., 2021). This sequence of events that results in tissue damage from sustained pressure or mechanical deformation is a cycle that occurs over time and is not a linear process (Gefen et al., 2021).

When pressure and deformation persist, a cascade of events transpires that intensifies the extent of tissue damage. At the cellular level, disruption of the cell wall results in cell death, the release of cellular byproducts into the extravascular space, inflammation, increased interstitial pressure, and interstitial edema. Capillary changes ensue resulting in endothelial cell damage, venous thrombus formation, increased capillary permeability, redistribution of blood supply in ischemic tissue, alteration in lymphatic flow, and alterations in interstitial fluid composition. With the inhibition of the normal movement of interstitial fluid due to mechanical deformation, protein is retained in the interstitial tissues, causing increased interstitial oncotic pressure, edema formation, dehydration of cells, and tissue inflammation.

While ischemic damage with pressure injuries primarily results from inflammatory changes, ischemia may be preexisting due to comorbidities such as arterial insufficiency or diabetes. In addition, ischemic changes may also be exacerbated by reperfusion injury. As blood returns to tissue following occlusion, an accumulation of damaged cellular byproducts and white blood cells obstructs the capillaries, and free radicals are released. These free radicals damage cellular proteins, DNA, and cell membranes and contribute to cell death (Mervis & Phillips, 2019). Once reperfusion begins, injury can be paradoxically exacerbated and proceed at an accelerated pace, and loss of additional cells occurs. As the endothelium is shed, platelets are activated by the underlying collagen, and clot formation is triggered. Furthermore, damaged endothelial cells lose their usual anticoagulant characteristics and release thrombogenic substances that exacerbate vessel occlusion and ultimately cause increased tissue ischemia. Tissue injury thus increases with each ischemia–reperfusion cycle, the duration of ischemia, and the frequency of ischemia–reperfusion cycles.

Related to capillary perfusion and indicators of pressure injury, it is important to understand the concepts of blanching and nonblanching erythema. At a superficial level, the effect of occluding superficial blood vessels can be observed by applying pressure to the skin for short periods of time. Upon release of the pressure, a phenomenon known as *reactive hyperemia* occurs. This is a compensatory mechanism whereby blood vessels in the pressure area dilate in an attempt to overcome the ischemic episode. Reactive hyperemia, by definition, is transient and may also be described as blanching erythema. As described in Chapter 10 and shown in Plate 24, *blanching erythema* is an area of erythema that becomes white (blanches) when compressed such as with a finger. The erythema promptly returns when the compression is removed. The site may be painful for the patient with intact sensation. Blanching erythema is an early indicator of inflammation and will usually resolve without tissue loss if pressure is reduced or eliminated. *Nonblanching erythema* is a more serious sign of sustained deformation and tissue damage and results from damage to cells and blood vessels and the extravasation of cellular byproducts into the tissues. The color of the skin can be an intense bright red to dark red or purple. It is important to delineate pressure-related nonblanching erythema from a hematoma or ecchymosis. When deep tissue damage is also present, the area is often either indurated or boggy when palpated.

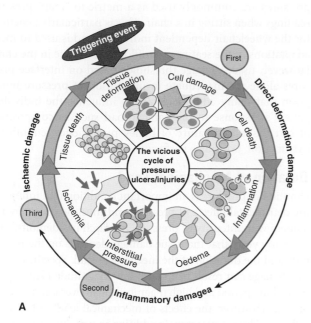

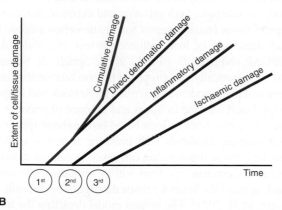

Fig. 11.4 (A) A schematic description of the vicious cycle of cell and tissue damage in pressure ulcers/injuries (PUs/PIs), resulting from sustained mechanical deformations (the triggering event), which inflicts the primary, direct deformation damage (first damage event), then leading to secondary inflammatory-oedema-related damage (second damage event), and finally to tertiary ischaemic damage (third damage event). (B) Each of these three factors contributes to the cumulative cell and tissue damage, which develops in an escalated manner as a result of the added contributions of the above factors. (From Gefen, A., Brienza, D. M., Cuddigan, J., Haesler, E., & Kottner, J. (2022). Our contemporary understanding of the aetiology of pressure ulcers/pressure injuries. *International Wound Journal, 19*(3), 692–704. doi: 10.1111/iwj.13667. Epub 2021 Aug 11. PMID: 34382331; PMCID: PMC8874092.)

In summary, sustained mechanical deformation precipitates inflammatory and edema-related tissue damage which then triggers ischemic changes. The interstitial fluid movement of wastes and fluid among the capillaries and lymphatic system becomes jeopardized. Tissues are deprived of oxygen and nutrients and exposed to toxic metabolic products and increased interstitial fluid which retains proteins that dehydrate cells and irritate tissues. The ensuing tissue acidosis, capillary permeability, and edema further aggravate cellular death.

Factors Influencing Susceptibility for Pressure Injury Development

Mechanical load, susceptibility and tolerance of the individual, and risk factors interact to result in the onset of a pressure injury (see Figs.11.3 and 11.8). Three conditions are identified to characterize mechanical load: (1) type of mechanical load, (2) magnitude or intensity of load, and (3) duration of mechanical load (Coleman et al., 2014).

Type of Mechanical Load

Mechanical load is the force applied to soft tissue (skin and underlying tissue) by an external object, surface, or device. This load will have a *normal* force, which is a force perpendicular to the skin, and a *shear* force. *Shear force* is a force parallel to the skin and is associated with the skin being dragged over a surface either laterally (e.g., during transfers from bed to stretcher) or vertically (e.g., sliding up or down in the bed or chair as seen in Fig. 9.1).

Vertical shear occurs due to the gravity pushing down on the body and resistance (friction) between the patient and a surface, such as the bed or chair. For example, when the head of the bed is elevated, the effect of gravity on the body is to pull the body down toward the foot of the bed (see Fig. 9.1). In contrast, the resistance generated by the bed surface tends to hold the body in place. However, what is actually held in place is the skin, while the weight of the skeleton continues to pull the body downward.

Shear causes much of the damage observed with pressure injuries. The primary effect of shear occurs at the deeper fascial level of the tissues overlying the bony prominence. For example, when the head of the bed is elevated more than 30 degrees, shear force occurs in the sacrococcygeal region. While the outer skin remains fixed against the surface of the bed, the body slides and pressure and deformation is exerted at the sacrum. As a result of the shear, blood vessels, which are anchored at the point of exit through the fascia, are stretched and angulated. This force also dissects the tissues, resulting in undermining in the pressure injury (see Plates 31 and 63). High shear forces at the interface between the body and the supporting surface may exacerbate the damage caused by normal stresses alone (EPUAP, NPIAP, & PPPIA, 2019) due to the thrombosis and undermining in the dermis.

The skin is also vulnerable to friction forces. Friction can cause minor to substantial skin impairment, and results from the sliding of two surfaces together. Continuous sliding of the skin against bed sheets or a shoe, for example, may result in inflammation, abrasion, or blisters and should be referred to as a friction injury, not pressure injury (Antokal, Brienza, Bryan, et al., 2012). Typically, skin damage caused by friction is confined to the epidermal and upper dermal layers and disturbs the barrier function of the stratum corneum (EPUAP, NPIAP, & PPPIA, 2019). In its mildest form, friction abrades the epidermis and dermis similar to a mild burn, and sometimes is referred to as "sheet burn." This type of damage most frequently develops in patients who are restless. To prevent friction when moving up in bed, a patient who can lift independently should do so with a lift device or with use of the hands and arms. A patient who is dependent in care may need multiple caregivers to assist with moving up in bed while using a lift sheet or lift device to prevent the body from dragging. When friction occurs in tandem with shear, the resulting damage is considered a pressure injury (Gefen et al., 2021).

Magnitude or Intensity of Mechanical Load

Historically, concepts of *capillary pressure, capillary closing pressure and interface pressures* were fundamental to the pathophysiologic process of pressure injury formation. *Capillary pressure,* the pressure within the capillary that moves fluid outward through the capillary membrane, was estimated via indirect measurement techniques, to be approximately 32 mmHg at the arterial end of a capillary bed and 12 mmHg at the venous end (Fig. 11.5) (Kumar, Fausto, & Abbas, 2005a). The mean colloidal osmotic pressure in tissue was approximated at 25 mmHg. *Capillary closing pressure,* or *critical closing pressure,* was the minimal amount of pressure required to collapse a capillary (Burton & Yamada, 1951) and it was inferred that the amount of pressure required to collapse a capillary exceeded the estimated capillary pressure; 32 mmHg became the numerical "standard" for capillary closing pressure.

Interface pressure is the pressure being applied externally to the skin. The implication was that interface pressures that exceeded the capillary closing pressure were sufficient to cause pressure injuries (Kosiak, 1961; Kosiak, Kubicek, Olson, et al., 1958; Lindan, 1961). Early research demonstrated that healthy people experience elevated interface pressures (as high as 300 mmHg) while in the sitting, supine, prone, or side-lying positions (Bennett, Kavner, Lee, et al., 1984; Kosiak, 1961; Lindan, 1961). Despite these high pressures, healthy people with normal sensation regularly shift their weight in response to the discomfort associated with capillary closure and tissue hypoxia and thus do not experience tissue destruction. Unfortunately, pathologic processes such as spinal cord injury or sedation impair the ability to recognize or respond to this discomfort. Today interface pressures are commonly used as a metric to "map" pressure readings when sitting in a chair. This is particularly beneficial for the wheelchair dependent individual and is used to make adaptations in the seating and offloading surface in the chair. However, tissue damage thresholds based on interface pressures alone are inadequate in prevention of pressure injury given that many additional factors influence the individual patient's response to mechanical load such as composition of soft tissues, curvature of boney prominence, endothelial dysfunction, arteriolar perfusion, etc.

Duration of Mechanical Load

Duration of pressure is an important condition that influences the detrimental effects of pressure and must be considered in tandem with intensity of pressure. Research has demonstrated for many years that the tissue damage depends on the magnitude and the duration of the mechanical load. Specifically, tissue damage can result from both low magnitude load applied over a long period and high magnitude load over a short period of time. However, the effects of mechanical load on tissue are influenced by many factors in addition to magnitude and duration. For example, both intrinsic and extrinsic factors such as type of tissue (muscle versus soft tissue versus adipose tissue) and size/shape of load influence extent of cellular damage (EPUAP, NPIAP, & PPPIA, 2019; Sprigle & Sonenblum, 2011). Historically, this proposed inverse relationship between time and magnitude was described by Reswick and Rogers in a graph based on time in hours and amount of pressure. However, these observations were based on the visual appearance of skin changes consistent with pressure. It is now understood that high tissue deformation can result in cellular damage visible at the microscopic level within minutes while sustained loading may take hours for tissue damage to be clinically visible (Gefen et al., 2021). The revised model depicting the tolerance of soft tissues to sustained mechanical load has been adapted to reflect these concepts (see Fig. 11.4).

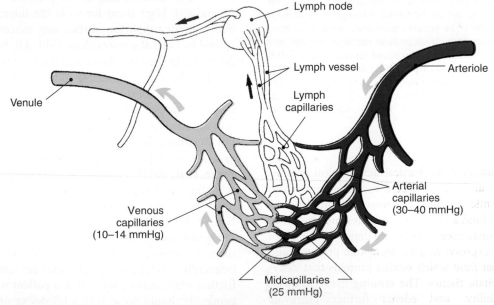

Fig. 11.5 Estimated pressures within the capillary bed.

Tissue Tolerance

Several patient level attributes will influence an individual's susceptibility to mechanical load or their "tissue tolerance" (ability of skin and its supporting structures to endure pressure without adverse sequelae). Tissue tolerance describes the condition or integrity of the skin and supporting structures that influence the skin's ability to redistribute the applied pressure. Compression of tissue against skeletal structures and the resulting cellular damage can be prevented by effective redistribution of pressure.

The concept of tissue tolerance was first discussed with the need to identify how much pressure skin could "tolerate." Later, Husain (1953) introduced the concept of sensitizing the tissue to pressure and consequently to ischemia. Rat muscle was sensitized with a pressure of 100 mmHg applied for 2 h. Seventy-two hours later, a mere 50 mmHg pressure applied to the same tissue caused muscle degeneration in only 1 h. This muscle destruction resulted during the second application of pressure, even though the intensity and duration of pressure were lower than the initial intensity and duration. This finding has significant implications for the patient population at risk for pressure injuries. It indicates that episodes of deep tissue ischemia can occur without cutaneous manifestations and that such episodes can sensitize the patient's skin. As observed by Hussain in 1953, deep

muscle tissue appears to be more susceptible to pressure damage than are skin and fat (Berlowitz & Brienza, 2007). In vitro findings show that relatively small loads cause structural changes to the dermal component of tissue. Human tissue exhibits changes visible at the surface that often are minor compared with damage seen in deeper tissue layers (Edsberg, 2007). Muscle tissue is the most vascularized tissue layer between bone and skin. It is the tissue with the highest metabolic demand and the lowest tolerance to mechanical compression (Gefen, 2008a). In addition, atrophied, scarred, or secondarily infected tissue has an increased susceptibility to pressure because of injured cells (Kumar, Fausto, & Abbas, 2005b).

Muscle damage may occur with pressure injuries and is more significant than cutaneous damage. Pressure is highest at the point of contact between the soft tissue (e.g., muscle or fascia) and the bony prominence. This cone-shaped pressure gradient as seen in Fig. 11.6 indicates that deep pressure injuries initially form at the bone–soft tissue interface, not the skin surface, and extend outward to the skin. Thus, deep tissue damage may occur with relatively little initial cutaneous or superficial evidence of damage. The skin damage seen with pressure injuries is often referred to as the "tip of the iceberg" because a larger area of necrosis and ischemia is present at the tissue–bone interface. Muscle and fat tissue loading over a

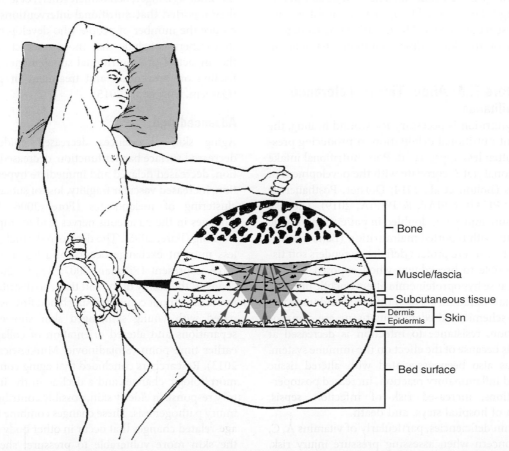

Bone

Muscle/fascia

Subcutaneous tissue

Dermis
Epidermis
Skin

Bed surface

Fig. 11.6 This cone-shaped pressure gradient indicates that deep pressure injuries initially form at the bone–soft tissue interface, not the skin surface, and extend outward to the skin.

bony prominence is substantially higher during sitting than lying down, so pressure injury and deep tissue injury development are likely to occur sooner while sitting versus lying down (Gefen, 2008a).

Tissue tolerance is influenced by the ability of the skin and underlying structures (e.g., blood vessels, interstitial fluid, collagen) to work together as a set of parallel springs that transmit load from the surface of the tissue to the skeleton inside (Krouskop, 1983). Several intrinsic and extrinsic factors can alter the ability of the soft tissue to perform this task.

Extrinsic Factors That Affect Tissue Tolerance

The environment between the skin and the support surface, referred to as microclimate, contributes to pressure injury formation. Microclimate includes moisture, temperature, humidity, and airflow. Moisture, specifically from incontinence, is as a predisposing factor to pressure injury development (Table 11.2). Persistent moisture alters the resiliency of the epidermis to external forces by weakening the lipid layer of the stratum corneum and collagen. Both shear and friction are increased in the presence of mild to moderate moisture but may be decreased in the presence of profuse moisture. The high-moisture environment created by urinary incontinence can affect the skin by alkalinizing the skin's pH, thereby altering normal skin flora. Persons with fecal incontinence are more likely to develop pressure injuries than are persons without this condition (Bergquist-Beringer & Gajewski, 2011). Clinicians need to be able to differentiate among lesions caused by moisture, moisture and friction, and pressure and shear. The negative impact of prolonged moisture on the skin is discussed in greater detail in Chapter 9.

Intrinsic Factors That Affect Tissue Tolerance
Nutritional Debilitation

Although good nutrition is necessary for wound healing, the role of significant nutritional debilitation in producing pressure injuries is often less appreciated. Poor nutritional intake and poor nutritional status correlate with the development of pressure injuries (Bolton et al., 2014; Dorner, Posthauer, & Thomas, 2009; EPUAP, NPIAP, & PPPIA, 2019). The risk of having a pressure injury was doubled in patients in a public health care facility with reported malnutrition (Banks, Bauer, Graves, et al., 2010). Severe protein deficiency renders soft tissue more susceptible to breakdown when exposed to local deformation because hypoproteinemia alters oncotic pressure and causes edema formation. Oxygen diffusion and transport of nutrients in ischemic and edematous tissue are compromised. In addition, resistance to infection is decreased at low protein levels because of the effect on the immune system. Malnutrition has also been associated with altered tissue regeneration and inflammatory reaction, increased postoperative complications, increased risk of infection, sepsis, increased length of hospital stays, and death.

Certain vitamin deficiencies, particularly of vitamins A, C, and E, are a concern when assessing pressure injury risk. Vitamin A has a role in epithelial integrity, protein synthesis, and immune function; therefore, a deficiency of vitamin A delays reepithelialization, collagen synthesis, and cellular cohesion. Vitamin C plays a role in collagen synthesis, enhanced activation of leukocytes and macrophages at a wound site, and immune function. Specific to wound healing, vitamin E aids in collagen synthesis, metabolism of fat, and stabilization of cell membranes (Posthauer, 2006). Vitamin D deficiency was not found to be an independent risk factor for pressure injuries but may be a marker of comorbid illnesses, which increase the risk of pressure injuries (Kalava, Cha, & Takahashi, 2011).

All nutrients have an important role in maintaining skin integrity. Cowan, Stechmiller, Rowe, et al. (2012) found that malnutrition, along with three other medical factors, had stronger predictive value for predicting pressure injuries in acutely ill veterans than Braden Scale total scores alone. Still, questions remain regarding how much supplementation of nutrients will positively affect outcomes. Metaanalyses of the clinical benefits of nutritional support in patients with or at risk for pressure injuries showed an oral nutritional supplement was associated with a significantly lower incidence of pressure injury development in at-risk patients of 25% compared with routine care (Stratton, Ek, Engfer, et al., 2005). A Cochrane evaluation of enteral and parenteral nutrition on pressure injury prevention and treatment was not able to draw conclusions about the effect of such nutrition because of the small number of studies and methodological issues with the studies (Langer, Schloemer, Knerr, et al., 2003). However, they reported that nutritional interventions may be able to reduce the number of people who develop pressure injuries. Researchers conclude that more research is needed about the impact of oral nutritional supplements and enteral tube feeding on prevention and treatment of pressure injuries (Qaseem, Mir, et al., 2015).

Advanced Age

Aging skin experiences decreased epidermal turnover, decreased surface barrier function, decreased sensory perception, decreased delayed and immediate hypersensitivity reaction, increased vascular fragility, loss of subcutaneous fat, and clustering of melanocytes (Fore, 2006; Pittman, 2007). Changes in the cutaneous nerves lead to impaired early pain warning (Fore, 2006). The dermoepidermal junction flattens, less nutrient exchange occurs, and less resistance to shear force is present (Pittman, 2007; Reddy, 2008). With these changes, the ability of the soft tissue to distribute the mechanical load without compromising blood flow is impaired. Compared with young skin, aged skin showed subepidermal separations and altered orientation of collagen fibers at an earlier time point (Stojadinovic, Minkiewicz, Sawaya, et al., 2013). Researchers concluded that aging contributes to rapid morphologic changes and a decline in the innate inflammatory response in elderly skin, possibly contributing to pressure injury pathogenesis. These changes combine with many other age-related changes that occur in other body systems to make the skin more vulnerable to pressure, shear, and friction (Pittman, 2007).

TABLE 11.2   Braden Scale for Predicting Pressure Sore Risk

Patient's Name: _____   Evaluator's Name: _____   Date of Assessment: _____

	1	2	3	4
Sensory Perception Ability to respond appropriately to pressure-related discomfort	**1. Completely limited** Unresponsive (does not moan, flinch, or grasp) to painful stimuli, due to diminished level of consciousness or sedation OR limited ability to feel pain over most of body	**2. Very limited** Responds only to painful stimuli. Cannot communicate discomfort except by moaning or restlessness OR has a sensory impairment that limits the ability to feel pain or discomfort over half of body	**3. Slightly limited** Responds to verbal commands, but cannot always communicate discomfort or the need to be turned OR has some sensory impairment that limits ability to feel pain or discomfort in one or two extremities	**4. No impairment** Responds to verbal commands. Has no sensory deficit that would limit ability to feel or voice pain or discomfort
Moisture Degree to which skin is exposed to moisture	**1. Constantly moist** Skin is kept moist almost constantly by perspiration, urine, etc. Dampness is detected every time patient is moved or turned	**2. Very moist** Skin is often, but not always, moist. Linen must be changed at least once a shift	**3. Occasionally moist** Skin is occasionally moist, requiring an extra linen change approximately once a day	**4. Rarely moist** Skin is usually dry; linen only requires changing at routine intervals
Activity Degree of physical activity	**1. Bedfast** Confined to bed	**2. Chairfast** Ability to walk severely limited or nonexistent. Cannot bear own weight and/or must be assisted into chair or wheelchair	**3. Walks occasionally** Walks occasionally during day, but for very short distances, with or without assistance. Spends majority of each shift in bed or chair	**4. Walks frequently** Walks outside room at least twice a day and inside room at least once every 2 h during waking hours
Mobility Ability to change and control body position	**1. Completely immobile** Does not make even slight changes in body or extremity position without assistance	**2. Very limited** Makes occasional slight changes in body or extremity position, but unable to make frequent or significant changes independently	**3. Slightly limited** Makes frequent though slight changes in body or extremity position independently	**4. No limitations** Makes major and frequent changes in position without assistance
Nutrition Usual food intake pattern	**1. Very poor** Never eats a complete meal. Rarely eats more than one-third of any food offered. Eats two servings or less of protein (meat or dairy products) per day. Takes fluids poorly. Does not take a liquid supplement OR is NPO and/or maintained on clear liquids or IVs for more than 5 days	**2. Probably inadequate** Rarely eats a complete meal and generally eats only about half of any food offered. Protein intake includes only three servings of meat or dairy products per day. Occasionally will take a dietary supplement OR receives less-than-optimum amount of liquid diet or tube feeding	**3. Adequate** Eats over half of most meals. Eats a total of four servings of protein (meat, dairy products) per day. Occasionally will refuse a meal, but will usually take a supplement when offered OR is on a tube feeding or TPN regimen, which probably meets most of nutritional needs	**4. Excellent** Eats most of every meal. Never refuses a meal. Usually eats a total of four or more servings of meat and dairy products. Occasionally eats between meals. Does not require supplementation
Friction & Shear	**1. Problem** Requires moderate to maximum assistance in moving. Complete lifting without sliding against sheets is impossible. Frequently slides down in bed or chair, requiring frequent repositioning with maximum assistance. Spasticity, contractures, or agitation leads to almost constant friction	**2. Potential problem** Moves feebly or requires minimum assistance. During a move, skin probably slides to some extent against sheets, chair, restraints, or other devices. Maintains relatively good position in chair or bed most of the time, but occasionally slides down	**3. No apparent problem** Moves in bed and in chair independently and has sufficient muscle strength to lift up completely during move. Maintains good position in bed or chair	

Total Score _____

Low Blood Pressure

When perfusion is decreased by hypotension, shock, or dehydration, blood flow to the skin is likely to be compromised, thus increasing ischemia; deep tissues may be particularly vulnerable because of their extensive vascular supply (Berlowitz & Brienza, 2007). Hypotension may shunt blood flow away from the skin to more vital organs, thus decreasing the skin's tolerance for pressure by allowing capillaries to close at lower levels of interface pressure. Hypotension was a significant factor in patients with pressure injuries in intensive care units (Terekeci et al., 2009). Man and Au-Yeung (2013) reported the odds of developing a pressure injury in a patient with hypotension in the acute care setting was 6.71 ($P = 0.001$). That said, vasopressor medications are a first-line treatment modality for hypotension (Cox, 2013). In a literature review, 7 of 10 studies reported significant associations among the broad category of vasopressors as a pressure injury risk factor (Cox, 2013). Research is needed to elucidate vasopressors as an independent risk factor for pressure injury development.

Stress

Hospitalization in acute or long-term care is stressful. In examining the relationship between stress and wound healing, stress has been negatively associated with healing. Cortisol may be the trigger for lowered tissue tolerance when a person is under stress. Cortisol is the primary glucocorticoid secreted when a person is exposed to a stressor and lacks appropriate coping mechanisms to mediate the stress-related hormonal response. Higher cortisol levels were related to longer time to heal (Ebrecht et al., 2004; Gouin & Kiecolt-Glaser, 2008). Cortisol may also alter the mechanical properties of the skin by disproportionately increasing the rate of collagen degradation over collagen synthesis. Glucocorticoids may trigger structural changes in connective tissue and affect cellular metabolism by interfering with the diffusion of water, salt, and nutrients between the capillary bed and the cells. Many factors affect cortisol: advanced age, immobility, body fat, recent surgery, stroke, and malnutrition.

Smoking

Smoking is associated with tissue hypoxia, nicotine-induced stimulation of the sympathetic nervous system resulting in epinephrine that causes peripheral vasoconstriction and decreased circulation, carbon monoxide shift of the oxygen dissociation curve, and hydrogen cyanide interference with cellular oxygen metabolism (Ahn, Mulligan, & Salcido, 2008). While the relationship between smoking and risk of pressure injury may be inconsistent, it is well known that smoking impairs wound healing.

Elevated Body Temperature

The body experiences a 10% increase in tissue metabolism with each 1°C (33.8°F) rise in skin temperature (Aronovitch, 2007). Elevated body temperatures increase metabolic rates and subsequently increase oxygen consumption rates. Elevated skin temperature exacerbates the effects of ischemia by increasing the need for oxygen (Berlowitz & Brienza, 2007). Findings on elevated body temperature are mixed. Dhandapani, Dhandapani, Agarwal, et al. (2014) reported prolonged fever had no significant association with pressure injury development in patients with severe traumatic brain injury. Systemic infection or fever was associated with mortality in 90 days for hospitalized patients with pressure injuries; it did not show a confounding effect on other variables (Flattau & Blank, 2014).

Rapp, Bergstrom, and Padhye (2009) examined skin temperature in a small sample of nursing facility residents. Skin temperature was lowest in those who developed pressure injuries and between low-risk and high-risk residents. They concluded the findings support skin temperature regulation as a component of tissue tolerance to pressure.

Miscellaneous Factors

Other conditions, such as those that create sluggish blood flow, anemia, blood dyscrasias, or poor oxygen perfusion, may be significant intrinsic factors jeopardizing tissue tolerance. For example, greater tissue damage has been associated with increased blood viscosity and high hematocrit level. This may explain why dehydration is sometimes mentioned as a contributing factor in pressure injury development.

CLASSIFICATION OF PRESSURE INJURIES

History and Purpose

Pressure injury staging system has undergone numerous revisions and updates. During the 1980s, the International Association for Enterostomal Therapy, now known as the WOCN Society, modified the Shea staging system, which originally was developed in 1975 (WOCN, 2016). It has subsequently been updated by the NPIAP to align with new evidence and improve clarity of descriptors (Box 11.2). There are several classification systems commonly used in the United States, Europe, and the Pan Pacific such as the WHO ICD-10, WHO ICD-11, ICD-11 Australian modified, NPUAP Classification System, U.S. CMS Long Term Care, U.S. ICD-10-CM, and the International Pressure Ulcer Classification System. Experts emphasize that staging provides increased uniformity of language, a basis for evaluation of protocols and treatment options, and potentially a method for predicting prognosis. International guidelines suggest verification of clinical agreement in pressure injury classification (e.g., interrater reliability, two clinician verification) (EPUAP, NPIAP, & PPPIA, 2019).

The NPIAP pressure injury staging system (Box 11.2) is based on the ability to assess the type of tissue in the wound bed. Therefore, it is essential to distinguish between cellular debris (i.e., slough) from nonviable or necrotic tissue in the wound bed. Task force members for the revised national pressure ulcer advisory panel (now NPIAP) pressure injury staging system (Edsberg et al., 2016) define slough as

BOX 11.2 NPIAP Pressure Injury Stages

Pressure Injury:

A pressure injury is localized damage to the skin and underlying soft tissue usually over a bony prominence or related to a medical or other device. The injury can present as intact skin or an open ulcer and may be painful. The injury occurs as a result of intense and/or prolonged pressure or pressure in combination with shear. The tolerance of soft tissue for pressure and shear may also be affected by microclimate, nutrition, perfusion, co-morbidities and condition of the soft tissue.

Stage 1 Pressure Injury: Nonblanchable erythema of intact skin

Intact skin with a localized area of nonblanchable erythema, which may appear differently in darkly pigmented skin. Presence of blanchable erythema or changes in sensation, temperature, or firmness may precede visual changes. Color changes do not include purple or maroon discoloration; these may indicate deep tissue pressure injury.

Stage 2 Pressure Injury: Partial-thickness skin loss with exposed dermis

Partial-thickness loss of skin with exposed dermis. The wound bed is viable, pink or red, moist, and may also present as an intact or ruptured serum-filled blister. Adipose (fat) is not visible and deeper tissues are not visible. Granulation tissue, slough and eschar are not present. These injuries commonly result from adverse microclimate and shear in the skin over the pelvis and shear in the heel. This stage should not be used to describe moisture associated skin damage (MASD) including incontinence associated dermatitis (IAD), intertriginous dermatitis (ITD), medical adhesive-related skin injury (MARSI), or traumatic wounds (skin tears, burns, abrasions).

Stage 3 Pressure Injury: Full-thickness skin loss

Full-thickness loss of skin, in which adipose (fat) is visible in the ulcer and granulation tissue and epibole (rolled wound edges) are often present. Slough and/or eschar may be visible. The depth of tissue damage varies by anatomical location; areas of significant adiposity can develop deep wounds. Undermining and tunneling may occur. Fascia, muscle, tendon, ligament, cartilage and/or bone are not exposed. If slough or eschar obscures the extent of tissue loss this is an Unstageable Pressure Injury.

Stage 4 Pressure Injury: Full-thickness skin and tissue loss

Full-thickness skin and tissue loss with exposed or directly palpable fascia, muscle, tendon, ligament, cartilage, or bone in the ulcer. Slough and/or eschar may be visible. Epibole (rolled edges), undermining and/or tunneling often occur. Depth varies by anatomical location. If slough or eschar obscures the extent of tissue loss this is an Unstageable Pressure Injury.

Unstageable Pressure Injury: Obscured full-thickness skin and tissue loss

Full-thickness skin and tissue loss in which the extent of tissue damage within the ulcer cannot be confirmed because it is obscured by slough or eschar. If slough or eschar is removed, a Stage 3 or Stage 4 pressure injury will be revealed. Stable eschar (i.e., dry, adherent, intact without erythema or fluctuance) on the heel or ischemic limb should not be softened or removed.

Deep Tissue Pressure Injury: Persistent nonblanchable deep red, maroon or purple discoloration

Intact or nonintact skin with localized area of persistent non-blanchable deep red, maroon, purple discoloration or epidermal separation revealing a dark wound bed or blood filled blister. Pain and temperature change often precede skin color changes. Discoloration may appear differently in darkly pigmented skin. This injury results from intense and/or prolonged pressure and shear forces at the bone-muscle interface. The wound may evolve rapidly to reveal the actual extent of tissue injury, or may resolve without tissue loss. If necrotic tissue, subcutaneous tissue, granulation tissue, fascia, muscle or other underlying structures are visible, this indicates a full thickness pressure injury (Unstageable, Stage 3 or Stage 4). Do not use DTPI to describe vascular, traumatic, neuropathic, or dermatologic conditions.

Additional pressure injury definitions.

Medical Device-Related Pressure Injury: This describes an etiology

Medical device-related pressure injuries result from the use of devices designed and applied for diagnostic or therapeutic purposes. The resultant pressure injury generally conforms to the pattern or shape of the device. The injury should be staged using the staging system.

Mucosal Membrane Pressure Injury

Mucosal membrane pressure injury is found on mucous membranes with a history of a medical device in use at the location of the injury. Due to the anatomy of the tissue these ulcers cannot be staged.

"inflammatory exudate composed of proteinaceous tissue, fibrin, neutrophils, and bacteria, rather than nonviable tissue. Slough is usually light yellow/cream colored and moist and soft." This distinction creates a dilemma when staging a pressure injury because the term *slough* is included in the definition of an unstageable pressure injury while unstageable pressure injuries are defined as full thickness (stage 3 or stage 4). However, the inflammatory phase of wound healing also occurs in patient thickness (e.g., stage 2 pressure injuries)

wounds as well which inherently results in "inflammatory exudate composed of proteinaceous tissue, fibrin, neutrophils, and bacteria." known as slough.

Accurate staging requires knowledge of the anatomy of skin and deeper tissue layers, the ability to recognize these tissue layers and the ability to differentiate among them. For example, the distinction between a Stage 2 and Stage 3 can be as little as one millimeter. Therefore, careful evaluation of the wound bed is essential. Pressure injury staging is a

BOX 11.3   Differential Diagnoses of Deep Tissue Pressure Injury (DTPI)

Bruise: Extravasation of blood in the tissues as a result of blunt-force impact to the body. Usually about 2 weeks is required for a bruise to heal under normal conditions. History of trauma is common.

Calciphylaxis: Vascular calcification and skin necrosis most common in patients with long-standing history of chronic renal failure and renal replacement therapy. Lesions may have a violaceous hue and be excruciatingly tender and extremely firm. Lesions are most commonly seen on the lower extremities, not over bony prominences. The incidence of these lesions is very low in general patient populations.

COVID-19 ischemic microangiopathy: Retiform, irregular, jagged shapes of purple discoloration the may occur over bony prominence or areas without pressure. Skin changes occur due to ischemia. Associated with hyper-coagulable states (e.g., prolonged PT and aPTT or elevated D-dimer).

Fournier's gangrene: Intensely painful necrotizing fasciitis of the perineum. May manifest initially as cellulitis.

Hematoma: Deep-seated purple nodule from clotted blood; usually associated with trauma.

Livedo reticularis: Cutaneous microvascular changes caused by spasms of capillary blood vessels or reduction in arteriolar blood flow to capillaries resulting in deoxygenated blood flow. The appearance of mottling or blue discoloration to skin typically in a net like distribution.

Perirectal abscess: First sign commonly is a dull, aching, or throbbing pain in the perianal area. The pain worsens when sitting and immediately before defecation; the pain abates after defecation. A tender, fluctuant mass may be palpated at the anal verge. These abscesses can open to reveal large cavities, which can be confused with a deep pressure injury.

Purpura: Purple colored spots or patches that occur on the skin generally caused by rupture of small blood vessels. May occur anywhere; not limited to pressure points.

Skin failure: Initial indications may present at mottling or blisters. Distinctive features include sudden appearance with rapid deterioration in critically ill patient or area does not correspond with pressure or shear.

---

complex skill that takes time to develop. Examples of Stage 1 to 4 pressure injuries, DTPI, and unstageable pressure injuries are provided in Plates 29, 31, 33, 34, 35A,E, 36–39. Box 11.3 provides a list of differential diagnoses for DTPI. Some experts have challenged the current staging system and proposed a paradigm that delineates superficial skin changes and deep pressure injuries (Sibbald, Krasner, & Woo, 2011). In people with darker skin tones, early pressure-related changes (i.e., erythema, purple discoloration, etc.) are difficult to detect and require additional scrutiny as discussed in Chapter 10. Checklist 10.1 describes important considerations for assessing pressure injuries on darkly pigmented skin. Box 7.1 lists unique characteristics of darker skin.

Device-Related Pressure Injuries

Pressure injuries can develop as a result of the use of diagnostic or therapeutic devices as well as personal care items such as a hearing aid. Pittman and Gillespie (2020) originally defined medical device-related pressure injury (MDRPI) as "a localized injury to the skin and/or underlying tissue including mucous membranes, as a result of pressure, with a history of an external medical device at the location of the ulcer and mirrors the shape of the device."

The device-related pressure injury conforms to the shape of the device. This was further refined and proposed by an international panel of experts as: "*…a device related pressure ulcer (DRPU) involves interaction with a device or object that is in direct contact with skin…or is transdermally implanted under the skin, causing focal and localized forces that deform the superficial and deep underlying tissues. A DRPU, which is caused by a device or object, is distinct form a PU, which is caused primarily by body-weight forces. The localized nature of the device's interaction with the patient's tissue results in*

the appearance of skin ad deeper tissue damage that mimics that of the device in sharpen ad distribution." (Gefen, Alves, Ciprandi, et al., 2022). Examples of medical devices that cause pressure injuries, factors associated with MDRPIs, differential diagnosis, prevention, and management are described later in this chapter.

Mucosal Pressure Injuries

Mucous tissues (i.e., lining of the gastrointestinal tract, oral cavity, nares, etc.) are also vulnerable to pressure injuries from the presence of medical devices such as oxygen tubing, endotracheal tubes, bite blocks, nasogastric tubes, urinary catheters, and fecal containment devices. These ulcers cannot be staged using the pressure injury staging system or classified as partial or full thickness because the histology of mucous membrane tissue is different from skin. Therefore, pressure injuries on mucous membranes should be documented simply as mucosal pressure injuries (EPUAP, NPIAP, & PPPIA, 2019).

Reverse Staging

The practice of reverse staging, in which the wound is described as progressing from a Stage 3 to a Stage 2 to a Stage 1 pressure injury, is incorrect. Once layers of tissue and supporting structures are gone (such as with full-thickness wounds), they are not replaced. Instead, the wound is filled with granulation tissue. This staging system is to be used for describing wounds in their most severe state, and once the wounds are accurately described, these descriptor levels endure, even in the presence of healing (Black, Baharestani, Cuddigan, et al., 2007). Negative outcomes of reverse staging can lead to (1) denial of acute or skilled care after Stage 4 injuries have been restaged as Stage 2 injuries; (2) withdrawal of pressure-reducing support surfaces when injuries have "healed" from Stage 3 or Stage 4 to Stage 2; and (3) lower fees paid to extended care facilities for care of patients with healing Stage 3 and Stage 4 injuries that have been reclassified as Stage 2 or Stage 1 pressure injuries. Therefore, a Stage 3 pressure injury that appears to be granulating and resurfacing is described as a healing Stage 3 pressure injury.

OPERATIONALIZING A PRESSURE INJURY PREVENTION PROGRAM (PIPP)

Every health care organization needs a pressure injury prevention program (PIPP). A PIPP consists of a *best-practice bundle* and organizational *infrastructure* (operations). The components of a PIPP have been widely adopted by WOC nurses for years (Bryant, Shannon, Pieper, et al., 1992) and were included in the 1992 AHCPR Pressure Injury Prevention Guideline. Historically, PIPPs have been demonstrated to be effective at reducing the incidence of pressure injuries. However, the implementation, maintenance, and survival of the PIPP were often dependent on WOC nurse involvement. Although the successful PIPP may be coordinated by the wound specialist, it should not be owned by or dependent on one individual or group. Rather, it must be adopted into the facility's overall patient safety culture, supported, and protected by the administration, and therefore integrated into the facility's infrastructure. Lack of infrastructure is frequently the reason for PIPP failure.

When creating a PIPP, both the structure of the program (i.e., best-practice bundle) and the operations of the program (i.e., organizational infrastructure) must be addressed. From a structural (bundle) perspective, the best-practice bundle components of the PIPP include skin inspection, risk assessment, pressure redistribution and offloading, skin health, nutrition and hydration, device-related pressure injury prevention, and patient and family education. For a PIPP to be successful, all caregivers and administration must share the belief that pressure injuries are a negative outcome and that all health care providers play a role in their prevention. In addition, the bundle must then be integrated into the culture and infrastructure of the health care system. Evidence suggests that the infrastructure components are often the missing link to implementation and maintenance of a PIPP. Common gaps include lack of interdisciplinary engagement and accountability (e.g., physician, nursing assistants, respiratory therapists, etc.) knowledge deficits and lack of resources including staff, adequate documentation templates, decision-making tools, and appropriate outcome measures (EPUAP, NPIAP, & PPPIA, 2019; Kaba, Kelesi, Stavropoulou, Moustakas, & Fasoi, 2017; Patrician et al., 2017; Tallier et al., 2017). In the following sections, we define and discuss the structure of a PIPP and steps for integration into the care delivery system to ensure ongoing viability and growth of the program. Special considerations for patients in perioperative, special procedures,

emergency services, and critical care environments are discussed in this chapter. Special considerations for pediatrics and neonates, individuals with obesity, and patients receiving palliative care are discussed in Chapters 36–38.

PIPP JUSTIFICATION

There are numerous reasons to justify a PIPP. Certainly, economics has heightened the interest of some, but the most important reasons stem from a concern for patient safety and quality care.

Demonstrated Effectiveness

The most compelling argument for implementing a PIPP is that high level studies (e.g., RCTs and systemic reviews) show that such programs are effective in reducing the incidence of facility-acquired pressure injuries in multiple countries and multiple health care settings (Beeckman et al., 2013; Chaboyer et al., 2016; Lin, Wu, Song, Coyer, & Chaboyer, 2020; Rantz, Zwygart-Stauffacher, Flesner, et al., 2013; Soban, Hempel, Munjas, et al., 2011; Tayyib & Coyer, 2016). These studies and many others describe a range of initiatives customized to facility or care setting and often increase as a quality improvement is demonstrated. Continued effectiveness and sustainability vary due to factors such as the baseline pressure incidence (EPUAP, NPIAP, & PPPIA, 2019).

National Priority to Eliminate Patient Harm

The national priority to reduce patient harm in the health care setting has increased in intensity over the past 20 years. In response to this focus of zero harm and federal and state mandates, quality tracking measures for pressure injury prevention, as described in Chapter 6, become central to a successful PIPP. Pressure injury prevention has been in the mission of the Wound, Ostomy and Continence Nurses Society™ (WOCN®) and has been included in the curriculum for WOC nursing education programs since 1982 (Alterescu, 1991; Goode, 1991; IAET, 1987; Wright, 1991). In 1992, the U.S. Agency for Healthcare Research and Quality (AHRQ), formerly the Agency for Health Care Policy and Research published clinical practice guidelines on preventing pressure ulcers. By the year 2000, the U.S. Department of Health and Human Services (2000a, 2000b) document, *Healthy People 2010: Understanding and Improving Health*, listed reducing pressure injury incidence as an objective for all health care providers. By fiscal year 2007, a preventable pressure injury was listed as a secondary diagnosis for 300,000 Medicare patients; adding up to $43,180 in costs to a hospital stay. Reports estimated about 60,000 patient deaths annually in the United States as a direct result of pressure injuries (AHRQ, 2011). These statistics are startling when we consider the fact that people come to the hospital when they are ill, trusting that they will be taken care of and protected from adversities. By 2008, the Centers for Medicare and Medicaid Services (CMS) ceased payment for hospital complications considered reasonably preventable, including Stage 3 or 4 pressure injuries, and released new codes for pressure injuries capturing wound severity forcing hospitals to incur the previously mentioned costs of hospital acquired pressure injuries (HAPIs).

Economic Burden of HAPI

Conservatively, it is estimated that a Stage 1 pressure injury will cost as much as $500, a Stage 2 as much as $3600, Stage 3 as much as $8800 and a Stage 4 as much as $44,000. A large part of the increased costs stems from the increased length of stay when a patient develops a pressure injury (AHRQ, 2011; Brem, Maggi, Nierman, et al., 2010; Trueman & Whitehead, 2010). More recently, Padula and Delarmente (2019) used economic simulation methods to estimate financial burden to US hospitals due to HAPI. Outcomes of hospitalized adults with acute illness were analyzed in 1-day cycles until discharge or death. Their analysis suggested that a HAPI could cost an average of $10,708 per patient with annual costs of treating HAPIs in the United States estimated to be greater than $26.8 billion.

In contrast to the high costs per patient for HAPI care, prevention of pressure injuries in hospitals is estimated to cost only $54.66 per day (Padula, Mishra, Makic, et al., 2011). Additionally, research suggests that 59% of the many billions spent on HAPIs in the United States are due to the small subset of patients with stage 3 and 4 pressure injuries (13.2%) further underscoring the cost effectiveness of prevention and early detection of pressure injuries (Padula & Delarmente, 2019).

Recognizing the Unavoidable Pressure Injury

Another key justification for a PIPP is the ability of the PIPP team members to recognize conditions that may be mis-interpreted as a pressure injury and in particular the avoidable and unavoidable pressure injury as well skin failure. By stating "hospital-acquired conditions (such as pressure injuries) could be *reasonably prevented* with evidence-based guidelines," the CMS introduces the possibility that some pressure injuries cannot be avoided (Schmitt et al., 2017; WOCN, 2017). Before the introduction of POA for hospitals, CMS defined the term *unavoidable pressure injury* (for the long-term care setting) as a pressure injury that develops in spite of the facility's best efforts at prevention (Checklist 11.1). However, a similar definition by the CMS for the hospital or home care setting does not exist. The WOCN® Society recognized the absence of a definition for acute care as a potential problem. To fill this gap, they released a position statement (*Avoidable Versus Unavoidable Pressure Injuries*) using the CMS definition of an unavoidable pressure injury and refuting the assumption that all pressure injuries are preventable (Schmitt et al., 2017; WOCN, 2017). There is also consensus from the National Pressure Injury Advisory Panel (NPIAP) that some conditions (e.g., hemodynamic instability worsened with movement) do *not* make pressure injuries inevitable but *may* lead to unavoidable pressure injuries. Further, consensus showed that the NPIAP continues to support the position that pressure injury avoidability is determined when

---

CHECKLIST 11.1 Avoidable and Unavoidable Pressure Injuries

Avoidable

The resident developed a pressure injury, and the facility did *not* do one or more of the following:
✓ Evaluate the resident's clinical condition and pressure injury risk factors
✓ Define and implement interventions that are consistent with the resident's needs and goals and with recognized standards of practice
✓ Monitor and evaluate the impact of interventions
✓ Revise the interventions as appropriate

Unavoidable

The resident developed a pressure injury even though the facility *did* the following:
✓ Evaluated the resident's clinical condition and pressure injury risk factors
✓ Defined and implemented interventions that were consistent with the resident's needs and goals and with recognized standards of practice
✓ Monitored and evaluated the impact of interventions
✓ Revised the interventions as appropriate

---

the outcome is known and preventive interventions are evaluated (Black et al., 2020; Black, Edsberg, Baharestani, et al., 2011).

A PIPP is based on evidence-based guidelines or best practices and therefore provides a structure in which unavoidable pressure injuries may be identified. Identifying a potentially unavoidable pressure injury may not assist with reimbursement in hospitals. However, it will help to identify whether a best practice was delivered and therefore may be useful in protecting against litigation.

In addition, this definition of avoidable and unavoidable is useful in the population of patients at the end of life or critically ill who may develop a pressure injury. CMS, International pressure injury guidelines (EPUAP, NPIAP, & PPPIA, 2019), and the WOCN Society (2016) have agreed that some pressure injuries are unavoidable. Under the current definition of "unavoidable," documentation is the only way to determine whether a pressure injury was or was not avoidable (Black, et al., 2011). See Checklist 11.2 for examples of relevant audit questions for the patient's medical record.

Skin Failure

Although there is support for the concept of skin failure, their is no universally agreed upon definition for the condition as yet (Levine, 2017; Mileski & McClay, 2021; Sibbald & Ayello, 2020). For example, in a recent systematic review, skin failure is described as the presence of skin or tissue damage in areas not subjected to pressure and shear (Dalgleish, Campbell, Finlayson, & Coyer, 2020). Later in a scoping review, the concept of skin failure is described as acute or chronic and may also be called Kennedy terminal ulcers, skin changes at life's end (SCALE) and Trombly-Brennan terminal tissue injuries (TB-TTI). Hill and Peterson (2020) suggest a unique feature

CHECKLIST 11.2   Hospital-Acquired Pressure Injury Prevention Best-Practice Audit

*Note best practice must be reflected in practice *and* in documentation

✓ Pressure injury risk assessment on admission and at least daily.

✓ Skin inspection on admission and at least daily.

✓ Removal of devices (e.g., stockings, splints, masks) at least twice a day (more frequently in the presence of edema).

✓ Devices that cannot be removed, such as indwelling tubes and drains, stabilized and repositioned at twice daily skin inspection (more frequently in the presence of edema).

✓ Care plan links risk assessment findings to specific preventive interventions.

✓ Impaired sensory perception, mobility, and activity as defined by the risk assessment has applicable MDRPI prevention (see Table 11.5) and offloading interventions in place while in the bed or chair including repositioning every 2 h, heels off bed (see Fig. 11.10), and appropriate support for mattresses and chair (see Chapter 12).

  ✓ Friction and shear risk as defined by pressure injury risk assessment is addressed including HOB ≤30 degrees with flex the knees (if not medically contraindicated) and put

pillows under arms to prevent slouching or sliding down in bed.

  ✓ If HOB ≤30 is medically contraindicated, interventions are in place to mitigate the effects (see Box 11.9).

✓ Nutritional deficiencies are addressed by dietary services once the deficit is identified.

✓ Incontinence is managed with cleansers, moisture barriers, collections devices designed for incontinence, underlying causes addressed.

✓ Patient and family skin safety education is addressed and readdressed as indicated.

✓ Best practice skin safety interventions determined to be medically contraindicated or inconsistent with the patient's overall goals are addressed by the provider and routinely reevaluated.

✓ Declination of skin safety interventions (previously referred to as refusal, nonadherence) is addressed by the care team through patient and family education and ongoing efforts to mitigate, reeducate, and modify plan of care (see Chapter 5, Fig. 5.2).

---

of skin failure is that they appear suddenly then rapidly deteriorate to necrosis or full-thickness tissue loss. Ultimately the delineation between skin failure and pressure injury requires further descriptive studies and research (EPUAP, NPIAP, & PPPIA, 2019).

Litigation Avoidance, Patient Trust, and Facility Reputation

Patient trust and facility reputation are other justifications for PIPP implementation as patient safety becomes transparent through published reports on the Internet and the ability of consumers to compare facility outcomes. More than 17,000 lawsuits are related to pressure injuries annually. It is the second most common claim after wrongful death and greater than falls or emotional distress (AHRQ, 2011; VanDenBos et al., 2011). As discussed in Chapter 5, pressure injuries often lead to significant and prolonged suffering including impaired physical and social function, self-care, and mobility and often require either long-term hospitalization or frequent hospital admissions. Beyond the financial, physical, and psychological impact, errors in patient care are costly in terms of loss of trust in the system by patients, diminished satisfaction by both patients and health professionals, and loss of morale by health care professionals who are not able to provide the best care possible.

A BEST-PRACTICE BUNDLE FOR PIPP

From a structural perspective, the best-practice bundle of the PIPP contains several components: skin assessment, risk assessment, skin health, nutrition and hydration, pressure redistribution and offloading, integration into specialty care environments, prevention of device related pressure injuries, and patient education. The best-practice bundle includes

research-based evidence and, when a higher level of evidence is not available, expert opinion.

Skin Inspection and Assessment

A skin inspection should be obtained for all patients upon admission. Because the admission inspection serves as a baseline for comparisons and pressure injuries can develop quickly, this skin inspection should be a high priority and obtained as soon as possible (EPUAP, NPIAP, & PPPIA, 2019). Physiologically a pressure injury can develop as early as within 1 h (Gefen, 2008b; Lustig, Levy, Kopplin, Ovadia-Blechman, & Gefen, 2018). Therefore, it may be reasonable to inspect the skin within the first few hours of admission, given the need for patient repositioning and other cares that are conducive to skin inspection (see Table 10.1). Subsequent inspection and monitoring by trained staff are recommended at least daily as part of every risk assessment when patients are deemed at risk for pressure injuries or have existing impaired skin integrity (NPIAP, 2020). The frequency of skin assessment should be increased if the patient's overall condition deteriorates. All skin assessment findings should be documented. Skin temperature, erythema, edema, and alterations in tissue consistency should be noted by comparing adjacent skin or contralateral body part. If erythema is noted, it should be determined whether it is blanchable (see Box 10.1 and Plate 24) or nonblanchable (EPUAP, NPIAP, & PPPIA, 2019).

Optimal visualization and palpation of skin changes require adequate lighting, removal of garments, repositioning of medical devices, and the spreading of skin folds, buttocks, and toes. Palpation of darker skin tones is particularly important, as identification of erythema in darkly pigmented skin (Bates-Jensen, McCreath, & Pongquan, 2009; EPUAP, NPIAP, & PPPIA, 2019; WOCN®, 2016). Studies report

---

BOX 11.4   Pressure Injury Risk Assessment Tools by Patient Population

Adults
- Braden Scale
- Norton Scale
- Waterloo Score

Critical Care
- Norton MI
- EVARUCI
- Cubben-Jackson Scale

Home Care
- Pressure Injury Primary Risk Assessment Scale

Hospice/Palliative
- Performance Palliation Score (PPS)

Neonatal
- Neonatal Skin Condition Score (Neonatal)

Pediatric
- Starkid skin scale
- Braden Q
- Pediatric Pressure Ulcer Prediction Tool (PPUPET)
- Glamorgan

Perioperative
- Munro Scale
- Scott Triggers Tool

Spinal Cord Injury
- Spinal Cord Injury Pressure Ulcer Scale (SCIPUS)

---

higher rates of full-thickness pressure injuries in patients with dark skin tones compared with patients with light skin tones which suggests the early indicators of pressure injury damage (e.g., blanching and nonblanching erythema) are not recognized in patients with dark skin tones (Oozageer Gunowa, Hutchinson, Brooke, & Jackson, 2018). Unique characteristics of darker versus lighter pigmented skin are described in Chapter 7 and Box 7.1. Teaching points and special considerations when inspecting darkly pigmented skin are provided in Chapter 10 and Checklist 10.1. Unlike inspection, skin *assessment* involves interpretation and synthesis of additional data gathered from the comprehensive holistic patient assessment, such as nutrition, perfusion, medications, and other comorbidities. A comprehensive review of skin assessment and proper technique is presented in Chapter 10.

Risk Assessment and Screening

Pressure injury risk assessments should be conducted in conjunction with the comprehensive skin assessment as soon as possible after admission followed by development of a risk-based prevention care plan. As with other assessments, pressure injury risk assessment includes identification of subjective, objective, and psychosocial factors to determine and assess the risk and care needs of the patient (EPUAP, NPIAP, & PPPIA, 2019; WOCN, 2016). Many of these risk factors at first glance seem intuitive. However, due to highly variable experiences and knowledge among caregivers, intuitive sense alone in identifying those at risk is not reliable, as demonstrated through many studies including metaanalysis (García-Fernández, Pancorbo-Hidalgo, & Soldevilla Agreda, 2014). Furthermore, the assumption that all patients are at risk and that preventive measures should be universally applied is difficult to defend due to the inefficient use of resources.

The WOCN Society (2016) recommends using a validated risk screening scale as part of the structured approach to risk assessment. International pressure injury guidelines (2019) cite valid and reliable risk assessment tools as an option for inclusion in a structured approach. Experts are

clear that regardless of structured method chosen, consideration of risk factors that are not included in most scales and clinical judgment rooted in up-to-date evidence-based knowledge are essential (EPUAP, NPIAP, & PPPIA, 2019; WOCN, 2016).

A risk assessment tool or scale is a noninvasive, cost-effective method for distinguishing between patients who are at risk for developing a pressure injury and those who are not. Scales identify the extent to which a person exhibits a specific risk factor and are useful for developing and implementing risk-based interventions to mitigate modifiable risk factors (EPUAP, NPIAP, & PPPIA, 2019; WOCN, 2016).

Box 11.4 provides a list of risk assessment tools described in recent literature organized by intended patient populations (Anthony, Papanikolaou, Parboteeah, & Saleh, 2010; Chen, Cao, Zhang, Wang, & Huai, 2015; García-Fernández et al., 2014; Kottner, Hauss, Schlüer, & Dassen, 2013; Lund & Osborne, 2004; Maida, Lau, Downing, & Yang, 2008; Moore & Cowman, 2014; Noonan, Quigley, & Curley, 2011; Sterken, Mooney, Ropele, Kett, & Vander Laan, 2015; Suddaby, Barnett, & Facteau, 2005; Wang et al., 2015). In selecting a scale for predicting a condition such as a pressure injury, the scale must have demonstrated reliability and validity. *Reliability* refers to the degree to which the results obtained by the measurement procedure can be replicated. For example, if two nurses administered a pressure injury risk scale on the same patient at the same time and their scores were the same, the reliability of the scale would be a perfect 1.0, or 100% agreement. *Validity* refers to accuracy. A screening test such as a pressure injury risk scale should provide a good preliminary test of which individuals are at risk and which are not. Validity has two components: *sensitivity*, which correctly identifies patients at risk, and *specificity*, which correctly identifies patients not at risk. An ideal risk scale would be 100% sensitive and 100% specific, so it does not overpredict (therefore no false-positive scores) or underpredict (no false-negative scores). However, 100% is rarely achieved due to an inverse

CHECKLIST 11.3 Recommendations for Frequency of Pressure Injury Risk Assesses

✓ Perform pressure injury risk assessment upon entry to a health care setting

✓ Repeat risk assessment on a regularly scheduled basis or when there is a significant change in condition

✓ Establish a schedule for reassessing risk based on acuity:
  • Acute care: At least every 24–48 h and whenever the patient's condition or deteriorates
  • Long-term care: Weekly for the first 4 weeks, then monthly, and when the patient's condition deteriorates
  • Home care: Every nurse visit

WOCN Society (2016).

BOX 11.5 Factors Associated With Medical Device–Related Pressure Injuries

• Sensory deficit and/or inability to communicate pressure-related discomfort (e.g., Diabetic neuropathy or "the strap too tight")
• Excess moisture and body secretions at the interface of the skin and medical device
• Edema near the device
• Inadequate equipment selection and/or fitting
• Inadequate positioning and stabilization of device
• Absence of routine skin inspection under and around the device
• Impaired perfusion at the interface of the skin and medical device

relationship between sensitivity and specificity; as the scale becomes more sensitive, specificity declines. Nevertheless, these measures of predictability are invaluable when comparing tools that attempt to predict a condition such as a pressure injury (Portney, 2020).

The validity and reliability of several pressure injury risk assessment scales have been reported in the literature and summarized in a meta-analysis (Anthony et al., 2010; Chen, Cao, Wang, & Huai, 2015; García-Fernández et al., 2014; Kottner et al., 2013; Lund & Osborne, 2004; Maida et al., 2008; Moore & Cowman, 2014; Noonan et al., 2011; Sterken et al., 2015; Suddaby et al., 2005; Wang et al., 2015). These tools identify risks so they can be targeted; they logically have poor predictability rates because once a risk is identified, interventions are put in place to reduce the likelihood of pressure injury development. Reassessment is intuitively logical because factors known to contribute to risk clearly fluctuate with medical condition and hospital course. Checklist 11.3 lists recommendations from the WOCN Society (2016) for frequency of pressure injury risk assessment. Using a pressure injury risk assessment tool to address modifiable risk factors is described in the following sections. Factors associated with medical device-related pressure injuries are listed in Box 11.5.

Risk Assessment of Modifiable Risk Factors

One of the most widely used and researched pressure injury risk tools is the Braden Scale for the Prediction of Pressure Injury Risk (García-Fernández et al., 2014; Huang et al., 2021). Translated into many languages, numerous reports attest to the reliability of the scale with adequately trained registered nurses and licensed practical nurses (Huang et al., 2021; Magnan & Maklebust, 2008).

The Braden Scale (Table 11.2) is composed of six risk factor subscales that conceptually reflect degrees of sensory perception, skin moisture, physical activity, nutritional intake, friction and shear, and ability to change and control body position. All subscales are rated from 1 (most risk) to 4 (least risk), except the friction and shear subscale, which is rated from 1 to 3. Each rating is accompanied by a brief description of criteria for assigning the rating. Therefore, the subscales identify which risk factors are present so that interventions can be targeted to reduce specific risk factors (Table 11.3) (EPUAP, NPIAP, & PPPIA, 2019; WOCN, 2016).

Braden Scale scores are grouped according to level of risk: not at risk (>18), mild risk (15–18), moderate risk (13–14),

TABLE 11.3 Skin Safety Interventions by Risk Factor

Risk Factor	Interventions (Skin Safety Precautions)

Impaired sensory perception, mobility, activity	1. Pressure redistribution support surface for patients with multiple intact turning surfaces and Braden score ≤18
	2. Obtain therapeutic pressure redistribution support surface (i.e., low air loss) for patients with:
	  • Full-thickness or suspected deep tissue injury on the trunk
	  • Wounds on multiple turning surfaces
	3. Reposition every 2 h in bed, *regardless* of bed/mattress type
	  • Avoid positioning directly on trochanter
	  • Collaborate with provider for pain control as needed to promote appropriate repositioning
	  • Use positioning devices (e.g., pillows, fluidized positioners) to keep bony prominences (including heels) from direct contact with potential pressure-inducing surfaces.
	  • Stabilize and position tubes to prevent them from creating pressure
	4. Reposition once every hour in chair
	  • Use pressure redistribution chair cushion
	  • Return to bed after 1 h if unable to reposition in chair

Continued

TABLE 11.3	Skin Safety Interventions by Risk Factor—cont'd
Risk Factor	**Interventions (Skin Safety Precautions)**
	5. Moisturize dry skin; do *not* massage reddened bony prominences
	6. Remove or reposition devices (stockings, masks, tubes) at least twice daily for skin inspection, and more frequently in the presence of fluid shifts and/or signs of localized/generalized edema. Note: patients with sensory deficit may not be able to identify or communicate that their device is too tight or causing discomfort
Moisture	1. Address cause and offer bedpan/urinal/toileting every 2 h
	2. Notify provider and registered dietitian if patient has loose stools
	3. Use absorbent pads with polymers that wick moisture away from the body (avoid diapers/briefs with plastic backing)
	4. Incontinence skin care twice per day and after each incontinent episode to include:
	• Incontinence cleanser and barrier in one
	• Moisture barrier skin protectant paste if stools are loose or perineal skin is red or open
	5. Consider containment devices for frequent loose stools (rectal pouches, FDA-approved indwelling fecal containment device)
Nutritional deficit	1. Consult nutritional services
	2. Maintain adequate hydration
	3. Monitor intake to consume at least the minimum recommended daily allowance of protein (0.8 g/kg)
Friction and shear	1. Limit head-of-bed elevation to 30 degrees or less, unless contraindicated
	2. Use knee gatch as needed to prevent sliding down in bed
	3. Use trapeze when indicated
	4. Use lift sheet or air transfer device to move (rather than drag) the patient to prevent shear injury
	5. Protect elbows and heels
	6. If head-of-bed elevation to 30 degrees or less is contraindicated, put interventions in place to mitigate effects (see Box 11.9)

high risk (10–12), and very high risk (≤9). After the total score is obtained, if other major risk factors are present (i.e., age, fever, poor dietary intake of protein, diastolic pressure <60 mmHg, and/or hemodynamic instability) advance the score to the next level of risk (WOCN, 2016).

For example, a patient with a Braden score of 12 would be considered at moderate risk but should be "upgraded" to the high-risk category if he or she also has a fever. When a patient has a pressure injury or a history of a pressure injury but is rated "not at risk" according to the tool creators, it is recommended to automatically place the patient in the "at-risk" category (WOCN, 2016). It is important to emphasize that a pressure injury prevention care plan is *not* based on total score alone; subscale scores, consideration of additional risk factors, and clinician judgment will serve as a more accurate guide (EPUAP, NPIAP, & PPPIA, 2019; WOCN, 2016).

Accurate use of the Braden Scale requires user training and retraining, even when nurses use the tool regularly and for a long period of time. A study involving more than 2500 nurses in Detroit Medical Center showed that only 75.5% of nurses correctly assigned Braden Scale scores (Maklebust, Sieggreen, Sidor, et al., 2005). Although the two extremes of risk levels, "not at risk" and "severe risk," were most often rated correctly, the subscales "moisture" and "sensory perception" were most often misunderstood. Therefore, ongoing education and competencies for risk assessment are justified to support reliability (EPUAP, NPIAP, & PPPIA, 2019; Magnan & Maklebust, 2008; Maklebust & Magnan, 2009; Pandhare, 2018). Similarly,

---

BOX 11.6 Recommendations to Improve Accuracy of Pressure Injury Risk Assessment

- Use risk assessment tool subscale (rather than total) scores to guide pressure injury prevention plan of care
- When using the Braden Scale adjust risk level to account for advancement for age, fever, poor dietary intake, diastolic pressure <60 mmHg and/or hemodynamic instability
- Implement a pressure injury prevention plan of care for the patient with an existing or history of pressure injury (regardless of pressure injury risk score)
- Implement a pressure injury prevention plan of care for the patients with a medical device (regardless of pressure injury risk score)
- Assign score based on subscale definitions rather than memory or recall
  - Sensory perception refers to the patient's ability to communicate pressure-related pain or discomfort (e.g., "my mask is too tight," or they have altered sensation or numbness due to diabetic neuropathy in the foot)
  - Mobility refers to the patient's ability to CHANGE and CONTROL body position

---

the definitions for risk factors and subscales for each risk factor are essential in both paper and electronic documentation systems. Box 11.6 offers recommendations to improve accuracy of pressure injury risk assessment. The following section uses the Braden Scale to clarify definitions of common modifiable risk factors.

Sensory Perception. With respect to pressure injuries, *sensory perception* refers to the patient's ability to respond meaningfully to pressure-related discomfort. The extent of the deficit depends on the degree to which a patient is able to feel or communicate pressure-related discomfort. Patients without a sensory impairment move or ask to be moved if they are lying on intravenous tubing or feel pain on their tailbone. They remove or request removal of shoes, stockings, or medical devices that feel uncomfortable or too tight. Examples of patients with sensory deficits who cannot adequately communicate discomfort include those with confusion, disorientation, oversedation, or unresponsiveness. Patients who are alert and oriented may be unable to communicate discomfort (e.g., "my mask is too tight") if they are on a ventilator, speak a different language than their caregivers, or cannot feel pain due to paralysis or neuropathy.

Moisture. The more the skin is exposed to moisture, especially near a bony prominence, the more vulnerable the skin becomes to the mechanical forces of pressure, friction, and shear. Clinical examples include the patient with incontinence who is exposed to pressure, the critically ill patient with fever and diaphoresis, or the bedbound patient with poorly contained wound exudate from a perirectal abscess.

Activity. Degree of activity refers to how much a patient is in the bed or chair or is ambulating. Again, reading the subscale definitions is important. For example, "walks occasionally" means the patient spends most of the time in the chair. Therefore, a few steps to the bedside commode should be scored as "walks occasionally."

Mobility. One of the problems encountered with this subscale is the tendency to confuse activity (e.g., getting up in the chair) with mobility. *Mobility* refers to the patient's ability to change or control body position. The score assigned is based on what the patient demonstrates, such as the degree to which he or she is able to change or control body position (i.e., shifting weight in the chair or turning or repositioning in bed). A patient may be able to sit in a chair (activity) but may not be able to shift his or her weight (mobility). In contrast, a patient who is agitated and moving frequently may still have a mobility deficit because the movements are not purposeful or controlled.

Nutrition. One mistake made with the Braden nutrition subscale is failure of the rater to consider "*usual* food intake pattern." For example, the patient who is NPO (nil per os [nothing by mouth]) after midnight does not constitute a low nutrition score if his or her usual food intake pattern is adequate. Conversely, the patient's nutritional status may be rated "adequate" when the patient is receiving total parenteral nutrition or a tube feeding documented to "meet nutritional needs" even though the patient is malnourished. This occurs because the regimen "that meets nutritional needs" requires time to reverse the malnutrition that existed before supplementation was initiated. Therefore, patients at risk for pressure injuries with an adequate nutrition score should be placed at a higher risk level in the presence of clinical evidence of malnutrition.

Friction and Shear. Friction occurs when the skin rubs against another surface. Patients who are restless or agitated commonly create friction on their elbows and heels from constant movement and rubbing against the bed surface. Friction also can occur with a brace or shoe as it slides back and forth during ambulation. *Shear* occurs when friction acts with gravity. Classic examples of actions that cause shear injury include a patient sliding down in bed after the head of the bed has been elevated for lunch or allowing the patient's buttocks to drag across the bed, stretcher, or procedure table during transfer. Using the Braden Scale with 7514 hospital patients Cabrejo, Ndon, Saberski, Chuang, and Hsia (2019) found friction and shear to be the most predictive risk factor for HAPI development ($P < 0.01$).

Mining Data From the Electronic Health Record (EHR)

It must be emphasized that use of a risk assessment must include consideration of risk factors not included in many tools. Fig. 11.7 lists key risk factors in the context of a proposed causal (direct and indirect) pathway to pressure injury development. Because so many risk factors are not included in traditional pressure injury risk assessment tools, mining data from EHR may be the future of pressure injury risk assessment. Advances in data mining have the exciting potential to provide a more accurate risk status by using a greater number of risk factors while offering a real time assessment as the patient's condition changes (Alderden et al., 2018; Cramer, Seneviratne, Sharifi, Ozturk, & Hernandez-Boussard, 2019; Feng, Zhou, & Tong, 2021; Kaewprag et al., 2017; Li, Lin, & Hwang, 2019). Currently, however, pressure injury risk assessment tools that include common modifiable risk factors are widely used in health care.

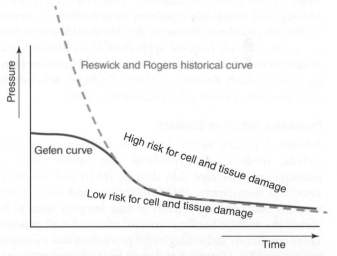

Fig. 11.7 Theoretical schema of proposed causal pathway for pressure ulcer development. The *solid arrows* show the causal relationship between the key indirect causal factors and direct causal factors and the outcome. *Interrupted arrows* show the causal relationship between other potential indirect causal factors and key indirect causal factors and between direct causal factors. *Interrupted arrows* also demonstrate interrelationships between direct causal factors and indirect causal factors. (From Coleman, S., Nixon, J., Keen, J., Wilson, L., McGinnis, E., Dealey, C., et al. (2014). A new pressure ulcer conceptual framework. *Journal of Advanced Nursing, 70*(10), 2222–2234. https://doi.org/10.1111/jan.12405.)

Optimize Skin Health

The third component of the PIPP's best-practice bundle is preserving the protective function of the skin. It is intuitive that maintaining skin integrity is important to prevent bacterial invasion and protect resilience of skin to deflect or absorb pressure, shear, or friction. There is growing evidence that *microclimate* (temperature, humidity, airflow around the skin surface) plays a role in pressure injury development. Excessively dry or moist skin as well as increased temperature weakens the skin (EPUAP, NPIAP, & PPPIA, 2019).

Moisturizers

Worldwide, overall prevalence of dry skin is estimated to be as high as 85% (Hahnel, Lichterfeld, Blume-Peytavi, & Kottner, 2017). Dry skin can lead to xerosis (as demonstrated by pruritic, erythematous, dry, scaly, cracked, or fissured skin) which results from loss of natural moisturizing factors, barrier abilities, and epidermal water. Xerosis may exist alone or cooccur with or be part of different conditions such as diabetes, HIV, hypothyroidism, and renal insufficiency, or pharmacologics such as statins, diuretics, or chemotherapeutic agents. Thus, dry skin is not only a common condition but may also be an indicator of a person's health status (Mekić et al., 2019). Lechner, Lahmann, Neumann, Blume-Peytavi, and Kottner (2017) analyzed data collected by trained RNs involving 3837 patients in 30 nursing homes and 13 hospitals in Germany. Researchers found 71.9% of patients with heel/ankle pressure injuries (Stage 2 and greater) were affected by dry skin on the legs or feet, compared with 42.8% of subjects without pressure injuries ($P < 0.001$). In the adjusted analysis, patients with dry skin had an 85% increased chance of developing a pressure injury on their legs or feet (adjOR = 1.85; 95% CI, 0.83–4.14). Although not statistically significant, these findings are viewed as clinically significant. Therefore, dry skin should be prevented or minimized with frequent application of moisturizers and emollients in addition, adequate hydration, and humidity management (Proksch, Berardesca, Misery, Engblom, & Bouwstra, 2020; Shannon, Coombs, & Chakravarthy, 2009).

Protective Moisture Barriers

Additional threats to the protective function of the skin include, medical adhesive-related skin injury (MARSI), incontinence-associated skin damage (IAD) and moisture-associated skin damage (MASD), friction, and shear. Interventions that minimize threats to skin integrity need to be part of the routine baseline standard of care for all patients. These conditions and strategies for prevention and treatment are presented in Chapter 9 and must be integrated into practice in order to optimize pressure injury prevention.

Prophylactic Dressings

Prophylactic dressings for managing friction, shear, and microclimate under pressure have been used for years and have become an important component of pressure injury prevention (EPUAP, NPIAP, & PPPIA, 2019; Sillmon, Moran, Shook, Lawson, & Burfield, 2021). A variety of dressings have been used for pressure injury prophylaxis including hydrocolloids,

---

BOX 11.7 Prophylactic Dressing: Selection and Use

Selection Considerations
- Appropriate size and thickness (e.g., avoid pressure or tension between dressing and medical device)
- Allows for frequently skin inspection without causing trauma to the skin
- Stays in place
- Safe to apply and remove
- Manages microclimate (especially under and around tube sites)
- Comfortable and safe for the patient (e.g., will not cause dislodgement of device or allergic reactions)
- Low friction between skin-dressing interface (e.g., multi-layer foam)
- Cost effective

Prophylactic Dressing Use:
- Use prophylactic dressings in combination with all other components of a pressure injury prevention program (e.g., offloading)
- Implement as soon as possible to vulnerable sites (e.g., ambulance, emergency room, preoperatively)
- Change dressings according to manufactures instructions, if dislodged, or soiled

---

transparents, hydrogels, and foams (Beeckman, Fourie, Raepsaet, et al., 2021; Clark, Black, Alves, et al., 2014; Fulbrook, Mbuzi, & Miles, 2019). Most recent published work focuses on foams and multilayer silicone foams (Beeckman et al., 2021; EPUAP, NPIAP, & PPPIA, 2019). Ongoing research suggests thermal conductivity found in other types of dressings more closely match the skin suggesting the "ideal" prophylactic dressing may not yet exist (Gefen, 2022).

Considerations for prophylactic dressing selection and use as one component of pressure injury prevention is presented in Box 11.7 (EPUAP, NPIAP, & PPPIA, 2019; Gefen, 2022). However, various dressings in different anatomical locations cause a variety of physiological responses during sustained pressure suggesting that several choices are needed and more importantly, there need to be consideration of the dressing features in order to make the best choice. In addition, universally recognized performance standards for prophylactic pressure injury prevention dressings do not yet exist. To address this gap, the International Prophylactic Dressing Standards Initiative involving multiple stakeholders including clinicians, bioengineers, industry, and test standard experts, professional societies (Brienza, Gefen, Clark, & Black, 2022; Gefen, 2022).

Optimize Nutrition and Hydration

The fourth component of a PIPP's best-practice bundle is maintenance of adequate nutrition and hydration. International evidence-based pressure injury guidelines (EPUAP, NPIAP, & PPPIA, 2019) report:
- Poor nutritional status and variables that indicate potential malnutrition, such as low body weight or poor oral intake, are independent risk factors for pressure injury development.

- Patients at risk and with existing pressure injuries often experience unintended weight loss.
- Inadequate nutrition and undernutrition are also associated with pressure injury severity and poor healing.

Hydration is vital to nutrition as water helps dissolve and transport nutrients through the body as well as eliminating waste products from the body. Therefore, providing and encouraging water and fluids for individuals with or at risk for pressure injuries is recommended. However, the amount must be compatible with the goals of care and clinical condition as fluid intake may need to be restricted for individuals with conditions such as renal or heart failure (EPUAP, NPIAP, & PPPIA, 2019). Chapter 29 discusses the details of nutritional assessment and support.

Redistribution and Offload Pressure

Pressure redistribution and offloading are required for the patient at-risk for pressure injuries, whether the individual is in a chair, on a transport or procedure cart, in the operating room, or in a bed. Pressure redistribution addresses *intensity* of pressure and is accomplished with the use of support surfaces (see Chapter 12). Offloading addresses the *duration* of pressure and is accomplished by turning and repositioning. Frequent turning and repositioning facilitate early mobilization by preventing an orthostatic response to movement. Drawn from a variety of key sources, Box 11.8 provides a compilation of evidence for early mobilization to address the serious complications that are associated with immobility (Barr, Fraser, Puntillo, et al., 2013; Brindle, 2013; Engel, Needham, Morris, et al., 2013; Schweickert, Pohlman, Pohlman, et al., 2009; Society of Critical Care Medicine, 2020; Vollman, 2010; Wu et al., 2018).

Repositioning Frequency and Reminder Methods

Repositioning is used to reduce the duration of pressure exerted over a bony prominence. In 1961, Kosiak recommended the frequency of repositioning to be hourly to every 2 h, based on the interface pressure readings from healthy, able-bodied subjects. There is widespread support for a repositioning schedule and documentation of positioning regimens, including selected positions, frequency, and outcomes. However, repositioning every 2 h as a standard of care to prevent pressure injuries continues to be debated (EPUAP, NPIAP, & PPPIA, 2019).

To date, there is a lack of evidence related to a standard process for determining an accurate individual turning frequency. For example, international guidelines (EPUAP, NPIAP, & PPPIA, 2019) continue to recommend a reposition frequency that is determined by skin and tissue tolerance, level of activity and mobility, general medical condition, overall treatment objectives, comfort, pain, and support surface. Although some of these factors are easily determined and remain constant (support surface), others cannot be measured with current technology (e.g., tissue tolerance) or may be unpredictable and labile (e.g., mobility, activity, medical condition, pain, comfort).

BOX 11.8 Evidence for Early Mobilization

- Immobility is an independent risk factor for several complications: pressure injuries, deep vein thrombosis (DVT), pneumonia, and urinary tract infection (UTI)
- Complications of immobility are associated with increased morbidity and mortality, prolonged length of stay, increased hospital cost, and contribution to global disease burden
- Frequent turning and repositioning facilitate early mobilization by preventing an orthostatic response to movement so the patient can progress to sitting or walking as soon as possible
- Early mobility programs have been shown to improve outcomes by decreasing the incidence of delirium, number of ventilator days, and length of stay while achieving a higher functional status at hospital discharge

Sources: Wu, X., Li, Z., Cao, J., Jiao, J., Wang, Y., Liu, G., et al. (2018). The association between major complications of immobility during hospitalization and quality of life among bedridden patients: A 3-month prospective multi-center study. *PLoS One, 13*(10), e0205729; Vollman, K. (2010). Introduction to progressive mobility. *Critical Care Nurse, 30*, 3–5; Brindle, C. T. (2013). Turning and repositioning the critically ill patient with hemodynamic instability: A literature review and consensus recommendations. *Journal of Wound, Ostomy, and Continence Nursing, 40*(3), 254–267; Schweickert, W. D., Pohlman, M.C., Pohlman, A. S., et al. (2009). Early physical and occupational therapy in mechanically ventilated, critically ill patients: A randomised controlled trial. *Lancet, 373*,1874–1882; Engel, H. J., Needham, D. M., Morris, P. E., et al. (2013). ICU early mobilization: From recommendation to implementation at three medical centers. *Critical Care Medicine, 20*(41), S69–S80; Barr, J., Fraser, G., L., Puntillo, K., et al. (2013). American College of Critical Care Medicine. Clinical practice guidelines for the management of pain, agitation, and delirium in adult patients in the intensive care unit. *Critical Care Medicine, 41*, 263–306; Society of Critical Care Medicine. (2020). ICU Liberation Bundle. Retrieved 4/7/2022 from: https://www.sccm.org/ICULiberation/ABCDEF-Bundles; Li, Z., Peng, X., Zhu, B., et al. (2013). Active mobilization for mechanically ventilated patients: A systematic review. *Archives of Physical Medicine and Rehabilitation*, 94, 551–561.

Much like determining frequency for pain medications, the effectiveness of an individualized repositioning schedule must be assessed, adjusting frequency as needed to achieve the desired outcome (e.g., no erythema). Specifically, when establishing a pressure injury prevention plan, positioning frequency might be determined by beginning with a schedule of every 2 h. Persistent redness noted during repositioning and inspection indicates that pressure is not adequately relieved. If it is difficult to differentiate between blanchable reactive hyperemia and nonblanchable erythema stage I pressure injury (see Plates 24 and 33), relieve the pressure for 30 min then reassess. Persistent pressure-related erythema indicates the need for an advanced support surface (see Chapter 12) or a more frequent repositioning schedule. A 4-h repositioning schedule may be warranted when the patient is on an appropriate support surface, the patient's skin has remained intact and without erythema, and the patient does not have an acute illness that would precipitate a sudden change in medical condition (e.g., hemodynamic instability). Although an every 4-h positioning schedule may be adequate in some situations for keeping the skin intact, it may be

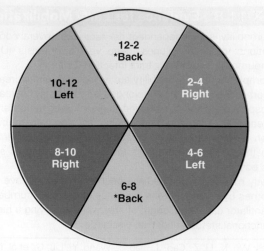

Fig. 11.8 Example of a turning schedule. *Consider omitting from schedule for patients that are already supine during activities throughout the day.

insufficient to prevent other immobility-related complications (see Box 11.8).

In contrast to positioning schedules customized for each individual patient, international pressure injury guidelines (EPUAP, NPIAP, & PPPIA, 2019) also recommend repositioning reminder strategies to promote staff adherence to positioning regimes citing evidence for the use of facility-based reminder systems customized to the *care setting* such as auditory or visual feedback systems (e.g., musical chimes every 2 h) (Yap et al., 2013) and continuous bedside pressure mapping (Behrendt, Ghaznavi, Mahan, Craft, & Siddiqui, 2014; Gunningberg, Sedin, Andersson, & Pingel, 2017; Siddiqui, Behrendt, Lafluer, & Craft, 2013). Regardless of choice between turning schedules customized to facility or an individual patient, reminder systems can be used. Options to consider range from advanced technologies such as

pressure mapping bed systems and overlays or wearable patient sensors to simple methods like alarms, notes, EMR prompts, and positioning clocks (Fig. 11.8) (Bales & Duvendack, 2011; Behrendt et al., 2014; EPUAP, NPIAP, & PPPIA, 2019; Gunningberg et al., 2017; IHI, 2022; Pickham et al., 2018; Shieh et al., 2018; Siddiqui et al., 2013; Yap et al., 2013).

Repositioning Techniques

Although repositioning does not reduce intensity of pressure, it does reduce the duration, which is a critical element of pressure injury formation (EPUAP, NPIAP, & PPPIA, 2019). In general, pressure-related discomfort will motivate an individual to reposition themselves. Therefore, it is critical to conduct frequent assessments to determine whether the patient:
(1) Can independently adjust their position to effectively achieve pressure-relief while in bed or up in chair.
(2) Can sense and communicate pressure-related discomfort before and after pain medication.

Repositioning techniques differ according to the patient's activity (chairbound, bedbound) and location (operating room, transport, emergency room, special procedures, and ICU). Patients receiving pain medication may benefit from a coinciding repositioning and pain medication schedule.

Turning. Turning the patient in bed is a universally accepted staple in preventing the complications associated with immobility, including pressure injuries. The proper technique for turning is to place the patient in a 30-degree side-lying position with a pillow between the knees as shown in Fig. 11.9. The patient should be turned alternately from right side, to back, to left side, to back. The proper technique avoids bony prominences, nonblanchable erythema, existing wounds, and medical devices such as tubes and catheters. For example, a 90-degree side-lying position is generally undesirable because it places the patient directly on the trochanteric bony prominence (EPUAP, NPIAP, & PPPIA,

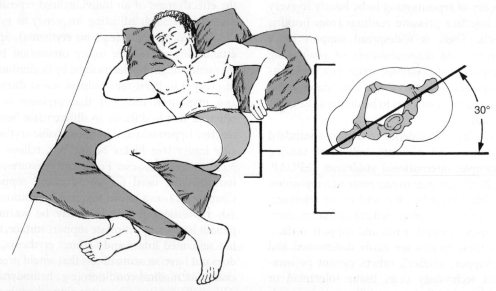

Fig. 11.9 Thirty-degree lateral position.

2019). When an injury is present on a turning surface, the turning schedule may be customized so that time spent on that turning surface is minimized.

Using wearable sensors, researchers were able to continuously monitor and record turning frequency and technique for 555 patients in intensive care units (ICUs) over a 5-month period recording 44 870 h of monitoring data (Pickham, Pihulic, et al., 2018). Clinical staff were not able to view the data. A qualified turn was defined as >20 degree angle and held for 1 min after turning. Out of 27566 turns recorded, only 39% of turns reached the minimum 20 degree angle. Compliance with turning frequency (every 2 h according to facility policy) was 54%. Unfortunately, low Braden scores and high body mass index (BMI) were factors associated with fewer turns; patients were recorded as supine for 72% of the observed time. A later study conducted in ICUs by Pickman and colleagues (2018) showed a statistically significant improvement in pressure injury incidence and turn frequency when clinical staff was allowed to receive the real-time data as feedback.

Limiting Head-of-Bed Elevation. The head of bed (HOB) should be kept as flat as possible to prevent shear injury (EPUAP, NPIAP, & PPPIA, 2019). Unfortunately, keeping the HOB flat is often contraindicated especially in acute care for a variety of reasons (e.g., respiratory distress, administering tube feedings). In those cases, an angle of 30 degrees or less continues to be recommended to minimize the pull of gravity, with the knee flexion adjusted to create a semi-Fowler's position (EPUAP, NPIAP, & PPPIA, 2019). When the HOB must be temporarily elevated over 30 degrees, such as when eating or drinking or during procedures, the caregiver should monitor the patient closely so that the head of the bed is not left in the elevated position longer than needed (e.g., 1 h). When having the head of the bed at 30 degrees or less is medically contraindicated, or the patient choses not to keep the HOB less than 30 degrees, (despite education and troubleshooting barriers), mitigation measures should be implemented (Box 11.9). Clinical practice guideline recommendations for HOB positioning to prevent VAP and aspiration are discussed in the critical care section of this chapter.

Transferring Without Lateral Shear. Lateral transfers, for example from the patient's bed to the OR surface, procedure table, or cardiac chair exposes the patient to lateral shear. Lateral transfer assist devices (e.g., mechanical lift with supine sling, mechanical lateral transfer device, or air-assisted lateral transfer devices, transfer sheets) are available to safely facilitate lifting, rather than dragging, the patient to facilitate transfer without skin injury while decreasing the risk of back injury for the staff. Patients who are able to move themselves laterally onto another surface should be instructed to do so without sliding. After transfer is complete, patients should move or be moved to release any tension or tangential forces created in the transfer (AORN, 2013). Transfer devices should not be left under the patient unless specifically designed for that purpose (EPUAP, NPIAP, & PPPIA, 2019).

> **BOX 11.9   Interventions to Help Mitigate the Effects of HOB Elevation**
>
> - Upgrade to a more advanced support surface with more effective pressure redistribution, shear reduction, and microclimate control (see Chapter 12)
> - Flex the knees (if not medically contraindicated) and position pillows under arms to prevent slouching or sliding down in bed
> - Apply prophylactic dressings to the sacral coccygeal region (see Box 11.7)
> - Inspect the sacral coccygeal region at least daily
> - Use fabrics/mattress covers designed to reduce pressure injury friction/shear
> - Use safe patient moving/handling equipment to lift rather than drag the patient up in bed or to another surface
> - Remove patient handling equipment from under the patient when not in use (unless specifically designed for that purpose)
> - Place a pressure redistribution cushion in the chair (including recliners)

> **BOX 11.10   Pressure Ulcer/Injury Knowledge and Attitude Assessment Tools**
>
> - Pressure Ulcer Knowledge Assessment Tool[a,b]
> - Pressure Ulcer Knowledge Assessment Tool 2.0[c,b]
> - Pieper Pressure Ulcer Knowledge Test[d,b]
> - Pieper Zulkowski Pressure Ulcer Knowledge Assessment Tool (see Appendix A)[e,b]
> - Attitudes Towards Pressure Ulcer Prevention Instrument[f]
>
> [a]Beeckman et al. (2010).
> [b]Kielo et al. (2020).
> [c]Manderlier et al. (2017).
> [d]Pieper and Mattern (1997).
> [e]Pieper and Zulkowski (2014).
> [f]Florin, Bååth, Gunningberg, and Mårtensson (2016).

Floating/Offloading Heels. The heels are one of the most frequent locations for pressure injuries and may be some of the most severe. The plantar aspect of the heel is well constructed to resist the forces of standing and walking. However, the posterior heel has only a thin layer of fat that is bound tightly to the underlying fascia and Achilles's tendon fibers and has limited ability to (1) redistribute pressure over the small area of skin overlying the posterior tubercle of the calcaneus and (2) absorb the compressive forces of shear generated during movement or transfers. Additionally, the small branches from the calcaneal and peroneal arteries and prolonged pressure on these relatively small vessels can lead to ischemia. Patients with diabetes and vascular disease are at increased risk for pressure injuries on the heel due to decreased perfusion and neuropathy (Bosanquet, 2017; Gefen, 2010). Therefore, experts recommend assessment of the perfusion status of the lower limbs, heel and feet during the skin assessment and pressure injury risk assessment (EPUAP, NPIAP, & PPPIA, 2019; Ramundo, Pike, & Pittman, 2018). As discussed in Chapter 17, sensory perception of the feet (ability to communicate pressure-related foot pain) is critical for patients with diabetes due to the prevalence of peripheral vascular disease and diabetic neuropathy.

Offloading products are used to "float" the heels off the surface of the bed. Options include pillows, support surfaces, and heel suspension devices. Selection considerations include patient condition, mobility status, skin condition (e.g., edema, wounds) presence of muscle spasms, hip foot and leg alignment, and patient's tolerance of the device. Offloading devices (fitted and used according to the manufacturer's instructions) and pillows should distribute the weight of the leg *without* putting pressure on the Achilles tendon while keeping the knees at a slight flexion 5–10 degrees. Devices with positioning blocks are available and should be considered for the patient that lacks optimal alignment and positioning of the foot (e.g., lateral or external rotation). When pillows are used, they should be positioned under the calf muscle with slight knee flexion (5–10 degrees) while preventing the heels from contacting the surface of the mattress (Fig. 11.10). Although pillows and foam cushions are inexpensive and readily available, they can be unreliable for maintaining the offloaded heel due to compression over time, or difficulty keeping them in place with the presence of contractures, restlessness, and spasms. Therefore, pillows and foam cushions are best used short term with patients

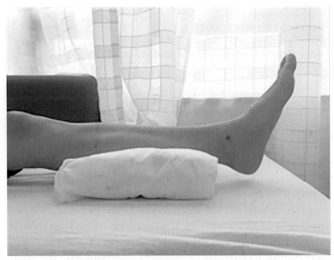

Fig. 11.10 Offloading or "floating" the heel with use of a pillow under leg to prevent contact with the bed surface. Positioned with slight knee flexion (e.g., 5–10 degrees) with the weight off the leg distributed along the calf without placing pressure on the Achilles tendon and the popliteal vein. (From Koh, S. Y., Yeo, H. L., Goh, M. L. (2018). Prevention of heel pressure ulcers among adult patients in orthopaedic wards: an evidence-based implementation project. *International Journal of Orthopaedic and Trauma Nursing, 31,* 40–47. https://doi.org/10.1016/j.ijotn.2018.08.003. Epub 2018 Aug 28. PMID: 30316760.)

who can reliably keep the heels floating off the bed (EPUAP, NPIAP, & PPPIA, 2019).

Several offloading medical devices for the heels have been found more effective than pillows and cushions however their is no "best" product as yet (Bååth, Engström, Gunningberg, & Muntlin, 2016; Gleeson, 2015; Meyers, 2017). Depending on the setting, collaboration with an occupational therapist or a physical therapist may be wise to select a device that will float the heels and be compatible with ambulation or address foot drop. Use of any device, especially with patients who have a sensory perception deficit, places the patient at risk of skin damage from the device. As with any removable device, it should be removed for skin inspection at least twice daily (more frequently in the presence of edema, peripheral vascular disease and neuropathy or reduced sensation). The product must be fitted and applied according to manufacturer's instructions (EPUAP, NPIAP, & PPPIA, 2019). Prophylactic dressings should be used to decrease pressure injuries by preventing friction and shear (Ramundo et al., 2018; Sillmon et al., 2021). Moisturizing dry skin on the feet and heels can improve overall skin health, resilience, and pressure injury prevention (Lechner et al., 2017).

Seating. For all patients at risk for a pressure injury, pressure injury prevention must consider (1) pressure redistribution seating cushions, (2) type of chair and seating position, (3) weight shifts, and (4) duration of sitting. A key component of the evaluation is the patients functional mobility. Moving from the bed to the chair thus increasing the level of activity may decrease the overall risk for pressure injuries. However, the patient in a seated position remains at risk for pressure injuries on the coccyx and develops new pressure points on the ischial tuberosities. Patients expected to be chairbound long term should be routinely reassessed by a seating specialist or team. To achieve appropriate alignment and posture the seating system will need to accommodate the patient's size, shape, mobility, and lifestyle needs (EPUAP, NPIAP, & PPPIA, 2019). Table 11.4 provides a reference for functional ability according to level of spinal cord injury (Nas, Yazmalar, Şah, Aydın, & Öneş, 2015).

Pressure redistribution seating cushions can be found in various mediums such as foam, air, gel, or mixed (discussed further in Chapter 9). They are available in a variety of sizes and contours to be individualized to the individual patient. Pressure redistribution seating cushions are also available for toilets, cars, and showers. Cushion covers need to stretch and fit loosely so the cushion can deform and immerse the patient for pressure redistribution. Research suggests that a rise in temperature and humidity can increase risk for pressure injury, a cushion and cover that can help manage microclimate should be considered. Cushions and covers wear out and require daily inspection and occasional maintenance according to manufacturer's instruction. Foam or rubber rings (i.e., donuts) are not indicated to redistribute pressure from sitting because they concentrate the intensity of the

TABLE 11.4 Examples of Functional Ability According to Level of Spinal Cord Injury

Level of Spinal Cord Injury	Functional Ability
C 1-3	• Breathing requires a ventilator or nerve stimulator to the diaphragm • Dependent for bed mobility and transfers • Weight shifts require power/tilt wheelchair with head, chin, or mouth controls for independence • Communication devices and environmental controls are often needed • Dependent for feeding, dressing, and bowel and bladder care
C 4	• Spontaneous respiration • Weight shifts require power/tilt wheelchair for independence • Dependent for bed mobility and transfers • Adaptive devices and environmental controls needed for communication • Dependent for feeding, dressing, and bowel and bladder care
C 5	• Moderate to maximum assist with bed mobility • Maximum assist for sliding board transfers (some exceptions) • Independent in electric wheelchair with hand drive • Independent in manual wheelchair with quad pegs and special gloved for indoor mobility • Independent in self-feeding with setup and adaptive equipment • Weight shifts side-to-side independently in wheelchair • Needs assist with upper body dressing • Dependent for bowel and bladder care
C 6	• Independent with bed mobility and level transfers, minimal assist with uneven transfers • Weight shifts side-to-side independently • Independent with lightweight manual wheelchair on level ground, mild slopes, and 2-inch curbs • Independently removes armrests and footplates • Independently drives adapted van • Independent in self-feeding with use of adaptive equipment • Independent with upper body dressing • Needs assist with lower body dressing • Dependent for bowel and bladder care
C 7-8	• Independent in uneven transfers over greater distances • Independent with wheelchair push-up • May be able to transfer floor to wheelchair • Independent in manual wheelchair on slightly uneven ground, low curbs, and standard ramps • Independent with all self-cares except some help for bowel care • May stand in parallel bars with braces
T 1-4	• Weight shifts and transfers independently • Independent with manual wheelchair on curbs, ramps, wheelies, and uneven ground • Able to load wheelchair into car and drive with hand controls • Able to walk short distances with leg braces locked straight and crutches or walker
T 5-12	• Walking with leg braces and walker possible • Wheelchair use is still needed due to the high energy needed
L 1-5	• Walking with leg braces, crutches, or straight canes • Wheelchair for sports or long distances

pressure on the surrounding tissue (EPUAP, NPIAP, & PPPIA, 2019).

The posture and position prescribed should minimize pressure and shear while maximizing safety, stability, and a full range of activities. For example, a reclining chair will off-load the ischial tuberosities but will place more pressure on the coccyx. In contrast, a commonly used straight-back chair facilitates an upright position, with most of the pressure on the ischial tuberosities, but the coccyx again becomes vulnerable to pressure damage if the patient slouches or slides. If the patient's feet do not touch the floor while seated, the feet should be positioned on a footrest. The footrest should be at a height that does not raise the knees above the patient's lap, which would create more pressure under the coccyx and ischial tuberosities (EPUAP, NPIAP, & PPPIA, 2019).

Weight shifts in the chair should be scheduled in routine intervals by standing up, performing pressure relief pushups, having the wheelchair tilted back 65% or more, leaning forward, or having the patient shift his or her weight from side to side enough to offload the ischial tuberosities and coccyx. Additional weight shifts can be incorporated into everyday functional activities such as reaching and leaning. Skin inspection should guide frequency of weight shifts. For instance, the patient who performs frequent weight shifts through functional activity may require fewer intentional weight shifts than the patient the patient who has less functional ability (EPUAP, NPIAP, & PPPIA, 2019).

Sitting duration should be limited for patients at risk for pressure injury if adequate pressure relief cannot be achieved in the chair (i.e., 2 h at a time). Even with the best pressure relief surface, patients with an existing coccyx or ischial tuberosity wound may need to limit sitting to 1 h or less, three times per day to heal their wounds and prevent deterioration. The location of the wound will help determine the position and posture that will minimize pressure to the wound. As with all interventions, risk and benefits to skin integrity and emotional well-being with limited sitting should be regularly evaluated and modified as indicated (EPUAP, NPIAP, & PPPIA, 2019).

PIPP in the Critical Care Environment

Critical care settings have some of the highest incidence rates for pressure injuries (Coyer et al., 2017; Zhou et al., 2018) often due to additional risk factors such as vasoactive medications, poor tissue perfusion and oxygenation, coagulopathy, and exposure to multiple life-sustaining medical devices (Alderden, Rondinelli, Pepper, Cummins, & Whitney, 2017; Alderden et al., 2018; Cox, Roche, & Murphy, 2018). All pressure injury preventive interventions apply to patients in critical care. However, with the additional risk factors, interventions often need to be intensified (EPUAP, NPIAP, & PPPIA, 2019).

Repositioning Unstable Critically Ill Patients

As previously stated, the effects of immobility can have serious consequences and early mobilization programs have shown significant outcomes (see Box 11.7). International pressure injury guidelines note that few individuals are truly too unstable to turn and recommend slow gradual turns to allow perfusion to the skin and time for hemodynamic and oxygenation stabilization; allowing 10 min to gain equilibrium before determining whether the position change can be tolerated. For the critically ill patient with a well-documented contraindication to slow turns, frequent small shift (also known as mini shifts) can be used including passive range of motion, floating the heels, head rotation, and lower angle "mini turns." Resume regular positioning frequency and techniques as soon as possible by conducting trials at least every 8 h (EPUAP, NPIAP, & PPPIA, 2019). After conducting a literature review for turning and repositioning critically ill patients, a multidisciplinary clinical medical and nursing group developed consensus recommendations for repositioning critically ill patients. The group identified examples of clinical conditions for miniturns and weight shifts instead of 30-degree lateral turns as a temporary intervention until the patient is stabilized. These conditions included: active uncontrolled bleeding, unstable open chest, sudden desaturation, or drop in blood pressure that does not recover or cannot be corrected with vasopressive agents (Brindle, 2013). Obviously, an advanced support surface (see Chapter 9) that provides more effective pressure redistribution, shear reduction, and microclimate control should

be implemented as soon as these conditions are anticipated and when clinically safe.

Head of Bed Positioning for VAP and Aspiration Prevention

As previously described, pressure injury prevention guidelines recommend HOB position less than or equal to 30 degrees for prevention of shear and pressure injury. Fortunately, best practice guidelines from the Centers for Disease Control and Prevention (CDC), the Infectious Diseases Society of America, the American Thoracic Society, and the Society for Healthcare Epidemiology of America (SHEA) all advocate HOB position from 30–45 degrees for aspiration and VAP prevention (American Thoracic Society & Infectious Diseases Society of America, 2005; Klompas, Branson, Eichenwald, et al., 2014; Tablan, Anderson, Besser, et al., 2004). More recently, a Cochrane review, Wang et al. (2016) and a literature review by the AHRQ (2017) reported the same recommendations. When the HOB cannot be maintained 30 degrees, either due to medical contraindication or patient refusal, mitigations to reduce their risk of shear injury should be implemented (see Box 11.9).

Prone Positioning in Critical Care. Prone positioning is used to improve oxygenations in patients with acute respiratory distress syndrome (ARDS). Proning allows better distribution and volume of air in the lungs and improves ventilation of the posterior lung regions. Systematic review and metanalysis comparing the mortality of patients with ARDS and mechanical ventilation when supine and prone shows a lower mortality for patients maintained in the prone position for at least 12 h (Munshi, Del Sorbo, Adjikan, et al., 2017). Not surprisingly, results of this study and several others show a higher rate of pressure injuries among patients in the prone position (Binda et al., 2021; Jahani, Soleymani, Asadizaker, Soltan,& Cheraghain, 2018; Luccini, Mattiussi, Elli, et al., 2020; Mora-Arteaga, Bernal-Ramirez, & Rodriguez, 2015). Assembling a protocol using an effective interprofessional team to ensure the safe transition of critically ill patients from supine to prone (e.g., critical care provider; respiratory therapist, critical care nurse, staff who move and position patients regularly) has been shown to decrease complications typically associated with prone positioning such as pressure injuries and accidental extubations (Johnson et al., 2022). Examples of skin protection strategies for the critically ill patient during pronation is presented in Checklist 11.4 (EPUAP, NPIAP, & PPPIA, 2019; Miguel et al., 2021). The recommended position during pronation of the critical care patient is illustrated in Fig. 11.11.

PIPP on the Emergency Services Environment

Emergency services entails the care of the patient enroute to the emergency department (such as in the ambulance and helicopter) as well as care while located in the emergency department (ED). Research suggests that patients at risk for pressure injuries can develop pressure injuries within a few

CHECKLIST 11.4 Skin Protection for the Critically Ill Patient During Pronation

✓ Multidisciplinary prone team with expertise in airway and positioning of the critically ill patient (e.g., respiratory therapy, physical therapy, critical care nurses, critical care provider)

✓ Upgrades support surface (e.g., low air loss)

✓ Offloading device for head, face, ear (e.g., fluidized positioner) molded to offload vulnerable areas

✓ Dry flow pads (avoid excessive layers)

✓ Prophylactic dressings (e.g., multilayer foam) to forehead, cheekbones, bony prominence of shoulders, breast/chest wall, medial elbows ileac crests knees and under devices on torso

✓ Secure medical devices to avoid pressure, when possible, e.g.:

• Place new EKG leads on the patient's back

• Secure indwelling urinary catheter to back of thigh without tension

✓ Avoid sliding with positioning

✓ Use positioning devices to offload toes, knees, penis, scrotum, breasts, and abdomen

✓ Position arms in modified swimmer's crawl position (see Fig. 11.11)

• Raise arm on same side patient is facing (shoulder is dropped, and elbow is below the level of the axilla)

• Opposite arm at patient's side with palm facing up

✓ Reposition head, arms, ETT, ventilator tubing, remold pillow every 2 h, lift head off pillow (slightly) each opposite hour

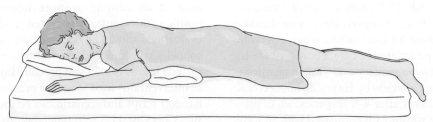

Fig. 11.11 Modified swimmer's crawl position for pronation. Raise arm on same side patient is facing (shoulder is dropped, and elbow is below the level of the axilla). Position opposite arm at patient's side with palm facing up. (From Sorrentino, S., Remmert, L. (2021). *Mosby's textbook for nursing assistants* (10th ed.). St. Louis: Elsevier.)

hours of entering an ED (Cereda, Neyens, Caccialanza, et al., 2017). Muntlin Athlin, Engström, Gunningberg, and Bååth (2016) noted that 9% of 169 patients assessed upon arrival and departure from ED developed pressure injuries of the heel during their ED stay. Researchers noted a 5.2% pressure injury prevalence in a random sample of 212 ED patients when inspected within 1 h of arrival (Fulbrook et al., 2019). These studies suggest that patients cared for in the ED for several hours may not receive a skin inspection until after admission to the hospital unit leading to the possibility that pressure injuries "present on admission" were acquired in the ED or before arrival to the hospital (Denby & Rowlands, 2010; Dugaret et al., 2014; Fulbrook et al., 2019). More recently, an observational study in the ED with 48, 641 adult patient admissions found that prolonged LOS in the ED (over 12 h was an independent risk factor for HAPI within a week of admission (adjOR = 1.51, 95% CI, 1.15–1.99) (Han et al., 2019). There are limitations to this study however, in that it was conducted in one setting, there was no adjustment for known pressure injury risk factors, and information about post ED stay events were not known. However, the study does suggest that promoting pressure injury prevention during the ED stay is important and may decrease facility-acquired pressure injuries (Han et al., 2019).

Although few EDs and ambulance services have pressure injury prevention protocols (Gamston, 2019; Stanberry,

Lahti, Kevin, & Delin, 2021), some strategies for the ambulance and ED have emerged including improved tracking methods, skin inspection, heel offloading, pressure redistribution support surfaces, and prophylactic dressings (Clark et al., 2014; Fulbrook et al., 2019; Muntlin Athlin et al., 2016).

Diagnostic and Ancillary Services Environment

Little has been published about pressure injuries among patients undergoing procedures in diagnostic and interventional ancillary units (e.g., radiology, renal dialysis, gastrointestinal, cardiac and vascular procedure labs) (Angmorterh et al., 2019; Messer, 2012). True incidence of pressure injuries in ancillary services is unknown. One prospective study using data from 80 patients found a 53.8% incidence of pressure injury development in patients undergoing lengthy radiology procedures (Messer, 2010). Haugen, Pechacek, Maher, et al. (2011) reviewed root-cause analysis reports for HAPIs over a 1-year time frame. Analysis showed that 76% of patients with HAPIs in that year had undergone three or more procedures prior to pressure injury development. Patients in ancillary services are frequently subjected to high interface pressures on procedure surfaces and exposed to shear during transfers and positioning. Procedures sometimes require prolonged immobilization and agents that may cause hypotension such as anesthesia and sedation (Messer, 2010). It has been reported that patients undergoing procedures ultimately could be in the same position on suboptimal support surfaces for 6–8 h (Haugen et al., 2011). Strategies to mitigate these risk factors include support surfaces designed for stretchers, advance notification, and handoff tools that communicate pressure injury risk, existing skin breakdown, and positioning tips. One rapid process improvement team even found ways to shorten scan time and provide breaks as needed for offloading (Haugen et al., 2011). Several strategies for pressure injury prevention in the perioperative environment are also appropriate in the perioperative environment (Messer, 2012) and will be discussed in the following section. An example of a handoff tool for ancillary services is located in Appendix A (Haugen et al., 2011).

PIPP in the Perioperative Environment

Pressure injuries identified within 72 h after a surgical procedure is commonly assumed to be an intraoperatively acquired pressure injury (Aronovitch, 2007; Kimsey, 2019; Primiano, Friend, McClure, et al., 2011). However, there is no standard definition or cutoff timeline for establishing when a pressure injury is attributable to perioperative care, because of the lag time that may occur between surgery and visable manifestation (AORN, 2022). Citing a review by Hayes, Spear, Lee, et al. (2015) involving 931 patients after 4-h surgeries, 5% of pressure injuries were visible within 24 h compared with 58% visible after the fifth hospital day. Regardless, the AORN (2022) recommends that health care organizations define a timeframe or criteria for determining perioperative-acquired pressure injuries (e.g., up to 5 days after surgery or in consultation with the interdisciplinary pressure injury team). This underscores the importance of examining preoperative history of exposure to pressure and shear as well as OR-specific risk factors since pressure injuries can also develop in emergency and ancillary services. This also reinforces the value in establishing the presence or absence of elevated subepidermal moisture measures (i.e., localized focal edema) prior to the surgical procedure.

The overall rate of intraoperatively acquired pressure injuries varies greatly due to the vast range of positions, equipment, and support surfaces used. For example, researchers (Shafipour, Ramezanpour, Gorji, & Moosazadeh, 2016) conducted a systematic review and meta-analysis of 19 articles available on the internet that included a total of 9527 patients. The prevalence of postoperative pressure injuries varied by study from 5.1% (N = 297 patients) to 64.1% (N = 53 patients). Due to the variability in data, a randomized effect model was used to report an overall prevalence of 18.96% Many perioperative pressure injuries are reported by specific patient populations. For example, an analysis from a scoping review conducted by Gefen, Creehan, and Black (2020) reported a pressure injury prevalence of at least 8.5% among patients having procedures lasting longer than 3 h. Incidence of pressure injury by surgical procedure include cardiovascular surgeries (9.2%–38%), orthopaedic surgeries (5.2%–36%) and 8.6% for patients with liver resections that lasted longer than 2 h.

Perioperative Specific Risk Factors

Risk associated by length of surgical procedure is: 6% for 3–4 h, 9% for 4–5 h, 10% for 5–7 h, and over 13% for more than 7 h. Additionally, A 2-h surgery translates into 6 h of immobility total including perioperative, intraoperative and post operative recovery. Therefore, procedures lasting more than 2 h should be considered high risk for pressure injury development (Gefen et al., 2020). The AORN advocates using a standardized, validated, and reliable risk assessment tool specific to perioperative patients (see Box 11.4) and age appropriate when possible (AORN, 2022).

Perioperative Preventive Interventions

According to the American Operating Room Nurses (AORN, 2022) perioperative pressure injuries are often preventable and require interdisciplinary collaboration for prevention beginning before the patient enters the operating or procedure room. Preoperative skin and risk assessments, the presence of an existing pressure injury, the surgical patient position, interventions provided, and postoperative patient evaluations should be documented and accessible to all personnel involved. Hand-over (also known as handoffs) should include results of skin and pressure injury assessments as well as interventions used to reduce pressure injury risk. A sample handoff script and scenario can be found at the AORN website. Checklist 11.5 recommendations perioperative pressure injury preventive interventions (AORN, 2022; EPUAP, NPIAP, & PPPIA, 2019). Common surgical and procedural positions within the context of a handoff communication tool are provided in Fig. 11.12.

Prevent Device-Related Pressure Injuries

Device-related pressure injuries can result from any device (medical or not) that exposes the patient's skin to pressure. Nonmedical devices that cause pressure can range from hair accessories to bed clutter such as phones, keys, remotes, and writing materials. The most common stages are 1 and 2 and common sites are ears, heels, and lower legs. Patients with a medical device are 2.4 times more likely to develop a pressure injury of any kind (Black, Baharestani, Black, et al., 2010).

Despite the wide variations in data collection and analysis, the majority of studies report the prevalence and incidence of MDRPI are high. A recent global systematic review reported an incidence of MDRPIs in adults within the acute hospital setting to be 28.1% (Brophy, Moore, Patton, O'Connor, & Avsar, 2021). Medical records of over 10,000 patients throughout US and Canadian hospitals revealed and prevalence of MDRPI of 0.6% (601 patients); 0.15% were present on admission (Kayser, VanGilder, Ayello, & Lachenbruch, 2018). The most frequently reported MDRPI was associated with respiratory equipment. An annual state department of health report (Minnesota Department of Health (MDH), 2019), revealed 44% of full-thickness hospital-acquired pressure injuries (HAPI) were associated with medical devices, predominantly respiratory devices. Critically ill patients have high rates MDRPI

CHECKLIST 11.5 Perioperative Pressure Injury Prevention

Patient Unit Prior to Surgery

✓ While on the preoperative unit, position the patient in a different position that anticipated during surgery

✓ Consider use of high-specification pressure redistribution support surface prior to surgery

✓ Remove braids, jewelry, or body piercing accessories it will cause potential pressure, injury or interfere with the surgical site

Perioperative Team Prior to Patient Arrival

✓ Identify and provide positioning equipment required for each procedure

✓ Prepare a support surfaces that reduces the potential for pressure injury

✓ Select, clean, inspect, and maintain position equipment devices, and support surfaces; ensure they are repaired or replaced when damaged, defective, or obsolete

✓ Use OR beds, positioning equipment and support surfaces correctly

✓ Identify potential positioning hazards and implement safe practices

Perioperative Team Once Patient Arrives

✓ Use a standardized, validated, and reliable PI perioperative risk assessment tool and when possible, age appropriate

✓ Ensure braids, jewelry, or body piercing accessories are removed before transferring to procedure bed if they will cause potential pressure, injury or surgical site interference

✓ Implement safe positioning practices for the anticipated surgical position (see Fig. 11.12 for common surgical/procedural positions)

✓ Implement measures to reduce injury while positioning patients who are pregnant

✓ Implement measures to reduce injury when positioning patients who are obese

✓ Float heels of surface with slight knee flexion, and supporting calves without pressure on the Achilles tendon or popliteal vein

✓ Apply prophylactic dressings to protect bony prominences or vulnerable skin (see Box 11.7)

✓ Consider and communicate need for high specification pressure redistribution support surface postoperatively

Perioperative RN and Perianesthesia RN

✓ Collaborate to identify patient injury caused by intraoperative positioning

✓ Document preoperative skin and risk assessments, the presence of an existing PI, the surgical patient position, interventions provided, and postoperative patient evaluations and make accessible to all personnel involved

Postoperative Unit

✓ Collaborate with OR staff to ensure Handover (AKA handoff) that includes position in OR (see Fig. 11.12), and results of skin and pressure injury assessments and interventions used to reduce risk

✓ Inspect skin including under and around medical devices, between buttocks, between skin folds

✓ Position the individual in a different posture than the posture adopted during surgery

✓ Provide ongoing evaluation of pressure redistribution support surface effectiveness

✓ In collaboration with provider, enhance perfusion and oxygenation (Chapter 31)

Health Care Organization

✓ Maintain records of patient care related to patient positioning and organizational processes related to positioning equipment and devices

✓ Develop policies and procedures for positioning, revise them as necessary, and make them readily available in the practice setting

✓ Ensure patient positioning is evaluated by the quality management program

✓ Patients who develop skin injury should be referred to wound specialist or their primary care provider post discharge

✓ Define in a policy and procedure a timeframe or method to determine how perioperative-acquired pressure injuries are identified (e.g., up to 5 days after surgery or in consultation with the interdisciplinary PI team)

✓ Monitor monthly incidence of perioperative pressure injuries and use the number as a quality indicator that informs performance improvement processes as part of the PI prevention program.

✓ Report perioperative PI incidence rates in a standardized method that enables comparison with published PI incidence rates (e.g., number of pressure injuries monthly [or annually] divided by the number of procedures performed monthly [or annually], # per 1000 procedures)

✓ Use root cause analysis to investigate reported and confirmed perioperative pressure injuries. A systems mindset should be used during root cause investigations to foster a culture of safety instead of blame.

✓ Report perioperative PI rates and any identified root causes to perioperative personnel to increase their awareness.

✓ Review root causes of perioperative pressure injuries for trends and use identified trends to inform quality improvement initiatives.

✓ Provide competency verification education related to positioning and PI prevention for perioperative personnel during initial orientation, annually, and as needed.

ranging from 11.3% to 68% in adult ICUs (Barakat-Johnson, Barnett, Wand, & White, 2017; Coyer, Cook, Doubrovsky, Vann, & McNamara, 2022; Mehta, Ali, Mehta, George, & Singh, 2019; Sala et al., 2021). Using a variety of sample sizes and methodologies, individual hospitals and organizations have reported MDRPI incidence (all stages) ranging from 27.9 % to 50% (Arnold-Long, Ayer, & Borchert, 2017; Barakat-Johnson et al., 2017).

The neonatal and pediatric populations are additional high risk for MDRPI (EPUAP, NPIAP, & PPPIA, 2019; Gefen et al., 2022). Immature skin is less resilient to pressure and as they grow, medical equipment may not fit properly and require frequent evaluation and refitting. Schlüer, Halfens, and Schols (2012) reported a 40% prevalence of MDRPI in the pediatric population using a multicenter, cross-sectional, point prevalence study in Switzerland. The literature for

PATIENT LABEL

AULTMAN

Surgical/Procedural Positioning Communication Tool
**Note Surgery Length In Hours _____

Circle affected area. Designate with an "I" for intraoperative or "P" for postoperative assessment. Describe the area in the comments section.

☐ **SUPINE**

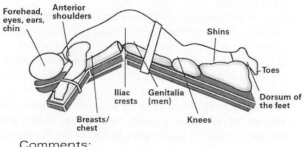

Occiput Arms and elbows Lumbar area Sacrum and coccyx Heels

Scapulae Thoracic vertebrae

Comments: _____

_____

☐ **PRONE**

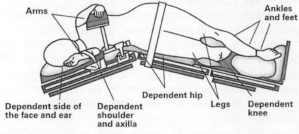

Forehead, eyes, ears, chin Anterior shoulders Knees Dorsum of the feet

Toes

Breasts/chest Iliac crests Genitalia (men) Shins

Comments: _____

_____

☐ **PRONE (JACKKNIFE)**

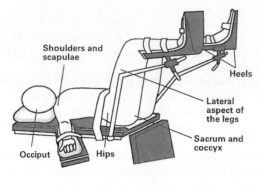

Forehead, eyes, ears, chin Anterior shoulders Shins

Toes

Iliac crests Genitalia (men) Dorsum of the feet

Breasts/chest Knees

Comments: _____

_____

☐ **LATERAL**

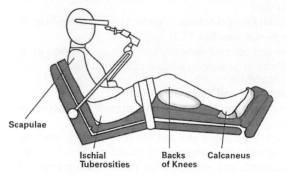

Arms Ankles and feet

Dependent hip Legs Dependent knee

Dependent side of the face and ear Dependent shoulder and axilla

Comments: _____

_____

☐ **LITHOTOMY**

Shoulders and scapulae

Heels

Lateral aspect of the legs

Sacrum and coccyx

Occiput Hips

Comments: _____

_____

☐ **SITTING**

Scapulae

Ischial Tuberosities Backs of Knees Calcaneus

Comments: _____

_____

Form 202504 D: 02/10

Fig. 11.12 Altman Surgical/Procedural Positioning Communication Tool.

MDPRI incidence in the neonatal and pediatric settings is most often reported by specific device rather than setting (Bakhshi, Kushare, Banskota, Nelson, & Dormans, 2015; Boesch et al., 2012).

MDRPI Risk Factors

A critical risk factor for MDRPI is the sensory perception or the inability to communicate pressure-related discomfort (e.g., "my mask is too tight") as defined by the Braden Scale for pressure injury risk assessment (see Table 11.2). Patients unable to communicate pressure-related discomfort include patients that are agitated, under anesthesia, receiving analgesia, unconscious or partially conscious and/or have a central nervous system injury (brain or spinal cord), respiratory or vascular disease where there is poor oxygenation and perfusion, neurological damage (stroke or multiple sclerosis), or peripheral neural damage (diabetic neuropathy) (Gefen, 2022). Box 11.5 lists factors associated with medical device-related pressure injuries.

MDRPI Differential Diagnosis

Device-related pressure injuries found inside the mouth (i.e., an endotracheal tube) or other areas lined with mucosa (Plate 35B, C) instead of skin are not staged; instead, they are called *mucosal pressure injuries* (EPUAP, NPIAP, & PPPIA, 2019; National Pressure Ulcer Advisory Panel [NPUAP], 2009). Because many devices are near anatomic locations without fatty tissue (e.g., nares, behind ears, occiput, bridge of nose), rapid deterioration to Stage 3 or 4, DTI, or unstageable pressure injuries is often seen.

It is important to distinguish DTPI from medical adhesive-related skin injury (MARSI) and moisture-associated skin damage (MASD) (Gefen et al., 2022), friction injury, and viral lesions especially around fecal containment devices and mouth. As with all lesions, a mixed etiology is possible. Key features of medical device-related pressure injuries being located under or near a medical device, not associated with a bony prominence, and often present in the shape of the device as shown in Plate 35A, B, and E.

MDRPI Prevention

MDRPI prevention includes improved design of devices; pressure relief through application of an alternative device; adequately designed prophylactic dressings or gel pads, strips or tubing (Gefen et al., 2022). Frequent assessment around and under medical devices assessment (e.g., twice daily) is necessary; more frequently in the presence of or at risk of edema (EPUAP, NPIAP, & PPPIA, 2019) such as with postoperative tracheostomy or endotracheal tubes while proning. Important parameters for assessing the skin under and around medical devices include color, moisture, dryness, temperature, texture, edema, turgor. Communication and collaboration with disciplines with expertise with the specific device (e.g., Respiratory therapist, orthotics specialist) is critical to effective and safe MDRPI prevention. Failure to follow manufacturer's application and instructions can result in harm

(e.g., skin damage) and can be a source of liability (EPUAP, NPIAP, & PPPIA, 2019). MDRPI preventive interventions for all medical devices and specific medical devices are found in Table 11.5. Samples of gap analysis for respiratory devices and cervical collars are found in Appendix A.

Provide Patient and Family Education

Tools for measuring patients' knowledge related to pressure injury prevention include the Patient Participation in Pressure Injury Prevention (PPPIP) tested with hospitalized adults (Ringdal, Chaboyer, Ulin, Bucknall, & Oxelmark, 2017) and Skin Management Needs Assessment Checklist (SMnac) tested with patient they have spinal cord injuries (Gélis et al., 2011). The results of patient education programs for pressure injury prevention are mixed (Carlson et al., 2019; Guihan et al., 2014; Kim & Cho, 2017; Mercier, Ni, Houlihan, & Jette, 2015) and may be dependent on factors such as delivery methods, patient characteristics, program content, follow up and outcome measurement methods (EPUAP, NPIAP, & PPPIA, 2019).

Both the WOCN® Society position statement and the CMS definition for unavoidable pressure injuries emphasize the importance of preventive interventions that are consistent with the patient's needs and goals: caregivers must respect *informed* choices of individuals who decline interventions (Schmitt et al., 2017; WOCN, 2017). For example, a patient facing the end of life may decline an intervention such as tube feeding to optimize nutrition. In this case, if a pressure injury develops, documentation of patient education and response could be sufficient to demonstrate *informed* refusal of care and thereby the pressure injury deemed to be unavoidable.

International guidelines for pressure injury prevention recommends assessing the health-related quality of life, knowledge, and self-care skill of individuals with or at risk for pressure injuries to facilitate the development of a pressure injury care plan and educational care plan (EPUAP, NPIAP, & PPPIA, 2019). Chapter 5; Patient Engagement Principles and Challenges, is dedicated to these topics within the framework of a health belief model. Chapter 5 includes but is not limited to Joint Commission standards for patient education, health literacy, barriers to learning, confirming patient learning and important factors to consider for documentation of *informed* declination of care. Sample patient education tools are available on the NPIAP website and in the AHRQ pressure injury prevention tool kit.

PIPP INFRASTRUCTURE AND ORGANIZATIONAL RESPONSIBILITIES

Creating the best-practice bundle for pressure injury prevention is only the first step of a PIPP. As mentioned, for a PIPP to be successful, the bundle must be integrated into the culture and infrastructure of the health care system. However, many hurdles have been identified that threaten the implementation and utilization of a PIPP. Even when a PIPP is implemented,

TABLE 11.5 Prevention of Medical Device–Related Pressure Injuries

Device	Preventive Interventions
All	Consider ALL individuals with medical devices to be at risk for pressure injuries Select medical devices that induce the least amount of skin damage Ensure correct size and fit to avoid excessive pressure Apply according to manufacturer's specifications[a] Ensure that medical devices are sufficiently secured to prevent dislodgement Inspect the skin and tension under and around medical devices at least twice daily and more frequently in the presence of fluid shifts and/or signs of localized/generalized edema Rotate or reposition medical devices when possible Avoid positioning the individual directly onto medical devices Reposition the individual and/or the medical device to redistribute pressure and decrease shear forces Remove as soon as medically feasible Keep skin under devices clean and dry If appropriate, use a prophylactic dressing (see Box 11.7), ensure the functionality of the medical device is not compromised by the dressing
Nasogastric tube	Consider commercial stabilizers to facilitate easier repositioning and inspection than possible with tape Proper application of stabilizers to keep clamp from touching skin Use liquid skin protectant and commercial feeding tube stabilizer to prevent accidental dislodgment Change stabilizer every other day; sooner if loose or leaking Document skin condition with site care
Noninvasive positive pressure ventilation (NIPPV) and bi-level positive airway pressure (BiPAP)	Consult with respiratory therapist for proper sizing and fitting Refitting may be indicated as edema changes Consider alternative masks such as full-face masks or masks with gel borders for select patients Apply minimal tension to mask strap required to create adequate seal Add skin checks under respiratory equipment to the workflow of the respiratory therapist
Nasal oxygen	Use commercially available nasal cannula with soft tubing High flow-use commercially available foam ear protectors that are preattached or can be attached to tubing Apply prophylactic dressing or liquid skin protectant to ears
Endotracheal tube and securement device	Combine endotracheal tube site care and inspection with oral care Reposition tube laterally to different locations in mouth while ensuring depth of tube is unchanged Consider commercial stabilizers instead of tape to facilitate easier repositioning and inspection Ensure proper application of stabilizers to keep clamp from touching mouth
Removable splint/protector/brace	Consult physical therapist/occupational therapist for proper selection, sizing, fitting Keep manufacturer's application instructions accessible Keep schedule accessible; if not available, ask for one Document device removal at least twice daily for skin inspection to documentation
Cervical collar	Consult with orthotics for proper sizing and fitting Palpate for skin changes within hairline Use soft collars as soon as medically indicated to lower levels of mandibular and occipital pressure
Tracheostomy flange and straps	Inspect under and around securement devices at least twice daily Apply prophylactic dressing to back of neck Use commercially available foam/collar-type adjustable straps instead of ties or twill tape for comfort, pressure redistribution, and easy adjustment and to prevent inadvertent extubating

[a]Note: Failure to follow the manufacturer's application instruction can result in harm (e.g., skin damage) to the individual and can be a source of liability.

time has shown that a PIPP is difficult to sustain. Because pressure injuries are a complex, multifactorial problem, a holistic view of the hospital system and a change in culture are required to reduce incidence. Barriers to implementation include staffing issues including skill mix, knowledge and attitudes of workforce, and access to resources including: (e.g., user friendly, decision-making tools, supplies) (EPUAP, NPIAP, & PPPIA, 2019; Kaba et al., 2017; Patrician et al., 2017; Tallier et al., 2017; Twigg, Gelder, & Myers, 2015; Twigg, Kutzer, Jacob, & Seaman, 2019). All caregivers and administrators must share the belief that skin safety is priority and all health care providers play a role in protecting the patient from pressure injuries. Implementation of a vital and enduring PIPP requires participation and oversight by management and critical scrutiny of the system's operations. The PIPP must become integrated into the day-to-day operations at the unit and systems level so that it is embedded into the infrastructure of education, documentation, decision making, and communication and handoffs. International guidelines provide evidence for many organizational-level recommendations (EPUAP, NPIAP, & PPPIA, 2019). Table 11.6 provides a summarized list of those recommendations, with implementation examples. Appendix A contains examples of polices, algorithms, gap analysis, and other tools designed to assist with the process.

Patient Handoffs

A hand-off (also known as handover) is a transfer and acceptance of patient care responsibility achieved through effective communication. It is a real-time process of passing patient-specific information from one caregiver to another or from one team of caregivers to another for the purpose of ensuring the continuity and safety of the patient's care (The Joint Commission, 2014).

It is estimated that a typical teaching hospital experiences more than 4000 hand-offs every day (Vidyarthi, 2006). Yet inadequate handoffs (e.g., not structured and focused to ensure continuity of care) result in part for 30% of malpractice claims, 1744 deaths and $1.7 billion in malpractice cost over 5 years. Contributing factors to hand-off communication breakdowns include insufficient information, absence of safety culture, ineffective communication methods, lack of time, poor timing between sender and receiver, interruptions or distractions, lack of standardized procedures, and insufficient staffing. A study by the Accreditation Council for Graduate Medical Education (ACGME) found that 69% of clinical learning environments did not have a standardized hand-off process, and only 20% had partial standardization (The Joint Commission, 2017).

The Joint Commission's care standards require a process for hand-off communication that provides opportunity for discussion between the giver and receiver of the handoff.

TABLE 11.6   Pressure Injury Prevention Program (PIPP)

Organizational and Operational Responsibilities

Responsibility	Implementation Tips and Examples
Assess/maximize workforce for PIPP	Ensure sufficient: • Clinical staff/patient ratio for patients at risk and safe patient handling for positioning • Clinical staff with competency-based PIP education • Support staff to facilitate clinical staff to work for PIP • Staffing for PIP education, unit-based initiatives, and quality tracking
Assess/maximize staff knowledge and improve staff attitudes about PIP	• Use knowledge and attitude assessment tools with good psychometric properties (Box 11.10) • Use assessment results to plan targeted education initiatives
Develop/implement a multifaceted staff education program for PIP	• Didactic education, competency-based education, bedside/hands on teaching, peer-to-peer teaching, e-learning • Mandated, attendance in employee record, continuing education credits
Assess/maximize equipment availability, quality, and standards for use (e.g., support surface, medical devices)	Ensure policies, protocols, procedures have a process in place to: • Stock medical devices that induce the least amount of skin damage while achieving the intended function • Include wound/skin specialist input for new product purchases that will interface with skin • Identify the fastest procurement of pip products including during nights, weekends, and holidays • Enforce manufacturer's instructions for indications, use, maintenance, and replacement of equipment
Engage all key stakeholders in oversight of PIPP	• See Chapter 1 for examples of key stakeholders • Strong leadership (director, administrator) engagement and support essential for success • Emphasize patient engagement (Chapter 5) • Promote interprofessional evidence-based team decision making

Continued

TABLE 11.6 Pressure Injury Prevention Program (PIPP)—cont'd

Organizational and Operational Responsibilities

Responsibility	Implementation Tips and Examples
Provide evidence-based policies, procedures, for PIPP	Include/describe responsibilities for all relevant disciplines and departments: • Support surface criteria, procurement, use, maintenance (Chapter 12) • Skin assessment (Chapter 10) and pressure injury risk assessment • Risk based preventive interventions (Table 11.3) • MDRPI prevention (Table 11.5, Box 11.5) • Proning and PIP • Patient refusal or declination of care (Chapter 5, Fig. 5.2), including reeducation, troubleshooting, and mitigation of risk strategies
Facilitate standard documentation systems for PIPP	Include access for all relevant disciplines • Skin and risk assessment (baseline, reassessments) • Offloading methods (e.g., bed, heels, chair) • Positioning and HOB elevation (time, position) • Incontinence care • MDRPI inspection and preventive intervention • Patient/family education • PIP care plan and patient response • Patient refusal or declination of care reeducation, troubleshooting, mitigation of risk strategies (Chapter 5, Fig. 5.2) and provider notification • Nutrition supplements • Tube site care
Provide clinical decision support tools and protocols for PIP	• Support surface algorithms for bed, chair, heel (Chapter 12) • Patient refusal or declination of care, reeducation, troubleshooting, mitigation of risk strategies, and provider notification (Chapter 5, Fig. 5.2) • MDRPI bundle • Repositioning clock reminders (Fig. 11.8) • Incontinence care product selection (Chapter 9) • Protocols and order sets instead of provider order for interventions within the domain of nonprovider clinical staff • Proning kit or checklist • Electronic medical record enhancements/reminders/prompts • Invest in technology (e.g., pressure mapping, subepidermal moisture scanner)
Provide clinical leadership in PIP	Include all relevant disciplines, units and departments (e.g., respiratory therapy, EEG, radiology, Perioperative, Emergency and ancillary settings): • Managers and assistant managers • PIP champions (facility, unit, department) • Clinical Nurse Specialists and Educators • Certified wound specialists
Regularly monitor, analyze, evaluate performance against quality indicators for PIP	• Collect and analyze (at least) ongoing incidence density data and periodic point prevalence/incidence data • Use point prevalence/incidence data to help assess reliability of incidence density data • Competency-based education for prevalence/incidence data collection • See Chapter 6 for measures, methodology, and rationale
Use feedback and reminder systems to promote PIP quality improvement program and outcomes to stakeholders	Facilitate transparent communication about quality improvement projects and outcomes with use of: • Brochures, flyers, posters • Recognition from directors and administrators • Awards, prizes

Data compiled from International Clinical Practice Guidelines European Pressure Ulcer Advisory Panel, National Pressure Injury Advisory Panel, & Pan Pacific Pressure Injury Alliance. (EPUAP, NPIAP, & PPPIA). (2019). In E. Haesler (Ed.). *Prevention and treatment of pressure ulcers/injuries.* Osborne Park: Cambridge Media.

Health care organizations must define, communicate to staff, and implement a process in which information about patient care is communicated in a consistent manner (The Joint Commission, 2017). Therefore, any handoff communication should include relevant information about the patient's risk of developing a pressure injury, locations and status of any existing pressure injuries, related interventions, and patient response. This information needed to be shared through discussion in handoffs during shift reports, interdisciplinary rounds, and transfers to other units and care settings.

Handoffs from the patient care unit to procedural settings (e.g., radiology department, OR) also necessitate communications concerning the patient's skin status and pressure injury risk. In particular, the staff of the receiving department should be made aware of the location of existing pressure injury, any positions that should be avoided, and the need for offloading (especially heels and sacrum). Appendix A provides an example of an interdepartmental handoff communication tool.

Formularies and Decision-Making Tools

A significant and valuable contribution the wound specialist can bring to any facility and any PIPP is to standardize and organize products available within his or her health care system. To bring order to the utilization of these products and enhance the quality of care provided, decision-making tools are used to facilitate the accuracy and efficiency of decision making, guide treatment selection, and educate the clinician concerning a particular disease entity. Annual review of these tools is recommended because changes in the pathophysiology of pressure injuries and product research and development are ongoing and quickly paced. Decision-making tools must use language that is consistent with policies, procedures, documentation, supply order menus, and current contracts for products. If any of these factors change, revisions are necessary to keep the tools accurate and user friendly. Examples of decision-making tools include interventions based on risk factors (see Table 11.3), support surface selection (see Chapter 12, Table 12.3), and skin care products (Table 9.4 and throughout this textbook).

Investing in Technology

Access to, and utilization of, appropriate technology involves not only patient care items (e.g., support surfaces or devices) but also medical record documentation so that information is always complete and readily available. In creating the documentation system, skin care, risk assessment, nutritional assessment, and the other critical elements of a best-practice bundle must be incorporated, which requires direct input of the certified wound specialist. As technological advances in existing PIPP tools, such as support surfaces, transferring devices, and heel offloading devices, occur, the advantages of these products should be methodically reviewed by the wound specialist and presented to the PIPP team members for discussion. Similarly, the team should have a mechanism for keeping abreast of new developments in technology that may improve efficiency and reliability of interventions and the PIPP and ultimately reduce the patient's risk of pressure injuries.

Staff Education and Competencies

All health care personnel providing care to the patient must appreciate the role they have in pressure injury prevention. In addition, it should not be assumed that the formal curriculum of the registered nurse, nurse practitioner, physician, physician assistant, physical therapist, and occupational therapist adequately incorporated pressure injury prevention and management (Barakat-Johnson, Barnett, Wand, & White, 2018; Demarr'e et al., 2011; Ebi, Hirko, & Mijena, 2019; Gunningberg et al., 2015; Simonetti, Comparcini, Flacco, Di Giovanni, & Cicolini, 2015; Usher et al., 2018). To keep the PIPP infrastructure strong, pressure injury education (including how to document) should be included in new employee orientation and annual competencies for nurses and nursing assistants. The content of the education is based on the scope of practice for the position. For example, the registered nurse should minimally demonstrate competency related to pressure injury etiology, skin inspection, risk assessment, wound assessment, and implementation of a full range of appropriate interventions to minimize or eliminate risk factors (EPUAP, NPIAP, & PPPIA, 2019). Nursing assistants may require education and competency related to monitoring the skin, reporting changes to the nurse, continence skin care, importance of nutrition, and appropriate positioning. To keep pace with the rapid changes in the science of pressure injury prevention and treatment, the health professional's knowledge and skills require routine and frequent updating through annual programs, at a minimum. Appendix A contains examples of wound and skin care competencies.

Staff Accountability/Ownership

Corporate culture must convey that facility-acquired pressure injuries are no longer tolerable or "acceptable" unless documentation indicates the pressure injury was unavoidable. Although it is important to encourage employees to "self-report," they still must be held accountable for any errors. Just as it is unhealthy to create a punitive environment where employees are fearful of admitting errors, so, too, is it unhealthy to create an environment of toleration of less than best practices, which can lead to errors and complications such as pressure injuries. Expectations for employees to meet this standard need to be communicated during orientation and annual education and through activities that encourage transparency and sharing of experiences (both successful and unsuccessful) and knowledge. Conducting good quality interdisciplinary, nonpunitive, and timely root-cause analysis (RCA) is critical for staff accountability, ownership, education, and problem solving. The NPIAP RCA template provides a systemic, structured, and evidenced-based method to collect data, identify potential gaps in care and drive action plans (available at NPIAP.org).

Quality Tracking and Evaluation

Once a program as extensive and system wide as the PIPP is implemented, feedback is needed that comes from routine measurements and quality tracking. Such feedback provides the affirmation participants need to reinforce the value of their efforts and investment in the program. Routine measurements and quality tracking will also identify areas for improvement.

Once a plan for reducing or eliminating pressure is developed and the plan is implemented, the effectiveness of the intervention (turning, support surface) should be evaluated at regular intervals. Daily skin inspection should provide the information needed to determine whether the PIPP is sufficient or requires modification. Generally, resolution of the intensity of erythema, if present, should become apparent within 24 h of placement upon a support surface. A patient's risk for pressure injury formation will vary as his or her overall condition changes; therefore, routine and regular reassessment and modification of the plan of care are warranted.

Quality tracking of the PIPP should include (1) facility-acquired pressure injuries, (2) process measures, and (3) outcome measures. Concurrent daily reporting of facility-acquired pressure injuries for all patients is perhaps a more important measure than are quarterly or annual incidence studies. A simple 24/7 mechanism for staff to report facility-acquired pressure injuries through quality tracking (e.g., event reports, incident reports) leads to more accurate reporting of facility-acquired pressure injuries, timelier RCA and action plans, and early identification of weakening infrastructure. For example, a rise in the number of pressure injuries secondary to oxygen masks may have resulted from a contract change to an inferior mask. Concurrent reporting of facility-acquired pressure injuries can uncover the problem quickly so that disciplines can unite, identify the root cause, and correct the problem quickly before more patients are injured. Conversely, a facility-wide incidence that is not reported daily cannot lead to problem resolution and pressure injury reduction as quickly. With an average length of stay in acute care of just a few days, countless patients are missed with such infrequent incident studies.

Process measures capture compliance with designated components of the PIPP, for example, pressure injury risk assessment within 8 h of admission, skin inspection upon admission, or daily risk assessments of "at-risk" patients. The value of process measures is heightened when correlated with concurrent self-reports. This will also be beneficial when targeting staff education.

The key outcome measure of a PIPP is the incidence of pressure injuries and can be tabulated to reflect unit-based incidence or system-wide incidence. Pressure injury incidence can be obtained quarterly or annually and compared with concurrent daily self-reporting data to essentially validate the accuracy of self-reported pressure injuries. However, these kinds of incidence calculations cannot be considered reliable data collection for mandated public reporting. Pressure injury incidence can be calculated and reported in many ways, which contributes to the confusion and the wide range of data when comparisons to other facilities are attempted. To be most relevant, incidence should be reported as pressure injuries per 1000 patient-days (IHI, 2008). Chapter 6 provides important information for understanding and implementing appropriate (and regulatory) quality tracking across the continuum of care.

CLINICAL CONSULT

A: Received referral for management of a DTPI on the left foot of 46-year-old Caucasian gentleman with type 2 diabetes, chronic kidney disease, and peripheral arterial disease admitted for congestive heart failure. Electronic medical record contains a photo of a dark-purple, intact lesion. Unable to discern exact location of lesion on foot by photo. Nurses consulted the dietician, placed patient on a low air loss support surface, and documented consistent repositioning and floating his heels off the bed with use of pillows under the legs. Patient denies pain in the foot or awareness of the lesions. He is up at pleasure and walking out of the bathroom. Visibly short of breath on 2 L of O_2 per nasal cannula; pulse oximetry 92%. Wound assessment reveals a generalized reticulate purple discoloration encompassing 4 × 4 cm on the lateral dorsal surface of the left foot. Epidermis is intact and nonblanchable. Periwound skin is intact, has no edema, and no local signs of infection. Lower extremities pulses palpable but diminished.
D: Overall assessment is not consistent with a pressure injury. Risk factors, patient history, distribution of lesion, and the appearance of the extremity are consistent with an arterial pathology.
P: Protect left foot from pressure and trauma to prevent break in skin integrity. Assess perfusion and circulation of lower extremity.
I: Nurse and patient understand and agree with the following plan of care: (1) Collaborate with primary care provider for further evaluation of vascular status. (2) Offloading: replace low air loss with standard pressure injury prevention static mattress to improve patient comfort and facilitate mobility and safety. Continue repositioning and floating heels while in bed. (3) Use appropriate footwear when up to protect from trauma. (4) Apply moisturizers daily to prevent skin dryness and maintain skin integrity. Topical dressing not indicted at this time. (5) Monitor lower extremities and lesion; notify provider for increased discoloration and size, pain, or change in temperature of extremity.
E: Will follow up to evaluate/monitor effectiveness and adapt plan as needed.

SUMMARY

- Pressure injuries present a significant economic, quality-of-life, and overall health care threat worldwide.
- Pressure injuries are a global health concern because, for the most part, they are a costly *preventable* complication.
- Once a problem considered a side effect of aging, pressure injuries have captured the attention of payers and regulators.

- Although not all pressure injuries are avoidable, pressure injuries now are more commonly considered preventable and unacceptable (in most cases) and are considered an indicator of quality care.
- As a consequence of unrelieved pressure, capillaries are occluded and tissue damage ensues, and the extent of tissue damage is influenced by numerous variables.

- Standards for assessment and care initially presented by the WOCN® Society have now been published by a number of dedicated disciplines and groups around the world.
- Pressure injury prevention requires a comprehensive interdisciplinary plan that includes risk assessment; regular and routine skin assessment; reducing risk factors; patient, family, and staff education; and evaluation.
- Ongoing maintenance of program infrastructure is critical to sustain a low incidence of pressure injuries. This is accomplished through (1) embedding education into patient education tools, staff orientation, and annual competencies; (2) ensuring thorough and user-friendly documentation methods and decision-making tools; (3) concurrent and reliable quality tracking; and (4) a team approach with safe handoffs and communication across settings.

SELF-ASSESSMENT QUESTIONS

1. Which of the following are major factors that contribute to pressure ulcer development?
   a. Shear, smoking, and friction
   b. Age, smoking, and blood pressure
   c. Nutrition and stress
   d. Shear, friction, and nutritional debilitation
2. Which of the following statements about blanching erythema is *false*?
   a. It resolves once pressure is removed.
   b. It indicates deep tissue damage.
   c. It is an area of erythema that turns white when compressed.
   d. It implies that pressure is not adequately relieved or reduced.
3. The undermining that is commonly observed with pressure ulcers may be the result of which of the following?
   a. Shear
   b. Friction
   c. Maceration
   d. Advanced age
4. Nonblanchable erythema of intact skin describes which classification of pressure ulcer?
   a. Deep tissue pressure injury
   b. Stage 1
   c. Stage 2
   d. Stage 3
5. Exposed tendon describes which classification of pressure ulcer?
   a. Stage 3
   b. Stage 4
   c. Unstageable
   d. Partial thickness
6. A brown, dry wound base on the right trochanter describes which classification of pressure ulcer?
   a. Deep tissue pressure injury
   b. Stage 3
   c. Stage 4
   d. Unstageable
7. A blood-filled blister on the heel describes which classification of pressure ulcer?
   a. Deep tissue pressure injury
   b. Stage 1
   c. Stage 2
   d. Unstageable
8. Intact, nonblanchable, persistent purple discoloration over the coccyx describes which classification of pressure ulcer?
   a. Deep tissue pressure injury
   b. Stage 1
   c. Unstageable
   d. None of the above
9. An intact, serous-filled blister on the heel describes which classification of pressure ulcer?
   a. Deep tissue pressure injury
   b. Stage 1
   c. Stage 2
   d. Stage 3
10. Keeping the head of the bed less than 30 degrees addresses which pressure ulcer risk factor?
    a. Impaired mobility
    b. Friction/shear
    c. Moisture
    d. Nutrition
11. Repositioning the patient every 2 h helps to address which pressure ulcer risk factor?
    a. Impaired mobility
    b. Nutrition
    c. Altered sensory perception
    d. Both a and c

REFERENCES

Agency for Healthcare Research and Quality (AHRQ). (2011). *Preventing pressure ulcers in hospitals: A toolkit for improving quality of care*. Rockville: AHRQ. Retrieved 4/15/2022 from: https://www.ahrq.gov/sites/default/files/publications/files/putoolkit.pdf.

Agency for Healthcare Research and Quality (AHRQ). (2017). *Estimating the additional hospital inpatient cost and mortality associated with selected hospital-acquired conditions. Results. Rockville*. Retrieved 4/1/2022: https://www.ahrq.gov/hai/pfp/haccost2017.html.

Ahn, C., Mulligan, P., & Salcido, R. S. (2008). Smoking—The bane of wound healing: Biomedical interventions and social influences. *Advances in Skin & Wound Care, 21*(5), 227–236.

Alderden, J., Pepper, G. A., Wilson, A., Whitney, J. D., Richardson, S., Butcher, R., et al. (2018). Predicting pressure injury in critical care patients: A machine-learning model. *American Journal of Critical Care, 27*(6), 461–468. https://doi.org/10.4037/ajcc2018525. PMID: 30385537; PMCID: PMC6247790.

Alderden, J., Rondinelli, J., Pepper, G., Cummins, M., & Whitney, J. (2017). Risk factors for pressure injuries among critical care patients: A systematic review. *International Journal of Nursing Studies, 71*, 97–114. https://doi.org/10.1016/j.ijnurstu.2017.03.012. Epub 2017 Mar 28. PMID: 28384533; PMCID: PMC5485873.

Alterescu, V. (1991). Reflections upon the history and future of the IAET. *Journal of ET Nursing, 18*(4), 126–131. https://doi.org/10.1097/00152192-199107000-00015.

American Thoracic Society & Infectious Diseases Society of America. (2005). Guidelines for the management of adults with hospital-acquired, ventilator-associated, and healthcare-associated pneumonia. *American Journal of Respiratory and Critical Care Medicine, 171*(4), 388–416. PMID: 21481251.

Angmorterh, S. K., England, A., Webb, J., Szczepura, K., Stephens, M., Anaman-Torgbor, J., et al. (2019). An investigation of pressure ulcer risk, comfort, and pain in medical imaging. *Journal of Medical Imaging and Radiation Sciences, 50*(1), 43–52. https://doi.org/10.1016/j.jmir.2018.07.003. Epub 2018 Aug 9. PMID: 30777247.

Anthony, D., Papanikolaou, P., Parboteeah, S., & Saleh, M. (2010). Do risk assessment scales for pressure ulcers work? *Journal of Tissue Viability, 19*(4), 132–136. https://doi.org/10.1016/j.jtv.2009.11.006.

Antokal, S., Brienza, D., Bryan, N., et al. (2012). *Friction induced skin injuries—Are they pressure ulcers?*. National Pressure Ulcer Advisory Panel white paper. Retrieved 4/16/2022 from: https://cdn.ymaws.com/npiap.com/resource/resmgr/white_papers/1c._npuap-friction-white-pap.pdf.

Arnold-Long, M., Ayer, M., & Borchert, K. (2017). Medical device-related pressure injuries in long-term acute care hospital setting. *Journal of Wound, Ostomy, and Continence Nursing, 44*(4), 325–330. https://doi.org/10.1097/WON.0000000000000347. PMID: 28682854.

Aronovitch, S. A. (2007). Intraoperatively acquired pressure ulcers: Are there common risk factors? *Ostomy Wound Manage, 53*(2), 57–69.

Association of periOperative Registered Nurses (AORN). (2013). Guidance statement: Safe patient handling and movement in the perioperative setting. In *Perioperative Standards and Recommended Practices* (pp. 553–572). Denver: AORN, Inc.

Association of periOperative Registered Nurses (AORN). (2022). Guideline for prevention of perioperative pressure injury. In *Guidelines for Perioperative Practice*. Denver.

Bååth, C., Engström, M., Gunningberg, L., & Muntlin, A.Å. (2016). Prevention of heel pressure ulcers among older patients—From ambulance care to hospital discharge: A multi-centre randomized controlled trial. *Applied Nursing Research, 30*, 170–175.

Bakhshi, H., Kushare, I., Banskota, B., Nelson, C., & Dormans, J. P. (2015). Pinless halo in the pediatric population: Indications and complications. *Journal of Pediatric Orthopaedics, 35*(4), 374–378.

Bales, I., & Duvendack, T. (2011). Reaching for the moon: Achieving zero pressure ulcer prevalence. An update. *Journal of Wound Care, 20*(8). https://doi.org/10.12968/jowc.2011.20.8.374. 374, 376–377. PMID: 21841712.

Banks, M., Bauer, J., Graves, N., et al. (2010). Malnutrition and pressure ulcer risk in adults in Australian health care facilities. *Nutrition, 26*(9), 896–901.

Barakat-Johnson, M., Barnett, C., Wand, T., & White, K. (2017). Medical device-related pressure injuries: An exploratory descriptive study in an acute tertiary hospital in Australia. *Journal of Tissue Viability, 26*(4), 246–253. https://doi.org/10.1016/j.jtv.2017.09.008. Epub 2017 Oct 4. PMID: 29050901.

Barakat-Johnson, M., Barnett, C., Wand, T., & White, K. (2018). Knowledge and attitudes of nurses toward pressure injury prevention: A cross-sectional multisite study. *Journal of Wound, Ostomy, and Continence Nursing, 45*(3), 233–237.

Barr, J., Fraser, G. L., Puntillo, K., et al. (2013). American College of Critical Care Medicine. Clinical practice guidelines for the management of pain, agitation, and delirium in adult patients in the intensive care unit. *Critical Care Medicine, 41*, 263–306.

Bates-Jensen, B. M., Anber, K., Chen, M. M., Collins, S., Esparza, A. N., Gieschen, K., Haglund, E., Lim, J. Y., Lin, C., Taw, E. J., Rodriguez, S., Truong, M., Tubillo, P., Xiao, A., & McCreath, H. E. (2021). Natural history of pressure injury among ethnically/racially diverse nursing home residents: The Pressure Ulcer Detection Study. *Journal of Gerontological Nursing, 47*(3), 37–46. https://doi.org/10.3928/00989134-20210210-03. PMID: 33626163.

Bates-Jensen, B. M., McCreath, H. E., & Pongquan, V. (2009). Subepidermal moisture is associated with early pressure ulcer damage in nursing home residents with dark skin tones: pilot findings. *Journal of Wound, Ostomy, and Continence Nursing, 36*(3), 277–284. https://doi.org/10.1097/WON.0b013e3181a19e53.

Beeckman, D., Clays, E., Van Hecke, A., Vanderwee, K., Schoonhoven, L., & Verhaeghe, S. (2013). A multi-faceted tailored strategy to implement an electronic clinical decision support system for pressure ulcer prevention in nursing homes: A two-armed randomized controlled trial. *International Journal of Nuring Studies, 50*(4), 475–486.

Beeckman, D., Fourie, A., Raepsaet, C., et al. (2021). Silicone adhesive multilayer foam dressings as adjuvant prophylactic therapy to prevent hospital-acquired pressure ulcers: A pragmatic noncommercial multicentre randomized open-label parallel-group medical device trial. *British Journal of Dermatology, 185*(1), 52–61.

Beeckman, D., Vanderwee, K., Demarré, L., Paquay, L., Van Hecke, A., & Defloor, T. (2010). Pressure ulcer prevention: Development and psychometric validation of a knowledge assessment instrument. *International Journal of Nursing Studies, 47*(4), 399–410.

Behrendt, R., Ghaznavi, A. M., Mahan, M., Craft, S., & Siddiqui, A. (2014). Continuous bedside pressure mapping and rates of hospital-associated pressure ulcers in a medical intensive care unit. *American Journal of Critical Care, 23*(2), 127–133. https://doi.org/10.4037/ajcc2014192. PMID: 24585161.

Bennett, L. M., Kavner, D., Lee, B. Y., et al. (1984). Skin stress and blood flow in sitting paraplegic patients. *Archives of Physical Medicine and Rehabilitation, 65*(4), 186–190.

Bergquist-Beringer, S., & Gajewski, B. J. (2011). Outcome and assessment information set data that predict pressure ulcer development in older adult home health patients. *Advances in Skin & Wound Care, 24*(9), 404–414.

Berlowitz, D. R., & Brienza, D. M. (2007). Are all pressure ulcers the result of deep tissue injury? A review of the literature. *Ostomy Wound Manage, 53*(10), 34–38.

Binda, F., Galazzi, A., Marelli, F., Gambazza, S., Villa, L., Vinci, E., et al. (2021). Complications of prone positioning in patients with COVID-19: A cross-sectional study. *Intensive and Critical Care Nursing, 67*, 103088.

Black, J., Baharestani, M., Black, S., et al. (2010). An overview of tissue types in pressure ulcers: A consensus panel recommendation. *Ostomy Wound Management, 56*(4), 28–44.

Black, J., Baharestani, M. M., Cuddigan, J., et al. (2007). National pressure ulcer advisory panel's updated pressure ulcer staging system. *Advances in Skin & Wound Care, 20*(5), 269–274.

Black, J., Cuddigan, J., Capasso, V., Cox, J., Delmore, B., Munoz, N., & Pittman, J. on behalf of the National Pressure Injury Advisory Panel. (2020). *Unavoidable Pressure Injury during COVID-19 Crisis: A Position Paper from the National Pressure Injury Advisory Panel.* Available at www.npiap.com.

Black, J. M., Edsberg, L. E., Baharestani, M. M., et al. (2011). Pressure ulcers: avoidable or unavoidable? Results of the National Pressure Ulcer Advisory Panel Consensus Conference (NPUAP). *Ostomy Wound Manage, 57*(2), 24–37.

Bliss, D. Z., Gurvich, O., Savik, K., Eberly, L. E., Harms, S., Mueller, C., et al. (2017). Racial and ethnic disparities in the healing of pressure ulcers present at nursing home admission. *Archives of Gerontology and Geriatrics, 72*, 187–194.

Boesch, R. P., Myers, C., Garrett, T., Nie, A., Thomas, N., Chima, A., et al. (2012). Prevention of tracheostomy-related pressure ulcers in children. *Pediatrics, 129*(3), e792–e797.

Bolton, L. L., Girolami, S., Corbett, L., et al. (2014). The Association for the Advancement of Wound Care (AAWC) venous and pressure ulcer guidelines. *Ostomy Wound Manage, 60*(11), 24–66.

Bosanquet, D. C. (2017). A review of the surgical management of heel pressure ulcers in the 21st century. *International Wound Journal, 13*(1), 9–16.

Braden, B. J., & Bergstrom, N. (1987). A conceptual schema for the study of the etiology of pressure sores. *Rehabilitation Nursing, 12*(1), 8–12.

Brem, H., Maggi, J., Nierman, D., et al. (2010). High cost of stage IV pressure ulcers. *American Journal of Surgery, 200*(4), 473–477.

Brienza, D., Gefen, A., Clark, M., & Black, J. (2022). The vision and scope of the prophylactic dressing standard initiative of the European Pressure Ulcer Advisory Panel and National Pressure Injury Advisory Panel. *International Wound Journal, 19*(5), 963–964. https://doi.org/10.1111/iwj.13859.

Brindle, C. T. (2013). Turning and repositioning the critically ill patient with hemodynamic instability: A literature review and consensus recommendations. *Journal of Wound, Ostomy, and Continence Nursing, 40*(3), 254–267.

Brophy, S., Moore, A., Patton, D., O'Connor, & Avsar, P. (2021). What is the incidence of medical device-related pressure injuries in adults within the acute hospital setting? A systematic review. *Journal of Tissue Viability, 30*, 489–498.

Bryant, R., Shannon, M. L., Pieper, B., et al. (1992). Pressure ulcer prevention and management. In R. Bryant (Ed.), *Acute and chronic wounds: Nursing management* (pp. 105–163). St. Louis: Mosby.

Burton, A. C., & Yamada, S. (1951). Relation between blood pressure and flow in the human forearm. *Journal of Applied Physiology, 4*(5), 329–339.

Cabrejo, R., Ndon, S., Saberski, E., Chuang, C., & Hsia, H. C. (2019). Significance of friction and shear in the prevention of contemporary hospital-acquired pressure ulcers. *Plastic and Reconstructive Surgery, 7*(4). https://doi.org/10.1097/GOX.0000000000002099. Global open, e2099.

Carlson, M., Vigen, C. L., Rubayi, S., Blanche, E. I., Blanchard, J., Atkins, M., et al. (2019). Lifestyle intervention for adults with spinal cord injury: Results of the USC–RLANRC Pressure Ulcer Prevention Study. *The Journal of Spinal Cord Medicine, 42*(1), 2–19.

Cereda, E., Neyens, J. C., Caccialanza, J., et al. (2017). Efficacy of a disease-specific nutritional support for pressure ulcer healing: A systematic review and meta-analysis. *The Journal of Nutrition, Health and Aging, 21*(6), 655–661. https://doi.org/10.1007/s12603-016-0822-y.

Chaboyer, W., Bucknall, T., Webster, J., McInnes, E., Gillespie, B. M., Banks, M., et al. (2016). The effect of a patient centred care bundle intervention on pressure ulcer incidence (INTACT): A cluster randomised trial. *International Journal of Nursing Studies, 64*, 63–71.

Chaboyer, W. P., et al. (2019). Incidence and prevalence of pressure injuries in adult intensive care patients: A systematic review and meta-analysis. *Critical Care Medicine, 46*, e1074–e1081.

Chen, H.-L., Cao, Y.-J., Wang, J., & Huai, B.-S. (2015). A retrospective analysis of pressure ulcer incidence and modified Braden Scale score risk classifications. *Ostomy Wound Management, 61*(9), 26–30.

Chen, H.-L., Cao, Y.-J., Zhang, W., Wang, J., & Huai, B.-S. (2015). Braden Scale is not suitable for assessing pressure ulcer risk in individuals aged 80 and older. *Journal of the American Geriatrics Society, 63*(3), 599–601. https://doi.org/10.1111/jgs.13303.

Clark, M., Black, J., Alves, P., et al. (2014). Systematic review of the use of prophylactic dressings in the prevention of pressure ulcers. *International Wound Journal, 11*(5), 460–471.

Coleman, S., Nixon, J., Keen, J., Wilson, L., McGinnis, E., Dealey, C., et al. (2014). A new pressure ulcer conceptual framework. *Journal of Advanced Nursing, 70*(10), 2222–2234. https://doi.org/10.1111/jan.12405.

Cowan, L. J., Stechmiller, J. K., Rowe, M., et al. (2012). Enhancing Braden pressure ulcer risk assessment in acutely ill adult veterans. *Wound Repair and Regeneration, 20*(2), 137–148.

Cox, J. (2013). Pressure ulcer development and vasopressor agents in adult critical care patients: A literature review. *Ostomy Wound Manage, 59*(4). 50–54, 56–60.

Cox, J., Roche, S., & Murphy, V. (2018). Pressure injury risk factors in critical care patients: A descriptive analysis. *Advances in Skin & Wound Care, 31*(7), 328–334.

Coyer, F., Cook, J. L., Doubrovsky, A., Vann, A., & McNamara, G. (2022). Exploring medical device-related pressure injuries in a single intensive care setting: A longitudinal point prevalence study. *Intensive & Critical Care Nursing, 68*, 103155. https://doi.org/10.1016/j.iccn.2021.103155. Epub 2021 Nov 1. PMID: 34736833.

Coyer, F., Miles, S., Gosley, S., Fulbrook, P., Sketcher-Baker, K., Cook, J. L., et al. (2017). Pressure injury prevalence in intensive care versus non-intensive care patients: A state-wide comparison. *Australian Critical Care, 30*(5), 244–250. https://doi.org/10.1016/j.aucc.2016.12.003. Epub 2017 Jan 4. PMID: 28063724.

Cramer, E. M., Seneviratne, M. G., Sharifi, H., Ozturk, A., & Hernandez-Boussard, T. (2019). Predicting the incidence of pressure ulcers in the intensive care unit using machine learning. *EGEMS (Washington, DC), 7*(1), 49. https://doi.org/10.5334/egems.307. PMID: 31534981; PMCID: PMC6729106.

Dalgleish, L., Campbell, J., Finlayson, K., & Coyer, F. (2020). Acute skin failure in the critically ill adult population: A systematic review. *Advances in Skin & Wound Care, 33*(2), 76–83.

Defloor, T. (1999). The risk of pressure sores: A conceptual scheme. *Journal of Clinical Nursing, 8,* 206–216.

Demarr'e, L., Vanderwee, K., Defloor, T., Verhaeghe, S., Schoonhoven, L., & Beeckman, D. (2011). Pressure ulcers: Knowledge and attitude of nurses and nursing assistants in Belgian nursing homes. *Journal of Clinical Nursing, 21,* 1425–1434.

Denby, A., & Rowlands, A. (2010). Stop them at the door: Should a pressure ulcer prevention protocol be implemented in the emergency department? *Journal of Wound, Ostomy, and Continence Nursing, 37*(1), 35–38. https://doi.org/10.1097/WON.0b013e3181c68b4b.

Dhandapani, M., Dhandapani, S., Agarwal, M., et al. (2014). Pressure ulcer in patients with severe traumatic brain injury: Significant factors and association with neurological outcome. *Journal of Clinical Nursing, 23*(7–8), 1114–1119.

Dorner, B., Posthauer, M. E., & Thomas, D. (2009). The role of nutrition in pressure ulcer prevention and treatment: National Pressure Ulcer Advisory Panel white paper. *Advances in Skin & Wound Care, 22*(5), 212–221.

Dugaret, E., Videau, M. N., Faure, I., Gabinski, C., Bourdel-Marchasson, I., & Salles, N. (2014). Prevalence and incidence rates of pressure ulcers in an emergency department. *International Wound Journal, 11*(4), 386–391. https://doi.org/10.1111/j.1742-481X.2012.01103.x. Epub 2012 Oct 8. PMID: 23043304; PMCID: PMC7950920.

Ebi, W. E., Hirko, G. F., & Mijena, D. A. (2019). Nurses' knowledge to pressure ulcer prevention in public hospitals in Wollega: A cross-sectional study design. *BMC Nursing, 18*(1), 1–12.

Ebrecht, M., Hextall, J., Kirtley, L. G., Taylor, A., Dyson, M., & Weinman, J. (2004). Perceived stress and cortisol levels predict speed of wound healing in healthy male adults. *Psychoneuroendocrinology, 29*(6), 798–809. https://doi.org/10.1016/S0306-4530(03)00144-6.

Edsberg, L. E. (2007). Pressure ulcer tissue histology: An appraisal of current knowledge. *Ostomy Wound Manage, 53*(10), 40–49.

Edsberg, L. E., Black, J. M., Goldberg, M., McNichol, L., Moore, L., & Sieggreen, M. (2016). Revised national pressure ulcer advisory panel pressure injury staging system: Revised pressure injury staging system. *Journal Wound, Ostomy, and Continence Nursing, 43*(6), 585–597.

Engel, H. J., Needham, D. M., Morris, P. E., et al. (2013). ICU early mobilization: From recommendation to implementation at three medical centers. *Critical Care Medicine, 20*(41), S69–S80.

European Pressure Ulcer Advisory Panel, National Pressure Injury Advisory Panel & Pan Pacific Pressure Injury Alliance. (EPUAP, NPIAP & PPPIA). (2019). In E. Haesler (Ed.), *Prevention and treatment of pressure ulcers/injuries.* Osborne Park: Cambridge Media.

Feng, Y., Zhou, M., & Tong, X. (2021). Imbalanced classification: A paradigm-based review. *Statistical Analysis and Data Mining: The ASA Data Science Journal, 14*(5), 383–406.

Flattau, A., & Blank, A. E. (2014). Risk factors for 90-day and 180-day mortality in hospitalized patients with pressure ulcers. *International Wound Journal, 11*(1), 14–20.

Florin, J., Bååth, C., Gunningberg, L., & Mårtensson, G. (2016). Attitudes towards pressure ulcer prevention: A psychometric evaluation of the Swedish version of the APuP instrument. *International Wound Journal, 13*(5), 655–662. https://doi.org/10.1111/iwj.12338. Epub 2014 Aug 14. PMID: 25124833; PMCID: PMC7950033.

Fore, J. (2006). A review of skin and the effects of aging on skin structure and function. *Ostomy Wound Manage, 52*(9), 24–35.

Fox, J., & Bradley, R. (1803). *A new medical dictionary.* London: Darton & Harvey.

Fulbrook, P., Mbuzi, V., & Miles, S. (2019). Effectiveness of prophylactic sacral protective dressings to prevent pressure injury: A systematic review and meta-analysis. *International Journal of Nursing Studies, 100,* 103400.

Gamston, J. (2019). Pressure induced skin and soft tissue injury in the emergency department. *Emergency Medicine Journal, 36*(10), 631–634. https://doi.org/10.1136/emermed-2018-207807.

García-Fernández, F. P., Pancorbo-Hidalgo, P. L., & Soldevilla Agreda, J. J. (2014). Predictive capacity of risk assessment scales and clinical judgment for pressure ulcers: A meta-analysis. *Journal of Wound, Ostomy, and Continence Nursing, 41*(1), 1–11.

Gefen, A. (2008a). Bioengineering models of deep tissue injury. *Advances in Skin & Wound Care, 21*(1), 30–36.

Gefen, A. (2008b). How much time does it take to get a pressure ulcer? Integrated evidence from human, animal, and in vitro studies. *Ostomy/Wound Manage, 54*(10). 26–28, 30–35.

Gefen, A. (2010). The biomechanics of heel ulcers. *Journal of Tissue Viability, 19*(4), 124–131.

Gefen, A. (2022). Alternatives and preferences for materials in use for pressure ulcer prevention: An experiment-reinforced literature review. *International Wound Journal,* 1–13. https://doi.org/10.1111/iwj.13784GEFEN13.

Gefen, A., Alves, P., Ciprandi, G., et al. (2022). Device-related pressure ulcers: SECURE prevention. Second Edition. *Journal of Wound Care, 31*(Suppl. 3), S1–S72.

Gefen, A., Brienza, D. M., Cuddigan, J., Haesler, E., & Kottner, J. (2021). Our contemporary understanding of the aetiolgy of pressure ulcers/pressure injuries. *International Wound Journal,* 1–13. https://doi.org/10.1111/iwj.13667.

Gefen, A., Creehan, S., & Black, J. (2020). Critical biomechanical and clinical insights concerning tissue protection when positioning patients in the operating room: A scoping review. *International Wound Journal, 17*(5), 1405–1423. https://doi.org/10.1111/iwj.13408.

Gélis, A., Daures, J. P., Benaim, C., Kennedy, P., Albert, T., Colin, D., et al. (2011). Evaluating self-reported pressure ulcer prevention measures in persons with spinal cord injury using the revised Skin Management Needs Assessment Checklist: Reliability study. *Spinal Cord, 49*(5), 653–658. https://doi.org/10.1038/sc.2010.177. Epub 2011 Jan 11. PMID: 21221117.

Gleeson, D. (2015). Pressure-ulcer reduction using low-friction fabric bootees. *British Journal of Nursing, 6,* S26–S29.

Goode, P. S. (1991). Pressure ulcer prevention and early treatment. *Journal of ET Nursing, 18*(5), 149–150.

Gouin, J. P., & Kiecolt-Glaser, J. K. (2011). The impact of psychological stress on wound healing: Methods and mechanisms. *Immunology and Allergy Clinics of North America, 31*(1), 81–93. https://doi.org/10.1016/j.iac.2010.09.010.

Gould, L., Stuntz, M., Giovannelli, M., Ahmad, A., Aslam, R., Mullen-Fortino, M., Whitney, J. D., Calhoun, J., Kirsner, R. S., Gordillo, G. M. (2016). Wound Healing Society 2015 update on guidelines for pressure ulcers. *Wound Repair & Regeneration, 24*(1), 145–162. https://doi.org/https://doi.org/10.1111/wrr.12396. Epub 2016 Mar 4. PMID: 26683529.

Guihan, M., Bombardier, C. H., Ehde, D. M., Rapacki, L. M., Rogers, T. J., Bates-Jensen, B., et al. (2014). Comparing multicomponent interventions to improve skin care behaviors and prevent recurrence in veterans hospitalized for severe pressure ulcers.

Archives of Physical Medicine and Rehabilitation, 95(7), 1246–1253.e3. https://doi.org/10.1016/j.apmr.2014.01.012. Epub 2014 Jan 30. PMID: 24486242.

Gunningberg, L., Mårtensson, G., Mamhidir, A.-G., Florin, J., Muntlin Athlin, Å., & Bååth, C. (2015). Pressure ulcer knowledge of registered nurses, assistant nurses and student nurses: A descriptive, comparative multicentre study in Sweden. *International Wound Journal, 12*(4), 462–468. https://doi.org/10.1111/iwj.12138.

Gunningberg, L., Sedin, I. M., Andersson, S., & Pingel, R. (2017). Pressure mapping to prevent pressure ulcers in a hospital setting: A pragmatic randomised controlled trial. *International Journal of Nursing Studies, 72*, 53–59.

Hahnel, E., Lichterfeld, A., Blume-Peytavi, U., & Kottner, J. (2017). The epidemiology of skin conditions in the aged: A systematic review. *Journal of Tissue Viability, 26*(1), 20–28.

Han, D., Kang, B., Kim, J., Jo, Y. H., Lee, J. H., Hwang, J. E., et al. (2019). Prolonged stay in the emergency department is an independent risk factor for hospital-acquired pressure ulcer. *International Wound Journal, 17*(2), 259–267. https://doi.org/10.1111/iwj.13266. Epub 2019 Nov 26. PMID: 31773872; PMCID: PMC7948751.

Harms, S., Bliss, D. Z., Garrand, J., et al. (2014). Prevalence of pressure ulcers by race and ethnicity for older adults admitted to nursing home. *Journal of Gerontological Nursing, 40*, 20–26. https://doi.org/10.3928/00989134-20131028-04.

Haugen, V., Pechacek, J., Maher, T., et al. (2011). Decreasing pressure ulcer risk during hospital procedures: A rapid process improvement workshop. *Journal of Wound, Ostomy, and Continence Nursing, 38*(2), 155–159.

Hayes, R. M., Spear, M. E., Lee, S. I., et al. (2015). Relationship between time in the operating room and incident of pressure ulcers: A matched case-control study. *American Journal of Medical Quality, 30*(6), 591–597.

Hill, R., & Petersen, A. (2020). Skin Failure Clinical Indicator Scale: Proposal of a tool for distinguishing skin failure from a pressure injury. *Wounds: A Compendium of Clinical Research and Practice, 32*(10), 272–278.

Hoh, D. J., Rahman, M., Fargen, K. M., Neal, D., & Hoh, B. L. (2016). Establishing standard hospital performance measures for cervical spinal trauma: A nationwide in-patient sample study. *Spinal Cord, 54*(4), 306–313.

Huang, C., Ma, Y., Wang, C., Jiang, M., Yuet Foon, L., Lv, L., et al. (2021). Predictive validity of the Braden Scale for pressure injury risk assessment in adults: A systematic review and meta-analysis. *Nursing Open, 8*(5), 2194–2207.

Husain, T. (1953). An experimental study of some pressure effects on tissues, with reference to the bedsore problem. *The Journal of Pathology and Bacteriology, 66*(2), 347–358.

Institute for Healthcare Improvement (IHI). (2008). *5 Million Lives Campaign. Getting started kit: Prevent pressure ulcers, Cambridge, MA*. Retrieved 4/16/2022 from: http://www.ihi.org/Engage/Initiatives/Completed/5MillionLivesCampaign/Pages/default.aspx.

Institute for Healthcare Improvement (IHI). (2022). *Pressure ulcers*. Retrieved 4/16/2022 from: http://www.ihi.org/Topics/PressureUlcers/Pages/default.aspx.

International Association for Enterostomal Therapy (IAET). (1987). *Standards of care. Dermal wounds: Pressure ulcers*. Santa Ana: IAET.

Jahani, S., Soleymani, Z. H., Asadizaker, M., Soltan, F., & Cheraghain, B. (2018). Determining the effects of prone position on oxygenation in patients with acute respiratory failure under

mechanical ventilation in ICU. *Journal of Medicine and Life, 1*(4), 274–280. https://doi.org/10.25122/jml-2018-0028.

Johnson, C., Giordano, N. A., Patel, L., Book, K. A., Mac, J., Viscomi, J., Em, A., Westrick, A., Koganti, M., Tanpiengco, M., Sylvester, K., & Mastro, K. A. (2022). Pressure injury outcomes of a prone-positioning protocol in patients with COVID and ARDS. *American Journal of Critical Care, 31*(1), 34–41. https://doi.org/10.4037/ajcc2022242.

Kaba, E., Kelesi, M., Stavropoulou, A., Moustakas, D., & Fasoi, G. (2017). How Greek nurses perceive and overcome the barriers in implementing treatment for pressure ulcers: "Against the odds". *Journal of Wound Care, 26*(Suppl. 9), S20–S26.

Kaewprag, P., Newton, C., Vermillion, B., Hyun, S., Huang, K., & Machiraju, R. (2017). Predictive models for pressure ulcers from intensive care unit electronic health records using Bayesian networks. *BMC Medical Informatics and Decision Making, 17* (Suppl. 2), 65. https://doi.org/10.1186/s12911-017-0471-z. PMID: 28699545.

Kalava, U. R., Cha, S. S., & Takahashi, P. Y. (2011). Association between vitamin D and pressure ulcers in older ambulatory adults: Results of a matched case-control study. *Clinical Interventions in Aging, 6*, 213–219.

Kayser, S. A., VanGilder, C. A., Ayello, E. A., & Lachenbruch, C. (2018). Prevalence and analysis of medical device-related pressure injuries: Results from the International Pressure Ulcer Prevalence Survey. *Advances in Skin & Wound Care, 31*(6), 276–285. https://doi.org/10.1097/01.ASW.0000532475.11971.aa.

Keast, D. H., Parslow, N., Houghton, P. E., et al. (2007). Best practice recommendations for the prevention and treatment of pressure ulcers: Update 2006. *Advances in Skin & Wound Care, 20*(8), 337–360.

Kielo, E., Suhonen, R., Ylönen, M., Viljamaa, J., Wahlroos, N., & Stolt, M. (2020). A systematic and psychometric review of tests measuring nurses' wound care knowledge. *International Wound Journal, 17*, 1209–1224. https://doi.org/10.1111/iwj.13417.

Kim, J. Y., & Cho, E. (2017). Evaluation of a self-efficacy enhancement program to prevent pressure ulcers in patients with a spinal cord injury. *Japan Journal of Nursing Science, 14*(1), 76–86.

Kimsey, D. B. (2019). A change in focus: Shifting from treatment to prevention of perioperative pressure injuries. *AORN Journal, 110* (4), 379–393.

Klompas, M., Branson, R., Eichenwald, E. C., et al. (2014). Strategies to prevent ventilator-associated pneumonia in acute care hospitals: 2014 update. *Infection Control and Hospital Epidemiology, 35*(8), 915–936. PMID: 25026607.

Kosiak, M. (1961). Etiology of decubitus ulcers. *Archives of Physical Medicine and Rehabilitation, 42*, 19–29.

Kosiak, M., Kubicek, W. G., Olson, M., et al. (1958). Evaluation of pressure as a factor in the production of ischial ulcers. *Archives of Physical Medicine and Rehabilitation, 39*(10), 623–629.

Kottner, J., Hauss, A., Schlüer, A. B., & Dassen, T. (2013). Validation and clinical impact of paediatric pressure ulcer risk assessment scales: A systematic review. *International Journal of Nursing Studies, 50*(6), 807–818.

Krouskop, T. A. (1983). A synthesis of the factors that contribute to pressure sore formation. *Medical Hypotheses, 11*(2), 255–267.

Kumar, V., Fausto, N., & Abbas, A. (2005a). Acute and chronic inflammation. In *Robbins and Cotran pathologic basis of disease* (7th ed.). Philadelphia: Saunders.

Kumar, V., Fausto, N., & Abbas, A. (2005b). Cellular adaptations, cell injury, and cell death. In *Robbins and Cotran pathologic basis of disease* (7th ed.). Philadelphia: Saunders.

Langer, G., Schloemer, G., Knerr, A., et al. (2003). Nutritional interventions for preventing and treating pressure ulcers. *The Cochrane Database of Systematic Reviews, 4*(4), CD003216.

Lechner, A., Lahmann, N., Neumann, K., Blume-Peytavi, U., & Kottner, J. (2017). Dry skin and pressure ulcer risk: A multi-center cross-sectional prevalence study in German hospitals and nursing homes. International Journal of Nursing Studies, 73, 63–69. https://doi.org/10.1016/j.ijnurstu.2017.05.011.

Levine, J. M. (2017). Unavoidable pressure injuries, terminal ulceration, and skin failure: In search of a unifying classification system. Advances in Skin & Wound Care, 30(5), 200–202.

Li, H. L., Lin, S. W., & Hwang, Y. T. (2019). Using nursing information and data mining to explore the factors that predict pressure injuries for patients at the end of life. *Computers, Informatics, Nursing, 37*(3), 133–141. https://doi.org/10.1097/CIN.0000000000000489. PMID: 30418245.

Lin, F., Wu, Z., Song, B., Coyer, F., & Chaboyer, W. (2020). The effectiveness of multicomponent pressure injury prevention programs in adult intensive care patients: A systematic review. *International Journal of Nursing Studies, 102*, 103483. https://doi.org/10.1016/j.ijnurstu.2019.103483. Epub 2019 Nov 21. PMID: 31835122.

Lindan, O. (1961). Etiology of decubitus ulcers: An experimental study. *Archives of Physical Medicine and Rehabilitation, 42*, 774–783.

Luccini, A., Mattiussi, S., Elli, E., et al. (2020). Prone position in acute respiratory distress syndrome patients: a retrospective analysis of complications. *Dimensions of Critical Care Nursing, 39*(1), 39–46. https://doi.org/10.1097/DCC.0000000000000393.

Lund, C. H., & Osborne, J. W. (2004). Validity and reliability of the neonatal skin condition score. *Journal of Obstetric, Gynecologic, & Neonatal Nursing, 33*(3), 320–327.

Lustig, M., Levy, A., Kopplin, K., Ovadia-Blechman, Z., & Gefen, A. (2018). Beware of the toilet: The risk for a deep tissue injury during toilet sitting. *Journal of Tissue Viability, 27*(1), 23–31.

Magnan, M. A., & Maklebust, J. (2008). The effect of web-based Braden Scale training on the reliability and precision of Braden Scale pressure ulcer risk assessments. *Journal of Wound, Ostomy, and Continence Nursing, 35*(2), 199–208.

Maida, V., Lau, F., Downing, M., & Yang, J. (2008). Correlation between Braden Scale and palliative performance scale in advanced illness. *International Wound Journal, 5*(4), 585–590.

Maklebust, J., & Magnan, M. A. (2009). A quasi-experimental study to assess the effect of technology-assisted training on correct endorsement of pressure ulcer preventive interventions. *Ostomy/Wound Management, 55*(2), 32–42.

Maklebust, J., Sieggreen, M. Y., Sidor, D., et al. (2005). Computer-based testing of the Braden Scale for predicting pressure sore risk. *Ostomy/Wound Management, 51*(4), 40–52.

Man, S. P., & Au-Yeung, T. W. (2013). Hypotension is a risk factor for new pressure ulcer occurrence in older patients after admission to an acute care hospital. *Journal of the American Medical Directors Association, 14*(8), 627.e1–5.

Manderlier, B., van Damme, N., Vanderwee, K., Verhaeghe, S., Van Hecke, A., & Beeckman, D. (2017). Development and psychometric validation of PUKAT 2·0, a knowledge assessment tool for pressure ulcer prevention. *International Wound Journal, 14*(6), 1041–1051.

Markova, A., & Mostow, E. N. (2012). US skin disease assessment: Ulcer and wound care. *Dermatologic Clinics, 30*(1), 107–111.

Mehta, C., Ali, M., Mehta, Y., George, J. V., & Singh, M. K. (2019). MDRPU-an uncommonly recognized common problem in ICU: A point prevalence study. *Journal of Tissue Viability, 28*(1), 35–39.

Mekić, S., Jacobs, L. C., Gunn, D. A., Mayes, A. E., Ikram, M. A., Pardo, L. M., et al. (2019). Prevalence and determinants for xerosis cutis in the middle-aged and elderly population: A cross-sectional study. *Journal of the American Academy of Dermatology, 81*(4), 963–969.

Mercier, H. W., Ni, P., Houlihan, B. V., & Jette, A. M. (2015). Differential impact and use of a telehealth intervention by persons with MS or SCI. *American Journal of Physical Medicine & Rehabilitation, 94*(11), 987–999. https://doi.org/10.1097/PHM.0000000000000291. PMID: 25888652.

Mervis, J. S., & Phillips, T. J. (2019). Pressure ulcers: Pathophysiology, epidemiology, risk factors, and presentation. *Journal of the American Academy of Dermatology, 81*(4), 881–890. https://doi.org/10.1016/j.jaad.2018.12.069.

Messer, M. (2010). PU risk in ancillary services. *Journal of Wound, Ostomy, and Continence Nursing, 37*(2), 153–158.

Messer, M. S. (2012). *Development of a Tool for Pressure Ulcer Risk Assessment and Preventive Interventions in Ancillary Services Patients*. Graduate Theses and Dissertations. Retrieved 4/16/2022 from: https://citeseerx.ist.psu.edu/viewdoc/download?doi=10.1.1.992.8302&rep=rep1&type=pdf.

Meyers, T. (2017). Prevention of heel pressure injuries and plantar flexion contractures with use of a heel protector in high-risk neurotrauma, medical, and surgical intensive care units. *Journal of Wound, Ostomy, and Continence Nursing*, 429–433. https://doi.org/10.1097/WON.0000000000000355. September/October 2017–Volume 44–Issue 5.

Miguel, K., Snydeman, C., Capasso, V., Walsh, M. A., Murphy, J., & Wang, X. S. (2021). Development of a prone team and exploration of staff perceptions during COVID-19. *AACN Advanced Critical Care, 32*(2), 159–168. https://doi.org/10.4037/aacnacc2021848. PMID: 33878151.

Mileski, M., & McClay, R. (2021). Natividad J. Facilitating factors in the proper identification of acute skin failure: A systematic review. *Critical Care Nurse, 41*(2), 36–42. https://doi.org/10.4037/ccn2021145. PMID: 33791763.

Minnesota Department of Health (MDH). (2019). Adverse health events in Minnesota. 15th Annual Public Report March 2019. Retrieved 1/28/2023 from: https://www.lrl.mn.gov/docs/2019/mandated/190370.pdf.

Moore, Z. E., & Cowman, S. (2014). Risk assessment tools for the prevention of pressure ulcers. *Cochrane Database of Systematic Reviews*, (2), CD006471. https://doi.org/10.1002/14651858.CD006471.pub3.

Mora-Arteaga, J. A., Bernal-Ramirez, O. J., & Rodriguez, S. J. (2015). The effects of prone position ventilation in patients with acute respiratory distress syndrome: A systematic review and meta-analysis. *Medicina Intensiva, 39*(6), 359–372. https://doi.org/10.1016/j.medin.2014.11.003.

Munshi, L., Del Sorbo, L., Adjikan, N. J., et al. (2017). Prone position for acute respiratory distress syndrome. *Annals of the American Thoracic Society, 14*(Suppl. 4), S280–S288. https://doi.org/10.1513/AnnalsATS.201704-343OT.

Muntlin Athlin, Å., Engström, M., Gunningberg, L., & Bååth, C. (2016). Heel pressure ulcer, prevention and predictors during the care delivery chain–when and where to take action? A descriptive and explorative study. *Scandinavian Journal of Trauma, Resuscitation and Emergency Medicine, 24*(1), 1–7.

Nas, K., Yazmalar, L., Şah, V., Aydın, A., & Öneş, K. (2015). Rehabilitation of spinal cord injuries. *World Journal of Orthopedics, 6*(1), 8–16. https://doi.org/10.5312/wjo.v6.i1.8.

National Pressure Injury Advisory Panel (NPIAP). (2020). *Pressure Injury Prevention Points*. Retrieved 4/11/2022 from: https://cdn.

ymaws.com/npiap.com/resource/resmgr/online_store/1a._pressure-injury-preventi.pdf.

National Pressure Ulcer Advisory Panel (NPUAP). (2009). *Mucosal pressure ulcers: An NPUAP position statement.* Retrieved 4/16/2022 from: https://cdn.ymaws.com/npuap.site-ym.com/resource/resmgr/position_statements/mucosal_pressure_ulcer_posit.pdf.

Noonan, C., Quigley, S., & Curley, M. A. (2011). Using the Braden Q Scale to predict pressure ulcer risk in pediatric patients. *Journal of Pediatric Nursing, 26*(6), 566–575. https://doi.org/10.1016/j.pedn.2010.07.006.

Ocampo, W., Cheung, A., Baylis, B., Clayden, N., Conly, J. M., Ghali, W. A., et al. (2017). Economic evaluations of strategies to prevent hospital-acquired pressure injuries. *Advances in Skin & Wound Care, 30*(7), 319–333.

Oozageer Gunowa, N., Hutchinson, M., Brooke, J., & Jackson, D. (2018). Pressure injuries in people with darker skin tones: A literature review. *Journal of Clinical Nursing, 27*(17-18), 3266–3275. https://doi.org/10.1111/jocn.14062.

Padula, W. V., & Delarmente, B. A. (2019). The national cost of hospital acquired pressure injuries in the United States. *International Wound Journal, 16,* 634–640. https://doi.org/10.1111/iwj.13071.

Padula, W., Mishra, M., Makic, M., et al. (2011). Improving quality of pressure ulcer care with prevention: A cost effective analysis. *Medical Care, 49*(4), 385–392.

Pandhare, P. (2018). Effectiveness of ptp regarding use of Braden Scale for pressure sore on knowledge and practices among staff nurses working in selected hospitals. *International Journal of Nursing Education, 10*(4), 139. https://doi.org/10.5958/0974-9357.2018.00120.4.

Patrician, P. A., McCarthy, M. S., Swiger, P., Raju, D., Breckenridge-Sproat, S., Su, X., et al. (2017). Association of temporal variations in staffing with hospital-acquired pressure injury in military hospitals. *Research in Nursing & Health, 40*(2), 111–119. https://doi.org/10.1002/nur.21781.

Pickham, D., Pihulic, M., Valdez, A., Mayer, B., Duhon, P., & Larson, B. (2018). Pressure injury prevention practices in the intensive care unit: Real-world data captured by a wearable patient sensor. *Wounds, 30*(8), 229–234. Epub 2018 May 29. PMID: 30212372.

Pieper, B. (2012). Long term care/nursing homes. In B. Pieper (Ed.), (with the National Pressure Ulcer Advisory Panel [NPUAP]): *Pressure ulcers: prevalence, incidence, and implications for the future* (pp. 65–88), Washington, DC: NPUAP.

Pieper, B., & Mattern, J. (1997). Critical care nurses' knowledge of pressure ulcer prevention, staging and description. *Ostomy/Wound Management, 43*(2), 22–31.

Pieper, B., & Zulkowski, K. (2014). The Pieper-Zulkowski pressure ulcer knowledge test. *Advances in Skin & Wound Care, 27*(9), 413–420. https://doi.org/10.1097/01.ASW.0000453210.21330.00.

Pittman, J. (2007). Effect of aging on wound healing: Current concepts. *Journal of Wound, Ostomy, and Continence Nursing, 34*(4), 412–415. https://doi.org/10.1097/01.WON.0000281658.71072.e6. quiz 416-417. PMID: 17667088.

Pittman, J., & Gillespie, C. (2020). Medical device related pressure injuries. *Critical Care Nursing Clinics of North America, 32*(4), 533–542. https://doi.org/10.1016/j.cnc.2020.08.004.

Ploumis, A., Kolli, S., Patrick, M., Owens, M., Beris, A., & Marino, R. J. (2011). Length of stay and medical stability for spinal cord-injured patients on admission to an inpatient rehabilitation hospital: A comparison between a model SCI trauma center and non-SCI trauma center. *Spinal Cord, 49*(3), 411–415. https://doi.org/10.1038/sc.2010.132.

Portney, L. G. (Ed.). (2020). *Foundations of clinical research: Applications to evidence-based practice* (4th ed.). McGraw Hill. https://fadavispt.mhmedical.com/content.aspx?bookid=2885&sectionid=243179474.

Posthauer, M. E. (2006). The role of nutrition in wound care. *Advances in Skin & Wound Care, 19*(1), 43–54. https://doi.org/10.1097/00129334-200601000-00015.

Primiano, M., Friend, M., McClure, C., et al. (2011). Pressure ulcer prevalence and risk factors during prolonged surgical procedures. *AORN Journal, 94*(6), 555–566.

Proksch, E., Berardesca, E., Misery, L., Engblom, J., & Bouwstra, J. (2020). Dry skin management: Practical approach in light of latest research on skin structure and function. *The Journal of Dermatological Treatment, 31*(7), 716–722.

Qaseem, A., Humphrey, L. L., Forciea, M. A., Starkey, M., Denberg, T. D., & Clinical Guidelines Committee of the American College of Physicians. (2015). Treatment of pressure ulcers: A clinical practice guideline from the American College of Physicians. *Annals of Internal Medicine, 162*(5), 370–379. https://doi.org/10.7326/M14-1568.

Qaseem, A., Mir, T. P., Starkey, M., et al. (2015). Risk assessment and prevention of pressure ulcers: A clinical practice guideline from the American College of Physicians. *Annals of Internal Medicine, 162,* 359–369.

Ramundo, J., Pike, C., & Pittman, J. (2018). Do prophylactic foam dressings reduce heel pressure injuries? *Journal of Wound, Ostomy, and Continence Nursing, 45*(1), 75–82. https://doi.org/10.1097/WON.0000000000000400. PMID: 29300293.

Rantz, J., Zwygart-Stauffacher, M., Flesner, M. H., et al. (2013). The influence of teams to sustain quality improvement in nursing homes that "need improvement." *Journal of the American Medical Directors Association, 14*(1).

Rapp, M. P., Bergstrom, N., & Padhye, N. S. (2009). Contribution of skin temperature regularity to the risk of developing pressure ulcers in nursing facility residents. *Advances in Skin & Wound Care, 22*(11), 506–513. https://doi.org/10.1097/01.ASW.0000305496.15768.82.

Razmus, I., & Berquist-Beringer, S. (2017). Pressure injury prevlanece and rate of hospital-acquired pressure injury among pediatric patients in acute care. *Journal of Wound Ostomy Continence Nursing, 44*(2), 110–117. https://doi.org/10.1097/WON.0000000000000306.

Reddy, M. (2008). Skin and wound care: Important considerations in the older adult. *Advances in Skin and Wound Care, 21*(9), 424–436.

Redelings, M. D., Lee, N. E., & Sorvillo, F. (2005). Pressure ulcers: More lethal than we thought? *Advances in Skin and Wound Care, 18*(7), 367–372.

Registered Nurses' Association of Ontario. (2016). Assessment and management of pressure injuries for the interprofessional team 3rd ed. Toronto, ON: Registered Nurses' Association of Ontario. Retrieved 01/30/2023 from: https://rnao.ca/bpg/guidelines/pressure-injuries.

Ringdal, M., Chaboyer, W., Ulin, K., Bucknall, T., & Oxelmark, L. (2017). Patient preferences for participation in patient care and safety activities in hospitals. *BMC Nursing, 16,* 69. https://doi.org/10.1186/s12912-017-0266-7

Sala, J. J., Mayampurath, A., Solmos, S., Vonderheid, S. C., Banas, M., D'Souza, A., et al. (2021). Predictors of pressure injury development in critically ill adults: A retrospective cohort study. *Intensive and Critical Care Nursing, 62,* 102924.

Schlüer, A. B., Halfens, R. J., & Schols, J. M. (2012). Pediatric pressure ulcer prevalence: A multicenter, cross-sectional, point prevalence study in Switzerland. *Ostomy Wound Management, 58*(7), 18–31.

Schmitt, S., Andries, M. K., Ashmore, P. M., Brunette, G., Judge, K., & Bonham, P. A. (2017). WOCN Society position paper: Avoidable versus unavoidable pressure ulcers/injuries. *Journal of Wound Ostomy, and Continence Nursing, 44*(5), 458–468. https://doi.org/10.1097/WON.0000000000000361. PMID: 28877112.

Schweickert, W. D., Pohlman, M. C., Pohlman, A. S., et al. (2009). Early physical and occupational therapy in mechanically ventilated, critically ill patients: A randomised controlled trial. *Lancet, 373,* 1874–1882.

Shafipour, V., Ramezanpour, E., Gorji, M. A., & Moosazadeh, M. (2016). Prevalence of postoperative pressure ulcer: A systematic review and meta-analysis. *Electronic Physician, 8*(11), 3170–3176. https://doi.org/10.19082/3170.

Shannon, R. J., Coombs, M., & Chakravarthy, D. (2009). Reducing hospital-acquired pressure ulcers with a silicone-based dermal nourishing emollient-associated skincare regimen. *Advances in Skin and Wound Care, 22*(10), 461–467.

Shieh, D. C., Berringer, C. M., Pantoja, R., Resureccion, J., Rainbolt, J. M., & Hokoki, A. (2018). Dramatic reduction in hospital-acquired pressure injuries using a pink paper reminder system. Advances in Skin and Wound Care, 31(3), 118–122. https://doi.org/10.1097/01.ASW.0000527966.72494.61. PMID: 29438145.

Sibbald, R. G., & Ayello, E. A. (2020). Terminal ulcers, SCALE, skin failure, and unavoidable pressure injuries: Results of the 2019 terminology survey. *Advances in Skin and Wound Care, 33*(3), 137–145. https://doi.org/10.1097/01.ASW.0000653148.28858.50. PMID: 32058439.

Sibbald, R. G., Krasner, D. L., & Woo, K. Y. (2011). Pressure ulcer staging revisited: Superficial skin changes & deep pressure ulcer framework. *Advances in Skin and Wound Care, 24*(12), 571–580.

Siddiqui, A., Behrendt, R., Lafluer, M., & Craft, S. (2013). A continuous bedside pressure mapping system for prevention of pressure ulcer development in the medical ICU: A retrospective analysis. *Wounds, 25*(12), 333–339. PMID: 25867745.

Sillmon, K., Moran, C., Shook, L., Lawson, C., & Burfield, A. H. (2021). The use of prophylactic foam dressings for prevention of hospital-acquired pressure injuries: A systematic review. *Journal of Wound, Ostomy, and Continence Nursing, 48*(3), 211–218.

Simonetti, V., Comparcini, D., Flacco, M. E., Di Giovanni, P., & Cicolini, G. (2015). Nursing students' knowledge and attitude on pressure ulcer prevention evidence-based guidelines: A multicenter cross-sectional study. *Nurse Education Today, 35*(4), 573–579. https://doi.org/10.1016/j.nedt.2014.12.020.

Soban, L. M., Hempel, S., Munjas, B. A., et al. (2011). Preventing pressure ulcers in hospitals: A systematic review of nurse-focused quality improvement interventions. *Joint Commission Journal on Quality and Patient Safety, 37*(6), 245–252.

Society of Critical Care Medicine. (2020). *ICU Liberation Bundle.* Retrieved 4/7/2022 from: https://www.sccm.org/iculiberation/abcdef-bundles.

Sprigle, S., & Sonenblum, S. (2011). Assessing evidence supporting redistribution of pressure for pressure ulcer prevention: A review. *Journal of Rehabilitation Research and Development, 48*(3), 203–213.

Stanberry, B., Lahti, N., Kevin, C., & Delin, J. (2021). Preventing pressure ulcers in emergency departments: Four simple and effective nurse-led changes. *Emerging Nurse.* https://doi.org/10.7748/en..e2119. Epub ahead of print. PMID: 34791839.

Sterken, D. J., Mooney, J., Ropele, D., Kett, A., & Vander Laan, K. J. (2015). Become the PPUPET Master: Mastering pressure ulcer risk assessment with the pediatric Pressure Ulcer Prediction and Evaluation Tool (PPUPET). *Journal of Pediatric Nursing, 30*(4), 598–610. https://doi.org/10.1016/j.pedn.2014.10.004.

Stojadinovic, O., Minkiewicz, J., Sawaya, A., et al. (2013). Deep tissue injury in development of pressure ulcers: A decrease of inflammasome activation and changes in human skin morphology in response to aging and mechanical load. *PLoS One, 8*(8), e69223.

Stratton, R. J., Ek, A. C., Engfer, M., et al. (2005). Enteral nutritional support in prevention and treatment of pressure ulcers: A systematic review and meta-analysis. *Ageing Research Reviews, 4*(3), 422–450.

Suddaby, E. C., Barnett, S., & Facteau, L. (2005). Skin breakdown in acute care pediatrics. *Pediatric Nursing, 31*(2). 132–138, 148.

Tablan, O. C., Anderson, L. J., Besser, R., et al. (2004). Guidelines for preventing healthcare-associated pneumonia, 2003: Recommendations of CDC and the Healthcare Infection Control Practices Advisory Committee. *MMWR Recommendations and Reports, 53,* 1–36. PMID: 15048056.

Tallier, P. C., Reineke, P. R., Asadoorian, K., Choonoo, J. G., Campo, M., & Malmgreen-Wallen, C. (2017). Perioperative registered nurses' knowledge, attitudes, behaviors, and barriers regarding pressure ulcer prevention in perioperative patients. *Applied Nursing Research, 36,* 106–110. https://doi.org/10.1016/j.apnr.2017.06.009.

Tayyib, N., & Coyer, F. (2016). Effectiveness of pressure ulcer prevention strategies for adult patients in intensive care units: A systematic review. *Worldviews on Evidence-Based Nursing, 13*(6), 432–444. https://doi.org/10.1111/wvn.12177. Epub 2016 Oct 6. PMID: 27712030.

Terekeci, H., Kucukardali, Y., Top, C., Onem, Y., Celik, S., & Oktenli, C. (2009). Risk assessment study of the pressure ulcers in intensive care unit patients. *European Journal of Internal Medicine, 20*(4), 394–397. https://doi.org/10.1016/j.ejim.2008.11.001.

The Joint Commission. (2017). *Inadequate handoff communication. Sentinel event Alert. A complimentary publication of the Joint Commission.* Retrieved 4/15/2022 from: https://www.jointcommission.org/-/media/tjc/documents/resources/patient-safety-topics/sentinel-event/sea_58_hand_off_comms_9_6_17_final_(1).pdf?db=web&hash=5642D63C1A5017BD214701514DA00139&hash=5642D63C1A5017BD214701514DA00139.

The Joint Commission Center for Transforming Healthcare. (2014). *Improving transitions of care hand-off communications.* Oakbrook Terrace: The Joint Commission.

Trueman, P., & Whitehead, S. J. (2010). The economics of pressure relieving surfaces: An illustrative case study of the impact of high-specification surfaces on hospital finances. *International Wound Journal, 7*(1), 48–54.

Twigg, D. E., Gelder, L., & Myers, H. (2015). The impact of understaffed shifts on nurse-sensitive outcomes. *Journal of Advanced Nursing, 71*(7), 1564–1572.

Twigg, D. E., Kutzer, Y., Jacob, E., & Seaman, K. (2019). A quantitative systematic review of the association between nurse skill mix and nursing-sensitive patient outcomes in the acute care setting. *Journal of Advanced Nursing, 75*(12), 3404–3423. https://doi.org/10.1111/jan.14194.

U.S. Department of Health and Human Services. (2000a). *Healthy People 2010: Understanding and improving health* (2nd ed.). Washington, DC: Government Printing Office.

U.S. Department of Health and Human Services. (2000b). *Healthy People 2010*. Washington, DC: HHS.

Usher, K., Woods, C., Brown, J., Power, T., Lea, J., Hutchinson, M., et al. (2018). Australian nursing students' knowledge and attitudes towards pressure injury prevention: A cross sectional study. *International Journal of Nursing Studies, 81*, 14–20.

VanDenBos, J., Rustagi, K., Gray, T., Halford, M., Ziemkiewicz, E., & Shreve, J. (2011). The $17.1 billion problem: The annual cost of measurable medical errors. *Health Affairs, 30*(4), 596–603. https://doi.org/10.1377/hlthaff.2011.0084.

Van Gilder, C. A., Cox, J., Edsberg, L. E., & Koloms, K. (2021). Pressure injury prevalence in acute care hospitals with unit-specific analysis: Results from the International Pressure Ulcer Prevalence (IPUP) Survey Database. *Journal of Wound, Ostomy, and Continence Nursing, 48*(6), 492–503. https://doi.org/10.1097/WON.0000000000000817.

Vidyarthi, A. (2006). *Triple handoff in cases and commentaries: Hospital medicine*. AHRQ Web M&M. Retrieved 4/16/2022 from: https://psnet.ahrq.gov/web-mm/triple-handoff.

Vollman, K. (2010). Introduction to progressive mobility. *Critical Care Nurse, 30*, 3–5.

Wang, L. H., Chen, H. L., Yan, H. Y., Gao, J. H., Wang, F., Ming, Y., et al. (2015). Inter-rater reliability of three most commonly used pressure ulcer risk assessment scales in clinical practice. *International Wound Journal, 12*(5), 590–594. https://doi.org/10.1111/iwj.12376.

Wang, L., Li, X., Yang, Z., Tang, X., Yuan, Q., Deng, L., et al. (2016). Semi-recumbent position versus supine position for the prevention of ventilator-associated pneumonia in adults requiring mechanical ventilation. *The Cochrane Database of Systematic Reviews, 2016*(1). https://doi.org/10.1002/14651858.CD009946.pub2. PMID: 26743945; PMCID: PMC7016937.

Wound, Ostomy and Continence Nurses Society. (2016). *Guideline for management of pressure ulcers, WOCN clinical practice guideline series #2*. Mt. Laurel: Wound, Ostomy and Continence Nurses Society.

Wound Ostomy and Continence Nurses Society. (2017). *WOCN Society position paper: Avoidable versus unavoidable pressure ulcers (injuries)* (p. 2017). Mt. Laurel: Wound Ostomy and Continence Nurses Society.

Wright, K. (1991). President's message: Pressure ulcer prediction, prevention, and early treatment. *Journal of Early Treatment Nursing, 18*(4), 115–116.

Wu, X., Li, Z., Cao, J., Jiao, J., Wang, Y., Liu, G., et al. (2018). The association between major complications of immobility during hospitalization and quality of life among bedridden patients: A 3-month prospective multi-center study. *PLoS One, 13*(10), e0205729.

Yap, T. L., Kennerly, S. M., Simmons, M. R., Buncher, C. R., Miller, E., Kim, J., et al. (2013). Multidimensional team-based intervention using musical cues to reduce odds of facility-acquired pressure ulcers in long-term care: A paired randomized intervention study. *Journal of the American Geriatric Society, 61*(9), 1552–1559. https://doi.org/10.1111/jgs.12422.

Zhou, Q., Yu, T., Liu, Y., Shi, R., Tian, S., Yang, C., et al. (2018). The prevalence and specific characteristics of hospitalised pressure ulcer patients: A multicentre cross-sectional study. *Journal of Clinical Nursing, 27*(3–4), 694–704.

FURTHER READING

Black, J. M., Cuddigan, J. E., Walko, M. A., et al. (2010). Medical device related pressure ulcers in hospitalized patients. *International Wound Journal, 7*(5), 358–365.

Cheng, F.-M., Jin, Y.-J., Chien, C.-W., Chuang, Y.-C., & Tung, T.-H. (2021). The application of Braden Scale and rough set theory for pressure injury risk in elderly male population. *Journal of Men's Health, 17*(4), 156–165.

Department of Health and Human Services, Centers for Medicare and Medicaid Services. (2007). Medicare program; changes to the hospital inpatient prospective payment systems and fiscal year 2008 rates; final rule. *Federal Register, 72*(162), 1–12.

Doughty, D., Junkin, J., Kurz, P., et al. (2012). Incontinence-associated dermatitis: Consensus statements, evidenced-based guidelines for prevention and treatment, and current challenges. *Journal of Wound, Ostomy, and Continence Nursing, 39*(3), 303–315.

Gray, M., Beeckman, D., Bliss, D. Z., et al. (2012). Incontinence-associated dermatitis: A comprehensive review and update. *Journal of Wound, Ostomy, and Continence Nursing, 39*(1), 61–74.

Gray, M., Black, J. M., Baharestani, M. M., et al. (2011). Moisture-associated skin damage: Overview and pathophysiology. *Journal of Wound, Ostomy, and Continence Nursing, 38*(3), 233–241.

Pickham, D., Berte, N., Pihulic, M., Valdez, A., Mayer, B., & Desai, M. (2018). Effect of a wearable patient sensor on care delivery for preventing pressure injuries in acutely ill adults: A pragmatic randomized clinical trial (LS-HAPI study). *International Journal of Nursing Studies, 80*, 12–19. https://doi.org/10.1016/j.ijnurstu.2017.12.012.

Rabadi, M. H., & Vincent, A. S. (2011). Do vascular risk factors contribute to the prevalence of pressure ulcer in veterans with spinal cord injury? *The Journal of Spinal Cord Medicine, 34*(1), 46–51.

12

Pressure Redistribution Support Surfaces

Denise P. Nix and Catherine T. Milne

OBJECTIVES

1. List four factors to consider when interpreting the significance of interface tissue pressure readings.
2. List three limitations to the reliance of capillary-closing values for support surface evaluation.
3. Define pressure redistribution, immersion, and envelopment.
4. Explain the difference between a reactive and an active support surface.
5. Compare the advantages and disadvantages of support surface categories and features.
6. List factors to consider for appropriate selection of a support surface.

A support surface is a specialized device for pressure redistribution designed for the management of tissue loads (European Pressure Ulcer Advisory Panel, National Pressure Injury Advisory Panel, Pan Pacific Pressure Injury Alliance (EPUAP/NPIAP/PPPIA), 2019). Depending on the composition of the support surface and its mechanism of action, additional therapeutic functions may include reduction of shear and friction as well as microclimate/moisture management. Support surfaces are available in different sizes and shapes for chairs, toilet seats, and horizontal surfaces, such as mattresses, examination and procedure tables, operating room (OR) surfaces, and emergency and transport stretchers or gurneys.

Four separate systematic reviews revealed insufficient evidence in terms of identifying one specific type of support surface as superior in the prevention or treatment of pressure injuries (Chou, Dana, Bougatsos, et al., 2013; McInnes et al., 2015; McInnes, Jammali-Blasi, Bell-Syer, & Leung, 2018; Saha, Smith, Totten, et al., 2013). However, static foam (Chou et al., 2013) and high-specification foam surfaces (McInnes et al., 2015) were associated with lower pressure injury incidence in nonoperating room settings when compared with standard hospital foam replacement mattresses. No comparative effectiveness support surface studies have been performed to examine specific wound type; nonpressure-related wounds or wound location. One systematic review (Junkin & Gray, 2009) examined pressure redistribution for patients at risk for heel pressure injuries found little evidence to suggest one device or surface was superior to another. It is generally agreed that individual patient characteristics guide support surface and offloading devices and may change as patient condition or care setting changes (EPUAP/NPIAP/PPPIA, 2019; Wound, Ostomy and Continence Nurses Society™ (WOCN®), 2016).

Although there is insufficient evidence to specify a particular brand of support surface (EPUAP/NPIAP/PPPIA, 2019; Whitney, Phillips, Aslam, et al., 2006; WOCN®, 2016), a variety of pressure-redistribution devices can help lower the incidence of pressure injuries up to 60% (Cullum, McInnes, Bell-Syer, & Legood, 2004; Whitney et al., 2006). This chapter reviews factors to consider for the (1) evaluation of support surfaces, (2) selection/evaluation of support surfaces based on individual patient assessment, and (3) creation/evaluation of a facility-wide or agency-wide support surface formulary. General guidance for the care of the patient requiring a support surface is given in Box 12.1.

INTERFACE TISSUE PRESSURES: PAST AND PRESENT

Interface tissue pressure is the force per unit area that act perpendicularly between the body and the support surface and is measured by a sensor placed between the skin and support surface. This process is also known as *pressure mapping* (Fig. 12.1). A review of 29 randomized controlled trials concluded that these measurements do not reliably predict support surface performance (Cullum et al., 2004). However, pressure mapping continues to be used to (1) produce images for product literature that appear to show pressure redistribution, (2) compare measurements from the same patient on two different surfaces, (3) assist with adjusting inflation of a chair cushion, or (4) teach a chairbound patient what type of position change will decrease pressure over an ischial tuberosity. Box 12.2 summarizes factors to consider when reviewing literature that includes interface tissue pressures (Miller, Parker, Blasiole, et al., 2013; Reger, McGovern, Chung, et al., 1988).

BOX 12.1 General Guidance for Care of Patient Requiring a Support Surface

- Support surfaces alone neither prevent nor heal pressure injuries and should be incorporated into a comprehensive individualized care plan.[a]
- Patient with or at risk[a] for pressure injuries should be placed on a support surface rather than on a standard hospital mattress.
- Patient with or at risk[a] for pressure injuries who sits should have a chair cushion and a sitting plan[a] that specifies frequency, duration, posture, and positioning needs.
- Support surfaces must be compatible with the care setting while meeting the individual needs of the patient.
- Support surfaces function best with minimal linens and pads under the patient.
- Patient must be able to assume a variety of positions on the selected surface (bed or chair) without bottoming out.
- When considering overlay use, it is important to assess risk for falls, entrapment, weight distribution, and potential for bottoming out.
- Patient should be turned and repositioned, regardless of support surface features.
- Multiple factors determine the frequency of repositioning[a] and must not be based solely on the features of the support surface.

- Use positioning devices and continence pads compatible with the support surface.
- A support surface that dissipates moisture (low air loss) may be indicated when moisture barriers, pouches, and dressings do not adequately protect the skin from moisture/incontinence.
- A reactive support surface with features and components such as low air loss, alternating pressure, or viscous or air fluids should be considered for patients who:
  - CANNOT be effectively positioned off their wound
  - Have pressure injuries involving multiple turning surfaces
  - Have pressure injuries that fail to improve despite optimal comprehensive management
- An active support surface (alternating pressure) should be considered when effective repositioning is determined by a provider to be medically contraindicated (frequent small shifts, reevaluation, and retrials at least every 8 h should be documented).
- Always follow manufacturers' instructions for appropriate use, contraindications, and precautions (see also Checklist 12.2).

[a] See Chapter 11 for details.

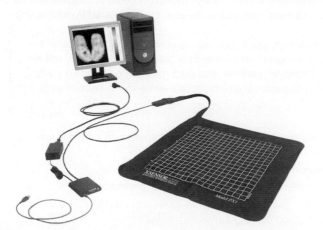

Fig. 12.1 Pressure-mapping device (XSensor pressure-mapping system). (Courtesy the ROHO Group, Belleville, IL.)

Historically, support surfaces have been categorized by comparing interface tissue pressure measurements obtained on a support surface to a standard capillary-closing value. Surfaces were then placed into categories called *pressure reduction* and *pressure relief* based on how close the interface tissue pressures were to the standard capillary-closing value; these terms have been considered invalid (EPUAP/NPIAP/PPPIA, 2019) for many years. However, because the concept of a standardized capillary-closing pressure is affected by many variables (see Box 12.2) and is unlikely to exist (Le, Madsen, Barth, et al., 1984), attempting to employ such a simplistic scheme to guide a process as complex as support surface selection is flawed. It is more useful to formulate a framework for support surface selection that is based on such traits as physical concepts, therapeutic functions, medium, forms, and features.

BOX 12.2 Capillary-Closing and Interface Tissue Pressures

A *capillary-closing* pressure value should not be used to compare support surfaces for the following reasons:
- Capillary-closing values are based on measurements obtained from the fingertips of young, healthy males.
- Pressure is three to five times greater at the bone than at the surface of the skin.
- Lower capillary-closing pressures have been reported in older patients.
- Tissue interface pressures do not ensure that blood flow through the capillaries is unimpeded.

Interface tissue pressure measurements (pressure mapping) should be reported with the following disclosures:
- Population tested (healthy subjects will demonstrate lower pressure readings than debilitated subjects because normal muscle mass supports and distributes weight more effectively)

- How often equipment was recalibrated (sensors are fragile and may malfunction)
- Number of readings conducted per site (range based on multiple readings is more reliable than one single reading per site)
- Factors known to affect results:
  - Stiffness of support surface
  - Composition of body tissue
  - Transducer size and shape
  - Method of equilibrium detection
  - Uniformity of measurement technique
  - Load shape and its interaction with support material
  - Skill of person taking measurements (uniformity of technique for measuring interface tissue pressure is necessary for accuracy)

PHYSICAL CONCEPTS AND THERAPEUTIC FUNCTIONS

Physical concepts are performance-related terms (Table 12.1) used to provide standard discussions about how support surfaces perform (Christian & Lachenbruch, 2007). *Life*

expectancy refers to the period during which a product can effectively fulfill its purpose. It may be affected by *fatigue* or a reduced capacity to perform due to intended or unintended use and/or prolonged exposure to chemical, thermal, or physical forces. These factors affect the ability of the support surface to redistribute pressure, control friction and

TABLE 12.1 Glossary of Support Surface Terms and Definitions	
Term	**Definition**
Active support surface	A powered support surface, with the capability to change its load distribution properties, with or without applied load
Air	A low-density fluid with minimal resistance to flow
Air fluidized	A feature of a support surface that provides pressure redistribution by forcing air through a granular medium (e.g., beads) producing a fluid state
Alternating pressure	A feature of a support surface that provides pressure redistribution via cyclic changes in loading *and unloading* as characterized by frequency, duration, amplitude, and rate of change parameters
Basic/standard hospital mattress	A term used to describe the mattress provided within a facility and generally used as the comparative intervention in research trials investigating the effectiveness of pressure redistribution support surfaces. As such, the qualities of a "standard" hospital mattress vary according to historical and clinical context and are rarely reported in detail in clinical trials. In most cases it is assumed that a "standard" hospital mattress is a non-powered foam or spring-based mattress NOTE: The term "Standard" hospital mattress should not be used without a full description. Commonly used mattresses have changed over time and no "standard" exists. Any reference, notation or category for standard hospital mattress, standard mattress or standard surface should describe the product using consistent and recognizable terms and definitions as listed in this document
Bladder	See Cell/bladder
Bottoming out	The state of a support surface deformation beyond critical immersion whereby effective pressure redistribution is lost
Cell/bladder	A means of encapsulating a support medium
Closed cell foam	A nonpermeable structure in which there is a barrier between cells, preventing gases or liquids from passing through the foam
Coefficient of friction	A measurement of the amount of friction existing between two surfaces
Constant/continuous low pressure	See Reactive Support Surface
Critical immersion	The threshold beyond which increased deformation of the support surface has the effect of concentrating and increasing localized pressure
Elastic foam	A chemically complex polymeric product having a broad range of load bearing capability and resiliency for comfort and cushioning typically characterized by an interconnected and open cell structure; the elastic nature of this foam causes it to resist deformation and return to its original shape after the stress (external force) that made it deform is removed
Elastomer	Various polymers having the elastic properties of natural rubber, being able to resume its original shape when a deforming force is removed
Envelopment	The ability of a support surface to conform, so as to fit or mold, around irregularities of the body
Fatigue	The reduced capacity of a surface or its components to perform as specified. This change may be the result of intended or unintended use and/or prolonged exposure to chemical, thermal, or physical forces
Friction (frictional force)	The resistance to motion in a parallel direction relative to the common boundary of two surfaces
Full-body support surface	A specialized device for pressure redistribution (e.g., mattress, mattress overlay, or integrated bed system) designed for management of tissue loads, microclimate, and/or other therapeutic functions
Gel	A semisolid system consisting of a network of solid aggregates, colloidal dispersions or polymers which may exhibit elastic properties. Gels can range from hard to soft

TABLE 12.1 Glossary of Support Surface Terms and Definitions—cont'd

Term	Definition
High specification foam support surface/mattress	A Reactive Support Surface meeting the specific requirements of density, support factor, depth, and type of mattress cover. Characteristics are found in The International Pressure Injury Guidelines under Support Surfaces
Immersion	Penetration (sinking) into a support surface, as measured by depth
Integrated bed system	A bed frame and support surface that are combined into a single unit, whereby the surface is unable to function separately
Lateral rotation	A feature of a support surface that provides rotation about a longitudinal axis as characterized by degree of patient turn, duration, and frequency
Life expectancy	The defined period of time during which a product is able to effectively fulfill its designated purpose
Low air loss	A feature of a support surface that uses a flow of air to assist in managing the heat and humidity (microclimate) of the skin
Mattress	A full-body support surface designed to be placed directly on the existing bed frame
Mechanical load	Force distribution acting on a surface
Microclimate	The temperature and humidity in a specified location. For purposes of support surfaces, microclimate refers to temperature and humidity at the support surface/body interface
Multizoned surface	A surface in which different segments can have different pressure redistribution capabilities
Nonpowered	Any support surface not requiring or using external sources of energy for operation. (Energy = DC or AC electrical current)
Open cell foam	A permeable structure with interconnection between the cells, the majority of which are open. The interconnectedness of the cellular matrix typically results in permeability to gases and liquids
Overlay	An additional support surface designed to be placed directly on top of an existing surface
Pad	A cushion-like mass of soft material used for comfort, protection, or positioning
Powered	Any support surface requiring or using external sources of energy to operate. (Energy = DC or AC electrical current)
Pressure	The force per unit area exerted perpendicular to the plane of interest
Pressure redistribution Deprecated: Pressure reduction pressure relief	The ability of a support surface to distribute load over the contact areas of the human body This term replaces prior terminology of pressure reduction and pressure relief surfaces
Pulsation	A feature of a support surface that provides repeating higher and lower pressures resulting in cyclic changes in stiffness of the surface, typically with shorter duration inflation/deflation, higher frequency, and lower amplitude than alternating pressure
Reactive support surface	A powered or nonpowered support surface with the capability to change its load distribution properties only in response to applied load
Safe working load	Maximum external mechanical load (mass) on equipment or an equipment part that is permitted in Normal Use (operation, including routine inspection and adjustments by any operator, and stand-by according to the instructions for use). *IEC 60601-1*
Shear (shear stress)	The force per unit area exerted parallel to the perpendicular plane of interest
Shear strain	Distortion or deformation of tissue as a result of shear stress
Solid	A substance that does not flow perceptibly under stress. Under ordinary conditions it retains its size and shape
Standard temperature and humidity environment	A test environment in which 23 ± 2°C and 50% ± 5% RH as specified in ISO 554 can be maintained
Support surface	A specialized device for pressure redistribution designed for management of tissue loads, microclimate, and/or other therapeutic functions. Support surfaces include but are not limited to mattresses, integrated bed systems, mattress replacements or overlays, or seat cushions and seat cushion overlays
Support surface loading indenter	An apparatus that is used to apply indentation forces to a support surface to determine its characteristics. Depending on test method, a partial or full body indenter will be used
Test dummy—full body	A physical analog of the human body used during testing
Therapeutic working load (weight range)	The rated load range at which the features of a support surface are functioning according to its intended use

Continued

TABLE 12.1   Glossary of Support Surface Terms and Definitions—cont'd

Term	Definition
Viscoelastic foam (memory foam)	A type of porous polymer material which conforms in proportion to the applied weight. The material exhibits dampened elastic properties when load is applied
Viscous fluid	A fluid having a molecular structure which produces sufficient internal friction to resist motion
Zone	A segment with a single pressure redistribution capability

Source: Terms and Definitions of Support Surfaces. Retrieved 3/13/2023 from http://www.resja.or.jp/sig-pmps/Support%20Surface%20Terms%20&%20Definitions%202006_current__1.pdf.

shear, and manage the microclimate (temperature and humidity) of the surface (EPUAP/NPIAP/PPPIA, 2019).

Pressure Redistribution (Immersion and Envelopment)

Support surfaces are designed to prevent pressure injuries and, through pressure redistribution, provide an environment more conducive to pressure injury healing. Support surfaces redistribute interface pressure by conforming to the contours of the body so that pressure is redistributed over a larger surface area rather than concentrated on a more circumscribed location. The therapeutic function of pressure redistribution is accomplished through immersion and envelopment. *Immersion* refers to the depth of penetration or sinking into the surface, allowing the pressure to be spread out over the surrounding area rather than directly over a bony prominence. Immersion is dependent on factors such as the stiffness and thickness of the support surface and the flexibility of the cover. *Envelopment* refers to the ability of the support surface to conform to irregularities (e.g., clothing, bedding, bony prominences) without causing a substantial increase in pressure (EPUAP/NPIAP/PPPIA, 2019; Soppi, Lehtio, & Saarinen, 2015) (Fig. 12.2). In contrast to the therapeutic functions of immersion and envelopment, *"bottoming out"* occurs when the depth of penetration or sinking is excessive, allowing increased pressure to concentrate over one area or bony prominence. Whitney et al. (2006) define bottoming out as less than 1 in of material between the surface and the skin when feeling under a support surface with the palm of a hand. Factors that may lead to bottoming out include (1) weight exceeds manufacturer's recommendations; (2) disproportionate weights and sizes, such as with bilateral lower extremity amputation; (3) tendency to keep the head of the bed greater than 30 degrees; and (4) inappropriate support surface settings, such as overinflation or underinflation. While many manufacturers' product information report hand checks by clinical staff should be performed routinely to evaluate bottoming out, the NPIAP position paper (2014) suggests that these are subjective measurements. Additionally, there may be associated safety issues in performing hand-checks, though evidence is very limited. Hand checks should not be performed with integrated mattress systems. All support surfaces function best with minimal linen and/or plastic-backed underpads and/or briefs between the patient and the surface (EPUAP/NPIAP/PPPIA, 2019; WOCN®, 2016).

Friction and Shear Reduction

Friction and shear are physical concepts associated with pressure injury formation. *Shear stress* refers to the perpendicular force on the tissue; *shear strain* refers to the resulting deformation (EPUAP/NPIAP/PPPIA, 2019; Levy & Gefen, 2017). A support surface reduces shear and friction by strategic placement of mediums and covers that allow for low-friction positioning without excessive sliding. However, the best support surface cover will not eliminate the need for additional interventions to minimize friction and shear, as described in Chapters 9 and 11.

Microclimate (Temperature and Moisture) Control

Microclimate control is a therapeutic function some support surfaces may provide. Excess moisture of the skin is a well-known factor associated with pressure injury development. Control of temperature at the interface surface (patient–bed boundary) helps to maintain normal skin temperature, which in turn inhibits sweating and lowers skin hydration (Mackey, 2005). A support surface should be designed to help maintain normal skin hydration and temperature

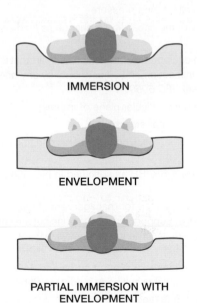

IMMERSION

ENVELOPMENT

PARTIAL IMMERSION WITH ENVELOPMENT

Fig. 12.2 An illustration of the differences between immersion and envelopment with regards to reactive therapy support surfaces. (Direct Healthcare Group.)

(Brienza & Geyer, 2005). Porous covers help reduce moisture by allowing air to transfer between the skin and surface so that moisture and body heat can dissipate. Some mediums may be nonpermeable and prevent liquid or air from escaping, whereas others interact with the body to affect microclimate, such as with continuously pumped air flowing across the skin.

COMPONENTS

Components of a support surface are manufactured from various mediums as a means of creating pressure redistribution. Mediums are solid, fluid, and air, either used alone or in combination. The means of encapsulating the medium is considered another component of the support surface and is called the *cell* or *bladder* (EPUAP/NPIAP/PPPIA, 2019). Multiple cells can be individual or interconnected, configured in a longitudinal or latitudinal pattern (Fig. 12.3 and 12.4).

Foam

Foam is available in chair cushions, overlays, mattresses for beds, transport gurneys, stretchers, and OR/procedure tables. Most foam overlays and cushions are indicated for single-patient use, whereas mattresses are intended for multiple-patient use. Both are designed for a specific weight limit

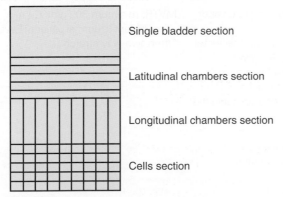

Single bladder section

Latitudinal chambers section

Longitudinal chambers section

Cells section

Fig. 12.3 Interconnected, single-bladder, longitudinal, or latitudinal cells.

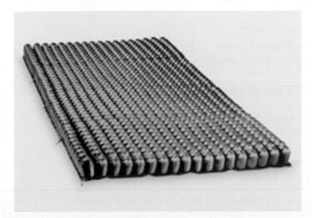

Fig. 12.4 Nonpowered static air support surface consisting of hundreds of individual air cells. (Courtesy the ROHO Group, Belleville, IL.)

and lifespan. Foam can be the sole medium or consist of hybrids that include composites of gel, air, or other more fluid materials to enhance envelopment in key areas. Benefits associated with foam support surfaces include their relatively low cost, light weight, and minimal maintenance. A disadvantage is the limited lifespan due to fatigue caused by flexion and compression over time.

Foam can be closed cell or open cell. *Closed-cell* foam is a nonpermeable formulation in which a barrier between cells prevents gases or liquids from passing through the foam (National Pressure Injury Advisory Panel (NPIAP), 2019), potentially increasing skin temperature by preventing dissipation of body heat (Nicholson, Scales, Clark, et al., 1999). *Open-cell* foam is higher-specification foam that is more effective in preventing pressure injuries than is closed-cell foam. Examples of higher-specification foams are elastic and viscoelastic. There is no evidence that one type of high-specification foam is better than high-specification foam (EPUAP/NPIAP/PPPIA, 2019; McInnes et al., 2018). Table 12.2 presents a consensus on minimum recommendations for high-specification foam mattresses (Australian Wound Management Association, 2012; EPUAP/NPIAP/PPPIA, 2019).

Elastic Foam

Elastic is high-specification foam made of porous polymer material that conforms in proportion to the applied weight. Air enters and exits the open-cell foam rapidly due to its greater density (NPIAP, 2019). The surface continues to conform until the resistance to compression exceeds the weight being applied (Christian & Lachenbruch, 2007). The combination of density and hardness determines compressibility and conformity, ultimately establishing the ability of the support surface to mechanically redistribute loading force. Density describes foam weight, reported as either pounds per cubic foot or kilograms per cubic meter. Greater density provides more durability.

Indentation force deflection (IFD), also known previously as indentation load deflection, is a measure of firmness or resistance to compression. In the United States IFD is reported as the force in pounds required to compress a prescribed size of foam by 25%. The more global foam industry tends to report the amount of force in "newtons" necessary to compress a prescribed size of foam by 40% after a process of preconditioning. Surfaces can be made with a combination of foams strategically placed to optimize pressure redistribution in targeted locations (Soppi et al., 2015)—for example, a relatively lower-density IFD foam located closer to the surface and therefore the patient to enhance conformation, and a higher-density IFD foam located more deeply in the mattress to prevent compression or bottoming out.

A foam overlay is a single-user form of support surface placed on top of a mattress. With the evolution of more affordable high specification foam mattresses, the use of most types of foam mattress overlays (e.g., egg crate foam) is not recommended in most settings. If a foam overlay is used for pressure redistribution, it should have a base height of at least 3 in measured from the base (or bottom) to the lower

TABLE 12.2 Consensus on Minimum Recommendations for High Specification Foam Mattresses

Characteristics	Explanation	High Specification Mattress
Classification	Classification according to the Australian Standards (AS2281-1993)	Type H/HR H—conventional resilience, heavy duty HR—high resilience LR—Low resilience
Multilayering	*Multilayering* of various grades/types of foam alters design features. Different density-hardness layers produce a harder base that increases upper weight limit *Slow recovery foam* increases the surface area contact, redistributes pressure, reduces peak pressures, and allows immersion of bony prominences. Has potential to increase skin surface temperature	Common feature
Density—hardness in single layer mattresses	*Density* is the weight of the foam in kilograms per cubic meter. *Hardness* is the ability of foam to "push back" and carry weight *Hardness* is defined as the amount of force (in Newtons) required to indent a sample of the foam by a specific percentage of the original thickness. This is known as the indentation force deflection (IFD). In Australia and Europe hardness is measured at 40% IFD *Density/hardness* defines the grade of foam and is stated with density followed by hardness	35–130 kg/m³ (minimum for single layer foam mattress) Variance in the hardness exists in top and middle layers of multilayer designs
Support factor	An indicator of foam comfort that is calculated as a ratio: IFD at 65% IFD at 25% = support factor A higher value usually indicates a softer feel and good base support	IFD: 1.6–2.6
Depth	Consider depth of the mattress alongside density/hardness. Different foam grades require different depth to manage upper body weight and prevent bottoming out	150 mm Mattress depth needs to be increased to support bariatric load
Mattress cover	*Vapor permeability:* the relevant measurement is moisture vapor transmission rate (MVTR) Increasing the MVTR potentially allows the trans-epidermal water loss (TEWL) of intact skin to transpire through the cover. Decreasing the MVTR of the cover protects the foam from moisture degradation. Changing the MVTR becomes a compromise between managing local climatic conditions and the patient's TEWL *Allows for partial immersion in foam* *Wrinkling:* may add additional pressure at skin surface *Shear resistance:* can be reduced with a low friction fabric. *Infection control:* • water proofing—prevents contamination of foam • welded seams prevent ingress of fluids • waterfall flap cover over zips • cleaning according to facility protocol and manufacturers guidelines *Fire retardant properties:* material must meet local standards	MVTR: minimum 300 g/m²/24 h (equivalent to normal patient TEWL) Often two-way stretch
Other considerations	*Castellated foam:* partial thickness cuts made in a regular block pattern on the top section of the foam increases surface contact area potentially reducing friction and shear. *Side walls:* a border or stiffener along the edge increases firmness and assists mobility and transfers *Safety sides (concave shape):* may reduce risk of falls but may also reduce bed mobility, need to consider facility restraint policy *Hinging system:* wedges removed on the inner border to allow for folding or bending of mattress to accommodate back rest and upper and lower leg sections to conform to profiling beds	Common features

level of convolution, suitable density to ensure durability (1.3–1.6 lbs/ft^3), IFD of 30, and ideally a ratio of 25%–40% for compression of 2.5 or greater (Whittemore, 1998). As described later in this chapter, when considering overlay use, it is important to assess risk for falls, weight distribution, and potential for bottoming out.

Viscoelastic (Memory) Foam

Viscoelastic is high-specification open-cell foam made of porous polymer material that conforms in proportion to the applied weight. Air enters and exits the foam cells slowly, which allows the material to respond slower than elastic foam. Viscoelastic foams are a subset of urethane polymer foams that exhibit a slow recovery (memory) property. A viscoelastic foam product generally has a higher density and a lower IFD. Because of their fluid nature, when an object is placed on a viscoelastic support surface, the viscoelastic tends to displace quickly and conform to the shape of the object, with low resistance. Viscoelastic foam is available in many grades and qualities, each having properties that affect pressure redistribution and microclimate performance in unique ways. Some viscoelastic foams are engineered to change hardness within a specific temperature range. These materials tend to get softer as the material warms to body temperature, resulting in conformation like that of a gel. Viscoelastic support surfaces are often used in the OR (Association of periOperative Registered Nurses (AORN), 2017; Oliveira, Nascimento, Nicolussi, et al., 2017) and have been shown to effectively decrease the incidence of pressure injuries in high-risk elderly patients with fractures of the neck and femur (Cullum, Nelson, Flemming, et al., 2001). One study of 838 patients at risk for pressure injuries found a significantly lower pressure injury incidence when patients were turned every 4 h on a viscoelastic surface compared with patients who were turned every 2 h on a standard mattress (Defloor, Bacquer, & Grypdonck, 2005). The review of higher specification mattresses by Soppi et al. (2015) suggests construction of a foam mattress using a viscoelastic layer on top of a high resilience foam best meets criteria for pressure redistribution while maintaining durability in the healthcare environment. As engineering and materials technology coupled with tissue deformation science progresses, further research will be needed.

Gel

Gel contains a network of solid aggregates, colloidal dispersions, or polymers that may exhibit elastic properties (National Clinical Guideline Centre (UK), 2014; NPIAP, 2019). Some gel products are called *viscoelastic gel* because they respond similarly to viscoelastic foam. Gel support surfaces are intended for multiple-patient use. Because of the consistency of the medium, gels have been found to be especially effective in preventing shear. Other advantages include easy cleaning and no need for electricity. Disadvantages of gel support surfaces are that they tend to be heavy and are difficult to repair. Skin humidity can increase due to the nonporous nature of the gel and the lack of air flow. Although the gel is cool upon initial contact, skin temperature may increase after hours of constant contact. Gel must be carefully monitored, and the material must be manually moved back to the areas under bony prominences if it has migrated (Brienza & Geyer, 2005).

Fluids (Viscous Fluid, Water, Air)

Fluids are considered substances whose molecules flow freely past one another. Fluids have no fixed shape, so they take on the shape of the load with less resistance than a gel or solid component, creating a high degree of immersion. Fluid mediums include viscous fluid, water, and air. Moisture control characteristics are dependent on the ability of the medium to conduct heat and the composition of the product's cover.

Viscous Fluid

Viscous fluid contains materials such as silicon elastomer, silicon, or polyvinyl (Brienza & Geyer, 2005). At first glance, viscous fluid can be mistaken for gel. Although many of its advantages and disadvantages are like those of gels, viscous fluid is free flowing and has a similar pressure redistribution response as air or water. Compared with air and water, viscous fluid is thicker, with a relatively higher resistance to flow (National Clinical Guideline Centre (UK), 2014; NPIAP, 2019).

Water

Water is a moderate-density fluid with moderate resistance to flow (NPIAP, 2019). Studies have demonstrated that water-filled support surfaces provide lower interface pressure than a standard mattress (McInnes et al., 2015). Although popular at home, water mattresses are undesirable in the hospital or long-term care setting due to multiple management concerns, including the following:
- Need for a heater to control the temperature
- Time and labor needed to drain and move the bed
- Potential for leaking
- Difficulty with repositioning and transferring and with performing cardiopulmonary resuscitation (CPR)

Air. Air is a low-density fluid with minimal resistance to flow. Air may be the sole redistribution medium, or it may be combined with other mediums (National Clinical Guideline Centre (UK), 2014; NPIAP, 2019). Support surfaces that incorporate air are available as chair cushions, toilet seat cushions, overlays, mattresses, and bed systems. Most air support surfaces are easy to clean and can be reused. Air products have the potential to leak if damaged and require adequate inflation so that the body can immerse into the product. Air mattresses and overlays have the advantage of being lightweight and easy to clean.

CATEGORIES AND FEATURES

Categories of pressure redistribution support surfaces include overlays, mattress replacements, and integrated bed systems. Pressure redistribution devices may be purchased in the form of a chair cushion or transport, procedure, emergency room, or perioperative surface. These surfaces may be powered or nonpowered, active or reactive. Features or functional components such as low air loss, air fluidization, lateral rotation, and alternating pressure may be used alone or in combination. A variety of pressure redistribution capabilities can exist in single or multizoned surfaces. A zone is a segment with a single pressure redistribution capability. Therefore, a multizoned surface has different segments with different pressure redistribution capabilities (National Clinical Guideline Centre (UK), 2014; NPIAP, 2019).

Mattress Overlays

The mattress overlay is a support surface that is placed on top of an existing mattress (National Clinical Guideline Centre (UK), 2014; NPIAP, 2019). Gel, water, and some air-filled overlays are intended for multiple-patient use and have the advantage of requiring much less storage space than mattresses and bed systems. Other overlays, such as foam and some air products, are for single-patient use and present environmental concerns relative to disposal of the product. Overlays are thinner than mattress replacements, so there is potential for the patient to bottom out onto the mattress below. Because they are applied over an existing mattress, mattress overlays increase the height of the bed and may complicate patient transfers, alter the fit of linens, or increase the risk for patient entrapment and falls (EPUAP/NPIAP/PPPIA, 2019; US Food and Drug Administration (FDA), 2006).

Mattresses

A mattress is composed of any medium or combination of mediums that is placed on an existing compatible frame. Mattresses reduce some of the high-profile-related disadvantages experienced with overlays and appear to have fewer issues with bottoming out. When first introduced, most support surfaces were integrated support surfaces or overlays that were rented or purchased. When support surfaces called *replacement mattresses* entered the marketplace, many facilities realized improved skin and wound outcomes by replacing their standard mattresses with replacement mattresses (Cullum et al., 2004; Gray, Cooper, & Stringfellowe, 2001). This investment reduced lead time and labor by eliminating the need to wait for delivery of bed systems or for staff to help move the patient once risk or pressure injuries were identified. Today, most companies no longer make mattresses that do not redistribute pressure, so their standard mattress *is* a support surface. Mattresses may include a variety of therapeutic functions such as shear and friction reduction and managing the microclimate between the patient and the support surface.

Transport, Procedure, Emergency Room, and Perioperative Support Surfaces

It stands to reason that patients who require a support surface in bed would benefit from a support surface during special procedures, surgeries, and long waits on emergency room and transport gurneys. In fact, patients on these surfaces may be more at risk for pressure injury development due to limited space for moving and repositioning, in addition to their potential need for sedation or anesthesia. Although limited in peer-reviewed publications, manufacturers now are creating support surface mattresses (sometimes called *pads*) with a pressure redistribution option for emergency room, transport, and procedure tables. Some companies will custom-fit their pressure redistribution products to fit surfaces other than beds. Chapter 11 provides information related to unique risk factors specific to patients in the OR. International guidelines recommend that the at-risk individual in the OR should have a mattress with pressure-redistributing properties (AORN, 2016; EPUAP/NPIAP/PPPIA, 2019).

However, a review of the literature suggests that, due to uncontrolled variables (e.g., reaction to anesthesia, discoveries leading to longer surgery), all surgical patients should be considered at risk and placed on a mattress with pressure-redistributing properties greater than those of the standard OR mattress (Walton-Geer, 2009).

Several support surface options are available for the perioperative environment including air, gel, and high-specification foam mattresses. The best OR surface for preventing pressure injuries has not been determined. McInnes et al. (2015) concluded that pressure redistribution overlays on the operating table reduce the incidence of postoperative pressure injuries. Selection of a support surface in the OR requires careful analysis of several factors to ensure the product provides pressure redistribution while demonstrating compatibility with the facility's most common surgical positions, safety procedures, transfer equipment, and budget (Box 12.3).

Two meta-analysis studies indicate that postoperative use of a pressure redistribution support surface reduces the incidence of surgery-related pressure injuries (Huang, Chen, & Xu, 2013; McNichol, Watts, Mackey, et al., 2015). Of note, the number of pads and blankets, including warming blankets placed beneath the patient and the mattress, interferes with the pressure redistribution properties of the mattress. Therefore, if a cooling blanket is placed between the patient and the OR mattress, a higher-grade surface should be considered to account for the change in pressure redistribution (AORN, 2017).

BOX 12.3 AORN Selection Recommendations for Operating Room Support Surfaces

- Facilitates ability to hold patient in desired position
- Available in variety of shapes and sizes
- Ability to support maximum weight requirements
- Durable material and design
- Evidence that it can disperse skin interface pressure
- Resistance to moisture
- Smooth and intact surfaces
- Low risk for moisture retention
- Radiolucent as needed
- Fire retardant
- Nonallergenic
- Promote air circulation
- Low risk of harboring bacteria
- Easy to use and store
- Cost effective

Integrated Bed Systems

An integrated bed system is a bed frame and support surface combined into a single unit. It is a rented or purchased unit whose components do not function separately (NPIAP, 2019); therefore, it is used in place of an existing bed. With the integrated bed system, the features of both the frame and the support surface must be evaluated. Frames come in different widths and lengths and support a specified amount of weight. Some frames can adjust or fold for storage or transport through narrow doors and elevators. Most frames today are electric, but alternatives are available. When selecting a frame, the population to be served and the setting in which it will be used should be considered. For example, frames with built-in bed exit alarms may be needed for patients who are confused or at risk for falls. Frames with built-in bed scales may be needed for the intensive care unit, where daily weights are a necessity, although many frames today include scales as standard operating equipment. Advantages and disadvantages mostly depend on whether the surface is rented (discussed later in this chapter).

Chair Cushions

Pressure redistribution in the chair often goes overlooked. Wounds that develop from sitting are located on the ischia during upright sitting and on the sacrum when slouching, sliding, or reclining. Pressure redistribution chair cushions should be used with seated individuals who are at risk for pressure injuries and have reduced mobility (EPUAP/NPIAP/PPPIA, 2019). Selecting a cushion of appropriate size for the seated patient is extremely important given the potential for the patient to "bottom out," as most of the weight is applied to a relatively small body surface. Chair cushions are available in foam, air, and gel, and alternating pressure (AP) therapy and bariatric sizes. Once implemented, chair cushions require routine and regular inspection to monitor for wear and tear. Improper inflation, over compression, or displaced gel can impair adequate pressure redistribution and lead to bottoming out.

Ring cushion (donut) devices increase venous congestion and edema and should not be used for pressure injury prevention and management (EPUAP/NPIAP/PPPIA, 2019; WOCN®, 2016). Chapter 11 provides additional discussion related to offloading and positioning in the chair.

Active (Alternating Pressure)

An *active* support surface is a powered mattress or overlay that changes its load distribution properties with or without an applied load (NPIAP, 2019). Therefore, an active support surface moves with or without a person in the bed (Christian & Lachenbruch, 2007). Active mattresses or overlays should be selected for high-risk patients when frequent repositioning is not possible (EPUAP/NPIAP/PPPIA, 2019). Active support surfaces on the market are those that include the feature of alternating pressure (AP) therapy alone or in a hybrid (a reactive foam surface in combination with alternating pressure) form. A meta-analysis of active support surfaces demonstrated a reduced pressure injury incidence when compared with a standard foam mattress (Shi, Dumville, & Cullum, 2018). An example of an AP therapy surface is shown in Table 12.3.

Alternating pressure is a weight-shifting feature found in overlays and mattress. Alternating pressure products have cells arranged in various patterns that are inflated and deflated with air. Rather than pressure being distributed by increasing the surface area through immersion and envelopment, pressure is periodically redistributed across the body by inflating and deflating the cells of alternating zones. *Pulsating pressure* refers to shorter-duration inflation and higher-frequency cycling for which there is less direct evidence of effectiveness (Gunther & Clark, 2000). The individual cell that composes the AP mattress or overlay must be 10 cm or greater to effectively redistribute pressure (EPUAP/NPIAP/PPPIA, 2019). Air cells can inflate and deflate in multiple stages resulting in relatively gradual transitions compared with single stage cycles. Experts agree that use of either stage (single vs multiple) will assist with the prevention of partial thickness wounds. However, mattresses with the multiple stage feature are more effective in the prevention of full thickness wounds (Demarré et al., 2012, 2013; McNichol et al., 2015; Vanderwee, Grypdonck, & Defloor, 2005).

International pressure injury guidelines (EPUAP/NPIAP/PPPIA) suggest the use of an active support surface (mattress or overlay) for patients at higher risk for pressure injury development where frequent manual repositioning is not possible. Both AP mattresses and overlays have similar efficacy in terms of pressure injury incidence; no significant difference in performance has been identified (EPUAP/NPIAP/PPPIA, 2019; Nixon et al., 2006).

TABLE 12.3	**Example of Support Surface Decision-Making Tool and Formulary**
Criteria	**Support Surface**
Weight < _____ lbs AND Braden score 13–18 AND one of the following: • Intact skin AND can be effectively positioned • Patient CAN be effectively positioned off wound	Reactive support surface Example: Viscoelastic foam mattress (Visco 1) (Image courtesy of Encompass TSS)

Continued

TABLE 12.3 Example of Support Surface Decision-Making Tool and Formulary—cont'd

Criteria	Support Surface
Weight < _____ lbs AND one of the following: • Intact skin with Braden score less than 13 • Intact skin but CANNOT be effectively positioned • Patient CANNOT be effectively positioned off wound • Patient has fewer than two intact turning surfaces	Reactive support surface with features and components such as low air loss, viscous fluid or air fluids, OR active support surface (alternating pressure) Example: Low-air-loss mattress (Flexicair Eclipse Low Airloss Therapy Unit) (Image courtesy of Hill-Rom Services, Inc., © 2005) 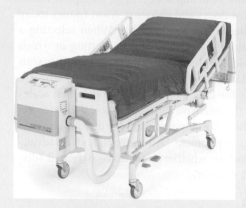
Weight > _____ lbs or BMI > _____ AND Braden score 13–18 (at risk to moderate risk) AND one of the following: • Intact skin AND can be effectively positioned • Patient CAN be effectively positioned off wound	Bariatric reactive surface Example: Bariatric with viscoelastic foam mattress (Image courtesy of Sizewise) 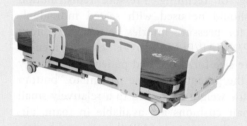
Weight > _____ lbs or BMI > _____ AND one of the following: • Intact skin with Braden score less than 13 • Intact skin but CANNOT be effectively positioned • Patient CANNOT be effectively positioned off wound • Patient has fewer than two intact turning surfaces	Bariatric reactive support surface with features and components such as low air loss, viscous fluid, or air fluids, OR active support surface (alternating pressure) Example: Bariatric with low-air-loss mattress (Image courtesy of Sizewise) 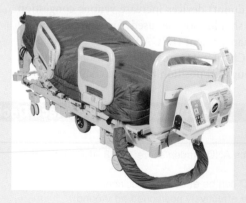

TABLE 12.3	Example of Support Surface Decision-Making Tool and Formulary—cont'd
Criteria	**Support Surface**
Effective repositioning is determined by a provider to be medically contraindicated (reevaluation/retrial at least every 8 h should be documented) *Specify bariatric option for weight > _____ lbs or BMI > ____*	Active support surface[a] Example: "Active" Therapy Mattress Replacement (Alternating) (Image courtesy of ArjoHuntleigh) 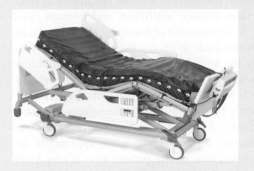
Extensive debridement or flap surgery OR patient is on bed rest and wound(s) have deteriorated on a low-air-loss surface despite optimal wound management	Air fluidized Example: Clinitron Air Fluidized Therapy (Image courtesy of Hill-Rom Services, Inc., © 2005) 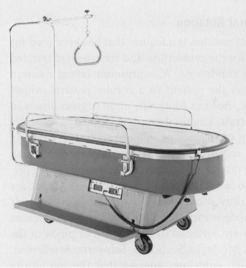
Patient meets three of the following criteria: artificial airway, PaO$_2$/FiO$_2$ <250 with FiO$_2$ >0.40, requires >10 PEEP (regardless of FiO$_2$), desaturates with manual turning, immobile/exhibits ineffective mobility, receiving neuromuscular blockade therapy or continuous IV sedation, difficulty mobilizing secretions, ventilated with sepsis/ARDS	Lateral rotation Example: TriaDyne Proventa Kinetic Therapy System (Image courtesy of KCI Licensing, Inc.) 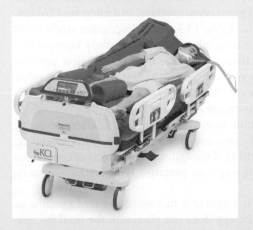

[a]Refer to active support surface (alternating pressure) section of chapter for explanation.
ARDS, acute respiratory distress syndrome; *BMI*, body mass index; *IV*, intravenous; *PaO$_2$/FiO$_2$*, ratio of arterial partial pressure to fractional inspired oxygen; *PEEP*, positive end expiratory pressure.

Reactive

A *reactive* support surface will move or change load distribution properties only in response to an applied load, such as the patient's body (Christian & Lachenbruch, 2007; NPIAP, 2019). Unlike active support surfaces that must be powered, reactive support surfaces are powered or nonpowered, with the potential to avoid the noise of a motor. Examples of reactive support surfaces include mattresses and overlays filled with foam, air, or a combination of foam and air. Gel surfaces, which may be in the form of chair cushions, overlays, mattresses and pads for stretchers, OR tables, and procedure tables, are nonpowered. Nonpowered air-filled support surfaces range from low-end prevention products that encapsulate air into a single bladder or cell to therapeutic products containing hundreds of individual interconnected cells (see Fig. 12.4). All reactive support surfaces are appropriate for pressure injury prevention in the patient who is frequently repositioned. Some are appropriate for patients with pressure injuries. With few exceptions, reactive support surfaces are compatible with long-term care facilities, hospitals, and home settings.

Continuous Lateral Rotation

Continuous lateral rotation is a feature that has been used for the past 35 years for the prevention and treatment of selected cardiopulmonary conditions. A continuous lateral rotation therapy bed rotates the patient in a regular pattern around a longitudinal (i.e., head to foot) axis of 40 degrees *or less* to each side. In contrast, kinetic therapy is defined as the side-to-side rotation of 40 degrees *or more* to each side. Drawing firm conclusions regarding effectiveness in the patient with cardiopulmonary disease is difficult, as these surfaces are primarily intended to facilitate pulmonary hygiene in the patient with acute respiratory conditions. Use of adult specialty beds in the rotation mode is ineffective for small children because their small bodies are confined to one section or pillow of the surface (McCord, Mcelvain, Sachdeva, Schwartz, & Jefferson, 2004). Additionally, guidelines suggest that the use of any adult-sized specialty bed is unsafe for neonates or children as well as ineffective (EPUAP/NPIAP/PPPIA, 2019).

Lateral rotation has been incorporated into some low-air-loss and air/foam mattresses, overlays, and integrated bed systems as shown in Table 12.3. One descriptive study of 30 patients on continuous lateral rotation therapy incorporated into a foam mattress replacement noted no new pressure injury development, with improvement of trunk and pelvis wounds (Anderson & Rappl, 2003). A Cochrane review comparing manual 30-degree repositioning to 90-degree continuous lateral rotation found no significant difference in the development of pressure injuries (Gillespie, Chaboyer, McInnes, et al., 2014). Knowledge of the effects of continuous lateral rotation therapy on pressure redistribution remains limited.

Therefore, it is important to emphasize that continuous lateral rotation therapy does not eliminate the need for routine manual repositioning. Staff will need to take extra precautions to prevent shear, including aligning and securing the patient with bolster pads that are provided by the manufacturer and frequent turning to inspect the skin for signs of shear. Optimally, if shear injury develops, the patient would be positioned off the injured area and an alternative support surface method used. However, if the patient is still in respiratory distress, the risks and benefits of continuous lateral rotation therapy should be carefully considered before making a change (EPUAP/NPIAP/PPPIA, 2019).

Low Air Loss

One commonly misunderstood feature related to support surfaces is low air loss. The NPIAP (2019) defines low air loss as a feature that provides a flow of air to assist in managing the heat and humidity (microclimate) of the skin. Low air loss consists of a series of connected pillows. A pump provides slow continuous air flow, allowing for even distribution into the porous mattress and continuous air flow across the skin (see Table 12.3). The amount of pressure in each pillow is controlled and can be calibrated according to height and weight distribution to meet the individual needs of the patient. As the patient settles down into the mattress, weight is distributed evenly for pressure redistribution. An additional component may be placed at the base of the product, such as foam or air pillows, when "bottoming out" is problematic. Low air loss can be found alone or in combination with AP, lateral rotation, and air-fluidized technology that is incorporated into overlays, mattresses, bed systems, and chair cushions.

The construction of a low-air-loss surface in addressing the microclimate of the skin can be achieved in two ways: with air flow under the cover or with an air-permeable cover. Most familiar to clinicians is the air-permeable cover that allows for the slow, evenly distributed release of air *through* the cover and directly to the skin. Low-air-loss surfaces with airflow *under* the cover address the skin microclimate by receiving heat, gas, and water molecules through a moisture vapor permeable cover (conducted downward from the skin) into the air stream inside the mattress, which eventually exits along the sides or ends of the mattress.

The smooth covers for low-air-loss surfaces are generally made of nylon or polytetrafluoroethylene fabric and have a low coefficient of friction. The covers are waterproof, impermeable to bacteria, and easy to clean. In order to receive the full benefits of low air loss, special underpads with a high level of moisture vapor permeability (rather than plastic-backed pads) should be used while minimizing the number and type of layers between the patient and the support surface (McNichol et al., 2015).

Low-air-loss support surfaces have been reported as an effective treatment surface and may improve healing rates of pressure injuries (Saha et al., 2013), while other conflicting data exists on its ability to prevent and treat pressure injuries (EPUAP/NPIAP/PPPIA, 2019). Because of the available two constructions (air-permeable cover vs air flow under the cover), low air loss is associated with decreasing moisture, thereby minimizing the risk of incontinence-associated dermatitis or maceration (Cullum et al., 2004; WOCN®, 2016). Wound desiccation, however, is also possible and may be prevented by using a moisture-donating rather than absorptive dressing if the wound begins to dry.

Low-air-loss surfaces have important safety features, such as controls that instantly inflate the cushions, thus facilitating patient positioning. Fowler boost controls help prevent bottoming out by adding more air under the buttocks when the patient's head is elevated. Controls that instantly flatten the air cushions are activated before administration of CPR so that effective chest compressions are possible.

Disadvantages to this type of surface exist. Due to the lack of stability compared with a firmer mattress, low air loss may be contraindicated for patients with an unstable spine (McNichol et al., 2015). Some patients lose their ability to effectively self-position on a low-air-loss surface, again due to the lack of firmness in the surface. Additional disadvantages of low-air-loss surfaces include increased risk of bed entrapment, especially if the device is not properly adjusted. It is imperative that clinicians and involved staff are familiar with the manufacturer's recommended instructions for use. Once the proper weight setting is established, it is prudent to record the setting to ensure consistency. Low-air-loss surfaces typically are more expensive and require electricity and special underpads costing more than the standard underpad.

Air Fluidized

The feature of air fluidization (AF) can only be found in an integrated bed system (see Table 12.3) and was initially developed to treat patients with burns. Also known as high air loss, the surface contains silicone-coated beads that become incorporated into both air and fluid support; by pumping air through the beads, the beads behave like a liquid. The person "floats" on a sheet, with one-third of the body above the surface and the rest of the body immersed in the warm, dry, fluidized beads. Body fluids flow freely through the sheet and cover, but contamination is prevented through continuous pressurization (Holzapfel, 1993). When the air-fluidized bed is turned off, it quickly becomes firm enough for repositioning or CPR.

Air-fluidized beds are commonly used for patients with burns, myocutaneous skin flaps, and multiple Stage 3 or 4 pressure injuries. Using a subset of retrospectively collected National Pressure Injury Long-Term Care Study data, Ochs, Horn, van Rijswijk, et al. (2005) compared pressure injury outcomes of 664 residents placed on several types of support surfaces, including air fluidized, low-air-loss, powered and nonpowered overlays, and hospital mattresses. Results indicated that residents placed on air-fluidized support surfaces had larger and deeper pressure injuries and higher illness severity scores than did residents placed on the other support surfaces. However, residents who used air-fluidized surfaces had better healing rates, fewer emergency visits, and fewer hospital admissions. Saha et al. (2013) reviewed five studies conducted in the 1980s and 1990s and found that air-fluidized beds produced better healing in terms of reduction in injury size compared with several nonair-fluidized surfaces. These findings, although significant, warrant more research on variables such as initial wound size, use of dressing, debridement, nutritional status, and presence of infection and incontinence.

In the institutional environment, these products are not ideally suited to facility ownership because of the complexity and the high costs of maintenance. An air-fluidized bed system is one of the most expensive support surfaces. Air-fluidized products have a warming feature for the pressurized air, which can be comforting or harmful depending on the overall condition of the patient. Hydration issues and dry skin may be more pronounced than that associated with low-air-loss surfaces. Because air-fluidized beds are heavy, they may not be safe for use in older homes. Traditional air-fluidized beds are not recommended for the patient with pulmonary disease or an unstable spine. However, air-fluidized therapy in the lower half of the bed has been combined with low air loss in the upper portion of the surface to create an adjustable bed for the patient who needs to be more upright. This bed is similar in size to a hospital bed, the head of the bed is readily adjustable, and the bed is lighter than a total air-fluidized system.

SUPPORT SURFACE SELECTION CRITERIA

Despite the lack of evidence specifying any brand of support surfaces, guidelines for selecting a support surface for specific patients are necessary to facilitate appropriate staff decision-making and proper product use. The WOCN Society offers an evidence and consensus-based algorithm. With pathways that guide clinical decision making for support surface use for pressure injury prevention or treatment. The interactive tool and related education It is available free of charge on the Internet (McNichol et al., 2015).

Because multiple forms of support surfaces with a full range of features are available, it is possible to create setting-specific formularies with options compatible with the individual needs of the typical patient population (Table 12.3). Having all stakeholders use the same glossary (Table 12.1) of terms for reference is helpful for developing formularies and site-specific algorithms.

Individual Patient Needs

Individuals with pressure injuries or those at risk for pressure injuries should be placed on a support surface rather than a standard hospital mattress (EPUAP/NPIAP/PPPIA, 2019; WOCN®, 2016). As described throughout this chapter, each support surface has disadvantages and contraindications. Therefore, support surfaces must not be selected based *solely* on the patient's wound assessment, but rather on the patient's individual needs (EPUAP/NPIAP/PPPIA, 2019; WOCN®, 2016). Individual needs of the patient with pressure injuries or who is at risk for pressure injuries are dependent on the condition and location of wounds (if applicable), activity and positioning, risk for falls and entrapment, size, weight, and patient response (McNichol et al., 2015).

For example, Rich, Shardell, Hawkes, et al. (2011) reported there was little or no preventive effect of pressure-redistributing support surfaces in the at-risk but nonbedbound ambulatory patient. The author concluded that the resources used to provide pressure-redistributing support surfaces to these individuals may be better allocated to other methods of pressure injury prevention. Critical analysis of these needs weighted with support surface indications, advantages, and disadvantages will lead to appropriate selection.

Condition and Location of Wounds

For the individual with large Stage 3 or 4 pressure injuries or pressure injuries involving multiple turning surfaces, a support surface should be considered that includes features and components such as low air loss, AP, viscous fluid, or air fluids. A support surface that dissipates moisture (low air loss) may be indicated when skin barriers and dressings do not adequately protect the skin from moisture/incontinence (Cullum et al., 2004; Whitney et al., 2006; WOCN®, 2016). As discussed in the chair cushion section of this chapter, patients with sitting-surface pressure injuries require a support surface for the chair.

Activity and Positioning

If frequent repositioning is not possible, an active support surface is indicated (EPUAP/NPIAP/PPPIA, 2019; WOCN®, 2016). Low-air-loss overlays may need to be changed to mattresses to prevent bottoming out if an elevated head of the bed for prolonged periods of time cannot be avoided. The patient who self-repositions, gets in and out of bed, or is attempting to increase and restore mobility and independence should use a support surface that facilitates rather than hinders activity and mobility.

Risk for Falls or Entrapment

A surface that raises the patient higher in the bed or creates more distance between the mattress and frame or side rails increases the risk for entrapment and falls. When possible, a pressure redistribution support surface that minimizes height and gaps should be selected for patients at risk for falls (EPUAP/NPIAP/PPPIA, 2019; US FDA, 2006). Some facilities are adding fall risk assessment scores to support surface selection criteria. If the patient becomes at risk for falls or entrapment on a selected pressure redistribution support surface, additional monitoring will be necessary or an alternative pressure redistribution support surface should be selected (McNichol et al., 2015).

Size and Weight

Bed frame and mattress specifications for weight capacity must be considered. Low-air-loss products designed for adults do not provide options to accommodate the height and weight of small children (WOCN®, 2016). Children and infants can sink into and between cushions, leading to risk for entrapment and falls (EPUAP/NPIAP/PPPIA, 2019; McLane, Bookout, McCord, et al., 2004).

Many adult hospital bed frames manufactured today hold up to 500 lbs. However, older frames may not be designed to hold more than 350 lbs and have a width that precludes the ability of obese patients to effectively reposition at any time.

Bariatric support surfaces are available in foam, air, gel, and water, with or without microclimate and moisture-control features. Care of the obese patient and bariatric support surface considerations are discussed in Chapter 36.

Patient Response

Once a product is selected, its effectiveness for any given patient must be reevaluated at regular intervals with the plan of care (Checklist 12.1, A). If expected outcomes are not achieved, an alternative support surface should be selected. Expected outcomes may include prevention of pressure injuries, patient comfort, or moisture control. Wound healing may not be an expected outcome if it is not realistic or consistent with the patient's overall goals. If wound healing is an expected outcome after support surface implementation, it must be used in conjunction with documented and comprehensive pressure injury management.

CHECKLIST 12.1   Evaluating Support Surface Effectiveness

A. Individual Needs

✓ Has there been an increase in factors that place a patient at risk for pressure injuries?
- Hemodynamic instability
- Frequent repositioning not possible
- Moisture management problems
- Increased need to keep head of the bed elevated

✓ Has the support surface caused any problems for the patient?
- Mobility impairment
- Pain or discomfort
- Sleeplessness
- Bottoming out
- Excessive dryness
- Skin breakdown

✓ Is the wound deteriorating despite appropriate care?
- Patient and caregiver education for pressure injury prevention and management
- Regular skin and risk assessment
- Appropriate turning and repositioning
- Appropriate wound care, including ongoing assessments and evaluation of healing
- Management of moisture and incontinence
- Nutritional support

B. Care-Setting Compatibility

✓ Does the formulary include enough options to meet the needs of the patient population?
✓ Do the formulary and selection criteria meet the fiscal needs of the setting?
✓ Is the staff competent with product procedures, such as set up, maintenance, and cleaning?
✓ Does the staff express overall satisfaction with the products?
✓ Is there an increase in entrapment, back injuries, or falls?
✓ Do the products conform to essential regulations?
✓ Are environmental concerns addressed?
✓ Does the company live up to promises for support and value-added services (see Table 12.4)?

The same factors that guided initial support surface selection should be reevaluated. Changes in patient status may guide the decision to discontinue or change a support surface. For example, the patient who once was comatose and hemodynamically unstable may require a different support surface to facilitate independence with self-positioning. Likewise, the patient on an overlay who was achieving expected outcomes may suddenly start bottoming out due to prolonged head-of-bed elevation because of respiratory distress. A patient on an overlay that previously was acceptable may be at increased risk for falling due to the onset of delirium.

Care Setting-Specific Formulary

A formulary of standardized products not only controls costs but also is necessary to minimize confusion and mistakes related to appropriate selection and safe use (Whittemore, 1998). Considerations for compatibility with care setting include reimbursement, renting vs owning, product maintenance, safety, and facility response and storage space capabilities. Once these considerations are analyzed, a formulary can be created with a range of products intended to meet the individual needs of the patient population. Attention must then turn to creating decision-making tools and educating staff for effective product selection and safe use. Table 12.3 provides an example of a decision-making tool to guide support surface selection. A content-validated consensus and evidence-based algorithm is available in both written form and in electronic form (McNichol et al., 2015). Two subscale scores from the Braden Scale (mobility and moisture) have been incorporated into the tool linking clinically relevant risk factors to the decision-making process.

Reimbursement

When patients covered by Medicare Part A need a support surface, hospitals and skilled nursing facilities are financially responsible for acquiring and supplying the appropriate product. Hospitals receive a diagnosis-related group payment based on patient diagnosis. Likewise, skilled nursing facilities receive payment based on the patient-driven payment model assignment for a Medicare Part A stay. Managed Medicare contracts vary in reimbursement but are inclusive of equipment and there is no extra payment to facilities or agencies using a support surface. Therefore, organizations must select the support surface that will provide the most cost-effective clinical outcome during a patient's stay.

When a patient is discharged to the home setting or converts from Medicare Part A to Medicare Part B, local coverage determination fee schedules for support surfaces take effect. According to a report from the Office of Inspector General (Levinson, 2009), inappropriate Medicare payments for group 2 support surfaces amounted to approximately $33 million during the first half of 2007. Of the 362 claims reviewed, 86% did not meet group 2 coverage criteria, 38% were undocumented, 22% were medically unnecessary, and 17% had insufficient documentation.

As a result, Medicare now requires prior authorization for support surfaces effective July 22, 2019, for California, Indiana, New Jersey, North Carolina, and all remaining states as of October 21, 2019. Support surfaces affected are outlined in Box 12.4. Prior authorization requests are submitted by a durable medical equipment (DME) to the Medicare Administrative Contractors (MACs). Chair cushions require a concomitant DME order for a wheelchair.

For approval and compliance, the provider must verify documentation in the medical record confirming that coverage requirements are met. In turn, many DME providers require signed attestation, sometimes with the actual medical record. Box 12.5 summarizes the necessary prior authorization information. In attempts to reduce fraud and waste, there is now significant preplanning required of providers and case

---

BOX 12.4 Support Surface Groupings by Durable Medical Equipment Medicare Administrative Contractors

HCPCS

Group 1 support surface
- A4640 — Replacement pad for use with medically necessary alternating pressure pad owned by patient
- E0181 — Powered pressure reducing mattress overlay/pad, alternating, with pump, includes heavy duty
- E0182 — Pump for alternating pressure pad, for replacement only
- E0184 — Dry pressure mattress
- E0185 — Gel or gel-like pressure pad for mattress, standard mattress length and width
- E0186 — Air pressure mattress
- E0187 — Water pressure mattress
- E0188 — Synthetic sheepskin pad
- E0189 — Lambswool sheepskin pad, any size
- E0196 — Gel pressure mattress
- E0197 — Air pressure pad for mattress, standard mattress length and width
- E0198 — Water pressure pad for mattress, standard mattress length and width
- E0199 — Dry pressure pad for mattress, standard mattress length and width
- E0272 — Mattress, foam rubber

Group 2 support surfaces
- E0193 — Powered air flotation bed (low air loss therapy)
- E0277 — Powered pressure-reducing air mattress
- E0371 — Nonpowered advanced pressure reducing overlay for mattress, standard mattress length and width
- E0372 — Powered air overlay for mattress, standard mattress length and width
- E0373 — Nonpowered advanced pressure reducing mattress

Group 3 support surface
- E0194 — Air fluidized bed

BOX 12.5   Support Surface Prior Authorization Requirements

- Patient's name, Medicare beneficiary number, date of birth, and address
- Supplier's name, National Supplier Clearinghouse (NSC) number, National Provider Identifier (NPI) number, address and phone number
- Provider (requestor) name, address, phone number, and NPI
- Submission date and associated Healthcare Common Procedure Coding System (HCPCS) code
- Indication of request type: initial or resubmission review and if expedited review is requested, the reason why
- A detailed written order
- Medical record documentation to support the necessity of requested item
- A prior authorization request cover sheet (available on the DME MAC website specific to the patient's coverage area)
- Documentation that the patient meets at least one of the three following criteria:
  - Multiple Stage 2 pressure ulcers on the trunk or pelvis failing to improve over the last 30 days, during which the

patient has been on a comprehensive ulcer treatment program including:
  - A Group 1 Support Surface and
  - Regular assessment by a nurse, physician, or other licensed healthcare professional and
  - Appropriate turning and repositioning and
  - Appropriate wound care and
  - Appropriate management of moisture/incontinence and
  - Nutritional assessment and intervention consistent with the plan of care
- Large or multiple Stage 3 or 4 pressure ulcer(s) on trunk or pelvis
  OR
  A myocutaneous flap or skin graft for a pressure ulcer on the trunk or pelvis within the past 60 days and having been on a Group 2 or Group 3 support surface immediately prior to discharge from a hospital or a nursing facility within the last 30 days.

---

managers when transitioning patients to the home health setting as well as from Medicare Part A to Medicare Part B stays to avoid delays or denials in support surface therapy, though expedited reviews are available. It is too early in the process to evaluate or perform research regarding the impact on outcomes as a result of this policy.

When possible, selecting a support surface that matches the needs of the patient *and* meets Reimbursement criteria would be ideal for patients making the challenging transition from the hospital or long-term care to home. Reimbursement criteria change as technology and knowledge about support surfaces and wounds evolve. It is important to contact insurance companies, health maintenance organizations/Managed Medicare, Medicaid, and Medicare and DME MACs for the most up-to-date information. Payer sources change as the patient moves through the continuum of care, and it is critical that the clinician work with the appropriate liaisons and provide documentation stating the rationale for product selections.

Renting (Leasing)

For many facilities, renting support surfaces is the best option. Renting enables access to the most current technology free of any concerns about the need to update equipment. Renting support surfaces places the responsibility of maintenance and much of the liability for malfunctioning equipment with the rental company. Companies that rent equipment must provide or facilitate in-services to educate the staff on safety issues and proper use of the equipment. Rental costs may be as variable as the technology and customer service, ranging from as little as a few dollars up to $150 per day. Some health care agencies negotiate individual contracts with manufacturers, based on the volume of product used. However, it is important to choose a rental company that is compatible with more than just the financial needs of the facility. Table 12.4

provides a list of customer service-related items to consider during contract negotiation.

Purchasing (Owning)

Advantages of owning support surface equipment include improved accessibility, decreased lead time for implementation, and potential decrease in rental expenses, particularly for critical care and bariatric surfaces. Before purchasing a product, the warranty information, guidelines for weight limit, set up, maintenance, and cleaning should be analyzed. Some frames of complete bed systems are not designed to accommodate certain mattresses. This will clearly restrict options for the facility's support surface formulary and usually more than once because frames tend to last longer than mattresses. However, many bed frame manufacturers have an "open architecture" design in which any mattress will fit the frame, allowing the clinician to choose the frame and the mattress that will best meet the needs of the patient population while opening up the possibility of mattress replacements as technology and patient needs evolve. Once the facility owns the equipment, it is responsible for storage, set up, cleaning, and maintenance, which can be resource intensive for certain products or a safety/liability issue when the product is inadequately executed. Any cost analysis before purchase should consider these potential and actual financial consequences.

Product Maintenance and Safety

Keeping patients safe on a support surface is accomplished by making appropriate equipment selections; establishing proper setup, monitoring, and maintenance; facilitating optimal pressure redistribution capacity; and maintaining the barrier to environmental hazards such as fire and infectious body fluids. Maintenance requirements of support surfaces

TABLE 12.4 Negotiating Rental Contracts/Service Expectations

Company Service Provided	Examples
Product standardization	All low-air-loss mattresses have the CPR lever in one standard place (e.g., left side of foot of bed)
Standardized delivery and pickup times	2–4 h
Safety and quality check on all units before product delivery	Flammability Product integrity (infection control/hygiene) Entrapment Labeling Biocompatibility Weight/weight capacity (maximum weight limits, safe working loads) Product expiration/lifespan
Conservation of the environment	Recycling of packaging materials Disposal and recycling of product Product is free from known harmful chemicals (PVC, DEHP, mercury, latex, etc.) Disclose all materials that compose product content/mattress core
Troubleshooting information accessible to all	Troubleshooting guides affixed to product 24-h Phone number for questions affixed to product
Daily rounds on beds by consistent and knowledgeable staff	Check whether product is in working order, appropriate labels/instructions are present and legible, patient is comfortable and is not bottoming out, timely staff education (review CPR procedures, appropriate linens, pads, etc.), interaction of surface to other products/supplies (frame, underpads, etc.)
Education	Timely in-services during daily rounds as previously described, education per 24/7 hotline calls, group in-services (orientation, yearly reviews)

CPR, cardiopulmonary resuscitation; *DEHP*, diethylhexyl phthalate; *PVC*, polyvinyl chloride.

vary by design, composition, and technology. For example, support surfaces with heel zones or head zones must be placed on the bed frame in a specific orientation. Others must be turned (or flipped) regularly to maintain efficacy and checked for wear, proper inflation, and resilience. Repairing or replacing loose or broken side rails, bed controls, and CPR levers (where applicable) will help to prevent some occurrences of entrapment and falls.

Inspecting and Replacing Support Surfaces

A system should be in place to verify that the support surface is being used within its functional lifespan, as indicated by the manufacturer's recommended test method (or industry-recognized test method) *before* use of the support surface (EPUAP/NPIAP/PPPIA, 2019). Due to infection-control concerns, the expected life of a support surface cover may differ from that of the mattress itself (US FDA, 2017).

Many facilities date the support surface before it is used for the first time with indelible ink and in a consistent location, so the date can be routinely checked for the manufacturer's specified lifespan. This process not only protects the patient from ineffective, damaged, or contaminated products, but it also may save money when a warranty for nonexpired products applies. Some warranties allow for full mattress replacement as indicated over a specified timeframe. Others are prorated according to the age of the product. Some of the more complicated support surfaces may require a different process that includes accessible personnel with bioengineering expertise to maintain, repair, and troubleshoot the product.

Irrespective of manufacturer's specified lifespan, staff who have ongoing exposure to support surfaces during bedding or room changes should practice continual awareness and opportunity-based observation of support surface life expectancy. This can include, but is not limited to, nursing staff, certified nursing assistants, housekeeping, engineering, and maintenance personnel. Indicators for expired lifespan include reduced height or thickness; discoloration; altered integrity of cover, seams, zipper/zipper cover flap, or backing; degradation of internal components; or presence of odor. If any of these are observed, it is recommended that the support surface performance verification is conducted by the manufacturer, or by hospital staff trained in the use of industry recognized test methods (EPUAP/NPIAP/PPPIA, 2019).

Additionally, the FDA is concerned that fluid ingress from worn or damaged medical bed mattress covers may be widespread and largely underrecognized by health care providers, health care facility staff, and caregivers. From January 2011 to January 2013, the FDA received 458 reports associated with medical bed mattress covers failing to prevent blood and body fluids from leaking into the mattress (fluid ingress). Fluid ingress may occur if mattress covers become worn or damaged from small holes or rips in the fabric or from incorrect cleaning, disinfecting, and laundering procedures. The zipper on the cover may also allow fluid to penetrate the mattress. Some reports indicate that if blood and body fluids from one patient penetrate a mattress, they can later leak out from the mattress when another patient is placed on the bed. Patients are at risk for infection if they encounter blood and body fluids from other patients. The FDA also recommends developing an inspection plan to (1) check the expected life of the medical bed mattress and the mattress cover; (2) create an inspection plan for all medical bed mattresses in the facility; and (3) contact the medical bed mattress cover manufacturer for any additional questions (Sivek & Davis, 2018). Checklist 12.2 contains items that may be used to identify reduced lifespan and infection-control concerns.

Evaluation of Outcomes

Factors to consider when evaluating a care setting-specific formulary are listed in Checklist 12.1, B. Successful implementation and ongoing use of any product will be dependent on compliance with standardization, manufacturer's customer service, effectiveness of staff education on selection criteria, and staff competency with product use, especially safety features such as CPR levers, maximum inflate mode, and other bed controls.

CHECKLIST 12.2 Inspection of Support Surfaces

Areas to inspect:
✓ On, around, and under support surface cover
✓ Mattress (over, under, and all sides)
✓ Seams
✓ Zippers
✓ Attached components if applicable (pumps, cords, plugs, etc.)

Indicators to look for:
✓ Reduced mattress height or height <_____ (as specified by the manufacturer)
✓ Reduced thickness
✓ Moisture or soiling (stains, odor, wet spots)
✓ Altered integrity (cuts, tears, cracks, pinholes, snags)
✓ Degradation of internal components
✓ Expired lifespan of mattress or cover according to manufacturer specification[a]

[a] Failure to follow the manufacturer's instructions may result in skin damage and may be a source of liability.

CLINICAL CONSULT

A: Referral received to evaluate redness on sacrum. Patient is a 66-year-old female on the geriatric unit with 12 × 20 cm area of mixed blanching and nonblanching sacral erythema. Noted bottoming out with head of bed consistently over 30 degrees due to choking and dysphagia following a mild cerebrovascular accident.
D: Stage 1 pressure injury due to pressure and shear.
P: Implement appropriate interventions to address pressure injury risk factors.

I: (1) Replace current support surface with low-air-loss mattress replacement (not an overlay) to reduce shear/pressure and provide moisture management. (2) Protect heels with offloading heel boots. (3) Encourage/engage family to notify the staff and the wound team if any further skin changes occur.
E: Nurses to reassess daily and reconsult wound specialist if erythema does not decrease in dimensions.

SUMMARY

- Well-designed clinical research on the effectiveness of various support surface devices is still needed.
- The NPIAP's Support Surface Initiative has focused efforts on the testing and reporting of criteria such as immersion, envelopment, and microclimate as they relate to support surfaces.
- Ideally, clinical trials should measure the effects of a specific support surface on outcomes such as incidence, comfort, cost, and satisfaction. Sample sizes should be appropriate to allow for the most relevant and meaningful type of statistical analysis.

- It is the responsibility of health care providers involved in product selection to maintain up-to-date knowledge regarding factors relevant to support surface selection. The prudent wound specialist must be familiar with the operation, indications, and contraindications and reimbursement/payment mechanisms of the specialty support surface products in the facility, the agency, or the patient's home.

SELF-ASSESSMENT QUESTIONS

1. Which is the best rationale for obtaining a pressure redistribution mattress?
   a. The patient has a pressure injury on both trochanters and sacrum.

   b. A nurse requests a lateral rotation low air-loss bed because he does not have enough time to turn his patient every 2 h.
   c. The patient is on a ventilator.
   d. Both a and c.

2. Which of the following is the most appropriate intervention for a Stage 2 ischial tuberosity pressure injury?
   a. Pressure redistribution mattress
   b. Pressure redistribution chair cushion
   c. Bed rest
   d. Wound culture

3. What patient safety item should healthcare providers assess when a patient is on a support surface?
   a. Entrapment
   b. Worn covers that may expose patient to infectious fluids via fluid ingress
   c. Mattress height affecting safe transfer
   d. All of the above

4. A key property of a reactive surface is:
   a. Only pertains to wheelchair support surfaces with an applied load
   b. Changes its pressure redistribution properties only in response to an applied load of a certain weight
   c. Changes its pressure redistribution properties only in response to an applied load
   d. Only pertains to powered support surfaces

5. Support surfaces come with different characteristics. These include:
   a. Physical components and nontherapeutic functions
   b. Physical components and therapeutic functions
   c. Nonphysical components and therapeutic functions
   d. Nonphysical components and therapeutic functions

REFERENCES

Anderson, C., & Rappl, L. (2003). Lateral rotation mattresses for wound healing. *Journal of wound, ostomy and continence. Nursing, 30*(3). https://doi.org/10.1097/00152192-200305000-00088.

Association of periOperative Registered Nurses (AORN). (2016). *Care of the older adult in perioperative settings [position statement].* https://www.aorn.org/docs/default-source/guidelines-resources/position-statements/patient-care/posstat-patients-older-adults373f019a-0a13-48f2-8f60-874dd4c5623b.pdf?sfvrsn=a1de65e2_1 (March 13, 2023).

Association of periOperative Registered Nurses (AORN). (2017). Guideline for positioning the patient. In *Guidelines for perioperative practice.* Denver, CO: AORN, Inc.

Australian Wound Management Association (2012). Pan Pacific clinical practice guideline for the prevention and management of pressure injury. Cambridge Media Osborne Park, WA: Retrieved 3/8/23 from: https://www.awma.com.au/files/publications/2012_awma_pan_pacific_guidelines.pdf.

Brienza, D. M., & Geyer, M. J. (2005). Using support surfaces to manage tissue integrity. *Advances in Skin & Wound Care, 18*(3), 151–157. https://doi.org/10.1097/00129334-200504000-00013.

Chou, R., Dana, T., Bougatsos, C., et al. (2013). *Pressure ulcer risk assessment and prevention: Comparative effectiveness.* Rockville, Maryland: Agency for Healthcare Research and Quality (US). 2013 May. (Comparative Effectiveness Reviews, No. 87.) https://www.ncbi.nlm.nih.gov/books/NBK143579/ (Retrieved: March 13, 2023).

Christian, W., & Lachenbruch, C. (2007). Standardizing the language of support surfaces. *Remington Rep, 15*(3), 11–14.

Cullum, N., McInnes, E., Bell-Syer, S. E., & Legood, R. (2004). Support surfaces for pressure ulcer prevention. *The Cochrane Database of Systematic Reviews, 3.* CD001735. ISSN 1469-493X https://doi.org/10.1002/14651858.CD001735.pub2.

Cullum, N., Nelson, E. A., Flemming, K., et al. (2001). Systematic reviews of wound care management: Beds; compression; laser therapy, therapeutic ultrasound, electrotherapy and electromagnetic therapy. *Health Technology Assessment, 5*(9), 1–221.

Defloor, T., Bacquer, D. D., & Grypdonck, M. H. (2005). The effect of various combinations of turning and pressure reducing devices on the incidence of pressure ulcers. *International Journal of Nursing Studies, 42*(1), 37–46. https://doi.org/10.1016/j.ijnurstu.2004.05.013.

Demarré, L., Beeckman, D., Vanderwee, K., Defloor, T., Grypdonck, M., & Verhaeghe, S. (2012). Multi-stage versus single-stage inflation and deflation cycle for alternating low pressure air mattresses to prevent pressure ulcers in hospitalised patients: A randomised-controlled clinical trial. *International Journal of Nursing Studies, 49*(4), 416–426. https://doi.org/10.1016/j.ijnurstu.2011.10.007.

Demarré, L., Verhaeghe, S., Hecke, A. V., Grypdonck, M., Clays, E., Vanderwee, K., et al. (2013). The effectiveness of three types of alternating pressure air mattresses in the prevention of pressure ulcers in Belgian hospitals. *Research in Nursing & Health, 36*(5), 439–452. https://doi.org/10.1002/nur.21557.

European Pressure Ulcer Advisory Panel, National Pressure Injury Advisory Panel, Pan Pacific Pressure Injury Alliance. (2019). In E. Haesler (Ed.), *Prevention and treatment of pressure ulcers/injuries.* Osborne Park, Western Australia: Cambridge Media.

Gillespie, B. M., Chaboyer, W. P., McInnes, E., et al. (2014). Repositioning for pressure ulcer prevention in adults. *Cochrane Database of Systematic Reviews, 4.* Art. No.: CD009958. https://doi.org/10.1002/14651858.CD009958.pub2.

Gray, D., Cooper, P. J., & Stringfellowe, S. (2001). Evaluating pressure-reducing foam mattresses and electric bed frames. *British Journal of Nursing, 10*(Sup 5). https://doi.org/10.12968/bjon.2001.10.sup5.12324.

Gunther, R. A., & Clark, M. (2000). The effect of a dynamic pressure-redistributing bed support surface upon systemic lymph flow and composition. *Journal of Tissue Viability, 10,* 10–15. https://doi.org/10.1016/s0965-206x(00)80033-9.

Holzapfel, S. K. (1993). Support surfaces and their use in the prevention and treatment of pressure ulcers. *Journal of Wound Ostomy & Continence Nursing, 20*(6), 251–260. https://doi.org/10.1097/00152192-199311000-00009.

Huang, H. Y., Chen, H. L., & Xu, X. J. (2013). Pressure-redistribution surfaces for prevention of surgery-related pressure ulcers: A meta-analysis. *Ostomy/Wound Management, 59*(4), 36–48.

Junkin, J., & Gray, M. (2009). Are pressure redistribution surfaces or heel protection devices effective for preventing heel pressure ulcers? *Journal of Wound Ostomy & Continence Nursing, 36*(6), 602–608. https://doi.org/10.1097/won.0b013e3181be282f.

Le, K. M., Madsen, B. L., Barth, P. W., et al. (1984). An in-depth look at pressure sores using monolithic silicon pressure sensors. *Plastic and Reconstructive Surgery, 74*(6), 745–756.

Levinson, D. (2009). *Inappropriate Medicare payments for pressure reducing support surfaces.* Department of Health and Human

Services, Office of Inspector General (OIG). https://oig.hhs.gov/oei/reports/oei-02-07-00420.pdf (Retrieved: March 13, 2020).

Levy, A., & Gefen, A. (2017). Assessment of the biomechanical effects of prophylactic sacral dressings on tissue loads: A computational modeling analysis. *Ostomy/Wound Management, 63*(10), 48–55.

Mackey, D. (2005). Support surfaces: Beds, mattresses, overlays—Oh my! *Nursing Clinics of North America, 40*(2), 251–265. https://doi.org/10.1016/j.cnur.2004.09.

McCord, S., Mcelvain, V., Sachdeva, R., Schwartz, P., & Jefferson, L. S. (2004). Risk factors associated with pressure ulcers in the pediatric intensive care unit. *Journal of Wound Ostomy & Continence Nursing, 31*(4), 179–183. https://doi.org/10.1097/00152192-200407000-00005.

McInnes, E., Jammali-Blasi, A., Bell-Syer, S. E. M., Dumville, J. C., Middleton, V., & Cullum, N. (2015). Support surfaces for pressure ulcer prevention. *Cochrane Database of Systematic Reviews, 9*. Art. No.: CD001735. https://doi.org/10.1002/14651858.CD001735.pub5.

McInnes, E., Jammali-Blasi, A., Bell-Syer, S. E. M., & Leung, V. (2018). Support surfaces for treating pressure ulcers. *Cochrane Database of Systematic Reviews, 10*. Art. No.: CD009490. https://doi.org/10.1002/14651858.CD009490.pub2.

McLane, K. M., Bookout, K., McCord, S., et al. (2004). The 2003 national pediatric pressure ulcer and skin breakdown prevalence survey: A multisite study. *Journal of Wound, Ostomy, and Continence Nursing, 31*(4), 168–178.

McNichol, L., Watts, C., Mackey, D., et al. (2015). Identifying the right surface for the right patient at the right time: Generation and content validation of an algorithm for support surface selection. *Journal of Wound, Ostomy, and Continence Nursing, 42*(1), 19–37.

Miller, S., Parker, M., Blasiole, N., et al. (2013). A prospective, in vivo evaluation of two pressure-redistribution surfaces in healthy volunteers using pressure mapping as a quality control instrument. *Ostomy/Wound Management, 59*(2), 44–48.

National Clinical Guideline Centre (UK). (April 2014). *The prevention and management of pressure ulcers in primary and secondary care*. London: National Institute for Health and Care Excellence (UK). (NICE Clinical Guidelines, No. 179.) 12, Pressure redistributing devices https://www.ncbi.nlm.nih.gov/books/NBK333135/ (Retrieved March 13, 2023).

National Pressure Injury Advisory Panel (NPIAP). (2019). *NPIAP support surface standards initiative: Terms and definitions related to support surfaces*. https://cdn.ymaws.com/npiap.com/resource/resmgr/terms_and_defs_nov_21_2019_u.pdf (Retrieved: March 13, 2023).

Nicholson, G. P., Scales, J. T., Clark, R. P., et al. (1999). A method for determining the heat transfer and water vapour permeability of patient support systems. *Medical Engineering & Physics, 21*(10), 701–712.

Nixon, J., Cranny, G., Iglesias, C., Nelson, E. A., Hawkins, K., Phillips, A., et al. (2006). Randomised, controlled trial of alternating pressure mattresses compared with alternating pressure overlays for the prevention of PRESSURE ulcers: PRESSURE (pressure relieving support surfaces) trial. *BMJ, 332* (7555), 1413. https://doi.org/10.1136/bmj.38849.478299.

Ochs, R. F., Horn, S. D., van Rijswijk, L., et al. (2005). Comparison of air-fluidized therapy with other support surfaces used to treat pressure ulcers in nursing home residents. *Ostomy/Wound Management, 51*(2), 38–68.

Oliveira, K. F. D., Nascimento, K. G., Nicolussi, A. C., et al. (2017). Support surfaces in the prevention of pressure ulcers in surgical patients: An integrative review. *International Journal of Nursing Practice, 23*(4). https://doi.org/10.1111/ijn.1255.

Reger, S. I., McGovern, T. F., Chung, K. C., et al. (1988). Correlation of transducer systems for monitoring tissue interface pressures. *Journal of Clinical Engineering, 13*(5), 365–371.

Rich, S. E., Shardell, M., Hawkes, W. G., et al. (2011). Pressure-redistributing support surface use and pressure ulcer incidence in elderly hip fracture patients. *Journal of the American Geriatrics Society, 59*(6), 1052–1059.

Saha, S., Smith, M. E. B., Totten, A., et al. (May 2013). *Pressure ulcer treatment strategies: Comparative effectiveness (AHRQ publication no. 13-EHC003-EF)*. Rockville, MD: Agency for Healthcare Research and Quality.

Shi, C., Dumville, J. C., & Cullum, N. (2018). Support surfaces for pressure ulcer prevention: A network meta-analysis. *PLoS One, 13*(2), e0192707. https://doi.org/10.1371/journal.pone.0192707re.

Sivek, A., & Davis, J. (2018). How wet is your patient's bed? Blood, urine, and microbiological contamination of mattresses and mattress covers. *Pennsylvania Patient Safety Advisory, 15*(4).

Soppi, E., Lehtio, J., & Saarinen, H. (2015). An overview of polyurethane foams in higher specification foam mattresses. *Ostomy/Wound Management, 61*(2), 38–46.

US Food and Drug Administration (FDA). (2006). *Hospital bed system dimensional and assessment guidance to reduce entrapment*. https://www.fda.gov/regulatory-information/search-fda-guidance-documents/hospital-bed-system-dimensional-and-assessment-guidance-reduce-entrapment (Retrieved: March 13, 2023).

US Food and Drug Administration (FDA). (2017). Covers for hospital bed mattresses: learn how to keep them safe. Retrieved 3/13/23 from: https://www.fda.gov/medical-devices/hospital-beds/covers-hospital-bed-mattresses-learn-how-keep-them-safe.

Vanderwee, K., Grypdonck, M. H. F., & Defloor, T. (2005). Effectiveness of an alternating pressure air mattress for the prevention of pressure ulcers. *Age and Ageing, 34*(3), 261–267. https://doi.org/10.1093/ageing/afi057.

Walton-Geer, P. S. (2009). Prevention of pressure ulcers in the surgical patient. *AORN Journal, 89*(3), 538–552. https://doi.org/10.1016/j.aorn.2008.12.022.

Whitney, J., Phillips, L., Aslam, R., et al. (2006). Guidelines for the treatment of pressure ulcers. *Wound Repair and Regeneration, 14* (6), 663–679.

Whittemore, R. (1998). Pressure-reduction support surfaces. *Journal of Wound Ostomy & Continence Nursing, 25*(1), 6–25. https://doi.org/10.1097/00152192-199801000-00005.

Wound, Ostomy and Continence Nurses Society™ (WOCN®). (2016). *Guideline for prevention and management of pressure ulcers/injuries. WOCN clinical practice guideline series 2*. Mount Laurel, NJ: WOCN®.

FURTHER READING

FDA. (2014). FDA warns of infection control risks from mattress covers. Retrieved 3/8/23 from https://www.linkedin.com/pulse/20141013093156-4574377-fda-warns-of-infection-control-risks-from-mattress-covers.

National Pressure Injury Advisory Panel. (2015). *Hand check method: Is it an effective method?*. Retrieved from https://cdn.ymaws.com/npuap.site-ym.com/resource/resmgr/position_statements/hand-check-position-statemen.pdf (Retrieved: March 8, 2023).

Polyurethane Foam Association. (1994). *Joint industry foam standards and guidelines. Indentation force deflection (IFD) standards and guidelines*. https://pfa.org/glossary/. https://pfa.org/industry-standards/ (Retrieved: March 8, 2023).

13

Lower Extremity Assessment

JoAnn Ermer-Seltun

OBJECTIVES

1. Identify critical assessment parameters of the lower extremity physical assessment.
2. For each indicator used to assess perfusion, describe the techniques and results.
3. Identify two methods for describing lower extremity edema.

4. Compare and contrast assessment parameters indicative of lower extremity venous disease (LEVD) and lower extremity arterial disease (LEAD).

More than 80%–90% of chronic lower extremity ulcers are linked to venous disease (Nelson & Adderley, 2016; WOCN®, 2019a, 2019b) and affect over 0.06%–2% of the global population (O'Donnell, Passman, Marston, et al., 2014). In the United States, Rice et al. (2014a, 2014b) reported that over $14 billion is spent annually for the care of venous leg ulcers (VLU) with the average direct expenditure to treat one VLU $15,732 (Ma et al., 2019). Individuals with diabetes have a 19%–34% incidence rate (Lazzarini, Pacella, Armstrong, & van Netten, 2018) of developing a diabetic foot ulcer (DFU) in their lifetime with a 40% reoccurrence within a year (Armstrong, Boulton, & Bus, 2017), leading to a substantial economic impact of $9–13 billion dollar cost to private and public payers (Rice et al., 2014a, 2014b). Moreover, those who develop a DFU, 50% will also suffer lower extremity arterial disease (LEAD) which often goes unrecognized until the individual presents with significant deterioration of the ulcer unfortunately, leading to hospitalization or even limb loss (Hinchliffe, Forsythe, Apelqvist, et al., 2019). These statistics are alarming and reflect a silent but major threat to public health and the financial system. Most of these wounds are chronic in nature, affect the individual's quality of life, drain monetary and health care resources, and may even progress to possible limb loss if not managed appropriately (Jarbrink, Ni, Sonnergren, et al., 2017; Olsson, Järbrink, et al., 2019; Sen, 2019). The key to successful prevention and management of any lower extremity ulcer is an insightful assessment to first identify individuals at risk for or with existing lower extremity ulcers and treatment modalities that properly address the

pathologic factors. The etiologic features of a lower extremity wound can include numerous diseases, infection, trauma, drugs, insect bites, pressure, or a combination thereof. Therefore, the wound specialist must be knowledgeable regarding clinical presentation and skilled in differential assessment. Critical assessment parameters are listed in Checklists 13.1 and 13.2 and described in this chapter.

GENERAL APPEARANCE OF THE LIMB

The wound specialist must become familiar with, and proficient in, using proper descriptive dermatologic terms to illustrate primary or secondary lesions, the pattern of distribution, and the arrangement of lesions or other abnormalities. Careful description often leads the examiner to a specific disease state. Limb appearance should be compared with that of the contralateral limb to identify or rule out trophic changes reflected in the wasting of the skin, hair, and nails. With the patient's shoes and socks off, the wound specialist should visually assess both extremities for varicosities, color, pigmentation, turgor, texture, dryness, fissures, hair distribution, calluses, abnormal nails, fungus, bunions, corns, bony deformities, and skin integrity (Botros, Kuhnke, Embil, et al., 2021; Bus, Lavery, Monteiro-Soares, et al., 2019; WOCN®, 2014, 2019a, 2019b, 2021). The web between the toes should be assessed for hygiene issues (Beuscher, 2019).

CHECKLIST 13.1 Lower Extremity Physical Assessment

General appearance
✓ Trophic changes
✓ Hair, nail, and skin patterns
✓ Veins
✓ Skin color, shape, texture, and integrity
✓ Edema

Functional sensory status
✓ Range of motion of ankle joint
✓ Protective sensation
✓ Vibration
✓ Deep tendon reflexes
✓ Pain

Perfusion
✓ Elevational pallor or dependent rubor
✓ Skin temperature
✓ Blood flow (bruit/thrill)
✓ Capillary refill
✓ Venous fill time
✓ Pulses
✓ Ankle-brachial index (ABI)

CHECKLIST 13.2 Diagnostic Tests for the Lower Extremities

Noninvasive tests for LEAD
✓ ABI
✓ Toe-brachial index (TBI)
✓ Transcutaneous partial pressure of oxygen (TcPO$_2$)
✓ Duplex imaging of arteries
✓ Skin perfusion pressure
✓ Pulse volume recording and Doppler waveform study
✓ Segmental limb pressure measurements
✓ Magnetic resonance imaging

Invasive tests for LEAD
✓ Computed tomographic angiography
✓ Arteriography

Noninvasive test for LEVD
✓ Duplex imaging of the veins

LEAD, lower extremity arterial disease; *LEVD*, lower extremity venous disease.

Trophic Changes

Trophic changes can occur when diminished blood flow can no longer support normal growth and development of the skin, hair, and nails. For example, thin and shiny epidermis, loss of hair growth, and thickened nails are often associated with, but are not diagnostic of, LEAD (WOCN®, 2014). Conversely, edema, hyperpigmentation scaly and eczematous skin, and varicosities (dilated, swollen, and torturous) may be indicative of lower extremity venous disease (LEVD) (WOCN®, 2019a, 2019b).

Trophic changes, however, are not definitive indicators of disease. Patterns of hair growth are affected by age, ethnicity, and perfusion status, as hair growth may be diminished or absent in the elderly and certain ethnic groups. Nail growth is also affected by factors other than perfusion, including age, nutritional status, and fungal infections.

Appearance of Veins

The leg should be visually inspected or palpated for dilated veins, especially along the saphenous vein, beginning at the medial marginal vein on the dorsum of the foot and terminating at the femoral vein (about 3 cm below the inguinal ligament). Normally, healthy distended veins can only be visualized at the foot and ankle; the presence of dilated veins anywhere else on the leg may imply venous pathology and often is the first sign of venous insufficiency. *Dilated veins*, or *varicose veins*, are dark blue to purplish, enlarged, and easily seen and palpated on the surface of the skin. Often described as tortuous or rope-like, varicose veins (diameter >3 mm) can be present from the upper thigh to the ankle but most often are found on the back of the calf or on the inner aspect of the leg. *Reticular veins* are smaller than varicose veins (1–3 mm diameter) and are frequently seen on the back aspect of leg especially in the popliteal region. Reticular veins have a ropey appearance and are bluish in color. These veins feed into even smaller vessels (*<1 mm diameter*), called spider veins or *telangiectasias* (Plate 6L). Telangiectasias are fine, dilated capillaries that look "spiderweb" like thus earning its spider vein nickname. The color varies from red to blue hues, lacking bulge or tenderness with palpation and can be located anywhere on the lower extremity. Corona phlebectatica (malleolar or ankle flare) consists of a cluster of intradermal red and blue dilated telangiectasias and venules usually near the medial ankle and may extend into the plantar arch that creates a fan shape or sunburst pattern, frequently perceived as an early sign of venous disease (Antignani, Carpentier, & Cornu-Thenard, 2012; Gohel, 2018).

Skin Color, Shape, and Integrity

The presence of any discoloration in the skin should be noted. For example, reddish-gray-brown (brawny) hyperpigmentation in the gaiter region, more specifically hemosiderin staining (see Plate 40), is another skin color change that should be noted. Hemosiderin staining or hemosiderosis is hailed as the "classic" sign of LEVD, but it also can be found if significant trauma has occurred to the lower extremity (WOCN®, 2019a, 2019b). This type of discoloration develops after extravasated red blood cells break down and release the pigment hemosiderin.

Atrophie blanche, also seen with LEVD, is an atrophic, thin, smooth, white plaque with a hyperpigmented border, often "speckled" with tortuous vessels, occurring near the ankle or foot. Due to its scar-like appearance, atrophie blanche is easily and often mistaken for a previously healed ulcer (see Plate 41). Its presence is considered high risk for impending ulceration.

Tiny individual reddish-purple, nonblanching discolorations on the lower extremity may be observed. When the individual discolorations are larger than 0.5 cm, they are called *purpura*; when they are smaller than 0.5 cm, they are called *petechiae*. Small blood vessels may leak under the skin and cause a blood or hemorrhagic patch that is a sign of some type of intravascular defect in individuals with normal or abnormal platelet counts. Purpura and petechiae (see Plates 42 and 43) are most often associated with LEAD (secondary to blood thinners) or vasculitis disorders such as systemic lupus erythematosus and polyarteritis nodosa. Purpura associated with vasculitis disorders is referred to as *palpable* purpura due to its raised manifestation that can be felt. Purpura that occurs in the elderly due to fragility of the vessels is known as *senile* purpura.

The presence of a condition known as *lipodermatosclerosis* (see Plate 44) should be noted as present or not present. Lipodermatosclerosis, a condition of the skin and soft tissues that develops in the presence of chronic swelling, is a progressive hardening or fibrosis of the soft tissues. Usually confined to the gaiter or "sock" area, lipodermatosclerosis may cause an inverted "champagne bottle" or "apple core" deformity of the lower extremity in sharp contrast to the unaffected leg (Beckman & Creager, 2019).

Dermatitis (see Plate 44) manifested by scaling, crusting, weeping, excoriations (linear erosions due to scratching) from intense pruritus, erythema, or inflammation should be noted. Often these symptoms of dermatitis are misdiagnosed as cellulitis (see Table 15.3). Ulcers on the lower extremity should be noted in terms of their appearance, location, size, pain, and duration (WOCN®, 2019a, 2019b).

Edema (Extent, Pattern, and Distribution)

Edema is a localized or generalized abnormal accumulation of fluid in the tissues (WOCN®, 2019a, 2019b). Numerous conditions can cause swelling of the lower extremity; examples include chronic venous disease, postphlebitic syndrome, iliac compression syndrome, lymphedema, and systemic disease such as chronic heart failure, pulmonary hypertension, and renal failure (O'Donnell et al., 2014; Trayes & Studdiford, 2013; WOCN, 2019a, 2019b). Edema causes swelling that may obscure the appearance of normal anatomy. To determine the presence of edema in the lower extremities, the appearance of one extremity should be compared with the other, noting the relative size and the prominence of veins, tendons, and bones. Edema is a significant finding in the examination of the lower extremity and should be further investigated.

Extent

Evaluating edema is challenging due to lack of objective measurement methods. One method is to have the patient sit or stand and, using a flexible tape, obtain measurements of the lower extremity at the calf and the ankle. For valid comparisons, subsequent measurements must be obtained with the patient in the same position and exact location. In order to establish a point of reference, calf circumference is obtained by first marking the largest part of the inner calf with a marker and then taking a measurement from the floor up to this mark (in centimeters). This is the floor-to-calf length, and all future measurements should occur at this level. Second, the calf circumference (in centimeters) at the largest portion of the calf that was previously marked is measured. The ankle circumference is measured 5 cm above the ankle. Similarly, the floor-to-ankle length is determined by placing the tape measure at 0 cm on the floor and making a dot on the skin 5 cm above the medial malleolus and then determining the circumference of the ankle (in centimeters).

The extent of edema can also be assessed by pressing firmly but gently with the index finger for several seconds on the dorsum of each foot, behind each medial malleolus, and over the shins. Edema is "pitting" when there is a visible depression that does not rapidly refill and resume its original contour (Fig. 13.1). Severity of edema can be categorized by either estimating the depth of the indentation or the length of time for the indentation to resolve. Fig. 13.1 and Box 13.1 provide examples and definitions for the assessment of edema. For clarity, the type of scale used should be recorded (e.g., 3+ pitting edema on a 4-point scale) (Nieman, Patten, & Chung, 2013).

The perometer, which is a computerized digital scanner, can be used to measure limb volume and is particularly useful with lymphedema and fitting compression garments. The perometer uses digital infrared technology to measure the girth and volume of an extremity (Sharkey, King, Kuo, et al., 2018).

BOX 13.1 Grading Scale for Severity of Edema

1+ Slight pitting, no visible distortion
    Disappears rapidly
2+ Somewhat deeper pit than in grade 1, but no readily detectable distortion
    Disappears in 10–15 s
3+ Pit is noticeably deep and may last more than 1 min
    Dependent extremity looks fuller and swollen
4+ Pit is very deep and lasts as long as 2–5 min
    Dependent extremity is grossly distorted

Ball, J. W., Dains, J. E., & Flynn, J. A. (2019). Blood vessels. In *Seidel's guide to physical examination* (9th ed., pp. 355–372). St. Louis, MO: Mosby.

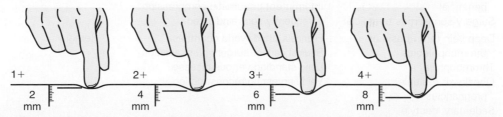

Fig. 13.1 Pitting edema may also be categorized by depth of depression. (Ball, J. W., Dains, J. E., & Flynn, J. A. (2019). Blood vessels. In *Seidel's guide to physical examination* (9th ed., pp. 355–372). St. Louis, MO: Mosby.)

Pattern and Distribution

The pattern and distribution of edema should be noted. For example, dependent edema is the accumulation of fluid in the lowest body parts, such as the feet and legs (WOCN®, 2019a, 2019b). With LEVD, dependent edema generally develops gradually, worsens with prolonged standing, and diminishes when the patient rests in a recumbent position with the legs elevated (WOCN®, 2019a, 2019b). However, the pattern of edema associated with lymphedema does not resolve with leg elevation and usually encompasses the entire leg. Another distinguishing feature of lymphedema is the presence of a positive Stemmer sign, in which a skin fold at the base of the second toe is too thick to lift. Differences in edema presentations are listed in Table 13.1. Chapter 16 provides an in-depth discussion of lymphedema.

FUNCTIONAL SENSORY STATUS

Functional assessment includes observation for impairments in ambulation, gait, balance, use of walking aids (walker, cane), and ability to remove shoes and socks. Because loss of function may be neuropathic in origin, a focused sensory examination is an essential component of any lower extremity assessment (ADA, 2019; Schaper, van Netten, Apelqvist, Bus, et al., 2019; WOCN®, 2021). Sensory assessment (the ability to feel pain, pressure, temperature changes, vibration, and friction in the lower extremities and feet) is particularly relevant to the patient with a lower extremity wound. Failure to detect touch indicates loss of protective sensation and warrants caution if compression wraps will be applied as the patient may not sense ischemic changes in a timely manner (WOCN®, 2019a, 2019b). Similarly, in patients with diabetes who also have neuropathy, motor neuropathy leads to flexion in the toes (hammer, claw, or mallet toes), flattening of the arch, fat pad loss, intrinsic or deep muscle wasting (atrophy) evidence by interdigit guttering of the dorsal foot and bones shifting that deteriorate into prominent plantar metatarsals (ADA, 2019; Botros et al., 2021). When combined with sensory (loss of sensation) and autonomic neuropathy (diminished capillary perfusion and sweat and oil gland production), a neuropathic ulcer may easily develop (ADA, 2019; Botros et al., 2021; WOCN®, 2021). In the case of LEAD, several studies confirmed peroneal nerve injury resulting in reduced nerve conduction velocity, poor functional outcomes, and loss of muscle strength in the lower extremities (WOCN®, 2014). These findings suggest that poor arterial flow has a direct harmful effect on peroneal nerve function (McDermott, Sufit, Nishida, et al., 2006). Signs of neuropathy include reduced sensation (detected by Semmes–Weinstein 5.07 monofilament) (HRSA, 2019), gait abnormalities caused by foot drop/drag, weakness of the ankles or feet, and loss of vibration (Boulton,

TABLE 13.1   Differences Between Edema, Lymphedema, and Lipedema

	Venous Edema	Lymphedema	Lipedema (Not True Edema)
Distribution	Ankle to knee May have limited foot involvement Usually unilateral	Toes to groin Usually unilateral	Ankle to groin Bilateral and symmetric
Characteristics	Pitting edema of variable severity In long-standing disease, nonpitting edema may result from tissue fibrosis	Brawny, nonpitting edema Skin and soft tissue changes common (e.g., papilloma formation and hyperkeratosis) Positive Stemmer sign (not possible to pinch fold of skin over dorsum of second toe) is early indicator Advanced disease: elephantiasis (loss of normal architecture/massive enlargement of limb)	Soft, rubbery tissue Pain on palpation common Painful bruising common Negative Stemmer sign Abnormal fat distribution from ankles to hips
Management	Elevation and compression (toes to knees) are primary approaches Intermittent pneumatic compression typically beneficial Surgery sometimes beneficial	Elevation and standard compression beneficial only in early stages Manual lymphatic drainage and inelastic compression are key elements of management Intermittent pneumatic compression frequently contraindicated	Weight loss, liposuction, but lack of evidence for long-term effect Management focus is treatment of any comorbidities, patient education, and support
Risk factors	Deep vein thrombosis or thrombophlebitis Thrombophilia Obesity or multiple pregnancies Sedentary lifestyle Calf muscle pump failure	Filariasis (third world countries) Radical cancer surgery plus radiation Long-standing venous disease Vein harvesting/reconstruction	Heredity

TABLE 13.2 Pain Assessment of Patient With Leg Ulcer

Factors to Be Assessed	TYPICAL FINDINGS		
	Venous	**Arterial**	**Neuropathic**
Characteristics	Dull Aching	Intermittent claudication Nocturnal pain Rest pain (see Box 14.3)	Burning/tingling "Shooting" "Pins and needles"
Severity	Variable Typically, moderate to severe	Variable Frequently severe	Variable Commonly severe
Exacerbating factors	Dependency Increased edema Infection	Elevation Activity Infection	Variable Inactivity sometimes a precipitating factor
Relieving factors	Elevation Edema control Reduction of bacterial burden	Dependency Rest Reduction of bacterial burden	Activity such as walking

Armstrong, Albert, et al., 2008) and deep tendon reflexes (ADA, 2019; Schaper et al., 2019). Sensorimotor assessment, foot deformities, and diabetic neuropathy are illustrated and discussed in detail in Chapters 17 and 18.

Range of Motion of the Ankle Joint

The calf muscle pump is a critical contributor to normal venous return. Normal function of the calf muscle pump is dependent on a normally moving ankle joint. A "normal" walking motion requires flexion of the ankle joint past the 90-degree position. Hence routine assessment of ankle range of motion should be incorporated into the physical assessment of a patient with known or suspected LEVD because elevated ankle stiffness has been associated with calf muscle pump impairment (Padberg, Johnston, Sisto, et al., 2004; WOCN®, 2019a, 2019b). Ankle stiffness due to edema and fibrosis should be quantified according to severity: 0 = none, 1 = reduced stiffness, and 2 = nonreducible or ankylosis (Carpentier, Cornu-Thénard, Uhf, et al., 2003). A goniometer device, often used by physical therapists to measure ankle flexion/stiffness, is an objective measurement of range of motion (Gatt & Chockalingam, 2017). Ankle joint equinus (the inability to dorsiflex the ankle joint less than 90 degrees) may occur with peripheral neuropathy. This loss of dorsiflexion can place extraordinary pressure on the sole of the foot, which in turn elevates the incidence of diabetic neuropathic ulceration (Searle, Spink, Ho, & Chuter, 2017).

Pain

Effective pain management is a critical aspect of care for any patient with an ulcer; thus the assessment must always include determination of the type and severity of pain (both baseline and procedural), exacerbating and relieving factors, and past and present attempts to manage the pain. For the patient with a lower extremity ulcer, the pain history provides additional important etiologic clues (Table 13.2). Chapter 14 describes ischemic pain that is relieved by placing the leg in a dependent position (see Box 14.3) (Gerhard-Herman, Gornik, Barrett,

et al., 2017; WOCN®, 2014). In contrast, leg pain that is relieved by elevation is more consistent with a venous etiology (WOCN®, 2019a, 2019b). The patient with diabetes who is complaining of leg pain described as "pins and needles," a shooting "electrical shock," or burning sensation that is relieved by walking probably is experiencing neuropathic pain (ADA, 2019; WOCN®, 2021). Because patients with lower extremity disease may limit walking and other activities due to discomfort and comorbidities, "classic" signs of pain may not be appreciated. Extreme pain that seems out of proportion to the type of ulcer present (hyperalgesia) or pain associated with nonpainful stimuli (allodynia) should alert the clinician to further investigate for other conditions that may lead to atypical leg wounds (Mufti, Maliyar, Syed, et al., 2020). Further discussion related to the assessment and management of pain is presented in Chapter 28.

PERFUSION

Extent of perfusion can be derived through inspection of leg temperature, position-related color changes; quality of pulses, and venous and arterial blood flow. Common noninvasive diagnostic tests used to assess perfusion include ABI, TcPO$_2$, and arterial or venous duplex ultrasound (Conte, Bradbury, Kolh, et al., 2019; Gerhard-Herman et al., 2017; Needleman et al., 2018).

Elevational Pallor and Dependent Rubor

The presence of permanent discoloration (cyanosis, dark brown to black, and pallor) of the digit and increased pain with or without ulceration may be evidence of critical digital ischemia and merits prompt investigation of the peripheral vascular system by a vascular specialist (Conte et al., 2019). Position-related color changes in one or both legs provide important information concerning adequacy of arterial perfusion.

Elevational Pallor

With the patient supine on the examination surface, the leg is raised to a 60-degree angle for 15–60 s. The color of the soles of the feet is observed. Normally, color should not change. When perfusion is impaired, pallor is observed in fair-skinned individuals and gray (ashen) hues in dark-skinned individuals (Conte et al., 2019). Box 13.2 correlates the severity of arterial occlusion with the amount of time needed for elevation pallor to occur (Ball, Dains, Flynn, & Solomon, 2019).

Dependent Rubor

As for the examination for elevational pallor, the leg is raised 60 degrees while the patient is supine on the examination surface for 15–60 ss then lowered to assess collateral blood flow (Beckman & Creager, 2019; Conte et al., 2019). The normal leg will remain a healthy color when dependent. Initially, the ischemic limb will slowly turn from white to pink and progress to a purple-red discoloration, referred to as *dependent rubor* or as reactive hyperemia. Color change occurs as a result of retention of deoxygenated blood in the dilated skin venules and arterioles. The amount of time it takes for the dependent rubor to subside reveals the severity of LEAD with >30 s suggestive of serious peripheral artery disease (Beckman & Creager, 2019). Venous fill time may be assessed simultaneously during the position-related color change assessment (see Box 13.3).

Venous Fill Time

Venous refill time is the measurement of venous blood return to the distal foot veins following leg elevation. Normal venous refill time is approximately 15–20 s (Beckman & Creager, 2019; Boyko et al., 1997). In venous disease where veins often exhibit dilation with valve incompetence, refill time may be grossly shortened, i.e., <10 s. In arterial disease, venous refill time may be normal to prolonged (>20 s) with >40 s suggestive of significant peripheral artery disease (Beckman & Creager, 2019; Boyko et al., 1997; McGee & Boyko, 1998). The test is easy to perform at bedside or in a clinic setting and is considered a significant clinical indicator for the presence of LEAD (Beckman & Creager, 2019; McGee & Boyko, 1998). Its utility may serve as a point of reference for noting abnormally fast venous refilling or grossly slow refill time as outlined in WOCN guidelines (2014, 2019a, 2019b) for venous and arterial disease. Currently, duplex ultrasound provides the most reliable diagnostic to detect venous reflux or obstruction and peripheral arterial disease if there is a high rate of suspicion. Chapters 14 and 15 discuss risk factors, assessment and management of LEVD and LEAD, respectively. Box 13.3 outlines the method of assessing venous fill time.

Skin Temperature

Skin temperature of the leg is assessed by palpating lightly with the palmar surface of the fingers and hands, moving from proximal to distal, and comparing each limb to the opposite limb (e.g., right leg with left leg). The findings of unilateral coolness and a sudden marked change from proximal to distal are possible indicators of LEAD (Conte et al., 2019). In contrast, patients with LEVD have been shown to have higher skin temperatures at the ankle (Kelechi, Good, & Mueller, 2010; WOCN®, 2019a, 2019b).

When localized inflammation occurs, a slight elevation in skin temperature (2.2°C [4°F]) at that location can be detected, referred to as *infrared dermal thermometry*. Such an elevation in skin temperature was reported to be highly predictive of impending ulceration in patients with LEVD (Sayre, Kelechi, Neal, et al., 2007) and lower extremity neuropathic disease within 7–10 days (Armstrong, Holtz-Neiderer, Wendel, et al., 2007). Numerous studies and guidelines have suggested that self-monitoring of skin temperature for patients with high-risk diabetes may reduce the incidence of ulceration by modifying activity to reduce the local inflammation (Armstrong et al., 2007; Armstrong, Lipsky, Polis, & Abramson, 2006; Bus et al., 2019; Hazenberg, van Netten, van Baal, & Bus, 2014; Lavery et al., 2004; Lavery, Higgins, Lanctot, et al., 2007; Liu, van Netten, van Baal, Bus, & van der Heijden, 2015; Schaper et al., 2019; Skafjeld et al., 2015; van Netten et al., 2016, 2014; WOCN®, 2019a, 2019b). However, further research is needed to support the use of home thermometry for patients with LEVD (Kelechi & Bonham, 2008; Kelechi, Haight, Herman, et al., 2003; Sayre et al., 2007; WOCN®, 2019a, 2019b). It should be noted that these devices are now more common in the clinical setting than when this correlation was first reported, thus making it more feasible to include this technology as a screening tool for leg ulcers.

Blood Flow (Bruit/Thrill)

Blood flow through the artery should move in a laminar flow pattern. Turbulence in the flow of arterial blood occurs when some pathology, such as a clot, compression, or fatty deposit, develops within the vessel. Velocity of blood flow will slow around the source of the turbulence and cause blood cells to adhere to the vessel lining, thus forming a clot. Turbulent blood flow through an artery may be auscultated with the bell of a stethoscope and is heard as a blowing or rushing sound, which is called a *bruit* (Beckman & Creager, 2019; Gerhard-Herman et al., 2017). The presence of a bruit is indicative of arterial narrowing. According to the American College of Cardiology and American Heart Association, the presence of a bruit is a strong indicator of LEAD (Gerhard-Herman et al., 2017). As the pitch of the bruit increases and continues through diastole so does the severity of the stenosis (Beckman & Creager, 2019). The low-frequency bruit sound may not always be heard however, turbulent blood flow may also be palpated, which is referred to as a thrill (Beckman & Creager, 2019; Gerhard-Herman et al., 2017).

Capillary Refill

The capillary bed consists of small-diameter vessels that lie between the arterial and the venous systems. The time needed for the capillary bed to fill after it is occluded by pressure (capillary refill time) gives some indication of the health of the system. Delayed capillary refill (<3 s) may indicate LEAD (Conte et al., 2019; WOCN®, 2014). However, the patient with LEAD may have normal capillary refill because the emptied vessels may refill in a retrograde manner from surrounding veins even if arterial inflow is markedly impaired or absent. Environmental factors such as temperature also may influence the speed of capillary refill; consequently, this assessment is vulnerable to considerable subjective interpretation and should be used only to confirm a clinical judgment (Gerhard-Herman et al., 2017). Box 13.4 explains how and why capillary refill time is assessed (Ball et al., 2019).

Assessment of Pulses

Pulses should be compared with the contralateral pulses and assessed in a proximal-to-distal direction. Normally pedal pulses can be palpated at both the dorsalis pedis and the posterior tibialis locations (Fig. 13.2). The presence or absence of palpable pulses is not diagnostic of LEAD (Conte et al., 2019). If pulses are palpable, the patient may still have LEAD. If pulses are not palpable, a handheld Doppler probe must be used to determine the presence or absence of pulses. This assessment tool may have the highest predictive value as to whether LEAD exists (Conte et al., 2019).

The absence of Doppler pulse usually should lead to referral. However, in healthy individuals, dorsalis pedis pulse is absent in 8.1% and posterior tibialis pulse in 2.9% and both are absent in less than 2%; hence, it is important to assess all dorsalis pedis and posterior tibialis pulses (Conte et al., 2019; Khan, Rahim, Anand, et al., 2006).

The best way to document pulses is to use descriptive terms such as *present* or *absent,* followed by clarifying terms such as *weak* or *bounding.* Box 13.5 presents a 4-point scale that describes the amplitude of the pulse (WOCN®, 2014). Because various 3- and 4-point scales are used in clinical practice, it is important to specify the type of scale used (e.g., 3+ pedal pulse on a 4-point scale).

DIAGNOSTIC TESTING

When the diagnosis is unclear or wound healing fails, diagnostic studies are indicated (WOCN®, 2014, 2019a, 2019b, 2021). Vascular referral and studies are indicated to identify the components of the vascular system involved in the disease process, the specific pathologic process, the anatomic level of the lesions or dysfunction, and the severity of dysfunction (Conte et al., 2019; WOCN®, 2014). With the exception of the ABI, these tests involve equipment that is reserved for use in a vascular laboratory by a trained technician and reviewed by a vascular radiologist or surgeon. Checklist 13.2 lists diagnostic tests used for the patient with a wound resulting from lower extremity disease. Diagnostic tests are described in detail in Chapters 14–17.

BOX 13.4 Assessment of Capillary Refill Time

- Blanch toenail bed with sustained pressure for several seconds
- Release pressure
- Observe time elapsed before nail regains full color
- In the presence of arterial occlusion, refill time will be longer than 2–3 s

Caution: Decreased temperature can prolong capillary refill time.
Ball, J. W., Dains, J. E., & Flynn, J. A. (2019). Blood vessels. In *Seidel's guide to physical examination* (9th ed., pp. 355–372). St. Louis, MO: Mosby.

BOX 13.5 Assessment of Amplitude of the Pulse

4	Bounding
3	Full, increased
2	Expected
1	Diminished, barely palpable
0	Absent, not palpable

Ball, J. W., Dains, J. E., & Flynn, J. A. (2019). Blood vessels. In *Seidel's guide to physical examination* (9th ed., pp. 355–372). St. Louis, MO: Mosby.

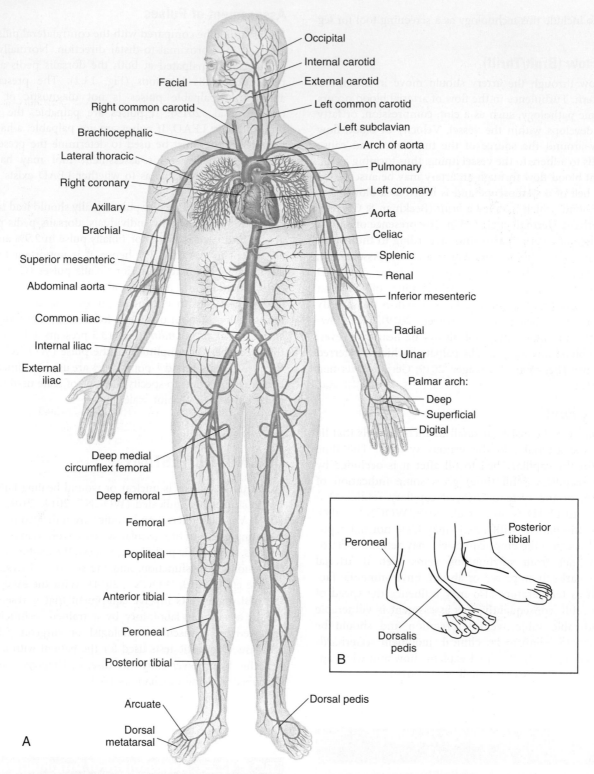

Fig. 13.2 (A) Arterial structure of lower extremity. (B) Delineates approximate location of peroneal artery, posterior tibialis, and dorsalis pedis pulses. (Ball, J. W., Dains, J. E., & Flynn, J. A. (2019). Blood vessels. In *Seidel's guide to physical examination* (9th ed., pp. 355–372). St. Louis, MO: Mosby.)

CLINICAL CONSULT

A: Referred to wound clinic by home care nurse for foot wound. Patient is a 58-year-old male, s/p colon resection, type 1 DM (A1c 7.8), coronary artery disease, hyperlipidemia, hypertension, retinopathy, and peripheral neuropathy. Patient was unaware of wound until nurse pointed it out. Patient reports previous callous in the same location. Right plantar aspect of the 5th metatarsal wound 2 × 2 cm punched out shape. Wound base 90% pale pink and 10% dry brown necrotic tissue, minimal exudate, calloused wound edges, and periwound skin intact. No local signs of infection. Bilateral legs warm, skin thin, dry, flaky, sparse hair growth below the knee, and nail discoloration. Capillary refill is >3 s. PT and DP pulses palpable but faint. No elevation pallor or dependent rubor noted. Bruit with high pitch was heard over the right femoral artery. Semmes–Weinstein 5.07 monofilament test shows loss of protective sensation. Patient states legs ache at night with periodic shooting pain that is relieved with walking. Patient reports a 10-lb weight loss since surgery.

D: Neuropathic ulceration with some level of arterial involvement. Inadequate nutrition and blood glucose management. High risk for amputation.

P: Protect feet from further pressure and trauma while minimizing potential for wound infection and ascertain level of arterial disease.

I: Home care nurse and patient understand and agree with the following plan of care: (1) Contact provider ASAP for further evaluation of arterial perfusion; recommend TBI testing due to type 1 DM causing vessel calcification. (2) Consult orthotics for custom insert and shoe to offload right 5th metatarsal; consider total contact casting if arterial perfusion is adequate. (3) Inspect feet daily, apply moisturizer to legs/feet daily, and keep toe web spaces clean and dry. (4) Conservative sharp debridement weekly to remove callous and nonviable tissue by certified wound care specialist. (5) Foam dressing for protection and exudate absorption, change three times per week. (6) Notify provider for changes in skin color, temperature, pain, or an increase size in wound size, drainage, or odor. (7) Dietary consult for assistance with blood glucose management and recent weight loss (importance of protein reviewed with patient).

E: Return to clinic in 1 week to continue callous debridement and to modify plan as needed based on consult recommendation and patient wishes.

SUMMARY

- Lower extremity ulcers are an increasingly common problem and may be caused by compromised function in any component of the circulatory system (e.g., arterial, venous, and lymphatic).
- Majority of the lower extremity physical assessment findings (general appearance, functional sensory status, and perfusion) reflect common disorders of the skin, veins, arteries, and nerves.
- Table 13.3 provides a brief summary of key assessment distinctions among arterial, venous, and neuropathic ulcers.
- Atypical leg ulcers with unique manifestations account for the minority of lower extremity ulcers (vasculitis,

autoimmune disorders, neuropathy, microthrombotic, and metabolic derangements) with clinical features that can be misidentified for more conventional etiologies (Mufti et al., 2020).
- Many patients have ulcers of mixed etiology or comorbidities that affect management and the potential for healing.
- The wound specialist must utilize astute physical assessment skills and clearly and accurately document findings to facilitate an appropriate differential assessment that leads to the correct diagnosis in a timely manner.

TABLE 13.3 Characteristics of Arterial, Venous, and Neuropathic Ulcers

	Arterial	Venous	Neuropathic
Location	Tips of toes (spontaneous necrosis) Pressure points (e.g., heel and lateral foot) Areas of trauma (nonhealing wounds)	Between ankles and knees; "classic" location is medial malleolus	Plantar surface over metatarsal heads Areas of foot exposed to repetitive trauma (toes and sides of feet)
Wound bed	Pale or necrotic	Dark red, "ruddy" May be covered with fibrinous slough	Typically red (if no coexisting ischemia)
Exudate	Minimal	Moderate to large amounts	Moderate to large amounts
Wound edges	Well defined	Poorly defined, irregular	Well defined Frequently associated with callous formation
Other	Infection common, but signs and symptoms muted Typically painful Typically associated with other indicators (ischemia, diminished/absent pulses, elevational pallor, dependent rubor, and thin fragile skin) See Plates 26–28	Edema common Hyperpigmentation surrounding skin common Feet typically warm with good pulses (if no coexisting arterial disease) See Plates 28, 40, 41, and 44	Infection common, but signs and symptoms may be muted May have coexisting ischemia See Plates 46 and 47

SELF-ASSESSMENT QUESTIONS

1. Refer to the case scenario presented in the Clinical Consult; which of the following assessment parameters is most indicative for LEAD?
   a. Diminished pedal pulses
   b. Presence of a high-pitch bruit
   c. Trophic changes
   d. Pain relieved by walking

2. Reviewing the case scenario, which two findings are the most alarming that indicated a need for a vascular specialist referral?
   a. Pain relieved with walking and loss of protective sensation
   b. Presence of a neuropathic ulcer and trophic changes
   c. Diminished pedal pulses and hair growth
   d. Diminished pedal pulses and femoral artery bruit

3. Which of the following terms best describes an assessment parameter that occurs due to diminished blood flow causing reduced growth and development of the skin, hair, and nails?
   a. Corona phlebectatica
   b. Bruit
   c. Trophic changes
   d. Atrophie blanche

4. The wound specialist is examining a patient with lower extremity edema and notes a brawny hyperpigmentation to the gaiter region. Which term best describes this assessment parameter?
   a. Trophic changes
   b. Telangiectasias
   c. Cellulitis
   d. Hemosiderosis

5. The wound clinician observes a smooth, atrophic, thin, white plaque in the medial malleolar region in a patient with chronic venous disease. Which dermatological term best describes this assessment finding?
   a. Purpura
   b. Atrophie blanche
   c. Venous ulceration
   d. Petechiae

6. A condition that reflects fibrosis of the soft tissues of the lower extremity due to chronic edema is recognized as?
   a. Palpable purpura
   b. Atrophie blanche
   c. Venous dermatitis
   d. Lipodermatosclerosis

7. An individual with chronic swelling of only one lower limb comes into the wound center for an evaluation. What two methods are available to measure the extent of edema?
   a. Perometer and scale to categorize depth of pitting edema
   b. 24-h fluid recall and a scale to categorize depth of pitting edema
   c. Goniometer device and perometer
   d. Venous fill time and goniometer device

8. Your patient is complaining of pain in their left lower extremity when they walk one block and subsides with rest. Which of the following parameters *best* assesses their perfusion status?
   a. Venous fill time following limb elevation
   b. Capillary refill with blanching the toenail
   c. Skin temperature of the lower limbs
   d. Handheld Doppler to check pedal pulses

9. The *best* method to reduce neuropathic ulcer reoccurrence in a patient self-monitoring home prevention program includes which of the following?
   a. Daily skin checks to the feet using a mirror
   b. Daily foot check for temperature changes with infrared dermal thermometry
   c. Palpate for any temperature changes to the feet daily
   d. Podiatry lower extremity assessment every 3 months

10. The wound specialist notes extreme pain that seems out of proportion associated with allodynia in a patient with a leg ulcer. This assessment finding *most often* reflects which of the following types of ulcers?
    a. Atypical
    b. Venous
    c. Arterial
    d. Neuropathic

REFERENCES

American Diabetes Association (ADA). (2019). Microvascular complications and foot care: Standards of Medical Care in Diabetes. *Diabetes Care, 42*(Suppl. 1), S124–S138.

Antignani, P. L., Carpentier, P. H., & Cornu-Thenard, A. (2012). UIP consensus on corona phlebectatica. *International Angiology, 31* (3), 217–218.

Armstrong, D. G., Boulton, A. J., & Bus, S. A. (2017). Diabetic foot ulcers and their recurrence. *New England Journal of Medicine, 376*, 2367–2375.

Armstrong, D. G., Holtz-Neiderer, K., Wendel, C., et al. (2007). Skin temperature monitoring reduces the risk for diabetic foot ulceration in high-risk patients. *American Journal of Medicine, 120*(12), 1042–1046.

Armstrong, D. G., Lipsky, B. A., Polis, A. B., & Abramson, M. A. (2006). Does dermal thermometry predict clinical outcome in diabetic foot infection? Analysis of data from the SIDESTEP* trial. *International Wound Journal, 3*, 302–307.

Ball, J. W., Dains, J. E., Flynn, J. A., Solomon, B. S., & Stewart, R. W. (Eds.). (2019). *Seidel's guide to physical examination. Blood vessels* (9th ed., pp. 355–372). St. Louis, MO: Mosby.

Beckman, J.A., & Creager, M.A. (2019). Part III. Principles of vascular examination: History and physical exam. In M. Creager, J. Beckman & J. Loscatzo, (Eds.): *Vascular medicine: A companion to Braunwald's heart disease*, (3rd ed.), St. Louis, MO: Elsevier, pp142–150.

Beuscher, T. L. (2019). Guidelines for Diabetic Foot Care. A template for the care of all feet. *Journal of Wound Ostomy & Continence, 46* (3), 241–245.

Botros, M., Kuhnke, J., Embil, J., et al. (2021). Best practice recommendations for the prevention and management of diabetic foot ulcers. In Foundations for Best Practice for Skin and Wound Management. A supplement of Wound Care Canada: 2017. 68pp. Retrieved from: www.woundscanada.ca/docman/public/health-care-professional/bpr-workshop/895-wc-bpr-prevention-andmanagement-of-diabetic-foot-ulcers-1573r1e-final/file. Last updated 2021.

Boulton, A. J., Armstrong, D. G., Albert, S. F., et al. (2008). Comprehensive foot examination and risk assessment. A report of the Task Force of the Foot Care Interest Group of the American Diabetes Association, with endorsement by the American Association of Clinical Endocrinologists. *Physical Therapy*, 88(11), 1436–1443.

Boyko, E. J., Ahroni, J. A., Davignon, D., et al. (1997). Diagnostic utility of the history and physical examination for peripheral vascular disease among patients with diabetes mellitus. *Journal of Clinical Epidemiology*, 50, 659–668.

Bus, S. A., Lavery, L. A., Monteiro-Soares, M., et al. (2019). *IWGDF guidelines on the prevention of foot ulcers in persons with diabetes.* International Working Group on the Diabetic Foot. Retrieved from https://iwgdfguidelines.org/wp-content/uploads/2019/05/02-IWGDF-prevention-guideline-2019.pdf. Accessed on February 29, 2020.

Carpentier, P. H., Cornu-Thénard, A., Uhf, J. F., et al. (2003). Appraisal of the information content of the C classes of CEAP clinical classification of chronic venous disorders: A multicenter evaluation of 872 patients. *Journal of Vascular Surgery*, 37(4), 827–833.

Conte, M. S., Bradbury, A. W., Kolh, P., et al. (2019). Global vascular guidelines on the management of chronic limb-threatening ischemia. *Journal of Vascular Surgery*, 69(6), 3S–125S.e40. Retrieved 8/10/2020 from https://www.jvascsurg.org/article/S0741-5214(19)30321-0/pdf.

Gatt, A., & Chockalingam, N. (2017). Assessment of ankle joint dorsiflexion: An overview. *Revista Internacional de Ciencias Podologicas*, 6(1), 25–29.

Gerhard-Herman, M. D., Gornik, H. L., Barrett, C., et al. (2017). 2016 AHA/ACC guideline on the management of patients with lower extremity peripheral artery disease. *Journal of American College of Cardiology*, 69(11), e71–e126.

Gohel, M. S. (2018). Varicose veins. In I. Loftus, & F. J. Hinchliffe (Eds.), *Vascular & endovascular surgery E-book: Companion to specialist surgical practice* (6th ed., pp. 266–270). St. Louis, MO: Elsevier.

Hazenberg, C. E., van Netten, J. J., van Baal, S. G., & Bus, S. A. (2014). Assessment of signs of foot infection in diabetes patients using photographic foot imaging and infrared thermography. *Diabetes Technology & Therapy*, 6, 370–377.

Health Resources and Services Administration (HRSA). (2019). *Lower extremity amputation prevention (LEAP).* Retrieved from http://www.hrsa.gov/hansensdisease/leap/index.html. Accessed February 29, 2020.

Hinchliffe, R. J., Forsythe, R. O., Apelqvist, J., et al. (2019). *International Working Group on the Diabetic Foot (IWGDF) on diagnosis, prognosis, and management of peripheral artery disease in patients with a foot ulcer and diabetes.* Retrieved 8/10/2020 from https://iwgdfguidelines.org/wp-content/uploads/2019/05/04-IWGDF-PAD-guideline-2019.pdf.

Jarbrink, K., Ni, G., Sonnergren, H., et al. (2017). The humanistic and economic burden of chronic wounds: A protocol for a systematic review. *Systematic Reviews*, 6, 15.

Kelechi, T. J., & Bonham, P. A. (2008). Lower extremity venous disorders: Implications for nursing practice. *Journal of Cardiovascular Nursing*, 23(2), 132–143.

Kelechi, T. J., Good, A., & Mueller, M. (2010). Agreement and repeatability of an infrared thermometer. *Journal of Nursing Measurement*, 19(1), 55–64. https://doi.org/10.1891/1061-3749.19.1.55.

Kelechi, T. J., Haight, B. K., Herman, J., et al. (2003). Skin temperature and chronic venous insufficiency. *Journal of Wound Ostomy & Continence Nursing*, 30(1), 17–24.

Khan, N., Rahim, S., Anand, S., et al. (2006). Does the clinical examination predict lower extremity peripheral arterial disease? *JAMA*, 295, 536–546.

Lavery, L. A., Higgins, K. R., Lanctot, D. R., Constantinides, G. P., Zamorano, R. G., Armstrong, D. G., et al. (2004). Home monitoring of foot skin temperatures to prevent ulceration. *Diabetes Care*, 27(11), 2642–2647.

Lavery, L. A., Higgins, K. R., Lanctot, D. R., et al. (2007). Preventing diabetic foot ulcer recurrence in high-risk patients: The use of temperature monitoring as a self-assessment tool. *Diabetes Care*, 30(1), 14–20.

Lazzarini, P. A., Pacella, R. E., Armstrong, D. G., & van Netten, J. J. (2018). Diabetes-related lower-extremity complications are a leading cause of the global burden of disability. *Diabetic Medicine*. https://doi.org/10.1111/dme.13680.

Liu, C., van Netten, J. J., van Baal, J. G., Bus, S. A., & van der Heijden, F. (2015). Automatic detection of diabetic foot complications with infrared thermography by asymmetric analysis. *Journal of Biomedical Optics*, 20, 26003.

Ma, K. F., Kleiss, S. F., Schuurmann, R. C. L., Bokkers, R. P. H., Ünlü, Ç., & De Vries, J. P. P. M. (2019). A systematic review of diagnostic techniques to determine tissue perfusion in patients with peripheral arterial disease. *Expert Review of Medical Devices*, 16(8), 697–710. Retrieved 8/10/2020 from https://doi.org/10.1080/17434440.2019.1644166.

McDermott, M., Sufit, R., Nishida, T., et al. (2006). Lower extremity nerve function in patients with lower extremity ischemia. *Archives of Internal Medicine*, 166(18), 1986–1992.

McGee, S. R., & Boyko, E. J. (1998). Physical examination and chronic lower-extremity ischemia: A critical review. *Archives of Internal Medicine*, 158, 137–1364.

Mufti, A., Maliyar, K., Syed, M., et al. (2020). Approaches to microthrombotic wounds: A review of pathogenesis and clinical features. *Advances in Skin & Wound Care*, 33(2), 68–75.

Needleman, L., Cronan, J. J., Lilly, M. P., Merli, G. J., Adhikari, S., Hertzberg, B. S., DeJong, M. R., Streiff, M. B., & Meissner, M. H. (2018). Ultrasound for lower extremity deep venous thrombosis: Multidisciplinary recommendations from the Society of Radiologists in Ultrasound Consensus Conference. *Circulation*, 137(14), 1505–1515.

Nelson, E. A., & Adderley, U. (2016). Venous leg ulcers. *BMJ Clinical Evidence*, 2016, 1902, PMID: 26771825.

Nieman, J., Patten, A., & Chung, E. S. (2013). A standardized method for assessing edema. *Journal of Cardiac Failure*, 19(8), S86.

O'Donnell, T. F., Passman, M. A., Marston, W. A., et al. (2014). Management of venous leg ulcers: Clinical practice guidelines of the Society for Vascular Surgery® and the American Venous Forum. *Journal of Vascular Surgery*, 60(2), 3S–59S. Retrieved from https://www.jvascsurg.org/article/S0741-5214(14)00851-9/pdf. Accessed February 29, 2020.

Olsson, M., Järbrink, K., Divakar, U., et al. (2019). The humanistic and economic burden of chronic wounds: A systematic review.

Wound Repair and Regeneration, 27(1), 114–125. https://doi.org/10.1111/wrr.1268.

Padberg, F. T., Johnston, M. V., Sisto, S. A., et al. (2004). Structured exercise improves calf muscle pump function in chronic venous insufficiency: A randomized trial. *Journal of Vascular Surgery, 39*(1), 79–87.

Rice, J. B., Desai, U., Cummings, A. K., Birnbaum, H. G., Skornicki, M., & Parsons, N. (2014a). Burden of venous leg ulcers in the United States. *Journal of Medical Economics, 17*(5), 347–356. https://doi.org/10.3111/13696998.2014.903258.

Rice, J. B., Desai, U., Cummings, A. K., Birnbaum, H. G., Skornicki, M., & Parsons, N. B. (2014b). Burden of diabetic foot ulcers for medicare and private insurers [published correction appears in Diabetes Care, Sep;37(9):2660]. *Diabetes Care, 37*(3), 651–658. https://doi.org/10.2337/dc13-2176.

Sayre, E. K., Kelechi, T. J., Neal, D., et al. (2007). Sudden increase in skin temperature predicts venous ulcers: A case study. *Journal of Vascular Nursing, 25*(3), 46–50.

Schaper, N. C., van Netten, J. J., Apelqvist, J., Bus, S. A., et al. (2019). *IWGDF practical guidelines on the prevention and management of diabetic foot disease* (p. 2019). IWGDF Guidelines: International Working Group on the Diabetic Foot. Retrieved from https://iwgdfguidelines.org/wp-content/uploads/2019/05/01-IWGDF-practical-guidelines-2019.pdf. Accessed on February 29, 2020.

Searle, A., Spink, M. J., Ho, A., & Chuter, V. H. (2017). Association between ankle equinus and plantar pressures in people with diabetes. A systematic review and meta-analysis. *Clinical Biomechanics (Bristol, Avon), 43*, 8–14. https://doi.org/10.1016/j.clinbiomech.2017.01.021.

Sen, C. K. (2019). Human wounds and its burden: An updated compendium of estimates. *Advances in Wound Care, 8*(2), 39–49.

Sharkey, A. R., King, S. W., Kuo, R. Y., et al. (2018). Measuring limb volume: Accuracy and reliability of tape measurement versus perometer measurement. *Lymphatic Research and Biology, 16*(2), 182–186. Retrieved 8/10/2020 from https://www.liebertpub.com/doi/full/10.1089/lrb.2017.0039?url_ver=Z39.88-2003&rfr_id=ori%3Arid%3Acrossref.org&rfr_dat=cr_pub%3Dpubmed&.

Skafjeld, A., Iversen, M. M., Holme, I., Ribu, L., Hvaal, K., & Kilhovd, B. K. (2015). A pilot study testing the feasibility of skin temperature monitoring to reduce recurrent foot ulcers in patients with diabetes—A randomized controlled trial. *BMC Endocrine Disorders, 9*(15), 55-015-0054-x.

Trayes, K. P., & Studdiford, J. S. (2013). Edema: Diagnosis and management. *American Family Physician, 88*(2), 103–110B.

van Netten, J. J., Price, P. E., Lavery, L. A., Monteiro-Soares, M., Rasmussen, A., Jubiz, Y., Bus, S. A., & International Working Group on the Diabetic Foot. (2016). Prevention of foot ulcers in the at-risk patient with diabetes: A systematic review. *Diabetes/Metabolism Research and Reviews, 32*(Suppl. 1), 84–98.

van Netten, J. J., Prijs, M., van Baal, J. G., Liu, C., van der Heijden, F., & Bus, S. A. (2014). Diagnostic values for skin temperature assessment to detect diabetes-related foot complications. *Diabetes Technology & Therapy, 16*, 714–721.

Wound, Ostomy and Continence Nurses Society™ (WOCN®). (2014). *Guideline for management of patients with lower extremity arterial disease* (WOCN® clinical practice guideline series no. 1). Mt. Laurel, NJ: WOCN®.

Wound, Ostomy and Continence Nurses Society™ (WOCN®). (2019a). *Guideline for management of patients with lower extremity venous disease* (WOCN® clinical practice guideline series no. 2). Mt. Laurel, NJ: WOCN®.

Wound, Ostomy and Continence Nurses Society™ (WOCN®). (2019b). *Venous, arterial, and neuropathic lower-extremity wounds: Clinical resource guide.* Mt. Laurel, NJ: WOCN®.

Wound, Ostomy and Continence Nurses Society™ (WOCN®). (2021). *Guideline for management of patients with lower-extremity wounds due to diabetes mellitus and/or neuropathic disease* (WOCN® clinical practice guideline series no. 3). Mt. Laurel, NJ: WOCN®.

FURTHER READING

Garcia, R., & Labropoulos, N. (2018). Duplex ultrasound for the diagnosis of acute and chronic venous diseases. *The Surgical Clinics of North America, 98*(2), 201–218. Retrieved 8/10/2020 from: https://doi.org/10.1016/j.suc.2017.11.007.

Nussbaum, S. R., Carter, M. J., Fife, C. E., DaVanzo, J., Haught, R., Nusgart, M., & Cartwright, D. (2018). An economic evaluation of the impact, cost, and medicare policy implications of chronic nonhealing wounds. *Value in Health, 21*(1), 27–32. https://doi.org/10.1016/j.jval.2017.07.007.

Sen, C. K., Gordillo, G. S., Roy, S., et al. (2009). Human skin wounds: A major and snowballing threat to public health and the economy. *Wound Repair and Regeneration, 17*, 673–771.

14

Arterial Ulcers

Karen L. Bauer and Munier Nazzal

OBJECTIVES

1. Describe etiologic factors, risk factors, pathophysiology, typical presentation, and principles of management for arterial ulcers.
2. Identify contributing comorbid factors such as coronary artery disease (CAD), diabetes mellitus (DM), and tobacco use to optimize holistic management.
3. Describe essential assessment and differential diagnosis for the patient with a suspected arterial ulcer, including history, pain assessment, physical assessment, and laboratory and imaging studies.
4. Outline a patient teaching plan for the individual with ischemic disease of the lower extremity, including Risk Factor Modification with lifestyle changes to maximize perfusion and measures to prevent trauma.
5. Distinguish between *critical* limb ischemia and *acute* limb ischemia, including assessment parameters and implications for management.
6. Identify indications and options for surgical revascularization and when amputation is needed.
7. Describe pharmacologic options for management of arterial ulcers.
8. Recommend appropriate topical therapy for each of the following: ischemic ulcer covered with dry eschar and no signs of infection; ischemic ulcer covered with dry eschar and mild erythema and fluctuance of surrounding skin; open ischemic ulcer with and without signs of infection.

INTRODUCTION

Arterial ulcers (also known as *ischemic ulcers*) occur as a result of severe tissue ischemia and are extremely painful in the absence of sensory neuropathy. Based on Rutherford classification of chronic ischemia, tissue loss represents class V and the presence of an ulcer or gangrene is classified as class VI (Rutherford et al., 1997). Ischemic ulcers can also cause limb loss. Ischemic ulcers are generally refractory to healing unless tissue perfusion can be improved, and they are prone to progress to invasive infection or gangrene, which may necessitate amputation (WOCN®, 2014). Based on the Wound Ischemia and Foot Infection classification system (Table 10.10), patients with advanced classes of ischemia involving tissue loss or infection have a higher rate of major compared with patients with lower composite scores (hazard ratio 1.6, 95% CI 1.1–2.3) (Darling et al., 2016). Of further concern is the likelihood of coexisting, and possibly unrecognized, cardiovascular or cerebrovascular disease. Thus, any patient with an ischemic ulcer requires risk factor evaluation including cardiac evaluation, timely physical assessment, and aggressive management. The treatment plan for these patients must be multifaceted, including measures to maximize perfusion, minimize risk of infection, evidence-based ulcer care, and ongoing assessment and management of ischemic pain. Patient education and counseling are essential elements of the management plan.

PERIPHERAL VASCULAR DISEASE

Peripheral vascular disease (PVD) describes numerous conditions affecting the arterial, venous, and lymphatic circulation. *Peripheral arterial disease* (PAD) specifically refers to a range of conditions caused by an alteration in the structure and function of the arteries that supply the brain, visceral organs, and limbs; it is the preferred term for stenotic, occlusive, and aneurysmal diseases (Hirsch, Haskal, Hertzer, et al., 2006). Peripheral arterial *occlusive* disease describes arterial disease resulting from varying degrees of atherosclerosis that affects different arterial segments in the body. When the arterial disease affects the lower extremities, the term *lower extremity arterial disease* (LEAD) is used (WOCN®, 2014). LEAD can be either acute or chronic. Both acute and chronic lower extremity ischemia are categorized by classification and grading systems such as the Rutherford Classification. Generally, LEAD is subdivided into four categories: asymptomatic, claudication, critical limb ischemia (CLI), and acute limb ischemia (ALI) (Hardman, Jazaeri, Yi, Smith, & Gupta, 2014). Most ischemic ulcers develop as a result of chronic LEAD. Chronic LEAD results in ischemic complications of variable severity; the disease process progresses over time and produces gradually worsening symptoms ending in ulceration, tissue loss, and potentially limb loss (Shu & Santulli, 2018).

ALI refers to ischemic changes that develop suddenly, or within 2 weeks of presentation. Acute ischemia can cause limb loss if not urgently treated (Hardman et al., 2014). Because of this, all patients with suspected ALI require urgent evaluation by a vascular specialist (Norgren, Hiatt, Dormandy, et al., 2007). Signs and symptoms of ALI are described as the six *P*s: pain, paralysis, paresthesias, pulselessness, pallor, and polar (cold extremity). ALI is further characterized in three categories: (1) viable, where there is no muscle weakness or sensory loss and distal pulses remain palpable, (2) threatened, where there is moderate muscle weakness or sensory loss and only venous pulses are dopplerable, and (3) irreversible, where there is significant tissue loss, motor deficit, and sensory loss, with absent arterial and venous flow by Doppler (Gerhard-Herman et al., 2017). Irreversible nerve and muscle damage may occur within hours.

ALI should be differentiated from CLI, which is the phrase used to describe the most advanced stage of chronic LEAD. Patients with CLI can present with chronic ischemic rest pain, ulcerations, or gangrene, in the presence of objective evidence of chronic ischemia such as low ankle or toe pressures or low transcutaneous oxygen (TcO_2) values (Farber & Eberhardt, 2016; WOCN®, 2014). Ankle pressure values less than 70 mm Hg, toe pressures less than 30, and TcO_2 less than 20 are consistent with CLI (Farber & Eberhardt, 2016). The goals in management of patients with CLI include ulcer healing, infection prevention, limb preservation, pain control, and improved quality of life (Farber & Eberhardt, 2016; Lambert & Belch, 2013; Gerhard-Herman et al., 2017).

Unfortunately, failure to diagnose LEAD early results in failure to treat until the disease is advanced and the patient becomes symptomatic. Patients with CLI have a higher rate of cardiovascular morbidity and mortality (Norgren et al., 2018). Because atherosclerotic disease is the most common disease process affecting the arterial system and is a systemic phenomenon, the patient with disease in one vascular bed (e.g., coronary artery bed) is at greater risk for disease in another vascular bed (Hirsch et al., 2006). Advanced (symptomatic) disease is associated with much greater risk of morbidity and mortality (e.g., myocardial infarction, cerebrovascular accident, and limb loss) and is much less amenable to effective treatment. Thus, the focus in management of patients with any form of vascular disease (e.g., CAD, cerebrovascular disease, LEAD) must shift to routine screening to detect asymptomatic disease in other arterial segments. Ankle-brachial index (ABI) testing with a handheld Doppler is an effective bedside screening procedure and an abnormal ABI (<0.9 or >1.4) is an independent predictor for increased risk of cardiovascular death. It is recommended that individuals with an abnormal ABI be referred for further assessment to rule out "silent but treatable" cardiac disease (Alzamora, Fores, Pera, et al., 2013; Bevc, Purg, Turnsek, et al., 2013; Jones, Patel, Rockman, et al., 2014).

As noted, a significant proportion of individuals with LEAD are asymptomatic. Patients who are symptomatic most commonly present with intermittent claudication (pain with walking that is relieved by rest). The diagnosis is frequently missed in these individuals who present with vague complaints of impaired mobility and leg weakness, because symptoms may be attributed to aging, musculoskeletal disorders, or sedentary lifestyle (Wennberg, 2013).

Epidemiology

Although ischemic ulcers are much less common than those resulting from venous insufficiency or neuropathy, the underlying disease process (LEAD) is quite prevalent, especially among the elderly. It is estimated that LEAD affects one third of adults from 40 to 70 years of age, and 40% of individuals over the age of 80 (WOCN®, 2014). The prevalence in African Americans is about twice that of non-Hispanic whites at any given age (Shu & Santulli, 2018). Men are more likely to suffer from PAD than women (Dua & Lee, 2016).

LEAD is the third leading cause of morbidity related to atherosclerosis, affecting approximately 202 million people worldwide (Bonham, 2011; Fowkes, Rudan, Rudan, et al., 2013; Gerhard-Herman et al., 2017). In spite of this high prevalence, CLI affects only about 1% of the population, while chronic limb ischemia affects about 10% of the population. Amputation rates in patients with CLI range from 35% to 67% (Farber & Eberhardt, 2016). Unfortunately, 50–80% of individuals with LEAD are undiagnosed or undertreated, especially when compared with patients with CAD (Haigh, Bingley, Golledge, et al., 2013; Shu & Santulli, 2018; Sigvant, Wiberg-Hedman, Bergqvist, et al., 2009; WOCN®, 2014). Many patients with CLI are also found to have carotid stenosis or CAD, and an annual rate of 5%–7% of CLI patients will experience a cardiovascular event such as a myocardial infarction or stroke (Farber & Eberhardt, 2016). Two-year mortality rates in patients with CLI are about 40%, with the risk of death increasing threefold in those with major tissue loss (Farber & Eberhardt, 2016).

The high prevalence of undiagnosed disease is explained by the fact that vascular disease is frequently asymptomatic until the disease process is advanced. The prevalence of asymptomatic PAD is between 3% and 10% in individuals below the age of 70 years, and 15% and 20% in patients over the age of 70 (Dua & Lee, 2016).

Costs

Management of PAD costs the United States' health care system $10–20 billion annually. With the expectation that the diabetic subgroup of PAD patients will double by 2030, costs are expected to continue to increase (Dua & Lee, 2016). The prevalence of PAD is steadily increasing, while scrutiny on clinicians to practice cost containment is constant. Cost may be driven by the need for repeat procedures, ancillary therapies to promote ulcer healing, and increased hospital length of stay or readmission (Dua & Lee, 2016). Clinicians must practice sound patient-selection practices for surgical intervention, be cost-aware in the choice of ancillary treatment of CLI and ischemic ulcers and ensure appropriate routine surveillance postsurgical intervention (Dua & Lee, 2016).

Classification of Chronic Lower Extremity Arterial Disease

LEAD secondary to atherosclerosis is a progressive disease course that spans from asymptomatic disease to spontaneous tissue necrosis and gangrene. The severity is sometimes classified according to the Fontaine system, which designates the following levels of progression: I = asymptomatic disease, II = intermittent claudication, III = nocturnal pain, and IV = tissue necrosis/gangrene (Gardner & Afaq, 2008). The Fontaine system is the first classification system used and is based on clinical symptoms only (Hardman et al., 2014). Another classification system, the Rutherford system, separates PAD into acute and chronic categories and specifies that each presentation requires different management protocols. The Rutherford system considers objective diagnostic testing (Hardman et al., 2014). The Society for Vascular Surgery also developed a CLI classification system that combines the Fontaine and Rutherford systems with diabetic ulcer classification systems to encompass the presence of a wound, ischemia, and infection (WIFI). See Table 17-10. It defines four stages that align with risk of amputation and revascularization benefit (Farber & Eberhardt, 2016; Hardman et al., 2014).

Risk Factors

Risk factors for LEAD (Box 14.1) include both modifiable factors and predisposing factors. The increased predisposition to PAD is multifactorial and complex. Studies have identified a number of "emerging" risk factors that appear to be associated with the development of atherosclerotic disease, but their impact is not yet well defined (Liapis, Avgerinos, Kadoglou, et al., 2009). Although some of these risk factors, such as age, gender, and family history, are irreversible, the majority are very responsive to lifestyle modifications and pharmacologic therapy. A clear understanding of current recommendations for management of risk factors is critical because effective management of the underlying

BOX 14.1 Risk Factors for Lower Extremity Arterial Disease (LEAD)

Causal Modifiable (see Table 14.1)
1. Smoking
2. Diabetes
3. Dyslipidemia
4. Hypertension
5. Chronic kidney disease

Predisposing
1. Modifiable factors (obesity, inactivity, social isolation, and stress)
2. Nonmodifiable factors (advanced age, male gender, postmenopausal status, family history, and African American ethnicity)

Emerging
1. Elevated homocysteine levels
2. Inflammation
3. Infection
4. Vitamin D deficiency, increased ALT/AST ratio

disease process is essential for ulcer healing, limb salvage, and long-term survival (Aronow, 2008; Liapis et al., 2009; WOCN®, 2014).

Risk factors may increase risk independently, but primarily increase the impact of primary causative factors. Predisposing risk factors include both modifiable factors (e.g., obesity, inactivity, social isolation, and stress) and nonmodifiable factors (e.g., advanced age, male gender, postmenopausal status, family history of PAD, heart disease, stroke, and African American ethnicity). Clinicians should work with patients and other providers to eliminate or minimize modifiable factors through diet, exercise, medication, and strategies that reduce stress and isolation. Clinicians should educate patients about the impact of nonmodifiable risk factors and the critical importance of attention to smoking cessation, glycemic control, BP control, and correction of dyslipidemia (Hopf, Ueno, Aslam, et al., 2008; Liapis et al., 2009; WOCN®, 2014).

Risk factors that appear to play a direct causal role in the development of atherosclerosis include smoking, diabetes mellitus, dyslipidemia, hypertension, and chronic kidney disease (CKD). All of these risk factors are modifiable, and all contribute to cardiovascular morbidity and mortality as well as to the progression of LEAD. Management of these factors is of utmost importance when caring for a patient with LEAD. Table 14.1 and Box 14.2 summarize goals and guidelines for the management of modifiable risk factors (Abdulhannan, Russell, & Homer-Vanniasinkram, 2012; Fowkes et al., 2013; Liapis et al., 2009).

Smoking

Smoking is a highly significant independent risk factor for atherosclerotic disease in general and for LEAD in particular. Smokers have a fourfold increased risk for LEAD. Current smoking is associated with the highest odds of PAD development (Farber & Eberhardt, 2016; Shu & Santulli, 2018). Most studies suggest a connection between pack-year history and the number and severity of vascular complications; however, the number of pack-years that constitutes a significant increased risk for vascular disease is unknown (Liapis et al., 2009; Sigvant et al., 2009; WOCN®, 2014). Smoking may be particularly harmful to women, who reportedly have a significant increase in risk with a 10-year pack history, compared with men, whose risk increases significantly with a 30-year pack history (Sigvant et al., 2009). The negative effects of tobacco on the vascular system are due to its byproducts: nicotine, carbon monoxide, and hydrogen cyanide. The most significant of these is nicotine, which is a potent vasoconstrictor and promotes platelet aggregation and clot formation. In addition to these negative effects, tobacco use potentiates the adverse effects of other risk factors for LEAD (Katsiki, Papadopoulou, Fachantidou, et al., 2013). Smoking cessation can significantly reduce the progression of LEAD, as well as mortality rates from other vascular complications. Because of this, smoking cessation (see Box 14.2) should be a primary target of therapy and should include patient education, patient support, nicotine replacement therapy, referral to a

TABLE 14.1 Management of Modifiable Risk Factors

Risk Factor	Management Goals/Guidelines
Tobacco use	*Goal:* Cessation of tobacco use *Guidelines:* See Box 14.2
Diabetes mellitus	*Goal:* HbA1c 6.5%–7.0% (8% for high-risk patient) *Guidelines:* • Patient education and counseling regarding diet and exercise • Oral hypoglycemics and/or insulin
Dyslipidemia	*Goals:* • LDL-C <100 mg/dL (<70 mg/dL for very-high-risk patient) • HDL-C >40 mg/dL for men, >45 mg/dL for women • Triglycerides <150 mg/dL *Guidelines:* • Patient education and counseling regarding diet and exercise • Statins
Hypertension	*Goals:* <130/80 mm Hg in patients with CVD or ASCVD 10-year risk of >10% 140/90 in patients with no CVD and <10% ASCVD 10-year risk *Guidelines:* • Patient education and counseling regarding diet and exercise • Antihypertensive medications • Thiazide diuretics as initial drug • Angiotensin-converting enzyme inhibitor or angiotensin receptor blocker for patient with diabetic renal disease (except patient with renal artery stenosis) or congestive heart failure • β-Adrenergic blocker for patient who also has CAD • Calcium channel blocker as needed for uncontrolled hypertension *Note:* Multiple agents should be used as needed to maintain blood pressure within accepted range.

ASCVD, atherosclerotic cardiovascular disease; *HDL-C,* high-density lipoprotein cholesterol; *LDL-C,* low-density lipoprotein cholesterol.

BOX 14.2 Interventions to Promote Cessation of Tobacco Use

1. General education concerning the negative effects of tobacco use on health status.
2. Specific and consistent advice from health care team to eliminate tobacco use.
3. Establishment of patient–provider contracts in which the patient commits to a date on which he or she will eliminate tobacco use.
4. Anticipatory guidance (e.g., counseling to help the patient identify triggers of tobacco use and specific strategies for managing triggering events and situations).
5. General stress management and support.
6. Appropriate use of adequate doses of nicotine replacement agents (nicotine replacement therapy) and/or medications for nicotine addiction.
7. Frequent follow-up during the critical weeks after initial termination of tobacco use (by phone or office visit).
8. Appropriate counseling after any relapse on recognition that most individuals who successfully stop smoking have one to four relapses.

formal smoking cessation program, and pharmacologic agents when needed (Farber & Eberhardt, 2016; Katsiki et al., 2013; Liapis et al., 2009; WOCN®, 2014). Smoking cessation should be addressed at each patient visit (Gerhard-Herman et al., 2017). Studies are inconclusive regarding novel tobacco product use such as electronic cigarettes or vaping devices (Gerhard-Herman et al., 2017).

Diabetes Mellitus

Diabetes mellitus (DM), especially type 2, is one of the strongest independent predictors of LEAD. Characteristically, LEAD in diabetics most often involves the below-knee tibial and peroneal arteries compared with the distribution in nondiabetic patients, whose occlusive disease involves more proximal segments (Farber & Eberhardt, 2016; Lowry, Saeed, Narendran, & Tiwari, 2018). Furthermore, atherosclerotic disease signifies the leading cause of morbidity and mortality in diabetics and significantly contributes to the cost of diabetes (Shu & Santulli, 2018). Patients with diabetes are at increased risk for death and limb loss caused by vascular disease. For each 1% increase in hemoglobin A1c (HbA1c), there is a 28% increase in risk of death, and individuals with diabetes are 10 times more likely to progress to CLI and amputation (Hirsch et al., 2006; Liapis et al., 2009; WOCN®, 2014). A large data review study of over 3.5 million participants aged 40–90 shows that diabetes, when concurrent cardiovascular risk factors (hypertension, hyperlipidemia, obesity, or smoking) are present, increases the chance of developing PAD threefold, even without comorbid CAD (Shu & Santulli, 2018). Patients with both DM and CAD also increase their risk of PAD development (Shu & Santulli, 2018). Patients with diabetes and two or fewer risk factors had decreased odds of PAD compared with nondiabetic patients with CAD, suggesting that diabetes in conjunction with other risk factors present a significantly increased threat in the development of PAD (Shu & Santulli, 2018).

Specific pathologic features associated with diabetes that contribute to LEAD include endothelial dysfunction (imbalance in production of vasoconstrictor and vasodilator substances), platelet overactivity (poor response to antiplatelet therapy), and possibly increased levels of profibrotic and proinflammatory cytokines such as endothelin-1 (Rollini, Franchi, Muniz-Lozano, et al., 2013; Saskin, Ozcan, Duzyol, Baris, & Koçoğulları, 2017). These pathologic processes result in vessel constriction, hypercoagulability, and overproduction of vascular smooth muscle. Insulin resistance and hyperinsulinemia may also contribute to hypertrophy of vascular smooth muscle, even in the early stages of the disease due to the vascular growth factor characteristic of insulin. Fortunately, tight glycemic control (HbA1c 6.5%) can significantly reduce the risk of vascular complications and amputation; thus, effective diabetes management (through diet, exercise, and pharmacologic therapy) is another key element of effective therapy for the patient with LEAD (Gerhard-Herman et al., 2017). Current guidelines suggest that the "usual" goal for glycemic control is an HbA1c of around 7.0%, which correlates with a mean plasma glucose level of 126 mg/dL (Farber & Eberhardt, 2016). For selected patients (those with newly diagnosed diabetes, long life expectancy, and no cardiovascular disease), tighter goals are appropriate (HbA1c of 6.5%). Conversely, a less stringent goal (HbA1c <8.0%) may be appropriate for patients with limited life expectancy, extensive comorbidities, a history of severe hypoglycemia, or long-standing disease that is very difficult to control despite aggressive management (American Diabetes Association, 2014).

Cardiovascular disease accounts for about 65% of deaths in diabetic patients. This mandates that the traditional glucocentric approach to DM management be reconsidered and has been expanded to promote aggressive, multifactorial strategies aimed at cardiovascular risk factors. Daily exercise, a nonatherogenic diet, and modification or elimination of atherosclerotic risk factors including hypertension, smoking, dyslipidemia, and diabetes are crucial in DM/PAD management (Shu & Santulli, 2018). Collaborative and multidisciplinary efforts are crucial to achieve weight management, optimal glycemic control, and preventative foot care. Communication among healthcare providers in the DM/PAD patient with an ischemic ulcer is paramount to limb preservation (Gerhard-Herman et al., 2017).

Dyslipidemia

Elevated levels of cholesterol, low-density lipoprotein cholesterol, triglycerides, and lipoprotein(a) are also independent risk factors for LEAD (Farber & Eberhardt, 2016). Each 10 mg/dL rise in total cholesterol is associated with a 10% increase in risk of LEAD (Hirsch et al., 2006; Liapis et al.,

2009; WOCN®, 2014). The ratio of total cholesterol to high-density lipoprotein cholesterol is the best predictor for the development of PAD (Dua & Lee, 2016). Recommended target levels for lipid management and strategies for maintaining normal lipid levels are provided in Table 14.1.

Hypertension

Elevated blood pressure (BP) is associated with up to a threefold increase in risk for LEAD, in addition to a significant increase in risk for cardiovascular disease. Although treatment with antihypertensive medication has not been shown to improve LEAD outcomes, it is an essential element of care because of its impact on morbidity from cardiovascular and cerebrovascular disease. There is no current evidence favoring one class of antihypertensives over another in the case of LEAD (Whelton et al., 2018). Current goals and guidelines for maintaining BP are listed in Table 14.1 (Aronow, 2008; Liapis et al., 2009; Mensah & Bakris, 2010).

Kidney Disease

CKD is also an independent risk factor for development of atherosclerotic disease (Arinze, Gregory, Francis, Farber, & Chitalia, 2019; Farber & Eberhardt, 2016; Luders et al., 2017). In addition, patients with CKD are at greater risk for cardiovascular-associated morbidity and mortality, including limb loss. The CKD-specific mediators in PAD are not fully understood. The pathophysiology of increased PAD in CKD may be related to albuminuria, which is a marker of generalized endothelial dysfunction and contributes to medial arterial calcification (Garimella & Hirsch, 2014). Systemic inflammation and hypoalbuminemia can also be contributing factors to developing LEAD in the chronic uremic state found in CKD patients (Garimella & Hirsch, 2014). The prevalence of PAD in patients with CKD ranges from 24% to 37%, although symptoms are often muted and ABI's falsely elevated due to calcinosis (Arinze et al., 2019). The presence of PAD has been shown to be one of the key mortality indicators in patients on hemodialysis (Matsuzawa, Aoyama, & Yoshida, 2015). The presence of higher stages of CKD in PAD caused more tissue loss and had more limb ulceration (Arinze et al., 2019). Additionally, the presence of CKD in PAD patients has been shown to negatively impact morbidity, hospital length-of-stay, in-hospital mortality, amputation, and the cost of treatment (Luders et al., 2017).

Revascularization for CLI is also less successful in these patients, with increased postoperative complications and increased need for early reintervention (Arinze et al., 2019). In addition, CKD patients are less likely to undergo revascularization. In one study, CKD patients represented 34% of the cohort, but represented only 28% of those who underwent revascularization and 45% of those who ended in amputation within 6 months of PAD diagnosis (Arinze et al., 2019). Another study showed a 1.8-fold higher amputation rate in CKD patients with PAD (Luders et al., 2017). Because of such findings, the importance of aggressive identification and management of all reversible risk factors for patients with

CKD, as well as prompt recognition and comprehensive treatment of PAD to minimize the risk of amputation cannot be overemphasized (Garimella, Hart, O'Hare, et al., 2012; Tamura, Tsurumi-Ikeya, Wakui, et al., 2013).

Emerging Risk Factors

Emerging risk factors include conditions such as elevated homocysteine levels, inflammation, and infection. Other emerging risk factors or contributors to PAD are not as well associated but still warrant mentioning, such as vitamin D deficiency and elevated aspartate aminotransferase (AST) to alanine aminotransferase (ALT) ratios. Results from the Chronic Renal Insufficiency Cohort study have also shown novel associations between markers of inflammation, pro-thrombotic state, oxidative stress, and insulin resistance with prevalent PAD among persons with CKD (Garimella & Hirsch, 2014).

Homocystinemia

Homocystinemia is a rare autosomal-dominant disease found in 30%–40% of individuals with LEAD. Studies suggest that elevated homocysteine levels are associated with atherosclerosis and may increase risk for LEAD; however, whether homocystinemia plays an etiologic role in LEAD is not clear. The abnormal metabolism of homocysteine (a thiol-containing amino acid) can be normalized through administration of vitamin B_6, vitamin B_{12}, and/or folic acid. Although some studies have shown significant improvements in ABI's following therapy to normalize homocysteine levels, there is no conclusive evidence that treatment leads to improved outcomes in ulcer healing, LEAD progression, or CV events (Andras, Stansby, & Hansrani, 2013; Gerhard-Herman et al., 2017; Liapis et al., 2009; WOCN®, 2014) More studies are needed before any definitive recommendations can be made.

Inflammation

Atherosclerosis is known to be a chronic inflammatory disease (Saskin et al., 2017). Endothelial injury triggers an inflammatory response that ultimately results in fibrosis. Some investigators suggest that repeated episodes of tissue ischemia (as evidenced by claudication) may trigger a low-grade inflammatory response that contributes to disease progression. Others have hypothesized that rapid progression of the disease process in a subset of patients may be the result of an underlying inflammatory disorder. The role of inflammation in the progression of the disease seems to be supported by studies demonstrating the presence of inflammatory markers such as C-reactive protein (CRP) within atherosclerotic plaque and by elevated levels of inflammatory markers such as CRP, fibrinogen, and interleukin-6 among patients with advanced PAD. In addition, the potential for therapeutic intervention seems to be supported by data showing an inverse relationship between patients' omega-3 values and inflammatory biomarkers; this suggests that dietary changes or fish oil supplements might possibly reduce the inflammatory process and improve outcomes in patients with LEAD.

However, the link between inflammation and the progression of PAD is unclear, and there are no current recommendations for routine assessment of inflammatory markers such as CRP levels or for intervention (Chaparaia et al., 2009; Grenon, Conte, Nosova, et al., 2013; Liapis et al., 2009; Van Wijk, Boekholdt, Wareham, et al., 2013; WOCN®, 2014).

Infection

Inflammation, specifically both periodontal disease and Chlamydia pneumoniae (CPN), has been associated with increased risk and severity of LEAD. Acute CPN infections have been associated with increased lipid abnormalities and endothelial dysfunction. Antibiotic treatment of LEAD resulted in better clinical outcomes in patients who were seropositive for CPN than in seropositive controls who did not receive antibiotic therapy. Although more research is needed, prompt treatment of any infectious process should be considered for all LEAD patients (Liapis et al., 2009; WOCN®, 2014).

Vitamin D Deficiency

It has been suggested that low vitamin D levels contribute to PAD and cardiovascular health overall (McDermott et al., 2014). While some studies have shown that vitamin D deficiency is associated with increased functional decline in patients with and without PAD, the link to cardiovascular mortality has been proposed but is not well established (McDermott et al., 2014). Meta-analyses have shown that patients with PAD have lower vitamin D levels than patients without PAD, and that both vitamin D deficiency and vitamin D insufficiency are associated with PAD, especially CLI. Reduced vitamin D levels might represent an independent risk factor for PAD and, in turn, for CV events (Iannuzzo, Forte, Lupoli, & Di Minno, 2018; Nsengiyumva et al., 2015). While the exact role of vitamin D in PAD cannot be ascertained at this time, this is of consideration for further investigation.

ALT/AST Ratio

An increased AST/ALT ratio has been reported in patients with CLI. Additionally, there are reports of higher AST/ALT ratio in patients with a previous myocardial infarction. Further studies are needed on this subject before recommendations are made (Rief et al., 2016).

PATHOPHYSIOLOGY OF ARTERIAL OCCLUSIVE DISEASE AND ULCERATION

The exact pathologic mechanisms producing ulceration in the ischemic limb have not been clearly defined. Spontaneous ulceration typically involves the toes or distal foot and is the result of progressive arterial occlusion, which leads to cellular ischemia and tissue necrosis. Arterial ulcers may also be precipitated by minor trauma, which results in nonhealing ulcers because the damaged vessels are unable to meet the increased demands for oxygen associated with tissue injury and the healing process (Hirsch et al., 2006; Wennberg, 2013). Patients with LEAD and compromised mobility are at greater risk for pressure ulcer development because they have an existing baseline of diminished blood flow. Arterial insufficiency and arterial ulcers are most common among older adults and middle-aged adults who have atherosclerotic risk factors (Fowkes et al., 2013). Other causes of arterial ulceration include thromboangiitis obliterans (TAO) (Buerger's disease), sickle cell disease (SCD), and vasculitis (see Chapter 32); these conditions are less common but can occur among younger as well as older adults. Least common are arterial ulcers that develop as a result of entrapment syndromes, acute embolic syndromes, and arterial trauma (Farber & Eberhardt, 2016).

Atherosclerosis

The most common cause of LEAD and arterial ulceration among older adults is atherosclerosis involving the peripheral circulation. Atherosclerotic disease can occur in any vessel in the body. In the peripheral circulation, the aortic, iliac, femoral, and popliteal arteries (see Fig. 13.2) are the vessels most commonly affected, although those with diabetes and renal disease typically experience infrapopliteal occlusive disease (Farber & Eberhardt, 2016).

The pathology of atherosclerotic disease is not completely understood but involves both macro- and microvascular dysfunction that results in oxygen and nutrient requirement of downstream tissue being unmet (Farber & Eberhardt, 2016). This leads to vasodilation and decreased vessel-wall thickness and consequently inflammation that causes endothelial damage and edema. While this tissue hypoxia may produce angiogenesis as a compensatory mechanism, it may also lead to destabilized proximal plaque. The cellular dysregulation and tissue edema create conditions that are not conducive to ulcer healing (Farber & Eberhardt, 2016).

Atherosclerosis is known to involve two primary processes: plaque formation, which causes narrowing of the vessel lumen, and endothelial injury triggering an inflammatory process that ultimately results in fibrosis and hardening of the vessel wall (Hirsch et al., 2006).

Plaque formation begins with the lesion known as a "fatty streak," which is a gray or pearly white lesion that adheres to the intima (inner layer of the arterial wall). This lesion consists of a lipid core and a connective tissue covering. As further lipid accumulation occurs, the plaque enlarges, which results in progressive narrowing of the vessel lumen. Over time the plaques harden as a result of deposition of calcium salts and cholesterol crystals, causing loss of vessel elasticity, which further compromises blood flow (Hirsch et al., 2006).

The second process contributing to vessel narrowing and hardening is triggered by damage to the vessel lining. Endothelial damage results in areas where the intimal lining is denuded. Platelets aggregate over these denuded areas, causing clot formation and the subsequent release of growth factors that stimulate mitosis of the vascular smooth muscle cells

and promote synthesis of connective tissue proteins such as collagen. The end result is thickening and fibrosis of the vessel wall, which further contributes to narrowing and hardening of the involved arteries. Clinically these changes result in a chronic reduction in blood flow to the tissues and a loss of the ability to respond with increased blood flow when metabolic demands are increased. In addition, acute vessel occlusion may occur as a result of sudden plaque enlargement or plaque rupture (Hirsch et al., 2006).

Thromboangiitis Obliterans (Buerger's Disease)

Thromboangiitis obliterans, previously known as Buerger's disease and arteriosclerosis obliterans, is a nonatherosclerotic disease process that involves the small- and medium-sized arteries and veins in both the upper and lower extremities (Shanmugam, Angra, Rahimi, & McNish, 2017). It most commonly affects men and young- to middle-aged adults and is predominantly found in those who are heavy smokers and of middle to low socioeconomic status (Fazeli, Moghadam, & Niroumand, 2018; Shanmugam et al., 2017). The prevalence of TAO in patients with PAD is as low as 0.5%–5.6% in Western Europe, but as high as 45%–63% in India and up to 80% in Israel (Shanmugam et al., 2017). The process is typically bilateral and frequently involves all four limbs. The pathology of the disease remains unclear, but suggests preserved vessel-wall structure, infiltration of inflammatory cells and thrombosis in the vascular walls, proliferation of endothelial cells in the intima layer, and fibrosis of the media layer (Fazeli et al., 2018; Shanmugam et al., 2017).

Both inflammation and hypercoagulability have been suggested as a possible etiology for TAO due to the higher levels of both prothrombotic factors and inflammatory cytokines compared with healthy controls. Inflammation can contribute to clotting by increasing the concentration of procoagulation factors, and clot formation can in turn contribute to inflammation, possibly due to the release of growth factors (Aksu, 2012; Dellalibera-Joviliano, Joviliano, Silva, et al., 2012; Hus, Sokolawska, Waleter-Croneda, et al., 2013). Erythrocyte sedimentation rate, CRP, serologic markers, and autoantibodies are usually normal on presentation (Shanmugam et al., 2017). Angiographic features may show distal occlusive lesions interspersed with normal appearing vessels. There may be areas of collateralization surrounding these lesions, a finding that is termed "corkscrew collaterals." Proximal atherosclerotic lesions are typically absent (Shanmugam et al., 2017).

Ulceration in patients with TAO may occur spontaneously but is more commonly precipitated by minor trauma (Shanmugam et al., 2017). TAO should be considered in any patient with CLI younger than 50 years (Shanmugam et al., 2017). There is no curative therapy for TAO, but elimination of tobacco use is the most critical management strategy. Nicotine replacement therapy is not recommended in this population (Shanmugam et al., 2017). Among individuals who continue to use tobacco, digit or limb amputations are common; however, mortality is not increased (Armstrong et al., 2014). Other treatments such as antiplatelet medications, autologous whole bone marrow stem cell transplantation, and in some cases, endovascular therapy have all been suggested as possible management techniques; however, studies are limited on these modalities (Shanmugam et al., 2017). In addition, selected prostacyclin analogs (e.g., iloprost) may provide improved healing and better pain relief, but only when combined with total elimination of tobacco use (Bozkurt, Cengiz, Arslan, et al., 2013).

Sickle Cell Disease

SCD is a hereditary disease that affects 90,000–100,000 Americans (Apanah & Rizzolo, 2013). Globally, it is most common among people with sub-Saharan African, Indian, Middle Eastern or Mediterranean ancestry (Martí-Carvajal, Knight-Madden, & Martinez-Zapata, 2014). During physiologic stress in a person with SCD, the red blood cells become deformed into a crescent moon or sickle shape. These abnormal blood cells clump together and cause vascular occlusion and tissue necrosis, a phenomenon known as vaso-occlusive crisis. In addition, there is increased expression of adhesion molecules on the endothelial surface during a vaso-occlusive crisis that causes the sickled cells to attach. This results in further occlusion and necrosis. One potential end result of this pathologic sequence is the development of lower extremity ulcers.

Sickle-cell related ulcers (SCLUs) typically occur in areas with minimal subcutaneous fat, with thin skin, and with decreased blood flow, including the medial and lateral malleoli (ankles), often becoming circumferential (Martí-Carvajal et al., 2014). In the United States, the average duration of SCLUs exceeds 3 years.

Ulcer development in SCD is essentially secondary to local ischemia and secondary defective immunity. Ulceration in SCD is correlated with ongoing hemolysis, demonstrated in low steady-state hemoglobin and high lactate dehydrogenase levels, suggesting that sickle cell ulceration may not be solely vaso-occlusive in nature but also related to a high inflammatory state (Shanmugam et al., 2017). Other factors in the pathogenesis of SCLU include decreased nitric oxide which leads to endothelial dysfunction, infectious processes as shown by increased bioburden in SCLU, and compromised immunity in SCD (Martí-Carvajal et al., 2014). Acquired antithrombin III deficiency is common in individuals with SCD, which creates a hypercoagulable state and further complicates ulcer healing. Many individuals with SCD also have chronic venous insufficiency (see Chapter 15), which also further delays healing.

Management of sickle cell ulcers begins with measures to reduce the risk of vaso-occlusive crisis, such as blood transfusions to replace the abnormal red blood cells with normal cells, and hydroxyurea, which increases the levels of fetal (normal) hemoglobin. A 2014 Cochrane Systematic Review identified systemic management to include vascular drugs such as pentoxifylline (blood-viscosity reducing agent), isoxsuprine hydrochloride (β-adrenergic receptor stimulant), xanthinol nicotinate (vasodilator), antioxidant agents (L-carnitine), recombinant agents (human erythropoietin or antithrombin

III), growth factors (bosentan), and oral zinc sulfate, however again, these agents are not adequately supported in the literature (Martí-Carvajal et al., 2014).

Additional treatment measures include pain management, prompt treatment of infection, and general health promotion. Ulcer care is based on moist ulcer healing, bioburden management with antiseptics and as-needed debridement, and advanced compression therapy to control edema (Apanah & Rizzolo, 2013; Delaney, Axelrod, Buscetta, et al., 2013; Martí-Carvajal et al., 2014). One topical therapy, RGD peptide therapy, did show decreased ulcer size however studies are limited secondary to bias (see Table 30.10 for a list of the characteristics and treatment for sickle cell ulcers).

Vasculitis

Another potential cause of ischemic ulceration is vasculitis, which is a general term for inflammation of vessel walls. The inflammation may produce defects in the vessel wall, allowing leakage of blood into the surrounding tissues, or it may produce vessel occlusion and tissue necrosis. The term "vasculitis" refers to a large number of conditions that vary significantly in clinical presentation and prognosis, depending on the size and location of the inflamed vessels. Vasculitic or autoimmune factors may play a role in about 20%–23% of chronic nonhealing ulcers, mandating consideration of such conditions if ischemic ulcers fail to respond to revascularization and appropriate ulcer therapy (Shanmugam et al., 2017). Vasculitic conditions producing lower extremity ulcers typically involve midsized and small arteries and are characterized by a petechial rash, purpura, tissue necrosis, and extreme pain. Diagnosis is suggested by patient history, clinical presentation, and high serum levels of inflammatory markers and is confirmed by biopsy demonstrating vessel inflammation.

Multidisciplinary care with consideration of rheumatology referral should occur to promote optimal ulcer healing and limb preservation (Shanmugam et al., 2017). Systemic management involves immunosuppressive and antiinflammatory agents, as well as effective pain management, but there are few RCT delineating best practice. Topical therapy is based on the principles of ulcer bed preparation (elimination of necrotic tissue and control of bacterial burden) and moist ulcer healing (Aksu, 2012; Gaffo, 2013). (See Chapter 32 and Table 32.3 for further discussion of vasculitis and vasculitic ulcers.)

ASSESSMENT OF LEAD

The presence of an ulcer should initiate an assessment plan that follows accepted guidelines in the management of ischemic ulcers (see Checklist 14.1). The first step in assessment of a suspected ischemic ulceration on the lower limb is to evaluate the ulcer clinically. The second step is to identify the potential cause of the ulcer using diagnostic studies. Some of the challenges related to etiology are that many ulcers are of mixed etiology and that expected presentation can be masked by other clinical conditions. Usually the arterial ulcer, if of purely ischemic cause, is extremely painful, tender, and in

CHECKLIST 14.1   Lower Extremity Arterial Disease (LEAD) Assessment

✓ General appearance
  • Trophic changes: thin, shiny epidermis
  • Hair and nail patterns: loss of hair growth, thickened nails
  • Edema: variable based on need to keep leg dependent and coexisting disease
  • Skin color: pale or ischemic colors (possibly purpura and petechiae secondary to blood thinners)
✓ Functional sensory status: may be diminished with deformities
✓ Range of motion of ankle joint: stiffness
✓ Pain: ischemic (see Box 14.3) or nonspecific limb symptoms
✓ Perfusion
  • Dependent rubor and elevational pallor: present (see Box 13.2)
  • Skin temperature: cool

  • Blood flow: abnormal turbulence (bruit)
  • Pulses: diminished or absent
  • ABI: diminished
  • TBI: diminished
✓ Diagnostic tests
  • ABI and TBI (see Table 14.3)
  • Transcutaneous partial pressure of oxygen
  • Skin perfusion pressure
  • Pulse volume recording and Doppler waveform study
  • Segmental limb pressure measurements
  • Magnetic resonance angiography
  • Duplex angiography
  • Computed tomographic angiography
  • Arteriography

ABI, ankle-brachial index; *TBI*, toe-brachial index

the distal portion of the extremity. Ulcer characteristics that are critical to differential assessment include ulcer location, ulcer contours, type of tissue in the ulcer bed, and characteristics and volume of exudate (WOCN®, 2014). The classic arterial ulcer (see Plate 45) is located distally at the point farthest from the heart (toes and forefoot). Arterial ulcers may also present as nonhealing traumatic injuries (because perfusion is insufficient to support healing). Arterial ulcers are frequently described as having a "punched out" appearance with well-defined edges. The ulcer bed is usually pale or necrotic, and there is minimal exudate. Arterial ulcers are frequently infected because ischemia compromises bacterial control, but the infection may be missed because the signs of inflammation are very subtle in ischemic tissue (faint halo of erythema, slight induration). Table 12.3 provides a comparison of arterial, venous, and neuropathic ulcer characteristics.

The features of arterial ulcers might be masked by the presence of venous disease, neuropathy, or localized infection. Only in a small percentage of patients is arterial insufficiency the sole etiologic factor. Often arterial insufficiency is a complicating factor for ulcers caused primarily by venous insufficiency, neuropathy, or combined pathologies. The clinician should always check for the presence of arterial disease, even if the presentation is not consistent with classic LEAD. This can be done using clinical exam and a number of diagnostic tests to identify the presence and severity of ischemic components. A comprehensive assessment provides the data needed for development of an appropriate management plan for any patient with a lower extremity ulcer (Checklist 14.1).

Simple noninvasive vascular studies should be conducted on all patients; select patients may require more complex or invasive vascular studies. It should be noted that palpable pulses alone do *not* rule out arterial disease; dependence on such unreliable assessment methods is a major contributing factor to the high incidence of unrecognized and untreated LEAD. Pulse assessment is, however, a crucial part of the lower extremity exam, especially if arterial disease is suspected.

Patient History

An extensive medical and surgical history should be taken in any patient with lower extremity ulcers. Emphasis on risk factors for arterial disease includes history of angina, myocardial infarction, cardiovascular procedures, or "problems with circulation." Smoking or tobacco use history, including any past attempts to stop smoking and willingness to consider smoking cessation is important. The clinician should ascertain if the patient has a history of diabetes, including onset, type, management, usual fasting glucose level, and most recent HbA1c. A history of hypertension, including onset, duration, management, and usual BP, as well as lipid levels (if known) and any measures in place to manage dyslipidemia should be delineated (Hopf et al., 2008). The history must include a review of all medications, including herbal agents, over-the-counter medications, and prescription drugs. The patient should be asked about ulcers, any associated events (e.g., trauma), past treatments, and ulcer response. See Checklist 14.1 for a list of LEAD assessment findings.

Evaluation of symptoms is essential to help identify the potential etiology of ulcers. As described in Chapter 13, a careful pain history must be obtained. Pain patterns are critical to differential assessment of ulcer etiology (see Table 12.2). Pain in the lower extremity is often the first indication of LEAD, and pain can progressively worsen from pain only with exercise to rest pain in severe ischemia. The location of the pain may suggest the level of occlusion; in general, the pain is one joint distal to the stenosis or occlusion (Table 14.2)

TABLE 14.2   Correlation Between Site of Occlusion and Location of Pain

Site of Occlusion	Location of Pain
Iliofemoral arteries	Thighs, buttocks, calves
Superficial femoral artery	Calf
Infrapopliteal artery	Foot

From Cimminiello, C. (2002). PAD: Epidemiology and pathophysiology. *Thrombosis Research*, 106(6), V295–V301.

BOX 14.3 **Categories of Ischemic Pain**

Intermittent claudication	Occurs with moderate-to-heavy activity; relieved by approximately 10 min of rest. Typically occurs when involved vessel is approximately 50% occluded.
Nocturnal pain	Develops as occlusion worsens. Occurs when patient is in bed. Caused by combination of leg elevation (to horizontal position) and reduced cardiac output. Relieved by placing limb in a dependent position.
Rest pain	Occurs in absence of activity and with legs in a dependent position. Rest pain signals advanced occlusive disease (typically >90% occlusion).

(Wennberg, 2013). As outlined in Box 14.3, pain characteristics may reflect ischemia severity. Unfortunately, the patient with LEAD does not always experience or report "classic" ischemic pain symptoms. Intermittent claudication, for example, is normally described as reproducible pain in the buttock, thigh, or calf muscle that is precipitated by exercise and that rapidly disappears within 10 min of rest (Hirsch et al., 2006). However, because the patient with LEAD may unconsciously limit walking or activities to avoid pain, signs of claudication may be absent or reported simply as "leg weakness." It is therefore helpful to query patients regarding usual activities and any pain experienced when performing activities of daily living (Wennberg, 2013). Patients with sensory neuropathy (e.g., mixed neuropathic and arterial disease) may have absent or blunted awareness of ischemic pain (Hopf et al., 2008).

Advanced LEAD is typically evidenced by rest pain, which is commonly described as a "constant, deep, aching pain." However, advanced LEAD may be associated with a shift in pain patterns, from nociceptive pain (described as "aching" or "throbbing") to neuropathic pain (described as "tingling, burning, and electric-shock" type pain). Further discussion related to the assessment and management of pain is provided in Chapter 28.

Lower Extremity Clinical Assessment

Comprehensive assessment of the patient with a lower extremity ulcer is described in detail in Chapter 13. A comprehensive lower extremity vascular examination should occur in all patients with increased risk for PAD (Gerhard-Herman et al., 2017; WOCN®, 2014). Signs of chronic tissue ischemia include thin, shiny skin, recent onset of diminished hair growth, purpura, thin, and ridged or thickened nails. It should be noted that absence of hair is a nonspecific finding and that ischemic changes in the nails are frequently obscured by fungal nail infections. There may be elevational pallor or cyanosis, and dependent rubor (WOCN®, 2014).

Diminished or absent pulses may be discernable on clinical exam. Absence of both pedal pulses mandates referral to a vascular surgeon. However, the presence or absence of pedal pulses cannot be used as a sole measure of arterial perfusion, because some individuals with normal perfusion lack one or both pedal pulses and many patients with arterial insufficiency retain palpable pulses. Audible Doppler signals, if triphasic, are effective for the exclusion of PAD (Federman et al., 2016). An abnormal ABI (see section on diagnostic testing) may be present. It should be noted that ABI greater than 1.4 is indicative of vessel calcification and mandates referral to a vascular laboratory for further testing if the clinical suspicion for PAD is significant. It should also be noted that patients with ABI of 0.50–0.90 have moderate-to-mild LEAD but retain the potential for healing and are unlikely to develop ischemic ulcers, though the LEAD could result in slower healing of ulcers caused by other pathologic processes. Functional and sensory deficits, especially if the patient has combined LEAD and lower extremity neuropathic disease, may be appreciated. Clinical examination findings of cool skin, pallor, or delayed capillary refill are not reliable for PAD diagnosis and all physical exam findings should thus be confirmed with diagnostic testing (Federman et al., 2016; Gerhard-Herman et al., 2017).

NONINVASIVE TESTING IN LEAD

Noninvasive evaluation of the lower extremities has two goals. The first goal is to objectively confirm the presence of arterial disease and the second goal is to decide on the severity of the arterial disease. Noninvasive evaluation of arterial disease should be part of the work-up in all patients with lower extremity ulcerations. The simplest noninvasive evaluation is based on pressure measurements of the legs divided by the arm pressure (the highest pressure of either arm) to produce the ABI. ABI testing should be done in all patients with lower extremity ulcers in order to determine whether or not arterial insufficiency is a contributing factor and to identify patients who require further vascular assessment. The lower the ABI, the higher the degree of arterial occlusive disease. Additional diagnostic tests are indicated when the diagnosis is unclear, the ulcer fails to improve, or surgical revascularization is being contemplated. The most common diagnostic tests for LEAD are listed in Checklist 14.1. With the exception of the ABI, these tests are performed in vascular laboratories by trained technicians; results are interpreted by vascular specialists.

Ankle-Brachial Index

The ankle-brachial index, also known as *ankle-arm index,* is a simple bedside test in which perfusion pressures in the lower leg are compared with those in the upper arm using a standard BP cuff and a handheld, battery-operated, continuous-wave, Doppler ultrasound device (Fig. 14.1). The ultrasound probe should utilize an 8–9-MHz frequency for accurate assessment of skin-level vessels (Bonham, Cappuccio, Hulsey, et al.,

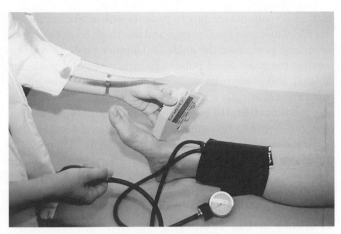

Fig. 14.1 Handheld Doppler probe being used to obtain an ankle-brachial index.

2007). The ABI has validity as a first-line test in suspected PAD, with sensitivities that range from 68% to 84% and specificities that range from 84% to 99% (Gerhard-Herman et al., 2017).

A "normal" ABI is considered to range from greater than 0.99 to 1.4. An ABI of 0.91–0.99 suggests PAD and may require further testing if the clinical suspicion for PAD is high (Gerhard-Herman et al., 2017). An ABI of 0.90 or less is approximately 95% sensitive for detecting LEAD compared with angiography-proven ischemic disease (Norgren et al.,

2007). An ABI value of more than 1.40 indicates vessel non-compressibility due to wall calcification, which is more common in diabetic and end-stage renal patients. An ABI of greater than 1.40 should lead to further testing if the clinical suspicion for PAD is high (Federman et al., 2016; Gerhard-Herman et al., 2017).

The ABI is also useful for detecting restenosis after revascularization and for monitoring LEAD progression; a 15% change from the baseline ABI is indicative of disease progression (Hirsch et al., 2006). The Wound, Ostomy and Continence Nurses Society™ (WOCN®, 2014) recommends conducting an ABI test every 3 months in patients suffering from LEAD and a nonhealing ulcer to identify severe or CLI that warrants referral or a change in the plan of care (see Table 14.3).

The procedure for conducting an ABI test is outlined in Box 14.4. Guidelines for interpretation of ABI and toe-brachial index (TBI) are provided in Table 14.3. A research-based protocol should be used to measure ABIs with a handheld Doppler; this approach has been shown to provide results that are valid and reliable compared with results obtained in a vascular laboratory (Bonham et al., 2007). At present, there is considerable variability in the approach and skill level of practitioners performing this test at the bedside; thus dissemination of evidence-based protocols and skills training is an urgent need (Sihlangu & Bliss, 2012).

ABI provides only an indirect measure of peripheral perfusion and cannot be considered accurate in patients with

TABLE 14.3 Interpretation of Noninvasive Tests for LEAD

Value	Interpretation/Clinical Significance
ABI	
	Abnormally high range, typically because of calcification of the vessel wall in patient with diabetes
	Renders ABI test invalid as a measure of peripheral perfusion
>1.4	TBI indicated
>0.9–1.3	"Normal" range
≤0.9	LEAD
0.6–0.8	Borderline perfusion
≤0.5	Severe ischemia; ulcer healing unlikely unless revascularization can be accomplished
TBI	
<0.70	
Or toe pressure <30 mm Hg	LEAD
TcPO₂	
(Obtain if ABI or TP cannot be performed due to calcification or amputations of ankle or toes)	
≥40 mm Hg	Normal
<40 mm Hg	Hypoxia with impaired ulcer healing
AP	
AP <40 mm Hg	Limb threatened
TP	
<30 mm Hg	Critical limb ischemia (<50 mm Hg in patient with diabetes)
SPP	
>30 mm Hg	Required for healing to occur

ABI, ankle-brachial index; *AP,* ankle pressure; *LEAD,* lower extremity arterial disease; *SPP,* skin partial pressure; *TBI,* toe-brachial index; *TP,* toe pressure; *TcPO₂,* transcutaneous partial pressure of oxygen.

BOX 14.4 **BOX 14.4   Procedure for Obtaining an ABI**

1. Place patient in supine position in warm, tranquil environment for at least 10 min before the test (prevents vasoconstriction of arteries). Provide blankets if necessary.
2. Obtain brachial pressure in each arm using Doppler probe and 12–14-cm cuff placed 3 cm above cubital fossa. Inflate cuff 20–30 mm Hg above the last sound; slowly deflate cuff until initial sound is heard. Record highest brachial pressure.
3. Place appropriately sized cuff (10–12 cm) around lower leg 3 cm above malleolus.
4. Apply acoustic gel over dorsalis pedis pulse location.
5. Hold Doppler probe over pedal pulse according to manufacturer's guidelines (e.g., pen-style Doppler devices should be held at 45-degree angle). Be careful not to occlude the artery with excessive pressure; hold the probe lightly!
6. Inflate cuff to level 20–30 mm Hg above point where pulse is no longer audible.
7. Slowly deflate cuff while monitoring for return of pulse signal. The point at which the arterial signal returns is recorded as the dorsalis pedis pressure.
8. Apply acoustic gel over posterior tibial pulse location and repeat procedure. The higher of the two values is used to determine the ABI.
9. Calculate ABI by dividing the higher of the two ankle pressures by the higher of the two brachial pressures.

ABI, ankle-brachial index.

noncompressible vessels (e.g., patients with diabetes, renal failure, and vessel calcification) (Bonham et al., 2007). In patients with elevated ABI (>1.3 or 1.4) and suspected calcification, the next step is to measure the TBI. It is believed that digital arteries are relatively spared from calcification. In case of normal ABI but clinical evidence of ischemia, further evaluation should be conducted starting with the TBI and other tests that can be done in a vascular laboratory; this may include treadmill exercise testing, segmental pulse volume recordings (PVRs), or others (Hirsch et al., 2006; Shu & Santulli, 2018; Wennberg, 2013).

Toe-Brachial Index

In patients with calcified arteries, the TBI is considered to be more accurate because the toe vessels are less likely to be calcified. The TBI is performed by a trained clinician and conducted in the same manner as the ABI test, with a small digit cuff placed around the great toe or the second toe and a photoplethysmography sensor placed on the tip of the toe. The test can be done either in the vascular laboratory or at the bedside with a portable photoplethysmograph (Bonham, 2011; Cao, Eckstein, DeRango, et al., 2011). A TBI less than 0.7 is generally considered indicative of LEAD. The likelihood of ulcer healing decreases with toe pressure less than 30 mm Hg (Gerhard-Herman et al., 2017).

Segmental Limb Pressure

Segmental limb pressure (SLP) measurements are used to determine the level of arterial occlusive disease, which helps

plan interventional therapy in patients with arterial occlusive disease. Cuffs are placed at high and low thigh level, below the knee, and just above the ankle. A Doppler probe is used to localize the most distal pulses (dorsalis pedis and posterior tibialis), and pressure us measured at different levels by inflating cuffs sequentially and obtain pressure each time the same way mentioned in ABI evaluation. A difference of 20 mm Hg or more between two adjacent cuff positions localizes the occlusion to the intervening vessels. A 20–30 mm Hg pressure difference between the contralateral positions suggests stenosis or an occlusive lesion in the extremity with the lower pressure (Gerhard-Herman et al., 2017).

Exercise Stress Testing

Exercise stress testing is an effective diagnostic study for symptomatic patients with normal ABI readings. It is used to assess the functional impact of LEAD. A baseline ABI is performed, and the patient then walks on a treadmill set at a constant speed and grade. A patient who is unable to walk on a treadmill can be asked to stand with knees fully extended and to repeatedly raise the heels off the floor. The stress activity (treadmill walking or repetitive heel raises) is continued until the patient becomes symptomatic or until a set limit is reached (e.g., 5 min on the treadmill or 50 heel raises). A repeat ABI is obtained 1 min after completion of the stress activity. Individuals with normal circulation exhibit no change or a slight increase in ABI, whereas individuals with LEAD exhibit a clear drop in ABI. Exercise treadmill stress testing can help rule out arterial occlusive disease if the test is normal. In addition, it helps guide individualized exercise programs (Gerhard-Herman et al., 2017).

Perfusion Evaluation

In patients with normal or borderline ABI with concurrent nonhealing ulcers or gangrene, especially when vessel calcification is suspected, CLI can be evaluated by use of Doppler waveforms known as pulse volume recording, transcutaneous oxygen pressure, or skin perfusion pressure (SPP) (Federman et al., 2016; Gerhard-Herman et al., 2017).

Pulse Volume Recording

The PVR provides a reflection of actual perfusion volume during the cardiac cycle. PVRs are obtained with cuffs that incorporate pneumoplethysmograph capability (i.e., the ability to detect changes in blood volume in the underlying arteries). The cuffs are inflated to a present level, and the machine provides tracings that reflect blood volume within the underlying arteries throughout the cardiac cycle. A similar tracing of flow within a single vessel may be obtained using a Doppler probe; this tracing is commonly referred to as a *Doppler waveform study.* Normal tracings for both PVRs and Doppler waveform studies are triphasic, showing a clearly defined systolic peak, followed by a dicrotic notch that represents reversal of blood flow during early diastole, and finally a diastolic wave (Fig. 14.2A). With mild LEAD, the waveform changes to a biphasic pattern, whereas with advanced LEAD, the

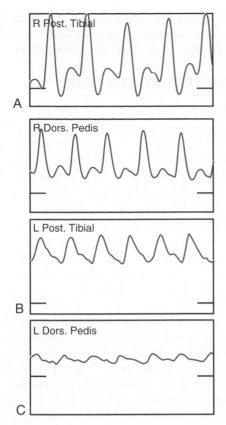

R Post. Tibial

A

R Dors. Pedis

L Post. Tibial

B

L Dors. Pedis

C

Fig. 14.2 Doppler wave forms.

waveform becomes monophasic or severely blunted (see Fig. 14.2B and C). Waveforms can also be obtained for the digital vessels by wrapping a cuff around the arch of the foot or the great toe; waveforms that are dampened or flat suggest small vessel disease. A monophasic waveform for the pedal arteries is predictive of lower extremity amputation in diabetic foot ulcers and dialysis patients (Aronow, 2008; Tsai, Chu, Wen, et al., 2013). However, results can be influenced by factors such as local edema and anemia (Tsuji, Hiroto, Kitano, et al., 2008).

SLP and PVR measurements are often obtained in combination. Each one is 85% accurate in detecting and localizing significant occlusive lesions, compared with angiography (see Fig. 14.2A). When SLP and PVR are used together, however, the accuracy is closer to 95%. Additionally, the patient with diabetes and calcified arteries who produces a falsely elevated SLP will be accurately assessed by PVR when the two tests are done in combination (Norgren et al., 2007).

Transcutaneous Oxygen Pressure

Transcutaneous partial pressure of oxygen ($TcPO_2$) measurements provides information about the adequacy of oxygen saturation in the skin and underlying tissues. This test is valuable for determining skin perfusion when an ulcer fails to improve or when ABI and TBI are not valid or are not possible due to incompressible arteries or amputation of feet or toes. $TcPO_2$ is a simple test that is usually performed in a vascular

laboratory, specialty clinic, or hyperbaric oxygen therapy (HBOT) center. To obtain a $TcPO_2$ measurement, an oxygen sensor and an electrode are attached to the skin in the area surrounding an ulcer and compared with that of a normal perfusion area such as the chest to quantify oxygen diffusion through the skin in both areas. The test should be done in a warm room to minimize arterial vasospasm in response to cold (Gerhard-Herman et al., 2017). Values greater than 30 mm Hg are predictive of ulcer healing. Values less than 20 mm Hg indicate that healing is unlikely (Wennberg, 2013). This diagnostic modality can also be used in angiosome-targeted assessment for revascularization and to assess patients for possible response to HBOT (Gerhard-Herman et al., 2017; Kaur, Pawar, Banerjee, & Garg, 2012).

Skin Perfusion Pressure

Laser Doppler SPP is another noninvasive measurement used for predicting successful ulcer healing in CLI or for planning amputation level for maximal preservation of functionality and mobility (Tsuji et al., 2008). SPP can be used in noncompressible arteries or in an already existing amputation of toes and legs. Unlike $TcPO_2$, SPP results are not influenced by factors such as local edema and anemia, and the procedure is less time consuming. An SPP value is obtained by using a laser Doppler probe and placing a cuff around the forefoot (including the 5 metatarsal and 14 phalange bones and surrounding soft tissues); the patient should be lying supine in a thermo-regulated room. An SPP greater than 30 mm Hg is requisite for ulcer healing (Gerhard-Herman et al., 2017).

Other Methods for Skin Perfusion Evaluation

Skin arterial ulceration healing is determined by the amount of oxygenation to the area of the ulcer. Perfusion to the area of an ulcer is more reflective of the amount of oxygen in the vicinity of the ulcer. All pressure measurement methods are considered surrogates for skin perfusion rather than a direct measurement of perfusion. In the absence of edema, infection, hypertension, renal failure, and diabetes, pressure might accurately reflect perfusion. This means that in the majority of patients, pressure measurements including toe pressure are not accurate in perfusion evaluation. Perfusion determinants include arterial pressure, venous pressure, lymphatic circulation, edema, cardiac output, outside temperature vessel diameter and autoregulation. Furthermore, based on the angiosome theory, a perfect pressure/perfusion in one area of the limb/foot does not mean an acceptable pressure/perfusion in another area of the extremity/foot. For that reason, local perfusion evaluation is gaining momentum in ulcer and ulcer management to guide both revascularization decisions and amputation decision.

These methods have yet to gain widespread acceptance by clinicians. Fluorescent angiography, transcutaneous oxygen measurement, hyperspectral oxygen saturation measurement, infrared oxygen saturation measurement, and laser Doppler flow are among the potential methods used to evaluate tissue perfusion that might a have future role in ulcer management

(De Silva, Saffaf, Sanchez, & Zayed, 2018; Fife, Smart, Sheffield, et al., 2009; Huang et al., 2011; Samies, Gehling, Serena, & Yaakov, 2015).

Duplex Angiography (Ultrasound Imaging), Magnetic Resonance Angiography, and Computed Tomographic Angiography

In patients with symptomatic PAD or CLI in whom revascularization is being considered, additional imaging is helpful to determine a patient-specific care plan and mapping (Federman et al., 2016). Ultrasonography, MRA, or CTA can be used to select vascular access sites for angiography or endovascular interventions. In addition, these diagnostic modalities identify significant lesion location and severity with different degrees of accuracy and help determine the modality for invasive or surgical management (Gerhard-Herman et al., 2017).

Ultrasonography uses sound waves to reveal characteristics of tissue or organs. Duplex angiography combines ultrasonographic imaging with Doppler assessment of blood flow. It provides direct imaging of arteries and the location and severity of stenosis, thrombi, or occlusive lesions, but offers lower spatial resolution than MRA or CTA (Cao et al., 2011; Gerhard-Herman et al., 2017; Wennberg, 2013). Duplex angiography has a sensitivity of 99% and 80% and specificity of 94% and 91% for the femoropopliteal and tibial segments, respectively, compared with arteriography. Results are comparable to contrast enhanced MRA with lower cost.

Magnetic resonance angiography (MRA), with or without gadolinium enhancement, can be helpful in determining the location and severity of stenosis and is a valid alternative to angiography for obtaining detailed anatomic information required for accurate decision making regarding surgical intervention (Gerhard-Herman et al., 2017; Shu & Santulli, 2018). Benefits of MRA include its noninvasive nature, minimal risk, and ability to show images of the smaller pedal arteries. MRA is not an option for patients with implanted defibrillators, permanent pacemakers, intracranial aneurysm clips, or claustrophobia. Gadolinium enhancement may be contraindicated in patients with chronic renal insufficiency. In addition, MRA does not reliably detect calcification and is not currently able to image endovascular stents constructed of metal alloys (Wennberg, 2013).

Computed tomographic angiography (CTA) utilizes iodinated contrast agent and X-rays to visualize arterial anatomy and to localize stenosis in patients who are candidates for surgical revascularization or endovascular procedures (Shu & Santulli, 2018). The use of CTA is increasing, due in part to improvements in image detail provided by new 64-channel "multidetector" channels, which can be used to image the arterial system all the way down to the pedal arteries and to evaluate the patency of bypass grafts (Schernthaner, Fleischmann, Stadler, et al., 2009). CTA is faster than MRA and safer than digital subtraction and is an alternative for patients with a pacemaker or implanted defibrillator who cannot undergo MRA. CTA has reduced accuracy in extensive vessel calcification and cannot be used in patients with compromised renal function or severe allergic reaction to dye (Gerhard-Herman et al., 2017; Wennberg, 2013).

INVASIVE TESTING FOR LEAD

Arteriography

Contrast angiography remains the gold standard when planning surgical intervention, especially for patients in whom MRA and multidetector CTA are contraindicated or would provide insufficient anatomic data. When performed, angiography utilizing digital subtraction technology is the usual choice. A plain film of the involved area is taken before injection of contrast material, and the computer then "subtracts" the plain film image from the postcontrast images. As a result, the final films show only the arteries, allowing for clear identification of the site and severity of stenotic lesions (Norgren et al., 2007; Wennberg, 2013). Angiography is an invasive procedure that can be associated with complications such as bleeding, hematoma, infection, vessel injury, thrombosis, dissection, and embolization. Because of this, it is performed only when surgical or endovascular intervention is anticipated. It is generally not a diagnostic test on its own, without potential for endovascular intervention. Most of the diagnostic information deducted from angiography can be provided by noninvasive evaluation including CTA and duplex ultrasound.

TREATMENT OF LEAD

The primary focus in the management of patients with an arterial ulcer is to improve perfusion to the ulcerated area. The ability to heal an ulcer is directly correlated with the ability to provide sufficient oxygen and nutrients to support the healing process. Secondary concerns include systemic support for ulcer healing, prevention and management of infection, appropriate topical therapy, and patient education and counseling regarding lifestyle changes and limb preservation. The patient must be monitored carefully for indicators of advancing necrosis, which may mandate some form of minor or major amputation.

Strategies for improving blood flow include surgical or endovascular revascularization, aggressive management of modifiable risk factors to prevent disease progression, pharmacologic therapy, HBOT, intermittent pneumatic compression devices, and lifestyle modifications. All patients with CLI/arterial ulceration should receive individualized but comprehensive, guideline-driven, management and therapy (Gerhard-Herman et al., 2017). This includes lifestyle modifications, structured exercise, smoking cessation, and pharmacotherapy (Gerhard-Herman et al., 2017). The importance of managing modifiable risk factors cannot be overemphasized, since this is the key to controlling disease progression and to prevention of cardiovascular-related morbidity and mortality. In one study, investigators found insufficient attention to this aspect of care; 1 month postendovascular intervention for advanced PAD, only 51% of patients had satisfactory control of systolic BP and the percentage of smokers had decreased only 17% (from 41% preop to 24% postop). The same study found that 89% of patients were receiving statins and 98% were receiving antiplatelet drugs or anticoagulants. The authors concluded that secondary prevention (e.g., Table 14.1) is an area where improvement is needed (Alhadad, Wictorsson, Alhadad, et al., 2013).

Patients with LEAD and cellulitis, osteomyelitis, intractable pain, or worsening ulceration with appropriate management should be referred for vascular or surgical intervention (WOCN®, 2014). An urgent vascular referral should be made if there are symptoms of ALI, ABI less than 0.40, or if gangrene is present (WOCN®, 2014).

Pharmacologic Therapy

In addition to risk factor modification by treatment of conditions including tobacco abuse, DM, dyslipidemia, hypertension, and CKD, the mainstays of pharmacologic therapy for LEAD include antiplatelet drugs, cilostazol, and statins (Farber & Eberhardt, 2016; WOCN®, 2014). Pharmacological agents can help healing of arterial ulcers indirectly by treating associated conditions such as infection or improve patency and longevity of treated occlusive disease. A detailed description is beyond the scope of this chapter.

Antiplatelet agents work primarily by reducing platelet aggregation. The most commonly used antiplatelet agent is low- to medium-dose aspirin (81–325 mg/day), which may delay the rate at which LEAD progresses and may improve long-term patency of bypass grafts. Until recently, the primary benefit of aspirin was considered to be reduction in morbidity and mortality related to cerebrovascular and cardiovascular disease (stroke and myocardial infarction), however a recent publication casted doubt on this long-term belief. In this study, the authors found that aspirin did not result in a significantly lower risk of cardiovascular disease than placebo (McNeil et al., 2018). Clopidogrel (75 mg/day) is currently recommended as an alternative to aspirin (Gerhard-Herman et al., 2017; WOCN®, 2014). The benefits of dual antiplatelet therapy (DAPT) to reduce the risk of cardiovascular ischemic events are not well established but may have a modest benefit in cardiovascular event risk reduction (Farber & Eberhardt, 2016; Gerhard-Herman et al., 2017). In a patient with a lower extremity or foot ulceration and concurrent ABI of less than 0.90, singular antiplatelet therapy is suggested. DAPT is a reasonable choice in patients with ischemic ulceration postrevascularization; however, studies are indeterminate on this recommendation (Gerhard-Herman et al., 2017).

Statins are lipid-lowering drugs used to treat systemic atherosclerosis. They slow disease progression, can improve the ABI, increase symptom free walking distance, reduce the risk of adverse cardiovascular events, improve limb outcomes, and may improve patency rates for bypass grafts (Farber & Eberhardt, 2016; Gerhard-Herman et al., 2017). In a systematic review and meta-analysis of 46 trials involving 2706 patients, Reriani et al. (2011) concluded that statin therapy is associated with significant improvement in endothelial function. Statins are currently considered to be standard

therapy for all patients with LEAD (Gerhard-Herman et al., 2017; WOCN®, 2014). Niacin or vitamin B_6 also may be helpful in reducing triglyceride levels and increasing HDL-C levels. The recommended dose of niacin is up to 3 g/day for as long as 60 weeks, as tolerated (WOCN®, 2014).

Hypertension is one risk factor for cardiovascular disease. Antihypertensives have been shown to reduce cardiovascular ischemic event risk in patients with PAD (Gerhard-Herman et al., 2017). There are no conclusive studies to differentiate among classes of hypertensives in PAD, but reduction of systolic blood pressure by at least 10 mm Hg in diabetics and patients with renal disease has been shown to reduce amputation risk (Farber & Eberhardt, 2016). Current guidelines should be referenced for the management of hypertension in PAD patients (Whelton et al., 2018). The PAD patient with an arterial ulceration should also be managed in collaboration with the patient's primary care provider and/or cardiologist in regard to hypertension.

Vasodilators used in LEAD include cilostazol and naftidrofuryl oxalate. Cilostazol has both antiplatelet and vasodilatory effects through its phosphodiesterase III inhibition and is the most commonly used drug for symptomatic LEAD. Benefits have included increased walking distance, improved ABI, and possibly a favorable impact on plasma lipoprotein levels (reduced triglyceride levels and increased levels of HDL-C). The recommended dose is 100 mg twice per day. Approximately one third of patients report mild side effects, which include headaches, abnormal stool, dizziness, and palpitations, which generally subside in about 6 weeks. New onset congestive heart failure is generally considered to be a contraindication to vasodilators (Bedenis, Lethaby, Maxwell, Acosta, & Prins, 2015; Rizzo, Corrado, Patti, et al., 2011). In a review of 26 RCTs addressing the efficacy of cilostazol, naftidrofuryl oxalate, and pentoxifylline, Stevens, Simpson, Harnan, et al. (2012) reported that in the studies they reviewed, both cilostazol and naftidrofuryl were effective, but naftidrofuryl was associated with the most significant improvement in pain-free walking distance. Squires, Simpson, Meng, et al. (2011) conducted a systematic review and concluded that both cilostazol and naftidrofuryl were effective and produced minimal side effects but noted that more studies are needed to assess long-term effectiveness of these agents. In 2014, a Cochrane review was conducted, which revealed improvement in claudication symptoms with cilostazol use, but no reduction of CV death or improvement in quality of life (Bedenis et al., 2015). Cilostazol may also be of benefit in reducing recurrent stenosis caused by intimal hyperplasia (Dindyal & Kyriakides, 2009). However, the Ulcer Healing Society's 2014 arterial ulcer guidelines state that the role of cilostazol in arterial ulcers remains to be evaluated (Federman et al., 2016).

Studies on pentoxifylline in the management of symptomatic LEAD are inconclusive. In one multicenter RCT comparing pentoxifylline, cilostazol, and placebo in moderate-to-severe claudication, there was no difference between pentoxifylline and placebo in maximal walking distance (Dawson et al., 2000). According to the American College of Cardiology/American Heart Association (ACC/AHA) guidelines and the Wound Healing Society (WHS) guidelines, pentoxifylline is not recommended to treat claudication or CLI. However, the 2014 WOCN guidelines recommend a trial of pentoxifylline as a second-line consideration in patients with intermittent claudication (Federman et al., 2016; Gerhard-Herman et al., 2017).

Analgesics may be required for patients with advanced ischemia to relieve chronic pain and thus improve quality of life. Effective pain management may also contribute to improved perfusion by preventing the vasoconstriction caused by sympathetic stimulation (Wipke-Tevis & Sae-Sia, 2004).

Oral anticoagulation is also being studied as adjunctive in the management of LEAD. There are few studies that suggest benefit of oral anticoagulation (AC) therapy postbypass to preserve bypass patency; however, a Cochrane Review (2015) showed no patency benefit. Many studies suggesting possible benefit also show increased bleeding complications and thus the use of AC in patients with PAD postsurgical intervention is uncertain (Gerhard-Herman et al., 2017).

Prostanoids is a family of medicines that can increase blood flow and dilate arteries. They are among the group of medications proposed to help heal arterial ulcers, especially those associated with conditions such as Buerger's disease. Based on a Cochrane review of 33 randomized studies with 4477 participants, the authors found that prostanoids provided a small benefit by improving rest pain and ulcer healing, but they did not improve amputation rates or reduce death. In addition, there was no increase in reported complications with prostanoids compared with placebo (Vietto et al., 2018).

Revascularization: Open and Endovascular Techniques

Ischemia is not the only reason for limb loss in patients with CLI. The presence of infection and ulceration adds to the potential of amputation has been described by Mills et al. (2014). Patients with pure ischemic ulceration secondary to occlusive disease can heal only with revascularization. While adjunctive therapies are important to improve ulcer closure, they do not correct the underlying causative ischemia and cannot replace revascularization (Federman et al., 2016). Since revascularization is not always successful or durable, however, ancillary treatment and interdisciplinary collaboration must occur to minimize tissue loss, close ischemic ulcers where possible, and preserve patient function (Federman et al., 2016).

Revascularization is the primary intervention for healing in patients with advanced LEAD and lower extremity ulcers. From 10% to 20% of individuals with LEAD will require revascularization (Federman et al., 2016). Regions with the most comprehensive vascular care in CLI also have the lowest amputation rates (Farber & Eberhardt, 2016). Patients who should be referred for surgical evaluation include those with CLI and those with ulcers that are not healing with appropriate therapy. According to the ACC/AHA guidelines for the management of patients with PAD, patients with incapacitating claudication should be evaluated for revascularization if there is a reasonable likelihood that symptoms will improve and there is an absence of another diagnosis that would limit exercise, such as angina or heart failure (Hennion & Siano, 2013; Hirsch et al., 2006). Appropriate evaluation is needed to ensure the patency of distal vessels and may involve MRA, multidetector CTA, or contrast angiography using digital subtraction techniques.

Revascularization can be achieved by a number of techniques that are beyond the scope of this chapter. Briefly, revascularization techniques include revascularization by endovascular repair or by open surgery. The risk of surgery should be weighed against the likelihood of success, with the patient's comorbidities being taken into account (Federman et al., 2016).

Endovascular Procedures

The goal of endovascular procedures in CLI is to establish in-line blood flow to the foot (Farber & Eberhardt, 2016; Federman et al., 2016; Gerhard-Herman et al., 2017). The technique chosen is dependent on the anatomic location of tissue loss, lesion characteristics, operator experience, and the overall clinical scenario (Federman et al., 2016; Gerhard-Herman et al., 2017). Endovascular procedures are advantageous because they are less invasive and therefore are associated with lower risk and have been shown to be an effective option for patients with CLI, compared with open surgery (Federman et al., 2016; Gerhard-Herman et al., 2017).

Endovascular procedures generally involve the use of a catheter and a wire to a target artery from a remote access site such as the contralateral groin (Farber & Eberhardt, 2016). The stenotic or occluded areas are crossed to treat the lesion using a variety of devices. Drug-eluting or plain ballooning, bare-metal or drug-eluting stenting, or atherectomy is then used to treat the lesion. While endovascular techniques have lower risk, there is also concern about longevity, durability, and over- or inappropriate use of these techniques (Farber & Eberhardt, 2016). Although there is no proof that endovascular techniques improve limb salvage compared with open surgery, there is agreement that it can be done repeatedly if needed, can revascularize more than one vessel at the same setting and is associated with shorter hospital stay compared with open surgery.

Angiosome targeted endovascular therapy in patients with nonhealing ischemic ulcers entails establishing direct blood flow to the infrapopliteal artery that perfuses the region of the leg or foot with the nonhealing ulcer (Gerhard-Herman et al., 2017; Soderstrom et al., 2013). This can be achieved better with endovascular techniques than with open surgery. Meta-analyses that looked at angiosome-directed endovascular therapy showed improved ulcer healing and decreased amputation rates, especially in diabetic patients, but study quality was low (Federman et al., 2016; Gerhard-Herman et al., 2017). One prospective study of 212 patients showed improved ulcer closure but little effect on amputation rates or 1-year amputation-free survival (Elbadawy, Ali, Saleh, & Hasaballah, 2017). Another study showed the most success in ulcer closure with direct bypass and the least success in ulcer closure with indirect endovascular repair and lower amputation rates with direct vs indirect endovascular therapy (Spillerova, Settembre, Biancari,

Alback, & Venermo, 2017). This is an area of inconclusive data that warrants further research and comparison of risk–benefit ratios, as angiosome-guided therapy may produce longer procedure times, need for more complex skill, and more exposure to contrast (Federman et al., 2016; Gerhard-Herman et al., 2017).

Open Surgery

There two main methods of improving blood flow to the lower extremities using open surgery: bypass and endarterectomy. The main technique is bypass surgery around the area of occlusive disease using a conduit that can be a native vein, a cryopreserved vein, or prosthetic graft. Bypass grafts are ideally done using the patient's own saphenous or other suitable vein (autologous saphenous vein bypass), and the greater saphenous vein has shown higher patency rates than the small saphenous vein, arm veins, or cryopreserved saphenous veins (Farber & Eberhardt, 2016). The most advantages of native veins occur when the bypass is below the knee (Fig. 14.3). If the saphenous vein is damaged or unavailable, a synthetic graft (e.g., heparin-bonded expanded polytetrafluoroethylene) or a cryopreserved vein may be used. Long-term results are generally good, especially in proximal bypass, with 5-year patency rates of approximately 70% in both diabetics and nondiabetics (Federman et al., 2016). Bypass procedures have up to an 80% limb salvage rate with 1%–2% amputation rates at 5 years (Federman et al., 2016). Distal bypass procedures involving smaller vessels below the knee have slightly lower long-term patency rates, with a primary patency rate of about 57% and secondary patency of 63% and limb salvage rate of 78% (Federman et al., 2016). Lower extremity bypass carries a risk of surgical site infection, especially in the groin, and might be complicated by graft thrombosis (Farber & Eberhardt, 2016). Smoking cessation can improve patency rates and is a key element of a comprehensive management program (Gerhard-Herman et al., 2017; WOCN®, 2014).

Open Surgery vs Endovascular Repair

Although the question is frequently entertained, neither is appropriate in all cases. Generally, the more extensive and multisegmented the disease, the more the chance the patient will need an open procedure. Many practitioners can offer surgical intervention, including vascular surgeons, cardiologists, and interventional radiologists, and there is a lack of uniformity in surgical treatment of CLI. There are ongoing randomized studies for the best treatment in patients with critical ischemia. One of them is the Best Endovascular vs Best Surgical Therapy for Patients with Critical Limb Ischemia (BEST-CLI) trial, which is a prospective multicenter study that is planned to, enroll 2100 patients (Menard et al., 2016). Two other studies falling at the foot of an earlier study (BASIL; Adam et al., 2005), both BASIL 2 and BASIL 3, are complementing the BEST study (Hunt et al., 2017; Popplewell et al., 2016). All of these studies are expected to shed more light on the endovascular vs open surgery options. Clinician experience and expertise and individual patient

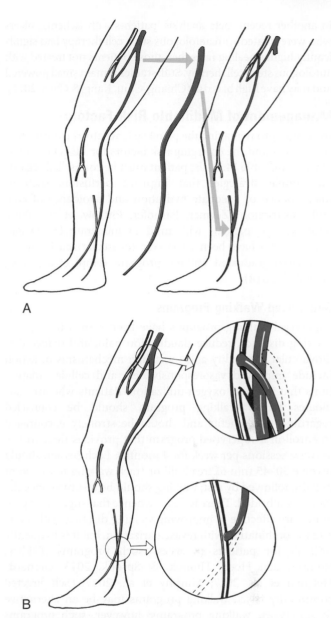

Fig. 14.3 Illustration of bypass grafts.

characteristics should be considered in this decision, as well (Federman et al., 2016).

Stem Cell Therapy

The use of stem cell therapy in small vessel revascularization is promising, but evidence remains indefinite (Federman et al., 2016). In one study in 2002, the TACT trial, autologous transplantation of bone marrow cells to promote angiogenesis displayed potential for this modality (Tateishi-Yuyama et al., 2002). In another more recent meta-analysis, a significant decrease was seen in amputation rates and rest pain, and increases seen in ulcer healing, amputation-free survival, ABI, and TcO_2 were demonstrated (Rigato, Monami, & Fadini, 2017). Interestingly, however, these results were minimized and insignificant in the placebo-controlled RCTs, suggesting study bias or low power in other studies. While results remain unclear, in another recent meta-analysis, patients with ischemic ulcers who were treated with autologous stem cell therapy had significantly higher healing rates than those patients not treated with autologous stem cell therapy. Still, studies remain small powered and may have high bias risk (Chiang, Chiu, Kang, & Chen, 2021).

Management of Modifiable Risk Factors

In addition to managing the primary (causative) contributing risk factors and the emerging risk factors for LEAD (as summarized in Table 14.1), the patient must be counselled regarding simple strategies that improve perfusion, such as maintenance of adequate hydration and avoidance of cold and constriction (Zeymer, Parhofer, Pittrow, et al., 2009). Strategies for patients with mild to moderate LEAD and patients who have been effectively revascularized include a supervised graduated walking program (Hopf et al., 2008; WOCN®, 2014).

Supervised Walking Programs

Supervised walking programs have been shown to improve walking distance, reduce claudication pain, and reduce cardiovascular morbidity and mortality; mechanisms of action include improved vasoresponsiveness and cellular adaptations that improve oxygen utilization. Patients who are candidates for a walking program should be counseled regarding the benefits and should be strongly encouraged to enroll in a supervised program that provides three to five exercise sessions per week for 4 months. Each session should involve 30–45 min of treadmill or track walking to the point of pain, followed by rest; walking should be resumed once the pain has subsided. There is clear evidence that supervised programs are effective in improving walking distance both alone and in combination with revascularization, but it is frequently difficult for patients to access such programs (Fakhry, Rouwet, den Hoed, Hunink, & Spronk, 2013; Gerhard-Herman et al., 2017; Murphy et al., 2015). Self-directed community-based walking programs may be an alternative to supervised walking programs; however, such programs have generally been shown to be ineffective compared with supervised programs, primarily due to their unstructured format. Interestingly, recent studies indicate that such programs can provide comparable outcomes to supervised programs only when they incorporate specific recommendations as well as active monitoring and feedback. Supervised walking programs are considered contraindicated in patients with CLI, due to the potential for development of new or worsening ulcerations (Diehm, Schmidli, Setacci, et al., 2011; Haas, Lloyd, Yang, et al., 2012; Mays, Rogers, Hiatt, et al., 2013).

Hyperbaric Oxygen Therapy

HBOT increases the amount of oxygen dissolved in the plasma, which results in the delivery of "oxygen-enriched" blood to the tissue. HBOT has been shown to increase tissue oxygen levels in ischemic tissue where positive plasma flow exists; it has also been shown to support angiogenesis and ulcer healing. Candidates for HBOT include patients with significant ischemic disease who are not candidates for revascularization and patients who have undergone revascularization but who still demonstrate significant tissue hypoxia and impaired healing. Patients should be evaluated carefully to ensure responsiveness to HBOT (i.e., reversal of tissue-level hypoxia). Responsiveness can be evaluated by obtaining $TcPO_2$ measurements while the patient is breathing room air and then repeating $TcPO_2$ measurements while the patient is breathing 100% oxygen. Normally the $TcPO_2$ level will rise to greater than 100 mm Hg when the patient is breathing 100% oxygen, which signifies a good potential for enhanced healing with HBOT. In contrast, a patient who demonstrates minimal response (<10 mm Hg increase) is not likely to benefit from HBOT (Fife et al., 2009).

HBOT is discussed in greater detail in Chapter 25. The effects of HBOT in CLI for ulcer healing are unknown and warrant further investigation, as most studies have been completed in mixed diabetic/arterial ulcers (Federman et al., 2016; Gerhard-Herman et al., 2017). Studies have shown modest decreases in amputation rates and increases in ulcer closure in concurrent DFU/AU, with RCTs showing more inconsistent results (Federman et al., 2016). Issues related to HBOT include patient compliance, time commitment, expense and insurance coverage by many carriers. CLI alone is not an FDA-approved indication for HBOT.

Intermittent Pneumatic Compression (Arterial Pumps)

While the hemodynamic effects of intermittent pneumatic compression (IPC) on the venous system are well known, IPC also exerts a modest beneficial impact on the arterial blood flow in the lower limb. (Federman et al., 2016; Gerhard-Herman et al., 2017). The hemodynamic effects of intermittent pneumatic compression on the venous system are commonly referred to, but positive effect on both arterial and venous blood flow in the lower limb can be attributed to the use of intermittent pneumatic compression. These devices are most successful in patients who are not candidates for revascularization and do not have serious arterial insufficiency, uncontrolled congestive heart failure, active phlebitis, deep vein thrombosis, localized wound infection, or untreated cellulitis.

Modified Compression for Patients With Mixed Arterial–Venous Disease

Because edema further compromises perfusion, strategies for edema control should be considered when managing the patient with LEAD complicated by lower limb edema. However, the use of sustained compression devices must be modified based on the severity of the arterial disease. Current evidence supports reduced or modified compression (23–30 mm Hg at the ankle) for patients with ABI greater than 0.5 and less than 0.8 (WOCN®, 2014).

Patients with ABI of 0.5 or less may be managed with intermittent pneumatic compression or low-level elevation (in collaboration with a vascular specialist) they should not receive sustained compression (WOCN®, 2014). Compression options including intermittent compression devices are discussed further in Chapter 15.

SYSTEMIC SUPPORT FOR ULCER HEALING

Long-term outcomes for CLI are great when complete ulcer healing can occur. It is imperative, then, that an interdisciplinary care team work together to optimize infection prevention, topical therapy, offloading, nutritional support, glucose control, and control of other comorbidities (Federman et al., 2016; Gerhard-Herman et al., 2017; WOCN®, 2014).

Management of Arterial Ulcer
Prevention and Management of Infection

Ischemia increases the risk for infection, and both ischemia and infection are significant impediments to the repair process. Thus, prompt recognition and aggressive treatment of infectious complications are critical to positive outcomes. However, this can be a challenge because signs of infection are frequently muted (and therefore easy to miss) in ischemic conditions. Clinicians must routinely assess for subtle indicators of infection, such as a faint halo of erythema extending circumferentially around the ulcer edge. In ulcers that present with signs of infection, systemic antibiotic therapy should be initiated. When viable tissue is present in the ulcer bed, a tissue culture should be obtained to ensure appropriate antibiotic selection. Effective management of infected ischemic ulcers involves revascularization when indicated and when possible, aggressive debridement of all necrotic tissue (including any necrotic bone), and appropriate antibiotic therapy should be instituted. Topical antimicrobial or antiseptic (see Chapters 19 and 21) dressings can be used in conjunction with systemic antibiotic therapy and may be helpful in controlling bacterial load as well as preventing infection in clean, open ulcers (Federman et al., 2016). However, antimicrobial dressings should not be used as sole therapy for infected ischemic ulcers (Gerhard-Herman et al., 2017; WOCN®, 2014).

Clinicians should have a high index of suspicion for infection in patients with LEAD or CLI, especially because infectious signs may be subtle in the presence of DM and LEAD (Gerhard-Herman et al., 2017). Those with LEAD and foot infection show a threefold higher risk of amputation than those with LEAD or foot infection alone, mandating that foot infection be treated promptly and comprehensively in this population (Gerhard-Herman et al., 2017).

Topical Therapy

Arterial ulcers typically have minimal exudate and are at very high risk for infection. For arterial ulcers that have marginal but adequate perfusion, hydrating dressings with sustained-release antimicrobial properties with a nonocclusive outer layer is likely to be of particular benefit. In addition, the periulcer skin is typically very fragile; thus, nonadherent dressings or those with silicone adhesive are preferable. The periulcer skin can be further protected with a skin sealant or moisture barrier ointment. According to a 2020 systematic review, there remains insufficient evidence to determine whether the choice of topical agent or dressing affects the healing of arterial ulcers (Broderick, Pagnamenta, & Forster, 2020; Normahani et al., 2021).

Management of Necrotic Ulcers

Although necrotic tissue is clearly a potential medium for bacterial growth, a dry, intact eschar also can serve as a bacterial barrier. A closed ulcer surface is advantageous when managing a very poorly perfused ulcer in which any bacterial invasion is likely to result in clinical infection and limb loss. Although research into optimal management of these ulcers is clearly needed, there is clinical consensus that a closed ulcer should be maintained.

Debridement

Debridement (either autolytic or sharp) should be avoided when (1) the involved limb is clearly ischemic with limited or no potential for healing, (2) no indications of infection are present, and (3) the ulcer surface is dry and necrotic (WOCN®, 2014). A sample topical therapy protocol for this type of ulcer is outlined in Box 14.5. Note that this protocol applies only to *uninfected* ulcers covered with dry, intact eschar. However, if the patient develops clinically significant ulcer infection, the patient should be promptly referred for surgical evaluation (for debridement and/or revascularization, or even amputation of the infected part to save the rest of the limb (WOCN®, 2014).

Ancillary Ulcer Healing Modalities

Revascularization is the first-line treatment for arterial ulceration and cannot be replaced by adjuvant agents. When revascularization is not possible, not successful, or ulcer closure does not result from revascularization, ancillary therapies may prove beneficial (Federman et al., 2016). Although ultrasound has been shown to assist ulcer closure in venous and pressure ulcers and there have been some studies showing potential in arterial ulcers, there is not enough evidence to recommend its use in this setting (Federman et al., 2016).

Spinal cord stimulation may assist with pain management in CLI; however studies do not show benefit in limb preservation or ulcer healing (Federman et al., 2016).

Negative pressure wound therapy has been shown to be a safe option in this population, but again has not been shown to affect clinical outcomes. Generally, patients with ischemic ulcers should not be treated with negative pressure dressing as this is likely to decrease perfusion and cause maceration of the skin in the vicinity of ulcer area.

BOX 14.5   Topical Therapy for Dry, Necrotic, Uninfected Ischemic Ulcer

1. Inspect for subtle indicators of infection. If any signs or symptoms of infection develop, immediate referral for debridement and initiation of antibiotic therapy are critical.
2. Paint with antiseptic solution (e.g., povidone-iodine 10% solution); allow to dry.
3. Apply dry gauze dressing and secure with wrap gauze.

BOX 14.6   Limb Preservation Strategies

Routine Skin Care
- Apply emollients after bathing to prevent cracking and fissures.
- Dry carefully between toes to prevent maceration.
- Use lamb's wool or foam toe "sleeves" to prevent interdigital friction and pressure.

Measures to Prevent Mechanical Trauma
- Avoid walking barefoot, even indoors; consistently use protective footwear (e.g., closed-toe shoes) to prevent inadvertent cuts or puncture ulcers.
- Inspect shoes before wearing.
- Carefully fit shoes to prevent pressure, friction, and shear injuries.
- If indicated, use protective shin guards when working around house or yard.

- Receive professional foot and nail care (or limit self-care of nails to conservative trimming and filing); no "bathroom surgery."

Measures to Prevent Thermal Trauma
- Wear warm socks during cold weather to prevent vasoconstriction.
- Do not use hot water bottles, heating pads, or other thermal devices.
- Check water temperature with hand or elbow before bathing.

Measures to Prevent Chemical Trauma
- Do not use antiseptic or chemical agents (e.g., corn removers).

General Measures
- Inspect feet and legs daily.
- Promptly report any minor injuries.

Topical oxygen has also received attention in the management of arterial ulcers, however the paucity of literature on this demonstrates a need for further investigation.

Amputation

Amputation is reserved as the "treatment of last resort" and is indicated primarily for patients with irreversible ischemia (i. e., tissue necrosis), invasive infection, or CLI and flexion contractures (Farber & Eberhardt, 2016). Healing is challenging in patients with ischemic ulceration. Different methods have been suggested to assist in choosing the level of amputation to achieve healing, including limb pressure measurement, toe pressures, waveform analysis, perfusion studies, and TcPO2 measurements (Aronow, 2008; Fife et al., 2009; WOCN®, 2014). It is likely that clinical examination with one or more of such methods can assist in choosing the level of amputation, which is also affected by the functional status of the patient. In some cases, limb preservation is important to the patient, thus eliminating the option of amputation and promoting attempts to preserve the limb as much as possible. In nonemergent cases where amputation is determined to be the optimal path, providers should openly discuss the risks and benefits with the patient prior to decision for amputation (Federman et al., 2016). Prosthetic professionals and physiotherapists should be involved as early as possible when the decision for amputation is made.

PATIENT EDUCATION

Lifestyle changes may be more difficult for the patient than either a surgical procedure or drug therapy; therefore, effective introduction of such changes requires in-depth education and supportive, goal-directed patient counseling. A team approach should be utilized in patient and family education (Federman et al., 2016). In addition to receiving education regarding the specific plan of care and rationale, the patient should be taught the importance (and specifics) of protective lower limb care (Box 14.6) (Aronow, 2008; WOCN®, 2014).

CLINICAL CONSULT

A: Consulted for nonhealing leg ulcer. 66-Year old Caucasian female with Type 2 diabetes × 32 years (HbA1c 8.2), atherosclerotic heart disease (stent placement × 3, 18 months ago), hypertension, obesity; 42-year history of cigarette smoking. Patient reports ulcer started as a tiny "nick" after bumping her leg 2 months ago. She rates rest pain with leg dependent as 3/10 and 9/10 with any significant activity. She sleeps in a recliner. Right lateral shin ulcer 4.5 cm (L) × 2.0 cm (W) × 0.3 cm (D). Ulcer bed 70% gray slough and 30% pale pink; minimal serious exudate; ulcer edges closed and "punched out" in appearance; periulcer skin mildly erythematous to 3 cm past ulcer edge circumferentially with slight induration. Lower extremities, absent of hair, with thin shiny skin and thickened fungal nails. Elevational pallor and dependent rubor (R > L), capillary refill of 6 s (R) and 5 s (L); venous filling time 30 s (R) and 26 s (L); diminished DP and PT pulses both feet; ABI 0.32 on right and 0.54 on left.

D: Arterial insufficiency, critical limb ischemia, infected right leg ulcer.

P: Implement interventions to maximize perfusion, eradicate infection and necrosis, promote healing, and prevent further injury.

I: (1) Urgent vascular consult. (2) Smoking cessation program. (3) Collaborate with provider for culture-based treatment of ulcer infection, effective pain management, and topical therapy that supports debridement and control of bioburden. (4) Collaborate with provider, patient, and dietitian for optimal glucose control. (5) Educate patient regarding preventive foot and lower extremity care.

E: Patient verbalizes understanding and agreement with plan of care. Will follow with care team, review vascular and dietitian consults, and modify topical management, as needed.

SUMMARY

- Arterial ulcers are most commonly caused by peripheral arterial occlusive disease and may progress to CLI and limb loss.
- Risk factors for peripheral arterial occlusive disease and arterial ulcers are the same as those for CAD and cerebrovascular disease. They include tobacco use, diabetes mellitus, dyslipidemia, hypertension, and CKD, as well as family history and age.
- Arterial ulcers typically present as spontaneous ulceration of the toes and distal foot or as a nonhealing traumatic injury.
- Typically, pure arterial ulcers are painful, with a pale or necrotic ulcer bed, well-demarcated edges, and minimal exudate.
- Arterial ulcers are commonly infected; however, the signs of infection are muted due to the underlying ischemia.
- Successful management of an arterial ulcer is dependent on measures to improve perfusion and oxygenation (revascularization, risk factor management, and lifestyle measures such as smoking cessation).
- Positive long-term outcomes are dependent on lifestyle modifications to correct reversible risk factors and a progressive walking program to improve lower limb perfusion, as well as measures to prevent injury.
- A multidisciplinary approach to ulcer healing is essential as patients might require offloading, nutritional support, glucose control, revascularization, and rehabilitation. In limb salvage programs, healing is achieved only through a team approach.
- Guideline adherence and optimal clinical outcomes are best achieved through collaboration among disciplines and in communication with the patient (Gerhard-Herman et al., 2017). Each patient's individual values and comorbidities should be considered, especially in complex conditions such as PAD.

SELF-ASSESSMENT QUESTIONS

1. Rest pain is indicative of which of the following?
   a. Mild occlusive disease, as occurs with 25% occlusion
   b. Moderate occlusive disease, as occurs with 50% occlusion
   c. Advanced occlusive disease, as occurs with 90% occlusion
   d. Need for amputation
2. Risk factors for lower extremity arterial disease include which of the following?
   a. Alcoholism
   b. Hypertension
   c. Elevated high-density lipoprotein levels
   d. Diabetes insipidus
3. What type of pain is claudication?
   a. Pain that exists without precipitating activity
   b. Pain that develops when the patient elevates the legs
   c. Pain that is triggered by moderate-to-heavy activity
   d. Pain that worsens with rest
4. Which of the following ankle-brachial index (ABI) values is indicative of calcification of the vessel wall in a person with diabetes?
   a. 0.95–1.1
   b. 0.5–0.95
   c. 0.5
   d. >1.3
5. Which of the following descriptions is classic for an arterial ulcer?
   a. Highly exudative
   b. Presence of red granulation tissue
   c. Common location above medial malleolus
   d. Dry ulcer bed
6. Which of the following describes the situation in which maintenance of an eschar-covered arterial ulcer is preferred?
   a. The involved limb can be revascularized.
   b. The TcPO$_2$ is 20 mm Hg.
   c. The ulcer is infected.
   d. Indications of infection are absent and potential for healing is limited.

REFERENCES

Abdulhannan, P., Russell, D., & Homer-Vanniasinkram, S. (2012). Peripheral arterial disease: A literature review. *British Medical Bulletin, 104*, 21–39.

Adam, D. J., Beard, J. D., Cleveland, T., Bell, J., Bradbury, A. W., Forbes, J. F., et al. (2005). Bypass versus angioplasty in severe ischaemia of the leg (BASIL): Multicentre, randomised controlled trial. *Lancet, 366*(9501), 1925–1934. https://doi.org/10.1016/S0140-6736(05)67704-5.

Aksu, K. (2012). Donmez A, Keser G: Inflammation-induced thrombosis: Mechanisms, disease associations, and management. *Current Pharmaceutical Design, 18*(11), 1478–1493.

Alhadad, A., Wictorsson, C., Alhadad, H., et al. (2013). Medical risk factor treatment in peripheral artery disease: Need for further improvement. *International Angiology, 32*(3), 332–338.

Alzamora, M., Fores, R., Pera, G., et al. (2013). Ankle-brachial index and the incidence of cardiovascular events in the Mediterranean low cardiovascular risk population ARTPER cohort. *BMC Cardiovascular Disorders, 13*, 119.

American Diabetes Association. (2014). Standards of medical care in diabetes—2014. *Diabetes Care, 37*(Suppl. 1), S14–S80.

Andras, A., Stansby, G., & Hansrani, M. (2013). Homocysteine-lowering interventions for PAD and bypass grafts. *Cochrane Database of Systematic Reviews, 7*, CD003285.

Apanah, S., & Rizzolo, D. (2013). Sickle cell disease: Taking a multidisciplinary approach. *Journal of the American Academy of Physician Assistants, 26*(8), 28–33.

Arinze, N. V., Gregory, A., Francis, J. M., Farber, A., & Chitalia, V. C. (2019). Unique aspects of peripheral arterial disease in patients with chronic kidney disease. *Vascular Medicine, 24*(3), 251–260. https://doi.org/10.1177/1358863XI8824654.

Armstrong, E. J., Wu, J., Singh, G. D., Dawson, D. L., Pevec, W. C., Amsterdam, E. A., et al. (2014). Smoking cessation is associated with decreased mortality and improved amputation-free survival among patients with symptomatic peripheral artery disease. *Journal of Vascular Surgery, 60*(6), 1565–1571.

Aronow, H. (2008). Peripheral arterial disease in the elderly: Recognition and management. *American Journal of Cardiovascular Drugs, 8*(6), 353–364.

Bedenis, R., Lethaby, A., Maxwell, H., Acosta, S., & Prins, M. H. (2015). Antiplatelet agents for preventing thrombosis after peripheral artery bypass surgery. *Cochrane Database of Systematic Reviews, 2*. https://doi.org/10.1002/14651858. CD000535.pub3.

Bevc, S., Purg, D., Turnsek, N., et al. (2013). Ankle-brachial index and cardiovascular mortality in nondiabetic hemodialysis patients. *Therapeutic Apheresis and Dialysis, 17*(4), 313–317.

Bonham, P. (2011). Measuring toe pressures using a portable photoplethysmograph to detect arterial disease in high risk patients: An overview of the literature. *Ostomy Ulcer Manage, 57*(11), 36–44.

Bonham, P., Cappuccio, M., Hulsey, T., et al. (2007). Are ankle and toe brachial indices (ABI-TBI) obtained by a pocket Doppler interchangeable with those obtained by standard laboratory equipment? *Journal of Wound Ostomy & Continence Nursing, 34*(1), 35–44.

Bozkurt, A., Cengiz, K., Arslan, C., et al. (2013). A stable prostacyclin analogue (iloprost) in the treatment of Buerger's disease: A prospective analysis of 150 patients. *Annals of Thoracic and Cardiovascular Surgery, 19*(2), 120–125.

Broderick, C., Pagnamenta, F., & Forster, R. (2020). Dressings and topical agents for arterial leg ulcers. *The. Cochrane Database of Systematic Reviews, 1*(1), CD001836. https://doi.org/10.1002/14651858.CD001836.pub4.

Cao, P., Eckstein, H., DeRango, P., et al. (2011). Diagnostic methods. *European Journal of Vascular and Endovascular Surgery, 42*(Suppl 2), S13–S32.

Chaparaia, R., et al. (2009). Inflammatory profiling of peripheral arterial disease. *Annals of Vascular Surgery, 23*(2), 172–178. https://doi.org/10.1016/j.avsg.2008.06.005 (Epub Jul 26, 2008).

Chiang, K. J., Chiu, L. C., Kang, Y. N., & Chen, C. (2021). Autologous stem cell therapy for chronic lower extremity wounds: A meta-analysis of randomized controlled trials. *Cells, 10*(12), 3307. https://doi.org/10.3390/cells10123307.

Darling, J.D., McCallum, J.C., Soden, P.A., Meng, Y., Wyers, M.C., Hamdan, A.D. Schermerhorn, M.L. (2016). Predictive ability of the SVS WIfI classification system following infrapopliteal endovascular interventions for CLI. *Journal of Vascular Surgery, 64*(3), 616–622. doi: https://doi.org/10.1016/j.jvs.2016.03.417.

Dawson, D. L., Cutler, B. S., Hiatt, W. R., Hobson, R. W., Martin, J. D., Bortey, E. B., et al. (2000). A comparison of cilostazol and pentoxifylline for treating intermittent claudication. *American Journal of Medicine, 109*(7), 523–530. https://doi.org/10.1016/s00029343(00)00569-6.

Delaney, K., Axelrod, K., Buscetta, A., et al. (2013). Leg ulcers in sickle cell disease: Current patterns and practice. *Hemoglobin, 37*(4), 325–332.

Dellalibera-Joviliano, R., Joviliano, E., Silva, J., et al. (2012). Activation of cytokines corroborate with development of inflammation and autoimmunity in thromboangiitis obliterans patients. *Clinical and Experimental Immunology, 170*(1), 28–35.

De Silva, G. S., Saffaf, K., Sanchez, L. A., & Zayed, M. A. (2018). Amputation stump perfusion is predictive of post-operative necrotic eschar formation. *American Journal of Surgery, 216*(3), 540–546. https://doi.org/10.1016/j.amjsurg.2018.05.007.

Diehm, N., Schmidli, J., Setacci, C., et al. (2011). Management of cardiovascular risk factors and medical therapy. *European Journal of Vascular and Endovascular Surgery, 42*(Suppl. 2), S33–S42.

Dindyal, S., & Kyriakides, C. (2009). A review of cilostazol, a phosphodiesterase inhibitor, and its role in preventing both coronary and peripheral arterial restenosis following endovascular therapy. *Recent Patents on Cardiovascular Drug Discovery, 4*(1), 6–14.

Dua, A., & Lee, C. J. (2016). Epidemiology of peripheral arterial disease and critical limb ischemia. *Techniques in Vascular and Interventional Radiology, 19*, 91–95. https://doi.org/10.1053/j.tvir.2016.04.001.

Elbadawy, M., Ali, H., Saleh, M., & Hasaballah, A. (2017). Editor's choice- A prospective study to evaluate complete ulcer healing and limb salvage rates after angiosome targeted infrapopliteal balloon angioplasty in patients with critical limb ischaemia. *European Journal of Endovascular Surgery, 55*, 392–397. https://doi.org/10.1016/j.evs.2017.12.003.

Fakhry, F., Rouwet, E. V., den Hoed, P. T., Hunink, M. M., & Spronk, S. (2013). Long-term clinical effectiveness of supervised exercise therapy versus endovascular revascularization for intermittent claudication from a randomized clinical trial. *British Journal of Surgery, 100*, 1164–1171.

Farber, A., & Eberhardt, R. T. (2016). The current state of critical limb ischemia: A systematic review. *Journal of the American Medical Association Surgery, 151*(11), 1070–1077. https://doi.org/10.1001/jamasurg.2016.2018.

Fazeli, B., Moghadam, M. D., & Niroumand, S. (2018). How to treat a patient with thromboangiitis obliterans: A systematic review. *Annals of Vascular Surgery, 49*, 219–228. https://doi.org/10.1016/j.avsg.2017.10.022.

Federman, D. G., Ladiiznski, B., Dardik, A., Kelly, M., Shapshak, D., Ueno, C. M., et al. (2016). Ulcer healing society 2014 update on guidelines for arterial ulcers. *Ulcer Repair and Regeneration, 24*, 127–135. https://doi.org/10.1111/wrr.12395.

Fife, C., Smart, D., Sheffield, P., et al. (2009). Transcutaneous oximetry in clinical practice: Consensus statement from an expert panel based on evidence. *Undersea & Hyperbaric Medicine, 36*(1), 43–53.

Fowkes, F., Rudan, D., Rudan, I., et al. (2013). Comparison of global estimates of prevalence and risk factors for peripheral arterial disease in 2000 and 2010: A systematic review and analysis. *Lancet, 382*(9901), 1329–1340.

Gaffo, A. (2013). Thrombosis in vasculitides. *Best Practice & Research. Clinical Rheumatology, 27*(1), 57–67.

Gardner, A., & Afaq, A. (2008). Management of lower extremity peripheral arterial disease. *Journal of Cardiopulmonary Rehabilitation and Prevention, 28*(6), 349–357.

Garimella, P., Hart, P., O'Hare, A., et al. (2012). Peripheral artery disease and CKD: A focus on peripheral artery disease as a critical component of CKD care. *American Journal of Kidney Diseases, 60*(4), 641–654.

Garimella, P. S., & Hirsch, A. T. (2014). Peripheral artery disease and chronic kidney disease: Clinical synergy to improve outcomes. *Advances in Chronic Kidney Disease, 21*(6), 460–471. https://doi.org/10.1053/j.ackd.2014.07.005.

Gerhard-Herman, M. D., Gornik, H. L., Barrett, C., Barshes, N. R., Corriere, M. A., Drachman, D. E., et al. (2017). 2016 AHA/ACC guideline on the management of patients with lower extremity peripheral artery disease: Executive summary: A report of the American College of Cardiology/American Heart Association task force on clinical practice guidelines. *Circulation, 135,* e686–e725. https://doi.org/10.1161/CIR.0000000000000470.

Grenon, S., Conte, M., Nosova, E., et al. (2013). Association between N-3 polyunsaturated fatty acid content of red blood cells and inflammatory biomarkers in patients with PAD. *Journal of Vascular Surgery, 58*(5), 1283–1290.

Haas, T., Lloyd, P., Yang, H., et al. (2012). Exercise training and peripheral arterial disease. *Comprehensive Physiology, 2*(4), 2933–3017.

Haigh, K., Bingley, J., Golledge, J., et al. (2013). Peripheral arterial disease screening in general practice. *Australian Family Physician, 42*(6), 391–395.

Hardman, R. L., Jazaeri, O., Yi, J., Smith, M., & Gupta, R. (2014). Overview of classification systems in peripheral arterial disease. *Seminars in Interventional Radiology, 31*(4), 378–387. https://doi.org/10.1055/s-0034-1393976.

Hennion, D., & Siano, K. (2013). Diagnosis and treatment of peripheral arterial disease. *American Family Physician, 88*(5), 306–310.

Hirsch, A., Haskal, Z. J., Hertzer, N. R., et al. (2006). ACC/AHA 2005 practice guidelines for the management of patients with peripheral arterial disease (lower extremity, renal, mesenteric, and abdominal aortic). *Circulation, 113*(11), 1474–1547.

Hopf, H., Ueno, C., Aslam, R., et al. (2008). Guidelines for the prevention of lower extremity arterial ulcers. *Wound Repair and Regeneration, 16*(2), 175–188.

Huang, C. L., Wu, Y. W., Hwang, C. L., Jong, Y. S., Chao, C. L., Chen, W. J., et al. (2011). The application of infrared thermography in evaluation of patients at high risk for lower extremity peripheral arterial disease. *Journal of Vascular Surgery, 54,* 1074–1080. https://doi.org/10.1016/j.jvs.2011.03.287.

Hunt, B. D., Popplewell, M. A., Davies, H., Meecham, L., Jarrett, H., Bate, G., et al. (2017). Balloon versus stenting in severe Ischaemia of the Leg-3 (BASIL-3): Study protocol for a randomised controlled trial. *Trials, 18*(224). https://doi.org/10.1186/s13063-017-1968-6.

Hus, I., Sokolawska, B., Waleter-Croneda, A., et al. (2013). Assessment of plasma prothrombotic factors in patients with Buerger's disease. *Blood Coagulation & Fibrinolysis, 24*(2), 133–139.

Iannuzzo, G., Forte, F., Lupoli, R., & Di Minno, M. N. (2018). Association of vitamin D deficiency with peripheral arterial disease: A meta-analysis of literature studies. *The Journal of Clinical Endocrinology and Metabolism, 103*(6), 2107–2115. https://doi.org/10.1210/jc.2018-00136.

Jones, W., Patel, M., Rockman, C., et al. (2014). Association of the ankle-brachial index with history of myocardial infarction and stroke. *American Heart Journal, 167*(4), 499–505.

Katsiki, N., Papadopoulou, S., Fachantidou, A., et al. (2013). Smoking and vascular risk: Are all forms of smoking harmful to all types of vascular disease? *Public Health, 127*(5), 435–441.

Kaur, S., Pawar, M., Banerjee, N., & Garg, R. (2012). Evaluation of the efficacy of hyperbaric oxygen therapy in the management of chronic nonhealing ulcer and role of periulcer transcutaneous oximetry as a predictor of ulcer healing response: A randomized prospective controlled trial. *Journal of Anaesthesiology Clinical Pharmacology, 28*(1), 70–75. https://doi.org/10.4103/0970-9185.92444.

Lambert, M., & Belch, J. (2013). Medical management of critical limb ischemia: Where do we stand today? *Journal of Internal Medicine, 274*(4), 295–307.

Liapis, C., Avgerinos, E., Kadoglou, N., et al. (2009). What a vascular surgeon should know and do about atherosclerotic risk factors. *Journal of Vascular Surgery, 49*(5), 1348–1354.

Lowry, D., Saeed, M., Narendran, P., & Tiwari, A. (2018). A review of distribution of atherosclerosis in the lower limb arteries of patients with diabetes mellitus and peripheral vascular disease. *Vascular and Endovascular Surgery, 52*(7), 535–542. https://doi.org/10.1177/1538574418791622.

Luders, F., Furstenberg, T., Engelbertz, C., Gebauer, K., Meyborg, M., Malyar, N. M., et al. (2017). The impact of chronic kidney disease on hospitalized patients with peripheral arterial disease and critical limb ischemia. *Angiology, 68*(2), 145–150. https://doi.org/10.1177/0003319716638797.

Martí-Carvajal, A. J., Knight-Madden, J. M., & Martinez-Zapata, M. J. (2014). Interventions for treating leg ulcers in people with sickle cell disease. *Cochrane Database of Systematic Reviews, 12.* https://doi.org/10.1002/14651858.CD008394.pub3.

Matsuzawa, R., Aoyama, N., & Yoshida, A. (2015). Clinical characteristics of patients of hemodialysis with peripheral arterial disease. *Angiology, 66*(10), 911–917. https://doi.org/10.1177/0003319715572678.

Mays, R., Rogers, K., Hiatt, W., et al. (2013). Community walking programs for treatment of peripheral arterial disease. *Journal of Vascular Surgery, 58*(6), 1678–1687.

McDermott, M. M., Liu, K., Ferrucci, L., Tian, L., Guralnik, J., Kopp, P., et al. (2014). Vitamin D status, functional decline, and mortality in peripheral arterial disease. *Vascular Medicine, 19*(1), 18–26. https://doi.org/10.1177/1358863X13518364.

McNeil, J. J., Wolfe, R., Woods, R. L., Tonkin, A. M., Donnan, M. B., Nelson, M. R., et al. (2018). Effect of aspirin on cardiovascular events and bleeding in the healthy elderly. *New England Journal of Medicine, 379*(18), 1509–1518. https://doi.org/10.1056/NEJMoa1805819.

Menard, M. T., Farber, A., Assmann, S. F., Choudhry, N. K., Conte, M. S., Creager, M. A., et al. (2016). Design and rationale of the BEST endovascular versus BEST surgical therapy for patients with critical limb ischemia. *Journal of the American Heart Association, 5.* https://doi.org/10.1161/JAHA.116.003219.

Mensah, G., & Bakris, G. (2010). Treatment and control of high blood pressure in adults. *Clinical Cardiology, 28*(4), 609–622.

Mills, J. L., Conte, M. S., Armstrong, D. G., Pomposelli, F. B., Schanzer, A., Sidawy, A. N., et al. (2014). *Journal of Vascular Surgery, 59,* 220–234. https://doi.org/10.1016/j.jvs.2013.08.003.

Murphy, T. P., Cutlip, D. E., Regensteiner, J. G., Mohler, E. R., Cohen, D. J., Reynolds, et al. (2015). Supervised exercise, stent revascularization, or medical therapy for claudication due to aortoiliac peripheral artery disease: The CLEVER study.

Journal of the American College of Cardiology, 65(10), 999–1009. https://doi.org/10.1016/j.jacc.2014.12.043.

Norgren, L., Hiatt, W., Dormandy, J., et al. (2007). Inter-society consensus for the management of peripheral arterial disease (TASC II). *Journal of Vascular Surgery, 45*(Suppl. S), S5–S67.

Norgren, L., Patel, M. R., Hiatt, W. R., Wojdyla, D. M., Fowkes, G. R., Baumgartner, I., et al. (2018). Outcomes of patients with critical limb ischaemia in the EUCLID trial. *European Journal of Vascular and Endovascular Surgery, 55*, 109–117. https://doi.org/10.1016/j.ejvs.2017.11.006.

Nsengiyumva, V., Fernando, M. E., Moxon, J. V., Krishna, S. M., Pinchbeck, J., Omer, S. M., et al. (2015). The association of circulating 25-hydroxyvitamin D concentration with peripheral arterial disease: A meta-analysis of observational studies. *Atherosclerosis, 243*, 645–651. https://doi.org/10.1016/j.atherosclerosis.2015.10.011.

Normahani, P., Mustafa, C., Shalhoub, J., Davies, A. H., Norrie, J., Sounderajah, V., et al. (2021). A systematic review and meta-analysis of the diagnostic accuracy of point-of-care tests used to establish the presence of peripheral arterial disease in people with diabetes. *Journal of Vascular Surgery, 73*(5), 1811–1820. https://doi.org/10.1016/j.jvs.2020.11.030.

Popplewell, M. A., Davies, H., Jarrett, H., Bate, G., Grant, M., Patel, S., et al. (2016). Bypass versus angioplasty in severe ischaemia of the leg-2 (BASIL 2) trial: Study protocol for a randomised controlled trial. *Trials, 17*(11), 2. https://doi.org/10.1186/s13063-015-1114-.

Reriani, M., Dunlay, S., Gupta, B., et al. (2011). Effects of statins on coronary and peripheral endothelial function in humans: A systematic review and meta-analysis of randomized controlled trials. *European Journal of Cardiovascular Preventative Rehabilitation, 18*(5), 704–716.

Rief, P., Pichler, M., Raggam, R., Hafner, F., Gerger, A., Eller, P., et al. (2016). The AST/ALT ratio: A novel marker for critical limb ischemia in peripheral arterial occlusive disease patients. *Medicine, 95*(24). https://doi.org/10.1097/MD.0000000000003843.

Rigato, M., Monami, M., & Fadini, G. P. (2017). Autologous cell therapy for PAD: Systematic review and meta-analysis of randomized, nonrandomized, and noncontrolled studies. *Circulation Research, 120*, 1326–1340. https://doi.org/10.1161/circresaha.116.309045.

Rizzo, M., Corrado, E., Patti, A., et al. (2011). Cilostazol and atherogenic dyslipidemia: A clinically relevant effect? *Expert Opinions in Pharmacotherapy, 12*(4), 647–655.

Rollini, F., Franchi, F., Muniz-Lozano, A., et al. (2013). Platelet function profiles in patients with diabetes mellitus. *Journal of Cardiovascular Translational Research, 6*(3), 329–345.

Rutherford, R. B., Baker, J. D., Ernst, C., Johnston, K. W., Porter, J. M., Ahn, S., et al. (1997). Recommended standards for reports dealing with lower extremity ischemia: Revised version. *Journal of Vascular Surgery, 26*, 517–538.

Samies, J. H., Gehling, M., Serena, T. E., & Yaakov, R. A. (2015). Use of a fluorescence angiography system in assessment of lower extremity ulcers in patients with peripheral arterial disease: A review and a look forward. *Seminars in Vascular Surgery, 28*, 190–194. https://doi.org/10.1053/j.semvascsurg.2015.12.002.

Saskin, H., Ozcan, K. S., Duzyol, C., Baris, O., & Koçoğulları, U. C. (2017). Are inflammatory parameters predictors of amputation in acute arterial occlusions? *Vascular, 25*(2), 170–177. https://doi.org/10.1177/1708538116652995.

Schernthaner, R., Fleischmann, D., Stadler, A., et al. (2009). Value of MDCT angiography in developing treatment strategies for critical limb ischemia. *American Journal of Roentgenology, 192*(5), 1416–1424.

Shanmugam, V. K., Angra, D. A., Rahimi, H., & McNish, S. (2017). Vasculitic and autoimmune ulcers. *Journal of Vascular Surgery. Venous and Lymphatic Disorders, 5*(2), 280–292. https://doi.org/10.1016/j.jvsv.2016.09.006.

Shu, J., & Santulli, G. (*2018*). Update on peripheral arterial disease: Epidemiology and evidence based facts. *Atherosclerosis, 275*, 379–381. https://doi.org/10.1016/j.atherosclerosis.2018.05.033 doi:10.1016/j.vs2012.07.057.

Sigvant, B., Wiberg-Hedman, K., Bergqvist, D., et al. (2009). Risk factor profiles and use of cardiovascular drug prevention in women and men with peripheral arterial disease. *European Journal of Cardiovascular Preventative Rehabilitation, 16*(1), 39–46.

Sihlangu, D., & Bliss, J. (2012). Resting Doppler ankle brachial pressure index measurement: A literature review. *British Journal of Community Nursing, 17*(7), 318–324.

Soderstrom, M., Alback, A., Biancari, F., Lappalainen, K., Lepantalo, M., & Venermo, M. (2013). Angiosome-targeted infrapopliteal endovascular revascularization for treatment of diabetic foot ulcers. *Journal of Vascular Surgery, 57*(2), 427–435.

Spillerova, K., Settembre, N., Biancari, F., Alback, A., & Venermo, M. (2017). *European Journal of Vascular and Endovascular Surgery, 53*, 567–575. https://doi.org/10.1016/j.ejvs.2017.01.008.

Squires, H., Simpson, E., Meng, Y., et al. (2011). A systematic review and economic evaluation of cilostazol, naftidrofuryl oxalate, pentoxifylline, and inositol nicotinate for the treatment of intermittent claudication in people with peripheral arterial disease. *Health Technology Assessment, 15*(40), 1–210.

Stevens, J., Simpson, E., Harnan, S., et al. (2012). Systematic review of the efficacy of cilostazol, naftidrofuryl oxalate and pentoxifylline for treatment of intermittent claudication. *British Journal of Surgery, 99*(12), 1630–1638.

Tamura, K., Tsurumi-Ikeya, Y., Wakui, H., et al. (2013). Therapeutic potential of low-density lipoprotein apheresis in the management of peripheral artery disease in patients with chronic kidney disease. *Therapeutic Apheresis and Dialysis, 17*(2), 185–192.

Tateishi-Yuyama, E., Matsubara, H., Murohara, T., Ikeda, U., Shintani, S., Masaki, H., et al. (2002). Therapeutic angiogenesis for patients with limb ischaemia by autologous transplantation of bone-marrow cells: A pilot study and a randomized controlled trial. *The Lancet, 360*, 427–435.

Tsai, C., Chu, S., Wen, Y., et al. (2013). The value of Doppler waveform analysis in predicting major lower extremity amputation among dialysis patients treated for diabetic foot ulcers. *Diabetes Research and Clinical Practice, 100*(2), 181–188.

Tsuji, Y., Hiroto, T., Kitano, I., et al. (2008). Importance of skin perfusion pressure in treatment of critical limb ischemia. *Ulcers, 20*(4), 95–100.

Van Wijk, D., Boekholdt, M., Wareham, N., et al. (2013). C-reactive protein, fatal and nonfatal coronary artery disease, stroke, and peripheral artery disease in the prospective EPIC-Norfolk cohort study. *Arteriosclerosis, Thrombosis, and Vascular Biology, 33*, 2888–2894.

Vietto, V., Franco, J. A., Saenz, V., Cytryn, D., Chas, J., & Ciapponi, A. (2018). Prostanoids for critical limb ischemia. *Cochrane Database of Systematic Reviews, 1*. https://doi.org/10.1002/14651858.CD006544.pub3.

Wennberg, P. (2013). Approach to the patient with peripheral arterial disease. *Circulation, 182*(20), 2241–2250.

Whelton, P. K., Carey, R. M., Aronow, W. S., Casey, D. E., Jr., Collins, K. J., Dennison Himmelfarb, C., et al. (2018). 2017 ACC/AHA/AAPA/ABC/ACPM/AGS/APhA/ASH/ASPC/NMA/PCNA guideline for the prevention, detection, evaluation, and management of high blood pressure in adults: Executive summary: A report of the American College of Cardiology/American Heart Association task force on clinical practice guidelines. *Hypertension (Dallas, Tex.: 1979), 71*(6), 1269–1324. Retrieved 8/10/2020 from https://doi.org/10.1161/HYP.0000000000000066.

Wipke-Tevis, D., & Sae-Sia, W. (2004). Caring for vascular leg ulcers. *Home Healthcare Nurse, 22*(4), 237–247.

Wound, Ostomy and Continence Nurses Society™ (WOCN®). (2014). *Guideline for management of patients with lower extremity arterial disease. (WOCN® clinical practice guideline series no. 1).* Mt. Laurel, NJ: WOCN®.

Zeymer, U., Parhofer, K., Pittrow, D., et al. (2009). Risk factor profile, management and prognosis of patients with peripheral arterial disease with or without coronary artery disease: Results of the prospective German REACH registry study. *Clinical Research in Cardiology, 98*(4), 249–256.

FURTHER READING

Kinlay, S. (2016). Management of critical limb ischemia. *Circulation. Cardiovascular Interventions, 9*(2). https://doi.org/10.1161/CIRCINTERVENTIONS.115.001946.

Yang, S., Zhu, L., Han, R., Sun, L., Li, J., & Dou, J. (2017). Pathophysiology of peripheral arterial disease in diabetes mellitus. *Journal of Diabetes, 9*(2), 133–140. https://doi.org/10.1111/1753-0407.12474.

15

Venous Leg Ulcers

Karen L. Bauer and Munier Nazzal

OBJECTIVES

1. Discuss venous ulcers in terms of etiologic factors, risk factors, assessment, diagnostic criteria, pathophysiology, typical presentation, and principles of management.
2. Describe Laplace's law in predicting subbandage pressure and the level of compression applied to the lower leg.
3. Explain the mechanism of action underlying effective compression therapy for the individual with chronic venous insufficiency.
4. Discuss considerations for use of inelastic compression, short-stretch bandages, long-stretch bandages, compression stockings, and intermittent pneumatic compression.
5. Identify adjunctive therapies that may be of benefit to the patient with a venous ulcer.
6. List three key points to include in patient education when managing patients with multilayer compression wraps.

Chronic venous disorders include a wide range of morphologic and functional abnormalities of the venous system. The term *chronic venous disease* (CVD) refers to a number of disorders including chronic venous insufficiency (CVI) and chronic venous occlusive disease. The term CVD includes conditions associated with arteriovenous malformations and other congenital problems that can result in venous hypertension, which manifests itself in a number of symptoms ranging from swelling to chronic venous ulcerations. CVI generally refers to damage to vein walls, incompetent venous valves, and/or failure of the calf muscle pump to promote venous return to the heart. The range of CVD has been classified using the CEAP system, which considers symptoms, etiology, and pathophysiology. The majority of chronic venous disorders exist in the healthy patient population.

Venous leg ulcers (VLUs) are the most common of lower extremity ulcers, accounting for about 70% of all leg ulcers (O'Donnell et al., 2014). VLUs are the most severe manifestations of CVD, with skin and soft tissue damage propagated by valvular dysfunction, venous hypertension, and chronic inflammatory processes that are not yet fully understood (Lim, Baruah, & Bahia, 2018).

Management of patients with venous ulcers must include measures to optimize wound healing through reduction of edema and prevention of complications. Compression therapy is a crucial component in the management of venous ulcers but is often not sufficient alone to achieve ulcer resolution. Appropriate topical therapy, leg elevation, and calf muscle pump activity are essential interventions to promote healing; procedural or surgical intervention may also be necessary (Alavi et al., 2016; O'Donnell et al., 2014). Once the ulcer is closed, emphasis shifts to long-term disease management and prevention of recurrence.

EPIDEMIOLOGY

The prevalence of VLUs in developed countries ranges from less than 1% to greater than 3% (O'Donnell et al., 2014). CVI affects approximately 2.5 million individuals in the United States; as many as 20% will develop ulcerations (O'Donnell et al., 2014). This contributes to 2 million lost workdays annually (Collins & Seraj, 2010; Morton, Bolton, Corbett, et al., 2013). Venous disease and venous ulcers occur in individuals as young as 20 years. "Peak" incidence occurs between the ages of 60 and 80 years (Kimmel & Robin, 2013). Although no racial predilection is apparent, most studies report female gender is a risk factor (Collins & Seraj, 2010; Olyaie, Rad, Elahifar, et al., 2013). In addition, an increased incidence of obesity is associated with venous ulcers (Milan, Gan, & Townsend, 2019; O'Donnell et al., 2014).

The impact of CVD is significant in terms of individual experience and economic burden. Individuals with CVD report pain, itching, anxiety, drainage, odor, social isolation, and reduced ability to perform usual activities as areas of greatest concern (Phillips et al., 2017; White-Chu & Conner-Kerr, 2014). Up to 60% of VLU remain nonhealing even after 12 weeks of compression therapy (Wound, Ostomy and Continence Nurses Society™ [WOCN®], 2019). Approximately $2.5 billion is spent annually in the United States on the management of VLUs (O'Donnell et al., 2014). In the United Kingdom, the estimated costs of VLU management range from £300 to £600 million per year (O'Donnell et al., 2014). The mean direct cost of treating one

VLU is estimated to be greater than $15,000, with the mean cost of surgical intervention for a VLU as high as $33,000 (WOCN®, 2019).

The negative impact of venous ulcers is compounded by recurrence rates. Some sources report about a 70% recurrence rate within 3 months after closure, while others show that as much as 40% recur in 5 years and about 50% of VLU will recur in 10 years (Dahm, Myrhaug, Stromme, Fure, & Bruberg, 2019; O'Donnell et al., 2014; WOCN®, 2019). Frequent recurrence is attributed to a failure to adequately address the primary problems of venous insufficiency and venous hypertension (WOCN®, 2019). Recurrence rates are reduced when ongoing daily compression is provided (Dahm et al., 2019). The implementation of clinical practice guidelines has been shown to decrease both healing times and recurrence of VLU, however, effective use of guidelines remains limited. Education, support, and access to compression devices are essential in the management of this patient population.

VENOUS STRUCTURE AND FUNCTION

A clear understanding of the anatomy and physiology of the lower extremity venous system provides the framework for determining the pathology of CVD, ambulatory venous hypertension, and venous ulceration. Veins are anatomically and physiologically different from arteries. The primary differences between arteries and veins are the thickness of the vessel walls and the presence of valves. The thinner media seen in veins allows the vein to stretch and creates a low-resistance vessel (Crawford, Lal, Duran, & Pappas, 2017). The lower extremity venous system consists of deep veins, superficial veins, perforator veins, and communicating veins. The deep veins are those veins that are deep to the muscular fascia and accompany the arterial system. In the calf, this includes the posterior and anterior tibial veins and the peroneal veins, which are adjacent to the calf muscle. The superficial venous system is known as the *saphenous system.* The two major superficial vessels are the greater saphenous vein (medial) and the small saphenous vein (lateral), which are located just below the superficial fascia and have multiple tributaries located in the superficial tissues (Fig. 15.1). The perforator veins connect the two systems, transporting blood from the superficial system into the deep system, from which point the blood is propelled back to the heart primarily by the activity of the calf muscle pump. The number of perforator veins varies by individual, with up to 200 perforator veins below the knee and 20 above the knee (Hussein, 2008). The three most important elements of normal venous function are competent valves, intact physical properties of the venous wall, and a functioning calf muscle pump.

Veins normally fill via slow capillary inflow. All veins are equipped with one-way valves that support a unidirectional flow of blood toward the heart. Because these valves prevent reflux of blood from the high-pressure deep venous system to the low-pressure superficial venous system, they play an essential role in normal venous function. Perforator veins follow an oblique course through the fascia and muscle layers, which provides additional support for the connecting veins

and their valves. The closed valves in the perforator veins prevent transmission of the high resting pressures from the deep system back into the superficial system, as long as the valves remain competent (Dolibog, Franek, Taradaj, et al., 2013). Approximately 50%–60% of patients with venous ulcers have incompetent superficial and perforator vein valves (Agren & Gottrup, 2007).

Venous return from the feet and legs to the heart is a major physiologic challenge because the blood must flow "uphill," against the forces of gravity. When an individual is standing upright, the gravitational force creates a column of hydrostatic pressure of approximately 90 mmHg at the ankle. The primary mechanisms by which venous blood is returned to the heart are the smooth muscle tone within the venous walls, the contraction of the calf muscles (gastrocnemius and soleus), and the negative intrathoracic pressure created during inspiration. Of these three mechanisms, contraction of the calf muscle pump is by far the most essential (Meissner, 2009).

The calf muscle pump and one-way valves normally work together to propel venous blood from the periphery to the heart. Calf muscle contraction forces the blood out of the deep veins and into central venous circulation. While blood is being pumped from the deep veins, the one-way valves in the perforator system are closed to prevent backflow of the venous blood into the superficial veins. As the calf muscle relaxes, the valves in the perforator veins open to permit the blood in the superficial system to flow into the deep veins. At the onset of calf muscle contraction, the pressures within the deep venous system peak at 120–300 mmHg. These pressures then fall rapidly as the veins empty and the calf muscle relaxes (Fig. 15.2). Thus, high resting (filling) pressures but low walking (emptying) pressures characterize normal venous function (Fig. 15.3).

PATHOPHYSIOLOGY OF CHRONIC VENOUS DISEASE

Venous hypertension is the result of venous reflux or obstruction. Either can occur in the distal extremity or centrally. Truncal obesity can also cause elevated vena cava pressure and calf muscle inactivity can contribute to venous hypertension and CVD (O'Donnell et al., 2014). Reflux is more prevalent in CVD, but patients with venous obstruction and subsequent valvular reflux are more likely to develop VLU (O'Donnell et al., 2014). Primary CVD results from structural or biochemical vein wall abnormalities secondary to reflux or congenital occlusion with or without truncal obesity or calf muscle inactivity. Secondary venous disease follows an episode of deep vein thrombosis and is called postthrombotic syndrome.

The pathophysiologic process of primary venous disease is complex and creates dilated and tortuous veins, varicose veins with incompetent valves, venous hypertension, and subsequent tissue hypoxia (de Carvalho et al., 2016). Incompetent valves can be caused by either direct damage to the valve leaflets or vein distension. Vein distention causes loss of valve leaflet coaptation when the vessel is mechanically stretched.

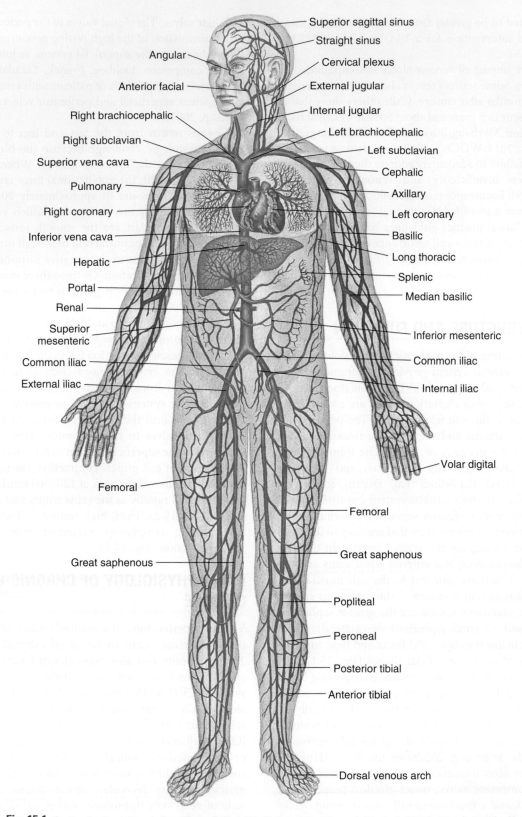

Fig. 15.1 Systemic circulation: veins. (From Ball, J. W., Dains, J. E., Flynn, J. A., et al. (2019). Blood vessels. In *Seidel's guide to physical examination* (9th ed.). St. Louis: Elsevier.)

Secondary venous disease involves thrombosis, recanalization or recanalization failure, vein wall damage, valvular insufficiency, and inflammation. The higher risk of VLU development seen in secondary CVD makes early and appropriate intervention in the case of deep vein thrombosis imperative (O'Donnell et al., 2014).

With the loss of valvular competence seen in both reflux and occlusion, veins no longer fill normally via slow capillary

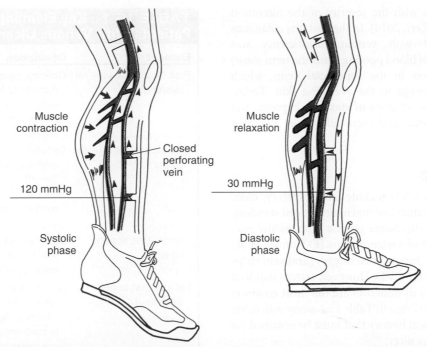

Fig. 15.2 Anatomy of the perforating (communicating) veins. During the systolic phase of calf muscle contraction, the one-way valves of the perforating veins are closed, which prevents deep-to-superficial blood flow. During the diastolic phase the valves of the perforating veins are open, allowing superficial-to-deep blood flow to refill the deep veins. (From O'Donnell, T. F., Jr., & Shepard, A. D. (1996). Chronic venous insufficiency. In F. Jarrett & S. A. Hirsch (Eds.), *Vascular surgery of the lower extremities.* St. Louis: Mosby.)

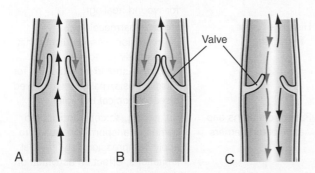

Fig. 15.3 Venous valves. (A) Open valves allow forward blood flow. (B) Closed valves prevent back flow. (C) Incompetent valves unable to fully close, causing blood to flow backward and producing venous insufficiency.

inflow. Normal, unidirectional venous blood flow becomes bidirectional and retrograde flow of venous blood occurs during calf muscle relaxation; thus, venous pressure remains high. Incompetent valves and the failure of the calf muscle pump to lower deep vein pressures causes incomplete emptying of the deep veins. High deep vein pressures then transmit to the perforator veins and the normally low-pressure superficial venous system (Meissner, 2009). The superficial veins and capillaries become distended and congested, causing edema. Venous ulceration is a result of ambulatory venous hypertension from CVD, complicated by endothelial damage and inflammatory cascade propagation at both the vessel and the tissue levels. As a result of venous hypertension, macrovascular and microvascular changes occur in the lower extremities, including basement membrane thickening,

endothelial damage, and capillary bed malformation (Gallelli, 2019).

The majority of patients with CVD have multisystem valvular incompetence (i.e., incompetent valves in at least two of the three venous systems) (Meissner, 2009). Perforator valve incompetence is particularly common and clinically significant. At least two-thirds of patients with venous hypertension and venous ulcers have incompetent perforator valves, which can result in supramalleolar pressures well above 100 mmHg and a "reflux rate" greater than 60 mL/min. When multiple valves become incompetent, the effect is magnified and clinically evident disease becomes much more likely (Meissner, 2009).

Contraction of the lower extremity muscles propels blood forward, acting as a second, peripheral heart (Crawford et al., 2017). Of the three leg muscle pumps responsible for venous return in lower extremities (foot, calf, and thigh), the calf muscle pump is of greatest importance and generates the highest pressure. Among the venous pumps, the ejection fraction of the calf muscle pump is 65% compared with only 15% from the thigh muscle. In a limb with active ulceration, the ejection fraction can decrease to 35% (Meissner, 2009).

The end result of prolonged ambulatory venous hypertension is damage to the skin and soft tissues that renders these structures vulnerable to minor trauma and susceptible to spontaneous ulceration. Venous ulcers are caused by high venous pressures, venous hypertension, dysfunctional valves, obstruction in veins, or failure of calf muscle pump (Comerota, 2011; Hunter, Langemo, Thompson, et al., 2013). However, the extent to which the calf muscle pump is impaired corresponds with the severity of the ulceration (White-Chu & Conner-Kerr, 2014). In the past, the cutaneous inflammation observed with venous insufficiency was believed to be the result of blood pooling (thus the term *stasis*) with low oxygen tension in the superficial veins, which precipitated hypoxic damage to the overlying skin. Today, no evidence supports the theories of stasis or hypoxia, and the terms *stasis dermatitis* and *stasis ulcers* are outdated (Hunter et al., 2013).

Risk Factors for CVD

Risk factors for primary CVD include family history, older age, female gender, pregnancy, estrogen, prolonged standing, sitting postures, and obesity. Some genetic diseases also predispose the development of varicose veins (O'Donnell et al., 2014). Major leg trauma, hip or knee surgery, and vein stripping are also risk factors for CVD. However, factors that lead to valvular or calf muscle dysfunction are the most common CVD risk factors; they are listed in Table 15.1 along with other key elements of the medical history that must be obtained for the patient with a venous ulcer.

Valvular Dysfunction

Numerous risk factors for valvular dysfunction have been identified and are listed in Box 15.1:

- Obesity, which creates resistance to venous return due to pressure on pelvic veins
- Pregnancy, especially multiple pregnancies or pregnancies that are close together, because of increased pressure against pelvic veins and compromised venous return
- Thrombophlebitis (e.g., deep vein thrombosis, pulmonary embolism), which triggers an inflammatory response that can cause direct damage to the valve leaflets, or chronic partial deep vein obstruction due to incomplete recanalization of the vein, which in turn causes venous distention and valvular compromise
- Leg trauma (e.g., fracture), which suggests undiagnosed damage to the vessel walls and valves
- Thrombophilic conditions (e.g., protein S deficiency, protein C deficiency, factor V [Leiden mutation]), which increase the coagulability of venous blood, thus increasing the risk of deep vein thrombosis and microvascular thrombosis; thrombophilic conditions have been identified in as many as 50% of patients with venous ulcers

Calf Muscle Dysfunction

The dynamics of the calf muscle pump can be adversely affected by changes that accompany major injuries, neurologic disease, and bone or joint pain. The calf muscle becomes weak with disuse; gait changes can exacerbate venous hypertension and calf muscle atrophy (Crawford et al., 2017). Risk factors for compromised calf muscle function (Box 15.2) include lifestyle, occupation, musculoskeletal conditions, age, mobility, arthroscopic surgery, extent of calf pump muscle contraction, and injection drug use (Pieper, Templin, Birk, et al., 2008).

TABLE 15.1   Key Elements of History for Patients With Venous Ulcers

Element	Description
Risk factors for valvular dysfunction	Obesity, pregnancy, thrombophlebitis, leg trauma (e.g., fracture), thrombophilic conditions, history of deep vein thrombosis
Risk factors for muscle dysfunction	Sedentary lifestyle, prolonged standing, advanced age, altered or "shuffling" gait, musculoskeletal conditions and surgeries that compromise calf muscle function (e.g., paralysis, arthritis)
Factors that impede healing	Diabetes, tobacco, malnutrition, unplanned weight loss, medications, immobility
Factors that impede treatment	Limited activity and mobility, cardiac disease, heart failure (clinically significant heart failure is contraindication to compression), moderate to severe arterial disease, patient tolerance
Ulcer history	Previous ulcers, onset, duration, precipitating event (duration >6 months is negative predictor for wound healing)
History of prior treatment	Surgical, pharmacologic, compression (venous ulcers that consistently fail to respond to treatment should be evaluated for misdiagnosis, malignant, or mixed disease), topical therapies
Patient concerns and anticipated barriers	Pain, itching, anxiety, anticipated barriers, transportation, ability to apply compression, job/financial limitations, effect on activities of daily living, treatment goals and priorities, appearance

BOX 15.1   Risk Factors for Valve Dysfunction

- Obesity
- History of deep vein thrombosis
- Pregnancy
- Thrombophlebitis
- Leg trauma
- Thrombophilic conditions (e.g., protein S deficiency, protein C deficiency, factor V [Leiden mutation])

PATHOPHYSIOLOGY OF VENOUS ULCERATION

The understanding of the pathophysiologic process of venous ulceration has significantly improved over the last 10 years because of more focused, VLU-specific research

> **BOX 15.2 Risk Factors for Calf Pump Muscle Dysfunction**
>
> - Sedentary lifestyle
> - Occupations that require prolonged standing
> - Musculoskeletal conditions that compromise calf muscle function (e.g., paralysis, arthritis)
> - Advanced age, which is associated with decreased elasticity of the calf muscle tendon
> - Reduced mobility
> - Altered or "shuffling" gait
> - Arthroscopic surgery
> - Injection drug use
> - History of ankle trauma or fusion

(Crawford et al., 2017). It has been established that the mechanisms contributing to VLU are a combination of macroscopic and microscopic pathologic processes. VLUs are the most severe manifestations of CVD. The presence of venous reflux, obstruction, or calf muscle pump dysfunction alone does not explain the occurrence of VLU, however (Lim et al., 2018). Although CVD is clearly precipitated by ambulatory venous hypertension, the reason for venous ulceration as a consequence of venous hypertension is not well understood, but likely involves activation of an inflammatory cascade (O'Donnell et al., 2014). This mystery is compounded by the fact that only about 20% of patients with CVD actually progress to ulceration (O'Donnell et al., 2014).

A VLU can be "pure," where there is greater saphenous vein reflux or an incompetent perforator in or near the ulcer bed, or "mixed," where there are other contributing factors such as local trauma, infectious processes, or autoimmune factors in addition to venous hypertension (O'Donnell et al., 2014). Recalcitrant VLUs may also be associated with compression of the iliac venous system or vena cava (May–Thurner syndrome) (Alavi et al., 2016). Other biochemical processes have also been postulated and must be understood to address the mechanisms of VLU development.

Browse and Burnand (1982) initially postulated that capillary bed distention permitted leakage of large molecules such as fibrinogen into the dermal tissue. This "fibrin cuff theory" proposes that the deposition of fibrin around cutaneous capillaries results in skin hypoxia and thus ongoing poor healing with further local inflammation (Lim et al., 2018). More recent theories on the progression of CVD indicate that chronic inflammation supersedes the "fibrin cuff" theory, however (Comerota, 2011; O'Donnell et al., 2014).

The "white blood cell activation and trapping theory" postulates that venous hypertension causes white blood cells to be sequestered in capillaries or postcapillary venules, subsequently activating them and stimulating release of inflammatory mediators. These inflammatory mediators then lead to tissue injury, poor healing, and ultimately necrosis (Lim et al., 2018). Leukocyte migration and activation and the interaction of leukocytes with the endothelium in the presence of venous hypertension play considerable roles in the pathophysiology of venous ulcerations (O'Donnell et al., 2014; Stana, Maver, & Potocnik, 2019).

It is most recently thought that the mechanism of VLU is best explained by the inflammatory cascade that occurs in both CVD and VLU development. Chronic extravasation of macromolecules, red blood cell degradation, and iron overload catalyze the inflammatory process. Chronic inflammation then causes white blood cell leakage into the dermis, with secretion of additional proinflammatory cytokines and matrix metalloproteinases. These cytokines change the morphology of fibroblasts, which increases tension in the dermis. Iron overload also affects the structure of macrophages, promoting tissue destruction instead of dermal repair (Crawford et al., 2017). Skin changes develop with this destruction of the dermal layer, eventually leading to VLU development (O'Donnell et al., 2014). A newer focus of research is also gene expression in the modulation of inflammatory processes and in nonhealing VLU (Stana et al., 2019). These theories are somewhat controversial, however, as a 2018 Cochrane review suggested there is only low-quality evidence of a correlation between proteases and VLU closure (Westby et al., 2018). Research continues on the complex and multifactorial nature of VLU pathophysiology.

Risk Factors for VLU

Risk factors for VLU development are not well understood (Meulendijks, de Vries, van Dooren, Schuurmans, & Neumann, 2019). Risk factors that have historically been associated with VLU include older age, higher body mass index, low physical activity, arterial hypertension, deep vein reflux, deep vein thrombosis, and family history of VLU (Meulendijks, de Vries, et al., 2019). Methodological differences in VLU research studies pose difficulty with quantifying risk factor analysis, but one systematic review identified that older age, higher body mass index, low physical activity, arterial hypertension, deep vein reflux, DVT, and family history of VLU were significantly associated with VLU development (Meulendijks, de Vries, et al., 2019). Another review further looked at obesity and immobility in the development of VLU and found that obesity and reduced mobility can lead to inadequate calf muscle pump function, increased abdominal pressure, and increased adipose tissue mass. These factors can lead to hemodynamic changes in the macro- and microcirculation of the lower extremities and thus contribute to VLU formation (Meulendijks, Fransen, Schoonhoven, & Neumann, 2019).

Gender, VLU duration, VLU-surrounding perforator vein diameter and reflux, and reflux time of the common femoral vein and the greater saphenous vein have also been found to be independent predictors of VLU size (Lim et al., 2018). Another study identified that 90% of patients with a VLU had at least one other chronic illness, 30% were obese, 30% were overweight, 22% had high cholesterol, and 22% had limited physical mobility (Kelly & Gethin, 2019). In a small 2018 study, risk factors associated with VLU failure to close at 1 year included deep venous disease, history of DVT, and depression. The same study identified race (nonwhite) as a novel risk factor (Melikian, O'Donnell, Suarez, & Iafrati, 2019).

TABLE 15.2 CEAP Classification for Lower Extremity Venous Disease

Clinical Classification*	Etiologic Classification	Anatomic Classification	Pathophysiologic Classification
C_0: No visible or palpable indicators of venous disease	E_c: Congenital	A_s: Superficial veins	P_r: Reflux
C_1: Telangiectasias	E_p: Primary	A_d: Deep system	P_o: Obstruction
C_2: Varicosities	E_s: Secondary (postthrombotic)	A_p: Perforator veins	P_{ro}: Combination of reflux and obstruction
C_3: Edema	E_n: No venous cause identified	A_n: No venous cause identified	P_n: No identifiable venous pathology
C_{4a}: Pigmentation (hemosiderosis) or eczema (dermatitis)		A: Asymptomatic	
C_{4b}: Lipodermatosclerosis or atrophie blanche			
C_5: Healed venous ulcer			
C_6: Active venous ulcer			

*Clinical Classification is further delineated as to where the patient is symptomatic (i.e., aches, pain tightness, skin irritation) or asymptomatic. For example: $C_{6s}E_pA_{pd}P_r$.

Classification

CVD is classified according to Clinical indicators, Etiologic factors, Anatomic location of the dysfunctional venous structures, and specific Pathophysiologic processes (CEAP). This system is presented in Table 15.2 (Eklöf, Rutherford, Bergan, et al., 2004; WOCN®, 2019).

ASSESSMENT

All patients with a VLU should undergo comprehensive systemic, regional, and local evaluation by a qualified provider (Franks et al., 2016). Key assessment parameters for patients with a leg ulcer include medical history, ulcer history, previous treatments, family history, medications, thorough clinical examination, lower extremity examination and inspection of the ulcer, and diagnostic imaging (Franks et al., 2016; Marston, Tang, Kirsner, & Ennis, 2016). Assessment of pulses is also key in assessing a patient with a VLU and is discussed in Chapter 13 Box 13.4 and illustrated in Fig. 13.2B. Although VLU compromise the majority of leg ulcerations, it is important to consider nonvenous causes such as vasculitis, pyoderma gangrenosum, infection, medication reactions, sickle cell anemia, or neoplasm (Marston et al., 2016; O'Donnell et al., 2014).

Patient History

Risk factors for CVD are identified by obtaining a thorough patient history. Of particular importance are factors that differentiate venous insufficiency and VLU from arterial disease and other pathologies that may cause ulceration in the lower extremity (see Table 13.3). Because of the contraindications to sustained compression, pretreatment evaluation must include a cardiac history and any indicators of uncompensated heart failure, as well as assessment for peripheral arterial disease (PAD).

History of Present Illness

It is important to ascertain subjective symptomatology in the patient with VLU. Symptoms that may be related to venous disease but are not limited to this condition are limb pain,

pruritus, cramping, fullness or heaviness, burning, aching, throbbing, limb fatigue, or restless legs (O'Donnell et al., 2014). Symptoms are usually made worse with limb dependent positioning and relieved with elevation or rest. They may be worse at the end of the day or after periods of prolonged standing or sitting.

It is also crucial to discern previous use of compression modalities and the presence of functional limitations that compromise calf muscle pump efficiency (such as ankle fusion or hemiparesis) (O'Donnell et al., 2014). Determine previous treatments used and ulcer duration as well as any trauma either locally or regionally (Dogra & Sarangal, 2014).

Past Medical, Surgical, Family, and Social History

Personal and familial history are also important in this population. The presence or history of obesity, immobility, congestive heart failure (CHF), diabetes, chronic lung, liver, or kidney disease, or other comorbid illnesses should be ascertained. It is additionally helpful to determine a history of inflammatory bowel disease, rheumatoid arthritis, other autoimmune disorders, or malignancy, to help differentiate a VLU from atypical causes of leg ulcerations.

Prior personal or family history of venous disease, varicose veins, DVT, pulmonary embolism, superficial thrombophlebitis, connective tissue disorders, or previous VLU should be investigated. In female patients, pregnancy history should be obtained. Surgical history should be thorough but should specifically include history of vein stripping, sclerotherapy, ablation, or other venous procedures, open or endovascular arterial repair, orthopedic surgeries, or reparative surgeries posttrauma.

A thorough social history specific to the patients with VLU should include dietary habits or nutrition, history of or current intravenous drug use, tobacco abuse, and hygiene practices (Dogra & Sarangal, 2014).

Medication Review

A thorough medication review is essential to identify venoactive drugs, cancer medications, blood thinners, immunosuppressants, steroid therapy, and other medications that may contribute to leg ulceration such as hydroxyurea (Marston et al., 2016).

Lower Extremity Assessment

In addition to a thorough physical exam, both legs need comprehensive examination by the trained clinician. This should include clinical assessment of arterial circulation. The lower extremity examination should be done while lying and standing (Lim et al., 2018). Visual signs of venous disease should be assessed, including edema, hemosiderin staining, lipodermatosclerosis, varicosities, atrophie blanche, and venous dermatitis, all of which can develop before ulceration (Lim et al., 2018). Other chronic venous skin changes include inflammation, eczema, hyperpigmentation, ankle flare, corona phlebectatica, and telangiectasias. Scar tissue or the presence of a healed VLU should be determined. Palpable signs of CVD include varicose veins, palpable venous cord, tenderness, induration, and edema. Ankle mobility and leg strength should be examined (O'Donnell et al., 2014). Checklist 15.1 gives a list of assessment findings unique to the lower extremity of a patient with CVI.

Arterial Perfusion

Coexisting arterial insufficiency is estimated in 10%–20% of patients with venous disease (WOCN®, 2019). Therefore an ankle–brachial index (ABI) should be obtained on all patients with venous ulcers to determine whether some degree of arterial insufficiency is present. An ABI of 0.8 or lower is interpreted to indicate coexisting arterial insufficiency; these ulcers are referred to as *mixed arterial/venous ulcers*. This is an important initial assessment because compression (critical for treatment of venous ulcers) must be modified or, in some cases, omitted. Venous ulcers can develop an arterial component, so monitoring for signs of arterial disease at regular intervals is necessary (WOCN®, 2019). See Chapter 13 and Checklist 13.1 for a list of lower extremity assessment tips.

CHECKLIST 15.1 Lower Extremity Assessment for Chronic Venous Insufficiency

General appearance
✓ Trophic changes: lipodermatosclerosis
✓ Edema: present from ankle to knee, often pitting
✓ Color: hemosiderin staining, atrophie blanche
✓ Dermatitis or varicosities may be present

Pain
✓ Dull aching, fatigue (see Table 13.2)
✓ Exacerbates with dependency, improves with compression

Ulcer characteristics
✓ Gaiter area (see Table 13.3)
✓ Exudative, ruddy, often with jagged edges

Perfusion
✓ Diminished only with coexisting arterial disease
✓ Diagnostic evaluation: duplex ultrasound, ABI

Edema is a classic indicator of venous disease because of the combination of capillary bed distention and elevated intracapillary pressures but can also be related to conditions such as CHF or chronic kidney disease. As described in Chapter 13, the severity of edema varies among patients and from time to time throughout the day. The classic pattern is pitting edema (see Fig. 13.1) that worsens with dependency and improves with elevation. Box 13.1 describes the assessment of pitting edema. With prolonged disease and gradual fibrosis of the soft tissues, edema may become "brawny," that is, nonpitting. Thus, the characteristics of the edema are a clue to the duration of the underlying disease process.

The distribution of edema is also indicative of the underlying process. Venous edema primarily involves the lower leg between the ankle and the knee. In contrast, lymphedema and lipedema involve the entire extremity. Table 13.3 gives a comparison of the edema associated with these three conditions. Measuring the circumference of the calf and gaiter area is another method for assessing edema, especially if it is unilateral. Changes in circumferential measurements provide an indication of the effectiveness of compression therapy (Kimmel & Robin, 2013). Circumferential measurements usually are taken weekly when the compression bandage is changed.

Hemosiderin Staining (Hemosiderosis)

Another "classic" indicator of venous insufficiency is hemosiderosis, which is the discoloration of soft tissue usually located in the gaiter area that results when extravasated red blood cells break down and release the pigment hemosiderin. The result is a gray-brown pigmentation of the skin known also as *hyperpigmentation, skin pigmentation changes,* or *hemosiderin staining* (Kimmel & Robin, 2013; WOCN®, 2019) (Plates 40, 41, and 44). Hemosiderin plays a significant role in the evolution of skin changes toward lipodermatosclerosis and ulceration (Caggiati, Rosi, Franceschini, et al., 2008; Kimmel & Robin, 2013).

Lipodermatosclerosis

Lipodermatosclerosis (see Plate 44) is a term used to denote fibrosis, or "hardening," of the soft tissue in the lower leg and is indicative of long-standing venous insufficiency. The fibrotic changes are typically confined to the gaiter, or "sock," area of the leg, which results in an inverted "champagne bottle" or "apple core" appearance of the affected lower leg (WOCN®, 2019). Lipodermatosclerosis can present acutely, even without other signs of CVD. In the acute phase, lipodermatosclerosis is typically painful. Acute lipodermatosclerosis is generally managed by intralesional corticosteroids, NSAIDs, and compression if tolerated (Alavi et al., 2016). In chronic stages, the fibrosis causes abnormal narrowing of the affected area, which contrasts sharply with the normal tissue in the proximal limb, and has a "woody," indurated texture when palpated. These fibrotic changes are thought to result from a combination of fibrin deposits, compromised fibrinolysis, and deposition of collagen in response to growth factors produced by activated white blood cells (Alavi et al., 2016). A body mass index greater than 34 has been found to predispose the patient to lipodermatosclerosis (Bruce, Bennett, Lohse, et al., 2002).

Varicosities

Varicose veins are swollen and twisted veins that appear blue, are close to the skin's surface, may bulge or throb, cause lower extremity edema, and precipitate a heavy feeling in the legs. They are most often seen in the back of the calf or the medial aspect of the leg. Varicosities precede valvular incompetence and appear to develop as a consequence of intrinsic structural and biochemical abnormalities of the vein wall. Varicosities in the groin, abdomen, or pelvis may indicate central venous outflow obstruction (Lim et al., 2018). Patients with varicosities should manage their weight, exercise, and avoid crossing their legs (WOCN®, 2019).

Atrophie Blanche Lesions

Atrophie blanche lesions (see Plate 41) can be found in as many as one-third of patients with CVD and are more common in women (Sreedharan & Siaha, 2011). These lesions are smooth, white plaques of thin, "speckled" atrophic tissue with tortuous vessels on the ankle or foot with hemosiderin-pigmented borders. Pathogenesis is unknown, and biopsy is not recommended (Alavi et al., 2016). These lesions were previously considered vasculitis but have since been thought to be related to hypercoagulability and inflammation, with cutaneous capillary occlusion that leads to microthrombosis, ischemia, and infarction (Vasudevan, Neema, & Verma, 2016). Sometimes mistaken for scars of healed ulcers, this clinical finding actually represents spontaneously developing lesions. Prompt recognition is important so that a plan can be established to protect these high-risk areas from ulceration due to the thin, atrophic epidermis. Ulcers occurring within these lesions are generally small, very painful, and difficult to close. Management of these lesions remains uncertain and based on anecdotal experience (Marques, Criado, Morita, & Garcia, 2018; Vasudevan et al., 2016).

Venous Dermatitis

In CVD, there is extravasation of inflammatory cells, making patients with CVD high risk for secondary dermatitis. About 80% of patients with VLU will have allergic dermatitis at some point (Alavi et al., 2016). Venous dermatitis is a common but distressing inflammation of the epidermis and dermis on the lower extremity of the patient with CVD (see Plate 44). Often the earliest cutaneous sequelae of CVD, venous dermatitis most commonly affects middle-aged to elderly patients. Manifestations of venous dermatitis include scaling, crusting, weeping, erythema, erosions, and intense itching. Symptoms may be acute or chronic, and this condition may occur on one or both lower legs. The cutaneous inflammation of venous dermatitis is often confused with cellulitis. Factors that distinguish between dermatitis and cellulitis are listed in Table 15.3 (WOCN®, 2019).

Venous dermatitis results from the release of inflammatory mediators from activated leukocytes that are trapped

TABLE 15.3 Distinguishing Between Dermatitis and Cellulitis

Dermatitis	Cellulitis
Afebrile	May have fever, lymphadenopathy
Pruritic	Painful
Usually chronic	Usually acute
Associated with chronic edema	Associated with symptoms of infection
Varicose veins/history of DVT	May have no venous symptoms
Normal white blood cell count	May have leukocytosis
Normal temperature	Elevated temperature
Erythema, inflammation	Erythema, inflammation
May be tender	Tenderness
May improve with compression alone	May not resolve with compression alone
Ulcers may be present	Red streaks/lymphangitis
Vesicles and crusting/scaling	Blisters/bullae may be present
May be unilateral or bilateral	Usually unilateral
May drain serous fluid	No crusting/scaling
May be excoriated, macerated	May have breaks in skin, ulcers, trauma

DVT, deep vein thrombosis.
Adapted from Simon, E. B. (2014). Leg edema assessment. *MedSurg Nursing, 23*(1), 44–53.

in the perivascular space. Dermal fibrosis, a hallmark of venous dermatitis, develops as a result of fibrin cuff formation, decreased fibrinolysis, and release of transforming growth factor-β_1 (a mediator of dermal fibrosis) by the leukocytes. Active leukocytes in the perivascular environment and perpetuate cutaneous inflammation with fibrosis.

Venous dermatitis increases the risk of developing contact sensitivity due to the presence of chronic inflammation of the skin. Contact with dressings, compression garments, or bandages may cause dermatitis in patients with VLU (Alavi et al., 2016). Exposure to usually benign topical substances (e.g., wound exudate, liquid skin protectants, adhesives, topical antibiotics) easily exacerbates venous dermatitis. Frequent contact allergens include lanolin, balsam of Peru, and fragrances (Alavi et al., 2016). Patients also can become sensitized to rubber products contained in some compression wraps and stockings. Allergic contact dermatitis due to topical antibiotics is very common. Neomycin and bacitracin are among the top 10 most common allergens to cause allergic contact dermatitis (Warshaw, Ahmed, Belsito, et al., 2007). The preservatives found in many hydrogels can also contribute to dermatitis (Alavi et al., 2016). Although less common, sensitization of the skin to topical corticosteroids can develop, triggering an allergic contact dermatitis. When the clinical manifestations of the limb affected with venous dermatitis worsen despite appropriate topical therapy, contact dermatitis should be considered.

To prevent venous dermatitis, product ingredients should be carefully scrutinized before topical therapy is selected, and products containing sensitizers should be avoided. Skin moisturizers such as bland, perfume-free topical emollients and white petrolatum can be used to maximize epidermal integrity. An essential component of prevention and treatment of venous dermatitis is graduated compression (discussed later in this chapter), which may require considerable patient education and encouragement due to the discomfort associated with an inflamed, edematous limb. Patients need reassurance that the discomfort should decrease as the edema resolves. Exudate-absorptive dressings are commonly indicated, often in combination with a secondary foam dressing to adequately absorb and contain exudate.

To reduce inflammation and itching, mild-potency topical corticosteroids (e.g., triamcinolone 0.1% ointment) can be used short term (i.e., 2 weeks) but sparingly because of the risk for skin atrophy. High-potency topical corticosteroids are rarely used because of the risk for skin atrophy and systemic absorption through open denuded skin. Systemic corticosteroids are seldom warranted for treatment of venous dermatitis. Fluocinolone acetonide ointment 0.025% is an example of an intermediate-potency steroid with no preservatives. Cool compresses with Burrow's solution (aluminum acetate) 30–60 min several times a day will soften the dry scaly skin and suppress inflammation (Hess, 2011). Patients with severe or nonresponsive dermatitis should be referred to dermatology for management.

Other Skin Changes

Local inflammation, hyperpigmentation, telangiectasias, reticular veins, and corona phlebectatica (ankle flare) are also associated with CVD and can precede or occur concurrently with VLU. See Chapter 13 and Plates 6L, 40, 41, and 44, for further description.

Ulcer Characteristics

The classic VLU is located in the gaiter area and around the medial malleolus, due to the greatest hydrostatic pressure at these sites. Typically, the ulcers are shallow, with moderate to high exudate. The wound bed can be ruddy red with adherent or loose yellow slough and granulation tissue (WOCN®, 2019). Ulcers that are deep and may have exposed tendon are likely not to be of pure venous origin. Venous ulcers usually have irregular edges and periwound maceration, crusting, scaling, edema, or hyperpigmentation (WOCN®, 2019) (see Plates 40, 41, and 44). See Table 13.3 for a comparison of features that distinguish venous, arterial, and neuropathic ulcers.

DIAGNOSTIC EVALUATION

Clinical evaluation of a patient with a suspected VLU should aim to determine whether there is venous reflux, obstruction, or both, and should include differentiation of primary, secondary, or congenital causes. To effectively diagnose and safely manage the patient with a VLU, the patient must also be evaluated for arterial insufficiency because standard therapy for venous ulcers (compression) may be contraindicated or may require modification in the presence of arterial disease (Marston et al., 2016; O'Donnell et al., 2014). The presence or absence of palpable dorsalis pedis and posterior tibial pulses alone should not be used to assess for arterial disease (WOCN®, 2019). In any patient with a VLU, an ABI or toe–brachial index is warranted. Chapter 14 describes other diagnostic tests for arterial disease.

CVI is the result of either venous reflux or venous obstruction. Noninvasive vascular tests are used to distinguish between these two conditions. Traditionally, tourniquet test, photoplethysmography, and venography were used. However, poor reliability and inability to provide visualization of the venous system compromise the utility of these tests. A hand-held noninvasive photoplethysmography instrument that measures venous filling time is also available but requires further testing of reliability. The duplex ultrasound imaging has largely replaced these tests, with the recommendation for photoplethysmography use only when venous duplex ultrasound does not provide sufficient diagnostic information (O'Donnell et al., 2014).

Duplex Ultrasound

Color duplex ultrasound scanning, including both supine and standing positions to identify anatomic and physiologic data related to venous reflux and/or obstruction, is the preferred method for confirming venous etiology (Marston et al., 2016). Duplex ultrasound imaging is noninvasive and has a high degree of sensitivity. Duplex imaging technology uses two-dimensional ultrasound and Doppler shift to produce images of blood flow through the superficial, deep, and perforating veins. This reveals incompetent perforating veins and pinpoints the anatomic site of reflux whether superficial or deep, previous venous thrombosis, or obstruction such as deep vein thrombus. Venous duplex ultrasound also shows vein wall abnormalities, as well as reflux through delicate venous valves (Coleridge-Smith, Labropoulos, Partsch, et al., 2006; Kelechi & Bonham, 2008; WOCN®, 2019). This is valuable in providing both anatomic detail and blood flow direction.

Other Venous Imaging

Computed tomography venography, magnetic resonance venography, contrast venography, or intravascular ultrasound is used to evaluate thrombotic or nonthrombotic iliac vein obstruction or for operative planning prior to open or endovenous intervention. These advanced studies are used selectively and should involve a vascular medicine specialist (O'Donnell et al., 2014).

Laboratory Data

Patients with chronic, early onset, or recurrent VLU should undergo laboratory testing to rule out thrombophilia. This should include a hypercoagulation profile. In some cases, a full blood count or basic metabolic panel can be useful to rule out anemia or systemic infection, and a glycated hemoglobin may be needed to rule out diabetes (Lim et al., 2018).

MANAGEMENT

As outlined in many clinical practice guidelines, key interventions for correcting the underlying cause of venous insufficiency and venous hypertension include lifestyle adaptations, compression therapy, and procedural intervention (Franks et al., 2016; O'Donnell et al., 2014; WOCN®, 2019). A multidisciplinary team must be involved to care for the VLU patient and may include clinicians from infectious disease, vascular surgery, physiotherapy, and others as needed. Current evidence supports treatment of VLU with compression therapy, exercise, dressings, pentoxifylline, tissue products, and procedural or surgical intervention (Milan et al., 2019). A comprehensive treatment plan for the patient with CVD and VLU is multimodal and includes nutritional assessment, exercise, compression therapy, vascular surgery, and advanced wound care modalities (White-Chu & Conner-Kerr, 2014). Other modalities, such as manual lymph drainage or ultraviolet light therapy are lacking solid evidential backing and thus not currently recommended (O'Donnell et al., 2014).

Primary Prevention

Studies that show benefit or lack of benefit of graduated compression in postthrombotic syndrome to treat venous changes or prevent ulceration are lacking (Azirar et al., 2019). However, adequate compression in patients presenting with clinical CEAP C1–C4 CVD should be implemented. Patients with chronic venous skin changes (Clinical CEAP C3–C4) should be encouraged to utilize 20–30 mmHg compression (O'Donnell et al., 2014). Evidence-based DVT prophylaxis is also warranted to prevent recurrence and negative sequela (e.g., postthrombotic syndrome, secondary CVD, and risk of ulceration). Patient and family education, regular exercise, healthy diet, leg elevation, meticulous skin care, and appropriate footwear should be addressed in patients with C1–C4 disease. Surgical intervention (see surgical options later in this chapter) is not recommended in C1–C2 disease but may be needed in symptomatic patients with skin changes, even pre-ulceration (O'Donnell et al., 2014).

Limb Elevation

Limb elevation is a simple but effective strategy for improving venous return by making use of gravitational forces. This is an important component of management for any patient with CVD, but it is an essential element of therapy for patients who are unable to adhere to a compression therapy regimen. Patients should be taught to lie down and elevate the affected leg above the level of the heart for at least 1–2 h twice daily and during sleep. This position may be difficult for the obese person to manage comfortably. In addition, patients should be taught to strictly avoid prolonged standing or prolonged sitting with the legs dependent. Periods of standing or sitting must be interspersed with walking.

Exercise

Normal function of the calf muscle pump is essential to venous return, and effective contraction of the calf muscle requires a mobile ankle and routine dorsiflexion beyond 90 degrees. Achieving VLU improvement or closure in a patient with a VLU and limited mobility can be challenging. Although evidence supporting improved VLU healing and quality of life (QOL) with supervised exercise therapy (e.g., three times per week) has limitations, most clinical practice guidelines recommend a supervised exercise program when feasible for patients with VLU (Jull, Slark, & Parsons, 2018; Marston et al., 2016; O'Brien, Finlayson, Kerr, & Edwards, 2017; O'Donnell et al., 2014; Smith et al., 2018; Tew et al., 2018; WOCN®, 2019). A 2022 systematic review exploring the effectiveness of exercise therapy on VLU healing found few studies, with no clear indication that exercise therapy is of benefit to ulcer healing and that further research may be warranted (Turner et al., 2023).

When patients are ambulatory, a walking program is recommended (Dissemond et al., 2016). Referral to a physical therapist could be beneficial in helping the patient adhere to the exercise program (White-Chu & Conner-Kerr, 2014). A patient with reduced ankle mobility or a "shuffling" gait should undergo a physical therapy evaluation to determine whether he or she can benefit from gait retraining and routine exercises to increase ankle strength and range of motion (Burrows, Miller, Townsend, et al., 2007).

Weight Control

All patients presenting with a VLU should be evaluated from a nutritional standpoint and when malnutrition is suspected, it should be addressed (see Chapter 29) (Marston et al., 2016). A 2017 systematic review showed that patients with VLU are more likely to be overweight or obese, with higher body mass index being associated with delayed wound healing (Barber, Weller, & Gibson, 2018). In addition, significant obesity makes it difficult for the patient to adhere to compression therapy and to avoid prolonged sitting. Overweight people also tend to be less mobile, which can affect calf muscle pump function and contribute to venous hypertension (White-Chu & Conner-Kerr, 2014). With the increase in obesity in younger people, the incidence of venous insufficiency and ulcers is anticipated to continue to rise. Therefore, it is important to educate patients regarding the relationship between weight and venous disease and to strongly encourage patients to reduce their weight to a healthy level. Patients who are morbidly obese may benefit from a referral to a dietician or a bariatric treatment center for evaluation and management.

Pharmacologic Therapy

Treating venous ulcers with pharmacologic means is based on the hypothesis of venous insufficiency pathogenesis. Inappropriate leukocyte activation, which has been shown to be present in CVD, can lead to the development of a venous ulcer (Coleridge-Smith, Lok, & Ramelet, 2005). Diuretics and topical corticosteroids reduce edema and pain in the short term but offer inadequate long-term treatment. There are herbal supplements that are touted to decrease the inflammatory response to venous hypertension, but these are not licensed by the U.S. Food and Drug Administration (FDA) and can vary in efficacy and safety. Pentoxifylline, aspirin, sulodexide, mesoglycan, flavonoids, thromboxane A2 antagonists (ifetroban), zinc, prostaglandin and prostacyclin analogs, and omega fatty acids have been studied, but only pentoxifylline shows evidential benefit in VLU management (Varatharajan, Thapar, Lane, Munster, & Davies, 2016).

Although aspirin has been suggested as an adjuvant to VLU management, it lacks sufficient evidence and is not routinely recommended (Marston et al., 2016). A 2016 Cochrane Database review downgraded the evidence to low quality based on selection bias and small sample size in studies on aspirin in VLU management (de Oliveira Carvalho, Magolbo, De Aquino, & Weller, 2016).

Several pharmacologic agents have demonstrated benefit in the management of venous disease. The three agents with potential efficacy in the management of venous disease are pentoxifylline (Trental), micronized purified flavonoid fraction (MPFF) (Daflon), and horse chestnut seed extract (HCSE).

Pentoxifylline (Trental)

In the United States, pentoxifylline (Trental) is the drug most commonly prescribed in CVD and appears to be an effective adjunct to compression therapy. Its mechanism of action is thought to alter microcirculation by reducing platelet aggregation and promoting leukocyte mobility, which reduces fibrin capillary plugging and decreases plasma viscosity. This reduces tissue ischemia (O'Donnell et al., 2014; Varatharajan et al., 2016). Dosages of 400 mg orally three times daily can accelerate healing of venous ulcers and should be considered for slow-healing venous ulcers (Varatharajan et al., 2016; WOCN®, 2019). The beneficial effects of pentoxifylline must be balanced against its potential adverse effects (e.g., diarrhea and nausea) and its cost. A Cochrane Review identified pentoxifylline to be an effective adjunct to compression therapy and may even be effective in the absence of compression therapy (Jull, Arroll, Parag, et al., 2012).

Micronized Purified Flavonoid Fraction

The phlebotropic drug known as MPFF (which consists of diosmin and flavonoids, diosmiplex) has recently become available for use in patients with CVD in the United States, but other formulations have already been used in European countries. The specific mechanisms of action of this medication include (1) enhanced venous tone, which promotes venous return; (2) reduced capillary permeability, which reduces edema; and (3) reduced expression of endothelial adhesion molecules, which reduces margination, activation, and migration of leukocytes (O'Donnell et al., 2014). These mechanisms decrease the release of inflammatory mediators, which is thought to be the primary pathologic event resulting in dermatitis, lipodermatosclerosis, and ulceration. MPFF has demonstrated clinical benefits in patients with C4–C6 venous disease (Bush et al., 2017; Marston et al., 2016). Adverse effects of flavonoids include gastrointestinal disturbance in a small percentage of patients.

The combination of MPFF with standard therapy (compression plus topical therapy) resulted in a statistically significant improvement in healing rates compared with standard therapy alone or to placebo in a double-blind trial, with a side effect profile comparable to that of placebo (Coleridge-Smith et al., 2005). A systematic review of MPFF as adjunct therapy for venous ulcers concluded that venous ulcer healing was accelerated and recommended MPFF use for large and long-standing ulcers as well as in patients with edema, with or without compression therapy (Bush et al., 2017). In addition, compared with conventional therapy, treatment with MPFF has demonstrated a significant reduction in cost of healing and a significant improvement in QOL scores (Coleridge-Smith et al., 2005; Nicolaides, 2020; Pompilio, Nicolaides, Kakkos, & Integlia, 2021).

Horse Chestnut Seed Extract

Rutosides are a group of compounds derived from horse chestnut (*Aesculus hippocastanum*), a traditional herbal remedy for treating edema formation in CVD (Morling, Yeoh, & Kolbach, 2018). The herbal agent HCSE, which contains escin, is commonly used in Europe as a method for managing CVD (Gallelli, 2019; Pittler & Ernst, 2012). The mechanism of action appears to be antiinflammatory and aid in decreasing hypoxic damage to endothelium. Escin has demonstrated antiedematous, antiinflammatory, and venotonic properties in various preparations (Gallelli, 2019).

Several placebo-controlled trials have demonstrated decrease in leg pain, edema, and pruritus (Pittler & Ernst, 2012). Preliminary evidence suggests comparable outcomes between HCSE and compression therapy. The recommended oral dosage is 300 mg twice daily (Pittler & Ernst, 2012). People with bleeding disorders, kidney disease, or liver disease should avoid HCSE and it is not recommended in combination with pentoxifylline, aspirin, or Coumadin (warfarin), unless under medical supervision. A recent Cochrane Review reported insufficient evidence to recommend the use of rutosides in the prevention of PTS or in DVT (Morling et al., 2018).

Antibiotics

Because of increasing bacterial resistance, antimicrobial drugs should be reserved only for cases of clinical infection or when bacteria are thought to be present in sufficient number to inhibit the healing process (Alavi et al., 2016). Tissue culture should be used to guide appropriate systemic antibiotic therapy in VLU management.

Smoking Cessation

Adequate tissue oxygenation is crucial to ulcer closure. Smoking cessation should be encouraged and assisted in any patient with VLU who smokes (Marston et al., 2016). Refer to Chapter 31 for a detailed discussion related to oxygenation, perfusion and wound healing which includes smoking tobacco and vaping.

COMPRESSION THERAPY

Compression therapy is the standard treatment for CVI (Alavi et al., 2016; Marston et al., 2016; O'Donnell et al., 2014). Compression systems that improve hemodynamics on the compromised calf muscle pump and that do not give way to the expanding muscle during ambulation are preferred (O'Donnell et al., 2014). Venous insufficiency is associated with increased hydrostatic pressure in lower extremity veins. Compression therapy is used to reduce hydrostatic pressure and aid venous return (Olyaie et al., 2013). A variety of wraps, bandages, garments, or devices are used to provide compression (Table 15.4). For the purpose of this chapter, compression modalities will be termed "compression therapy" when speaking generally or will be referred to by specific type when needed. Compression *wraps* are products that are applied by trained personnel and specifically wrap around the extremity. *Bandage* is the more common term used in European

literature in place of *wrap*. *Garment* refers to compression therapy that is a clothing item, such as compression stockings. The intermittent pneumatic compression (IPC) device is the only product that is powered.

Recognition of the difference between resting and working pressure is needed to understand the mechanisms of compression therapy. Resting pressure is the result of compression of the extremity at rest, when the legs muscles are relaxed. Working pressure is the pressure created by the interaction of muscle contraction and the compression therapy when the leg is moving, which is generated by resistance that counteracts muscle movement. The less the compression

TABLE 15.4 Indications for Type of Compression

Type	Examples	Indication	Self-application	Stiffness
Short-stretch bandages	Comprilan®, LoPress®	Decongestion phase; must be ambulatory	No	High
Long-stretch bandages	SurePress®, SetoPress®	Decongestion phase	No	Low
Tubular sleeve	Tubigrip®, Medigrip®, Comperm LF®, TG Grip®, Juzo® cotton stockinette, EdemaWear®, Compression Stockinettes	Maintenance phase Patients unable to tolerate or don other forms of compression	Yes	Low
Multicomponent (multilayer) systems	Coban 2®, Compri2®, Profore®, UrgoK2®, CoFlex®	Decongestion and maintenance phase in select cases as VLU or newly closed epithelial tensile strength improves Ulcer present Limb reshaping and edema reduction	No	High
Paste bandages	Viscopaste®, UNNA-Flex®	Decongestion phase; must be ambulatory	No	High
Layered ulcer stocking systems	Jobst UlcerCare®, Mediven ulcer kit®, Juzo Ulcer System®	Maintenance phase Intact skin with minimal skin changes and minimal shape distortion	Yes	Moderate
Reusable inelastic device	Circaid juxtalite®, ReadyWrap®	Decongestion and maintenance phase Fragile skin (provides friction free application and removal) Anticipated need for frequent readjustments and easy application to promote self-care Patients unable to tolerate or don other forms of compression	Yes	High
Compression stockings	JOBST UltraSheer/Classic®, Mediven plus®, Juzo Soft Series®	Maintenance phase	Yes	Moderate
Intermittent pneumatic compression	BioTAB®, Hydroven3®, Lympha Press®	Decongestion and maintenance phase	Yes	Variable
Hybrid systems (intermittent and sustained pneumatic compression)	Actitouch®	Decongestion and maintenance phase	Yes	Variable

Adapted from Dissemond, J., Assenheimer, B., Bultemann, A., Gerber, V., Gretener, S., Kohler-von Siebenthal, E., et al. (2016). Compression therapy in patients with venous leg ulcers. *Journal of the German Society of Dermatology.* https://doi.org/10.1111/ddg.13091 and Todd, M. (2014). Venous disease and chronic oedema: Treatment and patient concordance. *British Journal of Nursing, 23*(9), 466–470.

therapy yields, the higher the working pressure. The force of the compression applied, the material of the compression therapy, and the number of layers involved determine the level of resistance that the compression therapy provides (Dissemond et al., 2016).

Body positioning is also a factor in how well compression therapy improves venous return. In a lying position, pressure values as low as 15 mmHg are sufficient to constrict superficial and deep veins. To achieve adequate constriction while standing, significantly higher-pressure values (60–90 mmHg) are required. Compression with a stiff, rigid material provides stable support for the leg muscles when ambulating, thereby increasing the effects of the muscle pump, which in turn results in improved venous return (Dissemond et al., 2016).

Healing of VLUs occurs more rapidly with compression therapy (Alavi et al., 2016; Kimmel & Robin, 2013; O'Donnell et al., 2014). Compression therapy is used to apply pressure externally from the base of the toes to the knee, or above the knee, to support the calf muscle pump during ambulation and dorsiflexion. The consistent pressure to the veins results in decreased vessel diameter and reduced transmural pressure, thus increasing velocity of the blood flow almost twofold (Dissemond et al., 2016). The increased interstitial tissue pressure also serves to oppose leakage of fluid into the tissues and to return interstitial fluid to the blood and lymph vessels, thus eliminating edema. Additionally, compression of the superficial veins promotes coaptation and normal function of the valves. Better healing outcomes are associated with multilayer compression therapy vs single-layer compression therapy, due to increased external pressure, changes in the elasticity of the product, and friction between the layers (Kimmel & Robin, 2013; O'Donnell et al., 2014).

The objectives of compression therapy are classified into two phases: the *decongestion* phase and the *maintenance* phase. The goal of the decongestion phase is to reduce edema, improve microcirculation, and promote ulcer healing. In contrast, the goal of the maintenance phase is to prevent edema redevelopment. Therefore, patients with venous hypertension will need compression for life; compression is not a treatment that can be discontinued once the ulcer closes or the edema resolves (Dissemond et al., 2016). In the absence of maintenance compression, patients experience a 15%–70% recurrence rate of venous ulcers (Kimmel & Robin, 2013).

Diligent monitoring by the wound specialist is essential for continued follow-through with the plan of care (WOCN®, 2019). The wound specialist is challenged to recommend the most consistent, clinically effective, and patient-friendly compression therapy for each patient based on individual assessment, indications, contraindications, advantages and disadvantages, and special considerations.

Features

Compression therapies have many different features that guide optimal selection. Compression therapy can either be sustained (i.e., continuous) or intermittent. Compression therapy that remains in place and is removed after several days or only at night provides continuous pressure; the majority of compression therapies on the market provide

TABLE 15.5 Surgical Treatments for Chronic Venous Ulcers

Pathology	Surgical Treatment Options
Superficial vein reflux	Radiofrequency ablation (RFA) Endovenous laser therapy (EVLT) Vein stripping Chemical/nonthermal ablation
Perforator vein reflux	Subfascial endoscopic perforator vein surgery (SEPS) Radiofrequency ablation (RFA) Sclerotherapy Chemical/nonthermal ablation
Deep vein reflux	Valvuloplasty Valve transplantation

International Consolidated Venous Ulcer Guideline (ICVUG). (2015). *Update of AAWC Venous Ulcer Guideline, 2005 and 2010.* Retrieved 1/29/2023 from https://aawconline.memberclicks.net/assets/appendix%20c%20guideline%20icvug-textformatr ecommendations-final%20v42%20changessaved18aug17.pdf.

continuous compression (Tables 15.4 and 15.5). Compression therapy that provides intermittent compression is applied two to three times per day for 1- to 2-h intervals.

Another feature of compression therapy is the type of material used: elastic or inelastic. *Elastic compression* adapts to changes in limb volume. This form of compression therapy exerts external pressure while the leg is at rest and expands when the calf muscle expands during ambulation, thus continuing to provide external pressure, but with low resistance with muscle contraction. *Inelastic* (or *nonelastic*) *compression* will not expand during ambulation and provides less pressure at rest and high pressure with muscle contraction. Compression therapy can also be disposable or reusable. Many compression therapies, such as multilayer wraps, are disposable and are used early in treatment when significant edema or an ulcer is present. Reusable compression therapies, such as stockings, can be removed, cleaned, and then reused. The reusable forms of compression therapy are primarily used for *maintenance compression* once the ulcer is closed.

A key feature of compression therapy is that it can provide a range of pressures. In general, compression pressure considered most effective for maintaining optimal venous compression is 30–40 mmHg at the ankle (Marston, 2011; O'Meara, Cullum, & Nelson, 2009). This high pressure can make stockings difficult for the patient to apply independently. In these situations, lower levels of pressure are more appropriate, in the absence of ulceration (O'Meara et al., 2009; WOCN®, 2019). A general guide to categories of pressure is as follows: high pressure (30–40 mmHg), medium pressure (20–30 mmHg), and low pressure (14–17 mmHg) (WOCN®, 2019).

When a VLU is present, continuous, high-pressure, continuous compression should be achieved. One way to achieve this, especially in patients who have difficult donning or doffing compression stockings, is by the use of compression wraps. Antiembolism stockings used as compression therapy should be avoided in patients with VLU (WOCN®, 2019).

Many compression wraps have "indicators" to guide the amount of tension, or stretch, to use when applying the wraps, so that the desired amount of pressure can be attained. The use of a pressure-measuring device that measures applied subbandage pressures is available for clinicians treating patients with mixed arterial venous ulcers (Marston, 2011).

Contraindications

Compression therapy is contraindicated in the patient with a coexisting untreated DVT in the ulcerated extremity. It is also contraindicated in uncompensated heart failure when the patient's fluid status is not being monitored, as graduated compression of edematous lower legs facilitates mobilization of interstitial fluid back into the circulatory system, potentially increasing preload volume and precipitating pulmonary edema (Collins & Seraj, 2010; Dissemond et al., 2016). During the acute initial treatment of CHF, compression therapy may be used in conjunction with diuresis; however, fluid balance, electrolytes, and breath sounds should be monitored closely. In most cases, sustained compression is contraindicated in the presence of severe PAD (i.e., ABI ≤0.6) because sustained tissue pressure could further compromise tissue perfusion and potentially cause ischemic tissue death (Hopf, Ueno, Aslam, et al., 2006; Marston, 2011). However, the use of ankle perfusion pressure of greater than 60 mmHg as a cutoff, rather than ABI value, is favored because this better correlates with tissue perfusion pressure. Modified compression bandages can be used if the ankle systolic pressure is greater than 60 mmHg with an ABI of 0.5, but only in consultation with a vascular specialist (O'Donnell et al., 2014). See Chapter 14 for more about PAD.

Additionally, compression therapy should be used with caution for patients with polyneuropathy and mixed arteriovenous disease. Patients with polyneuropathy experience decreased sensation in the lower limb and will be less likely to detect indicators that the compression is too tight. These patients will require more frequent monitoring. External compression may also compromise blood supply to the skin.

If the patient expresses complaints about the extremity that are suggestive of device-related pressure damage, the compression will need to be removed so that the extremity can be assessed (Dissemond et al., 2016). Suggestions for correct compression are listed in Box 15.3.

COMPRESSION WRAPS

Wraps are one of the most commonly used compression therapies, especially during the initial (decongestive) phase of treatment when limb volumes are changing rapidly as a result of edema reduction. Compression wraps are referred to by the number of components in the wrap. Single-layer wraps contain a single component, whereas a multilayer wrap may have two, three, or four components that are applied to the extremity.

Generally, compression wraps are applied by trained professionals and left in place for 3–7 days. Most compression wraps are capable of providing modified, or lessened, compression. The most commonly used wraps are inelastic paste wraps, multilayer wraps, and single-layer inelastic (short-stretch) bandages (see Table 15.4). Systematic reviews of the literature conducted by the Cochrane Collaboration reported that multicomponent (multilayer) systems achieve better healing outcomes than single-component compression (Kimmel & Robin, 2013; O'Meara et al., 2009; O'Meara, Cullum, Nelson, et al., 2012). There are few studies to confirm optimal subbandage pressure, but some RCTs have shown that higher pressures lead to improved healing times (Karanikolic et al., 2018). However, the most effective compression is the compression that the patient is able to use consistently and comfortably.

APPLICATION TECHNIQUE

All compression wraps are designed based on *Laplace's law of physics,* which states that subbandage pressure is directly proportional to the tension and number of bandage layers, and inversely proportional to leg circumference and bandage

---

BOX 15.3 Suggestions for Correct Compression

- Follow manufacturer's instructions for application technique to ensure attaining the appropriate level of compression.
- Measure the extremity accurately when using compression garments.
- Assess patient mobility and activity carefully when selecting elastic vs inelastic compression products. Inelastic compression products will not be effective if the patient is unable to perform very frequent calf muscle pumps, such as with ambulation.
- Compression should be used with caution if the patient has decreased leg sensation, infection in the leg, or allergies to ingredients in the compression materials.
- Screen for arterial disease using a Doppler measurement of the ABI. Use modified or lower levels of compression (23–30 mmHg at the ankle) when coexisting arterial disease is present and ABI is >0.6.
- In most cases, compression is contraindicated when the patient with venous insufficiency has an ABI ≤0.6.

- Modified compression bandages can be used if the ankle systolic pressure is greater than 60 mmHg with an ABI of 0.5, but only in consultation with a vascular specialist.
- Ankle perfusion pressure of greater than 60 mmHg as a cutoff, rather than ABI value, is favored because it better correlates with tissue perfusion pressure.
- Obtain a toe brachial pressure when the ABI is >1.3 due to diabetes, arthritis, or renal failure.
- Monitor the skin around and under the compression wrap or device closely and particularly during dressing changes to prevent pressure ulcers.
- Multilayer wraps should be applied consistently and remain on continuously.
- Compression therapy choice should be based on the patient's ability to effectively utilize it. It should be as comfortable as possible, accessible, and financially feasible.

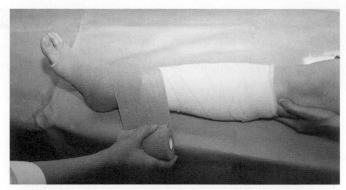

Fig. 15.4 Compression wraps: layered bandage system.

width (Box 15.4). Laplace's law explains why application of a wrap with constant tension will create graduated pressure. Bandage tension and subbandage pressure is highest at the ankle and lowest at the knee (de Carvalho et al., 2016).

Some compression wraps are designed to be applied with a spiral technique, whereas others require a figure-of-8 application to achieve optimal results. Application techniques must follow the manufacturer's instructions. Some layers require 100% stretch and others 50% stretch; some may incorporate a visual indicator to achieve the correct level of pressure.

The skill of the clinician applying the wrap will affect tension (Dissemond et al., 2016). Studies indicate that even when health professionals are experienced with application, they frequently wrap with insufficient tension to produce therapeutic pressure levels. Training has been shown to significantly improve accuracy, but further studies are needed to quantify the interval at which this training should be repeated (Dissemond et al., 2016). An accurate and precise subbandage pressure monitor may be an option for assessing the clinician's ability to apply safe, graduated pressure.

The patient with a large calf or uneven contours can experience difficulty in keeping the bandage in place. Slippage of the bandage can lead to a tourniquet effect, which can cause edema above the wrap and injury to the skin. The use of a topical roll-on-adhesive may help with preventing wraps from slipping. Compression wraps must be replaced when slippage occurs. Slippage of wraps is more common when wraps are initially applied due to fluids being shifted out of the tissue. Wraps need to be changed more frequently until edema has stabilized. Another technique for preventing slippage is the use of extra padding to recontour the leg to a normal shape. It has been found that bandages applied in a figure-of-8 configuration tend to stay in place better, especially for the person with a large leg. However, the manufacturer's instructions for wrapping must be followed to accommodate differences in product materials and layers, all of which affect the level of compression achieved. The best time of day to apply compression is when the least amount of edema is present: first thing in the morning before hanging the legs over the side of the bed. If this is not possible, elevate legs at 45 degrees for 10 min before application (WOCN®, 2019).

Multilayer Wraps

Multilayer wraps are disposable, provide sustained compression, and can be applied to provide either a modified or

therapeutic level of pressure (Fig. 15.4). Multilayer wraps cannot be reused and should be changed when they begin to loosen, slip, or become saturated (typically in 3–7 days). Although studies have shown that multilayer bandages promote ulcer closure better than their single-layer counterparts, research in this area has been limited by the challenge of controlling for consistent and appropriate application (Welsh, 2016). In many settings, multilayer wraps have become the product of choice for early intervention because of their ability to absorb exudate, adapt to changes in limb size, and provide sustained compression at rest and with activity. The use of cohesive bandages as the outer layer in multilayer wraps increases rigidity, thereby improving venous pump power while walking, even in case of low resting pressure (Dissemond et al., 2016). Some multilayer wraps contain both elastic and inelastic components and while these seem to compare to systems that contain layered elastic, medicated, or padded layers, the evidence is unclear whether one offer better healing times than the other (Welsh, 2016).

Paste Wraps

Paste wraps are inelastic wraps that cannot be reused and provide sustained compression. Dr. Paul Unna was the first to introduce use of a zinc paste bandage to create a conformable but inelastic "boot" around the leg; thus, a paste-type compression wrap is commonly referred to as an Unna's boot (Weingarten, 2001). Today, various inelastic paste wraps exist and are impregnated with any of the following products: zinc, glycerin, gelatin, or calamine (O'Connor & Murphy, 2014). These variations in paste wraps are not identical, and an adverse reaction to one does not predict a reaction to another. Nonelastic bandages such as zinc paste bandages are marked by very high working pressures and, even after a short period, only very low resting pressures. Paste bandages are best utilized in the early decongestion phase (Dissemond et al., 2016).

Inelastic paste wraps should be applied without tension, beginning at the base of the toes and extending to the tibial tuberosity below the knee. The patient must be reminded to maintain the foot in a dorsiflexed position while the paste wrap is applied (Box 15.5). Common and appropriate techniques used to ensure a smooth conformable fit include open or closed heel, pleating, reverse folding, and cutting and restarting. When left open to air, the paste layer dries to a

---

BOX 15.5   Procedure for Paste Bandage Application

1. Apply gloves after assembling supplies and washing hands.
2. Gently wash and dry extremity. Replace gloves.
3. Position patient with affected leg elevated and not in dependent position.
4. Foot should be dorsiflexed so foot and leg are at 90-degree angle while applying initial bandage layers around the foot and ankle.
5. Open all paste bandage wrappers and cover wrap. Estimate amount of material based on size of leg(s).
6. Hold paste bandage roll in nondominant hand. Begin to apply bandage at base of toes.
7. If an ulcer is present, apply appropriate topical dressing to ulcer and secondary dressing (if indicated) before applying paste bandage.
8. Treat periwound (if indicated) and moisturize rest of leg.
9. Wrap twice around base of toes without using tension.
10. Continue wrapping bandage around foot, ankle, and heel, using a circular technique, with each strip overlapping previous strip by approximately 50%–80%. Do not apply tension to the wrap.
11. Smooth paste bandage while applying and remove any wrinkles and folds (may pleat, reverse fold, or cut to ensure smooth bandage).
12. Wrap up to knee and finish smoothing.
13. Remove gloves.
14. Apply cover wrap using recommended amount of tension (e.g., 50% stretch) and 50% overlap.
15. Remove twice weekly or weekly as indicated by leakage, slippage, hygiene, wound care, complaint of numbness, or anticipated decrease in edema.

"semicast" consistency. The paste layer is then typically covered with an elastic self-adherent wrap. Paste bandages should be changed when they begin to slip, loosen, or become saturated (typically in 3–7 days). Problems associated with paste bandages include skin reaction to certain paste ingredients (e.g., calamine), maceration due to lack of an absorptive layer, slippage, poor fit, and inability to bathe (Davis & Gray, 2005; O'Connor & Murphy, 2014). As with all inelastic compression garments, paste bandages are most appropriate for actively ambulating patients and are not recommended for people in a wheelchair or bed.

In terms of effectiveness, a 2020 systematic review conducted to determine the effectiveness of inelastic, short stretch compression (i.e., Unna boot) compared to other types of compression, reported a moderate degree of evidence that there is no significant difference in VLU healing rates (Paranhos et al., 2021). However, these findings are limited by the considerable heterogeneity in the studies, variability in the control groups, and low number of studies. While compression garments and devices with better technology are more efficient that the paste dressings, advantages of the paste dressing include being low-cost and accessible in areas of reduced health care resources. The choice to use a paste wrap is often influenced by the availability of material, preference of the wound care specialist, and the unique situation and needs of patient situation.

Short-Stretch (Single-Layer) Reusable Wraps

Short-stretch reusable wraps are inelastic, single-layer wraps that provide sustained compression at a modified or therapeutic level. Because they are inelastic, they are most appropriate for the actively ambulating patient. Short-stretch wraps or single-layer wraps for compression must not be confused with typical elastic wrap bandages used primarily for splinting and securement (e.g., ACE™ brand elastic bandage) which provide low levels of compression and are not considered therapeutic for patients with venous hypertension or insufficiency.

A major advantage of short-stretch reusable wraps is their "wash and reuse" feature. This feature permits more frequent removal of wraps for bathing and dressing changes and contributes to cost-effective care. Short-stretch wraps provide low compression compared with a multilayer compression system. Many of these wraps incorporate a visual indicator of correct tension, such as printed rectangles that become squares when stretched and applied correctly. This feature is beneficial when teaching caregivers how to apply the wrap correctly to achieve the prescribed level of pressure. They are characterized by high working and low resting pressures and should be applied with a resting pressure of 40–60 mmHg. Because this pressure quickly drops to lower values, the bandages should be renewed prior to getting up in the morning and frequently throughout the day (Dissemond et al., 2016).

Long-Stretch Reusable Wrap

The long-stretch wrap is also a reusable, single-layer product that provides sustained compression at either a therapeutic or modified level of pressure. However, the distinctive feature of the long-stretch reusable wrap is that it is elastic so it can be used for both the sedentary and the actively ambulating patient. Much like the short-stretch wrap, the long-stretch wrap can be washed and reused and again, should not be confused with typical elastic wrap bandages used primarily for splinting and securement. With long-stretch wraps, active movement leads to bandage expansion, which results low resistance during muscle contraction and thus little aid in venous return. The use of long-stretch bandages for strong compression is not recommended. Given the high resting pressure, immobile patients in particular are at risk for severe constrictions when using long-stretch bandages, therefore, compression therapy exclusively consisting of long-stretch bandages should not be applied overnight (Dissemond et al., 2016).

COMPRESSION GARMENTS

Compression garments are cloth products that can be reused and may be in one of the following forms: stockings, layered stockings, tubular sleeves, and inelastic devices. These are generally used in the preventative or maintenance phases of VLU management.

Stockings

Compression stockings are reusable, elastic garments that are most commonly used for patients with stable venous insufficiency to prevent ulceration (either initial or recurrent). These garments are appropriate for sedentary and actively ambulating patients. Compression stockings must not be confused with *antiembolism* stockings, which provide 15–17 mmHg of pressure and are therefore not appropriate for therapeutic compression (WOCN®, 2019).

As described in Table 15.4, stockings are generally not a good choice for compression during the initiation of therapy because of the rapid changes in limb circumference associated with edema reduction. They should be used once the edema has been controlled and limb circumference has stabilized. Another relative contraindication for stocking use is severe lipodermatosclerosis because the "inverted champagne bottle" configuration of the leg typical of this condition makes obtaining a good fit difficult. If necessary, however, customized stockings can be made after a referral to a trained "stocking fitter."

Stockings are available in a variety of colors, styles, and sizes. To obtain a safe size, an accurate measurement of the leg should be obtained after the edema has resolved and with careful review of the manufacturer's instructions. Stockings may be knee high or thigh high; most patients with venous insufficiency are effectively managed with knee-high stockings. Compression stockings are classified according to the pressure produced at the ankle (Kline, Macias, Kraus, & et al., 2008): class I (light support), class II (medium support), class III (strong support), and class IV (very strong support). The actual amount of pressure (in mmHg) appointed to each classification varies by country and manufacturer. Compression stockings are produced as either a circular knit or a flat knit garment. The circular knit stocking is a thin, lightweight material without a seam; it is not available in high levels of compression (Moffatt, Partsch, & Clark, 2007). Compression stockings should generally be replaced at least once yearly

(Franks et al., 2016). While they can be machine washed, they should not be placed in the dryer and handwashing may help preserve stocking longevity. Mild detergents should be used, and compression stockings should never be chemically cleaned, self-repaired, or ironed (Dissemond et al., 2016).

Compression stockings are crucial to help prevent VLU recurrence (Dahm et al., 2019). Class 2 stockings perform better than class 1 stockings to prevent VLU recurrence (Dahm et al., 2019). Recurrence rates at 5 years have been shown to be statistically significantly lower when class 3 compression stockings are utilized compared with class 2 stockings. Noncompliance rates for class 3 stockings were slightly higher for class 3 stockings (10.23%) than class 2 stockings (6.25%) at 5 years (Milic et al., 2018).

Stockings are the "mainstay" of maintenance compression but are effective only if the patient wears them. Therefore, it is critical for the wound specialist to educate the patient and ensure that he or she understands the importance of lifelong compression and is able to correctly don the stocking (Moffatt et al., 2007). If barriers are identified, resources and devices to assist with application or other options for compression must be explored. Studies show that donning devices significantly improved elderly patients' ability to use compression stockings (Balcombe, Miller, & McGuiness, 2017; Sippel, Seifert, & Hafner, 2015). A 2016 Cochrane review determined that the evidence remains controversial that such devices contribute to improved management or prevention of VLU (Weller, Buchbinder, & Johnston, 2016). Other tips for applying compression stockings (including assist devices) and key points for patient education are outlined in Box 15.6. One example of a device that facilitates stocking application is shown in Fig. 15.5.

Layered Ulcer Stocking Systems

Ulcer stocking systems are recommended for the treatment of ulcers during the maintenance phase as an alternative to

---

BOX 15.6 Patient Education: Compression Stockings

Tips for Putting on Stockings
- Apply stockings immediately upon awakening, before getting out of bed. If this is not possible, elevate legs at 45 degrees for 10 min before application.
- For easier application of stockings, wear rubber gloves; apply talcum powder (light dusting) first to foot and leg.
- Apply heavy stockings over light silk stocking or silky stocking "liner."
- Use commercial device designed to facilitate stocking application:
  - Stocking butler or donning gloves
  - Easy-slide toe sleeves for open-toe stockings
  - Stocking donner
- Wash new stockings before wearing (follow manufacturer's directions) to reduce stiffness and difficulty in application.
- Use a "layered" approach: either two-piece stockings or two layers of lower-compression stockings (e.g., two layers of stocking, each of which provides 15 mmHg compression).

- Turn leg portion of stocking inside-out down to heel. With stocking stretched, slip foot in while pulling stocking by its folded edge over heel. Gently work stocking up leg, gradually turning stocking right-side out.
- Conduct foot exercises with stockings on: move toes in circular motion (make big circles) both clockwise and counterclockwise. Repeat exercise at least 10 times per day.

Care and Management
- Purchase two pairs of stockings to permit laundering.
- Launder with mild detergent and line dry (follow manufacturer's guidelines).
- Replace stockings every 3–6 months to maintain therapeutic efficacy.
- If stockings become too tight or too loose, contact trained professional for refitting.
- For person having problems with stocking sliding down, use roll-on adhesive applicator.

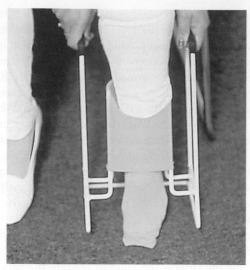

Fig. 15.5 Application of a therapeutic support stocking with a "stocking donner."

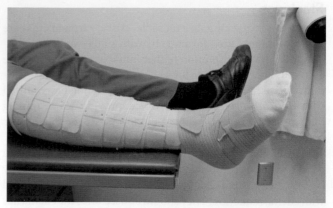

Fig. 15.6 Example of an inelastic reusable compression device with Velcro closures. Guides are available for adjusting the garment to prescribed compression range. (From Cameron, M. H., & Monroe, L. G. (2007). *Physical rehabilitation: Evidence-based examination, evaluation, and intervention.* St. Louis: Saunders.)

traditional compression stockings, especially in people who have difficulty donning and doffing high-pressure compression stockings (30–40 mmHg). Ulcer stocking systems typically consist of a light-compression understocking and a higher-compression overstocking. They are made to be easy to apply as the high-pressure overstocking slips more easily over the understocking than the skin (Balcombe et al., 2017). They are available as ready-to-use products in different sizes and lengths, or in made-to-measure models. In most models, the understocking already exerts a therapeutically effective resting pressure (Dissemond et al., 2016).

Following brief training, many patients are able to independently don and doff these stocking systems. Unlike compression bandages, where efficacy is dependent on the experience, skill, and technique of the individual applying them, appropriately fitted ulcer stocking systems ensure a constant pressure. Particularly in mobile patients, these stocking systems may be a reasonable alternative to compression bandages after initial decongestion (Dissemond et al., 2016).

Tubular Sleeve. The knit tubular sleeve is a reusable compression material that, when measured and applied correctly as a double layer, provides sustained compression at a modified level of pressure (18–25 mmHg) (O'Meara et al., 2009). A tubular sleeve may be selected when the patient cannot tolerate other types of compression. It also may be used as a temporary intervention while a more permanent solution is pending. Application and removal are easy and require minimal, if any, education. The tubular sleeve is an excellent option when simplicity is the top priority.

Reusable Inelastic Device (Velcro Wraps)

Many of the compression garments and devices used for managing lymphedema can also be used to manage the edema associated with venous hypertension. By securing the bands according to the pressure indicators, the device can provide therapeutic or modified levels of pressure (20–30, 30–40, or 40–50 mmHg) (Fig. 15.6). These can often be applied by

patients independently (Dissemond et al., 2016). The ability to easily apply and adjust the straps helps prevent slippage as edema fluctuates, allows for adjustment to maintain adequate compression, permits routine bathing, provides easy access to the wound for dressing changes, and allows the patient to wear shoes of his or her preference—all features that have been reported to improve adherence (Bianchi, Mahoney, Nugent, & et al., 2013; Todd, 2014). These products are washable, reusable, and have a 3–6-month warranty.

Intermittent Pneumatic Compression Devices. IPC is a reusable compression device that involves the use of an air pump to intermittently inflate a sleeve applied to the lower extremity (Fig. 15.7). The basic effects of IPC are to increase venous velocity, reduce edema, increase popliteal artery blood flow, and increase nitric oxide synthase (Comerota, 2009). Initially used to prevent deep vein thrombosis and pulmonary embolism (White-Chu & Conner-Kerr, 2014), this type of therapy is also used for lymphedema and arterial management. IPC may be used for patients with CVD who are mobile or for those who are immobile and need higher levels of compression than can be provided with stockings or wraps. Intermittent compression is particularly beneficial to the patient

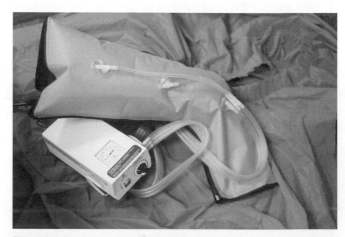

Fig. 15.7 Dynamic compression device: sequential compression therapy.

who cannot tolerate continuous compression or is unable to apply the continuous compression wraps or stockings (Marston et al., 2016).

Intermittent compression devices vary in terms of the inflation–deflation cycle, amount of pressure exerted against the leg, and number of compartments in the sleeve. Single-compartment sleeves simply inflate and deflate on a cyclic basis, whereas multicompartment sleeves provide sequential compression. Rapid IPC has been shown to have a greater rate of healing than slow IPC (Kimmel & Robin, 2013). Typically, patients are instructed to apply the therapy once or twice daily for 1–2 h each time.

Benefits of IPC include mobilization of interstitial (edema) fluid back into the circulation and enhanced venous return without impairing arterial flow (Nelson, Mani, Thomas, et al., 2011). Furthermore, IPC therapy may contribute to the healing of long-standing venous ulcers that have "failed" standard compression therapy. Advantages of IPC as a means of compression therapy include (1) ease of use, (2) provision of active and dynamic compression, and (3) the ability to be applied comfortably and consistently at home (Cervantes & Orphey, 2010). IPC is reimbursed in the home setting when the patient has one or more venous ulcers that have failed to heal after a 6-month trial of standard therapy (including adequate compression) directed by a provider. IPC replaces neither manual lymphatic drainage nor compression therapy for lymphedema (Dissemond et al., 2016).

IPC therapy serves as an adjuvant modality in VLU management and is particularly useful in nonmobile patients (Dissemond et al., 2016). The 2012 Wound Healing Society guidelines recommend the use of IPC, with or without compression, in patients unable to wear an adequate compression system (White-Chu & Conner-Kerr, 2014). One 2014 systematic review found that the use of IPC therapy may increase wound healing when compared with no compression use and limited evidence that IPC combined with compression stockings may improve wound healing (Nelson, Hillman, & Thomas, 2014). Similarly, Dolibog et al. (2013) conducted a pilot study and found that IPC demonstrated a faster reduction in wound surface area than ulcers treated with two-layer short-stretch wrap and standard care only. More research is needed to determine whether this therapy can increase healing of VLUs, manage edema, and reduce recurrence.

LOCAL WOUND CARE

Local wound management modalities must be used in combination with appropriate compression therapy or venous procedural intervention for optimal results. Debridement, either sharp, enzymatic, mechanical, or autolytic, should be considered in cases where necrosis or biofilm is present (see Chapter 20) (Alavi et al., 2016; Marston et al., 2016). As with all wounds, topical therapy for the venous wound is selected based on wound characteristics (see Chapter 21). Initially, the venous ulcer may present with copious amounts of exudate. Dressing selection should minimize potential allergens while effectively managing the exudate to prevent periwound maceration and control

bioburden (Alavi et al., 2016; Marston et al., 2016). A 2018 Cochrane review of 78 RCTs reported evidence is inconclusive for recommending a specific dressing in the management of VLU (Norman et al., 2018). Antimicrobial agents should only be used to treat clinical infection, not bacterial colonization; routine culture of VLU is not recommended (O'Donnell et al., 2014; O'Meara, Al-Kurdi, Ologun, et al., 2014) (see Chapter 19). Growth factors (Chapter 8) have shown promise in venous leg ulceration closure however evidence to recommend routine use is lacking (Marston et al., 2016). The pain associated with venous ulcers may be addressed with topical products such as lidocaine–prilocaine cream (Eutectic Mixture of Local Anesthetics) and ibuprofen slow-release foam dressings (available in some countries). Chapter 28 provides detailed information about managing wound pain.

Periwound skin requires protection from maceration that can accompany an exudative wound and from irritants such as adhesives and chemicals. Interventions to prevent and manage venous dermatitis were described earlier in the chapter. As edema decreases, the volume of exudate from the venous ulcer also will diminish, and the types of dressings will need to be modified.

Failure to Progress

Only 50%–75% of VLU will close within 6 months, with ulcers of larger size and longer duration being more likely to remain open (Marston et al., 2017). Patients with VLU who do not respond to appropriate initial treatment should be considered for more aggressive management or specialist referral (Marston et al., 2017). Serial VLU measurements (in cm) and ulcer characteristic should be completed at each patient evaluation for this purpose (Marston et al., 2016; O'Donnell et al., 2014).

Certain VLU characteristics are associated with poor healing potential, including large ulcer size (>5 cm^2), longer duration (>6 months), and failure to show significant progress toward healing during the first 3–4 weeks of compression therapy. In addition, the presence of deep vein reflux, perforator vein reflux, greater saphenous vein reflux, and history of DVT have been shown to be independent risk factors for nonhealing VLU (Liu et al., 2019a, 2019b; Melikian et al., 2019).

When an apparent venous ulcer fails to progress or worsens despite treatment, the treatment plan must be reevaluated. Many other causes of lower extremity ulcers can present similar to venous ulcers, such as mixed venous/arterial, lymphedema, vasculitis, pyoderma gangrenosum, autoimmune disease, and malignancy. Many clinical practice guidelines recommend tissue biopsy and histology when the venous ulcer does not improve after 6 weeks of adequate therapy (Marston et al., 2016; Morton et al., 2013; O'Donnell et al., 2014). If a biopsy and differential diagnosis confirm venous etiology, failure to heal may be due to biofilm, subclinical infection (discussed in Chapter 19), or the negative cellular environment of a chronic wound. In this case, deep tissue culture or validated quantitative tissue swab culture may be considered (Marston et al., 2016). If high levels of bacteria ($>1 \times 10^6$ CFU/g) or β-hemolytic streptococci are present, topical or systemic antimicrobial or topical antiseptic strategies should be utilized and promptly discontinued once bacterial levels are rebalanced or the ulcer shows improvement (Marston et al., 2016). Additionally, a product or therapy designed to convert the chronic wound environment into an environment that supports repair should be considered.

ADJUNCTIVE

Skin grafts, bioengineered human skin equivalents, negative pressure wound therapy (NPWT), modalities such as electrical stimulation and ultrasound, and hyperbaric oxygen therapy (HBOT) have shown varying degrees of success in the management of refractory venous ulcers once the underlying cause is appropriately addressed, host factors such as glycemic control or smoking are managed, and bacterial load in the ulcer bed is minimized (Marston et al., 2016).

Split-Thickness Skin Graft

Skin grafting is a form of surgical adjunctive therapy. Pinch grafts and split-thickness grafts have been studied, with healing rates of 45% for pinch grafts and 88%–90% for split-thickness grafts reported (Morton et al., 2013). However, recurrence rates after 4 months have been reported (Marston et al., 2016). Grafting along with compression therapy may improve the healing rate and recurrence rate but does not address the underlying venous hypertension (Marston et al., 2016). A 2017 systematic review reported that STSG remains a pivotal management technique in VLU, with one reviewed study also showing improved QOL after STSG in VLU (Serra et al., 2017). It is important to address the underlying venous pathology prior to STSG and to employ appropriate compression post-STSG (Serra et al., 2017).

Cellular and Tissue-Based Products

National guidelines for management of lower extremity venous ulcers recognize CTPs as a potential adjunctive therapy option (WOCN®, 2019). While there are many cell-based products that show promise in decreasing time to close in VLU, generalizability is limited by study design and sample size (Bianchi et al., 2018; Jones, Nelson, & Al-Hity, 2013; Marston et al., 2016; Serra et al., 2017; Towler, Rush, Richardson, & Williams, 2018). Biophysical and biologic agents are described in detail in Chapters 22–27.

NPWT is not recommended for routine management of VLU (Alavi et al., 2016; Dumville, Evans, & Peinemann, 2015; O'Donnell et al., 2014). However, NPWT has been reported by Society for Vascular Surgery (SVS) to be useful aid in skin graft healing of VLU (O'Donnell et al., 2014).

Electrical Stimulation and Ultrasound

The WOCN® guideline for management of lower extremity venous ulcers update (2014) identifies electrical stimulation as a potential adjunctive therapy but recommends against ultrasound therapy. The SVS guidelines recommend against routine use of electrical stimulation or ultrasound therapy in VLU, citing inconsistent and insufficient evidence (O'Donnell et al., 2014). A 2017 Cochrane review looked at 11 studies on both high- and low-frequency ultrasound in VLU management and determined the evidence to be of low quality (Cullum & Liu, 2017). This review cites high risk of bias, short follow-up time, and weak study design as limitations, and furthers that the evidence base does not currently support the use of ultrasound in the management of VLU.

Hyperbaric Oxygen Therapy

HBOT is not FDA approved for VLU management, but one RCT in 2018 showed that HBOT improved VLU healing (Thisttlewaite et al., 2018).

SURGICAL INTERVENTION

All patients with nonhealing VLU or other signs of PVD should be managed in consultation with a vascular specialist (Franks et al., 2016). There are two goals in the treatment of VLU: to heal the active ulcer and to prevent ulcer recurrence (O'Donnell et al., 2014).

The aim of any procedural intervention should be to manage the underlying causative factor: either primary reflux disease or secondary inflammatory thrombotic disease (Alavi et al., 2016; Marston et al., 2016; O'Donnell et al., 2014). More specifically, the underlying mechanism of venous ulceration is related to venous hypertension as a result of venous reflux in the deep or superficial veins, venous reflux in the perforator veins, or venous occlusive disease, which can be either congenital or acquired due to chronic thrombotic disease.

In a randomized study with a 10-year follow-up report on the same study, the authors found that surgery in addition to compression therapy improved healing and reduced both short-term and long-term recurrence. In this study, 58.9% of surgical patients were ulcer free after 10 years, compared with 39.6% after compression therapy only (van Gent et al., 2015).

Procedures to correct underlying causative factors may be open surgical procedures or endovascular procedures. Strength of evidence for open vs endovascular procedures in VLU management is primarily level "C," because there is a paucity of comparative, prospective, RCT.

Venous reflux affects the deep and superficial veins, and the perforators. Deep venous insufficiency is due to valvular incompetence. Surgical techniques available for deep valvular incompetence include venous valve insertion, direct valvuloplasty, and autogenous vein valve transplantation. Chronic vein occlusion, especially proximal occlusive disease, can be treated by either surgical intervention such as bypass procedures or via endovascular intervention. Endovascular occlusive therapy can be achieved by balloon angioplasty or bypass procedures such as the Palma procedure. Recently, stent recanalization of the iliac vein is recommended in chronic iliac vein obstruction associated with recalcitrant VLU (Marston et al., 2016). All patients with deep vein reflux and VLU should be evaluated and treated for any superficial vein abnormalities prior to consideration for these procedures (O'Donnell et al., 2014).

A number of surgical options are available that can be used to address superficial venous hypertension. Selection is based on the extent of valvular reflux (Table 15.5): subfascial endoscopic perforator vein surgery (SEPS), laser ablation, radiofrequency ablation (RFA), nonthermal venous closure, and sclerotherapy. There is good evidence to support the use of radiofrequency vein ablation and SEPS (Morton et al., 2013). A 2022 meta-analysis showed improved ulcer healing rates in patients who underwent foam sclerotherapy versus compression alone, making consideration of local sclerotherapy important in the management of VLU. Further studies are warranted in this area (Joyce et al., 2022). With the advancement of minimally invasive techniques there is a decrease in the number and size of incisions, procedure time, and recovery time (Kumar, Agarwal, & Garg, 2009).

Vein stripping was a treatment of choice in the early 20th century. This procedure was performed to prevent backflow of blood into the lower leg and involved physically removing the great saphenous vein. More current options have replaced this procedure. In the last decade vascular surgery options have increased to correct vein function (White-Chu & Conner-Kerr, 2014). These procedures are venous ablative surgery that is delivered by heat (laser or radiofrequency/sound waves), nonthermal closure using cyanoacrylate or polidocanol, or sclerotherapy that uses strong medications to destroy the saphenous vein without removal. Patients must have an intact deep venous system to be considered for surgical interventions. Within the past 10–15 years these treatments have replaced traditional vein stripping.

Subfascial Endoscopic Perforator Vein Surgery

The SEPS technique was introduced over 15 years ago and involves using an endoscopic video camera and instrumentation placed through small ports remote from the ulcer. All perforators in the vicinity of the ulcer that proved to be incompetent are ligated to prevent blood flow and reduce venous hypertension. This procedure is used as an alternative to ligation of the perforators, which uses a long incision on the leg. Healing rate of venous ulcers was reported in 8 weeks with no recurrence in 11.9 months using an ultrasonic scalpel in the SEPS procedure (Kumar et al., 2009). The Wound Healing Society Guidelines (Marston et al., 2016) recommend the SEPS procedure to address underlining venous etiology of the venous ulcer by preventing backflow from the deep to the superficial venous system.

A recent Cochrane review found inconclusive evidence the SEPS is more effective than compression alone in the treatment of VLU, and in comparison, with open surgical ligation (Linton procedure) the results were nonconclusive in favor one over the other (Lin, Loveland, Johnston, Bruce, & Weller, 2019). Additionally, patients treated with SEPS and saphenous surgery had no advantage over those treated with saphenous surgery only in relation to ulcer healing at 12 months. Complications with the SEPS procedure have been reported, including delayed wound healing (0%–11%), sural paresthesia (1.9%–3%), tibial nerve paresthesia (1%), and a recurrence rate of 8% at 3 years and 18% at 5 years (Di Battista, D'Andrea, Galani, et al., 2012).

Ablation Procedures

Ablation of the superficial veins can be achieved using either thermal or chemical ablation. The latter reduces procedure time and eliminates the need for tumescent anesthesia. Ablation is recommended in VLU if there is axial reflux or incompetent perforator veins directed to the ulcer bed or affected skin, for primary prevention, to promote wound healing, and to prevent recurrence. Evidence indicates effectiveness for open surgery, RFA, or sclerotherapy are comparable, however percutaneous or endovascular procedures are preferred to eliminate the need for incision (Marston et al., 2016; O'Donnell et al., 2014).

Two types of thermal ablation procedures for superficial venous reflux are used: endovenous laser ablation (EVLA) and RFA. Both procedures are performed in an outpatient setting with local anesthetic and usually no sedation. Patients are ambulatory after the procedure, and recovery time is short.

EVLA, also known as *laser surgery*, uses laser to create intense local heat in the incompetent vein. The goal of ELA is to deliver sufficient thermal energy to destroy the vascular endothelium layer of the wall of the incompetent vein segment to produce irreversible occlusion of the vein. The amount of thermal energy delivered corresponds with the success of ELA. A catheter is inserted into the vein to be treated, usually just below the knee. Using ultrasound, the surgeon injects a solution of saline and anesthetic agent along the length of the vein to be treated (tumescent anesthesia). After this, laser is applied. There may be some bruising over the treated site that can last up to 14 days and pain at the site.

Radiofrequency (RF) is delivered directly to the vessel wall; the RF energy is delivered both in and around the vessel to be treated. The amount of energy to be delivered is determined to ensure endothelial ablation by thermal sensors. The RF catheter repeats the process along the length of the vein (Subramonia & Lees, 2010). This is a longer procedure to perform, but the results have better outcomes compared with conventional surgery (Subramonia & Lees, 2010). It has been noted that patients have less postoperative pain and can return to their normal routine earlier than patients having the conventional open vein stripping surgery.

Venous intervention by vein ablation was reported to result in a healing rate ranging from 70% to 100% and recurrence from 0% to 49% based on a meta-analysis study recently published, while healing rates and recurrence rates were reported to be 59%–93% and 4%–33% in the perforator intervention group (Montminy, Jayaraj, & Raju, 2018). Another 2018 study found that early (2 weeks postidentification) endovenous ablation of superficial reflux lead to shorter healing times and reduced recurrence than deferred (6 months postidentification) ablation procedures (Gohel et al., 2018).

Chemical ablation can be achieved by delivering a chemical material within the lumen of the veins to be treated. Foam sclerotherapy (FS) is another vein ablating procedure. With this technique, a drug mixed with air is administered by a needle into the vein. This drug will burn and scar the inside of the saphenous vein. Ultrasound is used to direct where the drug will go in the vein. The addition of foam to the agent allows for decreased amounts of sclerosing agent injection and improved efficacy (Subramonia & Lees, 2010). Overall effectiveness of this procedure needs further studies, but one retrospective cohort study found that laser ablation with foam sclerotherapy in conjunction with compression therapy lead to shorter VLU closing time and reduced recurrence rates (Liu et al., 2019a, 2019b).

One 2018 RCT found that closure of the GSV using cyanoacrylate, an adhesive, showed similar QOL improvements and was found to be as safe and effective of RFA (Gibson et al., 2018). This 2-year noninferiority study was then extended to 5 years, and found that target veins remained closed, symptoms remained improved, and no serious adverse events occurred (Morrison, Gibson, Vasquez, Weiss, & Jones, 2019). These studies show potential for cyanoacrylate's use in the management of superficial and perforator reflux.

Surgical intervention of superficial venous reflux with compression therapy has been shown to reduce the recurrence of VLUs at 4 years (Gohel et al., 2018; Kimmel & Robin, 2013). *Effects of Surgery and Compression on Healing And Recurrence* (ESCHAR) studies suggest superficial vein surgery reduces venous ulcer recurrence and should be considered for all patients with chronic venous ulcers (Gohel et al., 2005, 2018, 2020; Howard, Howard, Kothari, et al., 2008; Wright, 2009). Although vein ablative surgery usually has minor complications, there have been some reported complications of nerve damage and deep vein thrombosis (Davies, Howard, Howard, et al., 2008). In addition, the chance of recanalization is high and requires follow-up to determine recurrence of reflux.

Quality of Life

The symptoms and associated treatments of VLU can have a negative impact on the patient's QOL, which may lead to limited adherence to recommended care plans. One systematic review identified common QOL themes such as physical impact, psychological effects, social factors, and other factors such as ulcer and treatment-related pain, odor, and exudate, all of which can have a negative impact on sleep, mobility, and mood (Phillips et al., 2017). Another study correlated delayed ulcer closure with overall QOL, suggesting the importance of assessing risk factors for decreased QOL with VLU patients (Finlayson et al., 2017). A 2016 review suggested that patients with VLU who underwent surgical procedures had improved QOL compared with patients who were treated with compression bandaging alone (Tollow, Ogden, & Whiteley, 2016). While studies on the QOL of VLU patients remain limited, this is an important factor in the management of VLU and warrants attention and further research. Plan of care with respect to VLU management should always be made in collaboration with patients and caregivers. Patient-centered care mandates collaboration among the entire care team, with the needs of patient at the forefront (Dissemond et al., 2016).

FOLLOW-UP AND LIFELONG MAINTENANCE

With recurrence rates of VLUs ranging between 15% and 71%, the emphasis of management must shift to prevention of recurrence once the ulcer is closed (Kimmel & Robin, 2013; Marston et al., 2016). Lifelong exercise, weight control, and compression therapy are ongoing challenges. Although compression garments have been demonstrated to increase healing rates (Marston et al., 2016) and reduce recurrence rates at 3 years compared with no compression, intolerance of compression is significant (Nelson & Bell-Syer, 2012). One of every two patients discontinue compression therapy due to pain and discomfort (Briggs & Closs, 2006). Patients also fail to utilize compression consistently for other reasons, including the patient's perception of the value of compression, lack of understanding of the mechanism of action of compression therapy, his or her level of comfort/discomfort with the stockings, challenges in application, and modified dress/shoe attire (Balcombe et al., 2017; Defloor, 2010; Shannon, Hawk, Navaroli, et al., 2013). Conditions that can affect the prognosis for invasive and noninvasive procedures are obesity, malnutrition, intravenous drug use, and coexisting medical conditions (Kimmel & Robin, 2013). These findings clearly speak to the importance of patient education regarding lifelong compression, ongoing support and encouragement, and identifying solutions to barriers that jeopardize the patient's adherence (Van Hecke, Beeckman, Grypdonck, et al., 2013).

Many different strategies can be employed to improve adherence. The patient may be able to tolerate a lower level of compression in terms of pain; he or she may also be able to apply the garment. Although evidence indicates high-level compression stockings are more effective in preventing recurrence, medium-level compression stockings are associated with significantly higher rates of adherence (White-Chu & Conner-Kerr, 2014). The wound specialist needs to recommend a compression device that the person can apply independently. There are more choices available than in the past—the clinician should offer options to meet the individual's needs. The choice may be based on cost issues and the patient's preference (Kimmel & Robin, 2013). Education that includes the families and caregivers, as well as the patient, is critical to achieving optimal outcomes (Burrows et al., 2007; Van Hecke et al., 2013). Chapter 5 provides more strategies for facilitating the patient's ability to adhere to a mutually agreeable plan of care.

In the United Kingdom there are community services, such as the Lindsay Leg Club, that provide quality care and empowerment for patients with leg ulcers, while also supporting and educating nursing staff (Clark, 2010; McKenzie, 2013). This model has been well accepted by patients and has been more economical than traditional visits from the home care nurse. Similarly, The Lively Legs program in the Netherlands is effective in promoting walking and leg exercises, potentially leading to decreased wound healing time (Heinen, Borm, van der Vleuten, et al., 2012). Total patient commitment is required for success in managing CVD.

CLINICAL CONSULT

A: Referral for leg ulcer recommendation. 60-Year-old Caucasian female with type 2 diabetes, obesity, and history of lower leg edema and venous ulcer of right leg.

Patient has edema of right lower leg, complains of pain with ambulation a short distance and when in bed. Wound assessment revealed a 2 cm × 2.5 cm wound, irregular wound margin, no depth, wound bed has 30% black necrotic tissue with 70% pale pink tissue. Hemosiderin staining present bilateral lower legs in gaiter area. ABI is 1.5.

D: Overall assessment is not consistent with venous ulcer. Risk factors: Diabetes, obesity, patient history. The appearance of the leg ulcer, patient history, and complaint of pain with leg elevation are consistent with mixed arterial venous ulcer. The ABI is a false high reading due to calcification.

P: Referral for vascular testing and vascular surgeon. Manage wound exudate and pain.

I: Plan of care will be as following: (1) Collaborate with vascular and primary provider for developing a treatment plan. (2) Patient and caregivers will be educated on the treatment plan. (3) Use of appropriate topical dressing to manage exudate, facilitate autolysis, and reduce/control pain. Light compression (less than 30 mmHg) or one-layer elastic tubular sleeve. (4) Gradual walking and weight loss program.

E: Will follow to evaluate treatment plan, assess tolerance of compression therapy, and revise interventions as needed.

SUMMARY

- Chronic venous disease is a potentially disabling condition accompanied by lower leg edema, venous hypertension, lower leg pain, and ulcerations.
- Venous ulcers are a common medical problem and are difficult to treat.
- Can be pure venous or mixed with concurrent illnesses or characteristics.
- There is no medical therapy that is proven to be effective in all VLU cases.
- There is no conclusive evidence that one type of topical therapy is better than others.
- Correcting the underlying venous problem and compression therapy are the keys for successful management.
- To prevent ulceration and to heal existing ulcers, graduated compression is required.
- Graduated compression therapy via single or multilayer wraps, stockings, or intermittent compression provides support to restore near normal vein and calf pump muscle function.
- Close monitoring with support and encouragement are important to facilitate continued use of these treatment modalities by the patient.

SELF-ASSESSMENT QUESTIONS

1. Describe how a competent venous system and the calf muscle pump work together to prevent venous hypertension.
2. Which of the following levels of pressure would be considered therapeutic for graduated compression when a patient has an ABI of 0.95 in the lower extremity?
   a. 20 mmHg compression at the ankle
   b. 25 mmHg compression at the ankle
   c. 30 mmHg compression at the ankle
   d. 50 mmHg compression at the ankle
3. Which of the following management options would be *best* for the patient with a venous ulcer complicated by arterial disease, as evidenced by an ABI of 0.5?
   a. Use leg elevation to control edema and 20 mmHg graduated compression wrap.
   b. Use pneumatic compression or graduated compression to provide pressures in the 25–30 mmHg range.
   c. Recommend Trental (pentoxifylline) as an alternative to compression.
   d. Delay any treatment until patient sees a vascular specialist or undergoes revascularization.
4. Distinguish between elastic and nonelastic static compression products and explain which is best for the sedentary patient.
5. Which of the following symptoms would indicate venous dermatitis instead of cellulitis?
   a. Erythema, elevated temperature
   b. Erythema, crusting, and itching
   c. Pain, fever, and bullae
   d. Inflammation, pain, and exudate
6. Venous contact dermatitis can be best managed with which of the following treatments?
   a. Antibiotic cream daily
   b. Lanolin cream twice a day
   c. Topical corticosteroid daily for 1 week
   d. Antifungal powder twice per day
7. Instructions to the patient being fitted for compression stockings for venous insufficiency include which of the following?
   a. Apply stockings first thing in the morning.
   b. Do not remove stockings at bedtime, only when bathing.
   c. Launder the stockings once per week.
   d. Do not perform ankle exercises while wearing the stockings.

REFERENCES

Agren, M., & Gottrup, F. (2007). Causation of venous ulcers. In M. Morison, C. J. Moffatt, & P. J. Franks (Eds.), *Leg ulcers: A problem-based learning approach*. Edinburgh: Elsevier.

Alavi, A., Sibbald, G., Phillips, T. J., Miller, O. F., Margolis, D. J., Marston, W., et al. (2016). What's new: Management of venous leg ulcers. *Journal of the American Academy of Dermatology, 74*, 643–664. https://doi.org/10.1016/j.jaad.2015.03.059.

Azirar, S., Appelen, D., Prins, M. H., Neumann, M. H., de Feiter, A. P., & Kolbach, D. N. (2019). Compression therapy for treating post-thrombotic syndrome. *The Cochrane Database of Systematic Reviews, 9*. https://doi.org/10.1002/14651858.CD004177.pub2.

Balcombe, L., Miller, C., & McGuiness, W. (2017). Approaches to the application and removal of compression. *Chronic Oedema,* S6–S14.

Barber, G. A., Weller, C., & Gibson, S. (2018). Effects and associations of nutrition in patients with venous leg ulcers: A systematic review. *Journal of Advanced Nursing, 74*, 774–787. https://doi.org/10.1111/jan.13474.

Bianchi, J., Mahoney, K., Nugent, L., et al. (2013). A fresh way to treat venous leg ulcers with measure compression. *British Journal of Community Nursing, Suppl. 34*, S36–S40.

Bianchi, C., Tettelbach, W., Istwan, N., Hubbs, B., Kot, K., Harris, S., et al. (2018). Variations in study outcomes relative to relative to intention-to-treat and per-protocol data analysis techniques in the evaluation of efficacy for treatment of venous leg ulcers with the dehydrated human amnion/chorion membrane allograft. *International Wound Journal, 16*, 761–767. https://doi.org/10.1111/iwj.13094.

Briggs, M., & Closs, S. J. (2006). Patients' perceptions of the impact of treatments and products on their experience of leg ulcer pain. *Journal of Wound Care, 15*(8), 333–337.

Browse, N. L., & Burnand, K. G. (1982). The cause of venous ulceration. *Lancet, 320*(8292), 243–245.

Bruce, A. J., Bennett, D. D., Lohse, C. M., et al. (2002). Lipodermatosclerosis: Review of cases evaluated at Mayo Clinic. *Journal of the American Academy of Dermatology, 46*(2), 187–192.

Burrows, C., Miller, R., Townsend, D., et al. (2007). Best practice recommendations for the prevention and treatment of venous ulcers: Update 2006. *Advances in Skin & Wound Care, 20*(11), 611–621.

Bush, R., Comerota, A., Meissner, M., Raffetto, J. D., Hahn, S. R., & Freeman, K. (2017). Recommendations for the medical management of chronic venous disease: The role of micronized purified flavonoid fraction (MPFF). *Phlebology, 32*(1 Suppl), 3–19. https://doi.org/10.1177/0268355517692221.

Caggiati, A., Rosi, C., Franceschini, M., et al. (2008). The nature of skin pigmentations in chronic venous insufficiency: A preliminary report. *European Journal of Vascular and Endovascular Surgery, 35*(1), 111–118.

Cervantes, C., & Orphey, S. (2010). Pneumatic compression and venous stasis ulcers and implications of lymphedema on delayed wound healing. *Today's Wound Clinic, 4*(11).

Clark, M. (2010). A social model for lower limb care: The Lindsay Leg Club Model. *European Medical Writer's Association Journal, 10*(3), 38–40.

Coleridge-Smith, P., Labropoulos, N., Partsch, H., et al. (2006). Duplex ultrasound investigation of the veins in chronic venous disease of the lower limbs: UIP Consensus Document: Part I. Basic principles. *European Journal of Vascular and Endovascular Surgery, 31*, 83–92.

Coleridge-Smith, P., Lok, C., & Ramelet, A. A. (2005). Venous leg ulcers: A meta-analysis of adjunctive therapy with micronized purified flavonoid fraction. *European Journal of Vascular and Endovascular Surgery, 30*(2), 198–208.

Collins, L., & Seraj, S. (2010). Diagnosis and treatment of venous ulcers. *American Family Physician, 81*(8), 989–996.

Comerota, A. (2009). Treatment of chronic venous disease of the lower extremities: What's new in guidelines? *Phlebolymphology, 16*(4), 313–320.

Comerota, A. (2011). Intermittent pneumatic compression: physiologic and clinical basis to improve management of venous leg ulcer. *Journal of Vascular Surgery, 53*(4), 1121–1129.

Crawford, J. M., Lal, B. K., Duran, W. N., & Pappas, P. J. (2017). Pathophysiology of venous ulceration. *Journal of Vascular Surgery. Venous and Lymphatic Disorders, 5*, 596–605. https://doi.org/10.1016/j.jvsv.2017.03.015.

Cullum, N., & Liu, Z. (2017). Therapeutic ultrasound for venous leg ulcers. *The Cochrane Database of Systematic Reviews, 5*. https://doi.org/10.1002/14651858.CD001180.pub4.

Dahm, K. T., Myrhaug, H. T., Stromme, H., Fure, B., & Bruberg, K. G. (2019). Effects of preventive use of compression stockings for elderly with chronic venous insufficiency and swollen legs: A systematic review and meta-analysis. *BMC Geriatrics, 19*(76). https://doi.org/10.1186/x12877019-1087-1.

Davies, A., Howard, A., Howard, D. P. J., et al. (2008). Surgical therapy for chronic venous insufficiency. In *Handbook of venous disorders: Guidelines of the American Venous Forum* (3rd ed., pp. 400–409). Boca Raton: CRC Press.

Davis, J., & Gray, M. (2005). Is Unna's boot bandage as effective as a four-layer wrap for managing venous leg ulcers? *Journal of Wound, Ostomy, and Continence Nursing, 32*(3), 152–156.

de Carvalho, M. R., de Andrade, I. S., de Abreu, A. M., Ribeiro, P. L., Peixotos, B. U., & Guitton, B. (2016). All about compression: A literature review. *Journal of Vascular Nursing, 34*(2), 47–53. https://doi.org/10.1016/j.jvn.2015.12.005.

de Oliveira Carvalho, P. E., Magolbo, N. G., De Aquino, R. F., & Weller, C. D. (2016). Oral aspirin for treating venous leg ulcers. *The Cochrane Database of Systematic Reviews, 2*. https://doi.org/10.1002/14651858.CD009432.pub2.

Defloor, M. (2010). Processes underlying adherence to leg ulcer treatment, A qualitative field study. *International Journal of Nursing Studies, 48*(2), 145–155.

Di Battista, L., D'Andrea, V., Galani, A., et al. (2012). Subfascial endoscopic perforator surgery (SEPS) in chronic venous insufficiency. A 14 year experience. *Il Giornale di Chirurgia, 33*(3), 89–94.

Dissemond, J., Assenheimer, B., Bultemann, A., Gerber, V., Gretener, S., Kohler-von Siebenthal, E., et al. (2016). Compression therapy in patients with venous leg ulcers. *Journal of the German Society of Dermatology*. https://doi.org/10.1111/ddg.13091.

Dogra, S., & Sarangal, R. (2014). Summary of recommendations for leg ulcers. *Indian Dermatology Online Journal, 5*(3), 400–407. https://doi.org/10.4103/2229-5178.137829.

Dolibog, P., Franek, A., Taradaj, J., et al. (2013). A randomized, controlled clinical pilot study comparing three types of compression therapy to treat venous leg ulcers in patients with superficial and/or segmental deep venous reflux. *Ostomy/Wound Management, 59*(8), 22–30.

Dumville, J. C., Evans, D., & Peinemann, F. (2015). Negative pressure wound therapy for treating leg ulcers. *The Cochrane Database of Systematic Reviews, 7.* https://doi.org/10.1002/14651858. CD011354.pub2.

Eklöf, B., Rutherford, R. B., Bergan, J. J., et al. (2004). Revision of the CEAP classification for chronic venous disorders: Consensus statement. *Journal of Vascular Surgery, 1248,* 40–52.

Finlayson, K., Miaskowski, C., Alexander, K., Liu, W. H., Aouizerat, B., Parker, C., et al. (2017). Distinct wound healing and quality-of-life outcomes in subgroups of patients with venous leg ulcers with different symptom cluster experiences. *Journal of Pain and Symptom Management, 53,* 871–879. https://doi.org/10.1016/j.jpainsymman.2016.12.336.

Franks, P. J., Barker, J., Collier, M., Gethin, G., Haesler, E., Jawien, A., et al. (2016). Management of patients with venous leg ulcer: Challenges and current best practice. *Journal of Wound Care, 25*(6), 1–67.

Gallelli, L. (2019). Escin: A review of its anti-edematous, anti-inflammatory, and venotonic properties. *Drug Design, Development and Therapy, 13,* 3425–3437. https://doi.org/10.2147/DDDT.S207720.

Gibson, K., Morrison, N., Kolluri, R., Vasquez, M., Weiss, R., Cher, D., et al. (2018). Twenty-four month results form a randomized trial of cyanoacrylate closure versus radiofrequency ablation for the treatment of incompetent great saphenous veins. *Journal of Vascular Surgery. Venous and Lymphatic Disorders, 6*(5), 606–613. https://doi.org/10.1016/j.jvsv.2018.04.009.

Gohel, M. S., Barwell, J. R., Earnshaw, J. J., Heather, B. P., Mitchell, D. C., Whyman, M. R., et al. (2005). Randomized clinical trial of compression plus surgery versus compression alone in chronic venous ulceration (ESCHAR study)—Haemodynamic and anastomical changes. *The British Journal of Surgery, 92*(3), 291–297. https://doi.org/10.1002/bjs.4837.

Gohel, M. S., Heatly, F., Liu, X., Bradbury, A., Bulbulia, R., Cullum, N., et al. (2018). A randomized trial of early endovenous ablation in venous ulceration. *The New England Journal of Medicine, 378,* 2105–2114. https://doi.org/10.1056/NEJMoa1801214.

Gohel, M. S., Mora, J., Szigeti, M., Epstein, D. M., Heatley, F., Bradbury, A., et al. (2020). Long-term clinical and cost-effectiveness of early endovenous ablation in venous ulceration: A randomized clinical trial. *JAMA Surgery, 155*(12), 1113–1121. https://doi.org/10.1001/jamasurg.2020.3845.

Heinen, M., Borm, G., van der Vleuten, C., et al. (2012). The Lively Legs self-management programme increased physical activity and reduced wound days in leg ulcer patients: Results from a randomized controlled trial. *International Journal of Nursing Studies, 49*(2), 151–161.

Hess, C. T. (2011). Venous dermatitis checklist. *Advances in Skin & Wound Care, 24*(2), 96.

Hopf, H. W., Ueno, C., Aslam, R., et al. (2006). Guidelines for the treatment of arterial insufficiency ulcers. *Wound Repair and Regeneration, 14*(6), 693–710.

Howard, D. P., Howard, A., Kothari, A., et al. (2008). The role of superficial venous surgery in the management of venous ulcers: A systematic review. *European Journal of Vascular and Endovascular Surgery, 36*(4), 458–465.

Hunter, S., Langemo, D., Thompson, P., et al. (2013). Observation of periwound skin protection in venous ulcers: A comparison of treatments. *Advances in Skin & Wound Care, 26*(2), 62–73.

Hussein, R. (2008). Chronic venous ulcer an end of long-term suffering. *Internet Journal of Plastic Surgery, 5*(1).

Jones, J. E., Nelson, E. A., & Al-Hity, A. (2013). Skin grafting for venous leg ulcers. *The Cochrane Database of Systematic Reviews, 1,* CD001737.

Joyce, D. P., DeFreitas, S., Woo, E. Y., Tang, T. Y., Tubassam, M., & Walsh, S. R. (2022). Ultrasound-guided foam sclerotherapy as a therapeutic modality in venous ulceration. *The Surgeon: Journal of the Royal Colleges of Surgeons of Edinburgh and Ireland, 20*(5), e206–e213. https://doi.org/10.1016/j.surge.2021.08.008.

Jull, A. B., Arroll, B., Parag, V., et al. (2012). Pentoxifylline for treating venous leg ulcers. *The Cochrane Database of Systematic Reviews, 12,* CD001733.

Jull, A., Slark, J., & Parsons, J. (2018). *JAMA Dermatology, 154*(11), 1304–1311. https://doi.org/10.1001/jamadermatology.

Karanikolic, V., Binic, I., Jovanovic, D., Golubovic, M., Golubovic, I., Djindjic, N., et al. (2018). The effect of age and compression strength on venous leg ulcer healing. *Phlebology, 33*(9), 618–626. https://doi.org/10.1177/0268355517749112.

Kelechi, T., & Bonham, P. (2008). Measuring venous insufficiency objectively in the clinical setting. *Journal of Vascular Nursing, 26*(3), 67–73.

Kelly, M., & Gethin, G. (2019). Prevalence of chronic illness and risk factors for chronic illness among patients with venous leg ulceration: A cross-sectional study. *The International Journal of Lower Extremity Wounds, 18*(3), 301–308. https://doi.org/10.1177/1534734619850444.

Kimmel, H., & Robin, A. (2013). An evidence-based algorithm for treating venous leg ulcers utilizing the Cochrane Database of Systematic Reviews. *Wounds, 25*(9), 242–250.

Kline, C., Macias, B., Kraus, E., et al. (2008). Inelastic compression legging produces gradient compression and significantly higher skin surface pressures compared with an elastic compression stocking. *Vascular, 16*(1), 25–30.

Kumar, A., Agarwal, P. N., & Garg, P. K. (2009). Evaluation of subfascial endoscopic perforator vein surgery (SEPS) using harmonic scalpel in varicose veins: An observational study. *International Journal of Surgery, 7*(3), 253–256.

Lim, C. S., Baruah, M., & Bahia, S. S. (2018). Diagnosis and management of venous leg ulcers. *British Journal of Medicine, 362.* https://doi.org/10.1136/bmj.k3115.

Lin, Z. C., Loveland, P. M., Johnston, R. V., Bruce, M., & Weller, C. D. (2019). Subfascial endoscopic perforator surgery (SEPS) for treating venous leg ulcers. *The Cochrane Database of Systematic Reviews, 3.* https://doi.org/10.1002/14651858. CD012164.pub2.

Liu, X., Zheng, G., Ye, B., Chen, W., Xie, H., & Zhang, T. (2019a). Factors related to the size of venous leg ulcers. *Medicine, 98*(5). https://doi.org/10.1097/MD.0000000000014389.

Liu, X., Zheng, G., Ye, B., Chen, W., Xie, H., & Zhang, T. (2019b). Comparison of combined compression and surgery with high ligation-endovenous laser ablation-foam sclerotherapy with compression alone for active venous leg ulcers. *Scientific Reports, 9.* https://doi.org/10.1038/s41598-019-50617-y.

Marques, G. F., Criado, P. R., Morita, T. C., & Garcia, M. S. (2018). The management of livedoid vasculopathy focused on direct oral anticoagulants (DOACs): Four case reports successfully treated with rivaroxaban. *International Journal of Dermatology, 57,* 732–741.

Marston, W. (2011). Mixed arterial and venous ulcers. *Wounds, 23*(12), 351–356.

Marston, W., Ennis, W. J., Lantis, J. C., Kirsner, R. S., Galiano, R. D., Vanscheidt, W., et al. (2017). Baseline factors affecting closure of venous leg ulcers. *Journal of Vascular Surgery. Venous and*

Lymphatic Disorders, 5, 829–836. https://doi.org/10.1016/j.jvsv.2017.06.017.

Marston, W., Tang, J., Kirsner, R. S., & Ennis, W. (2016). Wound healing society 2015 update on guidelines for venous ulcers. *Wound Repair and Regeneration, 24*, 136–144.

McKenzie, M. (2013). The Lindsay Leg Club: Supporting the NHS to provide leg ulcer care. *British Journal of Community Nursing, S2*, S16–S20.

Meissner, M. H. (2009). Pathophysiology of varicose veins and chronic venous insufficiency. In J. W. Hallett Jr., et al. (Eds.), *Comprehensive vascular and endovascular surgery*. Philadelphia: Mosby.

Melikian, R., O'Donnell, T., Suarez, L., & Iafrati, M. D. (2019). Risk factors associated with the venous leg ulcer that fails to heal after 1 year of treatment. *Journal of Vascular Surgery. Venous and Lymphatic Disorders, 7*, 98–105. https://doi.org/10.1016/j.jvsv.2018.07.014.

Meulendijks, A. M., de Vries, F. C., van Dooren, A. A., Schuurmans, M. J., & Neumann, H. M. (2019). A systematic review on risk factors in developing a first-time venous leg ulcer. *Journal of the European Academy of Dermatology and Venerology, 33*, 1241–1248. https://doi.org/10.1111/jdv.15343.

Meulendijks, A. M., Fransen, W. A., Schoonhoven, L., & Neumann, H. M. (2019). A scoping review on chronic venous disease and the development of a venous leg ulcer: The role of obesity and mobility. *Journal of Tissue Viability*. https://doi.org/10.1016/j.jtv.2019.10.002.

Milan, S. B., Gan, R., & Townsend, P. E. (2019). Venous ulcers: Diagnosis and treatment. *American Academy of Family Physicians, 100*(5), 298–305.

Milic, D. J., Zivic, S. S., Bogdanovic, D. C., Golubovic, M. D., Lazarevic, M. V., & Lazarevic, K. K. (2018). A randomized trial of class 2 and class 3 elastic compression in the prevention of recurrence of venous ulceration. *Journal of Vascular Surgery. Venous and Lymphatic Disorders, 6*, 717–723. https://doi.org/10.1016/j.jvsv.2018.06.009.

Moffatt, C. J., Partsch, H., & Clark, M. (2007). Compression therapy in leg ulcer management. In M. Morison, C. J. Moffatt, P. J. Franks, et al. (Eds.), *Leg ulcers: A problem-based learning approach*. Edinburgh: Elsevier.

Montminy, M. L., Jayaraj, A., & Raju, S. (2018). A systematic review of the efficacy and limitations of venous intervention in stasis ulceration. *Journal of Vascular Surgery. Venous and Lymphatic Disorders, 6*, 376–398. https://doi.org/10.1016/j.jvsv.2017.11.007.

Morling, J. R., Yeoh, S. E., & Kolbach, D. N. (2018). Rutosides for prevention of post-thrombotic syndrome. *The Cochrane Database of Systematic Reviews, 11*. https://doi.org/10.1002/14651858.CD005626.pub4.

Morrison, N., Gibson, K., Vasquez, M., Weiss, R., & Jones, A. (2019). Five-year extension study from a randomized clinical trial (VeClose) comparing cyanoacrylate closure versus radiofrequency ablation for the treatment of incompetent great saphenous veins. *Journal of Vascular Surgery. Venous and Lymphatic Disorders, 20*. https://doi.org/10.1016/j.jvsv.2019.12.080.

Morton, L. M., Bolton, L. L., Corbett, L. Q., et al. (2013). An evaluation of the Association for the Advancement of Wound Care venous ulcer guideline and recommendations for future research. *Advances in Skin & Wound Care, 26*(12), 553–561.

Nelson, E. A., & Bell-Syer, S. E. (2012). Compression for preventing recurrence of venous ulcers. *The Cochrane Database of Systematic Reviews, 8*, CD002303.

Nicolaides A. N. (2020). The benefits of micronized purified flavonoid fraction (MPFF) throughout the progression of chronic venous disease. *Advances in Therapy, 37*(Suppl. 1), 1–5. https://doi.org/10.1007/s12325-019-01218-8.

Nelson, E. A., Hillman, A., & Thomas, K. (2014). Intermittent pneumatic compression for treating venous leg ulcers. *The Cochrane Database of Systematic Reviews, 5*. https://doi.org/10.1002/14651858.CD001899.pub4.

Nelson, E. A., Mani, R., Thomas, K., et al. (2011). Intermittent pneumatic compression for treatment of venous leg ulcers. *The Cochrane Database of Systematic Reviews, 2*, CD001899.

Norman, G., Westby, M. J., Rithalia, A. D., Stubbs, N., Soares, M. O., & Dumville, J. C. (2018). Dressings and topical agents for treating venous leg ulcers. *The Cochrane Database of Systematic Reviews, 6*. https://doi.org/10.1002/14651858.CD012583.pub2.

O'Brien, J., Finlayson, K., Kerr, G., & Edwards, H. (2017). Evaluating the effectiveness of a self-management exercise intervention on wound healing, functional ability and health-related quality of life outcomes in adults with venous leg ulcers: A randomised controlled trial. *International Wound Journal, 14*, 130–137. https://doi.org/10.1111/iwj.12571.

O'Connor, S., & Murphy, S. (2014). Chronic venous leg ulcers: Is topical zinc the answer? A review of literature. *Advances in Skin & Wound Care, 27*(1), 35–44.

O'Donnell, T. F., Passman, M. A., Marston, W. A., Ennis, W. J., Dalsing, M., Kistner, R. L., et al. (2014). Management of venous leg ulcers: Clinical practice guidelines of the Society for Vascular Surgery and the American Venous Forum. *Journal of Vascular Surgery, 60*, 3s–59s. https://doi.org/10.1016/j.jvs.2014.04.049.

O'Meara, S., Al-Kurdi, D., Ologun, Y., et al. (2014). Antibiotics and antiseptics for venous leg ulcers. *The Cochrane Database of Systematic Reviews, 1*, CD003557.

O'Meara, S., Cullum, N. A., & Nelson, E. A. (2009). Compression for venous leg ulcers (review). *The Cochrane Database of Systematic Reviews, 1*.

O'Meara, S., Cullum, N., Nelson, E. A., et al. (2012). Compression for venous leg ulcers. *The Cochrane Database of Systematic Reviews, 11*, CD000265.

Olyaie, M., Rad, F., Elahifar, M., et al. (2013). High-frequency and noncontact low-frequency ultrasound therapy for venous leg ulcer treatment: A randomized, controlled study. *Ostomy/Wound Management, 59*(8), 14–20.

Paranhos, T., Paiva, C. S. B., Cardoso, F. C. I., Apolinário, P. P., Rodrigues, R. C. M., Oliveira, H. C., et al. (2021). Systematic review and meta-analysis of the efficacy of Unna boot in the treatment of venous leg ulcers. *Wound Repair and Regeneration, 29*(3), 443–451. https://doi.org/10.1111/wrr.12903.

Phillips, P., Lumley, E., Duncabn, R., Aber, A., Woods, H. B., Jones, G. L., et al. (2017). A systematic review of qualitive research into people's experiences of living with venous leg ulcers. *Journal of Advanced Nursing, 74*, 550–563. https://doi.org/10.1111/jan.13465.

Pieper, B., Templin, T. N., Birk, T. J., et al. (2008). Chronic venous disorders and injection drug use. *Journal of Wound, Ostomy, and Continence Nursing, 35*(3), 301–310.

Pittler, M., & Ernst, E. (2012). Meta-analysis of horse chestnut seed extract studies for chronic venous insufficiency. *The Cochrane Database of Systematic Reviews, 11*, CD003230.

Pompilio, G., Nicolaides, A., Kakkos, S. K., & Integlia, D. (2021). Systematic literature review and network Meta-analysis of sulodexide and other drugs in chronic venous disease. *Phlebology, 36*(9), 695–709. https://doi.org/10.1177/02683555211015020.

Serra, R., Rizzuto, A., Rossi, A., Perri, P., Barbetta, A., Abdalla, K., et al. (2017). Skin grafting for the treatment of chronic leg ulcers—A systematic review in evidence-based medicine. *International Wound Journal, 14*, 149–157. https://doi.org/10.1111/iwj.12575.

Shannon, M. M., Hawk, J., Navaroli, L., et al. (2013). Factors affecting patient adherence to recommended measures for prevention of recurrent venous ulcers. *Journal of Wound, Ostomy, and Continence Nursing, 40*(3), 268–274.

Sippel, K., Seifert, B., & Hafner, J. (2015). Donning devices (foot slips and frames) enable elderly people with chronic venous insufficiency to put on compression stockings. *European Journal of Endovascular Surgery, 49*, 221–229. https://doi.org/10.1016/j.ejvs.2014.11.005.

Smith, D., Lane, R., McGinnes, R., O'Brien, J., Johnston, R., Bugeja, L., et al. (2018). What is the effect of exercise on wound healing in patients with venous leg ulcers? A systematic review. *International Wound Journal, 15*, 441–453. https://doi.org/10.1111/iwj.12885.

Sreedharan, S., & Siaha, S. (2011). Atrophie blanche. *Wound Practice and Research, 19*(2), 74–80.

Stana, J., Maver, U., & Potocnik, U. (2019). Genetic biases related to chronic venous ulceration. *Journal of Wound Care, 28*(2), 59–65.

Subramonia, S., & Lees, T. (2010). Randomized clinical trial of radiofrequency ablation or conventional high ligation and stripping for great saphenous varicose veins. *British Journal of Surgery, 97*(3), 328–336.

Tew, G. A., Gumber, A., McIntosh, E., Kesterton, S., King, B., Michaels, J. A., et al. (2018). *European Journal of Applied Physiology, 118*, 321–329. https://doi.org/10.1007/s00421-017-3772-0.

Thistlewaite, K. R., Finlayson, K. J., Cooper, D., Brown, B., Bennett, M. H., Kay, G., et al. (2018). *Wound Repair and Regeneration, 26*, 324–331. https://doi.org/10.1111/wrr.12657.

Todd, M. (2014). Venous disease and chronic oedema: Treatment and patient concordance. *British Journal of Nursing, 23*(9), 466–470.

Tollow, P., Ogden, J., & Whiteley, M. S. (2016). The comparative impact of conservative treatment versus superficial venous surgery, for the treatment of venous leg ulcers: A systematic review of the impact on patients' quality of life. *Phlebology, 31*(2), 82–93. https://doi.org/10.1177/0268355515581278.

Towler, M. A., Rush, E. W., Richardson, M. K., & Williams, C. L. (2018). Randomized, prospective, blinded-enrollment, head-to-head venous leg ulcer trial comparing living, bioengineered skin graft substitute (Apligraf) with cryopreserved, human skin allograft (Theraskin). *Clinics in Podiatric Medicine and Surgery, 35*, 357–365. https://doi.org/10.1016/j.cpm.2018.02.006.

Turner, B. R. H., Jasionowska, S., Machin, M., Javed, A., Gwozdz, A. M., Shalhoub, J., et al. (2023). Systematic review and meta-analysis of exercise therapy for venous leg ulcer healing and recurrence. Journal of Vascular Surgery. *Venous and Lymphatic Disorders, 11*(1), 219–226. https://doi.org/10.1016/j.jvsv.2022.09.003.

van Gent, W. B., Catarinella, F. S., Lam, Y. L., Nieman, F. M., Toonder, I. M., van der Ham, A. C., et al. (2015). Conservative versus surgical treatment of venous leg ulcers: 10-year follow up of a randomized, multicenter trial. *Phlebology, 30*(1S), 35–41. https://doi.org/10.1177/0268355514568848.

Van Hecke, A., Beeckman, D., Grypdonck, M., et al. (2013). Knowledge deficits and information-seeking behavior in leg ulcer patients: An exploratory qualitative study. *Journal of Wound, Ostomy, and Continence Nursing, 40*(4), 381–387.

Varatharajan, L., Thapar, A., Lane, T., Munster, A. B., & Davies, A. H. (2016). Pharmacological adjuncts for chronic venous ulcer healing: A systematic review. *Phlebology, 31*(5), 356–365. https://doi.org/10.1177/0268355515587194.

Vasudevan, B., Neema, S., & Verma, R. (2016). Livedoid vasculopathy: A review of pathogenesis and principles of management. *Indian Journal of Dermatology, Venereology and Leprology, 82*, 478–488. https://doi.org/10.4103/0378-6323.183635.

Warshaw, E. M., Ahmed, R. L., Belsito, D. V., et al. (2007). Contact dermatitis of the hands: Cross-sectional analyses of North American Contact Dermatitis Group data, 1994–2004. *Journal of the American Academy of Dermatology, 57*(2), 301–314.

Weingarten, M. (2001). State-of-the-art treatment of chronic venous disease. *Clinical Infectious Diseases, 32*, 949–954.

Weller, C. D., Buchbinder, R., & Johnston, R. V. (2016). Interventions for helping people adhere to compression treatments for venous leg ulceration. *The Cochrane Database of Systematic Reviews, 3*. https://doi.org/10.1002/14651858.CD008378.pub3.

Welsh, L. (2016). What is the existing evidence supporting the efficacy of compression bandage systems containing both elastic and inelastic components (mixed-component systems)? A systematic review. *Journal of Clinical Nursing, 26*, 1189–1203. https://doi.org/10.1111/jocn.13611.

Westby, M. J., Dumville, J. C., Stubbs, N., Norman, G., Wong, J. K., Cullum, N., et al. (2018). Protease activity as a prognostic factor for wound healing in venous leg ulcers. *The Cochrane Database of Systematic Reviews, 9*. https://doi.org/10.1002/14651858.CD012841.pub2.

White-Chu, E., & Conner-Kerr, T. (2014). Overview of guidelines for the prevention and treatment of venous leg ulcers: A U.S. perspective. *Journal of Multidisciplinary Healthcare, 7*, 111–117.

Wound, Ostomy and Continence Nurses Society™ (WOCN®). (2019). *Guideline for management of patients with lower-extremity venous disease.* Mt. Laurel: WOCN®.

Wright, D. D. (2009). The ESCHAR trial: Should it change practice? *Perspectives in Vascular Surgery and Endovascular Therapy, 21*(2), 69–72.

16

Lymphedema

Catherine R. Ratliff

OBJECTIVES

1. Describe the pathophysiology of lymphedema.
2. Identify and describe two types of lymphedema.
3. Distinguish the difference between lymphedema and lipedema.
4. List two common diagnostic tests used to diagnose lymphedema.
5. Articulate important assessment features for the patient being evaluated for lymphedema.

6. Outline a treatment plan for a patient with lymphedema, including conservative measures and adjunctive therapies such as surgery.
7. Explain prevention and treatment measures for a patient with cellulitis.

Lymphedema is a chronic often progressive disease characterized by swelling of the affected body part, usually the upper and lower extremities, because of impaired lymph flow. Lymphedema—the accumulation of fluid in tissues, usually in the upper and lower extremities—often results from lymph node dissection or radiation and can cause painful and debilitating swelling that may interfere with a patient's daily living activities and quality of life. The swelling may be mild or severe so that the individual is unable to use the affected limb (Whitnell, 2020). The clinical presentation of lymphedema (see Plate 48) results from the subcutaneous accumulation of fluid. With interstitial fluid accumulation comes an inflammatory response; slowed lymphatic flow, which causes lipogenesis; and fat deposition. Patients develop firmer subcutaneous tissue in the limb as fibrosis, as well as hypertrophy of the adipose tissue. These physical changes present clinically as soft and pitting edema, but later progress to induration and fibrosis with nonpitting edema (Whitnell, 2020).

EPIDEMIOLOGY

As the third component of the vascular system, the lymphatic system receives the least attention. Lymphedema and related pathologies have received much less attention than the pathologies associated with venous and arterial ulcers. Chronic lymphedema has no cure, and long-term management with patient involvement is critical to control the lymphedema. Lymphedema is frequently undertreated with an insufficient number of lymphedema centers and specialists are addressing the problem. Lymphedema is a significant problem in the United States and throughout the world. It has been reported that lymphedema affects as many as 200

million people worldwide and approximately 3 million people in the United States. Lymphedema affects females more often than males (Cormier, Rourke, Crosby, et al., 2012; Grada & Phillips, 2017a). Lower extremity lymphedema is much more common than upper extremity lymphedema and is usually associated with infection, chronic venous insufficiency, and malignancies, such as uterine cancer, prostate cancer, lymphoma, and melanoma. Upper extremity lymphedema is most commonly associated with breast cancer. In patients undergoing postmastectomy irradiation therapy, the incidence of lymphedema is approximately 30% (Grada & Phillips, 2017a). For patients with breast cancer, the more lymph nodes the surgeon removes, the greater the risk for patients to develop lymphedema. A systematic review and meta-analysis found that the incidence of lymphedema in the upper extremities is approximately four times greater after axillary lymph node dissections than sentinel node biopsies (DiSipio, Rye, Newman, & Hayes, 2013; National Cancer Institute: Division of Cancer Control & Population Sciences. Office of Cancer Survivorship, 2019). With the increased survival of these patients, the numbers of patients with cancer and lymphedema are expected to increase. However, these patients may be sicker and less able to care for themselves, including managing their lymphedema.

PATHOPHYSIOLOGY

The lymphatic system is composed of lymphatic organs, such as lymph nodes, tonsils, thymus, and spleen, which are connected to lymphatic vessels that run parallel to the venous circulation. The lymphatic system has three main functions: drainage of excess interstitial fluid, fat absorption, and immune surveillance (Grada & Phillips, 2017a). The lymphatic system has an important immune surveillance function. Circulating lymph transports various antigens and activated antigen-presenting cells into the lymph nodes to promote the immune response. Skin has extensive lymphatic capillaries. Patients with lymphedema are prone to recurrent skin infections because of the accumulation of peripheral tissue antigens associated with autoimmunity. Chronic inflammation with soft tissue fibrosis in lymphedema has been attributed to T-helper 2 cells; a specialized group of T cells that are important for immune responses caused by lymphatic stasis (Grada & Phillips, 2017a; Li, Kataru, & Mehrara, 2020).

The lymphatic system transports fluid, delivers nutrients, and removes waste to defend against disease and maintain fluid balance in the body. When fluid from the interstitial space enters the lymphatic system, it is considered lymph fluid. Lymph fluid consists of protein, water, fatty acids, salts, white blood cells, microorganisms, and debris. It is absorbed from the interstitial spaces into the lymphatic vessels, where it is transported to the venous system (Whitnell, 2020). The major function of the lymphatic system is to return fluid and protein from interstitial spaces to the vascular system. Because lymphatic vessels often lack a basement membrane and have thinner vessel walls, they can reabsorb molecules too large for the venous system (Whitnell, 2020). Usually tissue fluid and protein macromolecules filtrated by the arterial capillaries are reabsorbed and returned to the circulation through the lymphatic system. From 50% to 100% of the intravascular proteins are filtered this way in the interstitial space. The lymphatic vessels absorb 2–4 L of protein-rich fluid retained in the interstitial space per day. This fluid is picked up by the lymphatic capillaries and returned to the circulation, thus maintaining normal plasma volume and preventing interstitial edema. If the system is overloaded, fluid and protein accumulate in the interstitial space, forming a high-protein edema that triggers an inflammatory response with deposition of collagen (Grada & Phillips, 2017a; Whitnell, 2020).

Two systems of lymphatic drainage work similarly to the venous system. The superficial system drains the skin and subcutaneous tissues, and the deep system drains the tissues to the fascia and below. The lymphatic vessels in the superficial system are located in the subcutaneous tissues, whereas those of the deep system are aligned with the blood vessels, especially the veins. These two systems of lymphatic drainage are connected by perforating vessels just like the veins (Lawenda, Mondry, & Johnstone, 2009). Unlike veins, which increase in size as they reach the center of the body, lymph-collecting vessels remain the same size as their proximity to the lymph nodes increases. The vessels pass through the interval lymph nodes (located in the limbs) and connect to the regional (e.g., axillary, supraclavicular) lymph nodes (Whitnell, 2020).

There are three types of lymphatic vessels: lymph capillaries, located in the dermis just beneath the epidermis;

precollector vessels, located below the lymph capillaries in the dermis; and lymph-collecting vessels, located in the subcutaneous and deep tissues. The network of lymph capillaries originates in the fingertips and palms for the upper extremities and the toes and soles of the feet for the lower extremities. The diameter of a lymph capillary ranges from 20 to 70 μm. They are composed of layers of overlapping endothelial cells connected to tissue by a fibrous filament. They do not contain any valves to direct the flow of fluid so lymph flows in the direction of the lower pressure. When the amount of fluid in the surrounding tissues increases, the filaments pull the endothelial cells apart and fluid flows into the lumen of the capillary (Whitnell, 2020).

The precollectors connect the lymphatic capillaries with the lymph collectors. The lymph collectors are similar to veins; they have valves and transport lymph fluid to the lymph nodes and lymphatic trunks. The precollectors and collectors are the principal vessels of the lymphatic system and eventually filter through to the lymph nodes (Suami & Scaglioni, 2018).

Lymph drains from the legs into the lumbar lymphatic trunk to the intestinal lymphatic trunk and cisterna chyli to the thoracic duct, which drains into the left subclavian vein (Fig. 16.1). The thoracic duct empties approximately 3 L of lymph fluid per day into the venous circulation (Lawenda et al., 2009). From the left side of upper body, the lymphatic vessels of the left arm drain into the left subclavian lymphatic trunk, which then drains into the left subclavian vein. Lymph is drained from the right side of the head, neck, thorax, and right arm into the right subclavian vein by way of the right thoracic duct (Lawenda et al., 2009).

Lymphedema is caused by dysfunction of the lymphatic system, where accumulation or pooling of lymph fluid into the interstitial space occurs. External forces such as surgery, radiation, or infection, can damage the lymphatic system causing the dysfunction. With an impaired lymphatic system, the amount of lymphatic fluid in the interstitial space becomes more than the body's lymph system can handle. Plasma oncotic pressure decreases, oncotic pressure of tissue fluid increases, and lymphatic blockage or obstruction occurs (Mehrara, 2019). With retention of fluid and large protein molecules within this interstitial space, the space swells (Mehrara, 2019). With swelling, the large protein molecules leak into the tissues, causing fibrosis. Over time, progressive obstruction to lymphatic flow occurs by distortion or obliteration of the lymphatic channels from the fibrotic changes in the tissues (Mehrara, 2019).

TYPES OF LYMPHEDEMA

Lymphedema is classified as primary or secondary. Primary lymphedema is caused by developmental lymphatic vascular anomalies. Secondary lymphedema is acquired and arises as a result of an underlying systemic disease, trauma, or surgery (Grada & Phillips, 2017a).

Primary lymphedema is rare, with an estimated prevalence of 1 in 100,000 individuals, and usually occurs during childhood,

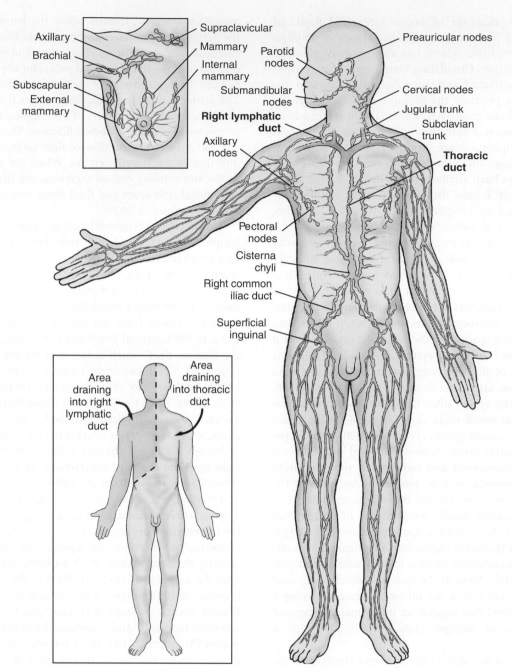

Fig. 16.1 Anatomy of the lymphatic system. (From Monahan, F. D., & Neighbors, M. (1998). *Medical surgical nursing: Foundations for clinical practice* (2nd ed.). Philadelphia: Saunders.)

but may present at any age. Approximately 99% of individuals with lymphedema have a secondary lymphedema (Grada & Phillips, 2017a). Secondary lymphedema is more common and occurs in 1 in 1000 individuals, with the mean age ranging from 50 and 58 years. In the United States and Western countries, secondary lymphedema is most commonly reported in patients undergoing lymphadenectomy or radiation therapy for breast cancer. It may occur after any malignancy that affects lymphatic drainage. Filariasis (described later in this chapter) is the most common cause of secondary lymphedema in the world (Grada & Phillips, 2017a).

Primary (Idiopathic) Lymphedema

Primary lymphedema is caused by congenital absence or abnormalities of lymphatic tissue which usually involves the leg (WOCN, 2019). There are three types of primary lymphedema based on the age of presentation: lymphedema precox typically presents at onset of puberty, congenital lymphedema typically presents before 2 years of age, and lymphedema tarda which typically presents after 35 years of age. Lymphedema precox is the most common form of primary lymphedema. Although it may occur between 2 and 36 years of age, it typically presents at the onset of puberty

TABLE 16.1 Types of Primary Lymphedema

Lymphedema precox
  Familial (Meige disease)

Congenital lymphedema
  Hereditary congenital lymphedema (Milroy disease)
  Other types—Noonan syndrome, Turner syndrome, and
    trisomy 13, 18, and 21

Lymphedema tarda

with unilateral foot and calf edema. Females are predominantly affected, and it is believed that estrogen may play a role because its onset at puberty (Rezaie et al., 2008). Ten percent of cases of lymphedema precox are familial (referred as Meige disease) with a mutation in the FOXC2 gene. Congenital lymphedema may be due to a congenital or inherited condition associated with pathologic development of the lymphatic vessels. Hereditary congenital lymphedema (Milroy disease) is transmitted as an autosomal dominant trait. Affected individuals develop bilateral lymphedema in both lower extremities after birth. Other conditions associated with congenital lymphedema include Noonan syndrome, Turner syndrome, and trisomy 13, 18, and 21 (Rezaie et al., 2008). Lymphedema tarda also occurs more commonly in women and affects the lower extremities (see Table 16.1).

Secondary (Acquired) Lymphedema

Secondary causes of lymphedema include cancer and cancer treatment, infection, inflammatory disorders (e.g., sarcoidosis, Crohn's disease), obesity, and chronic forms of lymphatic overload (e.g., chronic venous insufficiency, trauma, and burns) (Mehrara, 2019). The most common cause of secondary lymphedema in the United States is related to malignancy and its subsequent treatment (e.g., surgery, radiation). The types of cancers associated with secondary lymphedema include breast cancer, gynecologic cancer, lymphoma, melanoma, and urologic cancers. Secondary lymphedema is caused by dysfunction or obstruction of the lymphatic system that usually occurs at proximal limb segments (i.e., lymph nodes) due to surgery, radiation, trauma, infection, malignancy, or scar tissue. Surgery may include the removal of one or more lymph nodes. If the remaining lymph nodes and vessels cannot compensate for those that have been removed, then lymphedema can result. The current use of sentinel node biopsy (e.g., with cancer surgery) has helped reduce the risk of patients developing lymphedema because fewer lymph nodes are removed. Radiation can cause scarring and inflammation of the lymph system, which can restrict the flow of lymph fluid, thus increasing the risk for lymphedema. Cancer can block the lymphatic vessels, which also increases the risk for lymphedema. In addition to cancer, chronic diseases such as congestive heart failure, liver disease, and end-stage renal disease can cause chronic edema.

Infection from parasites can infiltrate the lymph vessels and block the flow. The cause of the most common form of infection, called *filariasis*, is the nematode *Wuchereria bancrofti*, which is transmitted to humans by mosquitoes (Mehrara, 2019). When the filarial larvae mature into adult worms in the lymphatic channels, they block the lymph hannels, causing severe lymphedema in the arms, legs, and genitalia, a condition also known as *elephantiasis*. It is estimated that as many as 36 million infected individuals are seriously disfigured by lymphatic filariasis (World Health Organization, 2020).

Once damage has occurred to the lymphatic system, transport capacity is permanently decreased, predisposing to lymphedema. The pelvic and inguinal nodes in the lower limbs and the axillary nodes of the upper limbs are the primary sites of obstruction. Lymphedema has been reported 20–30 years after the precipitating event (e.g., surgery).

With the rise in obesity rates comes an increase in the number of cases of secondary lymphedema in the morbidly obese. In a review of wound clinic data of approximately 15,000 patients from 17 wound centers in the United States, Fife and Carter (2008) found 74% prevalence of secondary lymphedema in morbidly obese patients. Morbidly obese patients also have been observed to have lymphedema in conjunction with venous ulcer disease. Obesity impedes lymphatic flow, leading to accumulation of lymphatic fluid in the subcutaneous tissue (Greene, Grant, & Slavin, 2012). The risk for lymphedema increases as body mass index (BMI) increases (Greene et al., 2012). Sizable weight gain has been shown to increase a woman's risk for lymphedema following breast cancer (Greene & Goss, 2018). With the increase of lymphatic fluid in the setting of decreased oxygen tensions, fibrosis with chronic inflammation and increased risk for infection result. In addition to occurring in the extremities, lymphedema can be seen in the overhanging abdominal pannus of the morbidly obese.

Severely obese patients with a BMI >50 can develop lower extremity lymphedema, termed "obesity-induced" lymphedema (Greene & Goss, 2018). Greene et al. (2012) studied 15 patients with BMIs of greater than 30 with bilateral lower extremity enlargement. Twelve of the 15 were women, and the mean age was 57.9 years; the mean BMI was 51.4 (range, 30.7–88.1). None of the patients had a history of primary lymphedema, inguinal lymphadenectomy or radiation, or lower extremity ulcers. The BMI range of the five patients with lymphedema (59.7–88.1) was significantly greater than the range of the BMI of the 10 patients without lymphedema; 30.7–53.3 ($P < 0.001$). The authors concluded that as BMI increases, there might be a threshold above which lymphatic flow becomes impaired.

STAGES OF LYMPHEDEMA

Although a variety of staging systems exist, providers often use the International Society of Lymphology staging system to gauge the severity of the disease. This system is based on the amount of swelling and the condition of the skin at each stage of the disease and provides a standard reference to evaluate the extent of lymphedema. Improving or worsening limb volume during each stage is based on excess volume in the affected extremity

TABLE 16.2   Stages of Lymphedema

Stage	Manifestations
0	Subclinical lymphedema with edema that is not evident despite impaired lymphatic function (Nonvisible, latency stage)
1	Reversible pitting edema that begins distally (at foot) Negative or borderline Stemmer sign No palpable fibrosis (Spontaneously reversible)
2	Minimally pitting or nonpitting (brawny) edema that is not reduced by conservative measures such as elevation Positive Stemmer sign Pronounced fibrosis Hyperkeratosis (thickening of skin) Papillomatosis (skin has rough cobblestone appearance and texture) (Spontaneously irreversible)
3	Lymphostatic elephantiasis (massive enlargement and distortion of limb caused by breakdown of skin's elastic components) Progressive fibrosis, acanthosis, hyperkeratosis, papillomatosis Ulceration (Spontaneously irreversible)

NLN Medical Advisory Committee. (2011). *Topic: The diagnosis and treatment of lymphedema. Position statement of the National Lymphedema Network* (pp. 1–19). https://lipedemaproject.org/pposition-statement-of-the-national-lymphedema-networkp-ptopic/. Accessed February 25, 2020.

compared with the contralateral extremity. The system includes the following four stages (Table 16.2): Stage 0 indicates a normal appearing extremity but with subclinical lymphedema in which swelling is not evident despite impaired lymphatic function. Stage 0 (reversible) may exist for months or years before edema occurs. Stage 1 (reversible) is early edema, which improves with limb elevation. Pitting may occur. Pitting edema is considered present when, after a finger is pressed into the edematous tissue, an indentation remains. In Stage 2 (irreversible), there is pitting edema that does not resolve with elevation. As Stage 2 progresses, tissue fibrosis develops. Stage 3 (irreversible) describes fibroadipose deposition and skin changes in the limb, such as acanthosis (increase in thickness of the epidermis), fatty deposits, and warty growths, may be present (Greene & Goss, 2018; Whitnell, 2020).

Within each stage, limb volume differences can be categorized as mild (<20% increase in size), moderate (20%–40% increase in size), and severe (>40% increase in size) (Greene & Goss, 2018).

LIPEDEMA

Lipedema, or adiposis dolorosa or painful fat, is an adipose tissue disorder often confused with lymphedema that affects about 11% of adult women worldwide (Buck & Herbst, 2016).

It is a syndrome of bilateral adipose deposition that almost always is seen in the lower extremities of overweight/obese women. It begins as abnormal depositions of body fat in the buttocks and hips and progresses gradually to include the thighs and calves but stops at the ankles. In those who are not overweight, the lower body shape is disproportionately larger than their upper body, producing a pear-shaped appearance (Canning & Bartholomew, 2018). Excess fatty tissue will affect the lymphatic system by constricting the flow of lymph fluid. It can affect the upper extremities in 30% of cases (Wagner, 2011).

The cause of lipedema is unknown. Some patients have affected female family members. Lipedema usually starts after puberty, pregnancy or menopause and is aggravated by weight gain. Symptoms include painful legs and symmetrical leg swelling ending just above the ankles, known as the "cut-off sign." The swelling does not typically indent with pressure ("nonpitting"). Swelling persists despite leg elevation or weight loss. Easy bruising and the presence of varicose or small spider veins near the skin surface are commonly reported. The feet are not involved, and the arms are less commonly affected. Women with lipedema may also complain of increased sensitivity to touch (Canning & Bartholomew, 2018).

The leg enlargement is frequently misdiagnosed as lymphedema even when no lymphatic malfunction is present. Lipedema may eventually result in secondary lymphatic dysfunction leading to lipolymphedema (Fife, Maus, & Carter, 2010). Features distinguishing lymphedema from lipedema are listed in Table 16.3 (Fife et al., 2010; Fonder, Loveless, & Lazarus, 2007; Warren, Janz, Borud, et al., 2007). Table 16.4 compares characteristics of venous edema to lipedema and lymphedema.

The diagnosis of lipedema usually is based on history and physical examination. Diagnostic tests, such as those done with lymphedema, may be conducted and usually only show subcutaneous fat hypertrophy. Lipedema has a tendency to progress over time such that disease severity can be described in stages. There are four stages of lipedema (see Table 16.5): stage 1 involves an even skin surface with an enlarged hypodermis, stage 2 involves an uneven skin pattern with the development of a nodular or mass-like appearance of subcutaneous fat, lipomas, and/or angiolipomas, stage 3 involves large growths of nodular fat causing severe contour deformity of the thighs and around the knee, and stage 4 involves the presence of lipolymphedema (Buck & Herbst, 2016).

The management of lipedema involves exercise, diet and nutrition, emotional support and management of other coexisting causes of lower extremity swelling. Exercise such as walking, swimming, cycling, and Pilates and a healthy diet are recommended to prevent progression of lipedema. Although weight loss may not help, prevention of additional weight gain is important. Water jet-assisted liposuction is a lymph-sparing procedure that removes excess fat and may be useful for patients who have not improved with conservative measures. This procedure is generally performed under local anesthesia and is less likely to damage lymphatic vessels when compared with standard liposuction procedures.

TABLE 16.3 Comparison of Lymphedema and Lipedema

	Lymphedema	Lipedema
Gender	Male and female	Female
Age	Any age	After or during puberty (10–30 years of age)
Edema	Pitting progresses to firm fibrotic	Nonpitting, soft
Epidermal skin changes	Common	Uncommon
Cellulitis	Common	Uncommon
Stemmer sign	Positive	Negative, but positive fat pad sign at ankle (fatty tissue just anterior to lateral malleolus and between Achilles tendon and medial malleolus)
Distribution	Unilateral or bilateral, toes to groin	Always bilateral legs, ends at ankles Feet usually spared, sometimes arms affected with hands spared
Tenderness	None usually	Tender to palpation Aching sensation
Bruising	No bruising	Bruising common
Leg elevation	Improvement with leg elevation	No improvement with elevation
Magnetic resonance imaging	Honeycomb pattern	Normal

TABLE 16.4 Lymphedema

Treatment Components

Intervention	Desired Effect	Action	Cautions
Complex decongestive therapy Therapeutic massage Compression bandages applied immediately after treatment	Mobilization of retained lymph	Mobilize lymphatic fluid in channels adjacent and proximal to involved site	Performed only by therapist trained in the technique Usually requires treatments daily for 1–3 weeks
Sequential compression therapy	Mobilization of retained lymph	Dynamic compression pumps with limb sleeves compress lymphatic fluid and mobilize lymph	Risk of displacing fluid to proximal leg or genitalia Risk of further damage to lymphatics
Limb elevation	Edema reduction	Counter effect of gravity on lymph flow	Effective only in early phase of disease
Compression bandaging	Critical component of maintenance therapy Nonelastic or short-stretch bandages and custom-fitted sleeves or stockings most effective	Apply pressure to tissues to facilitate compression of lymph channels and movement of lymph from interstitial space into circulation	Should provide 40–60 mm Hg subbandage pressure Replace regularly to prevent loss of therapeutic effectiveness
Exercise (light movement exercise with compression bandage or garment in place)	Maintenance of lymph reduction	Stimulate intact lymphatics to increase rate of lymph transport	Should not be strenuous or cause fatigue
Skin and nail care (avoid trauma, apply moisturizer, regular nail care)	Infection control during restorative and maintenance phases	Keep skin supple and prevent breaks in skin to reduce risk of infection	Recommend having standing prescription for antibiotic should signs of infection appear Do not cut cuticles

TABLE 16.5	Stages of Lipedema
Stage	**Manifestations**
1	Even skin surface with an enlarged hypodermis
2	Uneven skin pattern with development of nodular or mass-like appearance of subcutaneous fat, lipomas, and/or angiolipomas
3	Large growths of nodular fat causing severe contour deformity of the thighs and around the knee
4	Involves the presence of lipolymphedema

Other causes of leg swelling may coexist with lipedema and should not be overlooked during treatment. Skin care is important for patients with lipedema complicated by lymphedema or chronic venous insufficiency. Regular application of moisture barriers avoids dry skin, thus reducing the risk of infection (cellulitis). Compression stockings are useful when edema is present and may help prevent the progression of lipedema into lipolymphedema. Manual lymph drainage (MLD) and intermittent pneumatic compression therapy can be tried with varying degrees of success. Herbal medications such as horse chestnut or diosmin are often tried with varying results and are usually more effective when there is a venous component to the swelling. Emotional support is often overlooked. Information about patient support groups and counseling may be appropriate (Canning & Bartholomew, 2018).

DIAGNOSTIC TESTS

Diagnosis of lymphedema typically is made through clinical presentation and history. A difference of more than 2 cm in limb circumference or 200 mL in volume between the left and right extremities suggests lymphedema (Whitnell, 2020). Diagnostic confirmation can be made with isotopic lymphoscintigraphy, in which a radionuclide is injected into the lymphatic tissue between the first and second digits of the affected limb to identify abnormalities of the lymphatic pathways, including enlarged vessels and backflow problems due to obstruction. Lymphoscintigraphy is considered the gold standard for imaging studies for lymphedema (Grada & Phillips, 2017b). Lymphoscintigraphy is invasive and because radioactive dye must be injected into an already compromised limb, lymphoscintigraphy generally is indicated only if the patient is a surgical candidate and a definitive diagnosis is needed. Computed tomography scans or magnetic resonance imaging (MRI) can be performed to evaluate for the presence of lymphedema and to show lymph trunk anatomy and causes of obstructive secondary lymphedema. MRI can detect a honeycomb pattern of the subcutaneous tissue from fibrosis and lymph fluid, a finding that is not seen with other forms of edema, so it can be helpful for diagnosis (Grada & Phillips, 2017b). Lymph fluid analysis with protein content between 1 and 5.5 g/dL usually indicates lymphedema. Other laboratory studies, such as serum albumin and urinalysis, should

be performed to rule out other causes of edema, such as renal or hepatic impairment. Edema can be classified by protein content. Low-protein edema is composed of less than 1 g of protein per 100 mL of fluid; high-protein edema is composed of greater than 1 g of protein per 100 mL of fluid (Lawenda et al., 2009). Lymphedema is a high-protein edema. Ultrasound can provide an analysis of soft tissue changes but does not provide any information about the lymphatics. Duplex Doppler studies may be required if venous ulcer disease is also suspected. Genetic testing may be recommended for patients with primary lymphedema. Bioimpedance spectroscopy (BIS) is a procedure in which an electrical current is passed through the limb and impedance flow is measured. This technique, also known as *bioelectrical impedance analysis*, measures the composition of tissues, especially the presence of fluids such as lymph. Reduced impedance values are indicative of lymphedema. In lymphedema management, BIS can be used for early detection and ongoing measurements of fluid buildup in the affected limb to determine the effectiveness of therapy.

Ridner, Dietrich, Cowher, et al. (2019) conducted a randomized controlled trial (RCT) comparing lymphedema progression rates using volume measurements calculated from the circumference using a tape measure (TM) or BIS. Patients were randomized to either TM or BIS surveillance. The primary endpoint of the trial was the rate of progression to clinical lymphedema requiring complex decongestive physiotherapy (CDP), with progression defined as a TM volume change in the at-risk arm $\geq 10\%$ above the baseline. A total of 508 patients were included with 109 (21.9%) patients triggering prethreshold interventions. Compared with TM, BIS had a lower rate of trigger (15.8% vs 28.5%, $P < 0.001$) and longer times to trigger (9.5 vs 2.8 months, $P = 0.002$). Twelve triggering patients progressed to CDP (10 in the TM group [14.7%] and 2 in the BIS group [4.9%]), representing a 67% relative reduction and a 9.8% absolute reduction ($P = 0.130$). Results demonstrated that posttreatment surveillance with BIS reduced the absolute rates of progression of lymphedema requiring CDP by approximately 10%, a clinically meaningful improvement (Ridner et al., 2019).

Indocyanine green (ICG) lymphography is also used for lymphedema diagnosis. With lymphography, near-infrared fluorescence imaging allows for real-time imaging of lymph flow. The fluorescent agent (e.g., ICG) is injected into the web spaces in the hand or foot of the affected extremity. The lymph capillaries take in the dye and then an infrared camera is used to view the fluorescing-agent molecules as they flow through the lymphatic vessels. Normal, healthy lymph flow presents as smooth lines, whereas interrupted flow or blockages present as scattered, bright, constellation-like patterns. In a retrospective cohort study, Quin, Bowen, and Chen (2018) found that 58 patients had positive ICG lymphography results confirming the diagnosis of lymphedema consistently correlating with clinical examination. By contrast, BIS demonstrated a false-negative rate of 36%: 21 of 58 patients had normal BIS readings, but a positive ICG lymphography result. The 21 false-negative results occurred in patients with early-stage disease. The researchers concluded that ICG lymphography was a more accurate tool for diagnosing lymphedema (Quin et al., 2018).

ASSESSMENT

Assessment of the patient with limb enlargement should begin with a history of risk factors for lymphedema, such as surgeries (especially nodal dissections), radiation therapy, trauma, infection, malignancy, obesity, familial history, and travel to areas with endemic filariasis. To determine whether lymphedema is the cause of swelling, knowing the onset of limb enlargement and associated symptoms is important. Symptoms of lymphedema include feelings of heaviness, aching, and fatigue in the affected limb. A history of recurrent infections (e.g., cellulitis) is an important clue to lymphedema. Individuals may report less flexibility in the extremities and difficulty fitting into clothing, hardening of the skin, and paresthesias. Brown, Chu, Cheville, et al. (2013) surveyed long-term cancer survivors and found that 34.5% (37 of 107) reported one or more symptoms of lower leg lymphedema. Symptoms these patients reported included difficulty walking (100%), aching (86%), puffiness (76%), and pain (73%) (Brown et al., 2013).

Knowing if the patient has a history of comorbid conditions that can cause swelling of the extremities, such as cardiac disease, venous ulcer disease, renal disease, hepatic disease, trauma, and infection, also is important. Patients with rheumatoid arthritis, obesity, lipedema, and venous ulcer disease are at greater risk for lymphedema because these conditions further stress the already impaired lymphatics. Lymph nodes are located around most joints, so patients undergoing surgical procedures such as total knee replacements may be at greater risk for developing lymphedema because these nodes may become damaged during the surgery. Some relatively minor conditions, such as vein stripping may exacerbate mild lymphedema (Tiwari, Corridi, & Lamp, 2012). Yellow nail syndrome is an uncommon disorder that may be seen with lymphedema. The pathophysiology of the syndrome remains unclear, but lymphatic abnormalities, as well as chronic pulmonary disease and genetic predisposition, may play a role (Maldonada, Tazelaar, Wang, et al., 2008).

Physical Assessment

Physical assessment parameters for lymphedema include skin texture (soft vs hard), papillomatosis (cobblestone skin appearance), skin color (erythema, unusually dark), lymphangiomas (blisters containing lymph fluid), presence of skin fissures, presence of skin folds, presence of pedal pulses, edema, range of motion of the limb, neurologic deficits, and signs of venous ulcer disease. Mushroom-like papules may be present. In normal persons, leg circumference varies as the leg is measured from ankle to knee. However, in lymphedema patients, the circumference from ankle to knee is almost the same. The Stemmer sign (or Kaposi–Stemmer sign) is another clinical indication of lymphedema. In this test, the examiner is unable to pinch a fold of skin at the base of the second toe on the dorsal aspect of the foot or between the second and third finger. Skin

that does not fold up into a pinch is considered a positive sign of lymphedema (Goss & Greene, 2019). Goss and Greene (2019) conducted a study to determine the sensitivity and specificity of the Stemmer sign for lymphedema by comparing it with lymphoscintigraphy in 110 patients with a positive Stemmer sign ($n = 87$) who exhibited abnormal lymphoscintigraphy ($n = 80$). False-positive Stemmer signs included those with obesity ($n = 6$) or spinal muscle trophy ($n = 1$). The authors concluded that a positive Stemmer sign is a sensitive predictor for primary and secondary lymphedema (Goss & Greene, 2019). Physical examination and history usually are sufficient to make a diagnosis of lymphedema. Lymphedema is evaluated by visual inspection and palpation. Initially there will be soft, painless pitting edema, but over time fibrosis, nonpitting edema, and induration may be present in the affected limb. The characteristic lymphatic swelling in the lower extremity is edema from the ankle up toward the knee. Occasionally swelling includes the feet. Depending on the extent of the disease, the edema may extend into the groin. The skin has a roughened leathery appearance resembling an elephant's skin. Because of this appearance, the name *elephantiasis* was coined for the lymphedema caused by the filarial infection. The skin over the lymphedema does not usually have the darkened brown pigment skin changes seen with venous ulcer disease unless the patient has venous ulcer disease. Patients with lymphedema and venous ulcer disease may have a leathery appearance of the skin with dark-brown hemosiderin-pigmented skin changes.

Measuring Limb Size

Circumferential (>2 cm) and/or volume (>200 mL) differences between the affected and nonaffected extremity may be performed to diagnose lymphedema but can also be used to monitor effectiveness of therapies (Whitnell, 2020). Volume may be measured by tape, water displacement or perometry (Greene & Goss, 2018). Tape measurements are the least accurate but easiest method to determine extremity volume. It is difficult to use the exact reference points for future assessments and depending on how tight the clinician pulls the tape measure; the circumference can change significantly. It is important to measure the limb in the same position each time and try to measure the limb at the same time of day because girth may increase during the day because of swelling. Girth measurements should include 3 cm above the lateral malleolus, 12 cm above the lateral malleolus, and 18 cm above the lateral malleolus. Tape measurements are recommended to be performed by the same person at specific intervals. In children, extremity measurements may be inaccurate because the extremities are still growing.

Water displacement is an accurate method which is considered the gold standard for volume assessment on the extremities. For this method, a container is filled with tepid water and the limb is immersed in the water. The amount of overflow is measured to determine the volume of fluid displaced. Both limbs are assessed, and results are compared. A volume difference of 20% or more is considered significant.

Even though this method may be more precise than tape measurements, it is not user friendly and cannot be used if there is an open wound (Greene & Goss, 2018). Perometry is a computer-based study that calculates the volume of the affected limb via infrared optical electronic scanner and can demonstrate small changes, but it is expensive and may not be readily available in all settings.

To clinically define the presence of lymphedema, Spillane, Saw, Tucker, et al. (2008) assessed 66 patients who had undergone inguinal or ilioinguinal lymph node dissection for metastatic melanoma. They found that a change in limb volume of 15% or more and an increase of 7% or more in the sum of limb circumferences of the defined points on the limb provided a more standardized definition of lymphedema in those patients (Spillane et al., 2008).

PREVENTION

Prevention of lymphedema in high-risk individuals, especially those undergoing surgery and radiation for cancer, is paramount. The importance of skin integrity in preventing injury and infection cannot be overemphasized (Box 16.1).

BOX 16.1 Teaching Points for the Patient With Lymphedema

- Apply moisturizer to affected limbs daily to prevent dry/cracking skin.
- Protect exposed skin with sunscreen and insect repellent.
- Use care with razors by not shaving on dry skin or areas with skin folds.
- Avoid, if possible, blood draws and injections in affected limb.
- Provide good nail care and do not cut cuticles.
- If scratches in the skin occur, wash with soap and water, apply topical antibiotics, and monitor for signs of infection/cellulitis.
- Maintain ideal body weight since obesity is a known risk factor.
- Avoid prolonged (greater than 15 min) exposure to heat, such as saunas or hot tubs.
- Avoid exposure to extreme cold, which can cause chaffing and rebound swelling.
- Avoid prolonged standing, sitting, or crossing legs.
- Wear gloves when doing activities that may cause skin injury, for example, washing dishes, cleaning, using tools, and gardening.
- Protect lymphedema extremity and foot from all types of trauma.
- Avoid heavy lifting with affected limb (arm); do not carry handbag or other bags on shoulder of affected side.
- Do not restrict fluid or protein intake in attempt to prevent fluid buildup.
- Exercise in moderation wearing compression garment in place.
- Carry lymphedema alert card and wear lymphedema alert bracelet or necklace.

Skin Care

Skin care is important in the prevention of infection, dermatitis, and hyperkeratosis. Lanolin or fragrances can cause sensitization in this population and so should be avoided. Routine use of fragrance-free, lanolin-free emollients to prevent cracking and promote suppleness of the skin is encouraged. Emollients containing lactic acid, urea, ceramides, glycerin, dimethicone, olive fruit oil, or salicylic acid have been recommended to assist in hyperkeratotic skin desquamation. Salicylic acid is also a keratolytic agent that may or may not enhance the penetration of other topical agent's Salicylic acid ointment (6%), along with skin and nail care regimens, may reduce filariasis-related adenolymphangitis (Fife, Farrow, Hebert, et al., 2017). Any break in the skin can be an entry site for bacteria, and the protein-rich lymphedema fluid is a great medium for bacterial proliferation. Foot care with daily cleansing and drying of the toe web spaces will help to prevent fungal infections of the edematous feet.

A common symptom of lymphedema is pruritus. Scratching from pruritus can cause breaks in the skin, which contribute to infection and cellulitis. Pruritus is thought to be caused by factors in the lymphedematous skin that lower the threshold for degranulation of dermal mast cells. With the degranulation of mast cells comes a subsequent release of histamine, which potentiates the itch. McCord and Fore (2007) evaluated nine patients with mild to severe pruritus associated with lymphedema over a 6-month period that were treated with olivamine-based products. The average pruritus evaluation score before treatment with the products was 2, which corresponds to mild to moderate pruritus; after treatment the average score was 0.11, which corresponds to absent pruritus. Additional research is needed to determine which products work best for the management of pruritus associated with lymphedema (McCord & Fore, 2007).

Protect From Injury

Protecting the limb from injury is important to prevent infection. For example, using an electric razor and wearing gloves when gardening or washing dishes are advisable. Many of the interventions for protection are based on common sense to prevent injury to an already compromised limb.

Promote Lymphatic Flow

Placing limbs in gravity-dependent positions for long periods promotes swelling and should be avoided. The patient should avoid constricting garments, weight gain, heavy lifting, extreme heat (e.g., from heating pad or sauna), and rapid altitude changes seen with flying for 2 hours. Exercises that do not make the patient feel fatigued can increase movement of lymph fluid out of the limb and decrease the risk for lymphedema. Wrapping the limb with bandages can promote lymphatic flow and drainage.

MANAGEMENT

Chronic lymphedema has no known cure. Positive clinical outcomes depend on prompt recognition of lymphedema and initiation of treatment to interrupt the cycle of fluid retention, lymphatic obstruction, and soft tissue fibrosis. Effective management of the patient with lymphedema requires a comprehensive lifelong program of exercise, elevation, massage, prevention of infection, skin care, and compression garments and is most effectively carried out in a lymphedema center. Patients and care providers need to understand that conservative therapies are aimed at reducing symptoms and will not cure the underlying lymphatic dysfunction. Ridner, Fu, Wanchai, et al. (2012) conducted a systematic review from 2004 to 2011 on the benefit of specific interventions on lymphedema self-management. The studies on total body exercise, such as aerobics, showed that it may help to stabilize limb volume and may reduce exacerbations in those with lymphedema. Based on expert opinion, complete decongestive physiotherapy (CDT) benefits lymphedema patients. Compression garments and pneumatic compression devices did not have enough evidence to determine whether they would be effective as stand-alone therapy. Aromatherapy was found to be likely ineffective. However, few studies on lymphedema included clinical outcomes, and there were very few RCTs.

The goals of lymphedema management include (1) moving the "trapped" lymph from the interstitial space, (2) eliminating edema, (3) restoring normal limb contours, (4) maintaining the "restored" limb state, and (5) preventing infection. The components of treatment are highlighted in Table 16.4.

Complete Decongestive Therapy

Complete decongestive therapy (CDT) also known as Combined Physical Therapy or Complex Decongestive Physiotherapy is a nonsurgical two-phase treatment course that combines interventions with lifestyle changes and involves four components: manual lymphatic drainage (MLD), compression bandaging, exercise, and skin care (Whitnell, 2020).

CDT is the gold standard for management of moderate to severe lymphedema. Patients should be referred to a lymphedema therapist, who might be an occupational therapist, physical therapist, or nurse practitioner who is specially trained in CDT.

CDT is a specialized massage technique designed to stimulate the lymph vessels, break up subcutaneous fibrous tissue, and redirect lymph fluid to areas where lymph flow is normal. The therapy involves four steps: MLD, compression bandaging, exercises, and skin/nail care. CDT is administered in two phases. MLD is a hands-on technique and differs from standard massage by orienting the lymphedematous fluid to proper functioning lymphatics. In the initial reductive (restorative) phase, MLD involves daily to weekly sessions (3–8 weeks). The lymphedema therapist uses specialized massage techniques to (1) activate the lymphatic channels proximal to the affected limb, (2) mobilize lymph in the proximal tissues, and (3) mobilize lymph in the distal tissues. MLD is accompanied by range-of-motion exercises, short-stretch compression bandages (worn between treatments), and meticulous skin/nail care to prevent skin infections. When the extremity has been reduced in size, a

compression garment is ordered and the ongoing maintenance phase begins, which includes self-lymph drainage, exercise, skin care, and compression garments.

Compression wraps and stockings are an important component of therapy for all patients with lymphedema to prevent the reaccumulation of lymph fluid in the limb. Compression garments must be worn between MLD treatment sessions during the reductive phase and throughout the day and night thereafter. During the first phase of MLD, short-stretch bandages are used in multilayers. These bandages may be difficult to apply for some patients with physical impairments. There are also wraps with nonelastic Velcro straps that can be put on and taken off very easily. These products are especially beneficial for patients who cannot easily bend or have the strength to pull on elastic compression stockings (see Fig. 15.6). Intermittent pneumatic compression pumps (see Fig. 15.7) are another method for decreasing the volume of the affected limb. The pump which may be used in the home, consists of a sleeve with several compartments that are serially inflated to push the fluid out of the extremity from the distal to the proximal portion. After the daily or twice-daily treatments, which last for several hours, the patient should continue with compression through either a garment or bandaging. Reassessment determines frequency and duration of treatments. For example, if the treatments are not effective after 4 weeks of therapy, they should be discontinued.

Pneumatic compression devices are covered in the home setting for the treatment of lymphedema if the patient has undergone a 4-week trial of conservative therapy and the treating practitioner determines that there has been no significant improvement or if significant symptoms remain after the trial. The trial of conservative therapy must include use of an appropriate compression bandage system or compression garment, exercise, and elevation of the limb. The garment may be prefabricated or custom fabricated but must provide adequate graduated compression.

Preston, Seers, and Mortimer (2004) examined randomized controlled clinical trials that tested physical therapy modalities with a follow-up of at least 6 months. Only three studies with a total of 150 patients were included. Because none of the studies examined the same intervention, combining the data was not possible. One crossover study of MLD followed by self-administered massage vs no treatment concluded that improvements seen in both groups were attributed to compression sleeves and that MLD provided no extra benefit. Another trial of hosiery vs no treatment had a high dropout rate, with only 3 of 14 in the treatment group and 1 of 11 in the control group finishing the trial. Clearly more well-controlled clinical trials on the physical therapy modalities used to treat lymphedema are needed.

Lasinski, Thrift, Squire, et al. (2012) reviewed the research literature from 2004 to 2011 that pertains to the individual components of MLD and compression bandaging, as well as CDT. Ninety-nine articles related to lymphedema treatment were reviewed, but only 26 studies met inclusion criteria. CDT was found to be effective in reducing lymphedema, but the majority of the studies focused on CDT as a bundled intervention that included the two individual components, manual lymphatic drainage and compression bandaging. Additional studies are needed to determine the value and efficacy of the individual components of CDT.

Adjunctive Therapy

Forte, Boczar, Huayllani, Lu, and McLaughlin (2019) conducted a systematic review of publications assessing the potential use of pharmacotherapy agents in lymphedema treatment. They found studies that showed promising results for the oral administration of ketoprofen and selenium. Rockson et al. (2018) enrolled 21 patients with lymphedema in the open-label trial, from November 2010 to July 2011. Histopathology and skin thickness were significantly improved at 4 months compared with baseline. In the follow-up, double-blind, placebo-controlled trial, 34 patients were enrolled from August 2011 to October 2015: 16 patients received antiinflammatory drug ketoprofen and 18 received placebo. Patients taking ketoprofen demonstrated reduced skin thickness, as well as improved composite measures of histopathology and decreased plasma granulocyte CSF expression.

Selenium therapy for lymphedema is also currently being studied. The hypothesis is that lymphedema is caused by excessive generation of oxygen free radicals and that selenium, an antioxidant, consumes oxygen radicals, which might decrease the damage to the lymph system. Dennert and Horneber (2006) in a Cochrane systematic review on the effectiveness of selenium in the management for infective/inflammatory episodes in lymphedema patients reported that the effectiveness of selenium remains inconclusive in the absence of properly conducted RCTs.

Kinesio taping (KT) has become an alternative treatment for lymphedema volume reduction. Kinesio tape is a thin elastic tape invented by Kenzo Kase in 1996. The tape can be stretched up to 140% of its original length, making it very elastic (Fu et al., 2008). The wrapping technique with the Kinesio tape is thought to reduce swelling by improving blood and lymphatic fluid flow and is being used with lymphedema patients.

Kasawara, Mapa, Ferreira, et al. (2018) conducted a systematic review on KT effects on lymphedema related to breast cancer. They found seven studies which showed positive effects in reducing lymphedema (perimeter or volume) before vs after treatment. However, there were no studies that compared KT vs control group or others treatments. Pajero Otero et al. (2019) assessed the effectiveness of using Kinesio taping vs compression garments in 30 women with breast cancer-related lymphedema undergoing maintenance phase of complex decongestive therapy. The decrease in the RelativeVolume Change was greater in the Kinesio taping intervention (-5.7%, SD $= 2.0$) compared with that using compression garments (-3.4%, SD $= 2.9$) ($P < 0.001$). The range of motion of five upper-limb movements increased after applying taping (between 5.8 and 16.7 degrees)

($P < 0.05$), but not after compression ($P > 0.05$). Taping was perceived as more comfortable by patients and further reduced lymphedema-related symptoms compared with compression (between 0.96 and 1.40 points better in four questions with a six-point scale ($P < 0.05$)).

Surgery

The goals of surgery in the lymphedema patient are to alleviate pain, restore function, reduce swelling, and limit deformity. Procedures used for patients with early-stage lymphedema include lymphatic bypass procedures, flap transposition procedures, and vascularized lymph node transfers (VLNTs). The lymphatic bypass procedures are the most commonly used where the lymphatic vessels distal to the lymphatic obstruction are anastomosed to healthy lymphatic vessels or veins proximal to the obstruction. Procedures recommended for patients with more advanced lymphedema include direct excision and liposuction. Appropriate surgery can help reduce the size of an affected arm or leg, decrease the need for compression garments, and reduce the occurrences of infections or cellulitis.

Debulking or excisional surgical techniques involve the removal of lymphedematous adipose tissue down to the fascia, followed by skin grafting or skin flaps (Cormier et al., 2012). Resection or debulking procedures remove redundant skin folds and subcutaneous tissue to reduce the size and weight of the limb, resulting in good clinical outcomes with minimal complications (Tiwari et al., 2012). Salgado, Mardini, Spanio, et al. (2007) reported a 21% volume reduction in the upper extremity at 1 year postoperatively. Complications that have been reported include hematoma formation, skin/flap necrosis, infection, scarring, destruction of remaining lymphatic vessels, loss of limb function, and recurrence of the lymphedema (Cormier et al., 2012).

Microsurgical procedures for lymphatic reconstruction have included anastomosis between lymphatic channels and veins, between lymph nodes and veins, and between distal and proximal lymphatics. Lymphovenous bypass procedure such as the lymphatic-venous anatomosis (LVA) is a super-microsurgical procedure during which a surgeon makes direct connections subdermally between lymphatic vessels and nearby venules of less than 0.8 mm in diameter that are proximal to the obstruction and shunt the lymphatic fluid from the limb into the venous system. With the guidance of ICG lymphography, the surgeon can perform the anastomosis through a skin incision approximately 1 cm in size (Whitnell, 2020). It is believed that the subdermal lymphatics are less affected by lymphedema and the small venular pressure is low, decreasing the risk of backflow. The LVA procedures require less time than the debulking procedures since they require minimal dissections and can be performed under local anesthesia, shortening hospitalization times. At discharge, the patient is instructed not to use CDT (e.g., compression, massage therapy, exercise) nor fly on an airplane for 4 weeks to avoid injury to the bypasses (Whitnell, 2020). VLNTs involve the microsurgical transfer of lymph node containing tissue to a lymphedematous extremity with end-to-end anastomosis between the transplanted lymph tissue and the lymphedematous lymph node tissue.

Suction-assisted lipectomy, which is the removal of subcutaneous fatty tissue through circumferential liposuction of the affected limb, is less invasive and has been proven effective for volume reduction and increasing blood flow to the limb, decreasing the risk of cellulitis. The most common side effect of the liposuction is transient numbness (Tiwari et al., 2012). Patients undergoing all of these procedures are placed immediately postoperatively in compression garments (Warren, Brorson, Borud, et al., 2007).

Lamprou, Voesten, Damstra, and Wikkeling (2017) conducted a descriptive study of patients treated with circumferential suction-assisted lipectomy for unilateral chronic irreversible lymphedema of the leg. Compression therapy was resumed after surgery. Leg volumes were measured before surgery, and at 1, 6, 12, and 24 months after the procedure. A total of 47 patients with primary lymphedema had a median preoperative volume difference between affected and unaffected legs of 3686 (i.q.r. 2851–5121) mL. Two years after surgery, this volume difference was reduced to 761 mL, a 79% reduction. In the 41 patients treated for secondary lymphedema, the median preoperative volume difference was 3320 (i.q.r. 2533–4783) mL, decreasing after 2 years to −38 mL (101% reduction). The preoperative volume difference and the sex of the patient significantly influenced the final outcome after 2 years. The outcome was not related to BMI or other patient characteristics.

Salgado et al. (2007) reviewed 15 patients with lymphedema who had not responded to conventional therapy and were treated by surgical reduction of lymphedema tissue with preservation of perforating skin vessels from posterior tibial and peroneal arteries. This procedure allowed for reduction of lymphedema tissue in a single procedure while preserving blood supply to the skin. In these 15 patients, the average lymphedema reduction was 52%. At follow-up of 13 months, no cases of skin flap necrosis or incisional wound breakdown were seen. Three patients had cellulitis, and one patient had a seroma and hematoma (Salgado et al., 2007).

Campisi and Boccardo (2004) reviewed 676 patients with lymphedema treated with microsurgical LVAs. They found that of the 447 patients who were available for follow-up, 380 (85%) had been able to discontinue conservative methods for managing the disease, with an average reduction in limb volume of 69%. An 87% reduction in cellulitis after the microsurgery also was noted (Campisi & Boccardo, 2004). Koshima, Nanba, Tsutsui, et al. (2004) studied the effectiveness of LVAs for lower leg lymphedema in patients under local anesthesia and reported that 17 patients had a greater than 4 cm reduction in leg circumference.

Pharmacology

Few pharmacologic therapies have been found to be effective in the treatment of lymphedema. Case reports have suggested retinoid like agents (e.g., acitretin and topical tazarotene), topical skin products (e.g., ammonium lactate lotion and topical urea), and antibiotics (e.g., cefazolin, clindamycin, and penicillin) (Rockson, 2008). Diuretics are not beneficial for lymphedema because they may promote volume depletion. Diuretics draw off excess water, but not protein, from the interstitial spaces. As soon as the diuretic is stopped, the concentrated proteins pull more water back into the interstitial space, increasing the edema. Diuretics act to remove water from the cells. Lymphedema is a high-protein edema, and the high osmotic pressure from the increased protein in the interstitial space causes rapid reaccumulation of edema. In addition, the higher concentration of protein in the edema fluid causes increased fibrosis and induration of the skin. Diuretics are not contraindicated for treatment of other conditions in lymphedema patients, but they should not be used as primary treatment of lymphedema.

COMPLICATIONS

Common skin complications seen with lymphedema include lymphangitis and cellulitis. Lymphangitis has a distinctive erythematous linear pattern (red streak) that travels along the lymphatics. Fever, chills, headache, muscle aches, and loss of appetite are common presenting symptoms. Lymphangitis often results from a streptococcal or staphylococcal infection of the skin, which causes the lymph vessels to become swollen and tender. Antibiotics, analgesics, and antiinflammatory drugs may be prescribed, and elevation of the extremity recommended. Patients with recurrent lymphangitis and systemic signs of infection may require long-term, prophylactic, systemic antibiotics to reduce infectious episodes.

Cellulitis involves the subcutaneous tissue. It usually has an indistinct border and is characterized by pain, warmth, and edema, with red appearance of the skin. Fever, chills, headache, muscle aches, and fatigue may be presenting symptoms. Cellulitis occurs in approximately 50% of patients with lymphedema and usually occurs when a crack or fissure in the skin serves as the portal entry for bacteria. The most common pathogen is β-hemolytic streptococcus. Penicillin is the antibiotic of choice because streptococcus is believed to be the most common infecting organism. Antibiotics should be used at the first sign of cellulitis. In patients with recurrent cellulitis of the leg, penicillin has been shown to be effective in preventing subsequent attacks during prophylaxis, but the protective effect diminishes once drug therapy is stopped (Thomas et al., 2013).

Macdonald, Sims, Mayrovitz, et al. (2003) reported that compression bandaging is indicated for treatment of cellulitis. However, other sources do not recommend compression bandaging until the patient is afebrile and erythema is resolving (Feldman, 2005). Fungal infections with itching and burning between the toes increase the risk for cellulitis in the lower extremity (Feldman, 2005). Meticulous skin care, including washing with soap and water and applying emollients to dry skin areas, decreases the risk of cellulitis.

CLINICAL CONSULT

A: Referral from primary provider for wound management recommendations. 55-Year-old Caucasian male with leg edema, morbid obesity, type 2 diabetes (HbA1c pending), and coronary artery disease. Unemployed; spends most of his day at home computer with legs dependent. Complains of heavy achy legs. Right posterior calf wound 14 cm × 3 cm × 0.25 cm originated from bumping a chair 1 year ago. Wound base red with large amounts of serosanguinous exudate. No local signs of infection. Legs have leathery appearance with hemosiderin-pigmented skin changes and multiple mushroom papules. Edema nonpitting. Leg circumference measurements almost the same from ankle to knee (see flow sheet). Stemmer sign positive. Primary provider has also consulted a dietician and endocrinologist.

D: History, edema pattern, and positive Stemmer sign indicative of venous insufficiency and lymphedema.

P: Promote lymphatic flow, protect legs from additional injury, weight loss, and local wound care to promote healing and prevent infection.

I: (1) Referral to lymphedema clinic. (2) Educate on skin injury prevention strategies. Discuss the need for life style modifications such as weight loss, exercise, and diabetes management. (3) Calcium alginate followed by foam dressing changes every other day to manage moisture.

E: Wife demonstrates ability to change dressing and able to verbalize signs of infection. Patient states he is motivated to improve his health but is overwhelmed by all of the new information. No plans to return to wound clinic as lymphedema clinic will also help manage local wound care.

BOX 16.2 Lymphedema Resources

Circle of Hope Lymphedema Foundation	http://www.lymphedemacircleofhope.org accessed September 26, 2022
Lymphology Association of North America	http://www.clt-lana.org accessed September 26, 2022
Lymphatic Education and Research Network	http://lymphaticnetwork.org/ accessed September 26, 2022
Lymphedema Treatment Act (LTA)—Federal bill that aims to improve insurance coverage for the medically necessary compression supplies	http://lymphedematreatmentact.org/ accessed September 26, 2022
National Lymphedema Network	https://lymphnet.org/ accessed September 26, 2022
Lymphedema People	http://www.lymphedemapeople.com/ accessed September 26, 2022
Lymphedema Treatment Act	http://lymphedematreatmentact.org/ accessed September 26, 2022
Lymphedema Lifeline	https://lymphedemalifeline.org/ accessed September 26, 2022

SUMMARY

- Lymphedema is a chronic disease.
- Treatment focuses on managing the symptoms, mainly the high-protein edema and its effects on the limb.
- Lymphedema management crosses all care settings.
- The numbers of lymphedema patients, especially among the obese and the elderly, are increasing.
- Management of the disease relies on patients and caregivers assuming lymphedema care practices in the home

setting. Most care providers are not familiar with the specialized care required for patients with lymphedema, and local resources may be unavailable (Box 16.2).

- Health care providers need to become more knowledgeable about lymphedema practices because many lymphedema patients have comorbid conditions that necessitate their admission to acute and long-term care.

SELF-ASSESSMENT QUESTIONS

1. Lipedema occurs:
   a. in both sexes equally
   b. in the feet and the legs
   c. in both legs
   d. often in conjunction with cellulitis
2. Which of the following is the gold standard for diagnosing lymphedema?
   a. Isotopic lymphoscintigraphy
   b. Magnetic resonance imaging
   c. Computed tomographic scan
   d. Lymphangiogram
3. Comorbid conditions associated with lymphedema may include which of the following?
   a. Venous ulcer disease
   b. Obesity
   c. Hepatic disease
   d. All of the above

REFERENCES

Brown, J. C., Chu, C. S., Cheville, A. L., et al. (2013). The prevalence of lymphedema symptoms among survivors of long-term cancer with or at risk for lower leg lymphedema. *American Journal of Physical Medicine & Rehabilitation, 92,* 223–231.

Buck, D. W., 2nd, & Herbst, K. L. (2016). Lipedema: A relatively common disease with extremely common misconceptions. *Plastic and Reconstructive Surgery. Global Open, 4*(9), e1043. https://doi.org/10.1097/GOX.0000000000001043.

Campisi, C., & Boccardo, F. (2004). Microsurgical techniques for lymphedema treatment: Lymphatic-venous microsurgery. *World Journal of Surgery, 28*(6), 609–613.

Canning, C., & Bartholomew, J. R. (2018). Lipedema. *Vascular Medicine, 23*(1), 88–90. https://doi.org/10.1177/1358863X17739698.

Cormier, J. N., Rourke, L., Crosby, M., et al. (2012). The surgical treatment of lymphedema: A systematic review of the contemporary literature (2004-2010). *Annals of Surgical Oncology, 19*(20), 624–651.

Dennert, G., & Horneber, M. (2006). Selenium for alleviating the side effects of chemotherapy, radiotherapy and surgery in cancer patients. *Cochrane Database of Systematic Reviews,* (3), CD005037. https://doi.org/10.1002/14651858.CD005037.pub2.

DiSipio, T., Rye, S., Newman, B., & Hayes, S. (2013). Incidence of unilateral arm lymphoedema after breast cancer: A systemic review and meta-analysis. *The Lancet Oncology, 14*(6), 500–515.

Feldman, J. L. (2005). The challenge of infection in lymphedema. *Lymph Link, 17*(4), 1.

Fife, C. E., & Carter, M. J. (2008). Lymphedema in the morbidly obese patient: Unique challenges in a unique population. *Ostomy/Wound Management, 54*(1), 44–56.

Fife, C. E., Farrow, W., Hebert, A. A., et al. (2017). Skin and wound care in lymphedema patients: A taxonomy, primer, and literature review. *Advances in Skin & Wound Care, 30*(7), 305–318. https://doi.org/10.1097/01. ASW. 0000520501.23702.82.

Fife, C. E., Maus, E. A., & Carter, M. J. (2010). Lipedema: A frequently misdiagnosed and misunderstood fatty deposition syndrome. *Advances in Skin & Wound Care, 23*(2), 81–92.

Fonder, M. A., Loveless, J. W., & Lazarus, G. S. (2007). Lipedema, a frequently unrecognized problem. *Journal of the American Academy of Dermatology, 57*(2), 51–53.

Forte, A. J., Boczar, D., Huayllani, M. T., Lu, X., & McLaughlin, S. A. (2019). Pharmacotherapy agents in lymphedema treatment: A systematic review. *Cureus, 11*(12), e6300. https://doi.org/10.7759/cureus.6300.

Fu, T. C., et al. (2008). Effect of kinesio taping on muscle strength in athletes—A pilot study. *Journal of Science and Medicine in Sport, 11*(2), 198–201.

Goss, J. A., & Greene, A. K. (2019). Sensitivity and specificity of the Stemmer sign for lymphedema: A clinical lymphoscintigraphic study. *Plastic and Reconstructive Surgery. Global Open, 7*(6), e2295.

Grada, A. A., & Phillips, T. J. (2017a). Lymphedema: Pathophysiology and clinical manifestations. *Journal of the American Academy of Dermatology, 77*(6), 1009–1020.

Grada, A. A., & Phillips, T. J. (2017b). Lymphedema: Diagnostic workup and management. *Journal of the American Academy of Dermatology, 77*(6), 995–1006.

Greene, A. K., & Goss, J. A. (2018). Diagnosis and staging of lymphedema. *Seminars in Plastic Surgery, 32*(1), 12–16.

Greene, A. K., Grant, F. D., & Slavin, S. A. (2012). Lower-extremity lymphedema and elevated body-mass index. *The New England Journal of Medicine, 366,* 2136–2137.

Kasawara, K. T., Mapa, J. M. R., Ferreira, V., et al. (2018). Effects of Kinesio Taping on breast cancer-related lymphedema: A meta-analysis in clinical trials. *Physiotherapy Theory and Practice, 34*(5), 337–345. https://doi.org/10.1080/09593985.2017.1419522.

Koshima, I., Nanba, Y., Tsutsui, T., et al. (2004). Minimal invasive lymphaticovenular anastomosis under local anesthesia for leg lymphedema: Is it effective for stage III or IV? *Annals of Plastic Surgery, 53*(3), 261–266.

Lamprou, D. A., Voesten, H. G., Damstra, R. J., & Wikkeling, O. R. (2017). Circumferential suction-assisted lipectomy in the treatment of primary and secondary end-stage lymphoedema of the leg. *The British Journal of Surgery, 104*(1), 84–89. https://doi.org/10.1002/bjs.10325.

Lasinski, B. B., Thrift, K. M., Squire, D., et al. (2012). A systematic review of the evidence for complete decongestive therapy in the treatment of lymphedema from 2004 to 2011. *PM & R: The Journal of Injury, Function, and Rehabilitation, 4*(8), 580–601.

Lawenda, B. D., Mondry, T. E., & Johnstone, P. A. (2009). Lymphedema: A primer on the identification and management of a chronic condition in oncologic treatment. *CA: A Cancer Journal for Clinicians, 59*(1), 8–24.

Li, C. Y., Kataru, R. P., & Mehrara, B. J. (2020). Histopathologic features of lymphedema: A molecular review. *International Journal of Molecular Sciences, 21*(7), 2546.

Macdonald, J. M., Sims, N., Mayrovitz, H. N., et al. (2003). Lymphedema, lipedema, and the open wound the role of compression therapy. *The Surgical Clinics of North America, 83*(3), 639–658.

Maldonada, F., Tazelaar, H. D., Wang, C. W., et al. (2008). Yellow nail syndrome: Analysis of 41 consecutive patients. *Chest*, *134*(2), 375–381.

McCord, D., & Fore, J. (2007). Using olivamine-containing products to reduce pruritic symptoms associated with localized lymphedema. *Advances in Skin & Wound Care*, *20*(8). 441–442, 444.

Mehrara, B. (2019). Clinical Features of and diagnosis of peripheral lymphedema. UpToDate. Retrieved August 9, 2020 from: https://www.uptodate.com/contents/clinical-features-and-diagnosis-of-peripheral-lymphede-ma?search=lymphedema&source=search_result&selectedTitle=1~150&usage_type=default&display_rank=1.

National Cancer Institute: Division of Cancer Control & Population Sciences. Office of Cancer Survivorship (2019) Accessed February 25, 2020 from https://cancercontrol.cancer.gov/ocs/.

Pajero Otero, V., García Delgado, E., Martín Cortijo, C., Romay Barrero, H. M., de Carlos Iriarte, E., & Avendaño-Coy, J. (2019). Kinesio taping versus compression garments for treating breast cancer-related lymphedema: A randomized, cross-over, controlled trial. *Clinical Rehabilitation*, *33*(12), 1887–1897. https://doi.org/10.1177/0269215519874107.

Preston, N. J., Seers, K., & Mortimer, P. S. (2004). Physical therapies for reducing and controlling lymphoedema of the limbs. *Cochrane Database of Systematic Reviews*, (4), CD003141. https://doi.org/10.1002/14651858.CD003141.pub2.

Quin, E. S., Bowen, M. J., & Chen, W. F. (2018). Diagnostic accuracy of bioimpedance spectroscopy in patients with lymphedema: A retrospective cohort analysis. *Journal of Plastic, Reconstructive & Aesthetic Surgery*, *71*(7), 1041–1050.

Rezaie, T., Ghoroghchian, R., Bell, R., Brice, G., Hasan, A., Burnand, K., et al. (2008). Primary non-syndromic lymphoedema (Meige disease) is not caused by mutations in FOXC2. *European Journal of Human Genetics*, *16*(3), 300–304.

Ridner, S. H., Dietrich, M. S., Cowher, M. S., et al. (2019). A randomized trial evaluating bioimpedance spectroscopy versus tape measurement for the prevention of lymphedema following treatment for breast cancer: Interim analysis. *Annals of Surgical Oncology*, *26*, 3250–3259.

Ridner, S. H., Fu, M. R., Wanchai, A., et al. (2012). Self-management of lymphedema: A systematic review of the literature from 2004-2011. *Nursing Research*, *61*(4), 291–299.

Rockson, S. G. (2008). Diagnosis and management of lymphatic vascular disease. *Journal of the American College of Cardiology*, *52*, 799.

Rockson, S. G., Tian, W., Jiang, X., Kuznetsova, T., Haddad, F., Zampell, J., et al. (2018). Pilot studies demonstrate the potential benefits of antiinflammatory therapy in human lymphedema. *JCI Insight*, *3*(20), e123775.

Salgado, C. J., Mardini, S., Spanio, S., et al. (2007). Radical reduction of lymphedema with preservation of perforators. *Annals of Plastic Surgery*, *59*(2), 173–179.

Spillane, A. J., Saw, R. P., Tucker, M., et al. (2008). Defining lower limb lymphedema after inguinal or ilio-inguinal dissection in patients with melanoma using classification and regression tree analysis. *Annals of Surgery*, *248*(2), 286–293.

Suami, H., & Scaglioni, M. F. (2018). Anatomy of the lymphatic system and the lymphosome concept with reference to lymphedema. *Seminars in Plastic Surgery*, *32*(1), 5–11. https://doi.org/10.1055/s-0038-1635118.

Thomas, K. S., Crook, A. M., Nunn, A. J., Foster, K. A., Mason, J. M., Chalmers, J. R., et al. (2013). Penicillin to prevent recurrent leg cellulitis. *The New England Journal of Medicine*, *368*(18), 1695–1703.

Tiwari, P., Corridi, M., & Lamp, S. (2012). Lymphedema strategies for investigation and treatment. *Plastic Surgical Nursing*, *32*(4), 173–177.

Wagner, S. (2011). Lymphedema and lipedema—An overview of conservative treatment. *VASA*, *40*, 271–279.

Warren, A. G., Brorson, H., Borud, L. J., et al. (2007). Lymphedema: A comprehensive review. *Annals of Plastic Surgery*, *59*(4), 464–472.

Warren, A. G., Janz, B. A., Borud, L. J., et al. (2007). Evaluation and management of the fat leg syndrome. *Plastic and Reconstructive Surgery*, *119*(1), 9e–15e.

Whitnell, L. A. (2020). Lymphedema and lymphovenous bypass: Perioperative nursing implications. *AORN Journal*, *111*(2), 187–198. https://doi.org/10.1002/aorn.12924.

World Health Organization. (2020). *Lymphatic filariasis*. Retrieved 8/11/2020 from: https://www.who.int/news-room/fact-sheets/detail/lymphatic-filariasis.

Wound, Ostomy, and Continence Nurses Society. (2019). Guideline for the management of wounds in patients with lower-extremity venous disease. Mt. Laurel, NJ: Author.

FURTHER READING

Cheville, A. L. (2007). Current and future trends in lymphedema management: Implications for women's health. *Physical Medicine and Rehabilitation Clinics of North America*, *18*(3), 539–553.

NLN Medical Advisory Committee. (2011). *Topic: The diagnosis and treatment of lymphedema. Position statement of the National Lymphedema Network* (pp. 1–19). https://lipedemaproject.org/pposition-statement-of-the-national-lymphedema-networkp-ptopic/. Accessed February 25, 2020.

17

Neuropathic Wounds: The Diabetic Wound

Nanjin J. Park-McRae, Latricia Allen, and Vickie R. Driver

OBJECTIVES

1. Describe three types of neuropathy that may occur in the patient with diabetes.
2. Identify critical factors to be included in the history and physical examination of the patient with lower extremity neuropathic disease.
3. Describe the correlation of protective sensation with risk for diabetic foot ulcer.
4. Distinguish among the musculoskeletal foot deformities that lead to focal areas of high pressure in the patient with peripheral neuropathy.
5. Identify key components of a patient education program for the patient with lower extremity neuropathic disease.
6. Identify key concepts in effective and appropriate offloading.

Prevention and management of neuropathic foot ulcers requires risk identification, diligent surveillance, collaboration of a multidisciplinary team, adherence to best practices, and patient education. Clinician prevention and treatment choices must be driven by recent best practice guidelines in order to provide the most effective evidence-based therapy. The American Diabetes Association (ADA) recommends not only a multidisciplinary approach for high-risk patients but also long-term preventative visits with a foot specialist (ADA, 2014). The ADA's Standards of Medical Care in Diabetes are recommendations that are in the form of an evidence-based grading system to guide clinical practice (ADA, 2014).

Lower extremity neuropathic disease (LEND) develops as a result of damage to nerve structures. In the case of diabetic foot ulcers, lower extremity metabolic changes and peripheral arterial disease (PAD) exacerbate neuropathy. Diabetic foot ulcers are sometimes referred to as *neurotrophic, trophic, perforating,* or *mal perforans* ulcers. The presence of possible coexisting factors, such as impaired perfusion, susceptibility to infection, neuropathy, biochemical abnormalities, repeated or continual trauma, or a combination of these factors, in the patient with LEND who has diabetes creates a particularly challenging situation for ulcer healing (Frykberg, 2003). This chapter presents the assessment, prevention, and management of the diabetic foot ulcer.

EPIDEMIOLOGY

The prevalence of diabetes in the United States is 10.5% of the population, or 34.2 million people (Centers for Disease Control and Prevention [CDC], 2020), and is increasing.

Of these cases, 7.3 million are undiagnosed (CDC, 2020). The number of people with type 2 diabetes in the United States is steadily increasing. In the 34 years from 1980 to 2014, the prevalence of diagnosed diabetes increased almost 400% from 108 million to 422 million (CDC, 2020). Data from 2020 indicate that 88 million adults age 18 years and older qualify as prediabetic, that is, they have fasting glucose levels that are elevated but still below the threshold for a diagnosis of diabetes (CDC, 2020). The increasing prevalence of diabetes is due to various causes, with the obesity epidemic and an aging population heading the list. Although population-based prevalence data are lacking, statistics indicate that type 2 diabetes is on the rise among Americans 10–19 years old (American Academy of Pediatrics, 2013). An increase in type 2 diabetes is expected, with an estimated 1 of 5 adolescents in the United States meeting criteria of prediabetes during 2005–2016 (NCD Risk Factor Collaboration [NCD-RisC], 2016). These data lay the foundation for future research into the causative factors and lifetime risk of diabetes.

Using the Behavioral Risk Factor Surveillance System (BRFSS), a national survey database, the CDC (2003) estimated a 12.7% prevalence of patients with diabetes who had a history of foot ulcers. In the BRFSS, foot ulcers are defined as "any sores or irritations on the feet that took greater than 4 weeks to heal." Reiber (1995) estimated a slightly higher 15%–20% prevalence of diabetic foot ulcers during the lifetime of a patient with diabetes. Within a given year, the incidence of patients with diabetes who develop foot ulcers ranges from 1.0% to 4.1%, with a potential lifetime risk of 25% (Abbott, Carrington, Ashe, et al., 2002; Muller, De Grauw, Van Gerwen, et al., 2002; Singh, Armstrong, & Lipsky, 2005). More recently, Armstrong, Boulton, and Bus

(2017) estimated an even higher (19%–34%) lifetime prevalence of diabetic foot ulcers. After a diabetic foot ulcer has healed, recurrence is common with approximately a 40%, 60%, and 65% recurrence within 1 year, 3 years, and 5 years, respectively (Armstrong et al., 2017).

Foot ulcers precede lower extremity amputations in 85% of cases (Pemayun, Naibaho, & Minuljo, 2015). The leading nontraumatic cause of lower extremity amputations in the United States is attributed to diabetes. Of all the nontraumatic amputations in the United States, 50%–75% are caused by diabetic foot ulcers (Boulton, Vilekyte, Ragnarson-Tennvall, et al., 2005). The national average annual incidence of patients with diabetes having a lower extremity amputation was approximately 3.3 per 1000 (age-adjusted) for the year 2009 (CDC, 2014).

After decades of steady increase, the percentage of amputations in the diabetic population compared with total amputations appears to be decreasing. Department of Veterans Affairs data show that in 1986, 59% of all amputations were because of diabetes. In 1998, 66% of all amputations were because of diabetes (Mayfield, Reiber, Maynard, et al., 2000). In 1997, the total number of lower extremity amputations for patients with diabetes in the United States peaked at 84,000 (excluding military health care facilities), and the total figure remained above 80,000 annually until 2007 and then dropped to 68,000 in 2009 (CDC, 2014). Presumably, advancements in therapeutic modalities and diagnostics, implementation of multidisciplinary teams, and advanced wound care have supported this downtrend. Although overall lower extremity amputation rates are declining, they continue to rise with patient age (CDC, 2014). The rate of lower extremity amputation for patients with diabetes is 12 times greater than for individuals without diabetes (Fosse, Hartemann-Heurtier, Jacqueminet, et al., 2009). Furthermore, amputation of the contralateral limb within 2–3 years is 50%–84%, although implementation of a multidisciplinary foot care service has been shown to lower contralateral amputation rates to as low as 7% and to lower the odds for a lower extremity amputation in individuals with diabetes compared those without diabetes (Higorani, LaMuraglia, & Henke, 2016). Driver, Madsen, and Goodman (2005) reported an 82% reduction in amputations using a multidisciplinary approach, despite a 48% increase in patients diagnosed with diabetes. Three years after a patient with diabetes has a lower extremity amputation, the mortality rate is 20%–50% (Moulik, Mtonga, & Gill, 2003). Five-year survival rates among patients with diabetes who undergo above-knee and below-knee amputations are reported as low as 28% (Aulivola, Hile, Hamdan, et al., 2004; Corey, St Julien, Miller, et al., 2012).

Economic Burden

The economic burden of diabetes in the United States is enormous and is growing. Direct medical and indirect expenditures due to diabetes in 2017 were estimated to be $404 billion (Dall, Wang, Gillespie, et al., 2019). Lower extremity amputations in patients with diabetes and their consequences represent a significant portion of these costs (not to mention the cost in quality of life). According to Rice, Desai, and Cumming (2014), medical costs to care for a patient with a diabetic foot ulcer was reported to be $11,700 for Medicare patient and $16,883 for private insurance patient annually; a finding that is consistent with 1999 costs of the privately insured patients (Ramsey, Newton, & Blough, 1999). The 20-week healing rate for diabetic foot ulcers has been reported to be only 31% (Margolis, Kantor, Santanna, Strom, & Berlin, 2000) and the annual cost for lower extremity ulcer treatment in patients with diabetes to be $15,300, with 74% of the costs from inpatient charges (Harrington, Zagari, Corea, et al., 2000; Stockl, Vanderplas, & Tafesse, 2004).

The cost of care increases significantly when a diabetic foot ulcer proceeds to amputation. Using 2005 costs, the total event cost ranges from $43,800 for a toe amputation to $66,215 for an above-the-knee amputation (Boulton et al., 2005). An earlier comprehensive study of amputation costs from Sweden that includes all inpatient, outpatient, and home care costs over a 3-year period estimated a cost of $43,100 for a minor amputation and $63,100 for a major amputation (Apelqvist & Larsson, 2000). Shearer, Scuffham, and Gordois (2003) reported that the cost to treat an uninfected foot ulcer was $775 per month, increasing to $2049 per month for an ulcer with cellulitis and $3798 for an ulcer with osteomyelitis. Driver et al. (2005) found that hospitalizations involving patients with osteomyelitis were 2.5 times more expensive than hospitalizations involving patients noninfected diabetic foot ulcers. Economic data support early identification and intervention of diabetic foot ulcers to prevent not only amputations but also the vast increases in costs associated with recurring infections, comorbid disease progression, and hard-to-close wounds (ADA, 2007).

PATHOGENESIS

The origin and development of a diabetic foot ulcer has several components. An in-depth causal pathway study with two patient cohorts from different parts of the world identified 32 unique causal pathways for developing foot ulcers. The study found three components present in the majority (63%) of the identified pathways: peripheral neuropathy, structural foot problems, and minor trauma (Reiber, Vileikyte, & Boyko, 1999). In another study, peripheral neuropathy was the major contributing factor leading to the development of 90% of all foot ulcers (Lavery, 2013). The risk of developing a diabetic foot ulcer is seven times more likely in patients with neuropathy than in their nonneuropathic counterparts (Rathur & Boulton, 2007). Other less prevalent causes were edema, callus, and peripheral ischemia resulting from PAD. Patients with diabetes and PAD have been shown to have more distal disease coupled with poorer mortality and amputation outcomes than patients without diabetes (Lee, Rha, & Han, 2015). Infection is the most common factor that leads to lower extremity amputation and develops in over half of foot ulcers (Uckay, Gariani, & Dubois-Ferriere, 2016).

Neuropathy

Peripheral neuropathy is involved in 78% of diabetic foot ulcers (Reiber et al., 1999). The incidence of neuropathy in patients with diabetes appears to be linked to the duration of diabetes and, to some extent, to glycemic control. Prospective studies comparing patients with standard vs those with tighter control of blood glucose have shown that patients with better glucose control have better nerve conduction velocity and less retinopathy and nephropathy. Lowering hemoglobin A1c values has been shown to decrease the neuropathic and microvascular complications of diabetes (Nathan, Buse, Davidson, et al., 2009). The exact etiology of peripheral neuropathy is unknown. In the past, peripheral neuropathy was likely the result of metabolic events, including accrual of glucose, sorbitol, and fructose; reduction in myoinositol (needed for nerve conduction); and nerve ischemia due to reduction in the number and diameter of vessels in the vasa nervosum (Levin, 2002). Moreover, O'Brien, Hinder, and Sakowski (2014) implicate endoplasmic reticulum (ER) stress as a mechanism of diabetic peripheral neuropathy (DPN) and mouse studies show that an increased level of ER stress can cause abnormal metabolic events, which can play a role in cell injury. However, a study done by Hussain and Adrian (2017) shows that gene expression might be involved in this level of ER stress. Their study looked into the glutamate pathway in patients with neuropathy. Although several theories exist, the exact mechanism has yet to be established. The predominant structural mechanism affected by the various metabolic components may be the microvascular component. Under normal conditions, the arteriole–venule (AV) shunts in the sole of the foot are closed, and blood flows through the nutrient capillaries (capillary dermal papillae loops). With diabetic neuropathy, a decrease in the sympathetic innervation of the highly innervated AV shunts results in a greater dilation in the arterioles, which leads to a shunting away of blood from the capillary dermal papillae loops. This results in lower skin temperature and a decrease in transcutaneous oxygen tension at the skin. Theoretically, the metabolic components may be reversible, but structural component changes (shunting) apparently cannot be undone once changed (Tanenberg & Donofrio, 2008). However, recent advances and several randomized clinical trials in various areas of gene therapy and angiogenesis show promise in changing this long-standing convention and expanding our insight into the disease process (Driver & LeBretton, 2008). A more detailed explanation of the many etiologic pathways that lead to diabetic neuropathy is beyond the scope of this chapter.

Neuropathy can be either focal or diffuse. *Focal neuropathies* can be divided into ischemic and entrapment types. *Focal ischemic neuropathies* are caused by an acute event to the nerves. Examples include cranial and femoral neuropathies. These types of neuropathy are characterized by sudden onset and are asymmetric in distribution. Focal entrapment neuropathies occur when a nerve is compressed in a specific area of the body. These neuropathies tend to be more progressive in development and are also often asymmetrically located. Examples include carpal tunnel syndrome and tarsal tunnel syndrome.

Diffuse neuropathies can be divided into *distal symmetric polyneuropathy*, which includes motor and sensory neuropathies and *autonomic neuropathy* (Tanenberg & Donofrio, 2008). Diffuse neuropathies are caused by abnormal structural, vascular, and metabolic conditions. They have a symmetric distribution and are progressive in nature. Diffuse neuropathies are the type encountered frequently in patients with diabetes.

Neuropathy is a frequent risk factor for diabetic foot ulcers and can include (1) sensory nerves (controlling sensation), (2) motor nerves (controlling musculature), and (3) autonomic nerves (controlling functions, e.g., sweating and oil production, vascular flow, and heart rate) (Volmer-Thole & Lobmann, 2016). Sensory, motor, and autonomic neuropathies represent the most common complications affecting the lower extremities of patients with diabetes (Mulder, Armstrong, & Seaman, 2003; Nathan et al., 2009). Although diabetes is the most common cause of lower extremity neuropathy, other well-defined causes include uremia, acquired immunodeficiency syndrome, nutritional deficiencies, nerve compression, trauma, fractures, prolonged use of crutches, tumors, radiation and cold exposure, certain medicines, systemic lupus erythematosus, and rheumatoid arthritis (National Institute of Neurological Disorders and Stroke [NINDS], National Institutes of Health, 2003).

Sensory and Motor Neuropathy

Sensory and motor neuropathies are grouped under the frequently cited category of "peripheral neuropathy" rather than distal symmetric polyneuropathy. The vast peripheral nervous system connects the nerves running from the brain and spinal cord (the central nervous system) and transmits information to the rest of the body (arms, legs, hands, and feet). This distal and dying-back progression of neuropathy is often referred to as a "stocking and glove" pattern.

In *sensory neuropathy*, the loss of protective sensation leads to a lack of awareness of pain and temperature change, resulting in increased susceptibility to injury. However, the eventual lack of pain awareness is generally preceded by 8–10 years of painful neuropathy. Persons with this condition will have worse pain at night, and relief will come from movement rather than rest (Tanenberg & Donofrio, 2008). Once the painful phase ends, minor trauma caused by poorly fitting shoes or an acute injury can precipitate a chronic ulcer. Patients may not realize they have a foot wound for some time because of lack of sensation in their feet. The loss of pain sensation can reach to the knees.

Motor neuropathy affects the muscles required for normal foot movement and can result in muscle atrophy. The distal motor nerves are the most commonly affected and cause atrophy of the small intrinsic muscles of the foot. Often, wasting of the lumbrical and interosseous muscles of the foot will result in collapse of the arch (Alavi, Sibbald, Mayer, et al., 2014; Sumpio, 2000). Cocked-up or claw toes, hammertoes (Fig. 17.1), and weight redistribution from the toes to the metatarsal heads lead to increased pressures and subsequent ulceration (Alavi et al., 2014). Generally, patients with

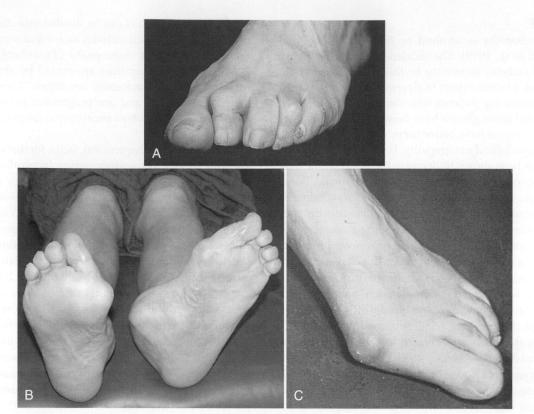

Fig. 17.1 (A) Hammertoes. (B) Charcot foot. (C) Hallux valgus (lateral deviation of hallux) and bunions. (Panel (A, C): From Ball, J. W., Dains, J. E., & Flynn, J. A. (2019). Musculoskeletal system. In: *Seidel's guide to physical examination* (9th ed.). St. Louis, MO: Elsevier. Courtesy Charles W. Bradley, DPM, MPA, and Caroline Harvey, DPM, California College of Podiatric Medicine. Panel (B): From Bowker, J. H., & Pfeifer, M. A. (2001). *Levin and O'Neal's the diabetic foot* (6th ed.). St. Louis, MO: Mosby.)

diabetes develop both kinds of distal symmetric polyneuropathy (Alavi et al., 2014; Sumpio, 2000).

Autonomic Neuropathy

Autonomic neuropathy—a disease of the involuntary nervous system—can affect a wide range of organ systems throughout the body. Diabetic autonomic neuropathy frequently coexists with other peripheral neuropathies and other diabetic complications (Zochodne & Malik, 2014). Autonomic neuropathy

results in decreased sweating and oil production, loss of skin temperature regulation, and abnormal blood flow in the soles of the feet. The resulting xerosis can precipitate fissures, cracks, callus, and finally ulceration (Alavi et al., 2014).

Musculoskeletal Abnormalities

Foot deformities (Table 17.1) are very common in patients with diabetes and peripheral neuropathy and lead to focal areas of high pressure. These deformities are also associated with

TABLE 17.1 Brief Descriptions for Selected Foot Malformations

Malformation	Characteristics
Plantar fasciitis	Heel pain caused by inflammation of long band of connective tissue running from calcaneus to ball of foot
Heel spurs	Bony growths on underside, forepart of calcaneus bone; may lead to plantar fasciitis
Bunions (hallux valgus)	First joint of large metatarsal slants outward, with tip angling toward other toes; may lead to edema, tenderness (see Fig. 17.1C)
Hammer (claw) toes	Toes appear bent into claw-like position, often seen in second metatarsal when bunion slants large metatarsal toward and under it (see Fig. 17.1A)
Neuromas	Enlarged, benign growths of nerves, most commonly between third and fourth toes; caused by bones or other tissue rubbing against and irritating the nerves
Charcot arthropathy	Disruption or disintegration of some foot and ankle joints; frequently associated with diabetes, resulting in erythema, edema, deformity (see Fig. 17.1B)
Pes cavus	High arch or instep
Pes planus	Flat foot

thinning of the fat pad under the metatarsal heads. Diabetic foot ulcers generally result from repetitive stress on "hot spots" that develop from bone deformities or callus buildup (Levin, 2002). The areas at the top of the toes, the tips of the toes, under the metatarsal heads, and the heels are vulnerable to ulceration and infection. Atrophied or dislocated fat pads beneath the metatarsal heads increase the pressure under them. This situation can lead to skin loss or callus development and increases the risk of ulceration (Alavi et al., 2014; Sumpio, 2000). A 28% incidence of ulcers among neuropathic patients with elevated plantar pressures has been observed compared with zero incidence of ulcers among patients with normal plantar pressures (Alavi et al., 2014; Boulton, 2004).

Associated callus can increase foot pressure by as much as 30% (Young, Cavanagh, & Thomas, 1992). Callus presence has been associated with a 77-fold increase in ulceration in one cross-sectional study. Further follow-up data showed that plantar ulcers in neuropathic patients formed only at callus sites, suggesting an infinite risk for ulcer development (Frykberg, Zgonis, Armstrong, et al., 2006; Murray, Young, Hollis, et al., 1996). In the absence of neuropathy, the patient can feel the presence of a fissure, blister, or bony prominence and will take corrective action. However, with neuropathy, the protective response is diminished or even nonexistent. Thus, foot ulcers can get progressively worse before any action is taken. Individuals with diabetic neuropathy have been known to walk around for days in shoes containing shoehorns. Abnormalities in foot biomechanics from the previously described deformities and possible ulceration often cause a dysfunctional gait, which leads to further damage to the structure of the foot.

Ankle Joint Equinus

Ankle joint equinus, defined as less than 0 degrees of ankle joint dorsiflexion, occurs in some patients with peripheral neuropathy. With ankle joint equinus the range of motion of the foot joint becomes limited, which increases pressure on the sole of the foot (Caselli, Pham, Giurini, et al., 2002). Of all patients with diabetes, 10.3% develop ankle joint equinus; this risk increases with duration of disease (Lavery, Armstrong, Boulton, et al., 2002). High plantar pressures from ankle equinus can increase the incidence of ulceration in patients with diabetes (Caselli et al., 2002).

Foot

Charcot foot or Charcot neuroarthropathy (or arthropathy) is a classic and increasingly common diabetic foot deformity affecting nearly 10% of diabetics with neuropathy and greater than 16% of those with a history of neuropathic ulcer (Reiber, 1995). Lavery, Armstrong, Wunderlich, et al. (2003) found the incidence of Charcot arthropathy for non-Hispanic whites with diabetes to be 11.7 per 1000 per year. A long duration of diabetes is an important factor in the development of Charcot neuroarthropathy (CN); greater than 80% of patients with Charcot foot had diabetes for more than 10 years (Cofield, Morrison, & Beabout, 1983; Rajbhandari, Jenkins, & Davies, 2002). The early stage of Charcot is characterized by erythema and edema. This can be similar to the early stage of infection; however, fever and pain can be absent in Charcot foot. Also, laboratory results show normal erythrocyte sedimentation rate (ESR) (Rogers, Frykberg, & Armstrong, 2011).

The precise neural mechanism causing Charcot foot is unknown, and a number of different theories have been proposed to explain the underlying etiology (Frykberg et al., 2006; Gerald & Hudson, 2002). Despite conventional thinking that many lower extremities of diabetics are ischemic, overwhelming evidence indicates that many patients with diabetic neuropathy have increased blood and pooling in their feet. This condition has been directly correlated with decreased bone density in Charcot foot, possibly as a result of autonomic neuropathy. Charcot foot may well be due to a combination of neurotraumatic and neurovascular mechanisms (Frykberg et al., 2006; Gerald & Hudson, 2002).

Progression of Charcot disease is divided into three radiographically different stages: development, coalescence, and reconstruction. *Development* represents the acute, destructive phase characterized by joint effusions, edema, subluxation, formation of bone and cartilage debris, intraarticular fractures, and bone fragmentation. This period is often initiated by minor trauma and is aggravated by persistent ambulation. The second stage, *coalescence*, is marked by a reduction in edema, absorption of fine debris, and healing of fractures. The final phase of bone healing is *reconstruction*, in which further repair and remodeling of bones take place, along with fusion and rounding of large bone fragments and decreased joint mobility. Early diagnosis and treatment (i.e., offloading) in the development stage are critical in the treatment of this disease (Sanders, 2008).

The Charcot foot is prone to increased pressures because of its deformity and possible bone or joint collapse. The patient with Charcot neuroarthropathy is four times more likely to develop a foot ulcer (Gerald & Hudson, 2002; Jeffcoate & Harding, 2003).

Peripheral Arterial Disease

PAD is a major risk factor for lower extremity amputation, particularly in patients who have diabetes, because the accompanying inadequate oxygenation and perfusion of tissues significantly impair wound healing (see discussion of PAD in Chapter 14) (Mulder et al., 2003). Patients with diabetes with PAD are five times more likely to have an amputation than patients without diabetes and PAD between 1992 and 1996 (Jude, Oyibo, Chalmers, et al., 2001). However, according to Lombardo, Maggini, and Anichini (2014), major amputation rate showed declining trend in diabetic patient compared to nondiabetic patient in Italy during 2001–2010, but minor amputation rate was showing inclination in patient with diabetes compared to nondiabetic patient. One of the reasons for declining of major amputation rate is due to quality of care in diabetic foot. A more recent report by Geiss et al. (2019) shows that after a two-decade decline in lower extremity amputations, the United States is experiencing a reversal in the progress.

The increase in diabetes-related NLEA rates between 2009 and 2015 was driven by a 62% increase in the rate of minor amputations (from 2.03 [95% CI 1.83–2.22] to 3.29 [95% CI 3.01–3.57], $P < 0.001$) and a smaller but also statistically significant, 29% increase in major NLEAs (from 1.04 [95% CI 0.94–1.13] to 1.34 [95% CI 1.22–1.45]). The increases in rates of total, major, and minor amputations were most pronounced in young (age 18–44 years) and middle-aged (age 45–64 years) adults and more pronounced in men than women.

The incidence of ischemic diabetic foot ulcers is relatively low. However, because more than half of people with PAD are asymptomatic, determining the true prevalence in patients with diabetes is difficult. Peripheral ischemia was present in 35% of ulcerations in a two-center causal pathway study (Reiber et al., 1999). Oyibo, Jude, and Voyatzoglou (2002) found that 11% of diabetic foot ulcers were ischemic (52.3% neuroischemic and 36% neuropathic). In contrast, a study from England found that only 16% of new diabetic foot ulcers were ischemic (24% neuroischemic). Incongruence in ulcer classification rates could indicate greater awareness spawned by the advent of multidisciplinary teams (Rathur & Boulton, 2007), as well as improvements in classification and stratification of ulcer presentation as diagnostic technology, research, and our understanding of causative factors continue to advance. Ischemic foot ulcers are relatively less common than neuropathic or neuroischemic diabetic foot ulcers. However, they lead to higher rates of amputation in patients with diabetes even in the absence of peripheral neuropathy (Moulik et al., 2003). Amputations of lower extremities in patients with diabetes are almost always due to multiple causes, including ischemia, infection, and neuropathy. Guis, Pellissier, Arniaud, et al. (1999) found that 55% of amputations required within a high-risk foot clinic were due to the combination of ischemia and infection. Their study supported the findings of Prompers, Schaper, and Apelqvist (2008) who showed a negative healing impact of infection among patients with PAD and infection compared with patients with infections and no PAD. Additionally, infection was the only predictor of healing in patients with PAD.

Relatively little is known about the biology of PAD in patients with diabetes; however, it is thought to be similar to other manifestations of atherosclerotic disease, such as coronary artery disease and carotid artery disease. The mortality risk of patients with PAD and diabetes is two times greater than it is for PAD patients without diabetes (Mueller, Hinterreiter, & Luft, 2014). PAD typically results from gradual diameter reduction of the lower extremity arteries and from the progression of atherosclerotic changes in arterial circulation in the lower extremities. Endothelial injury and resulting endothelial dysfunction occur in the earliest stages of the disease. The endothelial surface can be injured by various means, including hyperlipidemia and diabetes (Levy, 2002). The atherosclerotic plaque that develops in the patient with diabetes and PAD is no different from the plaque that develops in the patient without diabetes (Garcia, 2006; Levin, 2002). The pattern of PAD in patients with diabetes is such that medium-size arteries, mainly at the popliteal trifurcation, are affected. However, distal pedal vessels are spared (IWGDF, 2019).

Microvascular tissue perfusion, in contrast to macrocirculation, may present problems for patients with diabetes. Whereas PAD in persons with diabetes normally spares the small pedal arteries, microcirculation abnormalities in the foot as a result of neuropathy are common. Diabetic neuropathy impairs the nerve axon reflex and causes local vasodilation in response to a painful stimulus. The impaired vasodilation in diabetic neuropathic lower extremities can create a functional ischemia.

ASSESSMENT

The components of assessment for any patient with signs or symptoms of LEND include the patient history and risk factors, physical examination, and simple noninvasive tests. Select patients may require more complex studies.

Patient History

The patient history includes general state of health, a record of diabetic complications and treatments, walking difficulties, shoe problems, pain in the extremity, medications (prescribed and over-the-counter), glycosylated hemoglobin level, and risk factors for LEND and diabetic foot ulcers. Because diabetic foot ulcers can occur as a consequence of neuropathy and lower extremity arterial disease (LEAD), specific questions regarding any LEAD risk factors should be posed (see Table 14.1 and Box 14.1).

Risk Factors

A number of studies have quantified the relative significance of various risk factors associated with the presence of foot ulceration. Lavery, Armstrong, Vela, et al. (1998) reported that the relative risk (RR) for foot ulceration in the patient with diabetes increases according to the number and type of risk factor present:

- RR = 1.7 in persons with peripheral neuropathy.
- RR = 12.1 in persons with peripheral neuropathy *and* foot deformity.
- RR = 36.4 in persons with peripheral neuropathy, foot deformity, *and* a history of previous amputation.

In a large multicenter study that lasted 30 months, Pham, Armstrong, and Harvey (2000) analyzed the incidence of new foot ulceration in patients with diabetes and various measurable risk factors. Of the patients enrolled in their study, 29% developed one or more foot ulcers over the 30-month period (a very high incidence). Nearly all (99%) of these patients had a high neuropathy disability score and/or a poor score on the Semmes–Weinstein monofilament examination for sensation. Additional factors that yielded a statistically significant increased odds for foot ulceration during the study include the following:

- gender (male),
- ethnic background (Native American),
- duration of diabetes (long),
- palpable pulses,
- history of foot ulceration,

BOX 17.1   Diabetic Foot Ulcer Risk Factors

- Absence of protective sensation due to peripheral neuropathy
- Vascular insufficiency
- Structural deformities and callus formation
- Autonomic neuropathy causing decreased sweating and dry feet
- Limited joint mobility
- Long duration of diabetes
- Long history of smoking
- Poor glucose control
- Obesity
- Impaired vision
- Past history of ulcer or amputation
- Male gender
- Increased age
- Ethnic background with high incidence of diabetes (e.g., Native American)
- Poor footwear inadequately protecting skin from high pressures

BOX 17.2   Foot Risk Classification by the International Working Group on the Diabetic Foot

Category Ulcer risk Characteristics Frequency*

0: Very low no LoPS and no PAD once a year
1: Low LoPS or PAD once every 6–12 months
2: Moderate LoPS + PAD, or LoPS + foot deformity or once every 3–6 months
   PAD + foot deformity
3: High LoPS or PAD and one or more of the following: Once every 1–3 months
   - history of a foot ulcer
   - a lower extremity amputation (minor or major)
   - end-stage renal disease

International Working Group on the Diabetic Foot (IGWDF) (2019). *Practical guidelines on the prevention and management of diabetic foot disease.* www.iwgdfguidelines.org.
*LoPS, loss of protective sensation; PAD, peripheral arterial disease.

- high vibration threshold score, and
- high foot pressures.

Foot ulcers often have a multifactorial etiology. Although the earlier studies list the most commonly associated risk factors, the clinician must recognize many other risk factors in order to comprehensively assess a patient. Box 17.1 contains a list of the most commonly recognized risk factors for ulceration (Boulton, Rayman, & Wukich, 2020). As with the presence of infection, vascular insufficiency has a much more important role in delaying wound healing and subsequent amputation than as a risk factor contributing to ulceration (Okonkwo & Dipietro, 2017).

Classification of Risk. Many specialized foot treatment clinics use a foot risk classification system for patients with diabetes to allocate resources such as therapeutic shoes, education, and frequency of clinic visits (Frykberg et al., 2006; Peters & Lavery, 2001). The International Working Group on the Diabetic Foot (IWGDF, 2019) recommends the "international" system as listed in Box 17.2. Risk classification systems have been shown to be very effective in predicting future diabetic foot ulcers (Boulton et al., 2020). Additional risk classification systems are provided in Tables 17.2 and 17.3.

More recently, diabetic foot ulcer prevention research is shifting from the investigation of stratified health care interventions focused on classical risk factors such as PAD and neuropathy to personalized interventions focused on diabetic foot ulcer modifiable risk factors (van Netten, Woodburn, & Bus, 2020). Some examples of modifiable risk factor for diabetic foot ulcers are preulcerative lesions, foot deformities, plantar pressures, neuropathy symptoms, and joint range of motion (van Netten, Sacco, et al., 2020). According to van Netten, Sacco, et al. (2020), "modifiable risk factors are foot or person related characteristics that can be changed to reduce someone's risk of ulceration." A recent systematic review reported the following treatments that may improve diabetic foot ulcer modifiable risk factors: callus removal, custom therapeutic footwear, structured education (patient and provider), and foot and mobility-related exercises (Van Netten et al., 2020).

Lower Extremity and Foot Physical Examination

Chapter 13 describes how to conduct a comprehensive lower extremity assessment and should be carefully reviewed. The following section discusses the aspects of the lower extremity examination that are unique to the patient with LEND.

Protective Sensation

Screening for neuropathy can be done rapidly and reliably using a Semmes–Weinstein 5.07 (10-g) monofilament test or a vibration tuning fork test with the on–off method (ADA, 2007; Perkins, Olaleye, & Zinman, 2001). Biothesiometry expands on the traditional tuning fork, allowing for quantification of the vibration threshold (Fig. 17.2A). An electric oscillator is applied to the traditional assessment landmarks (see Fig. 17.2B) and "dialed in" until the patient is able to perceive the vibration (see Fig. 17.2C). The value obtained can be used to follow the progression of neuropathy and qualify future assessment findings. As shown in Fig. 17.3, the monofilament line used for the Semmes–Weinstein test is normally mounted on a rigid paper holder. The line has been standardized to deliver a 10-g force when pushed against an area of the foot. Regardless of which method is used, the patient should be relaxed and placed in a room that is quiet. Boxes 17.3 and 17.4 provide procedures for conducting these examinations.

Pain

A description of neuropathic pain is an important assessment parameter and may be specific to the disease state. In general, neuropathic pain varies in severity and is described as "burning," "tingling," "shooting," or "pins and needles." Activity can alleviate or exacerbate neuropathic pain. Because of the potential for LEAD, the patient should be assessed for ischemic pain (see Table 14.2, Box 14.3). Chapter 28 provides a detailed discussion on the assessment and management of wound-related pain including pharmacological interventions for neuropathic pain (see Table 28.4).

TABLE 17.2 Foot Risk Classification System and Management Considerations

Low-Risk Diabetes	Moderate-Risk Diabetes	High-Risk Diabetes
Classification		
Intact sensation (neurologic)	Intact sensation (neurologic)	Absence of sensation (neurologic)
and/or	and/or	and/or
Intact pulses (vascular)	Intact pulses (vascular)	Absence of pulses (vascular)
Absence of foot deformities	Presence of foot deformities	Presence or absence of foot deformities
Management		
Education emphasizing disease control, proper shoe fit/design, daily self-inspection, early reporting of foot injuries or breaks in skin	Education emphasizing disease control, proper shoe fit/design, daily self-inspection, early reporting of foot injuries or breaks in skin	Education emphasizing disease control, proper shoe fit/design, daily self-inspection, early reporting of foot injuries or breaks in skin
Proper fitting/design footwear with orthotics as needed	Proper fitting/design footwear with orthotics as needed; depth-inlay footwear, molded/modified orthosis may be required	May require modified or custom footwear
Annual follow-up for foot screening	Routine follow-up every 6 months for foot examination	Routine follow-up every 1–12 weeks for foot ulcer evaluation and callus/nail care
Follow as needed for skin/callus/nail care or orthosis	Referral to foot and ankle care specialist if deformity is causing pressure point and conservative measures fail	Referral to foot and ankle care specialist

Data from Driver, V. R., Madsen, J., & Goodman, R. A. (2005). Reducing amputation rates in patients with diabetes at a military medical center: The limb preservation service model. *Diabetes Care, 28*(2), 248–253.

TABLE 17.3 Lower Extremity Amputation Prevention (LEAP) Risk and Management Categories for the Foot

Risk Categories	Definition	Management Categories
0	Diabetes, but no loss of protective sensation in feet	Education emphasizing disease control, and daily foot inspection Foot and nail care as needed Follow-up annually for foot/shoe examination
1	Diabetes, loss of protective sensation in feet	Education emphasizing disease control, fit/design, daily inspection, skin/nail care, early reporting of foot injuries Properly fitting/design footwear with soft molded insoles Routine follow-up every 6 months for foot/shoe examination and nail care
2	Diabetes, loss of protective sensation in feet with high pressure (callout/deformity), or poor circulation	Education emphasizing disease control, daily inspection, skin/nail care, early reporting of foot injuries Proper footwear with possible modifications, custom molded insoles fitted into footwear Routine follow-up every 3 months with a foot specialist for foot/activity/footwear evaluation and callus/nail care
3	Diabetes, history of plantar ulceration or neuropathic fracture	Education emphasizing disease control, daily inspection, skin/nail/callus care, early reporting of foot injuries Extra depth footwear with custom modification, custom molded insoles with modifications to relieve pressure, offload with cast as necessary Routine follow-up every month with a foot specialist for foot/activity/footwear evaluation and callus/nail care

Note: "Loss of protective sensation" is assessed using a 5.07 monofilament at 10 locations on each foot.
Data compiled from International Diabetes Federation. (2022). Clinical practice recommendation on the diabetic foot: A guide for health care professionals.

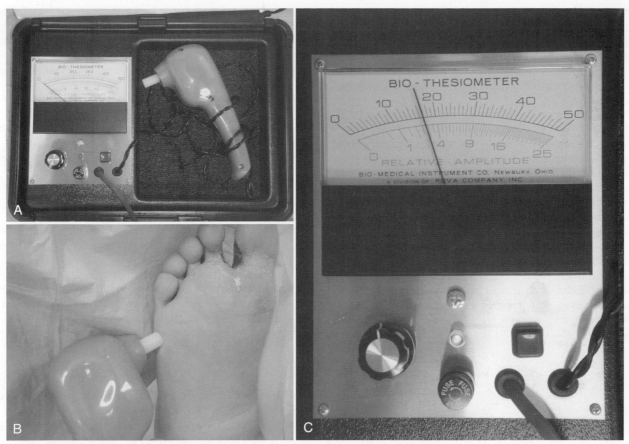

Fig. 17.2 (A) Biothesiometer. (B) Application of biothesiometer oscillator head to patient's foot during peripheral neuropathy assessment. (C) Oscillator amplitude knob to determine level of sensation. (Courtesy J. LeBretton and V. Driver.)

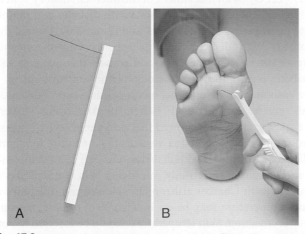

Fig. 17.3 (A) Monofilament. (B) Press the monofilament against the skin hard enough so that it bends. (Ball, J. W., Dains, J. E., & Flynn, J. A. (2019). Examination techniques and equipment. In: *Seidel's guide to physical examination* (9th ed.). St. Louis, MO: Elsevier.)

Musculoskeletal Abnormalities

Loss of motor nerve function affects the intrinsic foot muscles. When imbalances due to weakening of the intrinsic muscles occur, they can cause changes in foot structure and gait and muscle wasting. Plantar fat pads also become displaced,

and the metatarsal heads become prominent. These changes may predispose the patient to ulceration. Each foot has 26 bones, 29 joints, and 42 muscles; thus, there are numerous potential locations for problems. A few structural foot deformities are briefly described in Table 17.1. Fig. 17.1 provides illustrations of selected structural foot deformities.

Claw, hammer, and mallet toes are signs of distal muscle atrophy and foot neuropathy. When muscles weaken, other muscles can overpower them, leading to contractures. *Hammer toe* is a contracture of the proximal joint, which is further from the front (or top) of the toe. *Mallet toe* refers to the distal joint, closer to the end of the toe, and is almost identical to hammer toe. When both joints are contracted, the condition is called *claw toe*. Prominent metatarsal heads occur if one of the metatarsal bones is longer or lower than its neighboring bones. This may lead to uneven weight distribution between the heads and subsequent pain, callus, and ulceration. Bunions are caused by an enlarged head of the first metatarsal bone just below the first toe joint (ADA, 2008; IWGDF, 2019).

When changes in the gait or foot structure are observed, the patient should be referred for more testing. Patients with Charcot foot normally have a rocker-bottom foot that is hot, erythematous, and edematous with bounding pedal pulses and prominent veins (see Fig. 17.1). Pain is normally, but not always, minimal in the early stages. The foot may be

BOX 17.3   Procedure for Semmes–Weinstein 5.07 (10-g) Monofilament Examination (SWME)

1. Explain procedure to patient.
2. Position patient in sitting position, resting patient's lower leg on examiner's lap.
3. Demonstrate monofilament on patient's hand so that he or she knows what to expect.
4. Explain to patient that he or she should respond with a "yes" when he or she feels the filament touching the skin.
5. Have the patient close his or her eyes. The five key viability sites should be tested as shown in the illustration (fat pad of 1st and 4th toe, and metatarsal head of 1st, 3rd, and 5th toe).
6. Apply monofilament perpendicular to skin's surface. Apply sufficient force to cause the filament to buckle or bend in C-shape. Use a smooth, not jabbing, motion.
7. Total duration of the approach, skin contact, and departure of filament from each site should be approximately 1–2 s.
8. Apply filament along margin of callus, ulcer, scar, and/or necrotic tissue; do *not* apply filament over these lesions.
9. Record and, if appropriate, map the results on examination form.

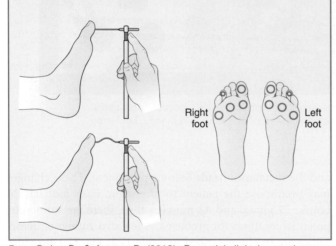

From Dehn, R., & Asprey, D. (2013). *Essential clinical procedures* (3rd ed.). St. Louis: Saunders.

BOX 17.4   Procedure for Biothesiometry Examination (Amplitude of Vibration)

1. Explain procedure to patient.
2. Position patient in sitting position, resting patient's lower leg on examiner's lap.
3. Demonstrate oscillator on patient's hand so that he or she knows what to expect.
4. Explain to patient that he or she should respond with a "yes" when he or she feels the oscillator vibrating.
5. Have the patient close his or her eyes. Sites to be tested should be shown on examination form.
6. Apply oscillator perpendicular to (flat against) skin's surface. Apply just enough force for the oscillator head to make total contact with skin. Use a smooth, not jabbing, motion.
7. The amplitude of the vibration should be slowly increased until the patient perceives the vibration and the value on the meter noted.
8. Apply oscillator along margin of callus, ulcer, scar, and/or necrotic tissue; do *not* apply oscillator over these lesions.
9. Record and, if appropriate, map the results on examination form.

with a Doppler device, a referral to a vascular specialist is warranted (WOCN Society, 2021).

In the absence of pedal pulses, additional noninvasive vascular tests may be conducted to obtain a better indication of the condition: (1) segmental pressures (i.e., taken at the thigh, calf, and ankle), (2) toe pressures, or (3) transcutaneous oxygen readings (WOCN Society, 2021). Transcutaneous oximetry ($TcPO_2$) is an assessment of the microcirculatory system, which can be impaired in persons with diabetes and peripheral neuropathy. Zimny, Dessel, and Ehren (2001) found that patients with diabetes and neuropathy had significantly higher sitting to supine $TcPO_2$ differences than patients with diabetes only, indicating microcirculatory impairment.

Vasodilation in diabetic, neuropathic lower extremities can create a functional ischemia. Armstrong, Lavery, Vazquez, et al. (2003) showed that skin temperature is a poor indicator of vascular status, neuropathy, or future foot complications in patients with diabetes. The only significant association found in their study was higher skin temperatures in patients with Charcot arthropathy. However, a difference in skin temperature may be an indication of trauma, fracture, and/or infection. Skin temperature should be assessed in both feet using the back of the examiner's hand or an infrared temperature scanner.

10–12°F warmer than the rest of the skin (Frykberg et al., 2006; Gerald & Hudson, 2002). A history including an absence of trauma, a portal of entry for infection, or other signs of infection is suggestive of an acute Charcot foot (Levin, 2002).

Vascular Status

The coexisting calcification of arteries that occurs with diabetes and PAD leaves the blood vessels difficult to compress and therefore difficult to assess (Levin, 2002). When pulses cannot be palpated, use of a Doppler probe will allow the skilled examiner to determine whether pulses are triphasic, biphasic, or monophasic. The absence of pedal pulses despite the presence of popliteal pulses is a classic finding for patients with diabetes who also have PAD. If pedal pulses are not detectable

Skin and Nail Condition

Skin and nail conditions are important components of assessment for the patient with LEND. Descriptions of foot lesions and nail disorders are given in Chapter 18. Loss of sweating and oil production may cause cracking of the skin and fissures that can become infected. The presence of eczema, dermatitis, and/or psoriasis should be noted. The web spaces between the toes should be examined for moisture and/or fungal problems. The patient's skin condition should be documented and any corns, calluses, preulcerative lesions (e.g., blisters and hematomas), or open ulcers measured and drawn on the documentation form. If the patient has coexisting vascular disease, additional skin changes may be apparent.

Callus formation is a natural protective response to repetitive stress. It is characterized by thickened hyperkeratotic skin. The problem with this buildup is that accumulation of callus can increase pressure by 25%–30%, resulting in an ulcer below the callused area that is not visible to the examiner and/or is not palpable. Hemorrhage into a callus is a principal indicator of ulceration (Aldana & Khachemoune 2020). A callus usually is painless but, in some cases, can cause pain because nerve endings close to the surface layers are irritated. Callus buildup is a result of a biomechanical problem. Unless the underlying cause is eliminated, callus will continue to occur. Based on the duration and amount of pressure applied, the skin may eventually breakdown and an ulcer will develop.

Thickened nails are common. In addition, any abnormalities under the nail and any sign of nail infections should be noted. Nails bear the brunt of daily activities: running, walking, participating in sports, and just wearing shoes. When feet are abused and/or injured, a portion or all of the nail plate can be damaged. Repeated trauma, improper trimming, and minor injuries can result in nail problems. If the toe box is pressing down on the nails, bleeding may occur under the nail. Some nail disorders are hereditary. Ingrown toenails (onychocryptosis) may have a convex deformity. As pressure is exerted on the tissues, callus builds up. Nails that are red, brown, or black may indicate trauma (acute or chronic). Any discharge from around the nail or under the nail may indicate an infection process. Fungal infections are common. A nail that curves inward in the corners is called a *paronychia.* If present, remove nail polish to better view the nails.

Footwear

Evaluation of the patient's shoes is as important as taking a good history or examining the patient's feet. The majority of injuries to the foot are not recognized by the person with diabetes because of neuropathy. Most skin injuries on the foot of the person with diabetes are located on either the dorsal or the plantar surface. Many ulcers on the dorsum are located at sites of high pressure where the patient's footwear creates a lesion, implying a biomechanical etiology. Due to the lack of clinical outcome studies guiding practice, assessment of footwear should follow a logical progression, observing for pressure points, wear, and areas of friction. Checklist 17.1 outlines the items that should be investigated when evaluating the patient's shoes. Box 17.5 provides tips for appropriate footwear selection.

Foot Imprints (Harris Mat)

Although a number of commercial devices exist for barefoot or in-shoe plantar pressure measurement, an inexpensive method that can be used to identify areas of increased pressure and unequal weight distribution of the patient's feet is the Harris mat (Tanenberg & Donofrio, 2008). The mat (foot

---

CHECKLIST 17.1   Items to Investigate When Evaluating Shoes in a Patient With Diabetes

✓ Bulges on outside of shoes
✓ Wear patterns on soles of shoes
✓ Wearing down on heels
✓ Worn lining inside shoes
✓ Shoe cushioning
✓ Foreign objects in shoes

---

imprint system) has two compartments. One side of the mat is inked. Paper is placed facing the inked surface. Two sheets are required, one for each foot. The inked side is closed, and the mat is reversed. The patient is asked to remove his or her shoes, leaving socks or hose on. The patient is asked to take a normal step down on the side that does not have ink. Stepping on the mat leaves an impression of the foot on the paper that indicates areas of high pressure and uneven weight distribution (Fig. 17.4A). Use of the mat identifies high-risk areas and is a good motivator for getting patients to wear their orthotics because they can see where problem areas exist.

Currently, there is new interactive insole system that has two parts which one measures the pressure points in the feet, and it will alert to the patient's smartphone device (Fig. 17.5). The results of this study showed that there was a 71% decrease in ulcer incidence with the interactive insole system when compared with standard of care alone (Abbott, Chawin, & Foden, 2019). This new device still needs further study, but it can be added as a secondary preventive measure for diabetic foot ulcer in the future.

Forefoot Test

The forefoot test shows patients how well their shoes fit their feet. First, have the patient remove his or her socks or hose. Instruct the patient to stand on a piece of paper with both feet. Trace the outline of both feet on the paper. Next, take the patient's shoes and just place the edge of the shoe over the traced outline. If any of the lines are visible, the shoes are too tight (see Fig. 17.4B). Again, this is a highly visual cue that helps the patient realize the importance of wearing shoes that fit his or her feet.

Diabetic Foot Ulcer Evaluation

The initial description of the foot ulcer is critical for mapping its development during treatment. Detailed wound assessment and evaluation of healing are described in Chapter 10.

Characteristics

Common locations and causes of diabetic foot ulcers are listed in Table 17.4. Ulcers with a LEND etiology may resemble a laceration, puncture, or blister with a rounded or oblong shape. The wound base may be necrotic, pink, or pale, with well-defined, smooth edges and small to moderate amounts of serous or clear exudate. The periwound skin often presents with callus.

BOX 17.5 Instructions for Care of Diabetic Feet

Inspection
- Inspect feet and toes daily for blisters, cuts, swelling, redness, and any other discolored areas. If you are unable to see the bottoms of your feet, use a mirror.
- Look for dry areas and cracks in the skin.
- Apply a thin coat of lubricating oil after bathing.
- If your vision is impaired, have a family member inspect your feet daily and trim nails and buff calluses when required.

Bathing
- Wash your feet daily. Dry them carefully, including between the toes. Test the water with hands or elbow to ensure it will not burn your feet.
- Do not soak your feet. Soaking actually dries the skin by removing natural oil and can cause maceration (wrinkled appearance).
- Apply moisturizing cream to feet top to bottom after bathing (not between toes).

Toenail Care
- Cut toenails after bathing, when they are soft and easier to trim.
- Never cut nails too short. Leave one-sixteenth to one-eighth inch of the nail. Nails should be cut straight across the top or shaped to follow the contour of the toe. Sharp edges should be filed smooth with an emery board to avoid cutting adjacent toes.
- Ingrown nails or other problematic nails should be cared for by a foot care provider.
- Avoid using sharp objects to clean under the toenail.

Corns and Calluses
- Do not use chemical corn or callus removers or corn pads. They can damage or burn the skin.

- When feet are dry, file away calluses with a pumice stone.
- Corns and calluses are a response to pressure from poorly fitting shoes. Change footwear to reduce these pressure "hot spots."
- Never use a razor blade yourself to reduce corns or calluses.

Shoes and Socks (Do not go barefoot)
- Wear clean socks every day. Avoid nylon socks as much as possible.
- Socks need to fit well, with no tight elastic at the top or seams.
- Do not walk barefoot, even in your home. Wear slippers with a rubber sole. Wear shoes and socks outside at all times.
- In winter, take special precautions to prevent foot damage from the cold.
- Inspect shoes for objects inside before you put them on.
- Buy shoes later in the day when feet are their largest. Do not depend on breaking in shoes.
- Shoes should be sufficiently wide for your feet and should have thick, flexible rubber soles, closed toes, and closed heels, as in running or walking shoes.
- Avoid pointed-toe shoes or boots. Do not wear sandals with a strap between your toes.
- Wear new shoes for short periods each day, from 1 to 2 h. Watch for signs of poor fit.

Circulation
- Do not smoke. If you do, stop!
- Exercise regularly.
- Put your feet up when you are sitting, and wiggle your toes for a few minutes several times throughout the day. If your feet are cold, wear socks to keep your feet warm.
- Do not use a heating pad or hot water bottle.

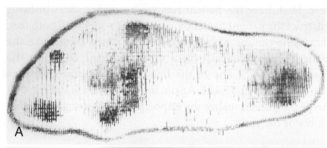
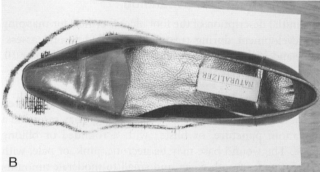

Fig. 17.4 (A) Example of Harris ink mat impression. (B) Patient's shoe laid over traced image of foot. (Courtesy David M. Osterman.)

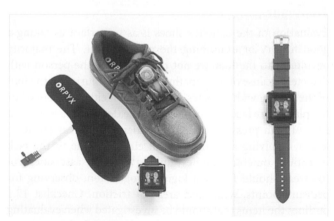

Fig. 17.5 Image of SurroSense RX smart insole system. (Image permission granted by Orpyx Medical Technologies Inc.)

Diabetic Foot Ulcer With Lower Extremity Arterial Disease

As previously mentioned, ischemic foot ulcers are relatively less common than neuropathic or neuroischemic diabetic foot ulcers. However, they are more serious and lead to higher rates of amputation in patients with diabetes (Moulik et al., 2003).

TABLE 17.4 Common Sites for Lower Extremity Wounds due to Diabetes Neuropathic Wounds Disease

Wound Location	Causative Factor(s)
Toe interphalangeal joints	Limited interphalangeal joint flexibility, rigid toe
Metatarsal heads	Increased prominence, limited ankle joint flexibility
Interdigital	Increased moisture, footwear too narrow, toe crowding, deformity
Bunion sites	Footwear too narrow, foot deformity
Dorsal toes	Hammer or claw toe deformity, footwear too shallow in toe box
Distal toes	Poor arterial perfusion, external force (heat); footwear too short, short, toe deformity
Midfoot plantar surface	Charcot foot/fracture; device- or footwear-related pressure; direct injury or other mechanical or thermal trauma; edema; moisture
Heel fissures	Unrelieved pressure, particularly during bedbound episodes

Wound, Ostomy and Continence Nurses Society. (2021). *Guideline for management of patients with lower extremity wounds due to diabetes mellitus and/or neuropathic disease.* WOCN Clinical Practice Guideline Series 3. Mt. Laurel, NJ: Author.

TABLE 17.5 Wagner Ulcer Classification System

0	At risk foot, preulcer, no open lesions, skin intact; may have deformities, callus, or cellulitis.
1	Superficial ulcer with partial—or full-thickness tissue loss.
2	Probing to ligament, tendon or joint capsule with soft-tissue infection.
3	Deep ulcer with abscess, osteomyelitis, or joint sepsis.
4	Ulcer localized to forefoot or heel gangrene.
5	Ulcer with gangrene involving entire foot, beyond salvage.

Wagner, F. W. (1981). The dysvascular foot: A system for diagnosis and treatment. *Foot & Ankle, 2*(2), 64–122.

A comparison of the characteristics of neuropathic, arterial, and venous wounds is given in Table 13.3. Trophic changes for arterial disease alone are not diagnostic of arterial insufficiency and should be interpreted with caution. Characteristics of ischemic foot ulcers include pain, absence of bleeding, presence of an underlying deformity, or history of a trauma (Sumpio, 2000). Ischemic ulcers on the dorsum are uncommon because perfusion usually is better and pressures are reduced at that location (Sumpio, 2000). Additional indicators of ischemia are discussed in detail in Chapter 14.

Diabetic Foot Ulcer Classification Systems

Numerous diabetic foot ulcer classification systems have been reported in the literature (Games, 2016; Ince, Abbas, Lutale, et al., 2008; Lipsky, Berendt, Cornia, et al., 2012; Wagner, 1981; Wound, Ostomy and Continence Nurses Society™ [WOCN®], 2021). These systems are useful for guiding treatment regimens, facilitating communication among care providers, predicting future outcomes, and conducting clinical trials. The various systems often include location, depth, necrotic characteristics, and presence of infection, ischemia, or neuropathy.

The *Wagner Foot Wound Classification System* (Wagner, 1981) is presented in Table 17.5. It divides foot ulcers into six grades based on the depth of the lesion and the presence of osteomyelitis or gangrene. It was later modified to include the presence of infection, ischemia, or neuropathy (WOCN®, 2021). Many experts do not advocate the use of the Wagner

classification system to assess the severity of a diabetic foot ulcer (Monteiro-Soares, Boyko, et al., 2020; National Institute for Health and Clinical Excellent [NICE], 2011). The system does not assess for PAD or infection and there are concerns regarding consistency (Bodsky, 2001; Bravo-Molina, Linares-Palomino, Vera-Arroyo, Salmerón-Febres, & Ros-Díe, 2016; Monteiro-Soares, Russel, et al., 2019).

The *S(AD) SAD Classification System* (Table 17.6) was designed primarily for clinical audit and consists of five elements: size (area and depth), infection (sepsis), ischemia (arteriopathy), and neuropathy (denervation) (Macfarlane & Jeffcoate, 1999). This system has undergone validation by seeking correlations with outcome in an internal and external setting (Abbas, Lutale, Game, & Jeffcoate, 2008; Parisi, Zantut-Wittmann, Pavin, et al., 2008; Treece, Macfarlane, Pound, Game, & Jeffcoate, 2004). Due to concerns about the lack of detail describing categories and the inclusion of Charcot foot, that system has been simplified to produce the SINBAD system (Games, 2016).

The *Site, Ischemia, Neuropathy, Bacterial Infection, Area and Depth (SINBAD) Classification System* is a simplified variation of the SAD. The SINBAD classification system (Table 17.7) appears to be the best validated system providing greater specification when compared with other classification systems (Games, 2016). The SINBAD classification has been recommended for communication among healthcare professionals by the IWGDF (2019).

The *University of Texas (UT) Classification system* (Table 17.8), utilizes a matrix structure with four grades of wound depth and four associated stages to specify ischemia, infection, both ischemia and infection, or neither (Lavery, Armstrong, & Harkless, 1996; NICE, 2011). When compared with the Wagner system, the UT system demonstrated superior prediction in healing time with each stage of the UT system ($P < 0.05$), and stage predicted healing ($P < 0.05$) (Oyibo, Jude, & Tarawneh, 2001).

The IWGDF and the Infectious Diseases Society of America (ISDA) developed the *IDSA/IWGDF Classification System* and integrated *Perfusion, Extent, Depth, Infection and*

TABLE 17.6 Size (Area and Depth) (SAD) Classification

Grade	Area	Depth	Sepsis	Arteriopathy	Denervation
0	Skin intact	Skin intact	No infection	Pedal pulses palpable	SWMT (Semmes–Weinstein monofilament test) normal (see Box 17.3 for procedure) VPT normal
1	<10 mm^2	Skin and subcutaneous tissue	Superficial slough or exudate	Diminution of both pulses or absence of one	Reduced or absent pinprick sensation VPT raised
2	10–30 mm^2	Tendon, joint, capsule, periosteum	Cellulitis	Absence of both pedal pulses	Neuropathy dominant, palpable pedal pulses
3	>30 mm^2	Bone and/or joint spaces	Osteomyelitis	Gangrene	Charcot foot

VPT, vibration perception threshold.
From Macfarlane, R., & Jeffcoate, W. (1999). Classification of diabetic foot ulcers: The size (area and depth) (SAD) system. *Diabetic Foot, 2*(4), 123.

TABLE 17.7 Site, Ischemia, Neuropathy, Bacterial Infection, Area, Depth (SIDBAD) Classification System

Category	Definition	Score
Site	Forefoot	0
	Midfoot and hindfoot	1
Ischemia	Pedal blow flow intact; at least one palpable pulse	0
	Clinical evidence of reduced pedal flow	1
Neuropathy	Protective sensation intact	0
	Protective sensation lost	1
Bacterial infection	None	0
	Present	1
Area	Ulcer <1cm^2	0
	Ulcer ≥1cm^2	1
Depth	Ulcer confined to skin and subcutaneous tissue	0
	Ulcer reaching muscle, tendon, or deeper	1

From Monteiro-Soares, M., Russesl, D., et al. (2019). *IWGDF guideline on the classification of diabetic foot ulcer.* Netherland, Australia, UK and USA: International Working Group on Diabetic Foot. Accessed 2/14/2020. Retrieved from www.iwgdfguidelines.org.

TABLE 17.8 University of Texas Diabetic Foot Classification System

	GRADE			
Stage	0	I	II	III
A	Preulcerative or postulcerative lesion completely healed	Superficial wound not involving tendon, capsule, or bone	Wound penetrating to tendon or capsule	Wound penetrating to bone or joint
B	Preulcerative or postulcerative lesion completely epithelialized with infection	Superficial wound not involving tendon, capsule, or bone with infection	Wound penetrating to tendon or capsule with infection	Wound penetrating to bone or joint with infection
C	Preulcerative or postulcerative lesion completely epithelialized with ischemia	Superficial wound not involving tendon, capsule, or bone with ischemia	Wound penetrating to tendon or capsule with ischemia	Wound penetrating to bone or joint with ischemia
D	Preulcerative or postulcerative lesion completely epithelialized with infection and ischemia	Superficial wound not involving tendon, capsule, or bone with infection and ischemia	Wound penetrating to tendon or capsule with infection and ischemia	Wound penetrating to bone or joint with infection and ischemia

From Lavery, L. A., Armstrong, D. G., & Harkless, L. B. (1996). Classification of diabetic foot wounds. *The Journal of Foot and Ankle Surgery, 35*(6), 528–531.

TABLE 17.9 IWGDF/ISDA Infection Classification System

Clinical Manifestation	Infection Severity	PEDIS Grade
Wound lacking purulence or any manifestations of inflammation	Uninfected	1
Presence of ≥2 manifestations of inflammation (purulence, or erythema, tenderness, warmth, or induration), but any cellulitis/erythema extends ≤2 cm around the ulcer, and infection is limited to the skin or superficial subcutaneous tissues; no other local complications or systemic illness	Mild	2
Infection (as above) in a patient who is systemically well and metabolically stable, but which has ≥1 of the following characteristics: cellulitis extending >2 cm, lymphangitic streaking, spread beneath the superficial fascia, deep-tissue abscess, gangrene, and involvement of muscle, tendon, joint or bone	Moderate	3
Infection in a patient with systemic toxicity or metabolic instability (e.g., fever, chills, tachycardia, hypotension, confusion, vomiting, leukocytosis, acidosis, severe hyperglycemia, or azotemia)	Severe	4

PEDIS, Perfusion, Extent, Depth, Infection and Sensation.
From Monteiro-Soares, M., Russesl, D., et al. (2019). *IWGDF guideline on the classification of diabetic foot ulcer*. Netherland, Australia, UK and USA: International Working Group on Diabetic Foot. Accessed 2/14/2020. Retrieved from www.iwgdfguidelines.org.

TABLE 17.10 Wound, Ischemia, and Foot Infection (WIfI) System

Wound Grade	DFU	Gangrene
0	No ulcer. *Clinical description: minor tissue loss. Salvageable with simple digital amputation (1 or 2 digits) or skin coverage.*	No gangrene
1	Small, shallow ulcer(s) on distal leg or foot; no gangrene exposed bone, unless limited to distal phalanx. *Clinical description: minor tissue loss. Salvageable with simple digital amputation (1 or 2 digits) or skin coverage.*	No gangrene
2	Deeper ulcer with exposed bone, joint or tendon; generally not involving the heel; shallow heel ulcer, without calcaneal involvement. *Clinical description: major tissue loss salvageable with multiple (≥3) digital amputations or standard transmetatarsal amputation (TMA) ± skin coverage.*	Gangrenous changes limited to digits
3	Extensive, deep ulcer involving forefoot and/or midfoot; deep, full-thickness heel ulcer ± calcaneal involvement. *Clinical description: extensive tissue loss salvageable only with a complex foot reconstruction or nontraditional TMA (Chopart or Lisfranc); flap coverage or complex wound management needed for large soft-tissue defect.*	Extensive gangrene involving forefoot and/or midfoot: full-thickness heel necrosis 6 calcaneal involvement

From Monteiro-Soares, M., Russesl, D., et al. (2019). *IWGDF guideline on the classification of diabetic foot ulcer*. Netherland, Australia, UK and USA: International Working Group on Diabetic Foot. Accessed 2/14/2020. Retrieved from www.iwgdfguidelines.org.

Sensation to assess the severity of infection (Table 17.9). IWGDF/ISDA classification is used as a guideline for management and is considered a strong predictor of the need for hospitalization (Bravo-Molina, et al., 2016; Monteiro-Soares, Russel, et al., 2019).

The *Wound, Ischemia and Foot Infection (WIfI) system* (Table 17.10) integrates the IWGDF/ISDA classification system for the patient with PAD to stratify amputation risk and the benefit of revascularization. A Delphi consensus of the members of the Society of Vascular Surgery Lower Extremity Guidelines Committee assigned a risk of intervention to each of the possible combinations of scores and created a WIfI spectrum score regarding the risk of limb amputation at 1 year (Mills, Conte, Armstrong, et al., 2014; Zhan, Branco, Armstrong, & Mills, 2015).

Infection

Infection rarely causes diabetic foot ulcers. Rather, ulcers provide a portal for the entry of pathogens, which often thrive because of the impaired host response of the person with diabetes. Infection is a causal component in 59% of diabetic limb amputations (Armstrong, Lavery, & Harkless, 1998; Pecoraro, Reiber, & Burgess, 1990). In a Swedish study, Eneroth, Apelqvist, and Stenström (1997) found that 42%

of patients with diabetes who had deep foot infections required lower extremity amputations and 86% required surgery. However, a recent study done by Frykberg et al. (2006) suggested that 20% of patients with foot ulcers will subsequently require an amputation.

The person with diabetes is more prone to infection than is the person without diabetes (Shah & Hux, 2003), most likely due to impaired leukocyte function in patients with chronic hyperglycemia. However, infected diabetic foot wounds often are less symptomatic than nondiabetic wounds, exhibiting only subtle or even a complete absence of signs (Frykberg, 2003; Lipsky et al., 2012). Recalcitrant hyperglycemia may be one of the clinical findings indicating a severe infection of a diabetic foot ulcer (Frykberg, 2002; Frykberg et al., 2006; Mendes & Neves, 2012). The presence of probable infection needs to be noted during the initial examination, although culturing is best done after surgical debridement.

Wound culture technique is important to ensure surface colonies are not included and therefore confused with infection (see Chapter 19). Wound cultures should be taken by obtaining tissue from the debrided wound base or by aspirating pus. If swabs are the only option, ensure they are taken from the wound base after cleansing. The gold standard for infection assessment is the quantitative biopsy (Frykberg, 2003). Evaluation does not end after initial culturing. Wounds must be continually monitored for bacterial colonization.

Like the classification of diabetic foot ulcers in general, the classification of diabetic foot infections can be useful for determining appropriate treatment. Diabetic foot infections are subdivided into either nonlimb-threatening or limb-threatening categories (Table 17.11), with the understanding that the latter classification can become life threatening (ADA, 1999). Research indicates that stratification is warranted to distinguish wounds with vascular insufficiency from those without. Prompers et al. (2008) suggest that diabetic foot ulcers with and without PAD be classified as different disease states due to vastly different predictors of healing between diabetic wounds with and those without concomitant PAD.

One of the most important assessments at this stage is wound depth and, more importantly, presence of osteomyelitis, which is surprisingly common. It is found in approximately 60% of moderate to severe diabetic foot ulcers (Berendt, Peters, Bakker, et al., 2008; Eneroth et al., 1997).

Bone biopsy gives a definitive diagnosis, but less invasive techniques are useful in establishing a diagnosis with a high degree of sensitivity and specificity. Appropriate diagnostic measures include probing the wound, serial X-ray films, magnetic resonance imaging, computed tomography, and radionuclide imaging. Either direct exposure of bone or a positive "probe to bone" test is used to determine the presence of osteomyelitis (WOCN Society, 2021). Probing can also detect sinus tract formations and undermining along the ulcer margins (Frykberg, 2002). X-ray studies are inexpensive, readily available, and useful for *excluding* an inflammatory process such as osteomyelitis. However, evidence of changes on X-ray films generally take about 2 weeks after bone infection, giving X-ray films a sensitivity of approximately 55% (Sinacore & Mueller, 2008a). Magnetic resonance imaging offers high-resolution views not only of bone but also of soft tissue; has a sensitivity and specificity of greater than 90% and 80%, respectively (Alaia et al., 2021); and, therefore, tends to be the diagnostic procedure of choice.

MANAGEMENT

The level of expertise and knowledge required to manage LEND and diabetic foot ulcers is constantly increasing. Because of the complex nature of diabetic foot ulcers and the numerous comorbidities that can occur in patients with diabetes, a multidisciplinary team approach to management is critical (ADA, 2007; Driver, Fabbi, Lavery, et al., 2010; Driver et al., 2005; Frykberg, 2002). An ideal foot care team should include: (1) podiatric/orthopedic surgeon, (2) vascular surgeon, (3) infectious disease specialist, (4) endocrinologist or family practice or internal medicine provider, (5) orthopedic/podiatric technician, (6) certified wound care nurse, (7) orthotist, (8) dietician, and (9) certified diabetes educator. Numerous references from the U.S. and European literature document improvements in patient outcomes, including reduction of lower extremity amputation rates, as a result of implementing a multidisciplinary approach to diabetic foot care (Driver et al., 2005; Sanders, Robbins, & Edmonds, 2010). Rates of avoidance of major amputation of lower extremity after implementation of a multidisciplinary team can be reduced from 40% to 76% (Weck et al., 2013). However, health care providers frequently work in situations without this level and various expertise; thus, patients with diabetes who develop a foot problem will often require referral to consultants. In fact, the standards of medical care in diabetes recommend the referral of high-risk patients to foot specialists for surveillance and preventative care (Bowen, 2015; Driver et al., 2005).

Diabetic neuropathy is associated with a reduced blood supply to the nerves, a microcirculatory network called the *vasa nervosum*. Currently, no prescription therapy in the United States is approved for the treatment of the underlying process of microvascular damage that leads to DPN, although lowering of HbA1c levels has been shown to decrease the microvascular complications of diabetes (ADA, 2007; Fowler, 2008). Research has demonstrated that capillary

TABLE 17.11 Signs of Limb-Threatening and Nonlimb-Threatening Diabetic Foot Infections

Nonlimb Threatening	Limb Threatening
Less than 2 cm of surrounding cellulitis	Greater than 2 cm of surrounding cellulitis
No systemic toxicity signs	Deep abscess or osteomyelitis, gangrene
No deep abscess, osteomyelitis, gangrene	

vascular perfusion is inversely correlated with the degree of peripheral neuropathy (Ostergard, Finnerup, & Andersen, 2015). Nerve ischemia leads to poor nerve function. Based on earlier research in which certain prostacyclins (vasodilators) or their analogs gained approval for the treatment of critical limb ischemia in Europe, Remodulin (treprostinil) is being tested in patients with diabetes and neuropathic ulcers. Mohler, Klugherz, Goldman, et al. (2000) demonstrated that treatment significantly increased lower limb blood flow in these patients. Furthermore, Berman, Quick, Yoder, et al. (2006) showed 62% reduction in mean worst rest pain during use of this medication, but study did not indicate the increase in blow flow. This study is open label and it suggested that further controlled studies are needed. At the time of publication, the FDA has not approved this medication for the limb ischemia. Remodulin is only approved for pulmonary hypertension treatment. Several phase 2/3 clinical trials for critical limb ischemia have been run with no success to market to date.

Another new area of investigation for neuropathy treatment of the patient with diabetes involves the enzyme protein kinase C-beta (PKC-β). Current hypotheses concerning the pathogenesis of diabetic neuropathy suggest that PKC-β (which is stimulated by hyperglycemia) may be involved in the process that leads to microvascular dysfunction, impairment of endoneural blood flow, and damage of nerves (Vinik, Bril, & Kempler, 2005). The PKC-β inhibitor LY333531 (Eli Lilly) is currently being tested and has shown encouraging results in improving DPN (Vinik et al., 2005). Advancements in gene therapy have shown promise as potential treatments of diabetic complications such as neuropathy and neuropathic wounds, and research continues to broaden our understanding of the biochemical and molecular bases of diabetes and associated complications (Driver & LeBretton, 2008; Park, Allen, & Driver, 2013).

Early Intervention (Prevention)

Careful and frequent inspection of the diabetic foot is the most effective and least expensive method for preventing diabetic foot ulcers and possibly lower extremity amputations. Abnormalities, whether age related, structural, or pathologic, can be assessed and documented. The ADA (2007) and Boulton, Armstrong, Albert, et al. (2008) recommend patients with a low-risk foot ulcer (no loss of protective sensation, no PAD, no deformity) with well-controlled diabetes undergo a comprehensive annual foot examination.

At least 50% of all amputations due to diabetic neuropathy are preventable with early intervention (Reiber, 1995). Given the life-altering and life-threatening risks associated with the development of a diabetic foot ulcer, it is incumbent upon the health care professional to identify patients with lower extremity peripheral neuropathy as early as possible so that preventive interventions can be implemented. Preventive interventions for the patient with LEND must become a routine that the patient incorporates into everyday life. Specific instructions concerning inspection of the foot, bathing, nail care, care of corns and calluses, shoes, socks, and circulation

should be enforced in writing and verbally as outlined in Box 17.5. Clearly, one of the most important components of the clinician's role is providing patient education.

Using the patient's foot risk classification, a management plan (i.e., education, diagnostic studies, footwear recommendations, referrals, and follow-up visits) can be developed in order to minimize the odds of developing a foot ulcer (Driver, 2004). Tables 17.2 and 17.3 list programs that correlate specific preventive interventions with each level of risk. Implementing these early interventions and adhering to preventive interventions (e.g., over-the-counter moisturizing cream to moisturize the foot and inspecting the shoe before putting it on) address the first two principles of wound management (i.e., control or eliminate causative factors, and provide systemic support to reduce existing and potential cofactors).

Glycemic Control

As many one in to Americans (37.3 million) have diabetes and one in five of those do not know they have it (CDC, 2022). In addition, of the more than 1 in 3 American adults (96 million) who have prediabetes, 8 in 10 do not know they have it (CDC, 2022). In some early research, Umpierrez, Isaacs, and Bazargan (2002) documented that one in three people with diabetes admitted to an urban hospital had no known history of the condition and were diagnosed during their stay.

Inadequate glycemic control is key in the development of neuropathy in the extremities of the person with diabetes (WOCN Society, 2021). Hyperglycemia results in leukocyte dysfunction and suppression of lymphocytes, high blood pressure, and impaired endothelial function, among other dangers. Because of their impaired immune response, persons with hyperglycemia will respond poorly to a severe foot infection. Armstrong, Perales, Murff, et al. (1996) found that 56% of persons being admitted for diabetic foot infections had normal white blood cell counts. Improved blood glucose levels will increase the immune defenses of patients and thus should be a component of clinical care of infected diabetic foot ulcers. Elevated HbA1c levels in a patient with diabetes who is infected may be the only sign alerting the provider to the problem (Frykberg, 2003). Thus, patients with diabetes must be managed with a high index of suspicion for soft-tissue infection, deep space infection, and osteomyelitis.

Offloading

Offloading and redistributing pressure is a basic principle involved in the prevention of foot ulcers and lower extremity amputations, as well as the healing of existing diabetic foot ulcers. Numerous books, references, and websites discuss the various offloading modalities used for patients with diabetic foot ulcers or at risk for developing foot ulcers. Orthotists and pedorthists are frequently consulted for assistance in managing foot problems. Orthotists and pedorthists are trained specifically to make and fit orthopedic footwear (and other appliances) that can accommodate the patient with diabetes. Table 17.5 lists various methods and considerations for offloading the foot. Options for offloading include bed rest, wheelchairs, crutches, surgical shoes, custom sandals, healing shoes, cast shoes, and foam dressings (WOCN Society, 2021). The following section discusses total-contact casts (TCCs), removable cast walkers (RCWs), felted foam dressings (FFDs), orthotics and orthopedic footwear, and surgical offloading procedures.

The TCC has been shown to be very effective at relieving pressure and healing diabetic foot ulcers. The cast is designed to equalize pressure loading of the plantar surface by equal "total contact" of the plantar skin with the cast material (Fig. 17.6). Repetitive injury to the wound site is reduced while the patient ambulates. Epidemiologic studies have shown that TCC healing rates are between 73% and 100%, with healing times between 30 and 63 days (Bus, Valk, van Deursen, et al., 2008). A study of the histologic features of patients undergoing ulcerectomy after 20 days in a TCC vs patients undergoing ulcerectomy at presentation showed marked increases in granulation and angiogenesis in the TCC group (Piagessi, Viacava, & Rizzo, 2003). TCCs are absolutely contraindicated for patients with acute deep infection, sepsis, or gangrene. Relative contraindications include patients with ulcers with depth greater than width, fragile skin, or excessive edema; noncompliant patients; and those who would be unstable with a cast (Sinacore & Mueller, 2008b).

A test of the effectiveness of TCCs, RCWs, and half-shoes in healing neuropathic diabetic foot ulcers demonstrated that patients with a TCC had significantly better healing rates at 12 weeks than did patients treated with the other two offloading modalities. Interestingly, patients with a TCC were significantly less active than were patients with half-shoes. No activity difference was noted between patients with the TCC and those with the RCW (Armstrong, Nguyen, Lavery, et al., 2001). Armstrong, Lavery, Kimbriel, et al. (2003) devised an activity test for patients with diabetic foot ulcers wearing RCWs. Total daily activity was recorded per patient. In addition, unbeknown to patients, the daily activity

of the RCW also was recorded. Results showed that patients wore the RCW only 28% of the time.

A study of 50 patients with neuropathic foot ulcerations compared healing rates of wounds offloaded with RCW to wounds offloaded with RCW wrapped with a cohesive bandage. Results showed that the wounds offloaded with the RCW wrapped with a cohesive bandage healed significantly sooner ($P < 0.05$) than did those with only the RCW, which could be removed more easily (Armstrong, Lavery, Wu, et al., 2005). These studies suggest that protective footwear that is less easily removed may increase the odds of healing diabetic foot ulcers by increasing patient compliance. Interestingly, a 2008 study showed that only 1.7% of the 895 clinical respondents used a TCC as a treatment modality for diabetic foot ulcer and 45.5% reported no use of a TCC. Patient tolerance and application requirements were the predominant reasons indicated for lack of TCC use (Wu, Jensen, & Weber, 2008).

Often described as a "poor man's TCC," the FFD has been shown to provide the offloading benefits of a TCC while allowing appropriate management of patients with typical contraindications (Fig. 17.7). A 2001 report from German researchers indicates that an FFD reduces plantar loading at the ulcer site while allowing for daily dressing changes (Zimny, Reinsch, & Schatz, 2001). Whether used as an adjunct to a surgical shoe, a healing shoe, or a walking splint, an FFD has been found to be equally as effective as a TCC in time to healing and healing proportion (Birke, Pavich, Patout, et al., 2002). An FFD requires less skill to apply and reduces or eliminates some of the inherent challenges and risks of a TCC, such as limited assessment ability (Wu et al., 2008) and edema-related compromise. An FFD helps to foster compliance levels while eliminating the bulk and relative immobility of TCCs. It also allows for direct offloading of a diabetic foot ulcer while permitting the use of orthotics to meet concurrent offloading needs. When felted foam is being applied, all edges must be beveled to prevent improper redistribution of forces (edge effect).

PPT and Plastazote (foam) inserts, custom-molded foot beds, and molded orthotics such as the Charcot restraint orthotic walker (Fig. 17.8) shoe modifications are the predominant methods of pressure management in the patients with diabetes (Fig. 17.9) (Wu et al., 2008). Patients who used a Plastazote arch filler in conjunction with an RCW showed healing of recalcitrant plantar ulcers within 4 months (Ritz, Rowland, & Rowland, 1996). Patients who used various foam inlays applied to their shoes and rocker-bottom outsoles demonstrated a reduction in peak plantar pressures (Praet & Louwerens, 2003).

Offloading can also be achieved with prophylactic and corrective surgical procedures such as Achilles tendon lengthening, sometimes referred to as tendo-Achilles lengthening (TAL), joint arthroplasty, and excision or resection of bony prominences. Patients who may be considered for TAL include those with peripheral neuropathy and equinus contracture. Equinus causes high forefoot pressure that contributes to plantar surface ulceration (Laborde, 2008). A randomized clinical trial of patients with plantar diabetic foot

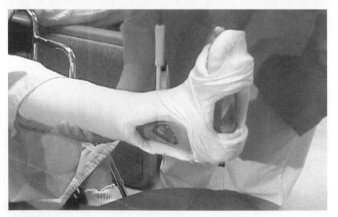

Fig. 17.6 Modified total-contact cast applied to offload pressure from neuropathic plantar ulcer that developed after prolonged use of a multipodus boot. A window around the wounds allows dressing changes without cast removal. The cutout portion of the cast is secured with self-adhering wrap. (Courtesy Ted Tomter, RN, CWOCN, St. Joseph's Candler Health System, Savannah, GA.)

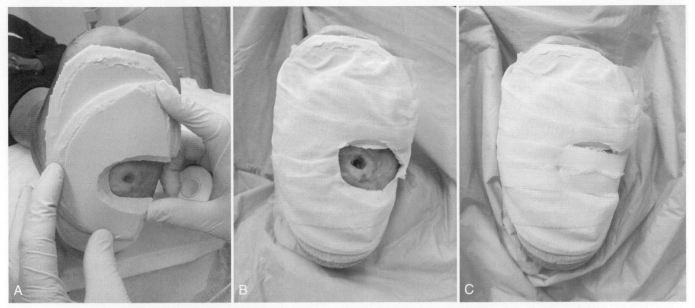

Fig. 17.7 (A) Felted foam applied to plantar aspect of foot to decrease loading forces directly over an ulcer. (B) Foam secured in place using cloth mesh tape and rubber cement. A cutout is made in the tape to allow for dressing changes between office visits. (C) Felted foam dressing with concurrent dressing applied. Gauze roll is used to further secure the dressing in place and then is covered in a sock or stockinette. (Courtesy J. LeBretton and V. Driver.)

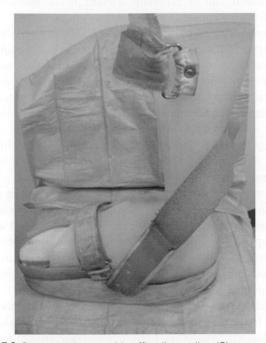

Fig. 17.8 Customized removable offloading walker (Charcot restraint orthotic walker) boot. (Courtesy J. LeBretton and V. Driver.)

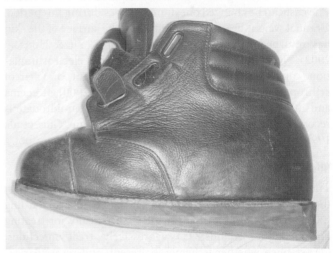

Fig. 17.9 Custom-molded shoe for a transmetatarsal amputation. (Courtesy J. LeBretton and V. Driver.)

ulcers compared TCC with and TCC without TAL. The study showed that all ulcers in the TAL plus TCC group healed with a risk of recurrence that was 75% less at 7 months and 52% less at 2 years than in the TCC-only treatment group (Mueller, Sinacore, Hastings, et al., 2003). However, a follow-up to this study found that patients who had undergone the TAL plus TCC procedure had decreased physical functioning compared with the TCC-only patients after

8 months (Mueller, Sinacore, Hastings, et al., 2004). Although joint arthroplasty in combination with TCC showed no difference in healing proportions compared with TCC alone, significantly shorter healing time was observed in the arthroplasty group (Armstrong, Lavery, Vazquez, et al., 2003; Finestone, Tamir, & Ron, 2018; Lin, Bono, & Lee, 2000). Metatarsal head resection has also been demonstrated to shorten healing time compared with a control group (Armstrong, Rosales, & Gashi, 2005). Increases in pressure in other areas of the foot have been observed with metatarsal head resection, necessitating a multidisciplinary approach and accommodative orthotics or other offloading to compensate for changes in pressure and to support prevention of new, recurrent, or recalcitrant ulceration.

TABLE 17.12	Stages of Charcot Foot	
Stage	**Radiographic Findings**	**Clinical Findings**
0 (prodromal)	Normal radiographs	Swelling, erythema, warmth
I (development)	Osteopenia, fragmentation, joint subluxation or dislocation	Swelling, erythema, warmth, ligamentous laxity
II (coalescence)	Absorption of debris, sclerosis, fusion of larger fragments	Decreased warmth, decreased swelling, decreased erythema
III (reconstruction)	Consolidation of deformity, joint arthrosis, fibrous ankyloses, rounding and smoothing of bone fragments	Absence of warmth, absence of swelling, absence of erythema, stable joint ± fixed deformity

Stages I–III were described by Eichenholtz (1966). Later Shibata et al. (1990) added Stage 0 to facilitate early diagnosis of Charcot neuropathy (CN) since clinical signs (increased temperature, edema, erythema) preceded radiographic changes. Today MRI and bone scans are used for early diagnosis of CN (Rosenbaum & DiPreta, 2015; WOCN Society, 2021).

Structural Foot Deformities

The traditional treatment for Charcot arthropathy (without ulceration) is cast immobilization. Few patients require surgery for this condition; however, exostectomy has been shown to be an appropriate method of treatment of Charcot prominences (Catanzariti, Mendicino, & Haverstock, 2000) should nonsurgical interventions fail. Before immobilization, compression bandages are applied at weekly intervals until all edema has subsided. This period can last 2–3 weeks. A short nonweight-bearing cast is generally required for 12–16 weeks. The cast can be changed one or more times during this period. Gradual weight bearing is started when the surface of the skin has returned to near-normal temperature (Yu & Hudson, 2002). Noninvasive bone stimulation such as electrostimulation can be a valuable adjunctive treatment of Charcot arthropathy (Grady, O'Connor, Axe, et al., 2000). If edema and inflammation persist, administration of pamidronate is recommended to prevent further deterioration (Guis et al., 1999). Table 17.12 lists the healing phases of Charcot foot.

Wound Management

The principles of wound management and goals of topical therapy are described in Chapter 21. Jeffcoate and Harding (2003) listed the following priorities specifically for treating diabetic foot wounds: (1) aggressively treat infections; (2) establish whether ischemia is present, and revascularization is required; (3) relieve pressure to the wound; and (4) improve the wound condition by debridement, dressings, and advanced care treatments where appropriate. Ultimately, the principal goal in the treatment of diabetic foot ulcers is wound closure.

Debridement and Callus Management

Wound and callus debridement is integral in the management of diabetic foot wounds. Key benefits of debridement in the diabetic wound include removal of free-living bacteria and biofilms, stimulation of growth factors (see Chapter 8), removal of senescent cells, and removal of hyperproliferative nonmigratory tissue (i.e., callus). Serial debridement of wounds for the first 4 weeks of treatment has been shown to reduce median wound area by as much as 54% compared with wounds not undergoing serial debridement. Notably, this was the first study to evaluate healing rates and debridement across multiple chronic wound etiologies (Cardinal, Eisenbud, Armstrong, et al., 2009). Methods of debridement may change over time or may be performed in combination as conditions change. Debridement is repeated as often as needed, depending on the formation of new necrotic tissue (Wilcox, Carter, & Covington, 2013). Weekly debridement is common and is generally referred to as *maintenance debridement* (Sibbald et al., 2021).

Hyperkeratotic callus buildup is frequently seen in the patient with diabetes due to the drying effects of autonomic dysfunction secondary to neuropathy and the natural response to repetitive minor trauma over pressure points. The callus development increases peak plantar pressures, fostering hematoma development and ulceration. A vicious circle is created in which high pressure causes callus buildup, which in turn leads to higher pressures and further callus development. Callus management is integral in the prevention and treatment of diabetic foot ulcer. Callus removal (see Plates 40 and 41) should be performed regularly and combined with effective orthotics or shoe modifications to better distribute pressures and prevent callus buildup. Supportive therapy, such as daily application of moisturizer, will assist in counteracting decreases in skin oil production seen in the patient with diabetes who has neuropathy.

Traditionally, callus has been removed by means of a scalpel or tissue nipper, but difficulty in smoothing the edges of the callus where tissue has been removed can result in areas of micropressure. Rotary files use a small drum covered with sandpaper or various burrs spun at rates of 1000–3000 rpm. Due to the high revolution, rotary files allow the skilled clinician to "shape" the callus rather than excise hyperkeratotic tissue, which can create minute pressure points and a potential portal of entry for infection. Removal of dry hyperkeratotic tissue decreases pressure and can reveal ulcerations and undermining of tissue under the callus that otherwise would not be visible.

When selecting a specific method of debridement of diabetic foot ulcers, many factors must be considered: pain, arterial insufficiency, antiembolic medications, patient setting, resources, characteristics of the wound, and the type of debridement. Methods of debridement and factors to consider for selection are discussed in detail in Chapter 20.

Considerations specific to patients with LEND and diabetic foot ulcers are highlighted by the IWGDF (2019):

- Revascularization and surgical removal of necrotic tissue from an infected wound on an ischemic leg or foot is the treatment of choice for limb salvage.
- All ulcers with extensive cellulitis and/or osteomyelitis should be debrided and referred for pharmacologic (intravenous) intervention.
- Evidence supporting the use of whirlpool or pulsatile jet irrigation in neuropathic ulcers is insufficient.
- Caution must be exercised to prevent immersion burns from whirlpools because of reduced sensitivity in the neuropathic leg.
- Maintain dry, stable eschar on noninfected, ischemic, neuropathic wounds.

Infection

The assessment and treatment of infection is discussed in detail in Chapter 19. The classification of the infection, allergies, medical condition of the patient, and culture results (often not available initially) usually guide antibiotic therapy (Frykberg, 2003). The ADA (1999) and Lipsky et al. (2012) cite categories of infection for the patient with diabetes as limb-threatening infections, nonlimb-threatening infections, and osteomyelitis.

No antibiotics are recommended for the patient with an ulcer that is not clinically infected. However, remember that the patient with diabetes often does not show common symptoms of infection and thus must be monitored closely. Limb-threatening infections (see Table 17.11) require immediate hospitalization. Additional conditions of limb-threatening infections may include necrotizing fasciitis, ischemia, hyperglycemia, and leukocytosis (ADA, 1999; Frykberg, 2003).

Patients with nonlimb-threatening infections require immediate antibiotic therapy, generally beginning the same day as the diagnosis is made. For mild and most moderate infections, therapy can be an oral agent, although certain patients may require parenteral therapy. Commonly used oral agents include cephalexin, clindamycin, and amoxicillin/clavulanate (Lipsky et al., 2012). Patients with mild or moderate infections may be treated on an outpatient basis, but only if certain criteria are met. Those who require surgical procedures, multiple diagnostic tests, or consultations or who are immunocompromised may be better treated and evaluated in a brief hospitalization.

Patients with limb-threatening infections need to be hospitalized and treated parenterally with antibiotics. Empirical therapy for these infections should be broad in spectrum, including aerobic, gram-positive, and gram-negative organisms, as well as resistant organisms. Examples of antibiotic therapies include imipenem/cilastatin or vancomycin plus aztreonam plus metronidazole. Antibiotics should be reassessed when culture results are available.

Healing osteomyelitis with antibiotics alone is difficult but possible. Treatment usually lasts 6 weeks or more, often with 1–2 weeks of parenteral therapy. Infected bones that can be easily resected should be removed to speed recovery and reduce the need for antibiotic therapy. Additional regimens for treating diabetic foot infections can be found in the new international consensus guidelines for diagnosing and treating infected diabetic feet (Lipsky et al., 2012; Richard, Sotto, & Lavigne, 2011).

Methicillin-resistant *Staphylococcus aureus* (MRSA) and other resistant bacteria are a major challenge in the treatment of diabetic foot ulcer infections (Frykberg, 2003). Using data from a multihospital study in the United States, Pfaller et al. (2002) reported that the percentage of MRSA of all *S. aureus* isolates increased from 22% to 34% from 1997 to 2000. In Korea, the number of MRSA cases was found to be 32% in 2008 and then it rebounded back to 63.7% in 2011 (Huh, Kim, Cho, et al., 2013). Vancomycin or linezolid is frequently prescribed for the control of MRSA. Vancomycin-resistant *S. aureus*, the evolution of MRSA in response to current practices in antibiotic therapy, has been reported (Holmes, Moore, & Sundsfjord, 2016; McGuinness, Malachowa, & DeLeo, 2017).

Topical Wound Care

Evidence does not support the use of one antimicrobial dressing over the other for the treatment of diabetic foot ulcers (Dumville et al., 2017). Topical therapy for diabetic foot ulcers is based on the principles outlined in Chapter 21, and a formulary of multiple dressing options is needed to accommodate the characteristics of the wound as they (e.g., size, depth, and exudate) change.

The increase in bacterial resistance to antibiotics has changed how clinicians view the use of topical antimicrobials. However, a recent meta-analysis reported more diabetic ulcers may heal with an antimicrobial dressing (e.g., silver, iodide) than a nonantimicrobial dressing (risk ratio = 1.28, 95% CI 1.12–1.45) (Dumville et al., 2017). Therefore, despite the low certainty of the evidence due to study design and small samples, the researchers recommended the use of antimicrobial dressings vs nonantimicrobial dressings for diabetic foot ulcers. This is particularly relevant given the fact that diabetic foot ulcers have a high prevalence of multispecies biofilm (Johani, et al., 2017; Malone, et al., 2017). See Chapter 19 for more details regarding topical management of biofilm and wound infection.

Advanced care has been described as "the use of drugs, devices, or treatment regimens that may be experimental, newly approved, or above and beyond treatment modalities routinely used in the general community for a specific medical problem." Advanced care may sometimes be the only means of rapidly and effectively attaining wound closure (Mulder et al., 2003). Diabetic foot ulcers that are limb threatening (based on ADA criteria) and require hospitalization, antibiotics, and debridement may not progress to this level (or any further) if early advanced care interventions are made. Early, advanced, or "appropriate" care practices may be more cost-effective than standard care practices in decreasing the incidence of lower extremity amputations (Apelqvist, Ragnarson-Tennvall, Larsson, et al., 1995; Warriner & Driver, 2006).

When confronted with a wound that fails to progress, the clinician must carefully reevaluate the entire treatment plan to ensure appropriateness and should consider biopsy to rule out malignancy. If the biopsy result is negative and the management plan is appropriate, the most likely reason for failure to heal is the negative cellular environment of a chronic wound. In this case, the clinician should consider implementing an interactive wound therapy, that is, a product or therapy designed to convert the chronic wound environment into an environment that supports repair (Driver, 2004). Specific therapies that have shown varying degrees of success in the management of diabetic foot ulcers include contact and noncontact ultrasound technologies, regenerative tissue matrix, electrical stimulation, negative pressure wound therapy, hyperbaric oxygen therapy, angiogenic stimulators, and protease inhibitors (Cullen, Smith, McCulloch, et al., 2002; Driver & Fabbi, 2010; Driver & LeBretton, 2008; Park et al., 2013). These therapies are discussed in Chapters 22–27.

Pain Control

Various interventions can be used for the treatment of neuropathic pain. Management of wound pain is discussed in detail in Chapter 28. In some cases, referral of the patient to a pain clinic and to neurologists for pain management may be necessary (American Society of Anesthesiologists [ASA], 2014).

Education

Basic knowledge assessment of patients with diabetes, regardless of the length of time since their diagnosis, often reveals a lack of understanding about the principles of diabetes self-management. Education must be relevant, simple, complete, and ongoing in order to assist the patient to achieve and maintain the highest possible level of functioning. However, education does not equal knowledge. Achieving understanding often requires presentation of material multiple times in different formats and by different health care team members.

Key components of the patient's education plan require behavioral change on the part of the patient, which can leave the patient feeling overwhelmed. The inability of the patient to follow through with a treatment plan should be carefully scrutinized and explored. The patient's behavior should not be assumed to be intentional nor should the patient be erroneously labeled as "noncompliant," as many factors can contribute to an individual's ability to succeed or fail in

adhering to the treatment plan. Key among these factors is expecting the patient to implement a therapy that he or she is physically unable to perform or that conflicts with another activity in his or her life. Probably the best advice to health care professionals was provided by Heisler and colleagues (Heisler, Bouknight, Hayward, et al., 2007; Heisler, Cole, Weir, et al., 2007), that to facilitate patients' self-management, there is a need for a paradigm shift in the relations between provider and patients from directive to a more collaborative interactive style in which problems, treatment goals, and management stratagems are defined together.

Studies have documented the success of diabetes and foot care education in reducing the incidence of diabetic foot ulcers (Al-Wahbi, 2010; Barshes, Saedi, & Wrobel, 2017; Dargis, Pantelejeva, Jonushaite, et al., 1999). However, many of the studies documenting success of educational efforts at reducing diabetic foot problems compared comprehensive programs that may not exist in more operational settings. In real-world situations, both patients and providers face significant challenges in the areas of diabetes and diabetic foot care education. A study in south Texas showed contextual factors such as time constraints, practice economics, and low reimbursement rather than physician knowledge and attitude affected caregivers' performance in delivering diabetes care education. The study also found that patients with a lower income had a decreased awareness of diabetic care principles (Larme & Pugh, 2001).

Appropriate measures should be implemented for patients who have limited mobility, cognitive problems, and visual difficulties. Other family members or friends can assist with visual assessments. Many patients diagnosed with diabetes participate in general diabetes self-management education programs through their primary health care provider (ADA, 2014). Some clinics include a preexamination and a postexamination test on diabetes and foot care knowledge, providing an opportunity to build on the patient's knowledge base. The test is scored at the time of the visit, and the patient was told that the test will be repeated at the end of the visit.

It is imperative that patients understand the importance of daily foot examinations, the implications of losing protective sensation, their risk for ulceration and amputation, and the methods for minimizing or eliminating factors that place them at risk for ulceration and amputation. Box 17.5 provides an example of general foot care instructions that can be given to patients (WOCN Society, 2021).

Teaching appropriate footwear selection is essential. All patients need to pay special attention to the fit and style of their shoes. Shoes need to fit the foot, so patients should avoid tight-fitting shoes, pointed-toe or open-toe shoes, flip-flops, and high heels. The shoes should be able to breathe; plastic shoes are inelastic and do not breathe. Finally, shoes should be adjustable with hook and loop closures, laces, or buckles. Shoes with soft insoles that cushion the feet may do well at reducing plantar pressure, but injury to the dorsum may result if the upper part of the shoes does not fit when the insole is inserted (Cavanagh & Ulbrecht, 2008).

CLINICAL CONSULT

A: Referral received for wound care consult for a 50-year-old male with diabetes presenting with a large demarcated ulceration on the posterior aspect of the plantar surface of the right calcaneus. Patient's type 1 diabetes first diagnosed at age 15 and appears to have overall good level of knowledge of DM and self-care needs. Lower leg without edema, hair present, warm to touch, all pedal pulses palpable. Small amount of callous present lateral to ulceration and over plantar surface of first metatarsal head. Loss of protective sensation present (0/10 with monofilament testing both feet). Reports walking barefoot in his home and in yard; often does not wear socks. Has never seen a podiatrist or foot specialist. Three days ago, a rock fell out of his shoe as it was being removed and he discovered a large, red, open wound on the plantar surface of his foot. Ulcer measures 4×3 cm $\times$ 1 cm. Wound base is 90% red, viable tissue with 10% yellow slough. No surrounding erythema or callous; minimal exudate present. Dry gauze in place over wound and adherent to wound bed.

D: Neuropathic diabetic foot ulcer in patient with high-risk diabetes; ulceration due to undetected object in shoe.

P: Promote moist wound healing, stimulate cellular activity, avoid repetitive stress and trauma to ulcer site, review essentials of foot care in insensate feet; refer to foot specialists to assess for appropriate footwear and provide ongoing routine monitoring.

I: (1) Review teaching materials for "Care of the Diabetic Foot" to include foot inspection before applying and after removing shoes, daily washing and drying well between toes, routine and appropriate nail care, no "bare-feet," and wear cotton socks. (2) Foot specialist to recommend appropriate footwear after ulcer heals. (3) TBI while in clinic and if >0.5 will notify mid-level provider to proceed with sharp debridement. (4) Apply thin layer of cadexomer iodine to nonadherent gauze and apply to the wound secure with roll gauze. Change three times weekly. (5) Return to wound clinic weekly to monitor for changes and debride as needed. (6) No weight bearing on right heel to protect ulcer from stress/friction. (7) Consult with PT to address ambulation needs. May use crutches.

E: Monitor wound dimensions weekly; anticipate at least 30% reduced size by week 10 and healed by week 20. Will reevaluate need for contact cast if unable to adequately offload wound site or healing slower than anticipated.

SUMMARY

- Peripheral neuropathy, structural foot problems, and minor trauma are the primary causative factors for a diabetic foot ulcer in the patient with LEND, and 25% of patients with a diabetic foot ulcer require lower extremity amputation.
- The ultimate goals of care of the patient with LEND and a diabetic foot ulcer are to reduce the incidence of lower extremity amputations and to increase the frequency of minor or partial foot amputations as a percentage of all lower extremity amputations.
- A team approach is required for comprehensive management of the patient with LEND to adequately address the complex needs of this patient population: prevention of injury or trauma, frequent inspection, diligent daily foot care, education and support, and appropriate offloading (i.e., use of shoes and orthotics).

SELF-ASSESSMENT QUESTIONS

1. 20% of patients with a diabetic foot ulcer (DFU) experience:
   a. Neuropathy
   b. Chronic inflammation
   c. Renal dialysis
   d. Amputation

2. DFUs result from a combination of:
   a. Neuropathy
   b. Hyperglycemia
   c. Ischemia
   d. All

3. Which of the following is the best intervention for the prevention of DFU and subsequent amputation?
   a. Adhering to oral medication therapy during hypoglycemic agents
   b. Controlling glucose through dietary measures

   c. Obtaining new footwear on yearly basis
   d. Obtaining regular foot examination

4. Which factors must be addressed in the management plan of a patient with a diabetic foot ulcer.
   a. Growth factors
   b. Hyperglycemia
   c. Offloading
   d. b and c

5. Routine teaching of the patient with lower extremity neuropathic disease include all but:
   a. Testing water with hands or elbow.
   b. Foot soaks.
   c. Apply moisturizing cream to feet, but not between toes.
   d. Proper footwear and inspecting inside shoes.

REFERENCES

Abbas, Z. G., Lutale, J. K., Game, F. L., & Jeffcoate, W. J. (2008). Comparison of four systems of classification of diabetic foot ulcers in Tanzania. *Diabetic Medicine, 25*(2), 134–137.

Abbott, C. A., Carrington, A. L., Ashe, H., et al. (2002). The North-West Diabetes Foot Care Study: Incidence of, and risk factors for, new diabetic-foot ulceration in a community-based patient cohort. *Diabetic Medicine, 19*(5), 377–384.

Abbott, C. A., Chawin, K. E., & Foden, P. (2019). Innovative intelligent insole system reduces diabetic foot ulcer recurrence at plantar sites: A prospective, randomized, proof of concept study. *Lancet, 1*(10), e308–e318.

Alaia, E. F., Chhabra, A., Simpfendorfer, C. S., Cohen, M., Mintz, D. N., Vossen, J. A., et al. (2021). MRI nomenclature for musculoskeletal infection. *Skeletal Radiology, 50*(12), 2319–2347. https://doi.org/10.1007/s00256-021-03807-7.

Alavi, A., Sibbald, R. G., Mayer, D., et al. (2014). Diabetic foot ulcers: Part 1: Pathophysiology and prevention. *Journal of the American Academy of Dermatology, 70*(1), e1–e18.

Aldana, P. C., & Khachemoune, A. (2020). Diabetic foot ulcers: Appraising standard of care and reviewing new trends in management. *American Journal of Clinical Dermatology, 21*(2), 255–264. https://doi.org/10.1007/s40257-019-00495-x

Al-Wahbi, A. M. (2010). Impact of a diabetic foot care education program on lower limb amputation rate. *Vascular Health and Risk Management, 6,* 923–934.

American Academy of Pediatrics. (2013). *Management of newly diagnosed type 2 diabetes mellitus (T2DM) in children and adolescents.* Accessed 2/14/2020. Retrieved from https://pediatrics.aappublications.org/content/pediatrics/131/2/364.full.pdf.

American Diabetes Association (ADA). (1999). Consensus development conference on diabetic foot wound care. *Diabetes Care, 22*(8), 1354–1360.

American Diabetes Association (ADA). (2007). Standards of medical care in diabetes—2007. *Diabetes Care, 30*(Suppl. 1), S4–S41.

American Diabetes Association (ADA). (2008). Comprehensive foot examination and risk assessment. *Diabetes Care, 31*(8), 1679–1685.

American Diabetes Association (ADA). (2014). Standards of medical care in diabetes. *Diabetes Care, 37*(Suppl. 1), S14–S80.

American Society of Anesthesiologists (ASA). (2014). *Standards, guidelines and statements and other documents.* Accessed 12/14/2019. Retrieved from https://www.asahq.org/For-Members/Clinical-Information/Standards-Guidelines-and-Statements.aspx.

Apelqvist, J., & Larsson, J. (2000). What is the most effective way to reduce incidence of amputation in diabetic foot? *Diabetes/Metabolism Research and Reviews, 16*(Suppl. 1), S75–S83.

Apelqvist, J., Ragnarson-Tennvall, G., Larsson, J., et al. (1995). Long-term costs for foot ulcers in diabetic patients in a multidisciplinary setting. *Foot & Ankle International, 16,* 388–394.

Armstrong, D. G., Boulton, A. J. M., & Bus, S. A. (2017). Diabetic foot ulcers and their recurrence. *The New England Journal of Medicine, 376*(24), 2367–2375.

Armstrong, D. G., Lavery, L. A., & Harkless, L. B. (1998). Validation of a diabetic wound classification system: The contribution of depth, infection, and ischemia to risk of amputation. *Diabetes Care, 21*(5), 855–859.

Armstrong, D. G., Lavery, L. A., Kimbriel, H. R., et al. (2003). Activity patterns with diabetic foot ulceration: Patients with active ulceration may not adhere to a standard pressure off-loading regimen. *Diabetes Care, 26*(9), 2595–2597.

Armstrong, D. G., Lavery, L. A., Vazquez, J. R., et al. (2003). Clinical efficacy of the first metatarsophalangeal joint arthroplasty as a curative procedure for hallux interphalangeal joint wounds in patients with diabetes. *Diabetes Care, 26*(12), 3284–3287.

Armstrong, D. G., Lavery, L. A., Wu, S., et al. (2005). Evaluation of removable and irremovable cast walkers in the healing of diabetic foot wounds: A randomized controlled trial. *Diabetes Care, 28*(3), 551–554.

Armstrong, D. G., Nguyen, H. C., Lavery, L. A., et al. (2001). Off-loading the diabetic foot wound: A randomized clinical trial. *Diabetes Care, 24*(6), 1019–1022.

Armstrong, D. G., Perales, T. A., Murff, R. T., et al. (1996). Value of white blood cell count with differential in the acute diabetic foot infection. *Journal of the American Podiatric Medical Association, 86*(5), 224–227.

Armstrong, D. G., Rosales, M. A., & Gashi, A. (2005). Efficacy of fifth metatarsal head resection for treatment of chronic diabetic foot ulceration. *Journal of the American Podiatric Medical Association, 95*(4), 353–356.

Aulivola, B., Hile, C. N., Hamdan, A. D., et al. (2004). Major lower extremity amputation: Outcome of a modern series. *Archives of Surgery, 139*(4), 395–399.

Barshes, N. R., Saedi, S., & Wrobel, J. (2017). A model to estimate cost-savings in diabetic foot ulcer prevention efforts. *Journal of Diabetes and Its Complications, 31*(4), 700–707.

Berendt, A. R., Peters, E. J., Bakker, K., et al. (2008). Diabetic foot osteomyelitis: A progress report on diagnosis and a systematic review of treatment. *Diabetes/Metabolism Research and Reviews, 24*(Suppl. 1), S145–S161.

Berman, S., Quick, R., Yoder, P., et al. (2006). Treprostinil sodium (Remodulin), a prostacyclin analog, in the treatment of critical limb ischemia: Open-label study. *Vascular, 14*(3), 142–148.

Birke, J. A., Pavich, M. A., Patout, C. A., Jr., et al. (2002). Comparison of forefoot ulcer healing using alternative off-loading methods in patients with diabetes mellitus. *Advances in Skin & Wound Care, 15*(5), 210–215.

Boulton, A. J. M. (2004). Pressure and the diabetic foot: Clinical science and offloading techniques. *American Journal of Surgery, 187*(5A), 17S–24S.

Boulton, A. J. M., Armstrong, D. G., Albert, S. F., et al. (2008). Comprehensive foot examination and risk assessment: A report of the Task Force of the Foot Care Interest Group of the American Diabetes Association, with endorsement by the American Association of Clinical Endocrinologists. *Diabetes Care, 31*(8), 1679–1685.

Boulton, A. J. M., Rayman, G., & Wukich, D. K. (2020). *Foot in diabetes* (5th ed.). Hoboken: John Wiley and Sons Ltd.

Boulton, A. J. M., Vilekyte, L., Ragnarson-Tennvall, G., et al. (2005). The global burden of diabetic foot disease. *Lancet, 366,* 1719–1724.

Bowen, G. C. (2015). Screening and treatment of early complications in the diabetic foot. In *Management of diabetic foot complications.* London: Springer-Verlag.

Bravo-Molina, A., Linares-Palomino, J. P., Vera-Arroyo, B., Salmerón-Febres, L. M., & Ros-Díe, E. (2016). Inter-observer agreement of the Wagner, University of Texas and PEDIS classification systems for the diabetic foot syndrome. *Foot and Ankle Surgery, 24*(1), 60–64. https://doi.org/10.1016/j.fas. 2016.10.009.

Bus, S. A., Valk, G. D., van Deursen, R. W., et al. (2008). The effectiveness of footwear and offloading interventions to prevent and heal foot ulcers and reduce plantar pressure in diabetes: A systematic review. *Diabetes/Metabolism Research and Reviews, 24*(Suppl. 1), S162–S180.

Cardinal, M., Eisenbud, D. E., Armstrong, D. G., et al. (2009). Serial surgical debridement: A retrospective study on clinical outcomes in chronic lower extremity wounds. *Wound Repair and Regeneration, 17*(3), 306–311.

Caselli, A., Pham, H., Giurini, J. M., et al. (2002). The forefoot-to-rearfoot plantar pressure ratio is increased in severe diabetic neuropathy and can predict foot ulceration. *Diabetes Care, 25*(6), 1066–1071.

Catanzariti, A. R., Mendicino, R., & Haverstock, B. (2000). Ostectomy for diabetic neuroarthropathy involving the midfoot. *The Journal of Foot and Ankle Surgery, 39*(5), 291–300.

Cavanagh, P. R., & Ulbrecht, J. S. (2008). The biomechanics of the foot in diabetes mellitus. In *Levin and O'Neal's the diabetic foot* (7th ed.). St. Louis: Mosby.

Centers for Disease Control and Prevention (CDC). (2003). History of foot ulcer among persons with diabetes—United States, 2000–2002. *MMWR. Morbidity and Mortality Weekly Report, 52*(45), 1098–1102.

Centers for Disease Control and Prevention (CDC). (2014). *Hospital discharge rates for nontraumatic lower extremity amputation per 1,000 diabetic population, by age, United States 1988–2009.* Accessed 2/14/2020. Retrieved from https://www.cdc.gov/mmwr/preview/mmwrhtml/mm5043a3.htm.

Centers for Disease Control and Prevention (CDC). (2020). *National diabetes statistics report, 2020.* Atlanta, GA: Centers for Disease Control and Prevention, U.S. Department of Health and Human Services. Accessed 8/10/2020. Retrieved from https://www.cdc.gov/diabetes/library/features/diabetes-stat-report.html.

Centers for Disease Control and Prevention (CDC). (2022). *The facts, stats, and impacts of diabetes.* Atlanta, GA: Centers for Disease Control and Prevention, U.S. Department of Health and Human Services. Retrieved 11/14/2022 from https://www.cdc.gov/diabetes/library/spotlights/diabetes-facts-stats.html.

Cofield, R. H., Morrison, M. J., & Beabout, J. W. (1983). Diabetic neuroarthropathy in the foot: Patient characteristics and patterns of radiographic change. *Foot & Ankle, 4*(1), 15–22.

Corey, M. R., St Julien, J., Miller, C., et al. (2012). Patient education level affects functionality and long-term mortality after major lower extremity amputation. *American Journal of Surgery, 204*(5), 626–630.

Cullen, B., Smith, R., McCulloch, E., et al. (2002). Mechanism of action of PROMOGRAN, a protease modulating matrix, for the treatment of diabetic foot ulcers. *Wound Repair and Regeneration, 10*(1), 16–25.

Dall, T., Wang, W., Gillespie, K., et al. (2019). The economic burden of elevated blood glucose level in 2017: Diagnosed and undiagnosed diabetes, gestational diabetes mellitus and prediabetes. *Diabetes Care, 42*(9), 1661–1668.

Dargis, V., Pantelejeva, O., Jonushaite, A., et al. (1999). Benefits of a multidisciplinary approach in the management of recurrent diabetic foot ulceration in Lithuania: A prospective study. *Diabetes Care, 22*(9), 1428–1431.

Driver, V. R. (2004). Treating the macro and micro wound environment of the diabetic patient: Managing the whole patient, not the hole in the patient. *Foot Ankle Quarterly. The Seminar Journal, 16*(2), 47–56.

Driver, V. R., & Fabbi, M. (2010). Recent advances in the use of ultrasound in wound care. In *Vol. 1. Advances in wound care.* New Rochelle: Mary Ann Liebert, Inc.

Driver, V. R., Fabbi, M., Lavery, L. A., et al. (2010). The costs of diabetic foot: The economic case for the limb salvage team. *Journal of Vascular Surgery, 52*(3), 17S–22S.

Driver, V. R., & LeBretton, J. M. (2008). "Gene therapy"-therapeutic angiogenesis—Does it have an impact for wound healing and limb preservation? *Podiatry Today,* 74–78.

Driver, V. R., Madsen, J., & Goodman, R. A. (2005). Reducing amputation rates in patients with diabetes at a military medical center: The limb preservation service model. *Diabetes Care, 28*(2), 248–253.

Dumville, J. C., Lipsky, B. A., & Cochrane Wound Group. (2017). Topical antimicrobial agents for treating foot ulcers in people with diabetes. *Cochrane Database of Systematic Reviews, 6,* CD011038. Accessed 8/5/2020. Retrieved from https://pubmed.ncbi.nlm.nih.gov/28613416/.

Eichenholtz, S. N. (1966). Charcot joints. Charles C Thomas, Springfield, III, pp. 3–10.

Eneroth, M., Apelqvist, J., & Stenström, A. (1997). Clinical characteristics and outcome in 223 diabetic patients with deep foot infections. *Foot & Ankle International, 18*(11), 716–722.

Finestone, A. S., Tamir, E., & Ron, G. (2018). Surgical offloading procedure for diabetic foot ulcers compared to best nonsurgical treatment: A study protocol for a randomized controlled trial. *Journal of Foot and Ankle Research, 11*(6). https://doi.org/10.1186/s13047-0180248-3.

Fosse, S., Hartemann-Heurtier, A., Jacqueminet, S., et al. (2009). Incidence and characteristics of lower limb amputations in people with diabetes. *Diabetic Medicine, 26,* 391–396.

Fowler, M. J. (2008). Microvascular and macrovascular complications of diabetes. *Clinical Diabetes, 26*(2), 77–82.

Frykberg, R. G. (2002). Diabetic foot ulcers: Pathogenesis and management. *American Family Physician, 66,* 1655–1662.

Frykberg, R. G. (2003). An evidence-based approach to diabetic foot infections. *American Journal of Surgery, 186*(5A), 44S–54S.

Frykberg, R. G., Zgonis, T., Armstrong, D. G., et al. (2006). Diabetic foot disorders—A clinical practice guideline. *The Journal of Foot and Ankle Surgery, 45*(Suppl. 5), S1–S66.

Games, F. (2016). Classification of diabetic foot ulcers. *Diabetes/Metabolism Research and Reviews, 32*(Suppl. 1), 186–194.

Garcia, L. A. (2006). Epidemiology and pathophysiology of lower extremity peripheral arterial disease. *Journal of Endovascular Therapy, 13*(Suppl. 2), II3–II9. https://doi.org/10.1177/15266028060130S204.

Geiss, L. S., et al. (2019). Resurgence of diabetes-related nontraumatic lower-extremity amputation in the young and middle-aged adult U.S. population. *Diabetes Care, 42*(1), 50–54.

Gerald, Y. V., & Hudson, J. R. (2002). Evaluation and treatment of stage 0 Charcot's neuroarthropathy of the foot and ankle. *Journal of the American Podiatric Medical Association, 92*(4), 210–220.

Grady, J. F., O'Connor, K. J., Axe, T. M., et al. (2000). Use of electrostimulation in the treatment of diabetic neuropathy. *Journal of the American Podiatric Medical Association, 90*(6), 287–294.

Guis, S., Pellissier, J. F., Arniaud, D., et al. (1999). Healing of Charcot's joint by pamidronate infusion. *The Journal of Rheumatology, 26*(8), 1843–1845.

Harrington, C., Zagari, M. J., Corea, J., et al. (2000). A cost analysis of diabetic lower-extremity ulcers. *Diabetes Care, 23*(9), 1333–1338.

Heisler, M., Bouknight, R. R., Hayward, R. A., et al. (2007). The relative importance of physician communication, participatory decision making, and patient understanding in diabetes self-management. *Journal of General Internal Medicine, 17*(4), 243–252.

Heisler, M., Cole, I., Weir, D., et al. (2007). Does physician communication influence older patients' diabetes self-management and glycemic control? *The Journals of Gerontology. Series A, Biological Sciences and Medical Sciences, 62*(12), 1435–1442.

Higorani, A., LaMuraglia, G. M., & Henke, P. (2016). The management of diabetic foot: A clinical practice guideline by the Society for Vascular Surgery in collaboration with the American Podiatric Medical Association and Society for Vascular Medicine. *Journal of Vascular Surgery, 62*(2), 3S–21S.

Holmes, A. H., Moore, L. S. P., & Sundsfjord, A. (2016). Understanding the mechanisms and drivers of antimicrobial resistance. *Lancet, 387*, 176–187.

Huh, K. M., Kim, J., Cho, S. Y., et al. (2013). Continuous increase of the antimicrobial resistance among gram-negative pathogens causing bacteremia: A nationwide surveillance study by the Korean Network for Study on Infectious Disease (KONSID). *Diagnostic Microbiology and Infectious Disease, 76*, 477–482.

Hussain, N., & Adrian, T. E. (2017). Diabetic neuropathy update on pathophysiological mechanism and the possible involvement of glutamate pathways. *Current Diabetes Reviews, 13*(5).

Ince, P., Abbas, Z. G., Lutale, J. K., et al. (2008). Use of the SINBAD classification system and score in comparing outcome of foot ulcer management on three continents. *Diabetes Care, 31*(5), 964–967.

International Working Group on the Diabetes Foot (IWGDF). (2019). *IWGDF guidelines*. Retrieved from https://www.iwgdfguidelines.org.

Jeffcoate, W. J., & Harding, K. G. (2003). Diabetic foot ulcers. *Lancet, 361*(9368), 1545–1551.

Johani, K., Malone, M., Jensen, S., Gosbell, I., Dickson, H., Hu, H., et al. (2017). Microscopy visualisation confirms multi-species biofilms are ubiquitous in diabetic foot ulcers. *International Wound Journal, 14*, 1160–1169.

Jude, E. B., Oyibo, S. O., Chalmers, N., et al. (2001). Peripheral arterial disease in diabetic and nondiabetic patients: A comparison of severity and outcome. *Diabetes Care, 24*(8), 1433–1437.

Laborde, J. M. (2008). Neuropathic plantar forefoot ulcer treated with tendon lengthenings. *Foot & Ankle International, 29*(4), 378–388.

Larme, A. C., & Pugh, J. A. (2001). Evidence-based guidelines meet the real world. *Diabetes Care, 24*(10), 1728–1733.

Lavery, L. A. (2013). Preventing the first or recurrent ulcers. *The Medical Clinics of North America, 97*(5), 807–820.

Lavery, L. A., Armstrong, D. G., Boulton, A. J., et al. (2002). Ankle equinus deformity and its relationship to high plantar pressure in a large population with diabetes mellitus. *Journal of the American Podiatric Medical Association, 92*(9), 479–482.

Lavery, L. A., Armstrong, D. G., & Harkless, L. B. (1996). Classification of diabetic foot wounds. *The Journal of Foot and Ankle Surgery, 35*(6), 528–531.

Lavery, L. A., Armstrong, D. G., Vela, S. A., et al. (1998). Practical criteria for screening patients at high risk for diabetic foot ulceration. *Archives of Internal Medicine, 158*, 157–162.

Lavery, L. A., Armstrong, D. G., Wunderlich, R. P., et al. (2003). Diabetic foot syndrome: Evaluating the prevalence and incidence of foot pathology in Mexican Americans and non-Hispanic whites from a diabetes disease management cohort. *Diabetes Care, 26*(5), 1435–1438.

Lee, M. S., Rha, A. Q., & Han, A. K. (2015). Comparison of diabetic and non-diabetic patients undergoing endovascular revascularization for peripheral arterial disease. *The Journal of Invasive Cardiology, 27*(3), 167–171.

Levin, M. E. (2002). Management of the diabetic foot: Preventing amputation. *Southern Medical Journal, 95*(1), 10–20.

Levy, P. J. (2002). Epidemiology and pathophysiology of peripheral arterial disease. *Clinical Cornerstone, 4*(5), 1–15.

Lin, S. S., Bono, C. M., & Lee, T. H. (2000). Total contact casting and Keller arthroplasty for diabetic great toe ulceration under the interphalangeal joint. *Foot & Ankle International, 21*, 588–591.

Lipsky, B. A., Berendt, A. R., Cornia, P. B., et al. (2012). Infectious Diseases Society of America clinical practice guideline for the diagnosis and treatment of diabetic foot infections. *Clinical Infectious Diseases, 54*(12), e132–e173.

Lombardo, F. L., Maggini, M., & Anichini, R. (2014). Lower extremity amputation in person with and without diabetes in Italy: 2001–2010. *PLoS One, 9*(1), e86405.

Macfarlane, R., & Jeffcoate, W. (1999). Classification of diabetic foot ulcers: The size (area and depth) (SAD) system. *Diabetic Foot, 2*(4), 123.

Malone, M., Johani, K., Jensen, S. O., Gosbell, I. B., Dickson, H. G., McLennan, S., et al. (2017). Effect of cadexomer iodine on the microbial load and diversity of chronic non-healing diabetic foot ulcers complicated by biofilm *in vivo. Journal of Antimicrobial Chemotherapy, 72*, 2093–2101.

Margolis, D. J., Kantor, J., Santanna, J., Strom, B. J., & Berlin, J. A. (2000). Risk factors for delayed healing of neuropathic diabetic foot ulcers: A pooled analysis. *Archives of Dermatology, 136*(12), 1531–1535.

Mayfield, J. A., Reiber, G. E., Maynard, C., et al. (2000). Trends in lower limb amputation in the Veterans Health Administration, 1989–1998. *Journal of Rehabilitation Research and Development, 37*(1), 23–30.

McGuinness, W. A., Malachowa, N., & DeLeo, F. R. (2017). Vancomycin resistance in *Staphylococcus aureus. Yale Journal of Biology and Medicine, 90*(2), 269–281.

Mendes, J. J., & Neves, J. (2012). Diabetic foot infections: Current diagnosis and treatment. *The Journal of Diabetic Foot Complications, 4*(2), 26–45.

Mills, J. L., Sr., Conte, M. S., Armstrong, D. G., et al. (2014). The Society for Vascular Surgery Lower Extremity Threatened Limb Classification System: Risk stratification based on Wound, Ischemia, and foot Infection (WIfI). *Journal of Vascular Surgery, 59*, 220–234.

Mohler, E. R., 3rd, Klugherz, B., Goldman, R., et al. (2000). Trial of a novel prostacyclin analog, UT-15, in patients with severe intermittent claudication. *Vascular Medicine, 5*(4), 231–237.

Monteiro-Soares, M., Boyko, E. J., Jeffcoate, W., Mills, J. L., Russell, D., Morbach, S., & Game, F. (2020). Diabetic foot ulcer classifications: A critical review. *Diabetes/Metabolism Research and Reviews, 36*(S1), e3272.

Monteiro-Soares, M., Russel, D., et al. (2019). *IWGDF guideline on the classification of diabetic foot ulcer*. Netherland, Australia, UK and USA: International Working Group on the Diabetic Foot. Accessed 2/14/2020. Retrieved from www.iwgdfguidelines.org.

Moulik, P. K., Mtonga, R., & Gill, G. V. (2003). Amputation and mortality in new-onset foot ulcers stratified by etiology. *Diabetes Care, 26*(2), 491–494.

Mueller, T., Hinterreiter, F., & Luft, C. (2014). Mortality rates and mortality predictors in patients with symptomatic peripheral artery disease stratified according to age and diabetes. *Journal of Vascular Surgery, 59*(5), 1291–1299.

Mueller, M. J., Sinacore, D. R., Hastings, M. K., et al. (2003). Effect of Achilles tendon lengthening on neuropathic plantar ulcers.

A randomized clinical trial. *Journal of Bone and Joint Surgery,* *85*(8), 1436–1445.

Mueller, M. J., Sinacore, D. R., Hastings, M. K., et al. (2004). Impact of Achilles tendon lengthening on functional limitations and perceived disability in people with a neuropathic plantar ulcer. *Diabetes Care, 27*(7), 1559–1564.

Mulder, G., Armstrong, D., & Seaman, S. (2003). Standard, appropriate, and advanced care and medical-legal considerations. Part one—Diabetic foot ulcerations. *Wounds, 15*(4), 92.

Muller, I. S., De Grauw, W. J., Van Gerwen, W. H., et al. (2002). Foot ulceration and lower limb amputation in type 2 diabetic patients in Dutch primary health care. *Diabetes Care, 25*(3), 570–574.

Murray, H. J., Young, M. H., Hollis, S., et al. (1996). The relationship between callus formation, high pressures and neuropathy in diabetic foot ulceration. *Diabetic Medicine, 13,* 979–982.

Nathan, D. M., Buse, J. B., Davidson, M. B., et al. (2009). Medical management of hyperglycemia in type 2 diabetes: A consensus algorithm for the initiation and adjustment of therapy. A consensus statement of the America Diabetes Association and the European Association for the Study of Diabetes. *Diabetes Care, 32* (1), 193–203.

National Institute for Health and Clinical Excellent (NICE). (2011). *Guideline; Diabetic foot problems.* Accessed 8/5/2020. Retrieved from http://www.nice.org.uk/guidance/CG119.

National Institute of Neurological Disorders and Stroke (NINDS), National Institutes of Health. (2003). *NINDS peripheral neuropathy information page.* Accessed 8/5/2020. Retrieved from https://www.ninds.nih.gov/Disorders/Patient-Caregiver-Education/Fact-Sheets/Peripheral-Neuropathy-Fact-Sheet.

NCD Risk Factor Collaboration (NCD-RisC). (2016). Worldwide trends in diabetes since 1980: A pooled analysis of 751 population-based studies with 4*4 millions participants. *Lancet, 387,* 1513–1530.

O'Brien, P. D., Hinder, L. M., & Sakowski, S. A. (2014). ER stress in diabetic peripheral neuropathy: A new therapeutic agent. *Antioxidants & Redox Signaling, 21*(4), 621–633.

Okonkwo, U. A., & Dipietro, L. A. (2017). Diabetes and wound angiogenesis. *International Journal of Molecular Sciences, 18*(7), 1419–1466.

Ostergard, L., Finnerup, N. B., & Andersen, H. (2015). The effects of capillary dysfunction on oxygen and glucose extraction in diabetic neuropathy. *Diabetology, 58*(4), 666–677.

Oyibo, S. O., Jude, E. B., & Tarawneh, I. (2001). A comparison of two diabetic foot ulcer classification systems: The Wagner and the University of Texas wound classification systems. *Diabetes Care, 24*(1), 84–88.

Oyibo, S. O., Jude, E. B., & Voyatzoglou, D. (2002). Clinical characteristics of patients with diabetic foot problems: Changing patterns of foot ulcer presentation. *Practical Diabetes International, 19,* 10–12.

Parisi, M. C. R., Zantut-Wittmann, D. E., Pavin, E. J., et al. (2008). Comparison of three systems of classification in predicting the outcome of diabetic foot ulcers in a Brazilian population. *European Journal of Endocrinology, 159,* 417–422.

Park, N., Allen, L., & Driver, V. L. (2013). Updating on understanding and managing chronic wound. *Dermatologic Therapy, 26*(3), 236–256.

Pecoraro, R. E., Reiber, G. E., & Burgess, E. M. (1990). Pathways to diabetic limb amputation. Basis for prevention. *Diabetes Care, 13* (5), 513–521.

Pemayun, T. G. D., Naibaho, R. M., & Minuljo, T. T. (2015). Risk factors for lower extremity amputation in patient with diabetic foot ulcers: A hospital-based case-control study. *Diabetic Foot and Ankle, 6,* 1–42.

Perkins, B. A., Olaleye, D., & Zinman, B. (2001). Simple screening tests for peripheral neuropathy in the diabetes clinic. *Diabetes Care, 24*(2), 250–256.

Peters, E. J. G., & Lavery, L. A. (2001). Effectiveness of the diabetic foot risk classification system of the International Working Group on the Diabetic Foot. *Diabetes Care, 24*(8), 1442–1447.

Pfaller, M. A., Diekema, D. J., Jones, R. N., Messer, S. A., Hollis, R. J., & SENTRY Participants Group. (2002). Trends in antifungal susceptibility of Candida spp. isolated from pediatric and adult patients with bloodstream infections: SENTRY Antimicrobial Surveillance Program, 1997 to 2000. *Journal of Clinical Microbiology, 40,* 852–856.

Pham, H., Armstrong, D. G., & Harvey, C. (2000). Screening techniques to identify people at high risk for diabetic foot ulceration: A prospective multicenter trial. *Diabetes Care, 23*(5), 606–611.

Piagessi, A., Viacava, P., & Rizzo, L. (2003). Semiquantitative analysis of the histopathological features of the neuropathic foot ulcer: Effects of pressure relief. *Diabetes Care, 26*(11), 3123–3128.

Praet, S. F., & Louwerens, J. W. (2003). The influence of shoe design on plantar pressures in neuropathic feet. *Diabetes Care, 26*(2), 441–445.

Prompers, L., Schaper, N., & Apelqvist, J. (2008). Prediction of outcome in individuals with diabetic foot ulcers: Focus on the differences between individuals with and without peripheral arterial disease. The EURODIALE Study. *Diabetologia, 51*(5), 747–755.

Rajbhandari, S. M., Jenkins, R. C., & Davies, C. (2002). Charcot neuroarthropathy in diabetes mellitus. *Diabetologia, 45*(8), 1085–1096.

Ramsey, S. D., Newton, K., & Blough, D. (1999). Incidence, outcomes, and cost of foot ulcers in patients with diabetes. *Diabetes Care, 22*(3), 382–387.

Rathur, H. M., & Boulton, A. J. M. (2007). The diabetic foot. *Clinics in Dermatology, 25,* 109–120.

Reiber, G. E. (1995). Lower extremity foot ulcers and amputations in diabetes. In *Diabetes in America* (2nd ed.). Bethesda: National Institutes of Health.

Reiber, G. E., Vileikyte, L., & Boyko, E. J. (1999). Causal pathways for incident lower-extremity ulcers in patients with diabetes from two settings. *Diabetes Care, 22*(1), 157–162.

Rice, J. B., Desai, U., & Cumming, K. (2014). Burden of diabetic foot ulcers for Medicare and private insurers. *Diabetes Care, 37*(3), 651–658.

Richard, J. L., Sotto, A., & Lavigne, J. P. (2011). New insights in diabetic foot infection. *World Journal of Diabetes, 2*(2), 24–32.

Ritz, G., Rowland, W. D., & Rowland, J. W. (1996). Use of the Cam Walker in treating diabetic ulcers, a case report. *Journal of the American Podiatric Medical Association, 86*(6), 253–256.

Rogers, L. C., Frykberg, R. G., & Armstrong, D. G. (2011). The Charcot foot in diabetes. *Diabetes Care, 34*(9), 2123–2129.

Rosenbaum, A. J., & DiPreta, J. A. (2015). Classifications in brief: Eichenholtz classification of Charcot arthropathy. *Clinical Orthopaedics and Related Research, 473*(3), 1168–1171. https://doi.org/10.1007/s11999-014-4059-y.

Sanders, L. J. (2008). The Charcot's foot (pied de Charcot). In J. H. Bowker, & M. A. Pfeiffer (Eds.), *Levin and O'Neal's the diabetic foot* (7th ed.). St. Louis: Mosby.

Sanders, L. J., Robbins, J. M., & Edmonds, M. E. (2010). History of the team approach to amputation prevention: Pioneers and milestones. *Journal of Vascular Surgery, 52*(Suppl. 3), S3–S16.

Shah, B. R., & Hux, J. E. (2003). Quantifying the risk of infectious diseases for people with diabetes. *Diabetes Care, 26*(2), 510–513.

Shearer, A., Scuffham, P., & Gordois, A. (2003). Predicted costs and outcomes from reduced vibration detection in people with diabetes in the U.S. *Diabetes Care, 26*(8), 2305–2310.

Shibata, T., Tada, K., & Hashizume, C. (1990). The results of arthrodesis of the ankle for leprotic neuroarthropathy. *Journal of Bone and Joint Surgery, 72*(5), 749–756.

Sibbald, R. G., Elliott, J. A., Persaud-Jaimangal, R., Goodman, L., Armstrong, D. G., Harley, C., et al. (2021). Wound bed preparation 2021. *Advances in Skin & Wound Care, 34*(4), 183–195. https://doi.org/10.1097/01.ASW.0000733724.87630.d6. PMID: 33739948; PMCID: PMC7982138.

Sinacore, D. R., & Mueller, M. J. (2008a). Infectious problems of the foot in diabetic patients. In J. H. Bowker, & M. A. Pfeiffer (Eds.), *Levin and O'Neal's the diabetic foot* (7th ed.). St. Louis: Mosby.

Sinacore, D. R., & Mueller, M. J. (2008b). Offloading for diabetic foot disease. In J. H. Bowker, & M. A. Pfeiffer (Eds.), *Levin and O'Neal's the diabetic foot* (7th ed.). St. Louis: Mosby.

Singh, N., Armstrong, D. G., & Lipsky, B. A. (2005). Preventing foot ulcers in patient with diabetes. *Journal of the American Medical Association, 293*(2), 217–228.

Stockl, K., Vanderplas, A., & Tafesse, E. (2004). Cost of lower-extremity ulcers among patients with diabetes. *Diabetes Care, 27*(9), 2129–2130.

Sumpio, B. (2000). Primary care: Foot ulcers. *The New England Journal of Medicine, 343*(1), 787–793.

Tanenberg, R. J., & Donofrio, P. D. (2008). Neuropathic problems of the lower limbs of diabetic patients. In J. H. Bowker, & M. A. Pfeiffer (Eds.), *Levin and O'Neals the diabetic foot* (7th ed.). St. Louis: Mosby.

Treece, K. A., Macfarlane, R. M., Pound, P., Game, F. L., & Jeffcoate, W. J. (2004). Validation of a system of foot ulcer classification in diabetes mellitus. *Diabetic Medicine, 21*, 987–991.

Uckay, L., Gariani, K., & Dubois-Ferriere, V. (2016). Diabetic foot infections: Recent literature and cornerstones of management. *Current Opinion in Infectious Diseases, 29*(2), 145–152.

Umpierrez, G. E., Isaacs, S. D., & Bazargan, N. (2002). Hyperglycemia: An independent marker of in-hospital mortality in patients with undiagnosed diabetes. *The Journal of Clinical Endocrinology and Metabolism, 87*(3), 978–982.

van Netten, J. J., Sacco, I. C. N., Lavery, L. A., Monteiro-Soares, M., Rasmussen, A., Raspovic, A., et al. (2020). Treatment of modifiable risk factors for foot ulceration in persons with diabetes: asystematic review. *Diabetes/Metabolism Research and Reviews, 36*(S1), e3271.

van Netten, J. J., Woodburn, J., & Bus, S. A. (2020). The future for diabetic foot ulcer prevention: A paradigm shift from stratified healthcare towards personalized medicine. *Diabetes/Metabolism Research and Reviews.* https://doi.org/10.1002/dmrr.3234.

Vinik, A. I., Bril, V., & Kempler, P. (2005). Treatment of symptomatic diabetic peripheral neuropathy with the protein kinase C β-inhibitor ruboxistaurin mesylate during a 1-year, randomized, placebo-controlled, double-blind clinical trial. *Clinical Therapeutics, 27*(8), 1164–1180.

Volmer-Thole, M., & Lobmann, R. (2016). Neuropathy and diabetic foot syndrome. *International Journal of Molecular Sciences, 17*(6), 917–928. https://doi.org/10.3390/ijms17060917.

Wagner, F. W. (1981). The dysvascular foot: A system for diagnosis and treatment. *Foot & Ankle, 2*(2), 64–122.

Warriner, R. A., & Driver, V. R. (2006). The true cost of growth factor therapy in diabetic foot ulcer care. *Wounds, 7*(Suppl), 1–11.

Weck, M., Slesaczeck, T., Paetzold, H., Muench, D., Nanning, T., & von Gagern, G. (2013). Structured health care for subjects with diabetic foot ulcers results in reduction of major amputation rates. *Cardiovascular Diabetology, 12*, 45.

Wilcox, J. R., Carter, M. J., & Covington, S. (2013). Frequency of debridements and time to heal: A retrospective cohort study of 312744 wounds. *JAMA Dermatology, 149*(9), 1050–1058. https://doi.org/10.1001/jamadermatol.2013.4960.

Wound, Ostomy and Continence Nurses Society. (2021). *Guideline for management of patients with lower extremity wounds due to diabetes mellitus and/or neuropathic disease.* WOCN Clinical Practice Guideline Series 3. Mt Laurel, NJ: Author.

Wu, S. C., Jensen, J. L., & Weber, A. K. (2008). Use of pressure offloading devices in diabetic foot ulcers. *Diabetes Care, 31*(11), 2118–2119.

Young, M. J., Cavanagh, P. R., & Thomas, G. (1992). The effect of callus removal on dynamic plantar foot pressures in diabetic patients. *Diabetic Medicine, 9*(1), 55–57.

Yu, G. V., & Hudson, J. R. (2002). Evaluation and treatment of stage 0 Charcot's neuropathy of the foot and ankle. *Journal of American Podiatric Medical Association, 92*(4), 210–220.

Zhan, L. X., Branco, B. C., Armstrong, D. G., & Mills, J. L., Sr. (2015). The Society for Vascular Surgery lower extremity threatened limb classification system based on Wound, Ischemia, and foot Infection (WIfI) correlates with risk of major amputation and time to wound healing. *Journal of Vascular Surgery, 61*(4), 939–944.

Zimny, S., Dessel, F., & Ehren, M. (2001). Early detection of microcirculatory impairment in diabetic patients with foot at risk. *Diabetes Care, 24*(10), 1810–1814.

Zimny, S., Reinsch, B., & Schatz, H. (2001). Effects of felted foam on plantar pressures in the treatment of neuropathic diabetic foot ulcers. *Diabetes Care, 24*(12), 2153–2154.

Zochodne, D. W., & Malik, R. A. (2014). Diabetic autonomic neuropathy. *Handbook of Clinical Neurology, 126*, 63–67.

FURTHER READING

Andes, L., Cheng, Y., Roik, D., et al. (2020). Prevalence of prediabetes among adolescents and young adults in the United States 2005–2016. *JAMA Pediatrics, 174*(2), e194498.

Armstrong, D. G., Lavery, L. A., Wunderlich, R. P., et al. (2003). Skin temperatures as a one-time screening tool do not predict future diabetic foot complications. *Journal of the American Podiatric Medical Association, 93*(6), 443–447.

Centers for Disease Control and Prevention. (2018). *Diabetes report card 2017.* Atlanta: Centers for Disease Control and Prevention, U.S. Department of Health and Human Services. Accessed 2/14/2020. Retrieved from https://www.cdc.gov/diabetes/pdfs/library/diabetesreportcard2017-508.pdf.

Creager, M. A., Luscher, T. F., & Beckman, J. A. (2003). Diabetes and vascular disease: Pathophysiology, clinical consequences and medical therapy: Part1. *Circulation, 108*, 1527–1532.

International Diabetes Federation. (2022). Clinical practice recommendation on the diabetic foot: A guide for health care professionals. Retrieved 11/26/2022 from https://www.idf.org/e-library/guidelines/119-idf-clinical-practice-recommendations-on-diabetic-foot-2017.html.

Joseph, W. S., & Lipsky, B. A. (2010). Medical therapy of diabetic foot infection. *Journal of Vascular Surgery, 52*(3), S67–S71.

Leibson, C. L., Ransom, J. E., Olson, W., et al. (2004). Peripheral arterial disease, diabetes, and mortality. *Diabetes Care, 27*(12), 2843–2849.

Lipsky, B. A. (2004). A report from the international consensus on diagnosing and treating the infected diabetic foot. *Diabetes/Metabolism Research and Reviews, 20*(Suppl. 1), S68–S77.

Maser, R. E., Steenkiste, A. R., Dorman, J. S., et al. (1989). Epidemiological correlates of diabetic neuropathy. Report from Pittsburg Epidemiology of Diabetes Complications Study. *Diabetes, 38*(11), 1456–1461.

Pecoraro, R. E., Reiber, G. E., & Burgess, E. M. (1990). Pathways to diabetic limb amputation. Basis for prevention. *Diabetes Care, 13*(5), 513–521.

Peters, E. J. G., & Lipsky, B. A. (2013). Diagnosis and management of infection in the diabetic foot. *The Medical Clinics of North America, 97*(5), 911–946.

Rosskopf, A. B., Loupatatzis, C., Pfirrmann, C. W. A., Böni, T., & Berli, M. C. (2019). The Charcot foot: A pictorial review. *Insights Into Imaging, 10*(1), 77. https://doi.org/10.1186/s13244-019-0768-9.

Schaper, N. C., van Netten, J., Apelqvist, J., Bus, S. C., Hinchliffe, R. J., & Lipsky, B. A. (2019). *IWGDF practical guidelines on the prevention and management of diabetic foot disease.* Netherland, Australia, UK and USA: International Working Group on the Diabetic Foot (IWGDF). Accessed 02/14/2020. Retrieved from www.iwdfguidelines.org.

Uçkay, L., Gariani, K., & Pataky, Z. (2014). Diabetic foot infection: State of the art. *Diabetes, Obesity & Metabolism, 16*(4), 305–316.

18

Foot and Nail Care

Sheila Howes-Trammel

OBJECTIVES

1. Correlate medical conditions with potential foot problems.
2. Describe the structure and function of the foot and nails.
3. Compare and contrast foot malformations addressing key features, prevention, and management.
4. Describe common foot lesions, including their etiology, manifestations, treatment, and prevention.
5. Distinguish between two toenail disorders and their treatments.
6. Develop an appropriate plan for routine care of the foot.

Foot problems occur in at least 75% of Americans (Menz & Lord, 2001). Several studies suggest foot problems affect 71–87% of the elderly population (Rodríguez-Sanz et al., 2018). The five most common foot problems in the elderly population are *toenail disorders* (75%); *toe deformities* (60%); *corns and calluses* (58%); *bunions* (37%); and *dry skin, fungal infections,* or *maceration between the toes* (36%). Most of these foot problems can be prevented by proper foot care performed on a regular basis (Badlissi, Dunn, Link, et al., 2005).

Age-related changes (e.g., impaired vision, inability to reach feet, thinning of epidermis and dermis), vascular-related skin changes (e.g., trophic, edema), and deformed hardened toenails affect foot hygiene. An age-related change in the foot and lower extremity is loss of hair, which leads to increased dry skin. Trophic changes in the skin are related to loss of vasculature (e.g., pigmentation changes; shiny, red skin; hair loss).

In a multiethnic sample of 784 community-dwelling adults over the age of 65, there was a minimal association between the prevalence of foot problems and level of education. The number of conditions was more common in certain racial/ethnic groups. Study participants had an average of four foot conditions. Women had more toe and arch conditions than men. Puerto Ricans had less orthopedic conditions versus non-Hispanic white and African Americans. African Americans had the highest incidence of dermatological conditions. The comorbidities assessed were obesity BMI > 30 (39%), diabetes (30%,) arthritis (57.9%), and LE vascular diseases (45%). The proportion of comorbid conditions varied by race/ethnicity in regard to diabetes and LE vascular diseases. Arthritis had the highest percentage with a mean of 57.9%. Compared with the other three comorbid conditions (Dunn, 2004).

Chronic foot problems (i.e., those lasting more than 2 weeks) are associated with diabetes, peripheral vascular disease, neuropathy, atherosclerosis, arthritis, and obesity. In fact, the signs and symptoms of many of these systemic disorders manifest initially in the feet. Improper shoe wear, overuse, or systemic disease can trigger chronic foot pain. These issues magnify the importance of a good foot assessment (Popoola & Jenkins, 2004).

Foot symptoms are associated with several aspects of impaired functional status: level of walking, stairs, and rising from a chair and balance. In Framingham foot study of 1544 community-dwelling older adults, the prevalence of foot pain was 19% in men and 25% women. Foot pain was associated with mobility limitations in both men and women (Menz et al., 2013). Regardless of the impact on function, the complaint of foot pain is undervalued in healthcare (Menz et al., 2013).

QUALITY OF LIFE

Foot diseases and their treatments have a tremendous impact on quality of life (Katsambas, Abeck, Haneke, et al., 2005). In fact, patients with diabetes who have foot ulcers report a poorer quality of life than patients with diabetes who have amputations (Price & Harding, 2000). In a large-scale, quality-of-life survey of 45,593 patients with various foot diseases representing 17 countries (the Achilles Project), the researchers found that 40.3% of the respondents experienced discomfort in walking, 30.7% had pain, 27.3% had embarrassment, and 19.6% experienced limitations in their activities of daily living (Katsambas et al., 2005).

Overall, foot disease has a significantly greater effect on the quality of life of women than of men with regard to their experience of pain, discomfort in walking, and embarrassment (Katsambas et al., 2005; Leveille, Gurainik, Ferrucci, et al., 1998; Awale, Dufour, Katz, Menz, & Hannan, 2016; López-López et al., 2018). One explanation is that the many types of shoes typically worn by women are tighter fitting, which increases their risk of developing toenail onychomycosis, which is associated with pain and discomfort in walking. In addition, symptoms of depression have been associated with foot pain. In The Framingham foot study mentioned previously, both the presence and severity of foot pain were associated with increased depression symptoms (Awale et al., 2016). Given the high prevalence of foot problems, foot care is an essential need to address before quality of life and the ability to self-manage is impaired. (López-López et al., 2018).

STRUCTURE AND FUNCTION

Feet are excellent at collecting information. Thousands of neurologic receptors in the feet send valuable feedback to the brain to tell your body where it is in space and what the terrain is like. Actively stimulating these receptors improves balance, increases circulation, and enhances overall foot health. There are three main elements of the body that send information to the central nervous system: the joints, skin, and muscles/tendons. Collectively they are otherwise called mechanoreceptors. When all three are firing properly and able to send accurate and precise information about pressure, joint orientation, rate of movement, and range of movement about the joint, the body works with greater synergy.

The foot is the foundation of the distal kinetic chain which maintains the contact with the ground. The kinetic chain is disrupted if the foot is not functioning properly. This dysfunction can lead to decreased mobility, balance, and decrease physical function (Oh-Park, Kirschner, Abdelshahed, & Kim, 2019).

The foot has two key functions: weight bearing and propulsion. To perform properly, the foot requires a high degree of stability and must be flexible to adapt to uneven surfaces. The numerous bones and joints in the foot provide flexibility; these bones also form the arch to support weight (Quinn, 2019). Each foot contains 26 bones; 33 joints; and a network of more than 100 tendons, muscles, ligaments, blood vessels, nerves, and nails. Together, the feet comprise a quarter of the 206 bones in the body. An average day of walking brings a force equal to several hundred tons to bear on the feet. As such, feet are more subject to injury than any other part of the body (Cavanagh & Ulbrecht, 2008; Mix, 1999).

Skeletal Components

The three functional units of the foot are the hindfoot (2 bones), midfoot (5 bones), and forefoot (19 bones). All units must work together to provide both flexibility and stability (Fig. 18.1).

Within the forefoot are the phalanges (toes) and the five metatarsal bones. Each toe (phalanx) is made up of several bones. The great toe (also called the hallux) consists of two phalanx bones: proximal and distal; these phalanges are larger than all the other phalanges. Phalanges two through five have three phalanx bones each: proximal, distal, and intermediate (an additional middle bone). Each phalanx is connected to a metatarsal at the metatarsophalangeal (MTP) joint; together the MTP joints form the ball of the foot. The proximal portion

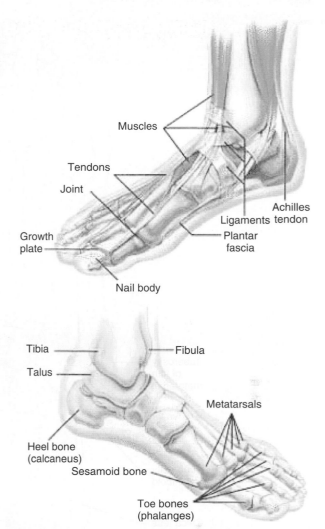

Fig. 18.1 Anatomic structures of the foot. (Courtesy Fort Worth Orthopedics.)

of a metatarsal is called the *base,* the middle is the *shaft,* and the distal is the *head* (Fig. 18.2). Each of the five metatarsals is unique in size. The first metatarsal is the shortest in length, the largest in diameter, bears the most weight, and plays the most important role in propulsion (Quinn, 2019). At the head of the first metatarsal bone on the plantar surface of the foot are two sesamoid bones that serve to attach small muscles and aid in stabilizing the first MTP joint. (A sesamoid bone is a bone imbedded within a tendon and functions to protect the tendon where it passes over a bony prominence.) The second, third, and fourth metatarsal bones are the most stable metatarsal bones. At the fifth metatarsal base is an eminence on the lateral aspect called the *tuberosity of fifth metatarsal* or *styloid process*. This area is easily palpated on the lateral aspect of the foot.

In the midfoot, five of the seven tarsal bones are located (see Fig. 18.2). These irregularly shaped tarsals (the navicular, cuboid, and three cuneiform) form the arch and contain multiple joints. The three cuneiform bones articulate with the navicular bone in the proximal midfoot. The midfoot connects with the forefoot at the five tarsometatarsal (TMT) joints and connects to the hindfoot by muscles and ligaments.

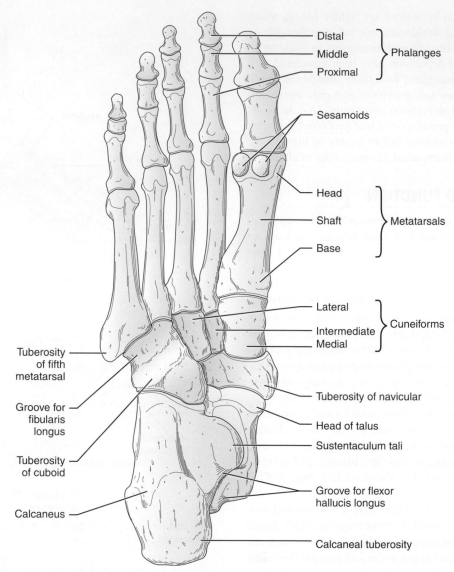

Fig. 18.2 Dorsal view of anatomic structures of foot. (From Jenkins, D. B. (2009). *Hollinshead's functional anatomy of the limbs and back* (9th ed.). St. Louis: Elsevier. p 333.)

The hindfoot links the midfoot to the ankle and consists of two of the seven tarsal bones: the talus and the calcaneus. The talus sits on top of the calcaneus and articulates with the tibia and fibula at the calcaneus and navicular bones, allowing the foot to move up and down. The calcaneus forms the heel and is the largest tarsal and the largest bone in the foot. It allows the foot to become rigid or loose to accommodate the process of walking. It is also the cause of numerous heel-related pains (Jolly, Zgonis, & Hendrix, 2005).

Ligaments hold the bones together at the joints. The Achilles tendon stretches from the calf muscle to heel and is the largest, strongest tendon in the foot. The planter fascia is the longest ligament and forms an arch on the sole of the foot from the heel to the toes. These long fibrous strands are vulnerable to injury (e.g., a strain or sprain in the foot or ankle) because the ligaments can overstretch, break, and curl back on themselves. Over time the strain heals with scar tissue; however, the scar is never as strong as the original fibers of the ligament.

Muscular Components

The foot is constructed of 20 muscles. These muscles hold the bones in place, providing the foot with its shape and contracting and relaxing to allow for movement. Key muscles are the anterior tibial (moves foot upward), posterior tibial (supports arch), peroneal tibial (controls lateral ankle movements), extensors (help ankle raise toes to begin walking), and flexors (stabilizes to the ground).

Neurovascular

The feet are innervated by the sciatic nerve, which branches off the spinal cord at the sacral level. As it descends, the sciatic nerve divides into the tibial and common peroneal nerves and further subdivides into numerous branches.

Branching off the popliteal artery in the lower leg are the anterior tibial artery and the posterior tibial artery. The anterior tibial artery becomes the dorsalis pedis (dorsum of the foot). The posterior tibial artery passes posterior to the medial malleolus, divides into the peroneal and plantar arteries, and

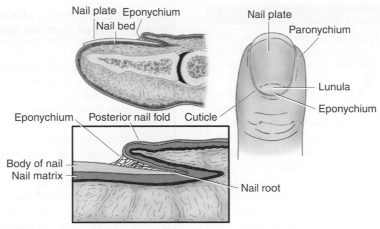

Fig. 18.3 Anatomic structures of the nail. (From Thompson, J. M., et al. (2002). *Mosby's clinical nursing* (5th ed.). St. Louis: Mosby.)

then feeds into the lateral plantar and medial plantar arteries. The two most dominant arteries in the foot are the dorsalis pedis and the posterior tibial artery. Two sets of veins drain the leg and foot: the deep veins and superficial veins.

As shown in Fig. 13.2, the dorsalis pedis pulse is palpated or auscultated over the navicular and middle cuneiform bones. The posterior tibial pulse is palpated over the medial malleolus of the tibia.

Cutaneous and Subcutaneous Components

The skin on the plantar surface of the foot is thick and hairless and contains numerous sweat glands. *Eccrine* sweat glands are densely populated on the soles of the feet, palms, and axillae. Their primary function is thermoregulation through evaporation of sweat. The sebaceous and apocrine sweat glands empty into the upper portions of the hair follicles. Sebaceous glands produce lipid-rich sebum that prevents the skin and hair from drying out. Because the foot has little hair growth and therefore very few *sebaceous* glands, the foot is extremely vulnerable to dryness and xerosis.

Three anatomic areas on the plantar surface of the foot have increased fat in the form of fat pads: the calcaneus, the metatarsals, and the lateral longitudinal arch. Contained by the subcutaneous tissue, the fat pad absorbs impact and tolerates weight bearing as a means of protecting the underlying bones. With age the foot becomes wider, t and there is progressive atrophy of fat pads which provides less shock absorbency, exposing the calcaneus and metatarsal heads (Oh-Park et al., 2019). More pressure is then exerted over the calcaneus and metatarsal subsequently causing callus formation, pain, and increased risk for ulceration. Thinning of the fat pad is accelerated by obesity, diabetes, and constant high impact. The thinning process begins as early as 30 years of age. An orthotic or insole cushioning can be used to provide additional shock absorption (Ozdemir, Söyüncü, Ozgörgen, et al., 2004).

Nail Structure

Nails are made of epidermal cells converted to hard plates of keratin. The function of the toenail is to provide protection to the soft tissue of the toe. The nail measures one-sixteenth of an inch in thickness and is composed of three layers: a dorsal thin covering, a thicker middle layer, and a deep inner layer derived from the nail bed. The nail bed, or the matrix, is made up of epithelium, a rough surface of longitudinal waves that interface with grooves on the underside of the nail plate, facilitating adherence of the plate to the bed. The distal aspect of the matrix is the lunula, or the moons, which is the crescent-shaped white area. Normal nail color is translucent with a pink tinge reflecting the highly vascular matrix. As the nail grows, extending beyond the nail root or matrix, the translucent color is lost and becomes white. The stratum corneum layer of the skin covering the nail root is the eponychium (cuticle), which forms a seal between the nail and the digit to prevent foreign matter from entering. The hyponychium smoothly seals the border between the distal end of the nail and the bed. The perionychium creates a seal on the lateral folds. These three parts of the nail prevent infection from occurring under the nail bed. The normal nail is composed of six parts: nail root (under the skin), nail bed (under the nail plate), nail plate, eponychium (cuticle), perionychium (nail fold), and hyponychium (skin under the front edge of the nail) as illustrated in Fig. 18.3 and described in Box 18.1.

Nails grow all the time, but their rate of growth slows with age and systemic disease. Fingernails grow faster than toenails. They grow at a rate of 3 mm per month and take 6 months to grow from root to free edge. Toenails grow approximately 1.5 mm per month and require 12 to 18 months to be completely replaced. Actual growth rate is dependent on age, gender, season, exercise level, diet, and hereditary factors (Lorizzo, 2015; Sinni-McKeehen, 2019).

PHYSICAL ASSESSMENT

Components of an initial evaluation of the patient with an actual or potential foot disorder are listed in Checklist 18.1. Because so many patients with foot disorders have concomitant lower extremity disease, perfusion and sensation must be assessed (see Chapters 13-17), and a baseline health history

BOX 18.1   Nail Anatomy

Nail Root (*Matrix*): Root of fingernail is also known as the matrix. The matrix begins 7–8 mm under proximal nail fold to lunula (white crescent at distal nail). Fingernail root produces most of volume of nail plate and nail bed.

Nail Bed: Part of nail matrix, under the nail plate. Extends from lunula (white crescent at distal nail) to hyponychium. Nail bed contains blood vessels, nerves, and melanocytes or melanin-producing cells. As nail is produced by root, it streams down along the nail bed, which adds material to the undersurface of the nail, making it thicker.

Nail Plate: The actual fingernail, made of translucent keratin. Pink appearance of nail comes from blood vessels underneath nail. Underneath surface of nail plate has grooves along length of nail that help anchor it to the nail bed.

Eponychium (*Cuticle*): Fold at proximal end of nail plate. Nail plate has very firm adhesion to the cuticle. Both epidermal structures are directly continuous with one another, overlapping the lunula. Fusing of these structures provides a waterproof barrier.

Perionychium: Skin that overlies nail plate on its sides. Also known as the paronychial edge. Site of hangnails, ingrown nails, and infection of skin called *paronychia*.

Hyponychium: Area between free edge of nail plate and epidermis of toe. Continuous fusing of these areas to epidermal structures provides waterproof barrier.

Periungual: Tissue around nail plate.

Subungual: Tissue under nail plate.

Ungual: Pertaining to the nail.

From Mix, G. (1998). *The salon professional's guide to foot care.* Albany: Milady Salon Ovations.

CHECKLIST 18.1   Components of Initial Evaluation of Patient With Foot Disorder

History

✓ Presenting complaint, including detailed description of pain
✓ General: vision, strength, dexterity, mobility
✓ Blood glucose readings for past month, HbA1c
✓ Personal or family history: skin, hair, or nail disease (especially rashes); lichen planus; psoriasis; diabetes; heart or vascular disease; obesity
✓ Specific history of foot problems: foot malformations, lesions, skin alterations, nail disorders, changes in sensation, foot/ankle strength
✓ Current and prior treatments and medications (including over the counter) used to treat nail and foot problems
✓ Health habits: smoking, exercise, hygiene, nutrition, weight management

Physical Assessment

✓ Overall skin condition
✓ Lesions on foot
✓ Foot malformations
✓ Condition of nails
✓ Perfusion and sensation, pulses, blanching, capillary refill, microvascular function (laser Doppler flowmetry), ankle-brachial index or toe-brachial index, temperature, hair growth
✓ Musculoskeletal function: gait, mobility, balance, hand strength and dexterity, visual cognition

Risk Assessment

✓ Ulceration risk (see Box 17.1)
✓ Amputation risk

Equipment

✓ Footwear (including socks)
✓ Mobility aids (canes, walkers)

---

is essential. The following discussion presents the unique assessment parameters for the foot and nail.

Specific information should be elicited about routine care of the foot, any history of foot and nail problems, and how these problems were treated either personally or by a health care provider. Effects of prior treatments, including prescription and over-the-counter medications, should be assessed (Piraccini, Iorizzo, Antonoucci, et al., 2004; Sprecher, 2005). Quality-of life-information should be solicited (Garrow, Silman, & Macfarlane, 2004; López-López et al., 2018; Vileikyte, Peyrot, & Bundy, 2003).

Musculoskeletal Function

Musculoskeletal function of the foot involves assessment of range of motion, deformities, and strength. Passive range of motion of the first MTP joint and the subtalar joint should be assessed. Limited ROM of the first MTP joint is high prevalent with age. Compensation of this limited ROM results in short step length and reduced push off time (Oh-Park et al., 2019). Maximal range of motion is determined from maximal inversion to maximal eversion of the subtalar joint of the foot (Fig. 18.4). If available, a goniometer can be used to quantify the arc or range of motion (Badlissi et al., 2005) (Fig. 18.5). Prolonged deformity of deformity of pronation or supination leads to limited ROM of subtalar joint (Oh-Park et al., 2019). Range of motion can also be tested by supporting the heel

with one hand, grasping the foot with the other hand, then moving the foot in dorsiflexion, plantar flexion, eversion, and inversion. The dorsiflexion position tests for shortening of the Achilles tendon. About 10% dorsiflexion is required for normal ambulation (Oh-Park et al., 2019). Inversion will be limited by a spasm of the peronei. Eversion will be limited with a rigid flat foot. Restrictions in range of motion of the ankle might limit the ability to correct a loss of balance (Duthie, 2007; Oh-Park et al., 2019).

Testing of muscle strength in the lower leg and foot is critical in foot care. To test the anterior leg muscles, the patient should be instructed to stand on their heels. Muscle strength can also be assessed by comparing both feet as the patient walks a few steps on the toes and then the heels. Toe flexor strength is a predictor of an older adult's balance and function (Fujii, 2019). In those patients who have difficulty with balance, cannot walk, or both, strength can be assessed in the sitting position. With the clinician's hand under the patient's foot, the patient is asked to flex and extend the foot against resistance by "pressing down on the gas pedal." Next, with the clinician's hand positioned on the top of the patient's foot and the clinician's thumbs underneath, the patient is instructed to pull the

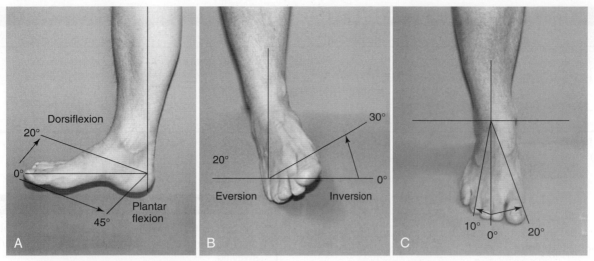

Fig. 18.4 Range of motion of the foot and ankle. (A) Dorsiflexion and planter flexion. (B) Inversion and eversion. (C) Abduction and adduction. (From Ball, J. W., Dains, J. E., Flynn, J. A. (2015). *Seidel's guide to physical examination* (8th ed.). St. Louis: Mosby.)

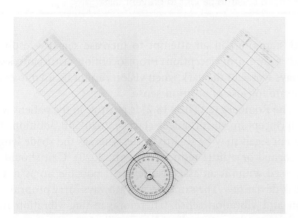

Fig. 18.5 Goniometer. (From Ball, J. W., Dains, J. E., Flynn, J. A. (2015). *Seidel's guide to physical examination* (8th ed.). St. Louis: Mosby.)

"toes toward the nose" while the clinician applies gentle pressure downward. Any differences in strength currently or in the past 6 months should also be recorded (Frey, 2005).

Foot and toe conditions will decrease the ROM, strength and plantar tactile sensation of the foot. Toes play an important role in lower extremity muscle strength, balance and weight distribution in the gait (Fujii, 2019). To assess toe flexibility, the patient can be instructed to pick up a marble or a small dishtowel with the toes (Table 18.1). To test ankle flexibility, the patient is instructed to stand on a stair step, hang his or her heel off a step, and let the heel drop below the level of the stair. If this motion causes pain, the exercise should be stopped. The heel should be able to drop below the level of the stair without causing strain in the calf. Foot and ankle

TABLE 18.1	Foot Flexibility Exercises		
	Exercise	**Instructions**	**Recommendations**
	Toe raise, toe point, toe curls	Hold each position for 5 s and repeat 10 times	Individuals with hammertoes or toe cramps
	Golf ball roll	Roll a golf ball under the ball of your foot for 2 minutes—great massage for bottom of foot	Individuals with plantar fasciitis (heel pain), arch strain, or foot cramps
	Towel curls	Place small towel on floor and curl it toward you, using only your toes. You can increase resistance by putting a weight on end of towel. Relax and repeat exercise five times	Individuals with hammertoes, toe cramps, and pain in the ball of the foot
	Marble pick up	Place 20 marbles on floor. Pick up one marble at a time with your toes and put it in a small bowl. Do this exercise until you have picked up all 20 marbles	Individuals with pain in the ball of the foot, hammer-toes, and toe cramps

Continued

TABLE 18.1	**Foot Flexibility Exercises—cont'd**		
	Exercise	Instructions	Recommendations
	Sand walking	Any chance you get, take off your shoes and walk in the sand at the beach. This not only massages your feet, but also strengthens your toes	Good for general foot conditioning Watch out for glass!

Modified from American Orthopaedic Foot & Ankle Society. (2022). *AOFAS FootCareMD. How to keep feet flexible.* Retrieved January 19, 2023 from: https://www.footcaremd.org/resources/how-to-help/how-to-keep-feet-flexible.

mobility and stability can be improved with flexibility exercises (Frey, 2005; Fujii, 2019).

The medial longitudinal arch can be examined by having the patient stand with feet parallel, separated by 4 inches. It is important to note if the arch flattens with weight bearing and if it resumes to normal shape without weight bearing. The evaluation of the gait should focus on the area of weight bearing of the feet, pronation and supination, varus and valgus, and step length and push off phase (Oh-Park et al., 2019).

Muscle strength reflexes (deep tendon reflexes) usually show no changes in the elderly patient, although nearly half have a diminished Achilles tendon reflex. This is likely due to slow nerve conduction and decreased tendon elasticity. Hyperactive deep tendon reflexes suggest upper motor neuron disease; hypoactive reflexes suggest lower motor neuron dysfunction. Tone is assessed through passive motion. Increased tone is suggestive of upper motor neuron dysfunction; decreased tone is suggestive of lower motor neuron dysfunction.

Functional Ability

The patient's functional ability is a significant factor influencing his or her ability for self-care and safety. Assessments of functional ability should address cognition, vision, strength–hand dexterity, coordination, balance, proprioception, and gait. Because key interventions in the prevention and management of foot and nail disorders are patient education and self-care, the patient will need adequate cognition to conduct self-care or communicate pain. Vision hand strength and hand dexterity are essential so that patients will be able to inspect their feet and remove footwear (Duthie, 2007). Many of these functional abilities can be assessed through observation and demonstration return.

Coordination can be determined with a rapid alternating movement that includes heel-to-shin testing. Another test in which the patient taps the feet rhythmically against the floor will assess the accuracy and reproducibility of endpoints, as well as the ability to maintain motor movements over time. The coordination testing is documented qualitatively because no quantification guidelines are available (Duthie, 2007).

Proprioception is the awareness of the body's position in context with the surrounding environment. Disturbed proprioception (loss of position sense) in the feet is disabling; the patient may be clumsy, bump into things, or have an abnormal gait. In practice, the patient often comes down hard on the heels and then slaps the sole of the foot (high stepping

BOX 18.2	**Romberg (Equilibrium) Test**

- Have patient stand with arms at side and feet together.
- Have patient maintain position for 20 s with only minimal swaying.
- Have patient perform initially with eyes open and then with eyes closed.
- Stand close to patient to prevent falls.

and stamping) in an attempt to increase sensory feedback and restore proprioception. Proprioception disturbances are always worse in the dark when vision cannot be used to compensate for loss of position sense.

The Romberg test (Box 18.2) is positive in the patient with proprioception disturbances (Jarvis, 2020). In addition, the patient's gait may be slightly wide, whereas the stride length is normal or a little reduced (Lowth, 2020). Gait should be assessed without an assistive device if possible, so as not to mask deviations. The same nerve pathways carry proprioception and vibration sense. Therefore, testing vibration may reveal proprioception disturbances. To test vibration sense, a low-pitch (128 Hz or 256 Hz) tuning fork is applied over a bony prominence such as the medial malleolus and the patient is asked to report when the vibration stops (Jarvis, 2020).

Condition of Legs, Feet, Toes, and Nails

Lower extremity assessment should include all of the components discussed in Chapter 13. In addition to examining skin integrity, color changes, sensation, pain, and vascular conditions, it is important to inspect for excessive dryness or moisture, evidence of fungal or bacterial infection, lesions, foot malformations, and nail conditions (Boulton & Armstrong, 2008). All surfaces of the heel (dorsal, plantar, medial, lateral, posterior), the interdigital spaces (i.e., between the toes), and each nail should be examined. Skin changes on the lower leg from the knee to the distal foot should be noted. When assessing the temperature and texture of the skin on the lower extremity and feet, the skin on the arms and hands can be used for comparison.

Ulceration and Amputation Risk

Data collected during the examination will assist in identifying risk for ulceration and amputation. Several risk factors for ulceration have been identified and include history of plantar ulcer, presence of foot deformity, presence of protective sensations, and presence of diseases that lead to decreased sensation. Risk categories for ulceration range from 0 (no risk) to 3 (greatest risk). The level of risk determines the patient's management strategy. Risk assessment tools with management strategies are given in Tables 17.2 and 17.3. The American Diabetes Association and the American Association of Clinical Endocrinologists (Boulton et al., 2008) endorses foot examinations every 3–6 months once loss of sensation develops, every 1–3 months once a callous also develops, and every 1–12 weeks when history of ulcer is present (see Table 17.3).

PREVENTION AND ROUTINE MANAGEMENT

Maintaining healthy nails and feet requires daily attention to the skin of the foot and ankle, nails, and footwear. Routine over-the-counter remedies can be used to correct common problems and hopefully prevent deterioration into a serious condition.

Routine Foot Hygiene

Routine foot care includes daily inspection and moisturizing. Daily cleansing or bathing should be based on the individual needs of the patient and should consist of mild skin cleansers and lukewarm water to minimize drying effects. After bathing, the feet must be dried completely, especially between the toes. The patient should use a mirror to view the bottom of the foot for inspection of any alterations in the skin. No moisturizers should be used between the toes. Patients should wear socks to provide extra padding to bony prominences and to wick away moisture from the skin. Socks may need to be changed more than once per day if feet sweat excessively. The use of an occlusive moisturizer can be applied to the feet at night and covered with socks for additional moisturizing.

Maceration between the toes (interdigital) and under the toes (subdigital) is a very common foot problem. Such overhydration of the skin, characterized by a white, "waterlogged" appearance, weakens collagen, promotes overgrowth of bacterial and fungal species of skin flora, and decreases the skin's ability to resist trauma (Stroud & Kelechi, 2006). *Pseudomonas* and Gram-negative organisms are common etiologic agents (Weidner, Tittlebach, & Elsner, 2017). Over hydration of the skin can occur with excessive perspiration (hyperhidrosis) related to endocrine, neurologic, or sweat gland disorders.

Keeping the skin dry and protected prevents maceration. After bathing, the patient should pay special attention to drying the interdigit spaces; using a hair dryer on a cool setting may be helpful. The treatment interventions include separating the toes with lamb's wool, dusting the skin with an absorbent foot powder (e.g., Zeasorb) twice per day, applying a skin sealant or an antiperspirant (e.g., Drysol) to protect the skin from moisture. If maceration persists after 1 week of care, interdigital tinea (Table 18.2) or superimposed bacterial infection should be considered. Treatment includes drying the interdigital web spaces, and applying topical econazole BID for 3 weeks for bacterial toe web infection, or 0.77%

ciclopirox gel BID for concomitant interdigit pedis and bacterial growth (Weidner et al., 2017).

Foot odor (bromhidrosis) is caused by excessive perspiration from the more than 250,000 sweat glands in the foot. Bacteria living in shoes and socks metabolize the sweat to form isovaleric acid, which is responsible for foot odor. In addition to washing the feet and changing shoes and socks even more frequently than daily, the patient can dust the feet with a nonmedicated spray, foot powder, or antiperspirant. Soaking feet in vinegar and water can help lessen odor (American Podiatric Medical Association, 2010). The shoes should be treated with freezing, washing in hot water, or discarding. Severe cases of foot odor may be caused by hyperhidrosis (excessive perspiration formation related to endocrine, neurologic, or sweat gland disorders). Aluminum chloride hexahydrate 20% (e.g., Drysol) antiperspirant can be used if over-the-counter antiperspirants or sprays fail (Fujimoto, 2016). In severe cases, the nerve controlling the sweat glands in the feet may be surgically severed, but compensatory sweating in other areas of the body may occur after surgery.

Anhidrosis (inability to produce sweat) is associated with autonomic dysfunction caused by endocrine or neurologic disorders, environmental conditions, and aging. Xerosis is a consequence of the skin's loss of natural moisturizing factors and loss of moisture from the stratum corneum and intercellular matrix (Hill, 2008; Parker, Scharfbillig, & Jones, 2017). Clinically, xerosis appears as excessively dry, rough, uneven, and cracked skin. Raised or uplifted skin edges (scaling), desquamation (flaking), chapping, and pruritus may be present. This condition occurs particularly on the heels and bottoms of the feet. A person who has a decrease or loss of function of the sweat glands on the plantar surface of the foot will experience xerosis or anhidrosis of the feet (Parker et al., 2017). *Xerosis* can lead to fissures (linear cracks in the skin), which may serve as a portal of entry for bacteria. Consequently, fissures are associated with increased risk of cellulitis and foot ulceration. *Fissures* are treated with humectants and exfoliant moisturizers or liquid adhesive bandage (e.g. Dermabond, Nexcare, or Liquiband) (Adelstein, Bray, & Schram, 2008; Vlahovic, Hinton, Chakravarthy, & Fleck, 2011). Prevention includes ongoing use of moisturizers and exfoliants and wearing shoes that do not flop at the heel. Hyperkeratotic tissue is common around fissures and often necessitates debridement and exfoliation. Table 18.3 provides a formulary of products for the prevention and treatment of dry skin.

Cuticles and Nails

About half of the foot care professional's activity is nail care and specifically nail debridement. Nail trimming can be performed by a nurse or caregiver when the nail is normal in thickness and appearance. The nail should be trimmed straight across, no lower than one-sixteenth to one-eighth of an inch from the end of the toe, to prevent ingrown toenails. After trimming, the nail should be smoothed with a rasp or file. The cuticle should not be trimmed or manipulated.

Nail debridement is often necessary but is only conducted by a nurse or provider who is qualified based on the individual

TABLE 18.2   Assessment, Prevention, and Management of Common Foot Lesions and Infections

Name	Description	Common Locations	Prevention	Treatment
Soft corn (heloma molle)	Enlarged interphalangeal joint causing friction to the opposing surface Aggravated by tight shoes and ambulation	Between fourth and fifth toes	Properly fitting shoes, offload with interdigit foam or gel pads, or lamb's wool	Pumice, file Wider shoes Surgically reshape phalange
Hard corn (heloma durum)	Toes curl inside of shoes, creating pressure between toes against the sole Aggravated by narrow-toed shoes	Sides and tops of toes	Offload pressure with pads (aperture or crest pads)	Use wider shoes or sandals Reduce corn with file, pumice, rotary tool Assess for underlying ulceration Offload and pad as needed Surgically straighten toes
Callus (keratoma or tyloma) generalized pressure (see Plate 47A)	Thickened areas of skin without distinct borders caused by repeated pressure Aggravated by narrow-toed shoes and high heels	Planter surface, heel, under metatarsal head	Padding, properly fitting shoes	Reduce with file, pumice, rotary tool, or paring Assess for underlying ulceration Moisturize and exfoliate (best applied to damp skin after bathing) Offload and pad as needed Use shoes with soft soles, lower heels, arch support, extra width
Planter wart (*Verruca plantaris*)	Caused by a contagious viral infection (human papillomavirus) Overproliferation of skin and mucosa growing downward (iceberg effect) Single lesion or clustered Yellow, brown, gray, or black Vesicular inclusion from dried capillary ends leads to black/red appearance	Pressure points on sole, heel, ball of foot	Change socks and shoes daily Do not share shoes Keep feet clean and dry Avoid direct contact with warts on other people Use water-resistant footwear in showers, locker rooms, pools	Reduce with file or pumice Salicylic acid podophyllin, or cryotherapy/electrocautery Surgical curettage or laser removal Human papillomavirus dies within 1–2 years and wart disappears
Tinea pedis (interdigital)	Dermatophyte infection White, macerated, denuded, vesicles, scales, or fissures	Between fourth and fifth toes		Topical antifungal twice daily for minimum of 1 week (gel product to reduce the moisture) Urea cream for scaling, itching
Tinea pedis (plantar)	Dermatophyte infection Itchy, hyperkeratotic scaling, cracking, peeling, dry patches Chronic, diffuse, noninflammatory	Sole, heel, side of foot (moccasin)		Topical antifungal twice daily for minimum of 1 week Urea cream for scaling, itching
Tinea pedis (vesiculobullous)	Dermatophyte infection Acute, highly inflammatory eruptions	Arch, side of foot		Topical or systemic antifungals and corticosteroids (depending on severity)

TABLE 18.3 Formulary of Moisturizing Products

Descriptions, Examples, and Indications

Moisturizer	Indications and Actions	Ingredient Examples[a]	Product Examples[a]
Emollients	Prevent dry skin Fill in cracks between clusters of desquamating corneocytes Not occlusive unless applied heavily	Lipids Oils Dimethicone	Keri Original (Bristol Myers Squibb) Cavilon Emollient Cream (3M) Cetaphil Lotion (Galderma Laboratories)
Occlusives	Treat dry skin Reduce transepidermal water loss by creating hydrophobic barrier over skin Has most pronounced effect when applied to slightly damp skin	Petrolatum Lanolin Mineral oil Dimethicone	Cetaphil Cream (Galderma Laboratories) Remedy Skin Repair Cream (Medline) Sween 24 Cream (Coloplast)
Humectants and exfoliants	Treat dry skin, xerosis, fissures, ichthyoses Contains urea, lactic acid, or both, which are naturally present in healthy skin and markedly reduced in dry skin Enhance water absorption by drawing and absorbing water from environment and retaining moisture within skin cells Keratolytic effects soften scales to be easily released from skin surface Urea has antipruritic effects	Urea Lactic acid	Eucerin 10% Urea Lotion (Beiersdorf) Lac-Hydrin Lotion (Bristol Myers Squibb) Atrac-Tain Lotion (Coloplast)

[a]Concentrations and total formulation determine actions and effectiveness. List is not all inclusive.
Data from Pham, H. T., Exelbert, L., Segal-Owens, A. C., et al. (2002). A prospective, randomized, controlled double-blind study of a moisturizer for xerosis of the feet in patients with diabetes. *Ostomy Wound Manage, 48*(5), 30–36; Milne, C. T. (2014). *Wound Source.* 17th ed. Hinesburg: Kerstel Health Information; Lodén, M. (2003). Role of topical emollients and moisturizers in the treatment of dry skin barrier disorders. *American Journal of Clinical Dermatology, 4*, 771–788.

state's practice act. Nail debridement begins with nipping small areas of the nail, starting at one edge and completing to the other side of the nail, following the contour of the top of the toe. The shape and length will depend on the individual patient history and assessment. A hyperkeratotic nail or areas of hyperkeratosis (corns or calluses) on the toes or bottom of the foot should be debrided and a treatment plan developed. Nail debridement and trimming can be accomplished with manual nippers (Box 18.3) or with a mechanical rotary tool (Box 18.4). The use of proper and professional-quality instruments is key to providing proper foot and nail care. Five basic instruments are recommended for providing foot and nail care: toenail nippers, curette, rasp, ingrown nail shaver, and cuticle nippers.

BOX 18.3 Basic Cuticle and Nail Trimming Using Toenail Nippers

1. Begin cuticle and nail care after bathing when nails are softer.
2. Examine nails.
   a. Observe for presence of hyponychium that has hypertrophied, hypergranulation tissue, in growing corners of nail borders, hyperkeratosis, or other abnormal findings. Patients with very thick or ingrown nails require referral to foot care professional.
   b. Define the free nail border by assessing the tissue underneath the nail, using beveled edge of orangewood stick.
   c. Unhealthy nails should be trimmed last to prevent the transmission of infection.
3. Remove any loose debris from under the nail.
4. Gently trim excessively thick or loose cuticles with cuticle nippers.
   a. Avoid excess manipulation of the cuticle, which may lead to infection.
5. Decide between slightly rounded cut and straight across cut:
   a. *Straight across* (not too short) for puffy or thick skin folds prone to ingrown toenails

   b. *Slightly rounded* for problems with nail corners curving and causing pain and thickening of skin at distal aspect of nail groove
6. Remove free edge of nail.
   a. Do not trim nail off in one clip; make small cuts.
   b. Begin at one edge of nail, nip smoothly working across entire nail border no lower than one sixteenth to one eighth of an inch from end of toe (lateral plate should extend beyond nail fold).
   c. Do not cut deeply into lateral corners of nail bed.
   d. Avoid cutting skin; openings in skin are avenues of entry for bacteria and other infectious agents. If small cuts occur, cleanse thoroughly and apply an antibiotic ointment while educating the patient on follow-up care.
7. Use fine point of nipper to trim out sharp edge of lateral aspect of nail that curves deeply in nail margin.
8. For hyperkeratotic nails, the use of either nippers or a Dremel is effective in debriding the thickened nail plate. Smooth the top and edges of nail with nail rasp or nail file.

BOX 18.4 Nail Debridement Using Mechanical Rotary Tool

1. Before using a Dremel drill, patients should be informed that they will feel a vibration while the nail is being debrided.
2. Don appropriate personal protective equipment.
3. Remove most of fungal nail with quality nippers before using drill to minimize dust.
4. Support toe between index finger and thumb of nondominant hand to prevent toe from moving during debridement. The other toes should be held away from the bur during the procedure.
5. Set grinder speed to 10,000–15,000 rpm.
6. Debride nail by slowly and gently applying pressure as grinder is moved from proximal to distal portion of plate.
7. Keep nail plate visible at all times. Frequently stop grinding to wipe away dust with a cloth (do not blow).
8. Stop grinding when nail is thin or when dust becomes very fine and is not visibly produced during debridement.
9. *Do not grind through nail plate!* Soft underlying layers of plate can be abraded, possibly resulting in subungual wound to nail bed.
10. Avoid surrounding tissue, which can become abraded.

Equipment Options
- Drill with attached vacuum
- Room air circulators with high-efficiency particulate air (HEPA) filters
- Tungsten carbide burs and bits are preferable because they run cold, do not abrade skin, and produce big particles rather than dust
- Ruby carvers and diamond bits are preferable to steel

Equipment Sterilization
- Proper cleansing of equipment between patients is single most important task in reducing or eliminating spread of infection
- Sterilize in autoclave or use antifungal cold soaking solution (glutaraldehyde, phenol, sodium hypochlorite, sodium bromide, iodophors)
- Alcohol does not kill fungus and should not be used for cleansing nail equipment

Personal Protective Equipment and Back Safety
- Gloves, mask, goggles, gown, hair covering
- Height-adjustable chair or examination table for patient
- Height-adjustable chair for clinician
- Change positions frequently; stretch back muscles

Toenail Nippers

Podiatry toenail cutters or pedicure nail nippers are best suited for trimming thicker toenails and lateral curves of the nail. This instrument should be used like scissors. The nail should be removed incrementally to avoid injuring the hyponychium and thus breaking the seal on the nail plate, which would open a portal of entry for fungal or bacterial infections (Godfrey, 2006). There is much debate regarding the best methods for debriding or trimming toenails: straight across versus rounding or following the shape or contouring of the top of the toe. If the patient has a problem with nail corners curving and causing pain and thickening of the skin at the distal aspect of the nail groove, it is recommended that the corners be slightly rounded. Patients who have puffy or a thick skin fold might require nails that are cut straight across so that the corners grow up out of the grooves to prevent ingrown toenails (Katoh, 2008). Box 18.3 gives a procedure for basic cuticle and nail trimming using a nipper.

Curette

The dull-edged curette is a small spoon-shaped instrument that allows for removal of debris under the nail margins. A scooping motion is used along the nail plate to remove debris from the nail groove. This process may need to be repeated until all the debris is removed.

Nail Rasp or Nail File

The medical field calls the nail file a *nail rasp.* It is used to smooth the distal edges of the nail in the nail groove. The file is placed gently in the nail groove against the free (distal) edges of the nail plate. The rasp is then pulled along the edges of the rough nail plate. Each nail should be smoothed with the nail rasp, beginning with healthy nails to prevent transmission of infection.

Ingrown Nail Shaver and Cuticle Nippers

These tools are used when a little more nail needs to be removed from the lateral nail margins. The nail shaver is shaped like a small paddle and has a slot in the middle of the paddle; the end of the slot is filed to a sharp cutting edge. The paddle portion of the nail shaver is placed in the nail groove so that the end of the nail edge is in the slot to trim the spicule of nail present (Mix, 1999).

Mechanical Rotary Tool

The mechanical rotary tool (Dremel drill, cordless, or plug-in) is a standard tool used for nail debridement. Use of a rotary tool disperses nail dust into the air, which can be inhaled by the patient and the clinician and can settle on surfaces throughout the room. Aerosol nail dust, particularly from onychomycotic toenails, can lead to conjunctivitis, rhinitis, asthma, coughing, hypersensitivity, and impaired lung function (Ward, 2005). Personal protection equipment reduces the risk of exposure to the resulting small particles. The hazards associated with these aerosolized small particles have resulted in a great deal of controversy related to the appropriate selection and use of mechanical nail avulsion and debridement tools (Rees, 2008). For example, a drill with an attached vacuum is available that will automatically contain large particles. Box 18.4 lists equipment options and sterilization tips that enhance safety and effectiveness.

Footwear

The main purpose of the shoe is to protect and cushion the foot. Incorrectly fitting footwear is common in older people and is strongly associated with forefoot pathology (hallux valgus, lesser toe deformities, corns, and calluses), foot pain, skin breakdown, abnormal foot pressures, ischemia, and inflammation from repetitive stress (Menz, 2016; Menz & Morris, 2005; Ward, 2005). Although foot size increases with age, surprisingly, many people continue to wear the same size shoe throughout their lifespan. As a result, the foot will take on the shape of the shoe, regardless of the fit. A proper shoe fit requires appropriate length and width measurements, as well as an assessment of the person's style of arch. The correlation between suboptimal shoes and foot pathology, proves the most effective intervention is to evaluate and recommend appropriate footwear (Menz, 2016). Box 18.5 provides several considerations for selecting and maintaining appropriate footwear.

Assessment parameters include wear pattern; a tracing of the weight-bearing foot; footprints; and use of heels, arch supports, and heel cushions. Normal wear patterns occur on the outsole and slightly medial at the great toe and lateral calcaneus. Different wear patterns may be indicative of underlying foot problems or problems with alignment and gait, as illustrated in Fig. 18.6. For example, wear on the ball of the foot may indicate that the heel tendon is tight, in which case heel-raising exercises can be recommended to release this tendon. Toe-shaped ridges on the upper toe box may indicate that the shoes are too small or that hammertoes are developing. A bulge and wear to the side of the great toe may indicate that the shoe is too narrow or that a bunion is present. Finally, unridged wear on the upper toe box generally indicates that the front of the shoe is too low (Ward, 2005).

A tracing of the weight-bearing foot is useful in assessing the fit of the shoe in terms of length and width. The foot tracing is compared with the current shoe to objectively reveal the flaw in the fitting, whether the foot is wider or longer than the shoe (see Fig. 17.4). For example, toe box width plays an enormous role in the development of bunions, toe deformities, and corns. This type of foot tracing will also reveal the source of any foot pain. This tracing can be used to reinforce teaching to the patient about proper shoe fitting. Because the proper fitting of shoes is not an exact science, the patient should be encouraged to take the tracing to the shoe store when purchasing new shoes.

BOX 18.5 Selecting and Maintaining Appropriate Footwear

Shoe Size
- Do not select shoes by size marked inside shoe; sizes vary among shoe brands and styles.

Measurement
- Measure *both* feet regularly; size of feet change with age.

Fitting
- Fit to larger foot.
- Fit at end of the day when feet are at their largest.
- Stand during fitting process.
- Hold new shoe over foot tracing to be certain entire tracing is covered by shoe.
- There should be $3/8$ inch to $1/2$ inch between longest toe and end of each shoe.
- Stand next to shoes to determine whether shoes are shaped like feet or if there are areas of constriction.
- Shoe should conform as much as possible to shape of foot.
- Heel should fit comfortably in shoe with minimum amount of slippage.
- Ball of foot should fit comfortably into widest part (ball pocket) of shoe.
- Do not purchase shoes that feel too tight, expecting them to "stretch" to fit.
- Examine inside of shoe by hand to check for seams, tacks, rough places.
- Walk in shoe to make sure it fits and feels right.

Shoe Type
- A healthy shoe is one that is shaped like the foot. Shoe has deep, roomy, and rounded or square toe box (area of shoe over toes).
- Shoe should be made of very soft material similar to glove leather.

- Flat shoes (with heel height of 1 inch or less) are the healthiest shoes for feet. If high-heeled shoes are needed, keep to heel height of 2 inches or less; limit wearing of shoes to 3 h at a time; and take shoes off coming to and from work, dinner, or church.
- Soles should be shock absorbing and skid resistant (rubber rather than smooth leather).
- Avoid shoes that have seams over areas of pain (e.g., bunion).
- Avoid shoes with heavy rubber soles that curl over top of toe area (e.g., some running shoes) because they can catch on carpets and cause accidental falls.
- Lace-up rather than slip-on shoes provide more secure fit and can accommodate insoles and orthotic devices.
- Select and wear shoe appropriate to activity (e.g., steel-toed boots for farm work, running shoes for running).

Additional Tips
- Wear new shoes initially for short intervals (e.g., 20 min twice per day) and check feet and toes upon removal.
- Indentations, skin discoloration, warmth may be signs of mechanical trauma (pressure points, friction, repetitive stress).
- Do not wear same pair of shoes every day.
- Before putting on shoes, shake them and feel inside them to remove any foreign objects
- Note lumpy insoles or torn linings. Replace worn-out shoes as soon as possible.
- White or light-colored socks are preferred so that any drainage (suggestive of ulceration) is readily apparent.
- Avoid walking barefoot, even at home, because feet are more susceptible to injury and infection.
- Apply sun block to feet when wearing sandals or at the beach.
- Discard socks with holes, socks that have been darned.
- Tops of socks should not restrict circulation.

Source: American Orthopaedic Foot and Ankle Society. (2003). FootCareMD. The National Shoe Retailers Association, and the Pedorthic Footwear Association.

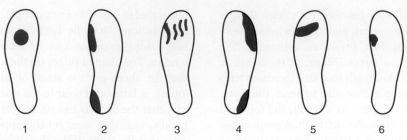

Fig. 18.6 How to "read" your shoes. (1) Wear on the ball of the foot. (2) Wear on the inner sole. (3) Toe-shaped ridges on the upper toe box. (4) Outer sole wear. (5) Bulge and wear to the side of the big toe. (6) Wear on the surface distal to metatarsal head and toes. (Modified from American Orthopaedic Foot and Ankle Society. (2020). *How to "read" your shoes imprint.* American Orthopaedic Foot & Ankle Society. Retrieved March 30, 2021 from: https://www.footcaremd.org/foot-ankle-health/adult-feet.)

To evaluate the arch, a footprint can be made by placing the foot into a bucket of water and making a footprint on a piece of brown paper (Fig. 18.7). A footprint that is very wide in the middle is indicative of flat feet (pes planus). With flat feet, the foot rolls excessively to the inside (i.e., overpronation), which leads to arch strain and pain on the inside of the knee. Adaptations to overcome flat feet and overpronation include molded leather arch supports (available over the counter) and athletic shoe styles. These types of shoes are designed with "control" features that aid in preventing the rolling-in motion of the ankle. If arch supports or sports shoes are ineffective, a foot specialist can fabricate a custom-molded orthotic shoe insert.

If the footprint shows little or no connectedness between the heel and the forefoot, the person has a high arch (pes

Normal foot

Flat foot

High arch

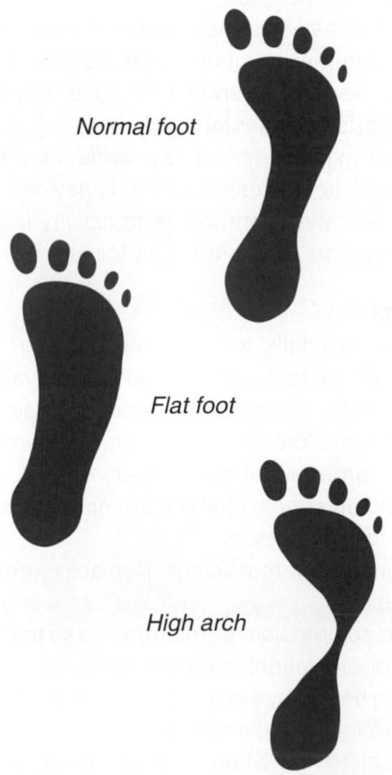

Fig. 18.7 How to "read" your footprint. (Modified from American Orthopaedic Foot & Ankle Society. (2022). Adult feet. *How to read your shoe imprint.* American Orthopaedic Foot & Ankle Society. Retrieved January 19, 2023 from: https://www.footcaremd.org/foot-ankle-health/adult-feet.)

cavus) (underpronation). In this case, the foot rolls too much laterally, with a lot of weight landing on the outside edge of the foot. With this type of situation, the ankle becomes more susceptible to sprains and stress fractures. Again, athletic shoes are most appropriate because (1) "stability" athletic shoes are built with extra cushioning and (2) high-top athletic shoes cover the foot and ankle snugly to reduce the risk of ankle sprains and minimize damage to the ankle from twists (American Orthopaedic Foot & Ankle Society, 2022). Foot pain may also need to have the addition of insert or orthosis inside the shoe. A pair of sneakers properly fitted may provide more room than other types of shoes. (Oh-Park et al., 2019) Several studies have demonstrated that foot orthosis reduce pressure in painful areas and improve balance (Menz, 2016).

High heels increase torque on the knee and increase pressure on the forefoot. In addition, women naturally pronate more than men and naturally rely heavily on heel cushioning and arch support to reduce pronation. Unfortunately, high heels and arch supports restrict the natural movement of the ankle. Furthermore, by reducing pronation, the natural function in ankle motion also increases torque on the knee (Godfrey, 2006; Menz, 2016).

Offloading and Padding

Offloading and padding are used to protect bony structures of the foot, such as prominent metatarsal heads, or toe deformities from mechanical trauma caused by seams in the socks or shoes. Offloading techniques such as those summarized in Table 18.4 and illustrated in Figs. 17.5–17.9 include total-contact casts; removable splints and casts; and customized shoes, pads, and inserts.

Over the counter and custom-molded padding and inserts can be used to redistribute pressure, reduce hyperkeratotic lesions, and eliminate repetitive stress and friction (Freeman, 2002; WOCN®, 2012). Pads can be used to protect diminished fat pads on the plantar surface of the foot. However, pads with aggressive adhesives should be avoided on fragile elderly skin. Nonadherent silicone pads should be used and can be held in place with socks over prominent metatarsal heads. Tubular pads can be fit on the tips of toes to protect at-risk areas or used between toes where interdigital calluses may form. Lamb's wool can be woven between all toes or placed

TABLE 18.4   Offloading Repetitive Stress for Foot and Nail

Anatomic Location	Offloading Method	Advantages/Disadvantages
All sites	Bed rest	Total non–weight-bearing
		Patient adherence is difficult
		Presents quality-of-life issues
		Promotes hyperglycemia
		Promotes patient debilitation
		Increases risk of posterior heel pressures (therefore must float heels)
All sites	Total contact cast (see Fig. 17.6)	Forces adherence
		Allows for limited ambulation
		Requires specialized skill to make
		Not advisable for infected or highly exudative wounds
All sites	Walking splints/removable casts (see Fig. 17.7)	Allows for daily wound surveillance and care
		Requires strict patient adherence
Forefoot ulcers	Football dressing	Forces compliance
		Ease of use with dressings
		Simple to make
		Inexpensive
		Can create balance issues
Forefoot sites	Wedge-soled shoe (aka custom molded shoe) (see Fig. 17.8)	Commercially available
		Can be customized
		May cause balance problems
Plantar/posterior heel ulcers	Heel sole shoe with removable offloading pegs	Commercially available
		Can be customized
		May cause balance problems
All wound sites	Healing shoe with large toe box and customized inserts	Provides offloading to specific wound locations
		Requires specialized equipment
		Requires specialized skill to make
Metatarsal head sites	Adhesive felt pad	Simple to make
		Inexpensive
		Easy to use with dressings
		Requires at least weekly dressing changes
Metatarsal head sites	Felted foam or gel pads	Simple to make
		Inexpensive
		Easy to use with dressings
		Requires replacement every 3–4 days
Toes	Crest pads	Simple to make
		Adjunct for hammertoes or claw toes
		Commercially available
		Inexpensive
		May be used for wound prevention
		Requires frequent replacement
Toes	Silicone or foam	Commercially available
	Interdigital pads	Especially useful for crowded toes and crossed toes and interdigital wounds
	Lamb's wool	May be used for wound prevention
		Ineffective if shoes are too narrow
		Monitor for toe constriction
		Inexpensive
Bony deformities all sites on foot	Padded socks	Commercially available
		May because of foot pressure and/or toe constriction if shoe fit does not allow for increased padding
All bony deformities	Ball and ring shoe stretcher	Simple to use
		Pressure relief on leather shoes at specific sites of deformity

between at-risk toes. The wool provides inherent moisturizing from the lanolin while also absorbing perspiration and excess moisture (Kelechi & Lukacs, 1996; Menz, 2016; Ozdemir et al., 2004).

MANAGEMENT OF SPECIFIC CONDITIONS

Many conditions and circumstances can greatly affect the integrity and function of the foot, such as obesity, anemia, renal insufficiency, impaired circulation, gout, warfarin therapy, Raynaud disease, immunosuppression, and recurrent cellulitis. The 33 joints in each foot must accommodate an extraordinary weight load, making the feet particularly susceptible to arthritic inflammation and swelling of the cartilage and lining of the joints. Individuals older than 50 years are at greatest risk for arthritis. Osteoarthritis is the most common form of arthritis and is associated with aging, injury, or overuse. The foot is one of the first places for osteoporosis to appear; a stress fracture of the foot is often its first sign. Various normal age-associated changes occur in the foot: the foot becomes wider, longer, and flatter; the fat pad on the bottom of the calcaneus thins; and the foot and ankle lose some degree of range of motion and become stiff, which contributes to some loss of balance with ambulation (Ozdemir et al., 2004; Lowth, 2020). Impaired circulation due to lower extremity arterial disease or lower extremity venous disease, as well as decreased foot sensation due to lower extremity neuropathic disease, syphilis, leprosy, myelomeningocele, syringomyelia, hereditary neuropathies, or traumatic nerve injury, contribute to problems with the foot (Adler, Boyko, & Smith, 1999; Younes, Albsoul, & Awad, 2004). Superficial as well as deep lesions and skin alterations can potentially lead to significant infection.

Skin Conditions

Various skin conditions (e.g., vesicles, bullae, or ulcers) can develop on the feet due to repetitive friction and prolonged pressure from ill-fitting shoes. Infection can develop in the foot triggered by a moist environment and require treatment with appropriate medications (antifungal, antibacterial, or antiviral). Hyperkeratotic lesions (corns and calluses) are among the most common foot problems in older people (Sanz, 2018) (Fig. 18.8). Ulcers can develop under these hyperkeratotic lesions with long-term, low-level insult and become particularly problematic in the person with loss of protective sensation (Spink, Menz, & Lord, 2009).

Warts (*Verruca papilloma*) are common dermatologic infections. Plantar warts, specifically, are caused by the human papillomavirus, affect persons of all ages, are contagious, and will spread to other people, especially where the epidermal barrier is disrupted (Watkins, 2006). Plantar warts can also spread to other histologically similar sites (Lichon & Khachemoune, 2007).

Fungal infections may develop and include candida (rarely seen on the feet) and dermatophytes (Ameen, 2010). More commonly called tinea, dermatophyte lesions are discussed in detail in Chapter 9. Dermatophyte symptoms may be less

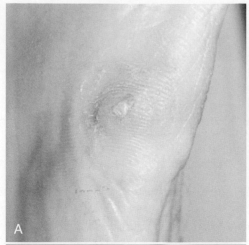

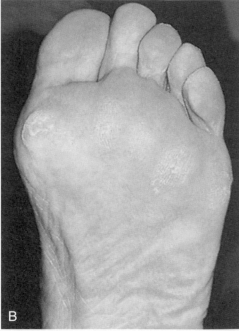

Fig. 18.8 Selected lesions and skin alterations. (A) Corn. (B) Callus. (From Ball, J. W., Dains, J. E., Flynn, J. A. (2015). *Seidel's guide to physical examination* (8th ed.). St. Louis: Mosby.)

pronounced in elderly individuals and in individuals with altered sensation (Hill, 2008). The moccasin type of tinea pedis is often mistaken for dry skin on the plantar surface of the foot but does not respond to emollient application (Crawford, 2004). Tinea pedis may coexist with a secondary bacterial infection (Erbagci, 2004).

Table 18.2 summarizes the assessment, prevention, and management of common foot lesions. Various interventions include properly fitting shoes; offloading; positioning; and topical agents such as emollients, antifungals, and, in some cases, corticosteroids. Offloading and padding, as described previously, is needed to interrupt the presence of the stressors causing vesicles, ulcers, and corns. In general, a vesicle or bulla should be left intact. Topical care of open lesions should be selected based on the needs of the wound, as described in Chapter 21.

As with all interventions, reevaluation of the effectiveness is needed. If the problem deteriorates or fails to respond to treatment within a reasonable period of time (i.e., 7 days), reassessment and modification of the treatment should be conducted. For example, topical antibiotics and corticosteroids may need to be delivered systemically rather than topically. However, use of these medications should be recommended only by a practitioner who is well informed of their potential complications and side effects, which can include conditions such as skin reactions, liver enzyme abnormalities, diarrhea, and visual and taste disturbances.

Foot Conditions (Malformations)

Foot malformations can affect all three sections of the foot: forefoot, midfoot, and hindfoot. Charcot arthropathy (see Fig. 18.1B) is a fairly rare but serious condition caused by the disruption or disintegration of some of the foot and ankle joints. Redness, swelling, and deformity may develop and may be misinterpreted as cellulitis. Charcot arthropathy is frequently associated with diabetes (discussed in greater detail in Chapter 17).

Forefoot

The forefoot area has the highest prevalence of foot malformations. The most common problems that arise in the forefoot are hallux valgus (bunions), bunionettes, hallux rigidus, claw toes, hammertoes and mallet toes, metatarsalgia, and interdigit neuromas (Morton neuroma). Forefoot problems are painful and are generally accompanied by ingrown toenail, calluses, and corns (Hsi et al., 2005). Forefoot problems occur nine times more often in women than in men and are most commonly associated with wearing shoes with high heels and a narrow toe box. Once forefoot problems develop, finding footwear can be difficult. Brief descriptions of forefoot malformations are provided in Table 18.5 and illustrated in Fig. 17.1 (Ferrari, Higgins, & Prior, 2004; Larson,

TABLE 18.5	**Types of Forefoot Malformations**	
Name	**Description**	**Common Location(s)**
Hallux valgus (bunion) (see Fig. 17.1C)	Lateral deviation of great toe (hallux)	First MTP joint
	Produces abnormal hypertrophic bursa over medial eminence of first metatarsal	
	Diagnostic testing includes examination and radiograph to determine degree of deviation	
	Symptoms include pain, redness, and swelling at or near the joint; as toe devastation progresses, bunion becomes more painful	
Bunionette (tailor's bunion)	Less common than bunion; see previous description	Fifth MTP joint
Hallux rigidus	Degenerative arthritis of MTP joint	First MTP joint
	Presents with pain in great toe with activity, especially in toe-off phase of gait	
	Stiffness of great toe and loss of extension at MTP joint	
	Toe in normal alignment	
	Radiographs show narrowing of MTP joint of great toe	
Interdigit neuroma (Morton neuroma)	Not a true neuroma	Metatarsal head
	Perineural fibrosis of common digital nerve as it passes through metatarsal head; fibrosis results from repeated irritation of nerve that may be caused by bones or other tissue rubbing against and irritating the nerves	
	Plantar pain in forefoot is most common presenting symptom	
	Pain usually is alleviated by rubbing ball of the foot after removing shoes	
Claw toe	Usually associated with neurologic disorder or inflammatory arthritis	Lesser toes
Hammertoe (see Fig. 17.1A)	Fixation of proximal dorsiflexion, middle joint is fixed in plantar flexion, distal joint is moveable	Lesser toes
	Usually bilateral	
	Often accompanied by hallux valgus	
Mallet toe	Distal interphalangeal joint is plantarflexed on intermediate phalanx with rest of joint in normal position	Lesser toes
Charcot arthropathy (see Fig. 17.1B)	Fairly rare but serious; associated with diabetes	Foot
	Caused by disruption or disintegration of some of the foot and ankle joints	
	Redness, swelling, and deformity may develop and may be misinterpreted as cellulitis	
	(Discussed in greater detail in Chapter 17)	

MTP, metatarsophalangeal.

Barrett, Battison, et al., 2005; Thomson, Gibson, & Martin, 2004). Forefoot pain, specifically metatarsalgia, results from an abnormal metatarsal length with alteration of the weight-bearing forces. Symptoms of metatarsalgia include callus formation and localized pain in the plantar aspect of the forefoot over the metatarsal heads. Treatment of forefoot pain involves the application of a metatarsal pad and paring down of calluses (Hsi et al., 2005).

Midfoot

The primary midfoot problem is pain. Midfoot pain is commonly caused by arthritis in the midfoot joints, including the TMT joint, subtalar joint, and talonavicular joint. The exact area of pain is easily pinpointed with palpation. The palpation of a bony prominence that is an osteophyte or dorsal bossing corresponds with the joint with the arthritis. Although less common, soft tissue pain can be present on the plantar aspect of the midfoot, which occurs with plantar fasciitis; this is discussed in more detail in the "Hindfoot" section (Frey, 2005).

Hindfoot

Heel pain, a typical hindfoot problem, is caused by stress on the calcaneus and results from poorly made footwear and walking or jumping on hard surfaces. Common causes include plantar fasciitis, heel spur, tarsal tunnel syndrome, and Achilles tendonitis (Labib, Gould, Rodriguez-del-Rio, et al., 2002). Additional causative factors include arthritis, gout, ankylosing spondylitis, Reiter syndrome, radiculopathy, inferior calcaneal bursitis, calcaneal fracture, foreign bodies, circulatory problems, and obesity. Calcaneus pain can be palpated directly over the plantar medial calcaneal tuberosity. A heel spur, an osteophyte bony growth on the underside, foremost part of the calcaneus bone, is commonly associated with plantar fasciitis, as illustrated in Fig. 18.9 (Frey, 2005).

Plantar fasciitis is the most common condition causing heel pain. This pain occurs with weight bearing or faulty biomechanics that place too much stress on the calcaneus bone, ligaments, or nerves in the area (Jolly et al., 2005; La Porta & La Fata, 2005). Plantar fasciitis is essentially an inflammation of the long band of connective tissue running from the calcaneus to the ball of the foot that forms the arch of the foot (Lemont, Ammirati, & Usen, 2003). Symptoms include pain on the plantar surface of the heel and pain that is worse upon arising or after sitting a long time and increases over a few months. Plantar fasciitis is most likely to develop in people with either overly flat feet or high arched feet.

Posterior heel pain causes symptoms behind the foot rather than underneath is likely related to irritation from shoes, and presents with a prominence over the superior process of the calcaneus. A common cause of posterior heel pain is Achilles tendonitis, considered a jumping injury. The Achilles tendon connects the calf muscle to the heel bone and facilitates walking by helping raise the heel off the ground. Symptoms of Achilles tendon pathology include pain along the tendon (aching, stiff, soreness) and pain that begins upon arising and after periods of rest, improves slightly with movement, then worsens with increased activity. Athletes are at high risk for developing Achilles tendon pathology. Tarsal tunnel syndrome causes heel pain similar to carpal tunnel syndrome in the hand and is a repetitive motion injury (Badlissi et al., 2005).

The cause of heel pain must be determined before a plan of treatment is initiated. General treatments include rest or avoiding the precipitating activity (e.g., jogging), icing the heel, exercises and stretches, and nonsteroidal antiinflammatory medications. An orthotic device, such as a silicone heel pad insert with shock-absorbing soles, is often key to successful treatment of calcaneus pain. Exercises such as "alphabet exercise," where the patient moves the ankle in multiple planes of motion by drawing both lowercase and uppercase letters of the alphabet with the foot, are particularly beneficial for heel spurs. Cortisone injections and over-the-counter heel cups or custom-made orthotics also may be warranted.

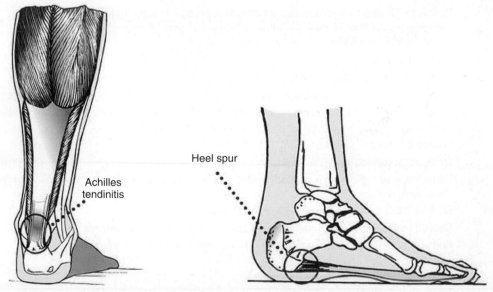

Achilles tendinitis

Heel spur

Fig. 18.9 Locations of Achilles tendonitis and heel spur. (From American Physical Therapy Association, 1996.)

Nail Conditions (Onychopathy)

Onycho means, "nail." Onychopathy is any disease or deformity of the nail. Abnormal nails are clues to multisystem diseases. The growth rate, discoloration, thickness, and structural changes can be equated to specific disease processes. Nails should be inspected for general appearance; nail plate for length, color, thickness, presence of subungual debris, odor, hyponychium or eponychium for separation from the nail plate; and paronychial edge for infection, ingrown nails, hangnails, and pain. The toenails should be assessed for changes in color, continuity of the nail plate, missing nails or nail malformations, and infection. Nail disorders are difficult to treat in part because of the slow growth rate of the toenail and the difficulty of getting the drug actives to penetrate the nail tissues (Lorizzo, 2015). The toenail can take up to 12–18 months for entire regrowth (Lipner, 2016). Selected nail disorders, descriptions, symptoms, and causes are listed in Table 18.6. This section describes management strategies.

Onychocryptosis (Ingrown Nail)

Management of onychocryptosis includes education on proper nail trimming and proper fitting of shoes. The lateral plate should be allowed to grow well beyond the nail fold before trimming horizontally in order to prevent trauma of the toenail edge to separate the nail plate from the nail fold which subsequently causes a painful inflammatory foreign body reaction. The mild to moderate ingrown nail with minimal pain and erythema and no discharge can be treated with the application of a cotton wedge or dental floss underneath the lateral nail plate. This separates the nail plate from the lateral nail fold, which relieves the pressure. The moderate to severe ingrown toenail with substantial erythema and pustular discharge (Fig. 18.10B) will require a digital block and removal of the involved nail wedge with a hemostat. Cleansing the area with 1:1 peroxide and water two to three times per day followed by the application of a topical antibiotic is recommended (Rounding & Bloomfield, 2005; Lomax, Thornton, & Singh 2016).

Onychomycosis (Fungal Infection of Nail)

Onychomycosis is an infection of the nail that includes the nail plate, nail bed and the peri-ungal tissue (Zeichner, 2018). Fungal infections account for only 50% of the dystrophic nails. Onychomycosis can affect 12% of the US population. The infection occurs more in men than women and the risk increases with age. Other predisposing factors include climate, lifestyle, and medical conditions, such as PVD, DM, and immune deficiencies (Zeichner, 2018).

Onychomycosis is a progressive disease and if left untreated can cause permanent nail dystrophy, cellulitis,

TABLE 18.6 Selected Nail Disorders

Name	Description	Symptoms	Cause
Paronychia (see Fig. 18.10A)	Painful infection of tissue around base of nail (perionychium)	Swelling and tenderness posterior or lateral to nail folds. May progress to superficial abscess	Bacteria enter break in skin caused by damage, trauma (e.g., nail biting, chemical irritants)
Onychocryptosis (ingrown nail) (see Fig. 18.10B)	Penetration of segment of nail plate into nail sulcus and subcutaneous tissue	Acute inflammation, edema, exudate, pain	Improper nail trimming / Shoe pressure
		Can evolve into infection (paronychia, cellulitis), ulceration, necrosis	Injury or fungal infection / Poor foot structure / Onychogryphosis
		Most commonly affects large toes	Higher risk: male, increasing age, immunosuppression, diabetes, PVD
Onychomycosis (fungal infection)	*Tinea unguium* or dermatophyte infection	Painless, dystrophic changes (thick, brittle discoloration) of one or many toenails	Infectious agent present on susceptible host / Chronic exposure to moisture
	Occurs in three distinct forms: distal subungual, proximal subungual, white superficial	Psoriasis, lichen planus, dermatitis, dyshidrosis may mimic onychomycosis	Hyperhidrosis / Tinea pedis / Poor hygiene
Onychogryposis (ram's horn nail)	Large, deformed, hypertrophic nail	Thick hard nails that curl like horn of ram	Nail was permitted to grow without trimming or debridement
Onychophosis	Localized or diffuse hyperkeratosis on lateral or proximal nail folds, in space between nail folds and nail plate	First and fifth toes are commonly affected	Poor-fitting shoes
Onychatrophia	Atrophy of nails	Softer, thinner, smaller nails. Nail detachment	Skin diseases, underlying diseases

PVD, peripheral vascular disease.

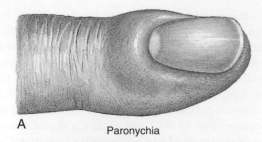

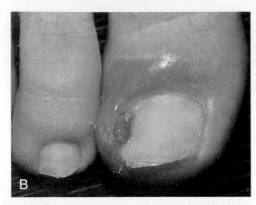

Fig. 18.10 Selected nail disorders. (A) Paronychia (B), Onychocryptosis (ingrown nail). (Panel A: From Ball, J. W., Dains, J. E., Flynn, J. A. (2019). *Seidel's guide to physical examination* (9th ed.). St. Louis: Mosby; Panel B: From White, G. M. (1994). *Color atlas of regional dermatology.* St. Louis: Mosby.)

distant spread of fungal infection to adjacent toenail, skin and interdigit plantar tinea. The compromised skin allows a port of entry for bacterial infections, which is why the risk of cellulitis is greater in a patient with onychomycosis. The combination of diabetes and onychomycosis puts the patient at higher risk for a bacterial infection (Zeichner, 2018).

Nail conditions such as psoriasis, lichen planus, dermatitis, dyshidrosis, and other infections may mimic onychomycosis (Baran & Kaoukhov, 2005). The nail becomes thick, discolored and can separate from the nailbed (Onycholysis) when infected with fungus (Zeichner, 2018). Therefore, culturing the nail has become a standard of practice before treatment with an antifungal. The antifungal chosen is usually driven by insurance reimbursement of the medication. The highest cure rates are associated with oral terbinafine and itraconazole. Topical nail lacquer containing ciclopirox is used for mild to moderate onychomycosis that does not involve the lunula (see Fig. 18.3). The lacquer is applied once daily to the affected nail, 5 mm of surrounding skin, the nail bed (hyponychium), and the undersurface of the nail plate. Once per week, the nail lacquer is wiped off with alcohol. Studies have shown increased efficacy with the combination treatment (Sidou & Soto, 2004). Despite the best treatment efforts, relapse occurs between 40% and 70% of cases (Zeichner, 2015).

Paronychia

Paronychia is an inflammation process involving the lateral and proximal nail fold and the cells that grow the nail (matrix) (see Fig. 18.10A), resulting in pain, edema and erythema with or without abscess formation caused from many of the disorders described in Table 18.6. For chronic paronychia, treatment consists of warm soaks and topical antifungal agents. Acute paronychia in toenails is usually associated with ingrown toenail or retronychia (Lomax et al., 2016). Treatment includes warm compresses for 20 min three times per day and topical antibiotics (triple antibiotic) applied after the warm soaks. For more severe infections, oral antibiotics with gram-positive coverage may be necessary (Billingsley & Vidimos, 2018) and treatment of the underlying cause such as: ingrown toenail (Lomax et al., 2016).

Referral

Numerous specialists (e.g., primary care provider, podiatry, orthopedics, dermatology, endocrinology, vascular surgery, general surgery, physical therapy, occupational therapy, orthotist, home health, pain management, diabetes education, smoking cessation, case/care manager, social worker, and wound specialist) may be required to provide comprehensive foot and nail care. The results of the foot screening must be communicated to the appropriate health care provider, along with the patient's foot ulceration risk and a record of the educational materials given to the patient and family (Boulton & Armstrong, 2008; Patout et al., 2001).

Patient and Caregiver Education

Involving patients in their own care decreases foot complications; therefore, it is important to provide education on foot and nail care to the patient and caregiver (Howell & Thirlaway, 2004). Box 18.6 lists the components of patient and family education related to foot care. Patients should be taught that they could protect the health of their feet by maintaining a normal weight to lessen changes due to osteoporosis (Neno, 2007; Woodrow, Dickson, & Wright, 2005).

BOX 18.6   Components of Patient and Family Education

- Foot care (hygiene, skin care, inspection, nail care)
- Anatomy and pathophysiology affecting the foot
- Age-specific foot changes
- Ulcer and amputation risk
- Lifestyle choices that affect health (exercise, smoking, nutrition, weight management)
- Plans for preventing foot disorders
- Proper footwear (see Box 18.5)
- Plan for follow-up
- Problems that should be reported:
  - Foot or ankle pain that is intense
  - Foot or ankle pain that persists for more than 72 h
  - Lower extremity pain that increases with exercise or ambulation, rest, or elevation
  - Swelling of one leg or foot that persists for more than 24 h
  - Sudden progression of a foot deformity
  - Unilateral flattening of foot arch
  - Infection
  - Loss of sensation
  - Blister or ulcer on foot that developed without the patient feeling it
  - Blister or ulcer on foot that is not healing

Additional foot care instructions can be found in Box 17.5. The patient should be taught to call the health care professional when problems listed in Box 18.6 arise (American Orthopaedic Foot & Ankle Society, 2022; Gemmell, Hayes, & Conway, 2005; van Os, Bierma-Zeinstra, Verhagen, et al., 2005).

Home Remedies

Many over-the-counter and home remedies are used for treatment of foot and nail problems. Four products are most commonly used: Vicks VapoRub, vinegar, vegetable oil, and Vaseline. Vaseline and vegetable oil (Crisco) are inexpensive options and can be used to moisturize the skin. Vegetable oil has a risk of bacterial growth while in the container and the risk of allergic dermatitis. Vaseline (petroleum) comes in different grades, which vary depending on composition, purity (depending on stock), production, and packaging. Petrolatum-based products have been identified as clinically effective and cost-effective. However, allergic dermatitis can occur from petroleum products (Kelechi & Stroud, 2004).

Vinegar, tea tree oil, and mentholated topical petrolatum-based gel (such as Vicks VapoRub) are used to treat fungal and bacterial infections. In various dilutions, vinegar is effective in reducing or eliminating growth of bacteria. Evidence for the use of vinegar in treating fungal infection is limited. The literature has reported vinegar (one-part vinegar and two parts water for 15 min per day) used as treatment of toenail fungus, athlete's foot, and foot odor and as an exfoliant. Long-term use of vinegar (regardless of concentration) is contraindicated, however, due to the drying effect and potential for skin irritation. Tea tree oil is an antiseptic/tinneacide. Anecdotally, Vicks VapoRub applied topically to the nail daily has been used for treatment of toenail fungus (Kelechi & Stroud, 2004).

Unsupervised home remedies for foot ailments should be avoided. Self-treatment has the potential for turning a minor problem into a major one. Persons with diabetes, poor circulation, or heart problems should not treat their own feet because they are more prone to infection. It is vital that older individuals see a foot care specialist at least once per year for a checkup (Neno, 2007; Woodrow et al., 2005).

CLINICAL CONSULT

A: Patient referred by nursing home nurse to evaluate a 63-year-old Caucasian male for scratching LE and open area on right great toe. Current medical history includes insulin-dependent diabetes, hypothyroid, hepatitis C, hypertension, major depression, and skin picking disorder. Upon exam patient states that he is not having any scratching, admits to picking/cutting his toenails. Ambulates independently. Wears orthotic shoes. Excoriation on bilateral lower extremities with no redness or drainage. Right great toe lateral nail fold has small purulent discharge, erythema, and edema present; painful to touch. Blood sugar 246, afebrile.
D: Paronychia, heel fissure, interdigit toe maceration.
P: Apply antibacterial ointment three times daily; cover with nonadherent dressing and secure with roll gauze. Start doxycycline 100 mg twice a day ×10 days.

I: (1) Use healing shoe until infection resolved to prevent further trauma. (2) Wear padded socks. (3) Schedule foot and nail care nurse visits for callus removal and nail debriding. (4) Remove nail-clipping tools from patient's room. (5) Education on diabetic foot care. (6) Apply Lac-Hydrin to lower extremities daily. Redirect if patient is seen scratching. (7) Lamb's wool between toes and changed daily. (8) Pedorthist to reevaluate orthotic shoes for proper fitting. (9) Joint collaboration with mental health care provider for potential antianxiety medications and behavior therapy to diminish picking behavior.
E: Recheck visit in 3 days.

SUMMARY

- Foot and nail disorders are predominantly a reflection of the patient's overall health status.
- Routine foot care should be integrated into everyday practice, thus keeping the skin healthy and intact and minimizing the risk of trauma or malformation thus by improving the overall health of the elderly.

- Conducting a regular and routine foot and nail assessment in conjunction with a routine skin assessment, preventive interventions can be identified that will prevent the discomfort and secondary complications that arise from foot and nail disorders.

SELF-ASSESSMENT QUESTIONS

1. Which of the following is *not* important information in gathering the patient's pertinent health history?
   a. Arthritis status
   b. Smoking habits
   c. Vision problems
   d. Nasal polyps

2. In assessing the anatomic level in the lower extremity at which arterial insufficiency becomes apparent, which of the following is diagnostically most useful?
   a. Segmental pressures
   b. Femoral bruit
   c. Venous refill time
   d. Ankle-brachial index

3. When instructing the patient and caregiver on proper shoe fit, which of the following is important to emphasize?
   a. Shoes should be selected based on the printed shoe size provided by the manufacturer.
   b. Shoes should be tested for fit early in the morning before the patient is too fatigued to adequately assess how it feels.
   c. Shoes should be fitted while the patient is sitting with the foot elevated on a slanted shoe-fitting stool.
   d. Shoes with heavy rubber soles that curl over the top of the toe area should be avoided.

4. Which of the following is *not* recommended when treating warts on the foot, particularly in younger individuals?
   a. Electrocautery
   b. Liquid nitrogen (cryotherapy)
   c. Salicylic acid
   d. Capsaicin ointment

5. Onychomycosis is:
   a. A bacterial infection
   b. Commonly painful
   c. A fungal infection
   d. Treatable with bleach solution soakings in persons with weak or frail skin

6. Options for toenail debridement should include the use of all of the following *except*:
   a. Manual nippers
   b. Mechanical rotary tools fitted with tungsten carbide burs
   c. Salicylate solutions
   d. Personal protective equipment to reduce exposure to dust

7. Which of the following causes foot odor?
   a. Fungi
   b. Isovaleric acid
   c. Foot powders
   d. Acetic acid

8. Natural, age-specific changes of the foot include which of the following?
   a. Bunions
   b. Narrowing of the foot
   c. Thickening of fat pad over calcaneus
   d. Decreased range of motion

9. The patient should notify his or her provider when any of the following develop *except*:
   a. Foot pain that persists for more than 72 h
   b. Foot pain that increases with elevation of the legs
   c. Swelling of one leg or foot that persists less than 8 hours
   d. Any sudden progression of a foot deformity

10. What causes maceration between the toes?
    a. Inflammation
    b. Allergy
    c. Excessively dry skin
    d. Excessively moist skin

11. Which of the following terms refers to a tinea infection of the nails?
    a. Tinea pedis
    b. Tinea cruris
    c. Tinea corporis
    d. Onychomycosis

12. Suggestions to prevent tinea infections include which of the following?
    a. Wash hair daily.
    b. Avoid wearing socks.
    c. Wear flip-flops or sandals in public places instead of going barefoot.
    d. Use antideodorant rather than antiperspirant.

REFERENCES

Adelstein, S., Bray, J., & Schram, A. (2008). Superglue for the treatment of heel fissures. *Journal of the American Podiatric Medical Association*, 89(8), 434–435.

Adler, A. L., Boyko, E. J., & Smith, D. G. (1999). Lower-extremity amputation in diabetes. The independent effect of peripheral vascular disease, sensory neuropathy and foot ulcers. *Diabetes Care*, 22(7), 1029–1035.

Ameen, M. (2010). Epidemiology of superficial fungal infections. *Clinics in Dermatology*, 28(2), 197–201. https://doi.org/10.1016/j.clindermatol.2009.12.005.

American Orthopaedic Foot & Ankle Society. (2022). *AOFAS FootCareMD. How to keep feet flexible.* Retrieved January 19, 2023 from: https://www.footcaremd.org/resources/how-to-help/how-to-keep-feet-flexible.

American Podiatric Medical Association. (2010). *Your podiatric physician talks about foot health.* Retrieved March 30, 2021 from: http://www.apma.org/files/ProductPDFs/Foot_Health.pdf.

Awale, A., Dufour, A. B., Katz, P., Menz, H. B., & Hannan, M. T. (2016). Link between foot pain severity and prevalence of depressive symptoms. *Arthritis Care & Research*, 68(6), 871–876. https://doi.org/10.1002/acr.22779.

Badlissi, F., Dunn, J. E., Link, C. L., et al. (2005). Foot musculoskeletal disorders, pain, and foot-related functional limitation in older persons. *Journal of the American Geriatrics Society*, 53, 1029–1033.

Baran, R., & Kaoukhov, A. (2005). Topical antifungal drugs for the treatment of onychomycosis: An overview of current strategies for monotherapy and combination therapy. *Journal of the European Academy of Dermatology and Venereology*, 19, 21–29.

Billingsley, E., & Vidimos, A. (2018). Paronychia treatment and management. Retrieved March 30, 2021 from: http://emedicine.medscape.com/article/1106062-treatment.

Boulton, A., & Armstrong, D. (2008). Comprehensive foot examination and risk assessment. *Diabetes Care*, 31, 1679–1685.

Boulton, A. J., Armstrong, D. G., Albert, S. F., Frykberg, R. G., Hellman, R., Kirkman, M. S., et al. (2008). Comprehensive foot examination and risk assessment: A report of the task force of the foot care interest group of the American Diabetes Association, with endorsement by the American Association of Clinical Endocrinologists. *Diabetes Care*, 31, 1679–1685.

Cavanagh, P. R., & Ulbrecht, J. S. (2008). The biomechanics of the foot in diabetes mellitus. In J. H. Bowker, & M. A. Pfeiffer (Eds.), *Levin and O'Neal's the diabetic foot* (7th ed.). St. Louis: Mosby.

Crawford, F. (2004). Athlete's foot and fungally infected toenails. *Clinical Evidence, 11*, 2128–2132.

Dunn, J. E. (2004). Prevalence of foot and ankle conditions in a multiethnic community sample of older adults. *American Journal of Epidemiology, 159*(5), 491–498. https://doi.org/10.1093/aje/kwh071.

Duthie, E. H. (2007). History and physical exam. In E. H. Duthie, et al. (Eds.), *Practice of geriatrics* (4th ed.). Philadelphia: Saunders.

Erbagci, Z. (2004). Topical therapy for dermatophytoses: Should corticosteroids be included? *American Journal of Clinical Dermatology, 5*, 375–384.

Ferrari, J., Higgins, J. P., & Prior, T. D. (2004). Interventions for treating hallux valgus (abductovalgus) and bunions. *Cochrane Database of Systematic Reviews, 1*, CD000964.

Freeman, D. B. (2002). Corns and calluses resulting from mechanical hyperkeratosis. *American Family Physician, 65*, 2277–2280.

Frey, C. (2005). Plantar fasciitis. In L. Y. Griffin (Ed.), *Essentials of musculoskeletal care* (3rd ed.). Rosemont: American Academy of Orthopaedic Surgeons.

Fujii, K. (2019). Effect of foot care interventions for older adults using day care services. *Nursing Open, 6*(4), 1372–1380. https://doi.org/10.1002/nop2.333.

Fujimoto, T. (2016). Pathophysiology and treatment of hyperhidrosis. *Current Problems in Dermatology, 51*, 86–93.

Garrow, A. P., Silman, A. J., & Macfarlane, G. J. (2004). The Cheshire foot pain and disability survey: A population survey assessing prevalence and associations. *Pain, 110*, 378–384.

Gemmell, H., Hayes, B., & Conway, M. (2005). A theoretical model for treatment of soft tissue injuries: Treatment of an ankle sprain in a college tennis player. *Journal of Manipulative and Physiological Therapeutics, 28*, 285–288.

Godfrey, J. R. (2006). Toward the optimal health. D. Casey Kerrigan, M.D., discusses the impact of footwear on the progression of osteoarthritis in women. *Journal of Women's Health (Larchmt), 15*, 894–897.

Hill, M. J. (2008). Fungal infections. *Dermatology Nursing, 20*, 137–138.

Howell, M., & Thirlaway, S. (2004). Integrating foot care into the everyday clinical practice of nurses. *The British Journal of Nursing, 13*, 470–473.

Hsi, W. L., et al. (2005). Optimum position of metatarsal pad in metatarsalgia for pressure relief. *American Journal of Physical Medicine & Rehabilitation, 84*, 514.

Jarvis, C. (2020). Neurologic system. In C. Jarvis (Ed.), *Physical examination and health assessment* (8th ed.). St. Louis: Elsevier.

Jolly, G. P., Zgonis, T., & Hendrix, C. L. (2005). Neurogenic heel pain. *Clinics in Podiatric Medicine and Surgery, 22*, 101–113.

Katoh, T. (2008). Outpatient foot care by dermatologist and specially trained nurse. *Japan Journal of Mycology, 49*, 173–174.

Katsambas, A., Abeck, D., Haneke, E., et al. (2005). The effects of foot disease on quality of life: Results of the Achilles project. *Journal of the European Academy of Dermatology and Venereology, 19*, 191–195.

Kelechi, T., & Lukacs, K. (1996). Intrapreneurial nursing: The comprehensive lower extremity assessment form. *Clinical Nurse Specialist CNS, 10*, 266–274.

Kelechi, T., & Stroud, S. (2004). The four V's of footcare. *Advance for Nurse Practitioners, 12*, 67–70.

La Porta, G. A., & La Fata, P. C. (2005). Pathologic conditions of the plantar fascia. *Clinics in Podiatric Medicine and Surgery, 22*, 1–9.

Labib, S. A., Gould, J. S., Rodriguez-del-Rio, F. A., et al. (2002). Heel pain triad (HPT): The combination of plantar fasciitis, posterior tibial tendon dysfunction and tarsal tunnel syndrome. *Foot & Ankle International, 23*, 212–220.

Larson, E. E., Barrett, S. L., Battison, B., et al. (2005). Accurate nomenclature for forefoot nerve entrapment: A historical perspective. *Journal of the American Podiatric Medical Association, 95*, 298–306.

Lemont, H., Ammirati, K. M., & Usen, N. (2003). Plantar fasciitis: A degenerative process (fasciosis) without inflammation. *Journal of the American Podiatric Medical Association, 93*, 234–237.

Leveille, S. G., Guralnik, J. M., Ferrucci, L., et al. (1998). Foot pain and disability in older women. *American Journal of Epidemiology, 148*, 657–665.

Lichon, V., & Khachemoune, A. (2007). Plantar warts: A focus on treatment modalities. *Dermatology Nursing, 19*(4), 372–375.

Lomax, A., Thornton, J., & Singh, D. (2016). Toenail paronychia. *Foot and Ankle Surgery, 22*(4), 219–223. https://doi.org/10.1016/j.fas.2015.09.003.

López-López, D., Becerro-De-Bengoa-Vallejo, R., Losa-Iglesias, M. E., Palomo-López, P., Rodríguez-Sanz, D., Brandariz-Pereira, J. M., et al. (2018). Evaluation of foot health related quality of life in individuals with foot problems by gender: A cross-sectional comparative analysis study. *BMJ Open, 8*(10). https://doi.org/10.1136/bmjopen-2018-023980.

Lorizzo. M. (2015). Tips to treat the 5 most common nail disorders: Brittle nails, onycholysis, paronychia, psoriasis, onychomycosis. *Dermatology Clinics, 3*(2), 175–183. https://doi.org/10.1016/j.det.2014.12.001.

Lowth, M. (2020). Abnormal gait. Retrieved January 19, 2023 from: http://www.patient.co.uk/doctor/Abnormal-Gait.htm.

Menz, H. B. (2016). Chronic foot pain in older people. *Maturitas, 91*, 110–114. https://doi.org/10.1016/j.maturitas.2016.06.011.

Menz, H. B., Dufour, A. B., Casey, V. A., Riskowski, J. L., Mclean, R. R., Katz, P., et al. (2013). Foot pain and mobility limitations in older adults: The Framingham Foot Study. *The Journals of Gerontology Series A: Biological Sciences and Medical Sciences, 68*(10), 1281–1285. https://doi.org/10.1093/gerona/glt048.

Menz, H. B., & Lord, S. R. (2001). The contribution of foot problems to mobility impairment and falls in community-dwelling older people. *Journal of the American Geriatrics Society, 49*, 1651–1656.

Menz, H. B., & Morris, M. E. (2005). Footwear characteristics and foot problems in older people. *Gerontology, 51*, 346–351.

Mix, G. (1999). *Salon professional's guide to foot care*. Albany: Milady Salon Ovations.

Neno, R. (2007). Feet for purpose? *Nursing Older People, 19*(8), 5–6.

Oh-Park, M., Kirschner, J., Abdelshahed, D., & Kim, D. D. (2019). Painful foot disorders in the geriatric population. *American Journal of Physical Medicine & Rehabilitation, 98*(9), 811–819. https://doi.org/10.1097/phm.0000000000001239.

Ozdemir, H., Söyüncü, Y., Ozgörgen, M., et al. (2004). Effects of changes in heel fat pad thickness and elasticity on heel pain. *Journal of the American Podiatric Medical Association, 94*, 47–52.

Parker, J., Scharfbillig, R., & Jones, S. (2017). Moisturisers for the treatment of foot xerosis: A systematic review. *Journal of Foot and Ankle Research, 10*, 9. https://doi.org/10.1186/s13047-017-0190-9.

Patout, C. A., Jr., Birke, J. A., Wilbright, W. A., et al. (2001). A decision pathway for the staged management of foot problems in diabetes mellitus. *Archives of Physical Medicine and Rehabilitation, 82,* 1724–1728.

Piraccini, B. M., Iorizzo, M., Antonoucci, A., et al. (2004). Drug-induced nail abnormalities. *Expert Opinion on Drug Safety, 3,* 57–65.

Popoola, M. M., & Jenkins, L. (2004). Caring for the foot mobile. *Holistic Nursing Practice, 19,* 222–227.

Price, P., & Harding, K. (2000). The impact of foot complications on health-related quality of life in patients with diabetes. *Journal of Cutaneous Medicine and Surgery, 4,* 45–50.

Quinn, E. (2019). Anatomy of the foot and common foot problems. *Sports Medicine.* About. ht. Retrieved March 30, 2021 from: https://www.verywellhealth.com/foot-anatomy-and-physiology-3119204.

Rees, H. G. (2008). World at work: Evidence-based risk management of nail dust in chiropodists and podiatrists. *Occupational and Environmental Medicine, 65,* 216–217.

Rodríguez-Sanz, D., Tovaruela-Carrión, N., López-López, D., Palomo-López, P., Romero-Morales, C., Navarro-Flores, E., et al. (2018). Foot disorders in the elderly: A mini review. *Disease-a-Month, 64*(3), 64–91. https://doi.org/10.1016/j.disamonth.2017.08.001.

Rounding, C., & Bloomfield, S. (2005). Surgical treatments for ingrowing toenails. *Cochrane Database of Systematic Reviews, 2,* CD001541.

Sidou, F., & Soto, P. (2004). A randomized comparison of nail surface remanence three nail lacquers, containing amorolfine 5%, ciclopirox 8% or tioconazole 28%, in healthy volunteers. *International Journal of Tissue Reactions, 26*(1–2), 17–24.

Sinni-McKeehen, B. (2019). Nursing assessment. Integumentary system. In S. L. Lewis, et al. (Eds.), *Medical-surgical nursing. Assessment and management of clinical problems.* St. Louis: Elsevier.

Spink, M. J., Menz, H. B., & Lord, S. R. (2009). Distribution and correlates of plantar hyperkeratotic lesions in older people. *Journal of Foot and Ankle Research, 30,* 8.

Sprecher, E. (2005). Genetic hair and nail disorders. *Clinics in Dermatology, 23,* 47–55.

Stroud, S., & Kelechi, T. (2006). Itching and sores between the toes. Maceration and fungal infection. *Advances for Nurse Practitioners, 16*(7), 26.

Thomson, C. E., Gibson, J. N., & Martin, D. (2004). Interventions for the treatment of Morton's neuroma. *Cochrane Database of Systematic Reviews, 3,* CD003118.

van Os, A. G., Bierma-Zeinstra, S. M., Verhagen, A. P., et al. (2005). Comparison of conventional treatment and supervised rehabilitation for treatment of acute lateral ankle sprains: A systematic review of the literature. *The Journal of Orthopaedic and Sports Physical Therapy, 35,* 95–105.

Vileikyte, L., Peyrot, M., & Bundy, C. (2003). The development and validation of a neuropathy- and foot ulcer-specific quality of life instrument. *Diabetes Care, 26,* 2549–2555.

Vlahovic, T. C., Hinton, E. A., Chakravarthy, D., & Fleck, C. A. (2011). A review of cyanoacrylate liquid skin protectant and its efficacy on pedal fissures. *The Journal of the American College of Certified Wound Specialists, 2*(4), 79–85. https://doi.org/10.1016/j.jcws.2011.02.003.

Ward, S. A. (2005). Diabetes, exercise, and foot care. *Physician Sports Medicine, 33,* 33–38.

Watkins, P. (2006). Identifying and treating plantar warts. *Nursing Standard, 20*(42), 50–54.

Weidner, T., Tittlebach, T., & Elsner, P. (2017). Gram-negative bacterial toe web infection—A systemic review. *European Academy of Dermatology and Venereology, 32*(39–47).

Woodrow, P., Dickson, N., & Wright, P. (2005). Foot care for non-diabetic older people. *Nursing Older People, 17*(8), 31–32.

Younes, N. A., Albsoul, A. M., & Awad, H. (2004). Diabetic heel ulcers: A major risk factor for lower extremity amputation. *Ostomy/Wound Management, 50,* 50–60.

Zeichner, J. A. (2015). *Onychomycosis to Fungal Superinfection: Prevention Strategies and Considerations.* Retrieved December 4, 2021 from https://www.ncbi.nlm.nih.gov/pubmed/26461832.

Wound Infection and Bioburden: Detection and Management

Jennifer Hurlow and Lindsay Kalan

OBJECTIVES

1. Describe each phase of the Wound Infection Continuum including signs/symptoms and treatment of wound bioburden.
2. Identify risk factors for wound chronicity and infection.
3. Describe the processes used in obtaining a wound culture by biopsy and swab including the strengths and limitations of each.
4. Interpret laboratory data indicative of a wound infection.
5. Review interventions for treatment of wound infection.
6. Propose interventions to treat wound biofilm and inhibit redevelopment.

Recognition and treatment of wound bioburden is essential to achieving wound healing and controlling costs. Management of an infected wound costs 70% more than an uninfected wound (Dowsett, 2015). As the body's primary environmental barrier, the skin provides protection from mechanical trauma, fluid loss and dehydration, and pathogens/infection. Further, the constant shedding of corneocytes, the final stage of keratinocyte differentiation, is a remarkable feature of the skin, allowing continual self-renewal. Thus, as the largest organ of the body, its waterproof barrier, acidic pH, and diverse microbial flora result in our greatest defense against infection. Therefore, one of the fundamental priorities of wound management is to support the skin's innate protective and self-renewing properties. Breaching this barrier provides an entrance for the invasion of microbes as well as an exit site for wound exudate. Disruptions to the delicate balance within the skin ecosystem may result in unwanted microbial *bioburden* within the wound, the effects of which are numerous and complex. This chapter will introduce a series of new terms and provide clarity on definitions of commonly used terms; an understanding of these terms is critical to fully understand biofilm and wound infection (Box 19.1).

MICROORGANISMS, PHENOTYPE, AND THE WOUND MICROBIOME

The term *microorganism* is a broad term used to refer to microscopic organisms, especially bacteria and fungi. Bacteria were the first life forms to appear on earth, possibly dating back as far as 4.28 billion years ago (Dodd, Papineau, Grenne, et al., 2017). Human beings have evolved in a microbial world and, as a result, have formed symbiotic relationships with microbes living in us and on us; some estimates say humans have 1.3–10 times the number of bacterial cells to human cells (Sender, Fuchs, & Milo, 2016). These bacteria line the human body inside and outside with an invisible armor that helps us to stay healthy. Bacteria digest food, produce vitamins, and actually educate the immune system to keep the potentially pathogenic bacteria out.

Microorganisms can be further described by phenotype. A *phenotype* is the observable characteristics or traits of an organism. These traits are directed by the genes and environment of the organism. An understanding of the phenotype of microorganisms is important because it can provide information on their ability to cause disease or susceptibility to antimicrobial agents. Scientists have primarily studied microorganisms in a laboratory setting as free-floating (i.e., unattached) organisms defined as the *planktonic phenotype*. But in nature, when viewed under a microscope, most microbial communities appear as aggregates attached to a surface. With commercial availability of scanning electron microscopy (SEM) in the 1970s, J.W. Costerton coined the term "biofilm" to describe these surface-attached microbes living either as single or multispecies aggregates encased within a protective extracellular matrix comprised of sugars, proteins, lipids, and DNA (Costerton, 1987). As more has been discovered about the properties of biofilms and how biofilm forms, this lifestyle

BOX 19.1   Definition of Terms

Antibiotic: Antibacterial chemicals produced either naturally (by a bacteria) or synthetically that in dilute solution inhibit or kill other bacteria. They usually act on one specific cell target, have a narrower spectrum of activity, are relatively nontoxic to a host, and are more susceptible to losing their effectiveness to bacterial resistance.

Antimicrobial Tolerance: General mechanisms that inhibit microbe susceptibility to antimicrobials (e.g., slowed metabolism).

Antibiotic Resistance: Results from a fundamental change in the microbe itself, leading to the loss of antibiotic effectiveness against a previously susceptible microbe.

Antimicrobial: General term for any agent that kills microorganisms or inhibits their growth. Antibiotics and antiseptics are both considered antimicrobials.

Antiseptic: Chemicals with broad spectrum multimodal activity against both bacteria and fungi. This simultaneous multimodal action, reduces potential to develop resistance. Silver and iodine dressings are antiseptic wound dressings.

Bioburden: Presence of microorganisms on or in a wound. Continuum of bioburden ranges from contamination, colonization, biofilm maturation, and infection. Bioburden includes the quantity of micro-organisms present, as well as their diversity, virulence, and interaction of the organisms with each other and with the body (synergism).

Biofilm: Complex three-dimensional community of bacteria in aggregates embedded in an extracellular matrix. Bacteria within biofilm can respond to signals from other bacteria in the community to change their phenotype. Microbes in the biofilm phenotype is protected from antimicrobial assault. Debridement can disrupt biofilm to expose microbes in the more susceptible planktonic phenotype.

Colonization: Replicating microorganisms' adherent to the wound surface without a host reaction. Topical antisepsis aids in prevention of progression to infection.

Contamination: Nonreplicating microorganisms on the wound surface without a host reaction. All open wounds are contaminated by normal skin flora. Aseptic practice can limit risk for progression to infection.

Debridement: removal of dead (necrotic), infected, senescent or foreign material from wound tissue.

Facultative Anaerobe: A microorganisms that can survive in the presence or absence of oxygen.

Infection: Wound infection is a host inflammatory response to interfering microorganisms that either directly or indirectly damage viable host tissue, hence preventing healing.

An acute wound infection involves invasion of metabolically active planktonic microorganisms that trigger a host inflammatory response and is clinically evidenced by classic, overt signs of infection.

A chronic wound infection is a prolonged destructive inflammatory state related to a persistent biofilm and is clinically evidenced by covert signs of infection.

Microorganism: A microscopic organism, especially a bacterium or fungus.

Microbiome: A defined microbial community not only referring to the microorganisms present but their combined activities.

Nonfastidious: Not requiring special nutrient supplementation to grow.

Obligate Anaerobe: A microorganism that cannot survive in the presence of oxygen.

Planktonic Bacteria: Free-floating (not anchored) bacteria, such as occurs with contamination and colonization.

Quorum Sensing: The regulation of gene expression in response to cell density.

---

appears to be the preferred state of many microorganisms (Costerton, Stewart, & Greenberg, 1999). The scientific and medical communities have come to appreciate the impact of the *biofilm phenotype.*

The skin itself is a complex ecosystem capable of supporting a diverse microbial community (i.e., a microbiome). The skin microbiome consists of bacteria, fungi, viruses, and even microeukaryote mites. Together the microbiome plays a protective role against invading pathogens both directly and indirectly. Members of the healthy microbiota directly inhibit pathogen growth via production of antimicrobial peptides and small molecule antibiotics (Zipperer et al., 2016). They fill the skin niche, preventing access to space and nutrients for pathogen colonization. Finally, they indirectly protect against infection by priming the immune system to discriminate commensal organisms from pathogens (Naik et al., 2015). The close symbiotic relationship between the skin and its microbiome acts to prevent massive microbial colonization by pathogens, allowing humans to exist and function within the extensive polymicrobial environment that characterizes our planet (Christensen & Brüggemann, 2014; Grice & Segre, 2011).

Since 2008, the use of culture-independent, DNA sequence-based genomic methods have resulted in a paradigm shift. It is now clear that wounds have a *microbiome* distinct from the surrounding skin and these microbiomes are highly diverse, comprise bacteria and fungi, and exhibit interindividual variation, even in the absence of classic or overt signs of acute infection (Plate 49A and B) (Chellan et al., 2010; Dowd et al., 2008, 2011; Kalan et al., 2016, 2019). Moreover, wound microbiomes are typically comprised of commensal microbes, skin pathogens, and environmental microbes. Numerous studies have also demonstrated that wound microbiomes are association with delayed wound healing (Chellan et al., 2012; Kalan et al., 2016).

Techniques also exist to show associations between microbiome community composition and specific host factors, such as glucose control, wound duration and size, and ischemia in diabetes. Chronic wound microbiomes that are "stable" (i.e., do not change over time) are significantly associated with longer healing times (Kalan et al., 2016; Loesche et al., 2017; Sloan et al., 2019; Tipton et al., 2017). These research data are consistent with the hypothesis that the microbiome contributes to persistent colonization and is suggestive of a link between biofilm formation and wound chronicity. Furthermore, specific types of bacteria have been correlated with wound healing outcomes, suggesting that microbial identification could play a predictive role in diagnosis and prognosis as wound healing biomarkers as well as leading to targeted approaches for treatment (Choi et al., 2019; Kalan et al., 2019; Min et al., 2020; Percival, Malone, Mayer, Salisbury, & Schultz, 2018; Sloan et al., 2019; Verbanic, Shen, Lee, Deacon, & Chen, 2020).

Finally, advances are being made in sequencing the entire microbial genetic content of microbiomes (i.e., metagenomics) rather than single marker genes. This approach allows the identification of microbial genes or pathways enriched in slow or fast healing wounds. For example, gene markers that are associated with adhesions and biofilm formation in *Staphylococcus* are more abundant in nonhealing wounds and mixed communities of anaerobic bacteria are highly predictive of an impaired healing trajectory (Kalan et al., 2019). Research has demonstrated that wounds with persistent colonization with multiple species of anaerobes even after aggressive sharp debridement did not heal (Kalan et al., 2019). In contrast, anaerobic communities were diminished after debridement in the healing wounds, providing additional support for the use of the microbiome as a potential prognostic marker to guide treatment. While these techniques are powerful, they are still highly specialized and costly, do not distinguish between live and dead cells, and cannot provide phenotypic data on antimicrobial susceptibility.

Biofilm Formation

Biofilms are pervasive in chronic wounds. Currently, data suggest that at least 78.2% of chronic wounds contain biofilm and multispecies biofilm is highly prevalent in diabetic foot ulcers (Johani, Malone, Jensen, et al., 2017; Malone, Bjarnsholt, McBain, et al., 2017). Much information about biofilm phenotype has been provided by laboratory studies on two common organisms: *Staphylococcus aureus* and *Pseudomonas aeruginosa*. For example, while *S. aureus* is often present in wounds with delayed healing, it is not always linked to *infection*. Recent studies have shown that strains of *S. aureus* with differing genetic content are associated with clinical outcomes. For example, strains with more antibiotic-resistance genes and genes encoding toxins have been associated with nonhealing or deteriorating wounds (Kalan et al., 2019). *P. aeruginosa* has been shown to be associated with larger pressure ulcers (Madsen, Westh, Danielsen, et al., 1996; Zhao, Hochwalt, Usui, et al., 2010). This organism produces rhamnolipids that impair neutrophil function. The combination of the influx of dead neutrophils, degradative enzymes (reactive oxygen species) and metalloproteinases (Fazli, Bjarnsholt, Kirketerp-Møller, et al., 2011), contributes to delayed healing.

Evidence suggests, however, that most wound biofilms are polymicrobial and contain many different species of microbes. Many wound isolates across diverse genera have the ability to form biofilm but the molecular processes driving biofilm formation within and between these organisms are less studied. This raises the question of how the biofilm contributes to the development of a chronic wound and its persistence. These studies have led to speculation that the combination of organisms present in a biofilm and their genetic background may be more important than the total number or organisms present

(Gottrup, Apelqvist, Bjarnsholt, et al., 2013; Kalan et al., 2019). The implications for virulence and wound healing are an active area of research.

Formation of a biofilm is a multistage process relying on communication in the form of microbial chemical messengers signaling proximity to surfaces and to each other. This communication is called *quorum sensing*. As biofilms mature, they become sophisticated three-dimensional structures, complete with water channels to cycle nutrients and metabolites across different pH and oxygen gradients (Costerton et al., 1999; Percival, Hill, Williams, et al., 2012). The resulting structure contains a mixture of active cells at the surface of the biofilm and more dormant cells in a low metabolic state in the oxygen-poor interior of the biofilm. Because most antibiotics target processes in the cell involved in active metabolism, the presence of both a protective matrix and slowed metabolisms creates a population of microbes that are more resistant to antimicrobials. The more mature a biofilm becomes, the more resistant it is to disruption and treatment (Daeschlein, 2013; Percival et al., 2012). This is relevant because if even a small number of these cells remain after removal of biofilm by mechanical or chemical means (i.e., debridement or antimicrobial treatment), dormant cells can transition toward a metabolically active state and begin growing and dividing once again, thus reseeding the biofilm and perpetuating the cycle of reinfection (Wolcott & Rhodes, 2008). The general consensus is that biofilms are not responsible for acute infective episodes. Instead, the planktonic microorganisms, which support dispersal then subsequent biofilm reseeding, are the major drivers of acute infections (Bjarnsholt, 2013).

Polymicrobial Biofilms

Chronic wounds are polymicrobial environment. In addition to differing bacterial phenotypes of planktonic and biofilm, interactions between different microbial species may drive differences in the pathogenicity of a microbial community as a whole. The differences between acute and chronic infections may be rooted in such microbial interactions that challenge traditional models of virulence (Ehrlich & Arciola, 2012; Percival, Thomas, & Williams, 2010). In the context of chronic wounds, Dowd et al. introduced the concept of functionally equivalent pathogroups, which are bacterial communities of many different species whose individual members may not cause infection when they occur alone, but when found together they act synergistically to cause an infection functionally equivalent to well-known pathogens like *S. aureus* (Dowd et al., 2008). These interactions suggest that polymicrobial communities warrant an approach that combines treatment. For example, using a laboratory model of mixed fungal-bacterial biofilms. Townsend et al. demonstrated that the use of both antibacterial and antifungal drugs was required to decrease the overall bioburden (Townsend et al., 2016, 2017). In addition, polymicrobial biofilms are known to have an increased tolerance to antimicrobials. For example, *S. aureus* coats itself with components from *C. albicans* that sequester and limit penetration of antibiotics, thus increasing drug tolerance in mixed fungal-bacterial biofilms (Kong et al.,

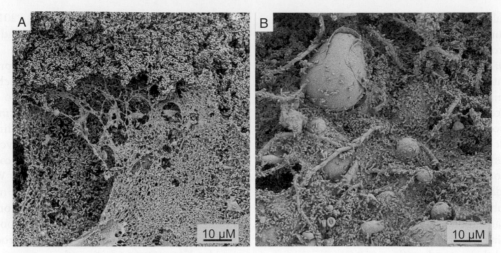

Fig. 19.1 Scanning electron micrograph of fungal and bacterial biofilms formed in ex vivo skin wounds. Wounds were either (A) mono-colonized with the Gram-negative bacterium *Citrobacter freundii* or (B) co-colonized with the fungus *Candida albicans* and *C. freundii*. Biofilms were allowed to form over a period of 48rs before imaging. In the co-colonized wounds aggregates of bacteria can be found coating the wound surface and host cells as well as fungal hyphae and cells. (Image courtesy of J.Z. Alex Cheong and Lindsay Kalan.)

2016). Reciprocally, *S. aureus* and *C. albicans* dual-species biofilms also increase tolerance to the antifungal drug miconazole (Carlson, 1982, 1983; Kean et al., 2017; Todd et al., 2019; Todd, Noverr, & Peters, 2019).

An additional mechanism of enhanced virulence in mixed-species biofilms may be via reinforcement of the structural integrity within biofilms. Visualization of fungal-bacterial biofilms in tissue structures by scanning electron microscopy reveal striking networks facilitated by fungal scaffolding. Bacteria take advantage of these scaffolds as additional sites within the wound tissue to colonize and begin replicating (Fig. 19.1). Beyond enhancement of antibiotic tolerance and virulence, biofilms can also enable growth of microbes that would not replicate on their own. For example, biofilms have lower oxygen tension that enable the growth of anaerobic bacteria even in oxygen-rich environments (Dalton et al., 2011; Fox et al., 2014; Sun, Smith, Wolcott, & Dowd, 2009). Finally, using advanced technology, it is evident that simple pairwise relationships between microbes during an infection can alter the expression of hundreds of genes. This implies that which species come together and how they interact with each other can change the course of infection and clinical outcomes (Ibberson et al., 2017; Lewin, Stacy, Michie, Lamont, & Whiteley, 2019). Understanding how this works will be critical for developing novel diagnostic tools and effective therapies. The potential translational aspects of these research avenues into a clinical wound care setting are exciting.

WOUND INFECTION CONTINUUM

The wound infection continuum (Ayton, 1985; Davis, 1998) is a theoretical concept which describes increasing microbial load in a wound. Although bacterial loads do not adhere to such an orderly progression in the clinical setting, this continuum provides the wound clinician with a tool for estimating the current quantity of or state of microbial presence. All wounds contain some amount of microbial burden within seconds of tissue disruption. As this bioburden grows, the impact on the wound healing trajectory becomes more pronounced with infection as the potential end result. Biofilm maturation is now recognized as a critical phase in increasing wound bioburden and is a potential precursor to acute infection. Biofilm is a microbe's preferred phenotype due to enhanced nutrient acquisition and protection from environmental stressors. Wound biofilm is now recognized to begin to form within an acute wound as soon as 4 days after injury (Bay, Kragh, Eickhardt, et al., 2018) and is present in the majority of chronic wounds (Malone et al., 2017). Attachment to an abiotic or biotic surface can triggers a microbe to begin to build a protective home and transition to the biofilm phenotype (Gaddy, Tomaras, & Actis, 2009). Revision of the wound infection continuum is likely to be ongoing as more is discovered regarding these concepts. Currently, the continuum is divided into the following progressive microbial states: contamination, colonization, biofilm maturation (sometimes labeled as a chronic infection and displaying covert or subtle signs of inflammation), and acute infection (exhibiting the classic, overt signs of infection).

Historically, the concept of critical colonization was used to describe a particular level of bacterial presence that affected skin cell proliferation and tissue repair in the absence of classic signs of infection (Landis, 2008). It was intended to describe wounds with delayed healing that responded to topical antimicrobial treatment (White and Cutting, 2006). However, the accuracy of the term "critical colonization" has been debated since it was first proposed in 1998 (Swanson et al., 2016). Scientists subsequently recommended this term be replaced by the phrase Biofilm Maturation (Percival & Bowler, 2004) and in 2019, the International Wound Infection Institute (IWII) formally agreed that the term *Critical Colonization* should be removed from the wound infection continuum (Haesler, Swanson, Ousey, & Carville, 2019).

Contamination

Contamination is the presence of nonreplicating microorganisms on the wound surface that do not trigger a host response (Swanson et al., 2016). Early contaminants of a wound surface may be endogenous (e.g., normal skin and gastrointestinal flora) or exogenous, present in the external environment (e.g., bed linen, devices, hospital personnel) (Woo & Sibbald, 2009). During the contamination phase, microbes are susceptible to a normal immune response at the site of the injury which destroys potential *invaders* as they advance. Microbes are unable to multiply or persist in this contamination phase; their presence is only transient. In this phase, hand washing, and other aseptic practices should be used to prevent cross contamination of pathogens in an attempt to halt an increase in wound bioburden (Swanson et al., 2016).

Colonization

Colonization is defined as the presence of proliferating or replicating bacteria that do not impair healing (Swanson et al., 2016). In this phase of the continuum, the microorganisms start to replicate to establish a microbial population, although this population remains under host control. Treatment strategies chosen to manage moist wound healing requirements and comorbid deficiencies will support uncomplicated wound resolution during this phase. However, knowing that small bacterial aggregates have been confirmed at the edge of the acute wound by day 4 (Bay et al., 2018), this phase may be a *critical turning point* on a high-risk patient when evidence-based healing strategies are not employed. A major limitation at the current time is the lack of biomarkers to identify this phase that could predict if a wound will continue along a healing trajectory or toward chronicity and acute infection.

Biofilm Maturation

In this phase of the wound infection continuum, colonizing microbes first attach to the wound surface. Then these bacteria and/or fungi undergo phenotypical changes with attachment and begin to form a biofilm (Percival, McCarty, Hunt, et al., 2014). An understanding of the characteristics of this biofilm phenotype best guides prevention of acute wound infection once a wound has progressed to this phase. During this third phase, the host begins to lose control over microbial proliferation. This loss of control may take place over days or weeks, depending on the host risk. As a biofilm matures, the host immune response, whether robust or diminished, declines in its ability to control biofilm growth leading to what has been referred to as a frustrated inflammatory response. Microbes become less susceptible to both host immune attacks and the action of topical antimicrobials. This phase has also been referred to as a state of *chronic infection* (Hurlow & Bowler, 2022; Wolcott, 2017) and is evidenced by the presence of covert, secondary signs of infection (i.e., friable or discolored granulation, increased exudate, odor and delayed healing) which were first reported by Gardner and colleagues in 2001. In their 2011 research with full thickness rabbit ear wounds, Gurjala et al. objectively confirmed that a biofilm related wound infection elicited a significantly lower host response than the host response in an acutely infected wound.

This acute infection response results from active tissue invasion by planktonic microbes (Bjarnsholt, 2013). Due to the protective nature of the biofilm, only the most sophisticated, focused strategies will allow reversal of infection trajectory at this point, especially when it involves a compromised host.

Clinical Manifestations of Biofilm

As biofilm matures, covert or secondary signs of chronic infection may be seen in the clinical setting (Plate 49A). These can include delayed healing, discolored or friable granulation, odor, serous exudate, and/or pocketing in granulation tissue (Gardner, Frantz, & Doebbeling, 2001). As a result of clinician attempts to manage biofilm maturation with strategies only confirmed to be effective on planktonic, free floating microbes, these covert signs of biofilm maturation may come and go. For example, a friable wound bed may redevelop even though covert signs of inflammation appear to resolve following a course of systemic antibiotics (Zhao, Usui, Lippman, et al., 2013). Although controversial, some experienced clinicians assert they can identify biofilm as translucent, shiny patches or layers of an opaque yellow-green or red substance on the wound surface (Metcalf, Bowler, & Hurlow, 2014). To further explore this hypothesis, researchers used scanning electron microscopy (SEM) to evaluate a specifically described wound bed substance for the presence of biofilm (Hurlow, Blanz, & Gaddy, 2016). They evaluated a gel-like substance that was *attached* to the wound bed similar to a suction cup bathmat. This substance was distinguished from free floating fibrinous exudate and from moist devitalized host tissue intimately attached to the underlying viable bed. Investigators reported the presence of biofilm in this gel-like substance in 15 of the 16 chronic wounds; 12 contained mature biofilm, 2 contained immature biofilm showing microbes not yet in a 3D structure, and 1 contained lysed bacterial cells, a dead biofilm from a wound on a patient receiving chemotherapy. Currently, biofilm is identified by scanning electron microscopy, confocal microscopy, and molecular modalities (Leaper, Schultz, Carville, et al., 2012; Percival et al., 2012). However, availability, technical complexity, and cost are roadblocks to their widespread use (Attinger & Wolcott, 2012; Jones & Kennedy, 2012). Point of care diagnostic is being developed to aid in clinical assessment (Blokhuis-Arkes, Haalboom, & van der Palen, 2015; Dargaville, Farrugia, Broadbent, et al., 2013).

Acute Infection

Acute infection is the result of tissue invasion by planktonic microorganisms (Costerton, 1987). This occurs when the host is no longer able to effectively resist microbe attack, whether due to host weakness, microbial virulence, or vulnerabilities in wound severity or treatment approach. The risk for a wound infection is multifactorial. Whether a wound heals or evolves to infection is dependent on interactions among three key elements: the resilience of the patient (i.e., host), the effectiveness of the wound treatment, and the numbers and virulence of the microorganisms present in the wound (Fig. 19.2). Evolution to wound infection involves deficits in host resistance that can be overcome or further aggravated

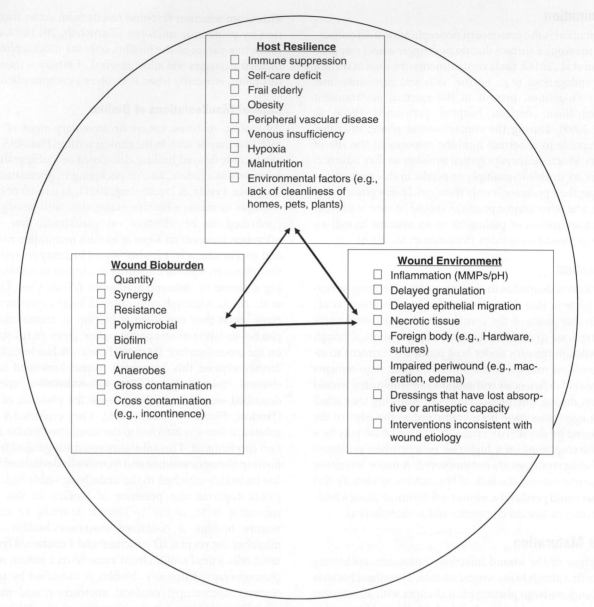

Host Resilience
- ☐ Immune suppression
- ☐ Self-care deficit
- ☐ Frail elderly
- ☐ Obesity
- ☐ Peripheral vascular disease
- ☐ Venous insufficiency
- ☐ Hypoxia
- ☐ Malnutrition
- ☐ Environmental factors (e.g., lack of cleanliness of homes, pets, plants)

Wound Bioburden
- ☐ Quantity
- ☐ Synergy
- ☐ Resistance
- ☐ Polymicrobial
- ☐ Biofilm
- ☐ Virulence
- ☐ Anaerobes
- ☐ Gross contamination
- ☐ Cross contamination (e.g., incontinence)

Wound Environment
- ☐ Inflammation (MMPs/pH)
- ☐ Delayed granulation
- ☐ Delayed epithelial migration
- ☐ Necrotic tissue
- ☐ Foreign body (e.g., Hardware, sutures)
- ☐ Impaired periwound (e.g., maceration, edema)
- ☐ Dressings that have lost absorptive or antiseptic capacity
- ☐ Interventions inconsistent with wound etiology

Fig. 19.2 Factors that interact to increase risk of infection.

by treatment adequacies, both of which may impact resistance to microbe tissue invasion.

Host frailty is a key risk factor for wound infection. Frailty is often associated with advanced age, diabetes, arterial insufficiency, obesity and malnutrition; all known to impact host resilience to infection (Gubbels Bupp, Potluri, Fink, & Klein, 2018). Elevated blood glucose, even in the short term, significantly impacts innate immune dysfunction common with diabetes (Jafar, Edriss, & Nugent, 2016; Kiselar, Wang, Dubyak, et al., 2015). The presence of arterial insufficiency will reduce access of the host's blood borne immunity (e.g., neutrophils) to the wound. Similarly, the presence of lower extremity edema and venous congestion such as with chronic venous insufficiency (CVI) will impair the delivery of nutrients and removal of cellular wastes from the wound site. Because adipose tissue is less vascularized than lean tissue (Landini, Honka, Ferrannini, & Nuutila, 2016), perfusion to a wound in a person who is overweight will be limited and

therefore reduce the host resilience to microbes. Additionally, obesity is a well-known risk factor for surgical site infection (Gurunathan, Ramsay, Mitrić, et al., 2017; Winfield, Reese, Bochicchio, Mazuski, & Bochicchio, 2016). Finally, malnutrition, directly linked to immunological alterations in children and increased risk for infection and death (Rytter, Kolte, Briend, Friis, & Christensen, 2014), impacts every phase of wound healing, from the inflammatory response to protein synthesis, further jeopardizing the potential for healing to occur (Quain & Khardori, 2015).

An inadequately managed wound environment may further exacerbate risk for wound infection. Inadequate dressing selection, management of underlying etiology, or wound bed preparation (Pilcher, 2016) will increase risk for wound infection by increasing likelihood for tissue invasion by pathogenic, multidrug-resistant organisms. The severity of the wound or the depth of any disruption in the protective epidermis logically increases this risk for infection by allowing microbial invasion into deeper tissue levels often not equipped to manage pathogenic bacterial load. For example, healing over structure (e.g., tendon or bone) or resolution of structure infection is a less predictable outcome than the same in generously perfused tissue. This is due to a more limited access to blood born immunity in such structures. Absence of timely dressing changes creates a situation in which there is prolonged contact between the wound and dressings that have lost absorptive and/or antiseptic action and therefore increase exposure of the wound to environmental contamination. Similarly, inadequate moisture management will promote tissue maceration and enhance microbial growth (Dannemiller, Weschler, & Peccia, 2017).

Finally, virulence and quantity of microbes will also impact wound infection risk. As discussed, chronicity naturally supports evolution from planktonic to the more ruggedly tolerant resistant biofilm phenotype. Current standard of wound care involves moist wound healing strategies which require balanced wound moisture control. Advanced wound care dressings, designed to absorb and/or donate moisture, facilitate achieving an optimally moist wound healing environment. However, it is important to change the dressing at appropriate time intervals to avoid prolonged contact between a dressing functioning at decreased capacity and a vulnerable wound bed. Additional sources of microbes and triggers for microbial proliferation include wound exudate and incontinence (urine and feces). Risk of wound infection is reduced by adequate exudate management and containment of incontinence.

The interplay among host resilience, wound environment and wound bioburden determines the likelihood of a wound infection. For example, inadequate wound management in a young healthy individual is sufficient to place the patient at risk for an acute infection. In contrast, ideal wound management may be insufficient to prevent an acute infection in the frail patient when a resistant organism is present. Yet, an individual with a robust immunity who is receiving ideal wound management may be sufficient to prevent an acute infection despite the presence of a resistant organism.

Clinical Manifestations of Acute Infection

Host response to an acute wound infection involves the overt, classic signs of infection which may include erythema, local warmth, edema, induration, and pain (Plates 49B and 50). These classic signs of infection result from the innate immune response to invasion which triggers vasodilation to facilitate entry of neutrophils into the tissue (Stevens, Bisno, Chambers, et al., 2014). Since several of these overt signs can be associated with nonmicrobial triggered inflammation (e.g., CVI), new or increasing pain has been found to be a sensitive marker for acute infection (Reddy, Gill, Wu, Kalkar, & Rochon, 2012). Although overt clinical signs of infection are promoted as critical to accurate diagnosis, these signs may be blunted, for example, in an immunocompromised patient or a patient with diabetes with concomitant neuropathy and peripheral arterial disease, therefore challenging the effort to establish an infection diagnosis. Infection must be diagnosed in the full context of patient history and risk factors.

Laboratory Tests and Cultures

Laboratory blood tests may reveal an increase in the number of white blood cells when infection is present. The differential may show an increase in bands or immature neutrophils. This "shift to the left," a term that arose during the days when white cells were counted by hand using a manual counting machine, denotes an increase in immature leukocytes being released from the bone marrow into the bloodstream to fight invading organisms. Ongoing evaluation of inflammation can be monitored with erythrocyte sedimentation rate (ESR) and C-reactive protein (CRP) levels, both of which are elevated with inflammation.

Wound cultures are indicated when overt or covert clinical signs of infection are present (see Plates 49A and B and 50) or when a clean wound does not show progress in healing following 2 weeks of appropriate topical therapy (Gould et al., 2016; Lavery et al., 2016; Marston, Tang, Kirsner, & Ennis, 2016). A wound culture can be obtained through either a swab of the wound or a tissue biopsy. Culture results typically underrepresent the number and type of organisms present, however (Gardner, Hillis, Heilmann, Segre, & Grice, 2013; Kalan et al., 2016; Leaper et al., 2012; Percival et al., 2016). A wound culture is performed primarily to identify the specific aerobic and anaerobic organisms present and their susceptibility to antibiotics, recognizing that only easily cultured organisms can be identified and the planktonic or biofilm phenotype in the wound is not known. Wound culture also is used to obtain a specimen for Gram staining, a rapid diagnostic technique for identifying infection (Duke, Robson, & Krizek, 1972; Levine, Lindberg, Mason, et al., 1976). For a Gram stain, the tissue fluid is placed on a slide, treated with stains that bind to the bacterial cell wall. This slide is then viewed under a microscope with the stain distinguishing gram-positive from gram-negative species and revealing cell morphology. Results from a Gram stain can be expected in 20 min, a preliminary culture report in 24 h, and a final culture and sensitivity within 48 h. A Gram stain provides information about the general type of organism present in the wound and allows the provider to prescribe a preliminary antibiotic. For example, the gram-positive wound pathogen *S. aureus* stains a deep purple and cells appear as round grape-like clusters.

The *swab technique* is the most commonly performed type of culture because it requires minimal clinical skills, and most laboratories are accustomed to performing the analysis. Two approaches have been used: the Levine technique and a Z technique. The Levine technique collects a sample by applying pressure to a $1\ cm^2$ area in the deepest part of the wound. The Z technique involves moving the swab back and forth over the entire surface at the base of the wound in a crisscross pattern. Sensitivity and specificity for the Levine technique is higher (91% sensitivity and 57% specificity) when compared with the Z technique (63% sensitivity and 53% specificity) (Levine et al., 1976). Consequently, the Levine technique is preferred over the Z technique (Leaper et al., 2012; Rondas, 2013). The procedure for the Levine technique is outlined in Box 19.2.

BOX 19.2   Procedure for Swab Wound Culture Using Levine Technique

1. Collect specimen before starting antibiotics.
2. Collect specimen using sterile technique. If a Gram stain will be performed, obtain a second swab from the same clean tissue site.
3. Identify 1 cm² of *clean wound tissue* (infection resides in viable tissue; culturing epidermis, periwound skin, or necrotic tissue will lead to false-positive results).
4. Clean wound with nonantiseptic sterile solution.
5. Moisten swab or applicator with normal saline without a preservative (moist swab provides more precise data than dry swab).
6. Apply pressure and rotate applicator within 1–2 cm² of clean wound tissue to elicit tissue fluid.
7. Insert tip of saturated swab into appropriate sterile container (do not contaminate specimen when placing it in sterile container).
8. Complete the laboratory slip to provide clinical data to the microbiologist, including wound site, time collected, and prior antibiotics.
9. Transport culture specimen quickly (within 1 h) to laboratory to keep the specimen stable.

The procedure used to obtain a swab wound culture is critical to obtain an accurate reflection of the bacteria present. A wound culture must be taken from clean, healthy-appearing tissue, rather than exudate, slough, eschar, or necrotic material (Gardner et al., 2006). The objective is to identify the organism present that is causing the infection. Cultures of wound exudate, slough, eschar or necrotic material will be apparent in the laboratory reports because a myriad of organisms will be present but will not provide an accurate profile of the microflora in the tissue nor the invasive organism. As a consequence, the reports will have one of the following types of errors: (1) false positive (organisms present in the area that is cultured but not present in the tissue), (2) false negative (organisms not present in the area that is cultured but present in the tissue), or (3) chance agreement (area that is cultured, and tissue have the same result). A false negative is problematic in that the patient actually has an infection which is not recognized and therefore will not be treated. A false positive is problematic in that the patient does not have an infection but will be treated unnecessarily thus exposing the patient to possible side effects from the antibiotics as well as increasing the chance for organisms to develop antibiotic resistance.

National guidelines recommend a *wound biopsy* or validated quantitative swab culture to determine the level of suspected infection in the chronic wound (EPIUAP, NPIAP, PPPIA, 2019; Gould et al., 2016; Lavery et al., 2016; Marston et al., 2016; WOCN®, 2016). While a tissue biopsy is considered the gold standard for wound culture (Gardner et al., 2006; Leaper et al., 2012; Robson & Heggers, 1969; WOCN®, 2016), the technique used to obtain a culture is determined by the provider with consideration of the available equipment, the speed with which the specimen can be transported to the laboratory, and the ability of the laboratory

to perform the requested culture. In general, a tissue biopsy for culture is the removal of a piece of tissue with a scalpel or punch biopsy. A physician, APP, or wound care specialist with appropriate training can perform the biopsy. The open wound is cleansed with a nonantiseptic sterile solution. A biopsy specimen is taken from clean tissue with a scalpel or punch biopsy, and bleeding is controlled. Caution should be exercised in the use of local anesthetic because local anesthetics may have antibiotic properties and thus result in false-negative results (Johnson, Swogger, & Wolcott, 2008). Once in the laboratory, the specimen is processed and plated (Gardner et al., 2006; Robson & Heggers, 1969). One of the limitations of the technique is that many facilities do not process tissue for culture, so the method cannot be used. In addition, obtaining a tissue biopsy requires disruption of the wound, which may cause the patient pain. Additionally, patients receiving anticoagulants are at risk of bleeding and will require application of pressure following biopsy or dusting with anticoagulant powder. And finally, a review of related literature reported since 1980 has shown little to no benefit of quantitative tissue biopsy analysis, with several studies showing only between 25% and 39% correlation between the wound microbiology and clinical signs and symptoms (Kallstrom, 2014). This surely puts into question the value of the wound care "Gold Standard."

Further complicating culture results is the fact that cultures are generally designed to detect organisms that rapidly grow in the laboratory and may only sample planktonic phenotypes (Daeschlein, 2013; Gardner et al., 2013; Leaper et al., 2012). This means that organisms present in very low numbers or representing only a small proportion of the wound microbiota may preferentially grow once in the lab, misrepresenting the true picture. Even within the same wound tissue, the number and types of organisms vary (Gardner et al., 2013; Leaper et al., 2012; Levine et al., 1976; Percival et al., 2012; Price et al., 2010). In general, a wound infection is present when the culture results show greater than 10^5 organisms or the presence of *any* β-hemolytic streptococcus (Gould et al., 2016; Lavery et al., 2016; Marston et al., 2016).

Species identification. Once a culture is performed, species are identified by a combination of phenotypic and molecular testing. Phenotypic testing evaluates classical features of pathogens, such as their Gram stain, colony morphology on selective media, blood hemolysis patterns and biochemical reactions. Molecular diagnosis involves extracting the total genomic DNA from isolated cultures and running a PCR to amplify the 16S rRNA marker gene followed by DNA sequencing. Other technologies such as MALDI-TOF (Matrix-Assisted Laser Desorption Ionization-Time of Flight) mass spectrometry have become commonplace to identify species directly from a pure culture grown on a nutrient agar plate.

There are limitations to these diagnostic methods. When culturing from a polymicrobial environment, the non-fastidious (defined in Box 19.1) will grow first, even if not present in high numbers. In addition, anaerobes are difficult to culture and require careful collection and transport to the laboratory. Finally, recent evidence suggests that some skin flora are opportunistic pathogens with multidrug resistance, for example, the emerging pathogen *Corynebacterium striatum* (Hahn, Werth, Butler-Wu, & Rakita, 2016). Newer technology permits direct visualization of microorganisms growing in the wound bed by taking advantage of the intrinsic properties of most bacteria to produce porphyrin molecules that fluoresce when placed under UV light. This device has a camera attached and can be used in a dark room to shine UV light onto the wound surface and visualize where the heavy bioburden is located across the spatial plane of the wound. This can then be used to target and direct debridement efforts at the bedside (Moelleken, Jockenhöfer, Benson, & Dissemond, 2020). This technology could revolutionize wound care. However, it is limited in the total number of different species of bacteria that can be detected.

Treatment of Wound Infection

When a wound infection is accompanied by systemic manifestations, systemic antibiotics will be required (Lavery, Peters, Armstrong, et al., 2009). Antibiotics should never be initiated prior to obtaining cultures so that the correct antibiotic is used, and resistant bacteria are identified. This is critical because microorganisms in the biofilm phenotype are tolerant to antimicrobials and the nonlethal exposure of microbes to antibiotics promotes the potential to develop antibiotic resistance, a growing global challenge (Hurlow, Humphreys, Bowling, & McBain, 2018; Song, Duperthuy, & Wai, 2016).

It is estimated that 65%–80% of all infections involve a biofilm (Lewis, 2001), rendering the microbes within this biofilm more tolerant to external threats, including host defenses and antimicrobial agents. Exposure of microorganisms to antibiotics can promote antibiotic resistance (Ciofu, Rojo-Molinero, Macia, & Oliver, 2017). This change in resistance can evolve in two ways: (1) mutation in the microbial genome resulting in protection and (2) acquired resistance via a process called Horizontal Gene Transfer (HGT). In contrast to the more familiar process of the transfer of genetic material from parents to offspring (i.e., Vertical Gene Transfer), Horizontal Gene Transfer involves the acquisition of resistance genes from the environment, often transferred from a resistant to a nonresistant organism, potentially existing in the same biofilm (Marcia, Roho-Molinero, & Oliver, 2014; Olsen, 2015).

Judicious use of antibiotics is essential to reduce the likelihood of these mutations. Key factors contributing to antimicrobial resistance include (1) over-prescription of antibiotics, (2) a failure to finish the entire antibiotic course, and (3) lack of appropriate infection control processes (e.g., universal precautions, etc.) (CDC, 2013; Lipsky, Dryden, Gottrup, et al., 2016; Spellberg, Srinivasan, & Chambers, 2016).

TOPICAL MANAGEMENT OF BIOBURDEN

Optimal topical wound care with specific interventions to control biofilm is a key objective in managing the patient with a wound. Removal of pathogenic organisms from the wound is essential to decrease risk of progressing to infection. Antiseptics are critical to provide broad antimicrobial coverage, including both bacteria and fungi. In addition, the delivery method of the antiseptic in combination with its antimicrobial activity creates a multimodal approach that is unlikely to promote resistance (Etebu & Arikekpar, 2016; Petchiappan & Chatterji, 2017).

Antimicrobials include both antibiotics and antiseptics; however, topical antibiotics are not recommended for use in wound care (Lipsky & Hoey, 2009). It is typically a challenge for antibiotics to reach adequate antibacterial concentrations in wounds (Daeschlein, 2013; Stewart, 2015; Stewart, White, & Boegli, 2019). For example, gentamicin 0.1% cream should be reapplied 3–4 times a day, a frequency often not practical for chronic wound care. This is now a more emphatic reality due to our growing understanding of biofilm tolerance and prevalence in wounds. As stated previously, microbes in the biofilm phenotype can be up to 1000 times less susceptible to antimicrobial action. Ultrahigh concentrations of gentamicin, over 1000 times the minimum inhibitory concentration, were required to effectively reduce bacterial levels in infected full-thickness porcine wounds (Junker, Lee, Samaan, et al., 2015). Further, the use of topical antibiotics can contribute to antimicrobial resistance due to their single mode of action which allows resistance with a single mutation. Interestingly this risk was understood by Alexander Fleming, the scientist who discovered penicillin back in 1928. Although he did not fully understand the mechanism, Fleming saw that bacteria previously destroyed by his penicillin developed resistance whenever too little antibiotic was used to adequately destroy the pathogenic bacteria.

Topical Antiseptic Wound Dressings

Antiseptics frequently used to manage bioburden are iodine, silver, polyhexamethylene biguanide (PHMB), or medical grade honey (Dissemond et al., 2017; Hurlow, 2017; Molan & Honey, 2015; Phillips, Yang, Davis, et al., 2015). These antiseptics are formulated into a foam, fiber, hydrocolloid, mesh, or gel (see Chapter 21). The appropriate media can then be chosen to meet the moisture control needs of a particular wound. Examples and descriptions of antiseptic wound dressings and wound cleansing solutions, including their potential impact on biofilms, are presented in Tables 19.1 and 19.2. Caution is advised in the use of antiseptics in the following conditions: neonates, pregnancy, and lactation. Clinicians are encouraged to check manufacturer's instructions regarding contraindications.

Iodine

Iodine is a very powerful antiseptic that was discovered by the French chemist Barnard Courtois in 1811 when it was accidentally isolated from seaweed. *Tincture of Iodine 2% to 7%* elemental iodine dissolved in a mixture of ethanol and water, was first used as a preoperative skin antiseptic in 1908 by surgeon Antonio Grossich (Block, 2001). However, it has since been found to hold risk for toxicity when absorbed through the skin. Elemental Iodine is also available as a sustained release preparation, known as an iodophor. For example, *povidone-iodine 10%* is an iodophor that is widely used as an antiseptic on intact skin. However, povidone-iodine 10% is toxic to fibroblasts in open wounds (Balin & Pratt, 2002).

TABLE 19.1 Antiseptic Wound Cleansers

Solution	Cytotoxicity	Effect on Biofilm	Comments
Polyhexanide (PHMB) & betain (e.g., Prontosan)	None (Leaper et al., 2012; Hübner & Kramer, 2010)	Disrupts attachment and Inhibits reformation (Davis, Harding, Gil, et al., 2017; Leaper et al., 2012)	Includes both a surfactant (to disrupt biofilm) and a noncytotoxic antiseptic
Sodium hypochlorite (NaOCL) (e.g., Dakins)	Concentrations as low as 0.025% NaOCL are bactericidal without impairing tissue viability (Georgiadis, Nascimento, Donat, Okereke, & Shoja, 2019)	0.01–0.16% NaOCL has antibiofilm effects against clinical S. aureus isolates (Eriksson, van der Plas, Mörgelin, & Sonesson, 2017)	Various concentrations have different effects on wounds
Hypochlorous Acid (HOCL) (e.g., Vasche)	None (Robson, Payne, Ko, et al., 2007)	Effective against bacterial and fungal biofilms with prolonged contact (Romanowski et al., 2018)	Manufacturers recommended contact time: 3–5 min per application 5–10 min for heavy amounts of necrotic tissue and slough
Acetic acid 0.025%	None (Bjarnsholt et al., 2015)	Eradication of both gram negative and gram positive biofilms (Bjarnsholt et al., 2015)	Various concentrations are cidal to various organisms and decreases wound pH (Agrawal et al., 2017)
Hydrogen peroxide (H_2O_2)	Toxic to keratinocytes and fibroblasts (Lu & Hansen, 2017)	Medical grade honey contains H_2O_2 but is safe to use for wound care (Sindi, Chawn, Hernandez, et al., 2019)	Reported cases of hydrogen peroxide causing oxygen embolism (Peng, Li, Cao, et al., 2020)
Gentian violet	Genotoxicity (Sun et al., 2018)	Fungal biofilms diminished (Traboulsi et al., 2011)	Antiseptic dye

Check manufacturers instructions for contraindications (e.g., neonates, pregnancy, lactation, long-term use) for all antiseptics.

TABLE 19.2 Antiseptic Wound Dressings

Dressing Type	(Not Inclusive)	Effect on Biofilm[a]	Comments
Cadexomer iodine	IODOSORB gel (Smith and Nephew) IoPlex foam (Medline)	Inhibits new biofilm, eradicates young biofilm colonies, reduces mature biofilm colonies	Broad spectrum
Gentian violet	DermaBlue Foam (DermaRite), Hydrofera BLUE (Hydrofera)	Fungal biofilms diminished	See Table 19.1
Medical grade honey (active Leptospermum or Manuka)	MANUKAhd gelling fiber (ManukaMed), MEDIHONEY Calcium Alginate (Integra LifeSciences), TheraHoney Foam (Medline)	Inhibits biofilm growth, colony formation, and ability to proliferate	Broad spectrum
Polyhexamethylene Biguanide (PHMB)	PHMB Antimicrobial Foam Border (Gemco), Curity AMD Antimicrobial Gauze (Cardinal Health), AMD kerlix, foam, telfa, foam (Cardinal Health)	Antibiofilm action not been confirmed	PHMB Wound Cleanser (with surfactant) may affect biofilm (see Table 19.1)
Silver	Kerracel Ag Gelling Fiber Dressing (3M), AQUACEL® Ag Foam (Convetec), BiatainAlginate Ag (Coloplast)	Denatures bacterialbiofilm in concentrations over 5 μg/mL	Broad spectrum, including *methicillin-resistant Staphylococcus aureus* and *vancomycin-resistant enterococcus*
Silver enhanced with ethylenediamine-tetraacetate (EDTA)	AQUACEL Ag Advantage hydrofiber (ConvaTec), ColActivePlus alginate (Covalon), DermaColAg Collagen (DermaRite)	Silver and antibiofilm (EDTA) disrupt biofilm	Broad spectrum, including *methicillin-resistant Staphylococcus aureus* and *vancomycin-resistant enterococcus*

[a]Effect on biofilm depends on the phase of the biofilm cycle the dressing is applied.
Check manufacturers instructions for contraindications (e.g., neonates, pregnancy, lactation, long-term use) for all antiseptics.

Another form of elemental iodine is a slow-release formulation, *Cadexomer iodine (CI)*, an iodophor of 0.9% elemental iodine. This significantly lower concentration of elemental iodine has not been associated with toxicities. The cadexomer bead is an absorbent polysaccharide starch matrix. As the cadexomer beads disintegrate with moisture, free iodine is slowly released into a wound (Milne, 2020). CI has been shown to have suppressive activity on in vitro biofilm (Phillips et al., 2015) although the mechanism of this action is not defined. A change in color from brown to a yellow/gray, sometimes referred to as "whiting out," indicates that the action of cadexomer iodine formulation is expired and a fresh application is required (Milne, 2020). Interestingly, Schwartz et al. (2012) treated 16 infected or "critically colonized" wounds for 6 weeks with CI and achieved a statistically significant median reduction in the bacterial load ($P = 0.025$) with a median reduction of 53.6% in ulcer surface area. To achieve optimal patient outcomes, frequency of dressing changes, as with all dressings, should be guided by the manufacturer's instructions and wound assessments such as exudate.

Silver

Silver, a naturally occurring element that has been used for centuries as an antimicrobial agent, is nonreactive in its elemental solid form. Silver must become ionized to exert its effect on killing microorganisms, which include bacteria and fungi. In addition to its antimicrobial action, there is some evidence that it may have antiinflammatory effects and promote neovascularization (International Consensus, 2012). Silver ions bind to proteins and other macromolecules in bacterial cells resulting in structural changes to the cell wall, membrane, and intracellular toxicity (Leaper et al., 2012). Given these highly diverse effects on various target structures, development of bacterial resistance to silver is very low (Landsdown & Williams, 2007). Although silver is highly toxic to bacterial cells, it has low toxicity toward human cells, making it an ideal antimicrobial.

Silver is available in a variety of compositions (e.g., nanocrystalline, silver sulfadiazine, metallic silver), concentrations and delivery mechanisms (e.g., embedded within a dressing vs. coated on the surface). Several comparative studies have been reported supporting the antibacterial effects and positive wound healing effects of silver dressings in a variety of wounds. In a study involving 619 patients with chronic venous ulcers, investigators reported faster healing when a sustained silver release foam dressing was used when compared with other silver dressing categories (Münter, Beele, & Russell, 2006). In a study of 110 patients following colorectal surgery, a high-risk population for postoperative surgical site infection, a statistically significant ($P = 0.011$) decrease in wound infection after 30 days was seen using a silver nylon dressing when compared with gauze (Krieger, Davis, Sanchez, et al., 2011).

Polyhexamethylene Biguanide (PHMB)

PHMB kills microbes when it enters through their cell wall where it can arrest cell division by harming chromosomal structure. Interestingly, PHMB cannot enter the nucleus of a human cell, which protects human DNA from this destruction. This results in a selective antiseptic action that is less toxic to human cells (Chindera et al., 2016). No acquired resistance to PHMB has yet been reported and it is generally thought to have good activity against a wide range of gram-positive and gram-negative bacteria, fungi and yeasts. PHMB impregnated dressings (e.g., PuraPly, AMD, Cellulose PHMD) appear to be very effective as a barrier to wound colonization and infection. This barrier is created by both topical protection of a currently stable wound or by PHMB action to control proliferation of bacterial in the dressing itself (Motta, Milne, & Corbett, 2004). While antibiofilm action of this chemical has not been confirmed (Gurjala et al., 2011; Seth et al., 2014), use of PHMB dressings may show antibiofilm *efficacy* when used within a strict protocol of biofilm-based wound care. Further, the addition of a surfactant to a PHMB containing wound cleanser shows some antibiofilm efficacy (Davis et al., 2017). PHMB is available as a solution, gel, and dressing. It can also be used with negative pressure wound therapy to reduce bioburden (Daeschlein, 2013).

Honey

Among the biologic agents, honey has been used to treat chronic wounds for millennia. It decreases the wound pH to a more acidic range, acts as an osmotic agent, and generates hydrogen peroxide to kill organisms. A Cochrane review concluded that topical honey may improve healing of partial thickness burns when compared with silver sulfadiazine (O'Meara, Al-Kurdi, Ologun, et al., 2014). However, compared with usual care in patients with venous ulcers, honey-based preparations showed no between-group differences in time to heal or complete healing. *Manuka-type honey* (commercially available in multiple wound dressing formulations) have been shown to penetrate biofilm and kill various strains of *S. aureus* and reduce biofilm CFU logs (Lu, Turnbull, Burke, et al., 2014). It is however important to use medical-grade honey (Lu et al., 2014) and apply it only to the wound, not to the skin surface. If Manuka honey is used in patients with thick eschar, scoring of the eschar allows the honey to penetrate the area, and an absorptive secondary dressing is required to contain the digested tissue (Sibbald, Goodman, Woo, et al., 2011).

Biofilm-Based Wound Care

Current and ongoing research into the prevalence of biofilm in wounds is revealing that biofilm is a major factor in wounds that are difficult-to-heal. Once host factors known to impair healing, such as ischemia, immunosuppression, and malnutrition, have been addressed, it is widely accepted that biofilm-based wound care is fundamental to chronic wound infection management. Further, if employed in a timely way can limit the inappropriate use of systemic antibiotics (Hurlow & Bowler, 2022). The goals of biofilm-based wound care are (1) disruption of the biofilm to expose the more vulnerable planktonic phenotype and (2) inhibition of its recurrence without causing tissue injury or development of drug resistance (Gottrup et al., 2013; Leaper et al., 2012; Murphy, Atkin, & Swanson, 2020; Sibbald et al., 2011) (Box 19.3).

Organisms protected in biofilm become from 100 to 1000 times more tolerant to antimicrobials than corresponding planktonic cells (Olsen, 2015; Stewart et al., 2019). This tolerance applies to both antibiotics and to the antiseptics in wound dressings. Therefore, disruption of the biofilm to expose these protected microbes is necessary to maximize efficacy of any chosen topical antimicrobial dressing.

Sharp debridement or at least sharp disruption is the cornerstone of biofilm-based wound care because it quickly and efficiently disrupts the integrity of the protective biofilm matrix. Wolcott and Rhodes (2008) offer a good model of the extent of sharp debridement. They describe opening all the surfaces of the wound (e.g., tunnels, undermining) and resecting them so no surfaces touch. Devitalized tissue should be debrided so that normal tissue with a good blood supply is visible. Interestingly, data show that the effectiveness of debridement is time dependent (Wolcott et al., 2010). Microbes exposed by debridement are most susceptible to antimicrobial treatment in the first 24 h, less susceptible in the 24- to 48-h period and become again tolerant by 72 h when biofilm has regained maturity; a state which again renders microbes tolerant to the action of any topical antiseptic wound dressings. Serial sharp debridement or disruption opens a potential window for breaking the biofilm growth cycle, but frequent sharp debridement can be a challenge in the outpatient setting where many wounds are managed. This is due to challenges with patient access to providers allowed to perform this sharp debridement procedure (Hurlow et al., 2016). The use of antibiofilm substances can, therefore, enhance wound management by both delaying biofilm maturation after disruption and by enhancing efficacy of any topical antiseptic wound dressing.

Antibiofilm Agents

Antibiofilm agents are not antimicrobials but instead impact biofilm by disrupting quorum sensing, degrading extracellular polymeric substance, or blocking attachments. Antibiofilm agents allow antimicrobials to act more effectively.

Ethylenediaminetetraacetic acid (EDTA) is a substance that has been and is used in a range of formulations. EDTA sequesters biofilm's stabilizing metal ions and, in so doing, can reduce the physical integrity of the biofilm matrix (Cavaliere, Ball, Turnbull, & Whitchurch, 2014; Finnegan & Percival, 2015; Fleming & Rumbaugh, 2017; Metcalf, Bowler, & Parsons, 2016). Commercially formulated antiseptic wound dressings with EDTA are available to enhance its antibiofilm efficacy (e.g., Aquacel AG Extra, ColActive Plus Collagen Matrix, and ColActive Plus Collagen Matrix). For example, a multicenter trial conducted by Walker, Metcalf, Parsons, and Bowler (2015) involved 113 patients with a stagnant or deteriorating wound. The 94.7% ($N = 107$) shifted toward healing when a silver fiber dressing containing EDTA and benzethonium chloride (a surfactant) was used.

Surfactants such as those used in many (not all) commercially available wound cleansers have been utilized for many years for their antimicrobial activity. Surfactants target the integrity of the protective biofilm matrix (Zölß & Cech, 2016) and therefore enhance the potency of antimicrobial compounds (Said et al., 2014). The action of surfactants is concentration-dependent, requiring attention to balance between efficacy and toxicity, and can be enhanced by physical disruption, such as with sharp or mechanical debridement (e.g., therapeutic irrigation (4–15 psi), monofilament fiber pads, low-frequency ultrasound, hydrosurgery) (Howell et al., 1993; International Wound Infection Institute (IWII), 2016; Kalel, Mora, Patro, Palit, & Nath, 2017; Li & Lee, 2017).

Lactoferrin and Xylitol have been reported to have potential antibiofilm activity but is not commercially available in topical wound care products. *Lactoferrin* is an important part of the innate immune system with a high affinity for iron. The potential antibiofilm activity of lactoferrin was originally reported by Singh and colleagues (Singh, Parsek, Greenberg, & Welsh, 2002). They hypothesized that it serves the innate immune system by specifically inhibiting biofilm formation on mucosal surfaces. The authors reported that lactoferrin demonstrates a concentration-specific ability to prevent *P. aeruginosa* biofilm formation by binding to essential iron and stimulating bacterial twitching motility, a mechanism by which the bacterium can spread across a surface instead of attaching to the surface which is a known precursor to matrix production and biofilm formation. *Xylitol* is a sugar alcohol that occurs naturally in low concentrations in fruits and can be used as a dietary sweetener with reported benefits for oral health. It has been claimed that xylitol will weaken biofilm matrix structure when used in combination with lactoferrin (Ammons, Ward, Fisher, et al., 2009). Xylitol has been shown to demonstrate enhanced antibiofilm activity when combined with farnesol, a naturally occurring acyclic sesquiterpene alcohol (Alves, Neves, Silva, Rôças, & Siqueira, 2013; Katsuyama, Ichikawa, Ogawa, & Ikezawa, 2005).

CLINICAL CONSULT

A: 69-year-old ambulatory female referred to the wound clinic 3 months ago with a 7-month-old, acutely infected hard-to-heal lateral calf wound. Her past medical history includes osteoporosis and bilateral total hip replacements. She is not obese and denies any problems with eating or recent weight loss. She has no history of kidney, thyroid disease or diabetes. The wound is shallow but profoundly inflamed and covered by an adherent opaque film (Plate 49B). There is no wound odor but periwound is inflamed and very tender to light touch. Her previous provider ordered a silver foam dressing secured with a short stretch layered compression system. The patient reports that she cares for her husband who is disabled and cannot regularly elevate her legs. A swab wound specimen for culture is obtained with Levine technique, the wound cleansed and a silver fiber dressing applied with the same brand of compression. Noninvasive arterial studies were conducted and revealed perfusion within normal limits. Based on the culture results, a 10-day oral antibiotic prescription, was subsequently called into the patient's pharmacy. Upon return to clinic one week later, the wound showed improvement including a decrease in periulcer erythema and new appearance of healthy granulation tissue.

Unfortunately, by week 3, the overt signs of infection returned. This patient was then referred to an infectious disease specialist who started IV antibiotics guided by original culture and again signs of infection abated. Two months after completing IV antibiotics, the signs of infection returned.

D: Acutely infected venous ulcer. Initial improvement after antibiotics related to killing of planktonic bacteria. Recurrent infection related to wound bacteria present in protective biofilm phenotype that survived systemic antibiotic treatment. Topical treatment strategy likely inadequate.

P: Disrupt wound bed biofilm to expose the more vulnerable planktonic microbes.

I: Treat wound with biofilm-based wound care (BBWC) strategies: debridement, cleanse with noncytotoxic antiseptic cleanser, apply topical absorptive antiseptic dressing which includes addition of antibiofilm agents especially if dressing cannot be changed within 3 days, educate patient on importance of elevation and elevation to promote venous return, consider elastic layered compression system.

E: Reevaluate weekly to bi-weekly for dressing changes based on wound exudate management needs.

SUMMARY

- Creating an optimal wound environment requires diligent management of the wound bioburden.
- The wound environment is usually polymicrobial and has a distinct microbiome from the surrounding healthy skin.
- Microorganisms in the wound exist as both planktonic and biofilm phenotypes.
- Failure to recognize and treat the manifestations of the continuum of bioburden conditions will lead to inflammation, delay of healing, and infection.
- Use of a noncytotoxic antiseptic wound management products during phases of contamination and colonization as well as after sharp debridement or disruption of wound biofilm will reasonably control bioburden progression.

SELF-ASSESSMENT QUESTIONS

1. All of the following factors contribute to recurrent wound infection EXCEPT:
   a. Inappropriate culture specimen collection technique
   b. Poorly controlled wound etiology
   c. Inattention to key concepts of Biofilm-Based Wound Care
   d. Colonization

2. What is the most appropriate consideration when choosing a systemic antibiotic?
   a. Cost
   b. Ease of administration
   c. Efficacy
   d. Patient preference

3. A "chronic" wound is best described as:
   a. Less of a problem to manage than an "acute" wound
   b. A wound on a noncompliant patient
   c. A Hard-to-Heal wound found to be associated with the presence of biofilm
   d. An incurable wound

4. Which is NOT an element of Biofilm-Based Wound Care?
   a. Biofilm disruption techniques
   b. Topical antibiotic ointment
   c. Noncytotoxic wound cleanser
   d. Antiseptic wound dressing to manage wound exudate

5. Which of the following statements is TRUE about the microbial state of the wound following debridement?
   a. The presence of bleeding into the wound prevents microbial reattachment to the wound surface.
   b. The wound is most susceptible to antimicrobial treatment in the first 24 hours.
   c. The wound is most susceptible to antimicrobial treatment after 48 hours.
   d. Biofilm reaches a mature state within 24 hours.

6. Information obtained from a Molecular (DNA sequence based) diagnostic report includes:
   a. The dominant species colonizing a wound
   b. All of the microbial species present in a wound
   c. All of the microbial species and their antibiotic susceptibility patterns
   d. The total quantity of bacteria in a wound

7. Which of the following statements about organisms in a biofilm is TRUE:
   a. They are more tolerant to antimicrobial agents
   b. They swim freely and spread across the wound surface
   c. They are metabolically very active
   d. They are anerobic only.

8. Which of the following techniques can be used to identify the presence of a biofilm?
   a. A swab cultures
   b. A tissue biopsy
   c. Electron microscope
   d. Serum blood test

9. To obtain the most accurate culture, it is important that the specimen be taken from:
   a. Healthy wound tissue
   b. Purulent material
   c. Necrotic tissue or slough
   d. Exudate

REFERENCES

Agrawal, K. S., Sarda, A. V., Shrotriya, R., Bachhav, M., Puri, V., & Nataraj, G. (2017). Acetic acid dressings: Finding the Holy Grail for infected wound management. *Indian Journal of Plastic Surgery: Official Publication of the Association of Plastic Surgeons of India*, 50(3), 273–280. https://doi.org/10.4103/ijps.IJPS_245_16.

Alves, F. R., Neves, M. A., Silva, M. G., Rôças, I. N., & Siqueira, J. F., Jr. (2013). Antibiofilm and antibacterial activities of farnesol and xylitol as potential endodontic irrigants. *Brazilian Dental Journal*, 24(3), 224–229. https://doi.org/10.1590/0103-6440201302187.

Ammons, M. C., Ward, L. S., Fisher, S. T., et al. (2009). In vitro susceptibility of established biofilms composed of a clinical wound isolate of Pseudomonas aeruginosa treated with lactoferrin and xylitol. *International Journal of Antimicrobial Agents*, 33(3), 230–236.

Attinger, C., & Wolcott, R. (2012). Clinically addressing biofilm in chronic wounds. *Advances in Wound Care*, 1(3), 127–132.

Ayton, M. (1985). Wound care: Wounds that won't heal. *Nursing Times*, 81(46), 16–19.

Balin, A. K., & Pratt, L. (2002). Dilute povidone iodine solutions inhibit human skin fibroblast growth. *Dermatologic Surgery*, 28(3), 2104.

Bay, L., Kragh, K. N., Eickhardt, S. R., et al. (2018). Bacterial aggregates establish at the edges of acute epidermal wounds. *Advances in Wound Care*, 7(4), 105–113.

Bjarnsholt, T. (2013). The role of bacterial biofilms in chronic infections. *APMIS. Supplementum*, 121, 1–58.

Bjarnsholt, T., Alhede, M., Jensen, P.Ø., Nielsen, A. K., Johansen, H. K., Homøe, P., et al. (2015). Antibiofilm properties of acetic acid. *Advances in Wound Care*, 4(7), 363–372. https://doi.org/10.1089/wound.2014.0554.

Block, S. S. (2001). *Disinfection, sterilization, and preservation* (5th ed., p. 922). Lippincott Williams & Wilkins. ISBN 978-0-683-30740-5.

Blokhuis-Arkes, M., Haalboom, M., van der Palen, J., et al. (2015). Rapid enzyme analysis as a diagnostic tool for wound infection: Comparison between clinical judgment, microbiological analysis, and enzyme analysis. *Wound Repair and Regeneration*, 23, 1–8.

Carlson, E. (1982). Synergistic effect of Candida albicans and Staphylococcus aureus on mouse mortality. *Infection and Immunity*, 38(3), 921–924. Retrieved 10/1/2020 from http://www.ncbi.nlm.nih.gov/pubmed/7152678.

Carlson, E. (1983). Effect of strain of Staphylococcus aureus on synergism with *Candida albicans* resulting in mouse mortality and morbidity. *Infection and Immunity*, 42(1), 285–292. Retrieved 10/1/2020 from http://www.ncbi.nlm.nih.gov/pubmed/6352497.

Cavaliere, R., Ball, J. L., Turnbull, L., & Whitchurch, C. B. (2014). The biofilm matrix destabilizers, EDTA and DNaseI, enhance the susceptibility of nontypeable Hemophilus influenzae biofilms to treatment with ampicillin and ciprofloxacin. *Microbiology*, 3(4), 557–567.

Centers for Disease Control and Prevention. Antibiotic resistance threats in the United States. (2013). Retrieved 9/1/2020 from: http://www.cdc.gov/drugresistance/threat-report-2013/pdf/ar-threats-2013-508.pdf.

Chellan, G., Neethu, K., Varma, A. K., Mangalanandan, T. S., Shashikala, S., Dinesh, K. R., et al. (2012). Targeted treatment of invasive fungal infections accelerates healing of foot wounds in patients with Type 2 diabetes. *Diabetic Medicine*, 29(9), 255–262.

Chellan, G., Shivaprakash, S., Ramaiyar, S. K., Varma, A. K., Varma, N., Sukumaran, M. T., et al. (2010). Spectrum and prevalence of fungi infecting deep tissues of lower-limb wounds in patients with type 2 diabetes. *Journal of Clinical Microbiology*, 48(6), 2097–2102.

Chindera, K., Mahato, M., Kumar Sharma, A. K., Horsley, H., Kloc-Muniak, K., Kamaruzzaman, N. F., et al. (2016). The antimicrobial polymer PHMB enters cells and selectively condenses bacterial chromosomes. *Scientific Reports*, 6, 23121.

Choi, Y., Banerjee, A., McNish, S., Couch, K. S., Torralba, M. G., Lucas, S., et al. (2019). Co-occurrence of anaerobes in human chronic wounds. *Microbial Ecology*, 77(3), 808–820.

Christensen, G. J., & Brüggemann, H. (2014). Bacterial skin commensals and their role as host guardians. *Beneficial Microbes*, 5(2), 201–215. https://doi.org/10.3920/BM2012.0062.

Ciofu, O., Rojo-Molinero, E., Macia, M. D., & Oliver, A. (2017). Antibiotic treatment of biofilm infections. *APMIS*, 125, 304–319.

Costerton, J. W. (1987). Bacterial biofilms in nature and disease. *Annual Review of Microbiology*, 41, 435–464.

Costerton, J. W., Stewart, P. S., & Greenberg, E. P. (1999). Bacterial biofilms: A common cause of persistent infections. *Science*, 284(5418), 1318–1322.

Daeschlein, G. (2013). Antimicrobial and antiseptic strategies in wound management. *International Wound Journal*, 10(Suppl 1), 9–14.

Dalton, T., Dowd, S. E., Wolcott, R. D., Sun, Y., Watters, C., Griswold, J. A., et al. (2011). An in vivo polymicrobial biofilm wound infection model to study interspecies interactions. *PLoS One*, 6(11), e27317. Retrieved 10/1/2020 from: https://doi.org/10.1371/journal.pone.0027317.

Dannemiller, K. C., Weschler, C. J., & Peccia, J. (2017). Fungal and bacterial growth in floor dust at elevated relative humidity levels. *Indoor Air*, 27(2), 354–363. https://doi.org/10.1111/ina.12313.

Dargaville, T. R., Farrugia, B. L., Broadbent, J. A., et al. (2013). Sensors and imaging for wound healing: A review. *Biosensors & Bioelectrons*, 41, 30–42.

Davis, E. (1998). Education, microbiology and chronic wounds. *Journal of Wound Care, 7*(6). 27–4.

Davis, S. C., Harding, A., Gil, J., et al. (2017). Effectiveness of a polyhexanide irrigation solution on methicillin-resistant Staphylococcus aureus biofilms in a porcine wound model. *International Wound Journal, 14*(6), 937–944. https://doi.org/10.1111/iwj.12734.

Dissemond, J., Böttrich, J. G., Braunwarth, H., Hilt, J., Wilken, P., & Münter, K. C. (2017). Evidence for silver in wound care—Meta-analysis of clinical studies from 2000–2015. *Journal der Deutschen Dermatologischen Gesellschaft, 15*(5), 524–535. https://doi.org/10.1111/ddg.13233.

Dodd, M. S., Papineau, D., Grenne, T., et al. (2017). Evidence for early life in Earth's oldest hydrothermal vent precipitates. *Nature, 543*(7643), 60–64. https://doi.org/10.1038/nature21377.

Dowd, S. E., Delton Hanson, J., Rees, E., Wolcott, R. D., Zischau, A. M., Sun, Y., et al. (2011). Survey of fungi and yeast in polymicrobial infections in chronic wounds. *Journal of Wound Care, 20*(1), 40–47.

Dowd, S. E., Sun, Y., Secor, P. R., Rhoads, D. D., Wolcott, B. M., James, G. A., et al. (2008). Survey of bacterial diversity in chronic wounds using pyrosequencing, DGGE, and full ribosome shotgun sequencing. *BMC Microbiology, 8*(1), 43. https://doi.org/10.1186/1471-2180-8-43.

Dowd, S. E., Wolcott, R. D., Sun, Y., McKeehan, T., Smith, E., & Rhoads, D. (2008). Polymicrobial nature of chronic diabetic foot ulcer biofilm infections determined using bacterial tag encoded FLX amplicon pyrosequencing (bTEFAP). *PLoS One, 3*(10), e3326. https://doi.org/10.1371/journal.pone.0003326. PMID.

Dowsett, C. (2015). Breaking the cycle of hard-to-heal wounds: Balancing cost and care. *Wounds International Journal, 6*(2), 4–53.

Duke, W. F., Robson, M. C., & Krizek, T. J. (1972). Civilian wounds, their bacterial flora and rate of infection. *Surgical Forum, 23*, 518–520.

Ehrlich, G. D., & Arciola, C. R. (2012). From Koch's postulates to biofilm theory. The lesson of Bill Costerton. *International Journal of Artificial Organs, 35*(10), 695–699.

Eriksson, S., van der Plas, M. J. A., Mörgelin, M., & Sonesson, A. (2017). Antibacterial and antibiofilm effects of sodium hypochlorite against *Staphylococcus aureus* isolates derived from patients with atopic dermatitis. *The British Journal of Dermatology, 177*(2), 513–521. https://doi.org/10.1111/bjd.15410.

Etebu, E., & Arikekpar, I. (2016). Antibiotics: Classification and mechanisms of action with emphasis on molecular perspective. *International Journal of Applied Microbiology and Biotechnology Research, 4*, 90–101.

European Pressure Ulcer Advisory Panel, National Pressure Injury Advisory Panel, Pan Pacific Pressure Injury Alliance. (EPIUAP, NPIAP, PPPIA). (2019). In E. Haesler (Ed.), *Prevention and treatment of pressure ulcers/injuries.* Osborne Park: Cambridge Media.

Fazli, M., Bjarnsholt, T., Kirketerp-Møller, K., et al. (2011). Quantitative analysis of the cellular inflammatory response against biofilm bacteria in chronic wounds. *Wound Repair and Regeneration, 19*, 387–391.

Finnegan, S., & Percival, S. L. (2015). EDTA: An antimicrobial and antibiofilm agent for use in wound care. *Advances in Wound Care (New Rochelle), 4*(7), 415–421.

Fleming, D., & Rumbaugh, K. P. (2017). Approaches to dispersing medical biofilms. *Microorganisms, 5*(15), 1–16.

Fox, E. P., Cowley, E. S., Nobile, C. J., Hartooni, N., Newman, D. K., & Johnson, A. D. (2014). Anaerobic bacteria grow within Candida albicans biofilms and induce biofilm formation in suspension cultures. *Current Biology, 24*(20), 2411–2416.

Gaddy, J. A., Tomaras, A. P., & Actis, L. A. (2009). The *Acinetobacter baumannii* 19606 OmpA protein plays a role in biofilm formation on abiotic surfaces and in the interaction of this pathogen with eukaryotic cells. *Infection and Immunity, 77*(8), 3150–3160. https://doi.org/10.1128/IAI.00096-09.

Gardner, S. E., Frantz, R. A., & Doebbeling, B. N. (2001). The validity of the clinical signs and symptoms used to identify localized chronic wound infection. *Wound Repair and Regeneration, 9*(3), 178–186.

Gardner, S. E., Frantz, R. A., Saltzman, C. L., Hillis, S. L., Park, H., & Scherubel, M. (2006). Diagnostic validity of three swab techniques for identifying chronic wound infection. Wound Repair & Regeneration. *14*(5), 548–557. doi:10.1111/j.1743-6109.2006.00162.x.

Gardner, S. E., Hillis, S. L., Heilmann, K., Segre, J. A., & Grice, E. A. (2013). The neuropathic diabetic foot ulcer microbiome is associated with clinical factors. *Diabetes, 62*(3), 923–930. https://doi.org/10.2337/db12-0771.

Georgiadis, J., Nascimento, V. B., Donat, C., Okereke, I., & Shoja, M. M. (2019). Dakin's Solution: "One of the most important and far-reaching contributions to the armamentarium of the surgeons". *Burns, 45*(7), 1509–1517. https://doi.org/10.1016/j.burns.2018.12.001.

Gottrup, F., Apelqvist, J., Bjarnsholt, T., et al. (2013). EWMA document: Antimicrobials and non-healing wounds—Evidence, controversies and suggestions. *Journal of Wound Care, 22*(Suppl. 5), S1–S92.

Gould, L., Stuntz, M., Giovannelli, M., Ahmad, A., Aslam, R., Mullen-Fortino, M., et al. (2016). Wound Healing Society 2015 update on guidelines for pressure ulcers. *Wound Repair & Regeneration, 24*(1), 145–162. https://doi.org/10.1111/wrr.12396. Epub 2016 Mar 4.

Grice, E., & Segre, J. (2011). The skin microbiome. *Nature Reviews. Microbiology, 9*(4), 244–253. https://doi.org/10.1038/nrmicro2537.

Gubbels Bupp, M. R., Potluri, T., Fink, A. L., & Klein, S. L. (2018). The confluence of sex hormones and aging on immunity. *Frontiers in Immunology, 9*, 1269. https://doi.org/10.3389/fimmu.2018.01269.

Gurjala, A. N., Geringer, M. R., Seth, A. K., Hong, S. J., Smeltzer, M. S., Galiano, R. D., et al. (2011). Development of a novel, highly quantitative in vivo model for the study of biofilm-impaired cutaneous wound healing. *Wound Repair and Regeneration, 19*, 400–410.

Gurunathan, U., Ramsay, S., Mitrić, G., et al. (2017). Association between obesity and wound infection following colorectal surgery: Systematic review and meta-analysis. *Journal of Gastrointestinal Surgery, 21*, 1700–1712.

Haesler, E., Swanson, T., Ousey, K., & Carville, K. (2019). Clinical indicators of wound infection and biofilm: Reaching international consensus. *Journal of Wound Care, 28*(Sup3b), s4–s12.

Hahn, W. O., Werth, B. J., Butler-Wu, S. M., & Rakita, R. M. (2016). Multidrug-resistant Cornyebacterium striatum associated with increased use of parenteral antimicrobial drugs. *Emerging Infectious Diseases, 22*(11), 1908–1914.

Howell, J. M., Stair TO, Howell, A. W., Mundt, D. J., Falcone, A., & Peters, S. R. (1993). The effect of scrubbing and irrigation with normal saline, povidone iodine, and cefazolin on wound bacterial counts in a Guinea pig model. *The American Journal of Emergency Medicine, 11*(2), 134–138.

Hübner, N. O., & Kramer, A. (2010). Review on the efficacy, safety and clinical applications of polihexanide, a modern wound antiseptic. *Skin Pharmacology and Physiology, 23*(Suppl), 17–27. https://doi.org/10.1159/000318264.

Hurlow, J. (2017). The benefits of using polyhexamethylene biguanide in wound care. *British Journal of Community Nursing, 22*(Suppl. 3), S16–S18. https://doi.org/10.12968/bjcn.2017.22.Sup3.S16.

Hurlow, J., Blanz, E., & Gaddy, J. A. (2016). Clinical investigation of biofilm in non-healing wounds by high resolution microscopy techniques. *Journal of Wound Care, 25*(Suppl. 9), S11–S22. https://doi.org/10.12968/jowc.2016.25.Sup9.S11.

Hurlow, J., & Bowler, P. G. (2022). Acute and chronic wound infections: Microbiological, immunological, clinical and therapeutic distinctions. *Journal of Wound Care, 31*(5), 436–445. https://doi.org/10.12968/jowc.2022.31.5.436.

Hurlow, J., Humphreys, G., Bowling, F., & McBain, A. (2018). Diabetic foot infection: A critical complication. *International Wound Journal, 2018*, 1–8.

Ibberson, C. B., Stacy, A., Fleming, D., Dees, J. L., Rumbaugh, K., Gilmore, M. S., et al. (2017). Co-infecting microorganisms dramatically alter pathogen gene essentiality during polymicrobial infection. *Nature Microbiology, 2*.

International Consensus. (2012). *Appropriate use of silver dressings in wounds. An expert working group consensus*. London: Wounds International. Retrieved 10/1/2020 from: www.woundsinternational.com.

International Wound Infection Institute (IWII). (2016). *Wound infection in clinical practice*. Wounds International.

Jafar, N., Edriss, H., & Nugent, K. (2016). The effect of short-term hyperglycemia on the innate immune system. *The American Journal of the Medical Sciences, 351*(2), 201–211.

Johani, K., Malone, M., Jensen, S., et al. (2017). Microscopy visualization confirms multi-species biofilms are ubiquitous in diabetic foot ulcers. *International Wound Journal, 14*, 1160–1169.

Johnson, S. M., Swogger, E., & Wolcott, R. (2008). Local anesthetics as antimicrobial agents: A review. *Surgical Infections, 9*(2), 205–213.

Jones, C. E., & Kennedy, J. P. (2012). Treatment options to manage wound biofilm. *Advances in Wound Care (New Rochelle), 1*(3), 120–126.

Junker, J. P., Lee, C. C., Samaan, S., et al. (2015). Topical delivery of ultrahigh concentrations of gentamicin is highly effective in reducing bacterial levels in infected porcine full thickness wounds. *Plastic and Reconstructive Surgery, 135*(1), 151–159.

Kalan, L., Loesche, M., Hodkinson, B. P., Heilmann, K., Ruthel, G., Gardner, S. E., et al. (2016). Redefining the chronic-wound microbiome: Fungal communities are prevalent, dynamic, and associated with delayed healing. *MBio, 7*(5), e01058-16.

Kalan, L. R., Meisel, J. S., Loesche, M. A., Horwinski, J., Soaita, I., Chen, X., et al. (2019). Strain- and species-level variation in the microbiome of diabetic wounds is associated with clinical outcomes and therapeutic efficacy. *Cell Host & Microbe, 25*, 1–15.

Kalel, R., Mora, A. K., Patro, B. S., Palit, D. K., & Nath, S. (2017). Synergistic enhancement in the drug sequestration power and reduction in the cytotoxicity of surfactants. *Physical Chemistry Chemical Physics, 19*(37), 25446–25455.

Kallstrom, G. (2014). Are quantitative bacterial wound cultures useful? *Journal of Clinical Microbiology, 52*(8), 2753–2756. https://doi.org/10.1128/JCM.00522-14.

Katsuyama, M., Ichikawa, H., Ogawa, S., & Ikezawa, Z. (2005). A novel method to control the balance of skin microflora. Part 1. Attack on biofilm of *Staphylococcus aureus* without antibiotics. *Journal of Dermatological Science, 38*(3), 197–205.

Kean, R., Rajendran, R., Haggarty, J., Townsend, E. M., Short, B., Burgess, K. E., et al. (2017). *Candida albicans* mycofilms support *Staphylococcus aureus* colonization and enhances miconazole resistance in dual-species interactions. *Frontiers in Microbiology, 8*(Feb), 1–11.

Kiselar, J. G., Wang, X., Dubyak, G. R., et al. (2015). Modification of β-defensin-2 by dicarbonyls methylglyoxal and glyoxal inhibits antibacterial and chemotactic function in vitro. *PLoS One, 10*(8), e0130533.

Kong, E. F., Tsui, C., Kucharíková, S., Andes, D., Van Dijck, P., & Jabra-Rizk, M. A. (2016). Commensal protection of *Staphylococcus aureus* against antimicrobials by *Candida albicans* biofilm matrix. *MBio, 7*(5), 1–12.

Krieger, B. R., Davis, D. M., Sanchez, J. E., et al. (2011). The use of silver nylon in preventing surgical site infections following colon and rectal surgery. *Diseases of the Colon and Rectum, 54*, 1014–1019.

Landini, L., Honka, M., Ferrannini, E., & Nuutila, P. (2016). Adipose tissue oxygenation in obesity: A matter of cardiovascular risk? *Current Pharmaceutical Design, 22*, 68.

Landis, S. J. (2008). Chronic wound infection and antimicrobial use. *Advances in Skin & Wound Care, 21*(11), 531–540. https://doi.org/10.1097/01.ASW.0000323578.87700.a5.

Landsdown, A. B., & Williams, A. (2007). Bacterial resistance to silver in wound care and medical devices. *Journal of Wound Care, 16*, 15–19.

Lavery, L. A., Davis, K. E., Berriman, S. J., Braun, L., Nichols, A., Kim, P. J., et al. (2016). WHS guidelines update: Diabetic foot ulcer treatment guidelines. *Wound Repair & Regeneration, 24*(1), 112–126. https://doi.org/10.1111/wrr.12391.

Lavery, L. A., Peters, E. J., Armstrong, D. G., et al. (2009). Risk factors for developing osteomyelitis in patients with diabetic foot wounds. *Diabetes Research and Clinical Practice, 83*(3), 347–352.

Leaper, D. J., Schultz, G., Carville, K., et al. (2012). Extending the TIME concept: What have we learned in the past 10 years? *International Wound Journal*, (Suppl. 2), 1–19.

Levine, N. S., Lindberg, R. B., Mason, A. D., Jr., et al. (1976). The quantitative swab culture and smear: A quick, simple method for determining the number of viable aerobic bacteria on open wounds. *The Journal of Trauma, 16*(2), 89–94.

Lewin, G. R., Stacy, A., Michie, K. L., Lamont, R. J., & Whiteley, M. (2019). Large-scale identification of pathogen essential genes during coinfection with sympatric and allopatric microbes. *Proceedings of the National Academy of Sciences of the United States of America, 116*(39), 19685–19694. Retrieved 10/1/2020 from: https://www.pnas.org/content/116/39/19685.

Lewis, K. (2001). Riddle of biofilm resistance. *Antimicrobial Agents and Chemotherapy, 45*, 999–1007.

Li, X. H., & Lee, J. H. (2017). Antibiofilm agents: A new perspective for antimicrobial strategy. *Journal of Microbiology, 55*(10), 753–766.

Lipsky, B., Dryden, M., Gottrup, F., et al. (2016). Antimicrobial stewardship in wound care: A position paper from the British society for antimicrobial chemotherapy and European wound management association. *The Journal of Antimicrobial Chemotherapy, 71*, 3026–3035.

Lipsky, B. A., & Hoey, C. (2009). Topical antimicrobial therapy for treating chronic wounds. *Clinical Infectious Disease, 49*(10), 1541–1549. https://doi.org/10.1086/644732.

Loesche, M., Gardner, S. E., Kalan, L., Horwinski, J., Zheng, Q., Hodkinson, B. P., et al. (2017). Temporal stability in chronic wound microbiota is associated with poor healing. *Journal of Investigative Dermatology, 137*, 237–244.

Lu, M., & Hansen, E. N. (2017). Hydrogen peroxide wound irrigation in orthopaedic surgery. *Journal of Bone and Joint Infection, 2*(1), 3–9. https://doi.org/10.7150/jbji.16690.

Lu, J., Turnbull, L., Burke, C. M., et al. (2014). Manuka-type honeys can eradicate biofilms produced by *Staphylococcus aureus* strains with different biofilm-forming abilities. *Peer J, 2*, e326.

Madsen, S. M., Westh, H., Danielsen, L., et al. (1996). Bacterial colonization and healing of venous leg ulcers. *APMIS, 104*, 895–899.

Malone, M., Bjarnsholt, T., McBain, A. J., et al. (2017). The prevalence of biofilms in chronic wounds: A systematic review and meta-analysis of published data. *Journal of Wound Care, 26*(1), 20–25.

Marcia, M. D., Roho-Molinero, E., & Oliver, A. (2014). Antimicrobial susceptibility testing in biofilm-growing bacteria. *Clinical Microbiology and Infection, 20*, 981–990.

Marston, W., Tang, J., Kirsner, R. S., & Ennis, W. (2016). Wound Healing Society 2015 update on guidelines for venous ulcers. *Wound Repair & Regeneration, 24*(1), 136–144. https://doi.org/10.1111/wrr.12394.

Metcalf, D. G., Bowler, P. G., & Hurlow, J. (2014). A clinical algorithm for wound biofilm identification. *Journal of Wound Care, 23*(3), 137–138. 140–142.

Metcalf, D., Bowler, P., & Parsons, D. (2016). In D. Dhanasekaran (Ed.), *Wound biofilm and therapeutic strategies, microbial biofilms—Importance and applications*. Rijeka, Croatia: InTech. Retrieved 5/9/2020 from: https://www.intechopen.com/books/microbialbiofilms-importance-and-applications/wound-biofilm-and-therapeutic-strategies.

Milne, C. T. (2020). *Wound source. The world's definitive source for wound care and product information* (23rd ed.). Atlantic Beach: Kestrel Health Information.

Min, K. R., Galvis, A., Nole, K. L. B., Sinha, R., Clarke, J., Kirsner, R. S., et al. (2020). Association between baseline abundance of Peptoniphilus, a Gram-positive anaerobic coccus, and wound healing outcomes of DFUs. *PLoS One, 15*(1), 1–20.

Moelleken, M., Jockenhöfer, F., Benson, S., & Dissemond, J. (2020). Prospective clinical study on the efficacy of bacterial removal with mechanical debridement in and around chronic leg ulcers assessed with fluorescence imaging. *International Wound Journal.* https://doi.org/10.1111/iwj.13345.

Molan, P., & Honey, R. T. (2015). A biologic wound dressing. *Wounds, 27*(6), 141–151.

Motta, G. J., Milne, C. T., & Corbett, L. Q. (2004). Impact of antimicrobial gauze on bacterial colonies in wounds that require packing. *Ostomy/Wound Management, 50*(8), 48–62.

Münter, K. C., Beele, H., Russell, L., et al. (2006). Effect of a sustained silver-releasing dressing on ulcers with delayed healing: The CONTOP study. *Journal of Wound Care, 15*(5), 199–206.

Murphy, C., Atkin, L., & Swanson, T. (2020). Defying hard-to-heal wounds with an early antibiofilm intervention strategy: Wound hygiene. *Journal of Wound Care, 29*(Sup3b), S1–S26. https://doi.org/10.12968/jowc.2020.29.Sup3b.S1.

Naik, S., Bouladoux, N., Linehan, J. L., Han, S.-J., Harrison, O. J., Wilhelm, C., et al. (2015). Commensal–dendritic-cell interaction specifies a unique protective skin immune signature. *Nature, 520* (7545), 104–108. https://doi.org/10.1038/nature14052.

O'Meara, S., Al-Kurdi, D., Ologun, Y., et al. (2014). Antibiotics and antiseptics for venous leg ulcers. *Cochrane Database of Systematic Reviews, 1*, CD003557.

Olsen, I. (2015). Biofilm-specific antibiotic tolerance and resistance. *European Journal of Clinical Microbiology & Infectious Diseases, 34*, 877–886.

Peng, Z., Li, H., Cao, Z., et al. (2020). Oxygen embolism after hydrogen peroxide irrigation during hip arthroscopy: A case report. *BMC Musculoskeletal Disorders, 21*, 58. https://doi.org/10.1186/s12891-020-3081-3.

Percival, S., & Bowler, P. (2004). Biofilms and their potential role in wound healing. *Wounds, 16*(7), 234–240.

Percival, S. L., Finnegan, S., Donelli, G., Vuotto, C., Rimmer, S., & Lipsky, B. A. (2016). Antiseptics for treating infected wounds: Efficacy on biofilms and effect of pH. *Critical Reviews in Microbiology, 42*(2), 293–309. https://doi.org/10.3109/1040841X.2014.940495.

Percival, S. L., Hill, K. E., Williams, D. W., et al. (2012). A review of the scientific evidence for biofilms in wounds. *Wound Repair and Regeneration, 20*(5), 647–657.

Percival, S. L., Malone, M., Mayer, D., Salisbury, A.-M., & Schultz, G. (2018). Role of anaerobes in polymicrobial communities and biofilms complicating diabetic foot ulcers. *International Wound Journal, 15*(5), 776–782.

Percival, S. L., McCarty, S., Hunt, J. A., et al. (2014). The effects of pH on wound healing, biofilms, and anti-microbial efficacy. *Wound Repair and Regeneration, 22*(2), 174–186.

Percival, S. L., Thomas, J. G., & Williams, D. W. (2010). Biofilms and bacterial imbalances in chronic wounds: Anti-Koch. *International Wound Journal, 7*(3), 169–175.

Petchiappan, A., & Chatterji, D. (2017). Antibiotic resistance: Current perspectives. *ACS Omega, 2*, 7400–7409.

Phillips, P. L., Yang, Q., Davis, S., et al. (2015). Antimicrobial dressing efficacy against mature Pseudomonas aeruginosa biofilm on porcine skin explants. *International Wound Journal, 12*(4), 469–483.

Pilcher, M. (2016). Wound cleansing: A key player in the implementation of the TIME paradigm. *Journal of Wound Care, 25* (3 Suppl), S7–S9. https://doi.org/10.12968/jowc.2016.25.Sup3.S7.

Price, L. B., Liu, C. M., Frankel, Y. M., Melendez, J. H., Aziz, M., Buchhagen, J., et al. (2010). Macroscale spatial variation in chronic wound microbiota: A cross-sectional study. *Wound Repair and Regeneration, 19*(1), 80–88. https://doi.org/10.1111/j.1524-475x.2010. 00628.x.

Quain, A. M., & Khardori, N. M. (2015). Nutrition in wound care management: A comprehensive overview. *Wounds, 27*(12), 327–335.

Reddy, M., Gill, S. S., Wu, W., Kalkar, S. R., & Rochon, P. A. (2012). Does this patient have an infection of a chronic wound? *JAMA, 307*, 605–611.

Rhoads, D., Wolcott, R. D., & Percival, S. (2008). Biofilms in wounds: Management strategies. *Journal of Wound Care, 17*(11), 502–508.

Robson, M. C., & Heggers, J. P. (1969). Bacterial quantification of open wounds. *Military Medicine, 134*(1), 19.

Robson, M. C., Payne, W. G., Ko, F., et al., et al. (2007). Hypochlorous acid as a potential wound care agent: Part II, stabilized hypochlorous acid: Its role in decreasing tissue bacterial bioburden and overcoming the inhibition of infection on wound healing. *Journal of Burns and Wounds, 2007*(6), 80–90.

Romanowski, E. G., Stella, N. A., Yates, K. A., Brothers, K. M., Kowalski, R. P., & RMQ, S. (2018). In vitro evaluation of a hypochlorous acid hygiene solution on established biofilms.

Eye Contact Lens, 44(Suppl. 2), S187–S191. https://doi.org/10.1097/ICL.0000000000000456.

Rondas, A. A. (2013). Swab versus biopsy for the diagnosis of chronic infected wounds. *Advances in Skin & Wound Care, 26*(5), 211–219.

Rytter, M. J. H., Kolte, L., Briend, A., Friis, H., & Christensen, V. B. (2014). The immune system in children with malnutrition—A systematic review. *PLoS One, 9*(8), e105017.

Said, J., Walker, M., Parsons, D., Stapleton, P., Beezer, A. E., & Gaisford, S. (2014). An in vitro test of the efficacy of an anti-biofilm wound dressing. *International Journal of Pharmaceutics, 474*(1–2), 177–181.

Schwartz, J. A., Lantis, J. C., II, Gendics, C., Fuller, A. M., Payne, W., & Ochs, D. (2012). A prospective, non-comparative, multicenter study to investigate the effect of cadexomer iodine on bioburden load and other wound characteristics in diabetic foot ulcers. *International Wound.* https://doi.org/10.1111/j.1742-481X.2012.01109.x.

Sender, R., Fuchs, S., & Milo, R. (2016). Are we really vastly outnumbered? Revisiting the ratio of bacterial to host cells in humans. *Cell, 164*(3), 337–340. https://doi.org/10.1016/j.cell.2016.01.013.

Seth, A. K., Zhong, A., Khang, T., Nguyen, K. T., Hong, S. J., Leung, K. P., et al. (2014). Impact of a novel, antimicrobial dressing on in vivo, Pseudomonas aeruginosa wound biofilm: Quantitative comparative analysis using a rabbit ear model. *Wound Repair and Regeneration, 22*, 712–719.

Sibbald, R. G., Goodman, L., Woo, K. Y., et al. (2011). Special considerations in wound bed preparation 2011: An update. *Advances in Skin & Wound Care, 24*(9), 415–436.

Sindi, A., Chawn, M. V. B., Hernandez, M. E., et al. (2019). Anti-biofilm effects and characterisation of the hydrogen peroxide activity of a range of Western Australian honeys compared to Manuka and multifloral honeys. *Science Reports, 9*(1), 17666. Published 2019 Nov 27 https://doi.org/10.1038/s41598-019-54217-8.

Singh, P. K., Parsek, M. R., Greenberg, E. P., & Welsh, M. J. (2002). A component of innate immunity prevents bacterial biofilm development. *Nature, 417*(6888), 552–555.

Sloan, T. J., Turton, J. C., Tyson, J., Musgrove, A., Fleming, V. M., Lister, M. M., et al. (2019). Examining diabetic heel ulcers through an ecological lens: microbial community dynamics associated with healing and infection. *Journal of Medical Microbiology, 68*(2), 230–240.

Song, T., Duperthuy, M., & Wai, S. N. (2016). Sub-optimal treatment of bacterial biofilms. *Antibiotics (Basel), 5*(2), 23. https://doi.org/10.3390/antibiotics5020023.

Spellberg, B., Srinivasan, A., & Chambers, H. (2016). New societal approaches to empowering antibiotic stewardship. *Journal of the American Medical Association, 315*, 1229–1230.

Stevens, D. L., Bisno, A. L., Chambers, H. F., et al. (2014). Practice guidelines for the diagnosis and management of skin and soft tissue infections: 2014 update by the Infectious Disease's Society of America. *Clinical Infectious Diseases, 59*(2), 147–159. https://doi.org/10.1093/cid/ciu296.

Stewart, P. S. (2015). Antimicrobial tolerance in biofilms. *Microbiology Spectrum, 3*(3), 1–30.

Stewart, P. S., White, B., Boegli, L., et al. (2019). Conceptual model of biofilm antibiotic tolerance that integrates phenomena of diffusion, metabolism, gene expression, and physiology. *Journal of Bacteriology, 201*(22), e00307-19.

Sun, Y., Smith, E., Wolcott, R., & Dowd, S. E. (2009). Propagation of anaerobic bacteria within an aerobic multi-species chronic wound biofilm model. *Journal of Wound Care, 18*(10), 426–431.

Sun, et al. (2018). Evidence on the carcinogenicity of gentian violet. *Office of Environmental Assessment.* Retrieved 10/1/2020 from: https://oehha.ca.gov/media/downloads/crnr/gentianviolethid081718.pdf.

Swanson, T., Angel, D., Sussman, G., Cooper, R., Haesler, E., Ousey, K., et al. (2016). *International Wound Infection Institute (IWII). Wound Infection in clinical practice: Principles of best practice.* Wounds International.

Tipton, C. D., Mathew, M. E., Wolcott, R. A., Wolcott, R. D., Kingston, T., & Phillips, C. D. (2017). Temporal dynamics of relative abundances and bacterial succession in chronic wound communities. *Wound Repair and Regeneration, 25*(4), 673–679.

Todd, O. A., Fidel, P. L., Harro, J. M., Hilliard, J. J., Tkaczyk, C., Sellman, B. R., et al. (2019). Candida albicans augments Staphylococcus aureus virulence by engaging the Staphylococcal agr quorum sensing system. *MBio, 10*(3), 1–16.

Todd, O. A., Noverr, M. C., & Peters, B. M. (2019). Candida albicans impacts Staphylococcus aureus alpha-toxin production via extracellular alkalinization. *MSphere, 4*(6), 1–12.

Townsend, E. M., Sherry, L., Kean, R., Hansom, D., Mackay, W. G., Williams, C., et al. (2017). Implications of antimicrobial combinations in complex wound biofilms containing fungi. *Antimicrobial Agents and Chemotherapy, 61*(9), e00672-17.

Townsend, E. M., Sherry, L., Rajendran, R., Hansom, D., Butcher, J., Mackay, W. G., et al. (2016). Development and characterization of a novel three-dimensional inter-kingdom wound biofilm model. *Biofouling, 32*(10), 1259–1270.

Traboulsi, R. S., Mukherjee, P. K., Chandra, J., Salata, R. A., Jurevic, R., & Ghannoum, M. A. (2011). Gentian violet exhibits activity against biofilms formed by oral Candida isolates obtained from HIV-infected patients. *Antimicrobial Agents and Chemotherapy, 55*(6), 3043–3045. Retrieved 10/1/2020 from: https://doi.org/10.1128/AAC.01601-10.

Verbanic, S., Shen, Y., Lee, J., Deacon, J. M., & Chen, I. A. (2020). Microbial predictors of healing and short-term effect of debridement on the microbiome of chronic wounds. *Npj Biofilms and Microbiomes, 6*(1), 21.

Walker, M., Metcalf, D., Parsons, D., & Bowler, P. (2015). A real-life clinical evaluation of a next-generation antimicrobial dressing on acute and chronic wounds. *Journal of Wound Care, 24*, 11–22.

White, R. J., & Cutting, K. F. (2006). Critical colonization—The concept under scrutiny. *Ostomy/Wound Management, 52*(11), 50–56. PMID: 17146118.

Winfield, R. D., Reese, S., Bochicchio, K., Mazuski, J. E., & Bochicchio, G. V. (2016). Obesity and the risk for surgical site infection in abdominal surgery. *The American Surgeon, 82*(4), 331–336.

Wolcott, R. (2015). Disrupting the biofilm matrix improves wound healing outcomes. *Journal of Wound Care, 24*(8), 366–371.

Wolcott, R. D. (2017). Biofilms cause chronic infections. *Journal of Wound Care, 26*(8), 423–425. https://doi.org/10.12968/jowc.2017.26.8.423. PMID: 28795886.

Wolcott, R. D., & Rhodes, D. O. (2008). A study of biofilm-based wound management in subjects with critical limb ischemia. *Journal of Wound Care, 17*(4), 145–155.

Wolcott, R. D., Rumbaugh, K. P., James, G., et al. (2010). Biofilm maturity studies indicate sharp debridement opens a time-dependent therapeutic window. *Journal of Wound Care, 19*(8), 320–328.

Woo, K. Y., & Sibbald, R. G. (2009). A cross sectional validation study of using NERDS and STONEES to assess bacterial burden. *Ostomy/Wound Management, 55*(8), 40–44.

Wound, Ostomy and Continence Nurses Society. (2016). *Guideline for management of pressure ulcers, WOCN clinical practice guideline series #2.* Mt. Laurel: Wound, Ostomy and Continence Nurses Society.

Zhao, G., Hochwalt, P. C., Usui, M. L., et al. (2010). Delayed wound healing in diabetic (db/db) mice with Pseudomonas aeruginosa biofilm challenge: A model for the study of chronic wounds. *Wound Repair and Regeneration, 18*(5), 467–477.

Zhao, G., Usui, M. L., Lippman, S. I., et al. (2013). Biofilms and inflammation in chronic wounds. *Advances in Wound Care, 2*(7), 389–399.

Zipperer, A., Konnerth, M. C., Laux, C., Berscheid, A., Janek, D., Weidenmaier, C., et al. (2016). Human commensals producing a novel antibiotic impair pathogen colonization. *Nature, 535* (7613), 511–516. https://doi.org/10.1038/nature18634.

Zölß, C., & Cech, J. D. (2016). Efficacy of a new multifunctional surfactant-based biomaterial dressing with 1% silver sulphadiazine in chronic wounds. *International Wound Journal, 13*(5), 738–743.

FURTHER READING

Brook, I. (1989). The concept of indirect pathogenicity by beta-lactamase production, especially in ear, nose and throat infection. *The Journal of Antimicrobial Chemotherapy, 24*(Suppl. B), 63–72.

Brook, I. (2007). Treatment of anaerobic infection. *Expert Review of Anti-Infective Therapy, 5*(6), 991–1006. https://doi.org/10.1586/14787210.5.6.991.

Health Canada. (2019). *Health Canada warns Canadians of potential cancer risk associated with gentian violet. Health Canada Recalls and Safety Alerts.* Retrieved 10/1/2020 from: https://

healthycanadians.gc.ca/recall-alert-rappel-avis/hc-sc/2019/70179a-eng.php.

Johnson, T. R., Gómez, B. I., McIntyre, M. K., Dubick, M. A., Christy, R. J., Nicholson, S. E., et al. (2018). The cutaneous microbiome and wounds: New molecular targets to promote wound healing. *International Journal of Molecular Sciences, 19*(9), 2699.

Kucisec-Tepes, N. (2013). Prevencija infekcije kronicne rane [Prevention of chronic wound infection]. *Acta Medica Croatica, 67*(Suppl. 1), 51–58.

O'Connell, H. A., Kottkamp, G. S., Eppelbaum, J. L., Stubblefield, B. A., Gilbert, S. E., & Gilbert, E. S. (2006). Influences of biofilm structure and antibiotic resistance mechanisms on indirect pathogenicity in a model polymicrobial biofilm. *Applied and Environmental Microbiology, 72*(7), 5013–5019.

Ovington, L. (2003). Bacterial toxins and wound healing. *Ostomy/Wound Management, 49*, 8–12.

Sen, C. K., Gordillo, G. M., Roy, S., et al. (2009). Human skin wounds: A major and snowballing threat to public health and the economy. *Wound Repair and Regeneration, 17*(6), 763–771. https://doi.org/10.1111/j.1524-475X.2009. 00543.x.

Sibbald, R. G., Woo, K., & Ayello, E. A. (2006). Increased bacterial burden and infection: the story of NERDS and STONES. *Advances in Skin & Wound Care, 19*(8), 447–461.

Thomas, D. W. W. (2003). Anaerobic cocci populating the deep tissues of chronic wounds impair cellular wound healing responses in vitro. *British Journal of Dermatology, 148*(3), 456–466.

Ugwu, E., Adeleye, O., Gezawa, I., Okpe, I., Enamino, M., & Ezeani, I. (2019). Predictors of lower extremity amputation in patients with diabetic foot ulcer: Findings from MEDFUN, a multi-center observational study. *Journal of Foot and Ankle Research, 12*, 34.

Wolcott, R., Hanson, J., Rees, E., et al. (2016). Analysis of the chronic wound microbiota of 2,963 patients by 16S rDNA pyrosequencing. *Wound Repair and Regeneration, 24*(1), 163–174.

20

Wound Debridement

Jacalyn Anne Brace

OBJECTIVES

1. Describe the role of debridement in the wound-healing process.
2. List contraindications to debridement.
3. Distinguish between selective and nonselective debridement.
4. Compare and contrast four methods of debridement: autolysis, chemical, mechanical, and sharp.
5. Describe the appropriate use of debridement using conservative sharp debridement and monofilament/microfiber pads.
6. List debridement options for the infected wound.
7. Describe at least five factors to consider when selecting a debridement approach.
8. For each method of debridement, list two advantages, disadvantages, and relevant special considerations.

Debridement is the removal of nonviable tissue and foreign matter from a wound and is a naturally occurring event in the wound repair process. During the inflammatory phase, neutrophils and macrophages digest and remove "used" platelets, cellular debris, and avascular injured tissue from the wound area. However, with the accumulation of significant amounts of damaged tissue, this natural process becomes overwhelmed and insufficient. Buildup of necrotic tissue then places considerable phagocytic demand on the wound, coupled with the continued presence of proinflammatory cells, both of which ultimately retard wound healing (Robson, 1997; Stotts & Hunt, 1997). Consequently, debridement of necrotic tissue is an essential objective of topical therapy and a critical component of optimal wound management. Debridement not only is an integral component of wound bed preparation but it also facilitates bacterial balance and moisture balance (Ousey et al., 2018; Sibbald et al., 2021).

Debridement is used to achieve several objectives:

1. Reduce the bioburden of the wound. Because devitalized tissue supports the growth of bacteria, the presence of necrotic tissue places the patient at risk for wound infection and sepsis. Using external measures to remove the necrotic tissue and foreign matter reduces the volume of pathogenic microbes present in the wound.
2. Control and potentially prevent wound infections, particularly in the deteriorating wound.
3. Facilitate visualization of the wound wall and base. In the presence of necrotic tissue, accurate and thorough assessment of the viable tissue is hampered.
4. Interrupt the cycle of the chronic wound at the molecular level, so that protease and cytokine levels more closely approximate those of the acute wound.

Necrotic tissue can appear in various forms. Eschar has the firm, dry, leathery appearance of desiccated, and compressed tissue layers (see Plates 26, 37A, 50, 72, 73, and 87A). When the tissue is kept moist, the devitalized tissue, referred to as nonviable tissue, remains soft and may be brown, yellow, or gray in appearance (see Plates 14, 27, 28, and 37A). Nonviable tissue may be adherent to the wound bed and edges or loosely adherent and stringy (see Plates 27 and 28). Slough may also be present in the wound bed. As described in Chapter 10, slough is the accumulation of the cellular byproducts from the inflammatory process and the continuous normal cycle of tissue breaking down and remodeling. During this inflammatory phase, matrix metalloproteinase levels increase and degrade the used growth factors and proteins resulting in the accumulation of slough (Angel, 2019; Edsberg et al., 2016). Components of slough include fibrin, microorganisms, intact leukocytes, cell debris, and serous exudate (Angel, 2019; Thomas, 1990). Once the eschar and nonviable tissue is removed, slough is often visible covering the wound bed. Maintaining a moist wound environment is essential because continued exposure to air dehydrates the wound bed and the nonviable tissue, causing it to return to a hard, leathery state.

Debridement is indicated for any wound, acute or chronic, when necrotic tissue, slough, and suspected or confirmed biofilm is present. Debridement is done initially and periodically (also known as serial or maintenance debridement). This is done as needed until the wound bed is free of suspected biofilm and nonviable tissue. The determination of whether to debride heel ulcers depends upon the clinical goals. In those patients with dry heel eschar who cannot be revascularized, have multiple comorbidities, and are immobile with no functional goals, the heel eschar may be left intact. Heel ulcers with dry eschar should be monitored closely and debrided if they develop signs of infection (European Pressure Ulcer Advisory Panel, National Pressure Injury Advisory Panel, Pan Pacific Pressure Injury Alliance [EPUAP, NPIAP, & PPPIA], 2019; Gould et al., 2016).

METHODS OF DEBRIDEMENT

Several methods of debridement are available for removal of devitalized tissue from necrotic wounds (Box 20.1). Debridement methods are classified as either selective (only necrotic tissue is removed) or nonselective (viable tissue is removed along with the nonviable tissue). More specifically, debridement is classified by the actual mechanism of action: autolysis, chemical, mechanical, biologic, or sharp (conservative or surgical). Although one method of debridement may be the primary approach selected to rid the wound of necrotic tissue, debridement typically involves a combination of methods.

Autolysis

Autolysis is a natural, highly selective, painless method of debridement. Specifically, autolysis is the lysis of necrotic tissue by the body's white blood cells and natural enzymes, which enter the wound site during the normal inflammatory process. The body's proteolytic, fibrinolytic, and collagenolytic enzymes are released to digest the devitalized tissue present in the wound while leaving the healthy tissue intact (Rodeheaver, Baharestani, Brabec, et al., 1994). As a naturally occurring physiologic process, autolysis is stimulated by a moist, vascular environment with adequate leukocyte function count. Therefore, autolysis is contraindicated in patients with compromised immunity. Autolysis as a sole method of debridement is not recommended for actively infected wounds or wounds with extensive necrotic tissue or significant tunneling and undermining (EPUAP, NPIAP, PPPIA, 2019; Nurses Specialized in Wound, Ostomy and Continence Canada [NSWOCC], 2021).

A moist environment is facilitated by the application of a moisture-retentive dressing left undisturbed for a reasonable length of time, typically 24–72 h. Maintaining a moist wound environment allows the cellular structures that are essential

BOX 20.1 Selective vs Nonselective Debridement Methods

Selective
Autolysis
Enzyme
Conservative sharp debridement
Biosurgical (maggot)
Ultrasound therapy

Nonselective
Surgical
Wet-to-dry gauze
Surgical sharp
Monofilament/microfiber pads

for phagocytosis (neutrophils and macrophages) to remain intact and avoid premature destruction through desiccation. An important role of macrophages is production of growth factors, so the presence of healthy macrophages in the wound fluid supports continued production of growth factors. Once autolysis is initiated, eschar will loosen from the edges, become soft, change to a brown or gray color, and eventually transform into stringy yellow slough. It is critical to monitor the wound closely during the autolysis process because as the wound is debrided, the full wound bed and walls are exposed and the true extent of the wound is revealed; consequently, the wound will increase in length, width, and depth, necessitating a change in topical therapy. Plate 28 shows the appearance of a wound before and after autolysis.

Clinicians, patients, and family members unfamiliar with the process of autolysis can misinterpret the collection of wound exudate and the accompanying odor as indicative of an infection. It is important to emphasize that the wound exudate contains enzymes and growth factors that are essential to wound repair. In fact, wounds treated with moisture-retentive dressings are less likely to become infected than are wounds treated with conventional dressings because moisture-retentive dressings are impermeable to exogenous bacteria. In addition, viable neutrophils and other natural substances in wound fluid inhibit bacterial growth (Hutchinson, 1989; Lawrence, 1994; Mir, Ali, Barakullah, et al., 2018).

The use of moisture-retentive dressings to create and maintain a moist wound environment launched the use of autolysis as an option for debridement. Moisture-retentive dressings attract enzyme-rich exudate to the wound site (Chen, Rogers, & Lydon, 1992; Mir et al., 2018), which is very effective at detaching nonviable tissue from the surrounding skin and wound base. Selection of dressings that promote autolysis is based on the condition of the wound base, depth of the wound, presence of tunnels or undermining, volume of wound exudate, and the patient's condition. When the wound base is dry, a dressing that will add moisture, such as a hydrogel, should be used. If absorption is needed, a dressing should be selected that will absorb excess exudate without dehydrating the wound surface. Chapter 21 provides an in-depth discussion on dressing selection to promote autolysis while matching the needs of the wound.

Experts agree that autolysis is slower than alternative methods of debridement such as mechanical and sharp (EPUAP, NPIAP, & PPPIA, 2019; NSWOCC, 2021). Generally, comparisons between different types of debridement demonstrate no statistically significant difference between methods in achieving improvement in wound surface area (Carter, Gilligan, Waycaster, Schaum, & Fife, 2017; EPUAP, NPIAP, PPPIA, 2019; McCallon & Frilot, 2015; Mearns et al., 2017; Waycaster & Milne, 2013). The time frame for the occurrence of autolysis varies depending on the size of the wound and the amount and type of necrotic tissue or slough. Generally, the softening and separating of necrotic tissue are observed within days. If significant debridement is not apparent in 1–2 weeks, another method of debridement should be used (Gould et al., 2016).

Autolysis can be used in combination with other debridement techniques. In fact, promotion of autolysis is an important adjuvant to all debridement modalities for ongoing maintenance debridement and prevention of tissue dehydration and cellular desiccation. For example, after surgical sharp debridement of a pressure injury, the application of a moisture retentive dressing maintains a moist wound environment, thus preventing tissue desiccation and promoting continued softening and loosening of residual necrotic tissue. It often becomes necessary to combine dressings to achieve debridement while meeting all the needs of the patient and the wound. For example, a transparent dressing is inappropriate for debridement of a wound that has depth or is heavily exudative. Instead, an absorptive dressing (e.g., alginate and Hydrofiber) with an absorptive cover dressing (e.g., foam) is warranted because it will fill the wound depth and absorb the exudate (see Chapter 21).

Chemical

Necrotic wound tissue can be removed through a chemical process using enzymes. Silver nitrate is another method of chemical debridement (also referred to as *chemical cauterization*); however, it is more commonly used on closed wound edges (described in Chapter 8 and shown in Fig. 8-6 and Plate 4) and hypergranulation tissue (described in Chapter 10 and shown in Plate 29).

Enzymes

Topical application of exogenous enzymes is a selective method of debridement. Over the years, various sources have been used to manufacture enzymes (e.g., krill, crab, papaya, bovine extract, and bacteria). There are enzymatic debriding agents available that contain collagenases (Onesti et al., 2016; Patry & Blanchette, 2017; Shoham et al., 2018). Collagenase digests collagen in necrotic tissue by dissolving the collagen "anchors" that secure the avascular tissue to the underlying wound bed (EPUAP, NPIAP, & PPPIA, 2019).

Similar to autolysis, enzymatic debridement is considered slower than mechanical or sharp debridement but is frequently used for initial debridement when anticoagulant therapy renders surgical debridement unfeasible (König, Vanscheidt, Augustin, et al., 2005; Ramundo & Gray, 2009). The length of time required to achieve debridement may range from several days to weeks. Historically, enzymes have been used to debride a wound with significant bacterial bioburden or infection (Ramundo & Gray, 2009). Today, sharp debridement is a critical intervention for removing biofilm. Immediate use of appropriate topical antiseptics is then indicated (see Chapter 19) to prevent the formation of new biofilm. *Alginogels* are antiseptics that combine alginates and antimicrobial enzymes (e.g., lactoperoxidase and glucose oxidase) to prevent formation of new and inhibit the growth of established biofilms (EPUAP, NPIAP, & PPPIA, 2019).

Although some topical antibiotics such as polymyxin B/bacitracin, mupirocin, or neomycin may be safely used in conjunction with collagenase, other antibiotics may inhibit the enzymatic activity (Carpenter & Shaffett, 2017; Jovanovic,

Ermis, Mewaldt, et al., 2012). Specific ions, including several commonly used antimicrobial dressings and antiseptic solutions, inhibit or inactivate collagenase. Silver dressings and cadexomer iodine have been reported to reduce collagenase activity by more than 50% and 90%, respectively. Antiseptic cleansers that have a pH level below 6.0 or above 8.0 also reduce the activity of collagenase. Most sodium hypochlorite-based cleansers may be safely used with collagenase (Carpenter & Shaffett, 2017; Jovanovic et al., 2012).

A secondary dressing is required when an enzyme is used and should be selected based on the needs of the wound. With the previously mentioned exceptions, manufacturers state that most dressings can be used safely with enzymes, including gauze, hydrogels, foams, petrolatum mesh dressing, and transparent film dressings; however, silver-impregnated dressings should be avoided. Iodine dressings or those containing zinc should not be used with collagenase (Shi, Ermis, Kiedaisch, et al., 2010). Frequency of enzyme application is at least daily and as need for soilage; therefore, the secondary dressing also should be appropriate for daily changes (Shi et al., 2010). Enzymatic debridement can be augmented by using a moisture-retentive dressing that will hold moisture at the wound bed. Enzymes require a prescription, so their use has cost and reimbursement implications. In addition, daily dressing changes dictate considerable commitment on the part of the caregiver (patient, family, or staff) that may not always be reasonable or acceptable.

When collagenase is used on a wound with intact eschar, the eschar must be cross-hatched to allow penetration of the enzyme, and the wound surface must be kept moist. Cross-hatching the eschar is achieved by using a no. 10 blade to make several shallow slits in the eschar without damaging the viable wound base. Once the eschar begins to separate or demarcate from the surrounding skin, the enzyme can be applied to the wound edges along the line of demarcation to hasten separation. At this point, conservative sharp debridement can be used to remove softened necrotic tissue. Enzyme treatment can then be continued, or another debridement technique such as autolysis can be instituted. Because these enzymes are selective, damage to viable tissue in the wound bed should not occur if the dressing is continued once debridement of the necrotic tissue is completed and viable tissue is exposed. However, enzyme application typically is discontinued when the wound bed is free of necrotic tissue. More appropriate dressings are available at a fraction of the cost and should be implemented once the wound is debrided. Patients may experience a transient stinging or burning sensation, particularly when the enzyme comes into contact with intact skin. Barrier ointments can be used to protect the periwound skin.

Biosurgical (Larval Therapy)

Originating from the battlefield, maggots have been used to achieve a biologic method of debridement. Providers noted anecdotal reports from medics who observed the rapid removal of necrotic tissue when maggots were present on the wound bed. Today, therapeutic maggot therapy involves sterilizing the eggs of *Lucilia sericata* (greenbottle fly). Once the eggs hatch (again, under sterile conditions), the sterile larvae are introduced into the wound bed. Larvae secrete proteolytic enzymes, including collagenase, allantoin, and other agents, which break down necrotic tissue (EPUAP, NPIAP, PPPIA, 2019). It is also believed that the larvae ingest microorganisms, which are then destroyed (Malekian, Esmaeeli Djavid, Akbarzadeh, et al., 2019; Shi & Shofler, 2014). In a study of 119 patients with slough-filled wounds, debridement was achieved faster with maggot therapy than wounds treated with sharp debridement and autolysis combined during the first week of treatment. However, no statistical significance was noted after 2 weeks of therapy (Opletalová, Patry, & Blanchette, 2017). Reviews and meta-analyses over the years have concluded that maggot therapy, although a promising therapy, offers no more overall effectiveness than other methods of debridement (Gray, 2008; Hoppe & Granick, 2012; Tian, Liang, Song, et al., 2013; Zarchi & Jemec, 2012).

Biosurgical therapy should not be used with wounds that are poorly perfused; require frequent inspection; or have exposed blood vessels, necrotic bone and tendon, or limb or life-threatening infections (Cowan, Stechmiller, Phillips, et al., 2013; EPUAP, NPIAP, & PPPIA, 2019). Care should be taken to prevent the larvae from coming in contact with healthy skin because the proteolytic enzymes can cause damage. Pain and bleeding have been reported, so the patient should be monitored for both, particularly with the widespread use of antiplatelet therapy (Bazaliński, Kózka, Karnas, & Więch, 2019; Steenvoorde & van Doorn, 2008). The main disadvantage to maggot therapy is the sensation of crawling that some patients experience, but confinement of the larvae to the wound bed decreases this sensation. Various dressings have been described to apply maggot therapy; most involve periwound protection with mesh or nylon net to contain the larvae and an absorbent pad to absorb exudate; some dressings incorporate the maggots into a layered dressing, which allows ease of application and removal, and eliminates concerns about containment (Opletalová et al., 2017).

Mechanical

Mechanical modes of debridement include monofilament/microfiber pads, low-frequency ultrasound (see Chapter 27), hydrosurgery, and wet-to-dry gauze dressings. These techniques represent selective and nonselective modes of debridement. Historically, whirlpool and pulsate lavage were used as a mechanical method of debridement. However, most recent wound management guidelines do not recommend or reference whirlpool and pulsate lavage as options (EPUAP, NPIAP, & PPPIA, 2019; Lavery et al., 2016; Sibbald et al., 2021; Wound, Ostomy and Continence Nurses Society, 2014, 2019).

Wet-to-Dry Gauze

Wet-to-dry gauze dressings are an age-old technique and require leaving the moist dressing in place in contact with the wound bed and alloying it to dry out before removal thus removing tissue as the gauze is removed. This technique can be painful and is nonselective, therefore removing healthy tissue and cells as well as nonviable tissue. Wet-to-dry dressings are associated with slower wound healing and higher cost due to the need for frequent wound dressing changes (EPUAP, NPIAP, & PPPIA, 2019; Sibbald et al., 2021; Woo, Keast, Parsons, et al., 2013). In addition, wet-to-dry dressings are not effective with removal of biofilm in a chronic wound (Phillips et al., 2015). If wet-to-dry debridement must be used, it is most appropriate with heavily necrotic and infected wounds without visible granulation tissue. Correct technique consists of lightly packing moistened (not dripping wet) open-weave cotton gauze in the wound bed and allowing it to dry in the wound to trap debris and necrotic tissue. Once dry, usually 6–8 h after application, the dressing is pulled off the wound along with the trapped debris and necrotic tissue; moistening the gauze before removal will not facilitate mechanical debridement. Finally, the wound is cleansed, and the process is repeated. If the procedure is performed correctly, wet-to-dry gauze debridement requires dressing changes for several days to weeks, two to three times per day.

Monofilament/Microfiber Pads

Monofilament wound debridement pads (Plate 51) are another type of mechanical debridement. The mechanism of action is that monofilament fibers detach, bind and remove debris, biofilm, slough and exudate from the wound bed and surrounding skin while protecting viable tissue (Dowsett, Swan, & Orig, 2013; EPUAP, NPIAP, & PPPIA, 2019; Strohal et al., 2013). This method of debridement has been described by the National Institute for Health and Care Excellence (NICE, 2014) as particularly effective for chronic sloughy wounds and hyperkeratotic skin around acute or chronic wounds. The monofilament fibers are cut at an angle to better penetrate irregularly shaped areas and remove devitalized skin and wound debris. The pad is moistened with tap water, sterile water, or saline and wiped across the wound with gentle pressure. The procedure averages 2–4 min. While pain has been reported during the procedure, it subsides after the debridement is completed and is generally tolerated without pain medicine (Atkin, 2014; Meads, Lovato, & Longworth, 2015; Schultz, Woo, Weir, & Yang, 2018).

Hydrosurgery

A *hydrosurgical water knife* is a fast method of surgical debridement that dispenses normal saline at a high power, enabling debridement and cleansing of the wound base. This water jet device is regulated so that the clinician is able to precisely control the depth of debridement. The high-velocity stream runs parallel to the wound surface and creates a vacuum, which then cleanses and removes debris into a collection container (Attinger et al., 2006; Ferrer-Sola et al., 2017).

Sharp Debridement

Sharp debridement is a rapid process that uses sterile instruments. Sharp debridement can be done sequentially in a conservative fashion (conservative sharp wound debridement), or it can be done surgically (surgical sharp debridement). Any method of sharp debridement requires that the practitioner is qualified and prepared to perform this procedure. Qualifications and preparations include: appropriate competency, scope of practice, the required equipment, support in the event of bleeding, and alignment with their facility's policies and procedures that are consistent with local legal and regulatory statutes (Sibbald et al., 2021).

Conservative Sharp Wound Debridement

Conservative sharp wound debridement, also known as *conservative instrumental debridement,* is a selective debridement method for the removal of loosely adherent, nonviable tissue using sterile instruments (e.g., forceps or "pick-ups," scissors, and scalpel with no. 10 or no. 15 blade). When done correctly, the procedure is not aggressive enough to harm viable tissue and is not likely to result in blood loss.

Conservative sharp debridement has several advantages. It removes the necrotic tissue more quickly than the previously discussed methods, and it can be accomplished in a serial manner. This method of debridement can be combined with other debridement techniques (autolysis or enzymatic) to shorten this phase of wound care. Theoretically, a more rapid approach to debridement decreases the body's expenditure of energy during a time of high resource use.

Because of the low risk involved, conservative sharp debridement in many states is a delegated medical function that can be performed in various settings by a clinician who is competent and credentialed in the technique. Therefore, conservative sharp debridement is a viable option for patients residing in nonacute care settings without the need for transfer to a hospital. Various requirements may need to be satisfied, depending on the nurse practice act specific to the state and the employer's requirements. Checklist 20.1 contains factors to consider before performing conservative sharp debridement. A sample policy, procedure and competency for conservative sharp debridement can be found in the Appendix A (Winnipeg Regional Health Authority, 2019).

A disadvantage of conservative sharp debridement is that, depending on the size of the ulcer and the amount of necrotic tissue involved, it could conceivably take weeks to remove all of the nonviable tissue. The procedure may be uncomfortable for the patient, so the need for analgesia should be considered. Blood loss is not expected during conservative sharp debridement but remains a possibility. As a result, the patient should be assessed for factors that place him or her at risk for clotting problems if a vessel is accidentally severed. Factors to consider include medications (e.g., anticoagulants, high-dose nonsteroidal antiinflammatory drugs) and pathologic conditions (e.g., thrombocytopenia, impaired hepatic function, vitamin K deficiency, and malnutrition). When any of these factors are present, the wound specialist should confer with the provider before proceeding with conservative sharp debridement.

There is the potential for transient bacteremia after debridement of a wound (Bryan, Dew, & Reynolds, 1983), particularly when the wound is infected. Therefore, wound bed and periwound should be prepped prior to debridement

---

CHECKLIST 20.1 Factors to Consider Before Performing Conservative Sharp Debridement

✓ Is conservative sharp debridement covered under the clinician's state practice act?

✓ Are specialty education, training, and credentials in conservative sharp debridement required by the state or the employer?

✓ What formal knowledge and skill updates are required and how often?

✓ Has the individual's professional organization or employer delineated specific guidelines related to conservative sharp debridement?

✓ Are policies, procedures, and protocols in place for conservative sharp debridement?

✓ Is conservative sharp debridement considered part of the clinician's clinical privileges, or is a provider's order required for each incident of conservative sharp debridement?

✓ What level of provider supervision, if any, is required for conservative sharp debridement?

✓ Does the employer provide malpractice insurance coverage for conservative sharp debridement?

✓ Does the clinician carry malpractice insurance to cover conservative sharp debridement?

---

for all debridement procedures and thoroughly cleaned after the debridement procedure (Murphy et al., 2020). Transient bacteremia in a patient who is nutritionally compromised, leukopenic, or otherwise immunocompromised can be devastating.

Surgical sharp debridement is the preferred method for debriding most infected wounds (EPUAP, NPIAP, & PPPIA, 2019). However, if surgical sharp debridement is not an option because of the patient's condition or the care setting, serial conservative sharp debridement can be conducted by the nonphysician wound care provider, but only in conjunction with appropriate antibiotic coverage. Although systemic antibiotics may not penetrate the necrotic tissue to reduce the bacterial load in the wound, they should reduce the potential for systemic dissemination of the pathogens. Topical antiseptic solutions may also be instrumental in reducing the bioburden of the wound. The wound specialist should be in compliance with the policies of the facility or agency on the management of infected wounds.

Surgical Sharp Wound Debridement

Surgical debridement is the fastest method for removing large amounts of necrotic tissue but is outside of the scope of practice of most providers. This method not only removes necrotic tissue and its attached bacterial burden but also can result in removal of senescent cells and bleeding, thus restarting the cascade of wound healing. In many cases, surgical debridement is performed at the bedside. However, international guidelines for the care of patients with a pressure injury recommend performing debridement in the operating room in the following cases (EPUAP, NPIAP, & PPPIA, 2019):

- Crepitus
- Fluctuance
- Presence of advancing cellulitis
- Wound-related sepsis
- Extensive necrotic tissue
- Inability to establish degree of undermining and tunneling
- Infected bone or hardware that may need to be removed

Disadvantages of surgical debridement include the potential for negative effects from anesthesia, excess bleeding, and transient bacteremia that may progress to systemic infection and patient death. The condition of the patient, aggressive nature of this procedure, and higher level of care required after debridement may require the patient to spend more time in the hospital.

Laser Debridement

Laser debridement, a form of surgical debridement, uses focused beams of light to cauterize, vaporize, or slice through tissue. Several light sources for lasers are available; each type of laser emits light at a specific wavelength, and different body tissues absorb different wavelengths. The part of the tissue that absorbs the light is called the *chromophore*. When the chromophore absorbs the light, it is quickly heated and vaporized. When the beam of light is tightly focused, it is capable of cutting through human tissue like a knife (Dinulos, 2021; Raz, 1995).

The use of lasers is well known for skin resurfacing, removal of hair, tattoo ink, and pigmented lesions as well as the treatment of vascular lesions (e.g., telangiectasias and spider leg veins). However, laser use in wound debridement is not yet recommended in recent wound-related clinical practice guidelines or presented in recent peer-reviewed literature beyond animal studies (Graham, Schomacker, Glatter, et al., 2002; Lam, Rice, & Brown, 2002), human case reports (Kazemikhoo, Hashemi Pour, Nilforoushzadeh, Mokmeli, & Dahmardehei, 2019) and pilot studies (Hajhosseini et al., 2020).

SELECTION OF DEBRIDEMENT METHOD

Three general parameters guide the selection of the most appropriate debridement process: (1) overall condition and goals for the patient, (2) status of the wound and urgency of the need for debridement, and (3) skill level of the care provider. Algorithms are available to guide the clinician in selecting the appropriate debridement method. Although they are based on expert opinion and have not been validated, these algorithms can serve as a useful starting point for decision making (Fig. 20.1).

Overall Condition and Goals for the Patient

Occasionally, it may be necessary to forgo debridement if it is not consistent with the patient's wishes and overall goals for care (EPUAP, NPIAP, & PPPIA, 2019). Such a decision must include input from the patient, the patient's significant others,

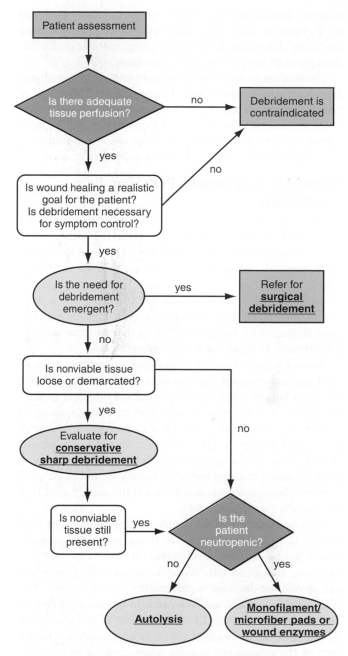

Fig. 20.1 Wound debridement algorithm.

and the primary care provider. Even if the goal is not to heal the wound, debridement of necrotic tissue will control infection and unpleasant wound odors, making the environment more comfortable for the patient, family, and caregivers.

The patient's history and coexisting morbidities affect the selection of debridement method. For example, awareness of any clotting disorders or anticoagulant medications used is critical when considering sharp debridement. When a patient has severe neutropenia (absolute count less than 500) and therefore at risk for severe sepsis, autolysis is not realistic or safe because of the insufficient number of neutrophils available to respond to the wound demands (Bodey, Buckley, Sathe, et al., 1966). Generally, the wound will appear stagnant during this time. Debridement by autolysis should be postponed until the neutrophil count climbs over 1000 mm^3. Chemical debridement using enzymes is an effective option in the presence of severe neutropenia.

The risk for transient bacteremia in conjunction with any debridement technique should be considered. The release of microorganisms from the necrotic tissue of even a noninfected wound may be sufficient to overwhelm the patient's immune system, and the procedure may need to be postponed for the patient who is critically ill or neutropenic.

Wound Status (Infection, Perfusion, Pain, and Biofilm)

When there is no urgent clinical need for debridement, then mechanical, autolytic, or enzymatic, methods of debridement can be used. Ulcer-related cellulitis, crepitus, or sepsis dictates rapid surgical debridement (EPUAP, NPIAP, & PPPIA, 2019). Surgical (or aggressive sharp) debridement is the cornerstone of biofilm management. Chapter 19 is a must read to understand the complexities and most recent management strategies for biofilm, including maintenance or serial debridement to break the biofilm growth cycle.

Wound pain is another critical determinant of debridement method selection. Patients who are experiencing wound pain may benefit from the less painful debridement modalities (autolysis or enzymatic). The other types of debridement (wet-to-dry, conservative sharp, and surgical sharp) may trigger or exacerbate pain. Therefore, patients need to be premedicated prior to the procedure. The patient's pain status during dressing changes and while resting should be assessed. Prophylactic analgesia should be administered topically or systemically (see Chapter 28).

As stated previously, dry, stable (i.e., noninfected or nonfluctuant) ischemic wounds or those with dry gangrene should not be debrided until perfusion to the extremity has. However, if the necrotic tissue becomes soft, demarcated and an odor or drainage is present, the necrotic tissue needs to be debrided, and blood flow needs to be restored urgently. As described in Chapter 13, measurement of vascular status, including an ankle-brachial index, is an important component of the assessment process when considering debridement in a patient with lower leg ulceration. Treatment goals should be consistent with the goals and lifestyle of the individual.

Clinician Experience and Competence

Although debridement methods such as autolysis, wound irrigation, wet-to-dry dressings, and enzymes ideally are initiated under the direction of the provider or wound care specialist, they are procedures that can be performed by nurses, physical therapists, the patient, and caregivers. However, the more aggressive methods of debridement, specifically sharp debridement, require a greater level of skill and competence. Conservative sharp debridement should be performed only by a wound specialist or provider with demonstrated and documented competence. Wound care specialists must be in compliance with their scope of practice, state nurse practice act, and institutional policies. Surgical sharp debridement and laser debridement are performed only by providers. See Appendix A for samples of a policy, procedure, and competency for conservative sharp debridement (Winnipeg Regional Health Authority, 2019).

Clinicians performing sharp debridement in the outpatient setting are encouraged to work closely with experienced coders and billing personnel. Accurate coding and billing will ensure the provider is adequately reimbursed and that errors are avoided. Guidelines are provided and should be followed carefully for the advanced practice provider, as well as certified wound care nurses who are billing "incident to" the licensed provider. A review by the Office of Inspector General (OIG) noted an error rate of 66% in Medicare claims from 2004 when the codes specific to debridement were examined (OIG, 2007).

Progression and Maintenance of Debridement

The methods of wound debridement typically used by the wound specialist do not immediately yield a completely clean wound; therefore, the wound must be closely monitored for indicators of progression of the debridement process. Deterioration of the wound requires reevaluation of the treatment selected. Assessment parameters include wound dimensions, volume of exudate, odor, type of tissue present, condition of the periwound skin, and the presence or increase of wound pain. Wound dimensions typically increase as the necrotic tissue is removed from the wound. Early in the debridement process, the wound is commonly exudative; this should decrease as the necrotic tissue is removed. As the underlying tissue is exposed, healthy viable tissue in the wound base should be present. When using autolysis, enzymes, or wet-to-dry dressings, a gradual transition in the type of necrotic tissue present in the wound base should be observed and documented. Hydrated eschar becomes gray and soft; firmly adherent slough becomes loose and stringy. When the wound is infected, a decrease in periwound erythema and induration should be observed after debridement. If the patient was febrile or had leukocytosis before initiating debridement, a decrease should be observed as the necrotic tissue is removed, and the bacterial load is reduced. However, these clinical changes may also be attributed to antibiotic therapy.

Traditionally, the clinician discontinues sharp or enzymatic debridement when the wound base is clean and free of necrotic tissue. At that point, moisture-retentive dressings are critical to the wound to maintain a clean vascular wound bed. Without this moist vascular wound environment, the wound bed will become dry, cellular desiccation will occur, and necrotic tissue and biofilm will begin to reform. Maintaining a moist wound environment with moisture-retentive dressings will prevent these negative consequences. In the case of recalcitrance and biofilm, further sharp debridement may be indicated even in the absence of necrotic tissue. Maintenance debridement for diabetic foot ulcers and biofilm management are discussed in Chapters 17 and 19, respectively.

CLINICAL CONSULT

A: Referred to wound care team for evaluation of an unstageable pressure injury present on admission. 84-year-old Caucasian female admitted from home with pneumonia and urinary tract infection. Cared for by elderly husband. History of congestive heart failure, hypertension, and type 2 diabetes mellitus. Weight 168 lbs, 5 ft 4 in, husband reports recent 15 lb weight loss. Currently febrile (oral temp 101°F). Altered mental status; restless in bed, does not respond to commands. Left trochanter pressure injury 5 cm × 4 cm; no measurable depth, wound base is 75% eschar beginning to lift from the wound; 25% adherent yellow slough. Mild periwound erythema and induration, small amount of yellow exudate.

D: Unstageable pressure injury with possible infection.

P: Remove nonviable tissue, confirm and treat infection, prevent further skin breakdown.

I: (1) Surgical consult for sharp wound debridement. (2) Collagenase ointment to wound to promote removal of slough and lifting of the eschar, cover with moisture retentive dressing and change daily. (3) Pressure redistribution mattress, turn and reposition every 2 h, repositioning off trochanter. (4) Float heels off mattress. (5) Nutrition consult. (6) Consult social work to assist with discharge planning.

E: Nurse and husband verbalize understanding of plan. Will meet with husband tomorrow for more teaching, review surgical consult and adjust local wound care as needed to control bioburden and promote moist wound healing.

SUMMARY

- Debridement is a critical component of topical therapy for necrotic wounds.
- The wound specialist should be knowledgeable about the various methods available for debridement and should discuss the options with the patient and with the patient's provider so that the most appropriate wound management choice can be made.
- Debridement methods are not used in isolation; rather, they are used in combination and are modified as the wound conditions change. For example, an eschar-covered, noninfected wound may be cross-hatched and covered with an autolytic or enzymatic dressing. As the eschar softens, a conservative sharp debridement to facilitate removal of the bulk of the residual eschar is needed and then continues use of the autolytic or enzymatic dressing, depending on the wound needs.
- Close supervision of the patient and accurate wound assessments during the debridement phase are essential to ensure an outcome consistent with the stated wound goals.

SELF-ASSESSMENT QUESTIONS

1. Which of the following methods of debridement is nonselective?
   a. Autolysis
   b. Chemical
   c. Enzymatic
   d. Surgical sharp
2. List three considerations in the use of enzymatic debridement.
3. Selection of debridement approach is guided by all of the following *except:*
   a. patient's age
   b. presence of wound infection
   c. extent and type of necrotic tissue
   d. clinician experience
4. The risk of transient bacteremia is associated with which of the following debridement techniques?
   a. Autolysis
   b. Conservative sharp
   c. Enzymes
   d. Wet-to-dry dressings

REFERENCES

Angel, D. (2019). Slough what does it mean and how can it be managed. *Wound Practice and Research, 27*(4), 164–167. https://doi.org/10.33235/wpr.27.4.164-167.

Atkin, L. (2014). Understanding methods of wound debridement. *British Journal of Nursing, 23*(Suppl. 12), S10–S15.

Attinger, C. E., Janis, J. E., Steinberg, J., Schwartz, J., Al-Attar, A., & Couch, K. (2006). Clinical approach to wounds: Debridement and wound bed preparation including the use of dressings and wound-healing adjuvants. *Plastic and Reconstructive Surgery, 117* (7S), 72S–109S.

Bazaliński, D., Kózka, M., Karnas, M., & Więch, P. (2019). Effectiveness of chronic wound debridement with the use of larvae of Lucilia Sericata. *Journal Clinical Medicine, 8*(11), 1845.

Bodey, G. P., Buckley, M., Sathe, Y. S., et al. (1966). Quantitative relationship between circulating leukocytes and infection in patients with acute leukemia. *Annals of Internal Medicine, 64*(2), 328–340.

Bryan, C. S., Dew, C. E., & Reynolds, K. L. (1983). Bacteremia associated with decubitus ulcers. *Archives of Internal Medicine, 143*(11), 2093–2095.

Carpenter, S., & Shaffett, T. P. (2017). Choosing the best debridement modality to "battle" necrotic tissue: Pros & cons. *Today's Wound Clinic, 11*(7).

Carter, M. J., Gilligan, A. M., Waycaster, C. R., Schaum, K., & Fife, C. E. (2017). Cost effectiveness of adding clostridial collagenase ointment to selective debridement in individuals with stage IV pressure ulcers. *Journal of Medical Economics, 20*(3), 253–265.

Chen, W. Y., Rogers, A. A., & Lydon, M. J. (1992). Characterization of biologic properties of wound fluid collected during early stages of wound healing. *The Journal of Investigative Dermatology, 99* (5), 559–564.

Cowan, L., Stechmiller, J., Phillips, P., et al. (2013). Chronic wounds, biofilms and the use of medicinal larvae. *Ulcers, 2013,* 487024. Retrieved 3/6/2022 from: https://doi.org/10.1155/2013/487024.

Dinulos, J. G. H. (Ed.). (2021). Habif's clinical dermatology: A color guide in diagnosis and therapy (7th ed.). Philadelphia: Elsevier.

Dowsett, C., Swan, J., & Orig, R. (2013). The changing NHS and the role of new treatments: Using a monofilament fibre pad to aid accurate categorization of pressure ulcers. *Wounds UK, 9*(4).

Edsberg, L. E., Black, J. M., Goldberg, M., McNichol, L., Moore, L., & Sieggreen, M. (2016). Revised national pressure ulcer advisory panel pressure injury staging system: Revised pressure injury staging system. *Journal of Wound, Ostomy, and Continence Nursing, 43*(6), 585–597. https://doi.org/10.1097/WON. 0000000000000281.

European Pressure Ulcer Advisory Panel, National Pressure Injury Advisory Panel, & Pan Pacific Pressure Injury Alliance (EPUAP, NPIAP, & PPPIA). (2019). In E. Haesler (Ed.), *Prevention and treatment of pressure ulcers/injuries.* Osborne Park: Cambridge Media.

Ferrer-Sola, M., Sureda-Vidal, H., Altimiras-Roset, J., Fontsere-Candell, E., Gonzalez-Martinez, V., Espaulella-Panicot, J., et al. (2017). Hydrosurgery as a safe and efficient debridement method in a clinical wound unit. *Journal of Wound Care, 26*(10), 593–599.

Gould, L., Stuntz, M., Giovannelli, M., Ahmad, A., Aslam, R., Mullen-Fortino, M., et al. (2016). Wound Healing Society 2015 update on guidelines for pressure ulcers. *Wound Repair and Regeneration, 24*(1), 145–162. https://doi.org/10.1111/wrr.12396. 26683529.

Graham, J. S., Schomacker, K. T., Glatter, R. D., et al. (2002). Efficacy of laser debridement with autologous split-thickness skin grafting in promoting improved healing of deep cutaneous sulfur mustard burns. *Burns, 28,* 719–730.

Gray, M. (2008). Is larval (maggot) debridement effective for removal of necrotic tissue from chronic wounds? *Journal of Wound, Ostomy, and Continence Nursing, 35*(4), 378–384.

Hajhosseini, B., Babak, C., Grace, J., Dori, G., Fukaya, E., Chandra, V., et al. (2020). Er:YAG laser vs. sharp debridement in management of chronic wounds: Effects on pain and bacterial load. *Wound Repair and Regeneration, 28*(1), 118–125.

Hoppe, I., & Granick, M. (2012). Debridement of chronic wounds: A qualitative systematic review of randomized controlled trials. *Clinics in Plastic Surgery, 39,* 221–228.

Hutchinson, J. J. (1989). Prevalence of wound infection under occlusive dressings: A collected survey of reported research. *Wounds: A Compendium of Clinical Research and Practice, 1*(2), 123–133.

Jovanovic, A., Ermis, R., Mewaldt, R., et al. (2012). The influence of metal salts, surfactants, and wound care products on enzymatic activity of collagenase, the wound debriding enzyme. *Wounds: A Compendium of Clinical Research and Practice, 24*(9), 242–253.

Kazemikhoo, N., Hashemi Pour, S., Nilforoushzadeh, M. A., Mokmeli, S., & Dahmardehei, M. (2019). The efficacy of carbon dioxide laser debridement along with low-level laser therapy in treatment of a grade 3 necrotic burn ulcer in a paraplegic patient (a case report). *Journal of Lasers in Medical Sciences, 10*(4), 338–341. https://doi.org/10.15171/jlms.2019.54.

König, M., Vanscheidt, W., Augustin, M., et al. (2005). Enzymatic versus autolytic debridement of chronic leg ulcers: A prospective randomized trial. *Journal of Wound Care, 14*(7), 320–323.

Lam, D. G., Rice, P., & Brown, R. F. (2002). The treatment of Lewisite burns with laser debridement—"Lasablation." *Burns, 28*(1), 19–25.

Lavery, L. A., Davis, K. E., Berriman, S. J., Braun, L., Nichols, A., Kim, P. J., et al. (2016). WHS guidelines update: Diabetic foot ulcer treatment guidelines. *Wound Repair and Regeneration, 24*(1), 112–126. https://doi.org/10.1111/wrr.12391. 26663430.

Lawrence, J. C. (1994). Dressings and wound infection. *American Journal of Surgery, 167*(1A), 21S–24S.

Malekian, A., Esmaeeli Djavid, G., Akbarzadeh, K., et al. (2019). Efficacy of maggot therapy on *Staphylococcus aureus* and *Pseudomonas aeruginosa* in diabetic foot ulcers: A randomized controlled trial. *Journal of Wound, Ostomy, and Continence Nursing, 46*(1), 25–29.

McCallon, S. K., & Frilot, C. (2015). A retrospective study of the effects of clostridial collagenase ointment and negative pressure wound therapy for the treatment of chronic pressure ulcers. *Wounds: A Compendium of Clinical Research and Practice, 27*(3), 44–53. https://www.ncbi.nlm.nih.gov/pubmed/25786076.

Meads, C., Lovato, E., & Longworth, L. (2015). The Debrisoft(®) monofilament debridement pad for use in acute or chronic wounds: A NICE medical technology guidance. *Applied Health Economics and Health Policy, 13*(6), 583–594. https://doi.org/ 10.1007/s40258-015-0195-0. 26315567. PMC4661219.

Mearns, E. S., Liang, M., Limone, B. L., Gilligan, A. M., Miller, J. D., Schaum, K. D., et al. (2017). Economic analysis and budget impact of clostridial collagenase ointment compared with medicinal honey for treatment of pressure ulcers in the US. *ClinicoEconomics and Outcomes Research: CEOR, 9,* 485.

Mir, M., Ali, M. N., Barakullah, A., et al. (2018). Synthetic polymeric biomaterials for wound healing: A review. *Progress in Biomaterials, 7,* 1–21. https://doi.org/10.1007/s40204-018-0083-4.

Murphy, C., Atkin, L., Swanson, T., Tachi, M., Tan, Y. K., Vega de Ceniga, M., et al. (2020). International consensus document. Defying hard-to-heal wounds with an early biofilm intervention strategy wound hygiene. *Journal of Wound Care, 29*(Suppl. 3b), S1–28.

NICE. (2014). The Debrisoft monofilament debridement pad for use in acute or chronic wounds. (Updated 2019). *National Institute for Health and Care Excellence. Medical technologies guidance [MTG17].* Retrieved 1/20/2023 from: https://www.nice.org.uk/guidance/mtg17.

Nurses Specialized in Wound, Ostomy and Continence Canada (NSWOCC). (2021). *Debridement: Canadian best practice recommendations for nurses* (1st ed.). Retrieved 3/5/2022 from: http://nswoc.ca/wp-content/uploads/2021/05/NSWOCC-Debridement-Best-Practice-Recommendations-April-2021.pdf.

Office of Inspector General (OIG). (2007). *Medicare payments for surgical debridement services in 2004.* OEI-02-05-00390. Retrieved 3/5/2022 from: https://oig.hhs.gov/oei/reports/oei-02-05-00390.pdf.

Onesti, M. G., Fioramonti, P., Fino, P., Sorvillo, V., Carella, S., & Scuder, N. (2016). Effect of enzymatic debridement with two different collagenases versus mechanical debridement on chronic hard to heal wounds. *International Wound Journal, 13*(6), 1111–1115.

Opletalová, K., Patry, J., & Blanchette, V. (2017). Enzymatic debridement with collagenase in wounds and ulcers: A systematic review and meta-analysis. *International Wound Journal, 14*(6), 1055–1065.

Ousey, K., Chadwick, P., Jawien, A., Tariq, G., Nair, H. K. R., Lázaro-Martínez, J. L., et al. (2018). Identifying and treating foot ulcers in patients with diabetes: Saving feet, legs and lives. *Journal of Wound Care, 27*(5 Suppl 5b).

Patry, E., & Blanchette, V. (2017). Enzymatic debridement with collagenase in wounds and ulcers: A systematic review and meta-analysis. *International Wound Journal, 14*(6), 1055–1065.

Phillips, P. L., Yang, Q., Davis, S., Sampson, E. M., Azeke, J. I., Hamad, A., et al. (2015). Antimicrobial dressing efficacy against mature Pseudomonas aeruginosa biofilm on porcine skin explants. *International Wound Journal, 12*(4), 469–483. https://doi.org/10.1111/iwj.12142.

Ramundo, J., & Gray, M. (2009). Collagenase for enzymatic debridement, a systematic review. *Journal of Wound, Ostomy, and Continence Nursing, 36*(Suppl. 6), S4–S11.

Raz, K. (1995). Laser physics. *Clinics in Dermatology, 13*, 11.

Robson, M. (1997). Wound infection: A failure of wound healing caused by an imbalance of bacteria. *The Surgical Clinics of North America, 77*(3), 637–650.

Rodeheaver, G. T., Baharestani, M. M., Brabec, M. E., et al. (1994). Wound healing and wound management: Focus on debridement. *Advances in Wound Care, 7*(1). 22–24, 26–29, 32–36.

Schultz, G. S., Woo, K., Weir, D., & Yang, Q. (2018). Effectiveness of a monofilament wound debridement pad at removing biofilm and slough: Ex vivo and clinical performance. *Journal of Wound Care, 27*(2).

Shi, L., Ermis, R., Kiedaisch, B., et al. (2010). The effect of various wound dressings on the activity of debriding enzymes. *Advances in Skin & Wound Care, 23*(10), 456–462.

Shi, E., & Shofler, D. (2014). Maggot debridement therapy: A systematic review. *British Journal of Community Nursing, 19* (Suppl. 12), S6–S13.

Shoham, Y., Krieger, Y., Tamir, E., Silberstein, E., Bogdanov-Berzovsky, A., Haik, J., et al. (2018). Bromelain-based enzymatic debridement of chronic wounds: A preliminary report. *International Wound Journal, 15*(5), 769–775.

Sibbald, R. G., Elliott, J. A., Persaud-Jaimangal, R., Goodman, L., Armstrong, D. G., Harley, C., et al. (2021). Wound bed preparation 2021. *Advances in Skin & Wound Care, 34*(4), 183–195.

Steenvoorde, P., & van Doorn, L. P. (2008). Maggot debridement therapy: Serious bleeding can occur: Report of a case. *Journal of Wound Ostomy Continence Nursing, 35*(4), 412–414.

Stotts, N., & Hunt, T. (1997). Managing bacterial colonization and infection. *Clinics in Geriatric Medicine, 13*(3), 565–573.

Strohal, R., Dissemond, J., Jordan O'Brien J., Piaggesi, A., Rimdeika, R., Young, T., et al. (2013). An updated overview and clarification of the principle role of debridement. *Journal of Wound Care, 22* (Suppl.), S1–S52. https://doi.org/10.12968/jowc.2013.22.Sup1.S1.

Thomas, S. (1990). *Wound management and dressings*. London: Pharmaceutical Press.

Tian, X., Liang, X. M., Song, G. M., et al. (2013). Maggot debridement therapy for the treatment of diabetic foot ulcers: A meta-analysis. *Journal of Wound Care, 22*(9), 462–469.

Waycaster, C., & Milne, C. T. (2013). Clinical and economic benefit of enzymatic debridement of pressure ulcers compared to autolytic debridement with a hydrogel dressing. *Journal of Medical Economics, 16*(7), 976–986.

Winnipeg Regional Health Authority. (2019). *Conservative sharp wound debridement (CSWD) in adults and children—Evidence informed practice tools*. Retrieved 3/5/2021 from: https://professionals.wrha.mb.ca/old/extranet/eipt/files/EIPT-013-017.pdf.

Woo, K., Keast, D., Parsons, N., et al. (2013). The cost of debridement: A Canadian perspective. *International Wound Journal, 12*, 402–407. https://doi.org/10.1111/iwj.12122.

Wound, Ostomy and Continence Nurses Society. (2014). Guideline for management of wounds in patients with lower-extremity arterial disease. In *WOCN clinical practice guideline series 1*. Mt. Laurel, NJ: Author.

Wound, Ostomy and Continence Nurses Society. (2019). Guideline for management of wounds in patients with lower-extremity venous disease. In *WOCN clinical practice guideline series 4*. Mt. Laurel, NJ: Author.

Zarchi, K., & Jemec, G. (2012). The efficacy of maggot debridement therapy—A review of comparative clinical trials. *International Wound Journal, 9*(5), 469–477.

FURTHER READING

Al-Waili, N., Salom, K., & Al-Ghamdi, A. A. (2011). Honey for wound healing, ulcers, and burns; data supporting its use in clinical practice. *Scientific World Journal, 11*, 766–787.

Attinger, C., & Wolcott, R. (2012). Clinically addressing biofilm in chronic wounds. *Advances in Wound Care, 1*(3), 127–132.

Bilgari, B., Moghaddam, A., Santos, K., et al. (2013). Multicentre prospective observational study on professional wound care using honey. *International Wound Journal, 10*(3), 252–259.

Burgos, A., Giménez, J., Moreno, E., et al. (2000). Cost, efficacy, efficiency and tolerability of collagenase ointment versus hydrocolloid occlusive dressing in the treatment of pressure ulcers: A comparative, randomised, multicenter study. *Clinical Drug Investigation, 19*(5), 357–365.

Caputo, W. J., Beggs, D. J., DeFede, J. L., et al. (2008). A prospective randomised controlled clinical trial comparing hydrosurgery debridement with conventional surgical debridement in lower extremity ulcers. *International Wound Journal, 5*(2), 288–294.

Flemming, A., Frame, J., & Dhillon, R. (1986). Skin edge necrosis in irradiated tissue after carbon dioxide laser excision of tumor. *Lasers in Medical Science, 1*, 263–265.

Gethen, G., & Cowman, C. (2009). Manuka honey vs. hydrogel—A prospective, open label, multicentre, randomized controlled trial to compare desloughing efficacy and healing outcomes in venous ulcers. *Journal of Clinical Nursing, 18*(3), 466–474.

Gravante, G., Delogu, D., Esposito, G., et al. (2007). Versajet hydrosurgery versus classic escharectomy for burn débridement: A prospective randomized trial. *Journal of Burn Care & Research, 28*(5), 720–724.

Jull, A. B., Walker, N., & Deshpande, S. (2013). Honey as a topical treatment for wounds. *Cochrane Database of Systematic Reviews, 2*, CD005083.

Klaus, K. (2015). Maggot debridement therapy: Advancing to the past in wound care. *MEDSURG Nursing, 24*(6), 407–411.

Leaper, D. J., Schultz, G., Carville, K., et al. (2012). Extending the TIME concept: What have we learned in the past 10 years? *International Wound Journal, Suppl. 2*, 1–19.

Milne, C. T. (2010). A comparison of collagenase to hydrogel dressings in wound debridement. *Wounds: A Compendium of Clinical Research and Practice, 22*(11), 270–274.

Müller, E., van Leen, M. W., & Bergemann, R. (2001). Economic evaluation of collagenase-containing ointment and hydrocolloid dressing in the treatment of pressure ulcers. *PharmacoEconomics, 9*(12), 1209–1216.

Murphy, C. A., Houghton, P., Brandys, T., Rose, G., & Bryant, D. (2018). The effects of 22.5 kHz low frequency contact ultrasound debridement (LFCUD) on lower extremity wound healing for a vascular surgery population: A randomized controlled trial. *International Wound Journal, 15*(3), 460–472.

Ramundo, J., & Gray, M. (2008). Is ultrasonic mist therapy effective for debriding chronic wounds? *Journal of Wound, Ostomy, and Continence Nursing, 35*(6), 579–583.

Rice, J. (2012). Conservative sharp debridement. *EWMA Journal, 12*(3), 33–38.

Schultz, G., Sibbald, R. G., Falanga, V., et al. (2003). Wound bed preparation, a systemic approach to wound bed management. *Wound Repair and Regeneration, 11*(Suppl. 1), S1–S28.

Shannon, M. K., Williams, A., & Bloomer, M. (2012). Low-frequency ultrasound debridement (Sonoca-185) in acute wound management. *Wound Practice and Research, 20*(4), 200–205.

Vallejo, A., Wallis, M., Horton, E., & McMillian, D. (2018). Low-frequency ultrasonic debridement and topical antimicrobial solution polyhexamethylene biguanide for use in chronic wounds: A case series. *Wound Practice and Research, 28*(1), 4–13.

Principles of Wound Healing and Topical Management

Ruth A. Bryant and Denise P. Nix

OBJECTIVES

1. Identify three guiding principles of wound management.
2. Describe the characteristics of a physiologic wound environment.
3. List at least seven objectives in creating a physiologic wound environment.
4. Describe the TIMERS framework and the Wound Bed Preparation paradigm for managing hard-to-heal wounds.
5. Define the terms occlusive, semiocclusive, moisture retentive, primary dressing, and secondary dressing.
6. List two indications and one contraindication for each dressing category.
7. Describe the factors to consider when selecting topical therapy.

PRINCIPLES OF WOUND MANAGEMENT

Numerous factors affect the process of wound healing, all of which must be addressed to achieve wound closure. Topical wound management is determined based on many of these factors. Topical wound management is the manipulation of the wound to positively influence the physiologic local wound environment. Three guiding principles of wound management provide a comprehensive and holistic framework to optimize the patient's ability to heal.

Wounds do not occur as an isolated event within a patient. Consequently, the guiding principles of effective wound management must incorporate a holistic approach that identifies and intervenes to minimize or abate the underlying etiology and any coexisting contributing factors. Box 21.1 lists the three guiding principles of wound management and examples of how these principles can be addressed: (1) control or eliminate causative factors, (2) reduce existing and potential cofactors, and (3) create and maintain a physiologic local wound environment. To control or eliminate causative factors requires astute history taking and physical assessment so that the correct underlying etiology is identified and addressed. Failure to address causative factors will result in delayed healing or a nonhealing wound despite appropriate systemic and topical therapies. No dressing can compensate for an uncorrected pathologic condition. To reduce potential cofactors known to delay healing or create hard-to-heal wounds, diagnostic or laboratory tests are often required. The various cofactors that impair wound healing are discussed throughout this textbook (e.g., diabetes, edema, hypoxia, pain, tobacco use, and obesity). This chapter focuses on the third principle of wound management: create a physiologic wound environment.

Characteristics of a Physiologic Wound Environment

Topical wound management is the manipulation of the wound to restore a physiologic wound environment; an environment that is "characteristic of an organism's healthy or normal functioning." Wound care dressings are used to mimic the skin so that a physiologic local wound environment can be created. Features of a physiologic local wound environment are adequate moisture level, temperature control, pH regulation, and control of bacteria (including removal of biofilm). With attention to these features, appropriate local wound care can be selected to best support expedient wound repair.

Dressing selection should be made with the goal of attaining undisturbed wound healing so that the microenvironment (i.e., pH, temperature, and growth factors) can be sustained (Brindle & Farmer, 2019). Therefore, the frequency of dressing changes must be minimized, wound cleansing solutions must be at room temperature, and dressings selected that provide adequate insulation, exudate control and moisture management (Brindle & Farmer, 2019; McGuinness, Vella, & Harrison, 2004).

Normal Body Temperature

One of the functions of the skin is to provide thermoregulation. All cellular functions are affected by temperature, including chemical reactions (e.g., metabolism, enzymatic catalysis, production of growth factors interleukin-1α and interleukin-2, protein synthesis, and oxidation) and processes. The consequences of local hypothermia on phagocytes include decreased phagocyte activity, decreased production of reactive oxygen products, impaired ability to migrate, and an increased risk of infection by causing vasoconstriction and increasing hemoglobin's affinity for oxygen, both of which result in a decreased availability of oxygen to phagocytes (MacFie, Melling, & Leaper, 2005).

In order for wound healing to occur without delay, a normal core body temperature and a body surface temperature above 33°C and below 42°C is needed. Studies show that each time a dressing is changed, the wound temperature drops and takes 30 min to restore after an appropriate dressing is reapplied.

Bacterial Control

The importance of bacterial control for a physiologic wound environment and interventions to control bioburden (including biofilm) are discussed in Chapter 19. Strategies include (1) debridement, (2) appropriate wound cleansing, (3) appropriate infection control precautions, (4) use of antimicrobials, and (5) moisture-retentive dressings.

Semiocclusive dressings reduce wound infections by more than 50% when compared with traditional gauze dressings. This finding supports the theory that semiocclusive dressings optimize the phagocytic efficiency of endogenous leukocytes by maintaining a moist wound environment and reduce airborne dispersal of bacteria during dressing changes. Semiocclusive dressings provide a mechanical barrier to the entry of exogenous bacteria. In contrast, bacteria have been reported

to penetrate up to 64 layers of gauze (Lawrence, 1994; Ovington, 2001).

pH

Initially the open wound pH will be acidic which is essential for many cellular activities (fibroblast proliferation, DNA cell synthesis, collagen formation, macrophage activity) and acidic associated with more rapid wound healing (Bennison et al., 2017). In contrast, the chronic wound tends to have an alkaline pH (7.2–8.9) which impairs the healing and immunological response by promoting bacterial growth, increased proteolytic activity, inhibiting fibroblasts and reducing oxygen supply (Bennison et al., 2017; Schneider, Korber, Grabbe, et al., 2007). The pH of a wound is a dynamic factor that fluctuates with therapeutic interventions; most notably, the kind of dressing applied to the wound affects the pH of the wound bed. Wound exudate under nonocclusive dressings is more alkaline than exudate under occlusive dressings. The more acidic environment under the occlusive dressing is thought to inhibit bacterial growth while promoting fibroblast growth. Any method of wound debridement is also known to raise the pH of the wound bed (Schneider et al., 2007).

Moisture Level

The human body is more than 65% water; the primary means of maintaining this level of moisture is located within the epidermis (Spruitt, 1972). The stratum corneum layer of the epidermis prevents loss of excessive amounts of water in the form of water vapor to the external environment. Therefore, moisture levels of healthy skin are maintained by an intact stratum corneum. When the stratum corneum has been removed or compromised, tissues and cells are subject to increased loss of moisture and may desiccate and eventually die. As shown in Fig. 8.2, wound healing slows significantly in a dry environment because epithelial cells must burrow below the dry surface to reach a moist surface over which they can migrate (Hinman & Maibach, 1963; Winter, 1962, 2006). As described in Box 21.2, a moist environment physiologically favors cellular migration and extracellular matrix formation, which facilitates healing of

TABLE 21.1   Objectives of a Physiologic Wound Environment

Objectives	Interventions
(1) Prevent and manage infection	Cover wound with dressings impermeable to bacteria to protect from outside contaminants, with the most appropriate dressing or combination of dressings based on wound assessment and overall goals for the patient Infection control precautions, no-touch dressing application Appropriate wound cleansing and debridement Antimicrobials when indicated Appropriate wound culture technique (see Chapter 19)
(2) Cleanse wound	Normal saline with 4–15 psi of pressure/force to remove debris without harming healthy tissue
(3) Remove nonviable tissue	Most appropriate debridement method or combination of debridement methods based on patient's condition and wound assessment (see Chapter 20) Method of debridement consistent with patient's overall goals
(4) Maintain appropriate level of moisture	Dressing with high moisture vapor transmission rate will allow moisture to escape and evaporate to manage minimally exudative wounds Moderate to heavily exudative wounds require absorptive dressings Select topical dressings that maintain moist wound environment to prevent tissue desiccation
(5) Eliminate dead space	Hydrating or absorbent-impregnated gauze for large, deep wounds Fluff packing material and loosely place into wound using cotton-tipped applicator Ensure packing material is in contact with wound edges and can be easily retrieved
(6) Control odor	Appropriate dressing change frequency Cleansing with each dressing change Debridement and antimicrobials as indicated Charcoal dressings
(7) Eliminate or minimize pain	Semiocclusive dressings Nonadherent dressings Dressings that require fewer changes Pain control interventions as described in Chapter 28
(8) Protect wound and periwound skin	Skin barriers (liquid, ointments, wafers) to protect the periwound skin from moisture and adhesives as described in Chapter 9 Appropriate interval for dressing changes so that exudate does not pool on surrounding skin or undermine adhesive of wound dressing

wounds, reduces pain and tenderness, reduces fibrosis, decreases wound infection, facilitates autolysis, and produces a better cosmetic outcome (Nuutilla & Eriksson, 2021). However, the moisture level of the wound surface can range from dry (particularly nonviable tissue) to an excessively moist surface.

Given the complexity if wound repair, using objectives to guide the selection of interventions provides the caregiver with a template of important issues to address to select the product that will best create a physiologic wound environment. Objectives and interventions for creating a physiologic wound environment are listed in Table 21.1.

A key strategy available to operationalize these objectives for local wound management is to use the TIMERS framework (Atkin et al., 2019). This acronym represents *tissue* management (wound bed preparation to remove nonviable tissue wound foreign material), *infection/inflammation* controlled (remove infection and reduce/prevent inflammation), *moisture* balance (remove excess moisture or donate moisture in dry wound), wound *edge* (optimal environment for epithelial edge migration), *repair* and regeneration of tissue (encourage wound closure using advanced therapy options when conservative therapy insufficient), and *social* factors

(patient engagement to enhance adherence, understanding, decisions, participation) (see Table 21.2).

Wound Dressing Selection

An optimal wound dressing should protect the wound (e.g., from bacterial invasion, trauma), provide a moist environment, and maintain an appropriate wound temperature that promotes tissue regeneration, and be easy to apply and remove (Nuutilla & Eriksson, 2021). Plain gauze is not an optimal wound dressing because unlike semiocclusive dressings, gauze lacks a mechanical barrier to the entry of exogenous bacteria and is not moisture retentive (see Table 21.3). Commercially available gauze impregnated with ingredients such as hypertonic saline or hydrogels are moisture retentive when used appropriately. When other forms of moisture-retentive dressings are not available, continuously moist gauze is preferable to dry gauze (European Pressure Ulcer Advisory Panel, National Pressure Injury Advisory Panel, & Pan Pacific Pressure Injury Alliance [EPUAP, NPIAP, & PPPIA], 2019). Box 21.3 provides a guide to appropriate use of gauze dressings in the absence of available moisture-retentive dressings.

TABLE 21.2 TIMERS

Principles of Wound Bed Preparation

Clinical Observations	Proposed Pathophysiology	WBP Clinical Actions	Effect of WBP Actions	Clinical Outcomes
Tissue nonviable or devitalized	Defective matrix and cell debris impair healing	Debridement (episodic or continuous) • Autolysis, sharp, surgical, enzymatic, mechanical, or biologic agents	Restoration of wound base and functional extracellular matrix proteins	Viable, clean wound base
Infection or inflammation	High bacterial counts or prolonged/chronic inflammation: ↑ Inflammatory cytokines (TNF-α; IL-1,6,8; CRP) ↑ Proteases ↑ ROS ↑ Cytotoxic exotoxins ↓ Growth factor activity	Remove biofilm and bacterial bioburden Implement topical/systemic • Antimicrobials • Antiinflammatories • Protease inhibition (MMP/TIMP management) • Bacterial binding dressings • Oxygen therapy • Surfactants	Low bacterial counts or controlled inflammation: ↓ Inflammatory cytokines ↓ Protease activity ↑ Growth factor activity	Bacterial balance and reduced inflammation
Moisture balance	Desiccation slows epithelial cell migration Excessive fluid causes maceration of wound margin	Apply moisture-balancing dressings Compression, negative pressure wound therapy, or other methods for controlling moisture	Restoration of epithelial cell migration, desiccation avoided Edema, excessive fluid controlled, maceration avoided	Moisture balance
Edge of wound (nonadvancing or undermined)	Nonmigrating keratinocytes Epibole Nonresponsive wound cells and abnormalities in extracellular matrix or abnormal protease activity	Reassess cause or consider corrective therapies • Debridement • Excise sclerosed margins • Biologic agents • Adjunctive therapies	Migrating keratinocytes and responsive wound cells Restoration of appropriate protease profile	Advancing edge of wound
Repair or regeneration	Healing stalled or slowed due to many of the above factors	CTPs Growth factors Platelet-rich plasma NPWT Oxygen Autologous skin graft	Overcome factors that created stalled wound environment	Decreasing wound size, closure
Social and patient related factors	Patient engagement enhances patients' ability to participate in care and adhere to treatment plan	Intentional and thoughtful social and family history to understand dynamics in patient's personal life that will impact their ability understand care and participate in self-care. Active listening, patient education, understanding belief system	Adherence to treatment plan, knowledge of patient's own goals	Patient satisfaction and consistency in care

TIMERS, Tissue, Infection, Moisture, Edge, Repair, Social; *WBP*, wound bed preparation.

TABLE 21.3 Disadvantages of Gauze Dressings

Disadvantage	Potential Consequences
Moisture evaporates quickly and dressing dries out	Painful removal Impaired cell migration Desiccation of viable tissue Impaired autolysis Removal of healthy tissue upon removal
Requires frequent dressing changes	Dispersal of bacteria with each dressing change Increased patient discomfort and need for pain medications Increased caregiver time and costs
Associated with increased infection rates compared with semiocclusive dressings	Increased cost for antimicrobials Slower healing rates Increased pain Decrease in patient satisfaction Increased caregiver time

BOX 21.3 Guide to Appropriate Use of Gauze Dressing

- Avoid gauze dressings for clean pressure injuries because these dressings are labor intensive and dry out easily, leading to painful removal and tissue desiccation.
- When other forms of moisture-retentive dressings are not available, use continuously moist gauze.
  - Loosely fill dead space to avoid pressure on the wound.
  - Fill dead space with single gauze piece or roll (small pieces may be left behind, creating a potential infection source).
- Use loosely woven gauze for highly exudative wounds.
- Use tightly woven gauze for minimally exudative wounds.

There are anywhere from 3000 to 6000 wound care dressings available today. This number alone can be intimidating to the novice wound care clinician. It becomes much more manageable to realize however that there are only 11 categories of wound care dressings and that all these dressings derive from those 11 categories. The challenge becomes understanding the features of each dressing category, their indications and how to assess their effectiveness. A central premise in dressing selection is aligning the current wound condition(s) and your objectives (Table 21.4). In general, most dressings are not intended to provide complete healing, from wound onset to healing. Rather, the dressing is selected to meet a specific objective which often changes as the needs of the patient and characteristics of the wound evolve (Gottrup & Apelqvist, 2010; Leaper & Drake, 2011; Rolstad, Bryant, & Nix, 2012; Sibbald et al., 2021; White, Cutting, Ousey, et al., 2010).

Wound Conditions That Effect Dressings Selection

Moisture Level. Wound dressings can be used to establish and maintain a moist—not wet—wound environment and promote autolysis and epithelial migration (Nuutila & Eriksson, 2021). In an open wound, a moist environment is maintained by one of three mechanisms: containing wound fluids, absorbing excess moisture, or donating moisture. Semiocclusive dressings can keep a wound moist, even when no additional moisture is supplied, by "catching" and retaining moisture vapor that is being lost by the wound on a continual basis. Their ability to maintain tissue hydration can be characterized by a measurement known as the moisture vapor transmission rate (MVTR). Dressings transmit less moisture vapor than the average wound loses, thus facilitating moisture retention in the tissue as opposed to desiccation. In general, if the dressing material transmits less moisture vapor than the wound loses, the wound will remain moist. If the dressing material transmits more moisture vapor than the wound produces, the wound may dry out. For this reason, transparent dressings designed for intravenous sites have a higher MVTR than the transparent dressings intended for wound management. In a wound that has excess moisture, the topical dressing must have moisture-absorptive capacity to prevent the wound from becoming overly saturated and the periwound skin macerated. In addition, the prolonged presence of excessive amounts of moisture in the wound may increase the patient's risk for developing hyperplasia or hypergranulation tissue in the base of the wound (see Plate 29). Methods of exudate management include moisture vapor transmission, as with transparent dressings, and wicking, as with alginate or foam dressings. The process of absorption physically moves drainage away from the wound's surface and edges and into the dressing material. At the other end of the hydration spectrum, wound tissue that is dry may need to be actively rehydrated using dressing materials that donate water to the tissue (e.g., hydrogel).

Frequency of dressing change can also impact moisture control. For example, if a wound has more exudate than the dressing can absorb, the wound specialist can either increase the frequency of dressing changes or choose a more absorptive dressing or combination of dressings. Conversely, a dressing that donates moisture to the wound could be changed more often if the wound becomes too dry or a moisture-retentive dressing may be changed less frequently.

TABLE 21.4 Wound Dressing Formulary

Dressing Examples	Description	Indications for Use	Contraindications/Considerations	Coverage Guidelines/HCPCS
Antimicrobial/ antibacterial/antiseptic dressing Cadexomer iodine, medical grade honey, silver, polyhexamethylene biguanide (PHMB), gentian violet/methylene blue foam Hydrofera Blue Antibacterial Foam Dressing (Essity) (see Plate 53)	Sustained release in lower concentrations to reduce toxicity potential Controls microbial overgrowth Broad spectrum Available as alginate, hydrogel, composite, gauze	Partial- or full-thickness wound with or without depth (depends on product selected) Microbial overgrowth as evidenced by increased exudate, odor, pain, confirmed infection or nonhealing wound Patient at high risk for infection (e.g., immunosuppression, diabetes) Biofilm management (select dressings only) See Chapter 19	Contraindicated with allergies (e.g., iodine, silver, bee stings, etc.) Contraindicated for MRI Avoid saline in nanocrystalline silver products Dressing change every 1–7 days, varies by product; see manufacturer's instructions Secondary dressing often required	Coded according to base composition of dressing (e.g., hydrogel, hydrocolloid, foam) Medical grade honey is not reimbursed
Calcium alginate: Algisite (Smith & Nephew) CalciCare (Hollister) Maxorb (Medline Industries, Inc.) AQUACEL Extra (ConvaTec) Tegaderm Alginate (3M Health Care) (see Plates 54 and 55)	Polysaccharide derived from brown seaweed Nonadhesive Absorbs 20 times their weight in exudate Converts to viscous, hydrophilic gel on contact with exudate Hemostatic properties for mild bleeding Flexible, conforming, can be cut to size of wound and layered to increase absorption capacity Used as primary dressing	Partial- or full-thickness without depth or with depth (add fillers) Moderate to heavy exudate	Contraindicated for narrow tunnels, third-degree burns, dry eschar, surgical implantation or heavy bleeding Not appropriate for dry wounds, or in combination with hydrogels If use inappropriately (minimal wound exudate) wound bed may become desiccated with embedded alginate fibers Requires a secondary dressing to secure and maintain moist wound environment without causing strike through of exudate	One dressing (enough for wound size) per day for moderate-to-heavy exudative wound Fillers up to 2 per day Coded as alginate or other fiber gelling/hydrofiber dressing A6196–A6199
Charcoal: Actisorb (3M) CarboFlex (ConvaTec) IoPlex (Medline Industries, Inc.)	Activated carbon (charcoal) Absorbs toxins and wound degradation products Absorbs volatile amines and fatty acids responsible for odor Used as "filter" for odor control	Malodorous wound (e.g., infected, fungating) Fecal fistula	May be reused if not soiled (e.g., if exudate does not strike through to the charcoal layer of dressing	Coded by predominant ingredient (i.e., CarboFlex is coded as an alginate, IoPlex is coded as a foam, Actisorb as miscellaneous)
Collagen: Puracol® Plus Collagen Dressings (Medline Industries, Inc.) Stimulen™ Collagen Powder (Southwest Technologies)	Processed from bovine, porcine, equine or avian sources Used to enhance deposition of organized collagen fibers Chemoattractant to granulocytes and fibroblasts Conformable, bioresorbable, nonadherent	Partial- or full-thickness without depth or with depth when wound fillers added Infected and noninfected wounds Minimal to heavy exudate varies by product (see manufacturer's instructions)	Contraindicated for sensitivities to collagen or bovine products and third-degree burns Inappropriate with dry or necrotic wounds Wear time at least 24 h; check manufacturer's recommendations	Collagen dressings A6021–A6024 Collagen fillers (once a day) A6010–A6011

Category / Products	Description	Indications	Considerations	Frequency / HCPCS Codes
Collagen matrix (deactivates MMPs): BIOSTEP Collage Matrix Dressings (Smith and Nephew Inc.) DermaCol Collagen Matrix Dressing (DermaRite) Promogran™ Prisma (Systagenix)	Collagen Matrix dressings also inactivates matrix metalloproteinases (MMPs) Available in gels, alginates, sheets, powders Used as a primary dressing		May require rehydration for removal Select a secondary dressing to promote moist wound healing without strike through exudate	
Composite: Alldress® Absorbent Composite Dressing (Mölnlycke Health Care US, LLC) Covaderm Plus® (DeRoyal) Tegaderm™ Absorbent Clear Acrylic Dressing (3M Health Care)	Combines physically distinct components into single dressing to provide multiple functions (e.g., bacterial barrier, absorptive layers, and adhesion) Generally, incorporate absorptive layers into a nonadherent or low-adherent pad for the wound with an adhesive border for securement May use over topical medications Used as primary or secondary dressing	Partial- or full-thickness without depth Surgical incision Dry-to-heavy exudate (depends on dressing components)	Contraindications dependent on product selected; check manufacturer's recommendations Do not cut dressings Dressing should extent as least 1 in larger than wound	Up to 3 per week A6203–A6205
Contact layer: Mepitel (Mölnlycke Health Care US, LLC) Profore WCL (Smith & Nephew) Cutimed® Sorbact WCL Dressing (Essity) Biatain® Contact (Coloplast Corp) Medipore (3M Health Care) UrgoTul™ (Urgo North America) VERSATEL™ Contact Layer Dressing (Medline Industries, Inc.)	Protects wound bed from direct contact with other agents and dressings Conforms to wound shape Porous to allow exudate to pass or medication to absorb into wound Available in pads, sheets, rolls Used as primary dressing	Partial- or full-thickness wounds, with or without depth Minimal to heavy exudate Infected wounds Donor sites Split-thickness skin grafts	Not recommended for Stage 1 PI and third-degree burns Not intended to be changed with each dressing change Can apply topical agent over contact layer Select a secondary dressing to promote moist wound healing without strike through exudate	One contact layer per week A6206–A6208
Foam: ALLEVYN Adhesive Foam (Smith & Nephew) Biatain® Silicone with 3DFit™ (Coloplast Corp) Hydrocell Non-Adhesive Foam Dressing (Derma Sciences)	Consists of hydrophilic polyurethane or film-coated layer Absorptive Adhesive or nonadhesive Available in pads, sheets, rolls, or filler dressing Used as primary or secondary dressing	Partial- or full-thickness without depth or with depth (add fillers) Moderate to heavily exudative wound Multilayer silicone foam dressings are often used to protect vulnerable skin and closed wounds but are not reimbursed for that purpose (see Chapter 11)	Contraindicated in ischemic wound with dry eschar and third-degree burns Dressing should extend at least 1 in larger than wound	Three dressings per week covered for full-thickness wound with moderate-to-heavy exudate Foam filler: one per day A6209–A6215

Continued

TABLE 21.4 Wound Dressing Formulary—cont'd

Dressing Examples	Description	Indications for Use	Contraindications/ Considerations	Coverage Guidelines/HCPCS
Mepilex® Border Silicone (Mölnlycke Health Care US, LLC) Optifoam® Gentle (Medline Industries, Inc.) PolyMem MAX® Non-Adhesive Dressing (Ferris Mfg. Corp.) (see Plates 56 and 57)				
Gelling/fiber: DURAFIBER Gelling Fibre Dressing (Smith and Nephew) Exufiber® (Mölnlycke Health Care US, LLC)	Carboxymethylcellulose Absorbs heavy exudate Converts to gel on contact with exudate Flexible, conforming, can be cut to size of wound Used as a primary dressing	Indicated to maintain moist environment and manage exudate Partial or full-thickness wounds; deep wounds that require filling Moderate to heavily exudative wound	Not appropriate for dry wounds, or in combination with hydrogels If used without enough exudate, the wound may become desiccated with embedded alginate fibers Select a secondary dressing to promote moist wound healing without strike through exudate	One dressing (enough for wound size) per day Fillers up to 2 per day Moderate-to-heavy exudate without use of hydrogels Coded as alginate or other fiber gelling/hydrofiber dressing A6196–A6199
Hypertonic saline gauze Curasalt™ Sodium Chloride Dressing (Tyco Healthcare/ Kendal) Mesalt® (Mölnlycke Health Care US, LLC)	Gauze impregnated with dry sodium chloride by the manufacturer Used as a primary dressing	Full thickness with or without depth Heavily exudating wounds Nonviable wound base or infection	Apply to the wound dry Select a secondary dressing to promote moist wound healing without strike through exudate	Coded as gauze impregnated with products *other than* water, normal saline, and hydrogel A6222–A6224
Hydrocolloid: DuoDERM (ConvaTec) Exuderm® Satin Hydrocolloid Wound Dressing (Medline Industries, Inc.) RepliCare Hydrocolloid Wound Dressing (Smith & Nephew) (see Plates 58–60)	Adhesive dressing with gel-forming agents (gelatin, pectin, carboxymethylcellulose) Adhesive, waterproof Impermeable to contaminants, reducing risk of infection Molds to body contours Prevents friction Used as a primary dressing	Partial- or full-thickness wound without depth Light to moderately exudative wound	Contraindicated in third-degree burns Avoid acutely infected wound or eschar Use with caution in persons with diabetes Dressing should extent as least 1 in larger than wound Apply light pressure while applying to allow body heat to promote adhesion Change every 3–5 days as needed Use a product to provide periwound skin protection from moisture	Three dressings per week per wound A6234–A6241

Dressing	Composition	Indications	Contraindications/Precautions	HCPCS Codes
Hydrogel amorphous: Skintegrity (Medline Industries, Inc.) Hydrogel Amorphous Wound Dressing (McKesson) AquaSite® Amorphous Hydrogel Dressing (Integra LifeSciences Corp.)	Formulations of water, polymers, and other ingredients to form a gel or impregnated gauze Nonadherent Donates moisture, little to no absorption Use as a primary dressing	Rehydrate wound Partial or full-thickness wounds Radiation tissue damage Wounds with necrotic tissue present Dry to lightly exudative wound	Contraindicated in third-degree burns Sterile gel for every 3-day dressing changes Nonsterile gel can be used for daily dressing changes Protect periwound skin Requires a secondary dressing	Hydrogel dressing, wound filler, gel, per fluid ounce A6248
Hydrogel sheets: Elasto-Gel™ (Southwest Technologies, Inc.) Vigilon Primary Wound Dressing (C.R. Bard, Inc.) Derma-Gel® Hydrogel Wound Dressing (Medline Industries, Inc.) AquaDerm™ Hydrogel Sheet (DermaRite Industries, LLC) (see Plates 62–64)	Cross-linked hydrophilic polymers that are insoluble in water Nonadherent Cooling effect Donates moisture; little to no absorption Available in various sizes, with and without adhesive borders Used as a primary or secondary dressing based on product selected	Partial- and full-thickness wounds, wounds with necrosis Dry to minimal exudate Minor burns Radiation tissue damage	Contraindicated in third-degree burns Caution with moving or dependent anatomical locations due to potential for the dressing to slide out of place Can macerate intact skin; protect periwound skin In the absence of an adhesive border, select a secondary dressing to maintain moisture against wound bed and prevent hydrogel from dehydrating	Hydrogel wound covers without adhesive border A6242–A6244 Hydrogel sheets or wound covers with adhesive border up to three times per week A6246–A6247
Impregnated wound dressings Adaptic (3M Health Care) Skintegrity Hydrogel Impregnated Gauze (Medline Industries, Inc.) (see Hypertonic gauze for additional examples)	Gauze and nonwoven sponge, rope, and strips saturated with various solution (e.g., oil, zinc, petrolatum, xeroform, saline, hydrogel)	Indications vary based on the composition of dressing	Contraindications vary based on the composition of dressing	Gauze, impregnated, water or normal saline or hydrogel A6228–A6233 Gauze, impregnated, with *other than* water, normal saline, hydrogel, or zinc paste (A6222–A6224, A6266)
Silicone gel sheet: CICA-CARE (Smith & Nephew, Inc.) Mepiform® (Mölnlycke Health Care US, LLC) Oleeva® Clear (Bio Med Sciences)	Composed of cross-linked polymers reinforced with or bonded to mesh or fabric Some products may be cut to size	Prevent or improve the appearance of hypertrophic and keloid scars	Contraindicated with silicone allergy or sensitivity Not for use on unhealed, open wounds May cause maceration or a rash May require a secondary dressing	Gel sheets for dermal or epidermal application (e.g., silicone, hydrogel, other) are codes A6025 Not reimbursed for the treatment of keloids or other scars does not meet the definition of the surgical dressing benefit and will be denied as noncovered

Continued

TABLE 21.4 Wound Dressing Formulary—cont'd

Dressing Examples	Description	Indications for Use	Contraindications/ Considerations	Coverage Guidelines/HCPCS
Superabsorbent dressing: OptiLock® (Medline Industries, Inc.) PRIMAPORE (Smith & Nephew, Inc.) Drawtex® (Urgo Medical North America) XTRASORB® Super Absorbent Dressing (Integra LifeSciences Corp.) Cutimed® Sorbion® Border (BSN Medical Inc.)	Multilayer wound covers that provide either a semiadherent or a nonadherent layer, combined with highly absorptive fibers such as cellulose, cotton, or rayon Designed to minimize adherence to the wound and manage exudate Used as a primary or secondary dressing	Surgical incisions, lacerations, abrasions, burns, donor or skin graft sites, or any other type of exudative wound Moderate to heavy exudate	Not appropriate for use in a wound with undermining	Without Border A6251–A6253 Without Border A6254–A6256
Transparent film: Opsite (Smith & Nephew) Suresite Window Transparent Film Dressing (Medline Industries, Inc.) Tegaderm™ Transparent Dressing (3M Health Care) (see Plates 65–67)	Polyurethane sheets coated on one side with acrylic Protects wound from environmental contaminants Waterproof, adhesive, nonabsorptive, impermeable to bacteria Semipermeable to oxygen and water vapor Reduces friction Used as a primary dressing	Shallow partial-thickness or closed wound Dry to minimally exudative wound May be used with necrotic tissue to stimulate autolysis	Contraindicated in third-degree burns Not recommended for acutely infected wound Do not use for autolysis on patient with compromised immune system or neutropenia Dressing should extent as least 1 in larger than wound Apply without stretching or tension Change every 4–7 days or as needed Use skin sealant around wound edges May be used to secure primary dressing but not reimbursed	Three dressings per week per wound A6257–A6259
Wound fillers: Dermagran (Integra LifeSciences Corp.) Multidex® Gel or Powder (DeRoyal) Triad™ (Coloplast)	Beads, creams, foams, gels, ointments, pads, pastes, pillows, powders, strands, or other formulations Nonadherent They may include a time-released antimicrobial Used as a primary dressing	Partial- and full-thickness wounds with depth Infected or noninfected Minimal to moderate	Contraindicated for third-degree burns and wounds with little to no exudate Usual dressing change is once per day Select a secondary dressing to promote moist wound healing without strike through exudate	Gel/paste A6261 Dry form A6262

HCPCS, Healthcare Common Procedure Coding System.
Examples of product brand names within this formulary are not inclusive or intended as a product endorsement.
Always screen for allergies prior to using all dressings.
Data compiled from Milne, C. T. (2021). Wound source product guide. In C. T. Milne (Ed.), Wound source the world's definitive source for wound care and product information (24th ed.). Pennsylvania: HMP Global. Retrieved 12/20/2021 from https://www.woundsource.com.

Extent of Tissue Loss. The extent of tissue loss, for example, depth or presence of undermining, is a key consideration in dressing selection. Wound tissue that is not exposed to treatment agents cannot be expected to respond to the regimen and proceed to healing (Gould et al., 2016). Once depth, tunneling, or undermining is identified, the dressing selected must be able to reach the extent of the wound base, as well as fill the dead space to prevent abscess and premature closure of the wound. For example, a hydrocolloid paste can fill a very small amount of depth, whereas a deeper wound may require layers or strips of packing agents such as impregnated gauze to adequately fill dead space. The size of the wound will also impact dressing selection based on the size of the dressing commercially available.

Type of Tissue in the Base of the Wound. When granulation is the primary tissue in the wound, a dressing that maintains a moist wound surface usually is ideal. The presence of slough or eschar in the wound will dictate the need for some form of debridement to decrease the bioburden in the wound and remove physical obstacles to wound closure. Moisture-retentive dressings promote autolysis by maintaining a moist wound dressing interface. The type of dressing moisture-retentive dressing used to achieve or assist with debridement varies depending on the wound characteristics described (see Table 21.5). For example, when the wound is minimally exudative and eschar covered, one option for autolysis is to apply an amorphous hydrogel over the wound. Once the eschar is rehydrated and loosening from the wound edges, sharp debridement may be indicated and the hydrogel may continue to be appropriate, or another dressing may be indicated if depth to the wound becomes apparent.

Condition of the Periwound Skin. The periwound skin can be intact, dry, cracked, macerated, erythematous, or infected (e.g., candidiasis). Dry and cracked skin may require a moisturizer before dressing application. Skin that is vulnerable to adhesives may require a nonadhesive dressing, a dressing with nonaggressive adhesives such as silicone, or protection from adhesives with the use of skin protectants, sealants, and barriers to prevent medical adhesive-related skin injury (MARSI). Because adhesive application and removal

technique can precipitate MARSI, it is critical to instruct caregivers on proper removal of adhesives to prevent skin stripping. When appropriate, less frequent dressing changes are preferred to prevent unnecessary exposure to potential trauma.

Exposure to wound exudate places the periwound skin at risk for moisture-associated skin damage (MASD) such as erythema, dermatitis, maceration, or candidiasis. Periwound maceration and prolonged contact with wound exudate can enlarge the wound and impede healing (Gould et al., 2016). The presence of maceration indicates that wound exudate is not adequately contained or managed. To correct this situation, the plan of care should include a more absorbent dressing or wound filler (see Tables 21.4 and 21.5), an increase in frequency of dressing changes, and inclusion of periwound skin protectants, sealants, or barriers. See Chapter 9 for more details about assessment, prevention, and treatment of MARSI and MASD, a product formulary with product examples, and a discussion of selection considerations for common periwound skin protection and management products.

Location of the Wound. The dressing selected should remain in place, minimize shear and friction, and not cause additional tissue damage (Lavery et al., 2016; Marston, Tang, Kirsner, & Ennis, 2016). Wound location combined with patient activity can significantly affect the ability of the dressing to remain intact. Challenging curved body parts will require tapering of the dressing to adhere or remain intact. Digit dressings are useful for the toes and fingers. Uniquely shaped flexible dressing options that contour to fit heels, elbows, and sacrum may provide better coverage and wear time than a standard square or rectangular dressing. Wounds in locations exposed to friction and shear from sheets, clothing, or braces may require thin adhesive dressings with smooth backings and tapered edges to keep from rolling. In the presence of incontinence, wounds close to the perineal region will benefit from waterproof dressings.

Inflammation, Infection, and Biofilm. Indicators of bacterial burden in the wound bed, such as inflammation, edema, induration, increased exudate and pain, are key considerations for selecting antimicrobial dressings.

	Dry to Minimal Exudate, Shallow	Moderate to Heavy Exudate, Shallow	Dry to Minimal Exudate With Depth	Moderate to Heavy Exudate With Depth	Periwound Skin, Vulnerable/ Painful	Eschar	Odor
Wound Characteristics							
Dressing options	Foam (thin) Hydrocolloid Hydrogel Transparent	Alginate Fiber gelling Foam Specialty absorptive	Impregnated hydrogel gauze	Alginate Foam cavity Hydrofiber Impregnated hypertonic saline gauze	Contact layer Foam (nonadhesive) Hydrogel	Hydrogel	Antimicrobial, antiseptic dressing Charcoal

TABLE 21.5 Dressing Options Based on Wound Characteristics

Perfusion and ability to heal must be established prior to dressing selection especially on lower extremities.

Furthermore, biofilm-based wound care (frequent debridement and antibiofilm dressings) is critical when managing a chronic wound, particularly since the presence of biofilm is typically not visible to the naked eye. Insufficient wound bed preparation to remove biofilm is sufficient to render a wound to be nonresponsive to appropriate topical therapy. In addition, only select topical antimicrobial dressings effectively remove biofilm. Chapter 19 addresses local wound care options for infection and biofilm-based wound care.

Healing Trajectory of the Wound. If a wound is not progressing despite optimal care, cellular senescence (a decrease in proliferation potential of dermal fibroblasts and inability of cells to respond to growth factors) as well as the presence of biofilm, should be considered. Collagen/matrix dressings, or biophysical and biologic agents (e.g., growth factors, electrical stimulation, and negative pressure wound therapy) may be warranted. These therapies are discussed in detail in Chapters 22–27.

Patient Factors That Impact Dressing Selection. A holistic assessment of the patient requires identifying who is (or will be) providing care and in what care setting. Box 21.1 shows the numerous variables that affect product selection and potential outcomes of care. Clearly, the caregiver has a significant impact on the ability to achieve positive wound-related outcomes. As the plan of care is being developed and dressing choices are being made, the availability, level of skill, and care-related concerns of the caregiver will be important to ascertain and explore. A primary concern of the caregiver is ease of use.

Reimbursement for supplies (and therefore access to products) is dependent on the type of health care setting and how the setting is paid for services. When the patient needs to pay out-of-pocket expenses for wound care supplies, the risk of nonadherence with the plan of care is increased. Therefore, treatment decisions should be made considering what is financially reasonable for the patient so that the patient is able to implement the plan of care. Wound care items that are not reimbursed are listed in Box 21.4. For more discussion of facilitating cooperation and establishing a sustainable plan of care, see Chapter 5.

Pain at the wound site must be adequately described and objectively quantified before the wound specialist can understand the origin of the pain and identify appropriate pain control measures. Chronic pain, as occurs with ischemia, requires maintenance pain control measures. Pain at the wound site may be relieved or minimized by the use of nonadhesive, moisture-retentive dressings. Analgesics given before the dressing change also may be indicated. However, pain that occurs during dressing changes should prompt a reevaluation of dressing change technique and wound care product choices. Liquid skin sealants will protect skin from mechanical forces during dressing removal. Nonetheless, caregiver technique in the removal of tape (i.e., proper use of adhesives and supporting the tissue during dressing removal) has a dramatic effect on the patient's pain experience. Wound pain and control measures are discussed in greater detail in Chapter 28.

BOX 21.4   Wound Care Items That Are Not Reimbursed

- Dressings for drainage from a cutaneous fistula that has not been caused by or treated by a surgical procedure
- Dressings for Stage 1 pressure injuries
- Dressings for first-degree burns
- Dressings for wounds caused by trauma that do not require surgical closure or debridement (skin tears or abrasion)
- Skin sealants or barriers
- Wound cleansers or irrigating solutions, solutions used to moisten gauze (e.g., saline), topical antiseptics, and topical antibiotics
- Gauze or other dressings used to debride a wound, but not left on the wound
- Dressing kits (all dressings must be individualized for each patient)
- More than one type of wound filler or wound cover in a single wound
- Use of some combinations of a hydrating dressing and an absorptive dressing (e.g., hydrogel, alginate) on the same wound at the same time
- More than a 1-month supply at a time

Note: If medically necessary and available by prescription, some of these items may be covered under the pharmacy benefit if ordered by a provider.
Data from Aetna. (2022). *Surgical dressings (wound care supplies). Clinical Policy Bulletin no. 0526.* Retrieved 7/8/2022 from: http://www.aetna.com/cpb/medical/data/500_599/0526.html.

Safety Issues That Impact Dressing Selection. Safety features of wound care dressings indicate that products be free from toxic chemicals and fibers and that product biocompatibility has been tested and reported by the manufacturers. Safety should also demonstrate that the product does not increase the patient's risk of morbidity or mortality. The wound specialist's role in safety includes correct use of the product as recommended by the manufacturer (including FDA-approved clinical indications) and proper education of the caregiver.

Sensitivities and Comorbidities. Allergy screening and potential sensitivities to wound care products and ingredients used by the patient in the past are important assessments for the wound care specialist. Early recognition of allergic contact dermatitis and removal of the suspected allergen are critical to minimize patient discomfort and optimize the healing environment. The majority of allergic reactions to wound care products present as allergic contact dermatitis. Patients with venous insufficiency are particularly vulnerable due to long-term repeated exposures to allergens under occlusion (dressings and compression wraps). As described in Chapter 9, differentiation between allergic dermatitis, irritant-related contact dermatitis, MASD and infection (e.g., cellulitis) can be challenging (Alavi et al., 2016).

Comorbid conditions must be taken into consideration and may prohibit use of some dressing ingredients. For example, cadexomer iodine is contraindicated in patients with

Hashimoto's thyroiditis, history of Graves' disease or non-toxic goiter, pregnancy, and lactation (Cunha, 2021). In addition, the patient with a wound on a limb with an ankle-brachial index of 0.6 that cannot be revascularized may not have enough blood flow to promote autolysis; thus, keeping the wound dry with Betadine treatments is a more appropriate plan than promoting moist wound healing.

Combining Products and Therapies. The wound specialist should be cautious about mixing different topical agents for use in a wound because ingredients in one agent may interact with ingredients in another. For example, the enzymatic activity of collagenase is adversely affected by certain detergents and heavy metal ions (e.g., mercury, silver), which are used in some antiseptics, and is inactivated by povidone-iodine. If the collagenase enzyme is used in combination with a secondary dressing containing silver ions, the silver ions would inactivate the enzyme, resulting in no enzymatic debridement and little or no antibacterial effect of the silver. Similarly, some foam dressings are degraded by hydrogen peroxide and should not be used sequentially. It is vitally important to thoroughly read product package inserts and instructions for use when dressings, ointments, and solutions are being used together or sequentially in the same wound.

Compatibility with adjunctive therapies and procedures is an important consideration in selecting the optimal dressing. For example, some products are not compatible with electrical stimulation, hyperbaric oxygen therapy, or radiation therapy. Because various compression therapy methods have change frequencies ranging from daily to weekly, the patient with a venous insufficiency wound requires a dressing with a compatible wear time. The patient with an ostomy close to a midline incision wound will require a dressing that does not interfere with the patient's ability to empty and change the ostomy pouch.

TYPES OF DRESSINGS

Wound dressings include both primary dressings and secondary dressings. The *primary dressing* is a therapeutic or protective covering applied directly to the wound bed to meet the needs of the wound. The *secondary dressing* serves a therapeutic or protective function and is used to increase the ability to adequately meet the wound needs and/or secure the primary dressing. For example, a hydrocolloid dressing is the primary dressing when it is used over a shallow, minimally exudative wound, but it functions as a secondary dressing when it is used over a wound filler.

Most wound dressings are semiocclusive rather than occlusive. Gauze, however, is neither. Semiocclusive dressings (also known as *moisture-retentive dressings*) emerged in the 1970s and currently are staples in the wound care portfolio. North America dominates the wound care market. Globally, the wound care market was valued at $ 20.59 billion in 2021. This growth is due to increasing number of surgical cases and rising prevalence of chronic diseases internationally. Advanced wound dressings experienced the largest revenue

share in 2021 in part due to the number of burn cases, increasing geriatric patient population, growing traumatic injuries, and increased number of Ambulatory Surgical Centers (Grand View Research, 2021). The wound care market is constantly changing with an extensive variety of dressings that vary by shape, size, and ingredients. They are selected based on the needs of the wound, the patient, and the care setting.

Common ingredients in wound dressings include glycerin, polymers, carboxymethylcellulose, collagen, alginate, cellulose, cotton or rayon, and polyurethane. Wound care dressings may be *single-component* dressings containing, for example, only alginate, hydrogel, or hydrocolloid, or *multi-component* dressings in which components are mixed together, such as an alginate and a hydrocolloid, to increase absorptive capacity. Multicomponent dressings are categorized and reimbursed according to the clinically predominant component (e.g., alginate, collagen, foam, gauze, hydrocolloid, hydrogel). Most of the dressing categories are available in an antimicrobial form such as silver (as discussed in Chapter 16); however, reimbursement is still based upon their clinically prominent component.

Wound care needs may change frequently throughout the various phases of wound healing. Therefore, a variety of products must be accessible. In general, dressing selection and utilization are guided by the Medicare Part B Surgical Dressing Policy (Centers for Medicare and Medicaid Services [CMS], 2017). Table 21.4 is a formulary of wound care products and provides examples in addition to the Medicare Part B utilization parameters and codes. Before using specific products, providers should refer to the manufacturer's product insert for the most current information on contraindications, interactions, and utilization. The policy also contains a category for pouching wounds. These products are described in Chapter 39.

COMPONENTS OF A DRESSING CHANGE

In general, the components of a dressing change are the same: infection control, atraumatic removal, cleansing, light filling or packing, periwound skin protection, dressing application, and securement.

Infection Control

Standard universal precautions (gloves, eye protection when splashes are possible, etc.) and handwashing should be routinely followed during dressing changes. Caregivers should wash their hands (1) before and after patient contact, (2) after contact with a source of microorganisms (e.g., body fluid and substances, mucous membranes, broken skin, soiled dressings), and (3) after removing gloves. In general, two sets of gloves should be used: one set for dressing removal and wound cleansing and another set for dressing application (Wound, Ostomy and Continence Nurses Society [WOCN] Wound Committee & Association for Professionals in Infection Control and Epidemiology, Inc. [APIC] 2000 Guidelines Committee, 2012).

Best practice is to use clean technique rather than sterile for changing dressings on chronic wounds. The preferred *no-touch* technique is a method of changing surface dressings without directly touching the wound or any surface that might come in contact with the wound. Sterile devices are used to hold and administer sterile irrigant solution. Sterile cotton-tipped applicators are used to probe the wound and insert wound fillers, gauze, or packing. Clean (rather than sterile) gloves are used to apply sterile dressings; however, the surface of the dressing that will contact the wound bed is not touched (WOCN Wound Committee & APIC 2000 Guidelines Committee, 2012).

Atraumatic Dressing Removal

During dressing removal, the periwound skin and the wound base must be protected from trauma. Adhesives are removed in the direction of hair growth. An edge of the dressing is gently rolled or lifted to obtain a starting edge. The tissue adjacent to the dressing is supported as the dressing is gently released from the skin. Moistened gauze can be used to support the skin during dressing removal to minimize the potential for stripping. If the dressing material is attached to the wound base, saline or a wound cleanser can be used to moisten the dressing and allow gentle release of the dressing material from the tissue. Difficult or painful removal must also facilitate an alternative wound care plan (i.e., skin sealant or nonadhesive product) to decrease pain and trauma to the wound with future dressing changes (McNichol, Lund, Rosen, et al., 2013). Dressing changes are performed on a scheduled basis depending on the type of dressing in use; dressings that are oversaturated or leaking should be changed promptly. Dressing materials and contaminated gloves are disposed of in accordance with agency policies and procedures.

Cleansing and Irrigation

Wound cleansing is necessary with each dressing change to physically remove surface bacteria and debris from the wound bed without damaging healthy tissue or inoculating the underlying tissue with bacteria (Gould et al., 2016; Lavery et al., 2016; Marston et al., 2016). For most chronic wounds, tap water (safe for drinking), normal saline, or low-toxicity antiseptic agents are appropriate. Cleansing with sterile products should be used with immunocompromised patients and deep postsurgical wounds (Sibbald et al., 2021).

Wound irrigation can be used with a force between 4 and 15 pounds per square inch (psi). This is accomplished with select commercially prepared wound irrigation and cleansing products or by delivering the irrigant with the following components:

- 19-gauge angiocatheter, and a 35-mL syringe (provides 8 psi);
- 28-gauge angiocatheter, and a 20-mL syringe (provides 12 psi); and
- a 22-gauge angiocatheter, and a 12-mL syringe (provides 13 psi) (EPUAP, NPIAP, & PPPIA, 2019).

Soaking the wound with gauze saturated with a wound cleansing solution can also be effective in removing debris (Sibbald et al., 2021) while allowing penetration of the antiseptic solution. Whirlpool therapy is no longer recommended due to increased risk for bacterial contamination, circulatory compromise and tissue maceration (Gould et al., 2016). Wound assessment should be completed after wound cleansing.

Periwound Skin Cleansing and Protection

After dressing removal and wound cleansing, the surrounding skin is gently cleansed and dried. If a moisture barrier is indicated, it is applied at this time. Skin sealants or films must be allowed to dry prior to dressing application, to prevent periwound MASD due to the dressing being applied over moist skin. As previously stated, Chapter 9 is a must read for assessment, prevention, and management of periwound MASD and MARSI. Examples and selection considerations for common periwound skin protectants, sealants, and barriers are presented.

Dressing Application

The selected dressing is applied according to manufacturer's instructions without stretching the skin. In the gluteal fold, wafer dressings are folded in half before application to ensure that the adhesive seals into the anatomic contours. Applications of dressings at the heel or elbow may require small slits to taper and shape the dressing to fit. Position the heel or elbow in the bent position during application so that the dressing does not pull the skin when the limb is extended.

Packing or Filling

The purpose of filling or packing the wound is to fill dead space and avoid the potential of abscess formation by premature closure of the wound. Packing materials should be conformable to the base and sides of the wound. In the presence of undermining, impregnated gauze, alginate rope, or fiber gelling/hydrofiber dressings may be used to gently pack the space. When tunneling is apparent in the wound, strip gauze packing may be used to fill narrow areas so that the complete dressing can be easily removed during dressing changes; packing should be one continuous piece of gauze with one end of the strip gauze coiled on top of the dressing for easy access during dressing removal. Absorbent packing dressings and wound fillers (e.g., alginate, fiber gelling/hydrofiber) are appropriate for wounds that are exudative. Conversely, for wounds that are dry, the packing material must be hydrating so that it provides moisture to the wounds (e.g., hydrogel-impregnated gauze, collagen dressings, continuously moist gauze). For large deep wounds, hydrating or absorbent-impregnated gauze is effective and usually requires fewer dressing changes than dry gauze. The packing material is fluffed and loosely placed into the wound with a cotton-tipped applicator so that the packing material is in contact with the wound edges and base. Gauze dressings may be necessary to act as an additional absorbent layer. "Overpacking" the wound should be avoided. A secondary cover dressing is then applied and secured.

Securing the Dressing

A method of securing nonadhesive dressings is necessary to keep such dressings in place. Self-adhesive wraps, tape, Montgomery straps, gauze wraps, or tubular mesh dressings may be used. If the wound is located on the leg, a gauze wrap can be taped upon itself to avoid applying tape to the skin. Again, see Chapter 9 for appropriate selection and use of medical adhesives (McNichol et al., 2013).

DOCUMENTATION OF MEDICAL NECESSITY

First and foremost, documentation should reflect evidence-based practice. Done accurately, the documentation will provide rational and justification for various dressing choices and will most likely be consistent with guidelines for utilization and Healthcare Common Procedure Coding System codes (Table 21.4). Additional guidelines for utilization as established by Medicare Part B require documentation of medical necessity as defined in Checklist 21.1 and Box 21.4 (CMS, 2017). Dressing size must be based on, and appropriate to, the size of the wound. For wound covers, the size of the wound pad should be approximately 2 in greater than the dimensions of the wound. No more than a 1-month supply of dressings may be provided at one time. If documentation is not consistent with these guidelines, wound care may be jeopardized if the patient is unable to pay out of pocket for their supplies.

CHECKLIST 21.1 Summary of Documentation Requirements for Coverage and/or Medical Necessity

✓ Maintained in the patient's medical record
✓ Legible signature provider responsible for and providing the care to the patient
✓ Accurate and specific diagnosis code(s)
✓ Appropriate evaluation and management of contributory medical conditions or other factors affecting the course of wound healing (such as nutritional status or other predisposing conditions)
✓ Status of the wound and response to the current treatment
✓ Description of wound location, size, depth, and stage (may be supported by a drawing or photograph of the wound)
✓ Debridement, complicating factors for wound healing and measures taken to control complicating factors, type of tissue removed
✓ Appropriate modification of treatment plans, when necessitated by failure of wounds to heal
✓ Improvement of tissue healing and viability, reduce or control tissue infection, remove necrotic tissue, or prepare the tissue for surgical management (except for patients with compromised healing from severe underlying debility or other factors documented)
✓ Appropriate palliative care standards if wound closure is not a reasonable goal
✓ Plan of care containing treatment goals and follow-up

Source: Centers for Medicare and Medicaid Services. (2017). *Local coverage determination (LCD): Wound care (L35125): General information.* Retrieved 7/18/2022 from: www.cms.gov/medicare-coverage-database/details/lcd-details.aspx?LCDId=35125.

CLINICAL CONSULT

A: Home care referral received to provide wound consult for a 78-year-old male who lives in a trailer with his son and his nursing assistant daughter-in-law. Patient was recently discharged following a lengthy hospital stay for pneumonia during which he required prolonged periods of head of bed elevation and supplemental oxygen. Respiratory status is much improved. He is afebrile and on oral antibiotics. Developed hospital-acquired pressure injury left buttock near gluteal cleft. Pressure injury encompasses a 5 × 6 cm area of nonblanchable erythema with a centrally located 2 × 1.5 × 0.5 cm full-thickness wound of red, viable tissue. Currently using a hydrocolloid dressing with instructions to change dressing twice weekly. Patient has noticed drainage from dressing onto underwear and tries to reduce this seepage by covering dressing with paper towels. Wound edges are open; periwound skin macerated; no periwound erythema. Patient spends much of his day on the couch reading or watching TV while his adult children are at work.

D: Stage 3 pressure injury with moderate exudate inadequately contained.

P: Implement absorptive wound filler and consult with PT regarding activity and seating surface support device.

I: (1) Calcium alginate rope into wound bed. (2) Cover with foam dressing with border adhesive. (3) Change every Monday and Thursday or if loosens. (4) Physical therapy to assess for pressure redistribution chair cushion, weight shifts, and safe use of his walker to stand and walk about the trailer each hour. (5) Dietary consult to assess nutritional needs and counsel patient/family.

E: Home care to continue to follow twice weekly. Wound care to return in 2 weeks to reassess wound progress and modify topical therapy as needed.

SUMMARY

- Wounded skin is a complex pathophysiologic condition that necessitates a specific and intricate knowledge base, which includes assessments and interventions to achieve appropriate outcomes for the wound.

- Nonphysiologic approaches and inappropriate product use remain commonplace and are likely to delay wound closure, thus increasing the overall cost of wound care.

- One treatment protocol is not appropriate for all wounds, and seldom does a wound progress to healing with only one type of dressing used. Most wounds require numerous modifications as wound characteristics change.
- Understanding the principles of wound management prepares the wound specialist to partner with interdisciplinary teams, to articulate underlying rationale, and to use a research-based approach to provide cost-effective care to the patient with a wound.

SELF-ASSESSMENT QUESTIONS

1. What are the three principles of wound management?
   a. Debridement, control of infection, and exudate management
   b. Establishment of a treatment goal, wound cleansing, and physiologic local wound care
   c. Assessment of the host, debridement, and physiologic local wound care
   d. Address the wound etiology, support the host, and maintain a physiologic local wound environment
2. Which of the following interventions indicates an attempt to control or eliminate the etiology of a venous ulcer?
   a. Resizing of shoe to include orthotics
   b. Applying an alginate and foam cover dressing
   c. Monitoring blood glucose levels
   d. Encouraging elevation of the leg three times daily
3. Which of the following statements about semiocclusive dressings is true?
   a. They are occlusive to liquids and gases.
   b. They are occlusive to liquids but transmit moisture vapor and gases.
   c. They are occlusive to gases and vapors but transmit liquids.
   d. They are inconsistent in their nonocclusive properties.
4. In the patient with a new approximated surgical wound, the primary wound care objective is:
   a. autolysis
   b. hydration
   c. cleansing
   d. protection
5. Dressing selection is primarily based on which of the following?
   a. Forms of the dressing
   b. Characteristics of the wound
   c. Product availability and cost
   d. Number of dressing changes required daily
6. In the patient with a highly exudative pressure ulcer, which category of dressings should be considered?
   a. Hydrocolloids
   b. Collagens
   c. Transparent dressings
   d. Alginates
7. Which of the following statements about wound care products is *true*?
   a. Hydrocolloids absorb more exudate than alginate dressings.
   b. Transparent dressings are contraindicated for Stage 2 pressure injuries.
   c. Wound fillers can be used to fill undermining and tunnels.
   d. Silver-impregnated dressings are indicated when critical colonization is suspected.
8. List seven objectives for local wound management.

REFERENCES

Alavi, A., Sibbald, R. G., Ladizinski, B., Saraiya, A., Lee, K. C., Skotnicki-Grant, S., et al. (2016). Wound-related allergic/irritant contact dermatitis. *Advances in Skin & Wound Care*, 29(6), 278–286. https://doi.org/10.1097/01.ASW.0000482834.94375.1e. 27171256.

Atkin, L., Bućko, A., Condo Montero, E., Cutting, K., Moffatt, C., Probst, A., et al. (2019). Implementing TIMERS: The race against hard to heal wounds. *Journal of Wound Care*, 23(Suppl. 3a), S1–S50.

Bennison, L. R., Miller, C. N., Summers, R. J., Minnis, A. M. B., Sussman, G., & McGuiness, W. (2017). The pH of wounds during healing and infection: A descriptive literature review. *Cambridge Media Journals*, 25(2), 63–69.

Brindle, T., & Farmer, P. (2019). Undisturbed wound healing: A narrative review of the literature and clinical considerations. *Wound International*, 10(2), 40–48.

Centers for Medicare and Medicaid Services (CMS). (2017). *Local coverage determination (LCD): Wound care (L35125): General information*. Retrieved 7/18/2022 from: www.cms.gov/medicare-coverage-database/details/lcd-details.aspx?LCDId=35125.

Cunha, J. (2021). *Cadexomer iodine*. RxList. Retrieved 7/18/2021 from: https://www.rxlist.com/consumer_iodosorb_cadexomer_iodine/drugs-condition.htm#what_are_warnings_and_precautions_for_cadexomer_iodine.

European Pressure Ulcer Advisory Panel, National Pressure Injury Advisory Panel, & Pan Pacific Pressure Injury Alliance (EPUAP, NPIAP, & PPPIA). (2019). In E. Haesler (Ed.), *Prevention and treatment of pressure ulcers/injuries*. Osborne Park: Cambridge Media.

Gottrup, F., & Apelqvist, J. (2010). The challenge of using randomized trials in wound healing. *The British Journal of Surgery*, 97, 303–304.

Gould, L., Stuntz, M., Giovannelli, M., Ahmad, A., Aslam, R., Mullen-Fortino, M., et al. (2016). Wound healing society 2015 update on guidelines for pressure ulcers. *Wound Repair and Regeneration*, 24(1), 145–162. https://doi.org/10.1111/wrr.12396. 26683529.

Grand View Research. (2021). *Wound care market size, share & trends analysis by produce (advanced, surgical) by application (chronic wounds, acute wounds), by end-use (hospitals specialty clinics), by region, and segment forecasts, 2022–2030. Report ID: GVR-3-68038-300-3.* Retrieved 6/3/2022 from: https://www.grandviewresearch.com/industry-analysis/wound-care-market.

Hinman, C. D., & Maibach, H. (1963). Effect of air exposure and occlusion on experimental human skin wounds. *Nature, 200,* 377–378.

Lavery, L. A., Davis, K. E., Berriman, S. J., Braun, L., Nichols, A., Kim, P. J., et al. (2016). WHS guidelines update: Diabetic foot ulcer treatment guidelines. *Wound Repair and Regeneration, 24*(1), 112–126. https://doi.org/10.1111/wrr.12391. 26663430.

Lawrence, C. L. (1994). Dressings and wound infection. *American Journal of Surgery, 167*(1A), S21–S24.

Leaper, D., & Drake, R. (2011). Should one size fit all? An overview and critique of the VULCAN study on silver dressings. *International Wound Journal, 8*(1), 1–4.

MacFie, C. C., Melling, A. C., & Leaper, D. J. (2005). Effects of warming on healing. *Journal of Wound Care, 14*(3), 133–136.

Marston, W., Tang, J., Kirsner, R. S., & Ennis, W. (2016). Wound healing society 2015 update on guidelines for venous ulcers. *Wound Repair and Regeneration, 24*(1), 136–144. https://doi.org/10.1111/wrr.12394. 26663616.

McGuinness, W., Vella, E., & Harrison, D. (2004). Influence of dressing changes on wound temperature. *Journal of Wound Care, 13*(9), 383–385.

McNichol, L., Lund, C., Rosen, T., et al. (2013). Medical adhesives and patient safety: State of the science: Consensus statements for the assessment, prevention, and treatment of adhesive-related skin injuries. *Journal of Wound, Ostomy, and Continence Nursing, 40*(4), 365–380.

Milne, C. T. (2021). Wound source product guide. In C. T. Milne (Ed.), Wound source the world's definitive source for wound care and product information (24th ed.). Pennsylvania: HMP Global. Retrieved 12/20/2021 from https://www.woundsource.com.

Nuutilla, K., & Eriksson, E. (2021). Moist wound healing with commonly available dressings. *Advances in Wound Care, 10*(12), 685–698.

Ovington, L. G. (2001). Hanging wet-to-dry dressings out to dry. *Home Healthcare Nurse, 19,* 477–484.

Rolstad, B. S., Bryant, R. A., & Nix, D. P. (2012). Topical management. In R. A. Bryant, & D. P. Nix (Eds.), *Acute & chronic wounds. Current management* (4th ed., pp. 289–306). St. Louis: Elsevier.

Schneider, A. K., Korber, A., Grabbe, S., et al. (2007). Influence of pH on wound-healing: A new perspective for wound-therapy? *Archives of Dermatological Research, 298,* 413–420.

Sibbald, R. G., Elliott, J. A., Persaud-Jaimangal, R., Goodman, L., Armstrong, D. G., Harley, C., et al. (2021). Wound bed preparation 2021. *Advances in Skin & Wound Care, 34*(4), 183–195. https://doi.org/10.1097/01.ASW.0000733724.87630.d6. 33739948. PMCID: PMC7982138.

Spruitt, D. (1972). The water barrier and its repair. In H. Maebashi, & D. Rovee (Eds.), *Epidermal wound healing.* Chicago: Yearbook Medical.

White, R., Cutting, K., Ousey, K., et al. (2010). Randomized controlled trial and cost-effectiveness analysis of silver-donating antimicrobial dressings for venous leg ulcers (VULCAN trial) (*Br J Surg* 2009, 96, 1147–1156). *The British Journal of Surgery, 97*(3), 459–460.

Winter, G. D. (1962). Formation of the scab and the rate of epithelization of superficial wounds in the skin of the young domestic pig. *Nature, 193*(4812), 293–294.

Winter, G. D. (2006). Some factors affecting skin and wound healing. *Journal of Tissue Viability, 16*(2), 20–23.

Wound, Ostomy and Continence Nurses Society (WOCN) Wound Committee, & Association for Professionals in Infection Control and Epidemiology, Inc. (APIC) 2000 Guidelines Committee. (2012). Clean vs. sterile dressing techniques for management of chronic wounds: A fact sheet. *Journal of Wound, Ostomy, and Continence Nursing, 39*(2 Suppl), S30–S34. https://doi.org/10.1097/WON.0b013e3182478e06. 22415169.

22

Cellular- and/or Tissue-Based Products for Wounds

Scott Ellis and John C. Lantis, II

OBJECTIVES

1. Describe the indications and role of cellular- and tissue-based products (CTPs) for wounds.
2. Identify the significance of a CTP being cellular or acellular.
3. Differentiate the function and composition of epidermal, dermal, extracellular matrix (ECM) scaffolds, and bilayer CTPs.
4. Outline the guiding principles for the process of patient and wound bed preparation, CTP application, method of securement, and frequency of follow-up and reapplication.
5. Discuss the issues related to regulatory and reimbursement policies by CMS and insurance carriers that must be addressed/explored when planning CTP utilization.

It would appear that in roughly 50% of wounds, despite optimum care utilizing moist wound-healing dressings and comprehensive systemic support (i.e., offloading, trauma reduction, compression, bacterial balance, glucose management, and nutritional support); there is failure to close in a timely fashion. Furthermore, a conservative approach may be inadequate for wounds with ongoing significant tissue loss, or that have been present for greater than 1 year. When confronted with these difficult-to-heal wounds tissue-engineered products may be indicated. Tissue engineering is defined as "the use of methods that promote biological repair or regeneration of tissues or organs by providing signaling, structural or cellular elements with or without systems that contain living tissue or cells" (Hashimoto, 2000). Historically, a variety of names have been used to describe these products: bioengineered skin equivalents, tissue-engineered skin, biologic skin substitutes, and living skin replacements. For clarity, accuracy, and consistency, the term *cellular-and tissue-based products (CTPs)* for wounds is recommended for the discussion around a permanent replacement for lost or damaged skin. Bioengineering is defined as the application of engineering principles and techniques to problems in medicine and biology, as the design and production of artificial limbs and organs. However, for convention, ease of use or scientific rigor the term is not currently applied to the field of CTPs. This chapter will not be discussing the use of patient autologous tissue therapies.

INDICATIONS FOR USE

CTPs act as protective dressings that limit bacteria colonization, mitigate fluid loss, and/or stimulate healing (Greaves, Iqbal, Baguneid, et al., 2013). These products are designed to mimic aspects of native tissues in order to promote healing. Over 74 CTPs are available in the US health care market (dependent upon the time of publication this will have most likely increased), and appropriate utilization requires an understanding of their composition and function. For example, a large number of CTPs are a scaffold (or matrix) product created from a collagen source and used as a temporary extracellular matrix (ECM) implant. These ECMs provide a structure into which native blood vessels, cytokines, and growth factors can migrate. A much smaller number of CTPs deliver keratinocytes to the wound bed and are described as epidermal CTPs. Bilayer CTPs exist that contain live keratinocytes on a dermal matrix seeded with fibroblasts; these may be bioengineered or cadaveric.

No matter the composition, all CTPs must be safe for the patient (nontoxic, nonimmunogenic, minimal to no inflammation, and no or low level of transmissible disease risk), clinically effective, and convenient in handling and application (Shevchenko, James, & James, 2009). Ideally, CTPs should also be biodegradable, support reconstruction of normal tissue that has similar function to the skin it replaces, provide pain relief, and be readily available with a long shelf life. Just as topical dressings are selected based on wound manifestations and needs that change over the healing time period, CTPs are selected to achieve specific objectives: (1) protection by providing a mechanical barrier to microorganisms and vapor loss; (2) provision of a temporary wound covering while awaiting permanent wound closure either innately or via skin grafting; (3) delivery of dermal matrix components, cytokines, and growth factors to stimulate and enhance wound-healing activity of host cells; and (4) delivery of structures (i.e., dermal collagen or cultured cells) that are integrated into the wound (Catalano, Cochis, Varoni, et al., 2013; Shevchenko et al., 2009). When trying to navigate and categorize the multiple CTPs it is convenient to categorize CTPs into products that (1) primarily deliver living viable cells, (2) ECMs, or (3) derivatives derived from amniotic products. Despite some degree of overlap, these categories ease the selection process in the clinical setting.

CTPs are used as adjuncts to appropriate standard wound and patient care, with the goal of improving patient outcomes by facilitating closure of chronic wounds and acute wounds or large areas of skin loss. Ultimately, the success in using these products depends on several factors: (1) appropriate product selection for the wound condition; (2) meticulous wound bed preparation; (3) diligent patient preparation and correction of systemic cofactors that impair healing; (4) aggressive correction of the underlying wound etiology; (5) proper CTP application; (6) appropriate cover dressings; and (7) consistent, regular monitoring of both the cover dressings and the wound bed. It is critical that the wound bed be debrided of nonviable tissue, sinus tracts, or tunnels and that there are no gross signs of clinical infection. Many CTPs require reapplication, and this should be anticipated when planning CTP use. Checklist 22.1 lists essential steps in the appropriate use of CTPs.

Food and Drug Administration (FDA)-approved indications for CTPs in chronic wound management vary by the specific CTP, as shown in the tables of this chapter. The range of indications includes burns, diabetic foot ulcers, venous ulcers, and epidermolysis bullosa. Contraindications to the use of CTPs include known allergy to bovine collagen or hypersensitivity to components in the CTP product shipping or packaging ingredients. In preparation for utilization, patients should be adequately informed of the source and composition of bioengineered skin out of respect for personal, cultural, ethnic, or religious preferences.

Another decision point when considering a CTP is the cost of the product and reimbursement. The Centers for Medicare & Medicaid Services (CMS) 2014 Hospital Outpatient Prospective Payment System rule bundled the widely diverse CTPs used in surgical procedures into a high- and low-cost group (Schaum, 2014). It is important to be familiar with this ruling and the impact on product selection and reimbursement for CTP utilization in hospital outpatient departments and ambulatory surgery centers. However, this makes the erroneous presumption that a very significant majority of wounds are treated in such facilities or that such facilities are a repository of actual wound expertise.

CHECKLIST 22.1 Essential Steps to Using CTPs

1. Address underlying pathology.
   ✓ Revascularize patients with peripheral arterial disease.
   ✓ Correct peripheral edema.
   ✓ Offload plantar ulcers.
   ✓ Redistribute pressure in patients with pressure injuries.
2. Correct systemic factors interfering with wound healing.
   ✓ Ensure adequate nutrition.
   ✓ Normalize blood glucose.
   ✓ Encourage smoking cessation.
   ✓ Collaborate with other clinicians on systemic medication changes to promote wound healing (e.g., decreasing steroid dose, if possible).
3. Identify and treat clinical infection.
4. Debride all necrotic tissue, fibrinous slough, and surrounding callus.
   ✓ Many wounds may require surgical debridement in the operating room.
5. Ensure complete contact of product with wound bed.
   ✓ Eliminate any bubbles or wrinkles.
   ✓ Use pressure dressings/bolsters to maintain contact.
6. Fenestrate product (if not already packaged that way) to allow wound fluid to escape and prevent accumulation of fluid under product.
7. Keep products without synthetic backings moist.
8. Follow package insert for directions specific to individual products.

Unfortunately, at times this requires that the wound care clinician is aware of the various insurance carrier's policy for CTP utilization (including frequency of reapplication), reimbursement, and medical necessity. In addition, although there are many CTPs on the market, not all are covered for use by Medicare and insurance companies. CTPs that are ruled as experimental or investigational by that insurance carrier or Medicare will not be reimbursed. It is recommended that all CTPs application be preauthorized with appropriate insurance verification. In addition, products that require multiple applications for efficacy should be preauthorized for a minimum of 5 applications. The local coverage determination (LCD) outlines appropriate utilization to optimize reimbursement and should be closely reviewed and followed for all Medicare patients. These LCDs are updated frequently and require close monitoring. In general, physicians and podiatrists with special training, surgeons, and advanced practice nurses are approved providers for the application of CTPs, although this should be verified with the insurance provider. Documentation should clearly address medical necessity, outline the treatment plan, and ideally include serial photographs to span the time period before application until the wound has healed. If a CTP application is denied for reimbursement, the provider may need to consider billing the patient for the service, which involves asking the patient to sign an advanced beneficiary notice. Once again preauthorization is recommended so that the financial aspect of providing optimal wound care is not a burden to the patient or health care provider.

CLASSIFICATION OF PRODUCTS

Several classification schemes are used to describe CTPs: cellular composition, anatomic structure, duration of product, source of CTP components, and processing (Box 22.1).

CTPs are either *cellular* (i.e., containing living cells) or *acellular*. Cellular CTPs contain cultured keratinocytes and/or fibroblasts situated on a "delivery system," usually a bioabsorbable matrix, and derived from either autologous or allogeneic sources. The majority of cellular products used in chronic wound care are produced with allogeneic cells. The primary purpose of allogeneic CTPs is to deliver healthy living cells to the wound, where they secrete multiple growth factors and other ECM proteins that stimulate the host cells to proceed with wound repair. However, there is the potential that cryopreserved tissue—both amniotic and allogenic split-thickness tissue—may contain "nonengineered" live endogenous cells.

Anatomically, *cellular* CTPs are designed to stimulate or function as specific skin layers: epidermal, dermal, or bilayered (or composite). Epidermal CTPs consist of keratinocytes; dermal CTPs contain fibroblasts that are embedded in a matrix; and bilayered skin substitutes have some type of both keratinocytes and the matrix-embedded fibroblasts to form epidermal and dermal layers. Cellular skin substitutes do not contain skin structures such as blood vessels, hair follicles, sweat glands, or many skin cells such as melanocytes, Langerhans cells, macrophages, and lymphocytes. Human neonatal foreskin grown is tissue banks are a common source for allogeneic cellular products (Ter Horst, Chouhan, Moiemen, & Grover, 2018).

In general, acellular CTPs act as *ECM scaffolds*. In addition to providing a moist wound environment, these products can actively interact with the wound environment to reduce high levels of matrix metalloproteinases (Límová, 2010). These products all contain collagen that is commonly derived from nonhuman sources known as a Xenograft (e.g., porcine, bovine, equine, and avian), biosynthetic sources (a combination of biologic and manufactured materials), or synthetic (manufactured materials) (Ågren & Werthén, 2007; Shores,

---

BOX 22.1   Classification Schemes for CTPs

Cellular composition
  Cellular
  Acellular
Anatomic structure
  Epidermal
  Dermal
  Bilayer (composite, dermoepidermal)
  Scaffold
Duration of product
  Temporary
  Permanent
Source of CTP components
  Biologic (autologous, allogeneic, xenogeneic)
  Synthetic
Processing
  In vitro
  In vivo

Gabriel, & Gupta, 2007). However, a whole host of acellular CTPs are also derived from human dermal sources, which have been decellularized in their commercialization process. Acellular CTPs are available as sheets (which may have to be rehydrated), gels, or granules. Some acellular CTPs retain native growth factors and other polypeptides, such as fibronectin, while most deliver some component of proteoglycans and glycosaminoglycans. It must be remembered that growth factors do not work without proteoglycans and glycosaminoglycans. While autologous skin grafts are expected to "take," or survive, allogeneic cell-based CTPs are temporary and biodegrade (Griffiths, Ojeh, Livingstone, et al., 2004; Metcalfe & Ferguson, 2007). Allogeneic fibroblasts have been reported to survive in the host for 3–8 weeks, whereas the host will reject and slough allogeneic keratinocytes within a few weeks (i.e., 2–3) (Shevchenko et al., 2009). However, CTPs that are engineered to resist degradation will more likely evoke an inflammatory response and, while enhancing wound closure, can result in scar tissue formation. In contrast, products that provide controlled degradation while allowing infiltration of and replacement by native tissue may have the potential to reduce scar formation (Badylak, 2007; Greaves et al., 2013; Shores et al., 2007; van Winterswijk & Nout, 2007). The tables in this chapter provide examples, descriptions, and indications for known cellular and acellular products, including those that are not available in the United States. In the following sections, products that are available in the US market are presented.

Dermal and Bilayered Cellular- and Tissue-Based Products: Living Cellular

Epidermal CTPs (Table 22.1) are insufficient for optimal wound healing when the dermis is absent because the dermis provides elasticity and mechanical resistance. In the absence of the dermis, the epidermis is fragile and vulnerable to blistering, scar formation, and contractures (Greaves et al., 2013). Dermal CTPs contain fibroblasts seeded and cultured on a three-dimensional bioabsorbable matrix, along with the ECM proteins and growth factors that they produce. The presence of viable cells seeded onto the matrix ensures that important growth factors are secreted into the wound bed and incorporated into the wound-healing process (Greaves et al., 2013; Jang, Choi, Han, et al., 2015). They may be delivered fresh or cryopreserved, although only the latter is available in the United States.

Dermagraft is a cryopreserved, allogeneic dermal substitute with fibroblasts seeded on a bioabsorbable polyglactin mesh (Roberts & Mansbridge, 2002). Once thawed at the bedside in an easy step-by-step process, a 5 × 7.5-cm living dermal substitute can be applied onto clean, debrided wounds that are free of infection.

The FDA approves dermagraft for the treatment of full-thickness diabetic foot ulcers at least 6 weeks' duration that extend through the dermis and are without tendon, muscle, joint capsule, or bone exposure. In a randomized controlled trial of 314 patients with diabetic foot ulcers of over 6 weeks' duration, 30% of Dermagraft-treated patients were healed at

TABLE 22.1 Epidermal CTPs

Product	Description
CellSpray XP[a] (Avita Medical, Cambridge, UK)	Autologous preconfluent keratinocytes in suspension, sprayed on wound. Requires larger biopsy. Suspension ready in 2 days
CellSpray[a] (Avita Medical, Cambridge, UK)	Autologous preconfluent keratinocytes in suspension, sprayed on wound. Requires small biopsy. Suspension ready in 5 days
Epicel (Genzyme, Cambridge, MA, USA)	Cultured from autologous keratinocytes obtained from skin biopsy of patient. Delivered as 30-cm^2 sheets, attached to a petrolatum gauze backing. Autologous cells; therefore, no risk of rejection; high incidence of uptake. Fragile. One-day shelf life. Inferior cosmesis in many patients. FDA approved for deep partial- and full-thickness burns
Keragraf[a] (Smith & Nephew Inc., FL, USA; Advanced Tissue Sciences Inc., La Jolla, CA, USA)	Cultured from autologous adult stem and precursor cells derived from hair plucked from the patient
Laserskin[a] (Fidia Advanced Polymers, Abano Terme, Italy)	Sheet of biodegradable matrix composed of a benzyl esterified hyaluronic acid derivative with laser-created perforations seeded with autologous keratinocytes that are cultured directly on the matrix. The graft can be removed from culture without disturbing the arrangement of basement membrane proteins. Duration of contact permanent

Products listed are not inclusive, and other products may be available.
FDA, Food and Drug Administration.
[a]Currently not available in the United States.

12 weeks vs 18.3% in the control group ($P = 0.023$) (Marston, Hanft, Norwood, et al., 2003). The very low healing rate noted in both arms may in part be attributed to very poor offloading in the trial. The Wound Healing Society (Lavery et al., 2016) also recommends dermagraft for the treatment of nonhealing diabetic foot ulcer. Of note its trial in the treatment of venous leg ulcer was not a significant clinical success (Harding, Sumner, & Cardinal, 2013).

Dermagraft is used as an adjunctive therapy to standard care, which includes offloading the ulcer, debridement, treatment of infection, glucose control, and assurance of adequate blood flow for healing. Optimal healing rates are associated with aggressive offloading. Dermagraft is applied with either side toward the wound bed and is covered with a nonadherent contact layer. To ensure good contact of Dermagraft with the wound bed, it may be bolstered with saline-moistened gauze or a soft foam dressing. In clinical trials Dermagraft was applied weekly for up to 8 weeks, yet this dosing regimen may not be necessary in clinical practice.

Apligraf (Plate 68), a living, allogeneic, bilayered CTP, consists of keratinocytes and fibroblasts. Fibroblasts are cultured in a Type I bovine collagen gel. Keratinocytes are then seeded on this gel, cultured, and air exposed to stimulate differentiation into the layers of the epidermis, including the stratum corneum. This process results in a 44-cm^2, 0.75-mm-thick skin substitute delivered fresh on a Petri dish containing nutrient medium and sealed in an airtight bag. Since this product may be considered to be the first in class in the late 1990s, it has been widely adopted as a covered entity by most commercial insurance payors.

Apligraf, when used in conjunction with compression therapy, has been demonstrated to achieve closure of hard-to-heal venous ulcers at a significantly higher rate than seen with compression alone (Falanga, Margolis, Alvarez, et al., 1998; Falanga & Sabolinski, 1999). Apligraf is FDA approved for the treatment of venous ulcers of greater than 1 month's duration that have not adequately responded to standard care, including debridement, infection control, assurance of adequate arterial flow, and compression therapy. National guidelines support the use of bilayered skin substitutes in conjunction with compression bandaging to improve healing rates of venous ulcers (Robson, Cooper, Aslam, et al., 2006). By far the greatest benefit seen in this VLU trial was the products benefit in patients that had venous leg ulcers with a duration of greater than 1 year.

In addition, Apligraf has also demonstrated efficacy in the treatment of diabetic foot ulcers. In a trial of 208 patients with diabetic neuropathic foot ulcers, Veves, Falanga, Armstrong, et al. (2001) found that 56% of patients treated with Apligraf were healed at 12 weeks vs 38% in the control group, a statistically significant difference ($P = 0.0042$). Apligraf is FDA approved for the treatment of diabetic neuropathic foot ulcers of at least 3 weeks' duration that extend through the dermis without tendon, muscle, joint capsule, or bone exposure and that have not adequately responded to standard care, including debridement, infection control, glucose control, offloading, and assurance of adequate arterial flow.

Like Dermagraft, Apligraf is an adjunct to standard wound care. Apligraf is applied to the wound with the dermal side contacting the wound bed. Many clinicians fenestrate Apligraf with a scalpel before application to allow exudate to pass through it onto bandages because pooled exudate under the product may decrease its efficacy. Once applied, it may be anchored with Steri-strips, staples, or skin adhesive. Negative pressure wound therapy (NPWT) can also be used to not only stabilize the graft to the wound bed but also enhance the direct contact and adherence of these fragile grafts to the wound bed. Apligraf should be covered with a nonadherent contact layer and a secondary bandage of choice. Foam dressings work well over venous ulcers because they absorb exudate and apply local pressure under the compression wrap to keep the Apligraf in good contact with the wound bed. Secondary dressings are changed as needed based on the amount of exudate; the contact layer over the Apligraf can be replaced in 7–10 days, being careful to cleanse the surface without disrupting any attached retained Apligraf. Best practice algorithms guiding the use of Apligraf in the treatment of diabetic foot ulcers and venous leg ulcers have been published (Cavorsi, Vicari, Wirthlin, et al., 2006).

OrCel is a bilayered allogeneic product first developed by an Australian physician in the 1980s to treat his son, who suffered from epidermolysis bullosa. This bilayered cellular matrix is made of human dermal cells (containing neonatal foreskin-derived cultured keratinocytes and fibroblasts) cultured in bovine collagen sponge. Fresh and cryopreserved OrCel is FDA approved under a humanitarian device exemption for the treatment of surgical wounds and donor sites in patients with epidermolysis bullosa undergoing reconstructive hand surgery. In a study of split-thickness autograft donor site treatment in burn patients, donor sites treated with OrCel healed an average of 7 days faster vs treatment with Biobrane-L ($P < 0.0006$) and were ready for recropping for more autografts an average of 5 days faster (Still, Glat, Silverstein, et al., 2003). This has also been used in combination with split-thickness autografts (Eisenberg & Llewelyn, 1998) (see Table 22.2).

Theraskin is a bioactive cryopreserved human skin allograft; harvested from viable donor sites at the time of organ donation.

TABLE 22.2 Dermal and Bilayered CTPs

Trade Name	Description	US FDA-approved indications
Apligraf (Organogenesis Inc., Canton, MA, USA) (see Plate 68)	Allogeneic Bilayered fibroblasts mixed with bovine collagen gel and cultured keratinocytes seeded and cultured on gel 44 cm^2 Delivered fresh Apply dermal side toward wound Five-day shelf life	Venous ulcers over 1-month duration Full-thickness diabetic neuropathic foot ulcers >3 weeks' duration but without tendon, muscle, capsule, or bone exposure Venous/diabetic ulcers
CDS (Cultured Dermal Substitute) (Kitasato University, Japan)	Allogeneic dermal fibroblasts seeded onto two-layered sponge of lyophilized hyaluronic acid and bovine collagen, then cryopreserved	None
Dermagraft (Organogenesis, Canton, MA, USA)	Allogeneic dermal fibroblasts obtained from neonatal foreskin seeded and cultured on bioabsorbable polyglactin mesh for several weeks then cryopreserved; delivered on dry ice 5 × 7.5 cm Apply either side to wound Duration of contact permanent Mimics function of dermis	Nonhealing full-thickness diabetic foot ulcers >6 weeks' duration, extending through dermis, but without tendon, muscle, joint, or bone exposure Ulcers secondary to epidermolysis bullosa
GammaGraft (Promethean LifeSciences, Pittsburgh, PA, USA)	Gamma-irradiated human cadaver skin Stored at room temperature up to 2 years May stay in place until wound heals if it remains adherent to wound bed Left in place while new host skin grows in under dressing Gradually dries out and edges peel away	Chronic wounds and burns
OrCel (Ortec International Inc., New York, NY, USA)	Allogeneic Bilayered fibroblasts seeded on porous side of bovine collagen sponge; keratinocytes seeded on nonporous side Has been used fresh or cryopreserved Duration of contact permanent Mimics cytokine expression of healing skin Nine-month shelf life Cryopreserved; requires cryopreserved storage	Hand reconstruction surgery in patients suffering from recessive dystrophic epidermolysis bullosa and for healing of autograft donor sites in burn patients

Products listed are not inclusive, and other products may be available.

Much like an autograft, Theraskin contains living cells—including fibroblasts and keratinocytes—and takes advantage of their inherent ability to produce cytokines, growth factors, and a native ECM and is indicated in a variety of wound types as long as the underlying wound bed is amenable to providing support (Gurtner, Garcia, Bakewell, & Alarcon, 2019). Multiple studies have demonstrated Theraskin's efficacy in healing wounds of various etiologies; two head-to-head studies showed increased wound healing of venous leg ulcers after application of Theraskin vs Apligraf (DiDomenico, Landsman, Emch, & Landsman, 2011; Towler, Rush, Richardson, & Williams, 2018).

Acellular Extracellular Matrix Scaffolds

Acellular scaffolds (also referred to as acellular dermal replacements) do not contain living cells and thus minimize the risk of an immunologic response (Greaves et al., 2013). Components of these products originate from allogeneic, xenographic, biosynthetic, or synthetic materials. Although most acellular products are commonly referred to as *ECM scaffolds,* those with a synthetic epidermal layer are considered to be bilayer or composites (Table 22.3). The goal in using ECM scaffolds in chronic wound care is to promote rapid healing while minimizing scar tissue formation (Kahn, Beers, & Lentz, 2011). The ideal ECM scaffold provides for host cell attachment and migration of keratinocytes, fibroblasts, endothelial cells, and other cells involved in wound healing. Depending on the signaling that occurs in response to the type of ECM scaffold used, marrow-derived stem cells may be recruited to the area, differentiating into various cell types that manufacture original host tissue instead of scar (Clark, Ghosh, Tonnesen, et al., 2007). Angiogenesis and neovascularization occur as the implanted scaffold is infiltrated by new host tissue the scaffold undergoes controlled degradation. Products such as noncross-linked "simple" collagen-based dressings, which degrade almost immediately, do not last long enough to function as a scaffold for cell ingrowth. Products that have been altered to withstand degradation for many months may elicit a chronic inflammatory response and result in worsened scar tissue formation (Badylak, 2007). Although the goal in the use of ECM scaffolds is the regeneration of architecturally normal tissue, most products available today result in varying degrees of regenerated and repaired (scarred) tissue. There is a continuum of the biologic effect of the wound of engraftment which may be interpreted as a modulatory effect on the wound to a more structural or template effect on the wound; these are usually but not directly proportional to the number of times the ECM must be applied to the wound.

The products presented here are used primarily for wound management. Many may also be used for surgical indications such as hernia repair, breast reconstruction, and other reconstructive surgeries. However, it is not within the prevue of this chapter to discuss these products may also be used for surgical indications such as hernia repair, breast reconstruction, and other reconstructive surgeries.

TABLE 22.3 Acellular ECM Scaffolds

Trade Name	Description	US FDA-Approved Indications
AlloDerm (LifeCell Inc., Woodlands, TX, USA)	Allogeneic Derived from cadaveric human skin from tissue banks Epidermis and all cellular components removed, leaving dermal matrix Freeze-dried; rehydrate to use Contains intact collagen fibers to support ingrowth of new tissue, elastin filaments to provide strength, and hyaluronan and proteoglycans for cell attachment and migration Duration of contact permanent Two-year shelf life Lacks cellular components	Burns, traumatic, or oncologic wounds with deep structure exposure, hernia repair, breast, and other tissue reconstruction
Cymetra (LifeCell)	Allogeneic injectable micronized particulate form of AlloDerm Dry form, packaged in syringe, rehydrated before use with either normal saline or lidocaine for injection	Cosmetic soft tissue augmentation and treatment of vocal cord paralysis by injection laryngoplasty
GraftJacket Regenerative Tissue Matrix (Wright Medical Technology, Inc., Arlington, TN, USA) (licensed to KCI USA, Inc.)	Allogeneic Same as AlloDerm, but meshed 1:1 to allow wound exudate to pass through; available in two sizes (4 × 4 cm and 4 × 8 cm) and one thickness (0.4–0.8 mm) for chronic wound care Available nonmeshed and thicker for tendon and ligament repair	Diabetic foot ulcers and other chronic wounds, ligament and tendon repair

Continued

TABLE 22.3   Acellular ECM Scaffolds—cont'd

Trade Name	Description	US FDA-Approved Indications
EZ Derm (Molnlycke Health Care, US, LLC, Norcross, GA, USA)	Porcine-derived xenograft (nonhuman skin graft) of collagen that has been chemically cross-linked with aldehyde to provide strength and durability Relatively long shelf life Potential immune response and/or disease transmission	Partial-thickness burns, venous ulcers, diabetic ulcers, pressure injuries
GraftJacket Xpress (Wright Medical Technology Inc., Arlington, TN, USA) (licensed to KCI USA, Inc.)	Allogeneic Same as Cymetra Available in a prefilled 5-cc syringe Once rehydrated, is injected to fill the entire dead space of a sinus tract or deep wound	Deep wounds, tunnels, or sinus tracts
DermaMatrix (Synthes CMF, West Chester, PA, USA)	Allogeneic Cadaver human skin from tissue banks Donor skin is processed to remove all cellular components, including epidermis, and then is freeze dried Rehydrate to use	Similar to indications for AlloDerm: soft tissue repair, breast reconstruction, abdominal hernia repair, head and neck reconstruction
Biovance (Alliqua Biomedical, Langhorn, PA, USA)	Allogeneic Derived from the placenta of a healthy, full-term human pregnancy Supplied as a single dehydrated sterile sheet to be applied and secured to a clean wound followed by a secondary, nonadherent dressing Five-year shelf life Store at room temperature Contains no antigens	Acute and chronic wounds
Oasis Matrix (Smith & Nephew Inc., FL, USA; Advanced Tissue Sciences Inc., La Jolla, CA, USA)	Xenographic and acellular Porcine small intestinal submucosa (SIS) with complex matrix of collagen, glycosaminoglycans, proteoglycans, cell adhesive glycoproteins, and growth factors; freeze dried Available in multiple sizes, fenestrated, or meshed Acts as a wound covering One-and-a-half-year shelf life Potential immune response	Partial- and full-thickness wounds, chronic ulcers, traumatic wounds, superficial and second-degree burns, surgical wounds
MatriStem (ACell Inc., Columbia, MD, USA)	Xenographic porcine urinary bladder matrix (UBM) with intact basement membrane; composed of collagen matrix, glycosaminoglycans, glycoproteins, and proteoglycans Available as fenestrated sheets of variable sizes or as powder Must be rehydrated before use and cut to size of wound	Partial- and full-thickness wounds, traumatic wounds, surgical wounds, chronic wounds
PriMatrix (TEI Biosciences, Boston, MA, USA)	Xenographic fetal bovine dermis that has been decellularized, freeze dried, and sterilized Must be rehydrated Available nonfenestrated in various sizes and thicknesses Must fenestrate for high-exudative wounds	Skin ulcers, second-degree burns, surgical wounds

TABLE 22.3 Acellular ECM Scaffolds—cont'd

Trade Name	Description	US FDA-Approved Indications
Xelma (Mölnlycke, Göteborg, Sweden)	Xenographic Consists of amelogenin proteins derived from the enamel matrix of developing porcine teeth, mixed with propylene glycol alginate and water Administered as a gel Promotes cell migration via ECM and cell adhesion properties	None
MatriDerm (Dr. Suwelack Skin & Health Care, Billerbeck, Germany)	Xenographic Engineered three-dimensional matrix consisting of native structured collagen from bovine dermis and elastin from bovine nuchal ligament Available in three sizes with 1- or 2-mm thickness, based on grafting needs of wound	None
Biobrane (UDL Laboratories, Sugar Land, TX, USA)	Biosynthetic very thin sheet of semipermeable silicone bonded to a knitted trifilament nylon or monofilament nylon (Biobrane-L) coated with Type I porcine collagen, which creates hydrophilic coating that facilitates adherence to wound Silicone membrane has water vapor loss rate similar to that of intact skin; once Biobrane has adhered to a wound, it provides moist, protected environment that minimizes water loss	Partial-thickness burns, skin graft donor sites, superficial wounds after surgery, laser resurfacing, dermabrasion Lesions secondary to toxic epidermal necrolysis and pemphigus, as coverage for chronic wounds
Integra (Integra LifeSciences Corp., Plainsboro, NJ, USA)	Bilayered (two layers) membrane system made of a porous matrix of fibers that cross-link bovine tendon collagen and glycosaminoglycan The epidermal substitute layer is made of a thin polysilicone layer to control moisture Duration of contact permanent Moderate shelf life Operative removal of silicone layer required	Deep partial- or full-thickness burns, contracture release procedures, reconstructive surgery of complex wounds and surgical defects
Hyalomatrix PA (Fidia Anika Therapeutics Inc., Bedford, MA, USA)	Synthetic Bilayered with thin moisture vapor-permeable silicone sheet adhered to nonwoven pad composed of the benzyl ester of hyaluronic acid (Hyaff-11) Provides matrix for cell migration, and silicone maintains protected moist environment	Most chronic wounds, partial- and full-thickness burns, surgical wounds, traumatic wounds Widely used in Europe
Suprathel (BioMed Sciences, Allentown, PA, USA)	Synthetic epidermal substitute composed of copolymer of polylactide, trimethylene carbonate, and ε-caprolactone Completely dissolves within 4 weeks	Used in Germany since 2004 for deep partial-thickness burns, superficial full-thickness burns, skin graft donor sites, abrasions, scar revision

Products listed are not inclusive and other products may be available.
ECM, extracellular matrix.

Allogeneic ECM Scaffolds

AlloDerm is an acellular dermal matrix derived from cadaveric human skin. It has a distinct basement membrane side and a dermal side. It is used to serve as a scaffold for normal tissue remodeling. The collagen framework provides strength to the skin and contains no cells that can cause rejection or irritation. AlloDerm is available in multiple sizes and thicknesses. The orientation of AlloDerm into a defect and the thickness chosen to depend on what is being treated (e.g., hernia vs soft tissue defect); therefore, the package insert should be checked for application instructions. AlloDerm has been studied for treatment of multiple surgical defects and wound repair procedures. No randomized controlled trials have examined the use of AlloDerm in chronic wound care. In a recent report describing AlloDerm use in over 200 patients with chronic wounds, the majority of patients treated with wide debridement, NPWT and AlloDerm, required an intermediate procedure (i.e., further debridement prior to skin grafting) when compared with using products such as Fetal Bovine Dermis (Lantis & Polanco, 2016).

Allopatch is an allograft dermal matrix constructed from donated human dermis that is subsequently processed to remove dermal cells prior to packaging in an ethanol solution. During the manufacturing process, the tissue undergoes removal of the epidermis while the underlying ECM remains present. As is common for dermal ECMs, it supports cellular migration, proliferation, and neovascularization via architectural scaffolding.

Cymetra is an injectable, micronized particulate form of AlloDerm. Only case reports and case series on the use of Cymetra in chronic wounds unresponsive to conventional therapy have been published. Although these cases are interesting and appear to indicate that Cymetra stimulates healing in chronic ulcers, no randomized controlled trials have compared this product to standard care in the treatment of chronic wounds. Therefore, no strong conclusions regarding its efficacy can be made.

GraftJacket regenerative tissue matrix is very similar in composition as AlloDerm. Unlike AlloDerm, however, GraftJacket is meshed and is available in only two sizes and one thickness for chronic wound care. GraftJacket is applied to clean, debrided ulcers with the dermal reticular side against the wound bed. It should cover the entire wound and be sutured or stapled in place. GraftJacket must be kept moist with mineral oil-soaked gauze packing, which is used to ensure that the product does not dry out and maintains good contact with the wound base. The dressing is left in place for 5 days without being disturbed and then changed every 3–5 days after that. Two small pilot studies have demonstrated enhanced healing of diabetic foot ulcers compared with control (Brigido, 2006; Brigido, Boc, & Lopez, 2004). A study of 86 patients with diabetic foot ulcers demonstrated complete healing at 12 weeks in 67% of patients treated with GraftJacket vs 46% in the control group, a statistically significant difference ($P = 0.03$) (Reyzelman, Crews, Moore, et al., 2009). More recently, a pooled analysis of three prospective clinical trials involving a total of 154 patients with lower extremity diabetic foot ulcers receiving application of GraftJacket, had a statistically significant reduction in mean healing time of 1.7 weeks compared with standard of care (Reyzelman & Bazarov, 2015).

Graft Jacket Xpress is described as a flowable soft tissue scaffold (Williams & Holewinski, 2015). It is processed by LifeCell for Wright Medical and is marketed for the treatment of wounds with depth and/or tunneling. The cover dressing should maintain a moist environment and apply gentle pressure to keep the matrix in place. It should be left in place for 3–5 days and then changed as needed to manage exudate. No randomized controlled trials have examined the use of GraftJacket Xpress in the treatment of chronic wounds, but case series using a combination of GraftJacket Xpress with GraftJacket have shown encouraging results for healing of wounds with tunneling (Williams & Holewinski, 2015). It

should be noted that "flowable" technologies, which are in general quite efficacious, thus far have no reimbursement strategy outside the operating room in the current (2020) US reimbursement strategy.

Dermal and Bilayered Cellular- and Tissue-Based Products: Nonliving Cellular

Cadaveric human skin has been used for years as temporary wound coverage in burn care (Britton-Byrd, Lynch, Williamson, et al., 2008; Kagan, Robb, & Plessinger, 2005). This nonliving product facilitates the short-term coverage of large tissue defects when autografts are not yet available, leading to reduced loss of fluid, electrolytes, and protein; decreased risk of infection; decreased wound desiccation and pain; and improved success of later autografting. One disadvantage of using cadaveric skin is the possibility of disease transmission, despite donor screening regulations by the FDA and quality control standards developed by the American Association of Tissue Banks (Humphries & Mansavage, 2006). Another disadvantage is the fact that the host rejects cadaveric skin within 2–4 weeks. Cadaveric human skin is available fresh (used within 14 days of harvesting), cryopreserved (stored in a freezer for 3–6 months or in liquid nitrogen for up to 10 years), or irradiated (stored at room temperature).

GammaGraft is gamma-irradiated human cadaver skin that provides wound coverage for chronic wounds or burns. It can remain in place until the wound is healed, depending on wound size and depth of tissue damage. GammaGraft is placed on a clean, debrided wound that is free of infection and is covered with a nonadherent dressing for 1–2 days. At that time, the graft should be adherent to the wound base. If the graft is not adherent, the wound may be infected and the graft should be removed. If GammaGraft is adherent, it should be left uncovered; it will dry out and appear much like a scab. It is left in place while new host skin covers the wound underneath. As the wound heals, the edges of the GammaGraft will peel away and can be cut off. Treatment of the underlying wound etiology, utilizing techniques such as compression for edema or offloading for pressure redistribution, must be continued throughout the treatment period. GammaGraft may be used on any chronic wound. However, although there are case reports of GammaGraft use in chronic wounds (Rosales, Bruntz, & Armstrong, 2004), no randomized controlled trials have demonstrated the efficacy of this product in wound healing compared with standard care.

Xenographic Extracellular Matrix Scaffolds

Oasis Wound Matrix is the 510K predicate product in the United States for almost all Xenograft ECM products. It is derived from porcine small intestinal submucosa, which was originally intended to be used for vascular (aortic) replacement. It has been examined in numerous preclinical studies; in the clinical treatment of soft tissue defects, wounds, and hernias; and in urologic, gynecologic, and orthopedic reconstructive surgeries (Badylak, 2007; Cook Biotech, 2010; Hodde, Ernst, & Hiles, 2005). In a prospective randomized controlled trial, 55% of 120 patients with venous ulcers healed at 12 weeks compared with 34% in the control group ($P < 0.02$) (Mostow, Haraway, Dalsing, et al., 2005). In clinical practice, Oasis acts as a very active easily incorporated wound covering. It should be applied to clean, debrided wounds that are free of infection; cut slightly larger than the wound; secured with Steri-strips, glue, staples, or sutures; and then moistened with normal saline. A nonadherent contact layer is then applied, and the cover dressing is based on the amount of exudate. Foam dressings work well to absorb exudate and provide local compression to maintain good contact of Oasis to the wound bed. Secondary dressings may be changed as needed, but any remnants of Oasis, which may appear as an amber gelatinous material in the wound, should be left undisturbed. Additional Oasis can be reapplied weekly as needed. In review of most papers 5–8 applications of the product are necessary. It exists in a single- and three-layer form. Unfortunately, in the current CMS wound care dressing policy, this product is placed in the lower reimbursement category and is therefore being used much less than it should be in the outpatient wound care setting.

Cytal Wound Matrix is comprised of Acell's proprietary MatriStem UBM technology and derived from porcine urinary bladder. Although animal studies indicate potential for this product to stimulate tissue regeneration (Gilbert, Nieponice, Spievack, et al., 2008; Nieponice, Gilbert, & Badylak, 2006), and it has been used with burns (Ryssel, Gazyakan, Germann, et al., 2008) and necrotizing fasciitis defects (Ryssel, Germann, Czermak, et al., 2010), additional clinical trials in chronic wounds are needed to establish efficacy. That being said, a 2013 case report investigated MatriStem's use in the healing of recalcitrant nonhealing radiation-induced wounds with complete wound closure demonstrated in the three patients presented (Rommer, Peric, & Wong, 2013). Also, in 2017, a prospective single-center study evaluating Cytal in diabetic foot ulcers in 17 patients showed that UBM, in addition to adequate offloading, could significantly shorten wound-healing time (Alvarez et al., 2017). In general, MatriStem was actually developed by a large state academic facility in the United States which also developed Oasis, however it has been commercially held by a company that engages in less prospective randomized data than *Oasis*.

PriMatrix is derived from fetal bovine dermis and is processed to preserve the natural structure and biologic properties of its native collagen. It should be applied with either side down to clean, debrided wounds, with a 1-mm overlap onto surrounding skin, and then secured with the clinician's choice of fixation. It can be fenestrated for exudative wounds. After application, PriMatrix should be covered with a nonadherent contact layer and then moist dressings, based on the amount of exudate. A prospective multicenter study led by the Mayo Clinic examined the use of PriMatrix in 55 patients with chronic diabetic foot ulcerations. At 12 weeks, an average of 76% of patients had wound closure; average time to healing was 7.5 weeks and 2 applications (Kavros et al., 2014). A retrospective study of "hard to heal" venous leg ulcers by the senior author and colleagues, has shown very favorable healing characteristics (Yang, Polanco, & Lantis, 2016).

EZ Derm is a porcine xenograft that has been used for years for temporary coverage of burns, surgical wounds, and partial- and full-thickness wounds of variable etiologies (Davis & Arpey, 2000). It is applied to freshly debrided wounds and is left in place until it sloughs, usually 1–2 weeks. During that period, the underlying tissue granulates, and potentially upon removal of the xenograft, a split-thickness skin graft can be applied. No large randomized controlled trials have demonstrated the efficacy of EZ Derm in chronic wounds, but multiple studies have demonstrated its robustness in the care of burn wounds (Burkey, Davis, & Glat, 2016; Troy et al., 2013).

Excellagen is an ECM made of a purified fibrillar bovine Type I collagen. It comes as a flowable, conformable, gel that is indicated in many types of wounds—including chronic ulcers, surgical wounds, and traumatic wounds, partial or full thickness. The provision of an ECM scaffold allows for increased rates of granulation in the wound bed via cellular migration and proliferation, as well as platelet activation and theoretical increases in PDGF (Chandler et al., 2020). Multiple case studies have demonstrated Excellagen's use in wound closure, with some chronic wounds completely closing within 4 weeks. It may also be used in conjunction with compression dressings in venous ulcerations; reapplication of Excellagen in the wound bed may be performed as necessary.

Biosynthetic Extracellular Matrix Scaffolds

Biobrane consists of a very thin sheet of semipermeable silicone bonded to nylon fabric. It has been used for over 25 years in the treatment of superficial burns as a biosynthetic wound dressing and has good data supporting its use for this indication (Whitaker, Prowse, & Potokar, 2008). Because of its ease of use, Biobrane may be particularly useful in pediatric burn care (Mandal, 2007). Ongoing studies in its efficacy in pediatric wound care are currently being performed (BRACS trial).

Biobrane should be applied to freshly debrided, noninfected wounds with the dull fabric side down and then secured with staples, sutures, or tape. It should be covered firmly with a gauze bolster to prevent movement of the dressing for 24–36 h. The gauze dressing should be removed at 24–36 h for assessment and again at 48–72 h. Adherence of Biobrane to the wound bed is the goal. After 72 h, if the Biobrane is loose or fluid or purulence is present under the dressing, the Biobrane may need to be removed, the tissue debrided, and a new piece of Biobrane applied, if no infection is present. Once there is good adherence, after 3 days, the secondary dressings can be removed, and the patient may be able to resume normal activity and bathing as desired. Biobrane should be removed once the underlying tissue is healed, typically 7–14 days later. Removal should be delayed if excessive pain or bleeding occurs when attempting to take the Biobrane off an apparently healed area. Further studies are needed before wide use of Biobrane can be recommended in chronic wound care.

Kerecis Omega3 intact fishskin is an acellular dermal matrix rich in Omega-3 fatty acids derived from fish skin (North Atlantic Cod), approved by the FDA in 2013 for the treatment of wounds—including diabetic foot ulcers; burns, pressure injuries, and venous leg ulcers (Michael, Winters, & Khan, 2019). A notable advantage of piscine vs mammalian xenografts stems from the fish skin's inherent resistance to the transmission of disease to a human host. Therefore, the sterilization process differs from that of mammalian sources, not requiring harsh detergents, which allows for the retention of more lipid cells and thus a more robust source of Omega-3 fatty acids. The presence of Omega-3 fatty acids downregulate the production of proinflammatory cascades, can remove the wound from a chronic inflammatory state, as well as modulates the inflammatory response in human keratinocytes. Ongoing investigations into dosing are being performed, but currently multiple reapplications of the product may be utilized. Multiple studies have demonstrated potential increased wound healing in chronic wounds, including diabetic foot ulcers. One retrospective single-center study examined 51 patients with 58 diabetic foot ulcers status postapplication of acellular fish skin dermal matrix followed until wound closure or 16 weeks. Overall, 35 of 58 wound had closure, and mean reduction in wound size was 87.5%. Patients received, on average, 4 applications of the product during their 16 weeks of follow-up (Michael et al., 2019).

Integra Dermal Regeneration Template (IDRT) is a bilayered product composed of an outer semipermeable silicone sheet and an inner ECM scaffold. The outer layer provides protection from bacterial invasion and significant fluid loss. The inner layer facilitates cell migration and tissue ingrowth, which leads to dermal regeneration, usually within 2–3 weeks of application. It was designed in the 1990s as a burn dressing but has become a "go to" product for large degloving injuries, and traumatic injuries. This product is designed to degrade as the neodermis develops. Once the new dermis is present, the silicone layer is removed and a very thin autograft can be applied, if required. It appears for wounds under 4 cm^2 that autografting is not typically necessary. However, wounds between 4 and 10 cm^2 this is variable. For those greater than 40 cm^2 a reepithelialization strategy is needed. There are multiple observational studies of IDRT for atypical wounds and in comparison, to local flaps and standard of care. While there are no randomized controlled trials of IDRT as named in chronic wounds, for almost inexplicable reasons, none of them clinical nor legitimate, Integra (Princeton, NJ) renamed their IDRT product and studied it in an elegant outpatient study (Driver et al., 2015). *Integra Omnigraft* is IDRT—the exact same product that is available in the operating room; bilayer silicone and bovine collagen ECM scaffold marketed in chronic wound care largely for diabetic foot ulcers. In the outpatient setting this product is only available in 7 and 4 cm^2 sizes, and at almost half the cost of the inpatient product. As for the inpatient product the wound must be thoroughly debrided to achieve achieved before application of Omnigraft. The product is rinsed in normal saline for 1–2 min before application and applied to the wound bed with the ECM side down. All air bubbles and wrinkles should be eliminated from the dressing to achieve intimate contact of the product with the wound. It then should be secured with either staples or sutures. The secondary dressing may include bolstering if necessary, to insure contact of the product with the underlying wound bed. In the inpatient setting the product is available in a fenestrated form, in the outpatient setting it is not available in that form and we tend to recommend fenestration with a 15 blade prior to application. It is not uncommon to use NPWT in the inpatient setting. In the outpatient setting, the product can only be used for Wagner 1 and 2 diabetic foot ulcers, therefore applied with a foam bolster and patellar weight bearing brace. Generally, the matrix will be completely vascularized in about 3 weeks. At this point, the silicone can be removed and if needed, an autograft can be applied. That being said, the underlying wound may completely heal within 3–4 weeks. As healing progresses, the silicone portion of the product will loosen and can be removed. *Integra Matrix Wound Dressing* is the ECM without the second layer of silicone coverage and is used alone or with IDRT for deeper wounds. *Integra Flowable Wound Matrix* has the same core composition as the aforementioned Integra products; however, the ECM is provided in a syringe as dry granules that require hydration with saline before use. It has the same indications as Omnigraft, but its use focuses on application to wounds with deep tunneling or undermining. It is available for one-time use in a 3-cc syringe. It is injected directly into wounds with depth or undermining until the wound is filled and then is covered with a dressing of choice to hold the matrix in place and absorb exudate. Dressing change frequency is based on the amount of exudate. A prospective clinical study in 2015 demonstrated that tunneled and/or undermined wounds may be particularly well served by application of Integra Flowable Matrix; of the 18 patients treated, 14 of which were chronic wounds, all but 1 patient experienced wound closure (Campitiello, Della Corte, Guerniero, & Canonico, 2015). The senior author has considerable anecdotal experience filling wounds up to 15 cm^3 with flowable matrix.

Hyalomatrix PA is a bilayered product consisting of a thin moisture vapor-permeable silicone sheet adhered to a nonwoven pad composed entirely of the benzyl ester of hyaluronic acid (Hyaff-11). It does not contain any animal-derived products. When the Hyaff-11 contacts the wound bed, it provides a scaffold for cell attachment and migration, and the silicone backing maintains a moist wound bed and protects against bacterial contamination (Price, Das-Gupta, Leigh, et al., 2006). The Hyaff-11 degrades over time as host tissue infiltrates the matrix. Case series have been published on the use of Hyalomatrix PA in deep partial-thickness burns and diabetic foot ulcers (Caravaggi, Sganzaroli, Pogliaghi, et al., 2009; Gravante, Delogu, Giordan, et al., 2007). It is intended for one-time use and is indicated for the treatment of most chronic wounds, partial- and full-thickness burns, surgical wounds, and traumatic wounds.

Novosorb Biodegradable Temporizing Matrix is a fully synthetic bilayer product comprised of a dermal layer made of porous 2 mm thick biodegradable polyurethane foam as well as an epidermal barrier layer in the form of a nonbiodegradable polyurethane sealing membrane, adhered together. Novosorb BTM has been indicated in management of an array of wound types, including chronic ulcers, surgical wounds, traumatic wounds, and burns. Novosorb BTM may be applied to large wound surface areas and fixation is commonly with staples. After 2–3 weeks of integration, the superficial barrier layer may be removed leaving behind a neovascular dermal layer. Closure method via STSG or other methods are at the clinician's judgment. The Novosorb wound matrix fully dissolves over a period of approximately 18 months (Wagstaff et al., 2015). In 2018, a study of Novosorb BTM in significant burn wounds (20%–50% TBSA full-thickness burns) demonstrated its efficacy: 5 study subjects had over 120% TBSA in wounds covered with BTM. It was left intact for 7 weeks prior to secondary grafting. BTM failed to adhere/integrate into <7% of TBSA, and secondary graft take over BTM was described as rapid with minimal need for regrafting (Greenwood, Schmitt, & Wagstaff, 2018).

Cryopreserved Umbilical Cord/Amniotic Membrane Matrix

Placental derived amnion/chorion and/or umbilical cord based wound care products have become a significant focus of novel wound care product development. Interest and use of amniotic membrane have been recorded as remotely as 1910 for tissue transplantation. In the later 20th century, it was notable in the field of ophthalmic surgery, as inherent properties of potentially scar-less healing were investigated. Amniotic membrane is the innermost layer of the fetal membranes and consists of an epithelium, basement membrane, and avascular stroma. The basement membrane contains Type IV, V, and VII collagen, in addition to laminin and fibronectin. The amnion demonstrates antiinflammatory, antifibrotic, immune-privileged, and antimicrobial properties (Malhotra & Jain, 2014). The umbilical cord is composed of amniotic epithelium, three vessels, and a gelatinous substance known as Wharton's Jelly (WJ). This substance, WJ, is a collagenous matrix rich in Hyaluronic Acid and mesenchymal stem cells (Bullard et al., 2019).

In terms of wound-healing products, the amniotic membrane/umbilical cord products tend to be stratified by their composition (isolated AM or UC or combination), and preservation technique (cryopreserved vs dehydrated)—implying an associated presence of living or nonliving cells.

NEOX Cord 1K is a proprietary matrix of cryopreserved umbilical cord and amniotic membrane. The umbilical cord,

during gestation, transports nutrient and oxygen rich blood from the placenta to the fetus. The umbilical cord is composed of three vessels, amnion, and Wharton's Jelly. Due to fetal wound healing with minimal scarring, the inherent composition and wound-healing properties of amniotic membrane (AM) and umbilical cord (UC) have long been of interest, and prior to chronic wound applications were most often being investigated for ophthalmologic procedures. The associated ECM of UC and AM is rich in hyaluronic acid, collagen, mesenchymal stem cells, and a variety of other cytokines and growth factors. Notably, a glycoprotein complex known as HC-HA/PTX3 has been identified, which may be active in the antiinflammatory and antiscarring properties of UC/AM. Like many CTPs, NEOX is applied to the properly debrided wound bed free of active infection, with a secondary dressing placed over the product. Reapplication may be applied if clinically necessary when there is no remaining product left in the wound bed.

Multiple small single-center studies have examined the use of NEOX in chronic wounds. One such retrospective study evaluated 57 patients with 64 chronic wounds, which after application of the product demonstrated an overall wound-healing rate of 79.7% (51 of 64 wounds healed) (Couture, 2016).

Biovance is a dehydrated, acellular, human derived amniotic membrane that provides an ECM for wound-healing processes to occur. Biovance is harvested from placentas of full-term pregnancies, and components include multiple collagens, fibronectin, laminin, GAGs, and proteoglycans. It purports to require no preparation, is bidirectional, and can be stored at room temperature for up to 5 years. Multiple studies have investigated the use of specifically dehydrated amniotic products in wound care, with several showing promising results (Forbes & Fetterolf, 2012).

Similarly, Amnioband is a minimally processed dehydrated allograft that undergoes MTF Biologics proprietary aseptic processing methods in order to retain an intact ECM. It is also flexible, able to be stored at ambient temperatures for up to 3 years, and available in multiple sizes.

CLINICAL CONSULT

A: Referral received for a 50-year-old female with diabetes who has an ulcer on the dorsal surface of her right foot. Moderate Charcot deformity present. The wound bed is not grossly infected, yet it has failed to close with serial debridements. The patient has an insensate foot; she is able to detect 2/9 points with monofilament testing. Her assessed ABI is 0.8. The wound bed is mostly clean, with presence of healthy granulation tissue under fibrinous slough. Palpable metatarsal head directly underlying the wound bed. Pressure points also noted surrounding ulceration due to a poorly fitted shoe and last appointment with orthotic specialist was 8 months ago. HbA1c is 5.6 indicating good glycemic control. No pedal or lower leg edema.

D: Nonhealing foot ulcer due to repetitive internal and external pressure related stresses in a patient with DM2. Level 1 LEAP risk category and high-risk diabetes due to absence of sensation in foot. Circulation in foot adequate for healing.

P: Plan for OR for wound bed debridement and internal offloading through associated metatarsal head bony resection. Will also plan for placement of bilayer acellular CTP with silicone and bovine collagen components; placement of temporary negative pressure wound therapy.

I: (1) Procedure will be explained patient scheduled for elective OR. (2) Procedure consent will be obtained. (3) Patient to OR for aforementioned debridement. (4) Patient to remain on temporary bed rest for 4 days at which time negative pressure wound therapy will be removed and wound assessed. (5) Patient to work with physical therapy to assess needs. (6) Continued glucose control

E: Return to clinic at 10–14 days for evaluation and if appropriate fixation removal of the silicone sheet component of the CTP. In addition to standard wound care, continued offloading imperative: arrange for appropriate offloading orthotic shoe to manage external pressure relief.

SUMMARY

- Standard wound care including light debridement, wet to dry dressing changes, and infection control may be inadequate for some chronic hard-to-heal wounds.
- When a wound does not heal appropriately or within a timely manner, despite optimal care and treatment, advanced modalities such as application of a cellular- and tissue-based product may be indicated.
- Clinicians should be knowledgeable about the variety of products available on the market, how the products function, its proper application and secondary dressing, and frequency of reapplication.

- Clinicians should also be aware of any patient moral, ethical, or religious implications of products due to their manufacturing and/or tissue source.
- Although many of these products would benefit from additional scientifically rigorous clinical studies, many of them, when used within the context of proper standard of care, have demonstrated potential efficacy in healing chronic wounds.

SELF-ASSESSMENT QUESTIONS

1. Which of the following statements about cellular- and tissue-based products (CTPs) best describes them?
   a. All CTPs provide an extracellular matrix (ECM).
   b. All CTPs provide growth factors.
   c. All CTPs are derived from animal sources.
   d. All CTPs mimic aspects of native tissues to promote healing.
2. Acellular CTPs are designed to:
   a. deliver living cells to the wound bed
   b. replace the need for a split-thickness skin graft
   c. function as an extracellular matrix (ECM) scaffold
   d. provide a dermal and epidermal covering
3. Which CTP is derived from the patient's own body?
   a. autologous
   b. allogeneic
   c. xenographic
   d. biosynthetic (biologic and manufactured materials)

4. Which CTP is derived from humans other than the patient?
   a. autologous
   b. allogeneic
   c. xenographic
   d. biosynthetic
5. Living bilayered CTPs provide:
   a. keratinocytes and fibroblasts
   b. blood vessels and fibroblasts
   c. melanocytes and keratinocytes
   d. macrophages and blood vessels
6. True or False: Allogeneic cell-based CTPs are temporary and biodegradable.
7. List at least three essential steps to using CTPs successfully.

REFERENCES

Ågren, M. S., & Werthén, M. (2007). The extracellular matrix in wound healing: A closer look at therapeutics for chronic wounds. *The International Journal of Lower Extremity Wounds, 6,* 82–97.

Alvarez, O. M., Smith, T., Gilbert, T. W., Onumah, N. J., Wendelken, M. E., Parker, R., et al. (2017). Diabetic foot ulcers treated with porcine urinary bladder extracellular matrix and total contact cast: Interim analysis of a randomized, controlled trial. *Wounds, 29*(5), 140–146.

Badylak, S. F. (2007). The extracellular matrix as a biologic scaffold material. *Biomaterials, 28,* 3587–3593.

Brigido, S. A. (2006). The use of an acellular dermal regenerative tissue matrix in the treatment of lower extremity wounds: A prospective 16-week pilot study. *International Wound Journal, 3,* 181–187.

Brigido, S. A., Boc, S. F., & Lopez, R. C. (2004). Effective management of major lower extremity wounds using an acellular regenerative tissue matrix: A pilot study. *Orthopedics, 27,* 145–149.

Britton-Byrd, B. W., Lynch, J. P., Williamson, S., et al. (2008). Early use of allograft skin: Are 3-day microbiologic cultures safe? *The Journal of Trauma, 64,* 816–818.

Bullard, J. D., Lei, J., Lim, J. J., Massee, M., Fallon, A. M., & Koob, T. J. (2019). Evaluation of dehydrated human umbilical cord biological properties for wound care and soft tissue healing. *Journal of Biomedical Materials Research. Part B: Applied Biomaterials, 107*(4), 1035–1046.

Burkey, B., Davis, W., & Glat, P. M. (2016). Porcine xenograft treatment of superficial partial thickness burns in paediatric patients. *Journal of Wound Care, 25*(2), S10–S15.

Campitiello, F., Della Corte, A., Guerniero, R., & Canonico, S. (2015). Efficacy of a new flowable wound matrix in tunneled and cavity ulcers: A preliminary report. *Wounds, 27*(6), 152–157.

Caravaggi, C., Sganzaroli, A. B., Pogliaghi, I., et al. (2009). Safety and efficacy of a dermal substitute in the coverage of cancellous bone after surgical debridement for severe diabetic foot ulceration. *EWMA Journal, 9,* 19–22.

Catalano, E., Cochis, A., Varoni, E., et al. (2013). Tissue-engineered skin substitutes: An overview. *Journal of Artificial Organs, 16,* 397–403.

Cavorsi, J., Vicari, F., Wirthlin, D. J., et al. (2006). Best-practice algorithms for the use of a bilayered living cell therapy (Apligraf) in the treatment of lower-extremity ulcers. *Wound Repair and Regeneration, 14,* 102–109.

Chandler, L. A., Alvarez, O. M., Blume, P. A., Kim, P. J., Kirsner, R. S., Lantis, J. C., et al. (2020). Wound conforming matrix containing purified homogenate of dermal collagen promotes healing of diabetic neuropathic foot ulcers: Comparative analysis versus standard of care. *Advances in Wound Care, 9*(2), 61–67.

Clark, R. A., Ghosh, K., Tonnesen, M. G., et al. (2007). Tissue engineering for cutaneous wounds. *The Journal of Investigative Dermatology, 127,* 1018–1029.

Cook Biotech. (2010). Lafayette, Indiana, United States. https://www.cookbiotech.com/products/.

Couture, M. (2016). A single-center, retrospective study of cryopreserved umbilical cord for wound healing in patients suffering from chronic wounds of the foot and ankle. *Wounds, 28*(7), 217–225.

Davis, D. A., & Arpey, C. J. (2000). Porcine heterografts in dermatologic surgery and reconstruction. *Dermatologic Surgery, 26,* 76–80.

DiDomenico, L., Landsman, A. R., Emch, K. J., & Landsman, A. (2011). A prospective comparison of diabetic foot ulcers treated with either a cryopreserved skin allograft or a bioengineered skin substitute. *Wounds, 23*(7), 184–189. PMID: 25879172.

Driver, V. R., Lavery, L. A., Reyzelman, A. M., Dutra, T. G., Dove, C. R., Kotsis, S. V., et al. (2015). A clinical trial of Integra Template for diabetic foot ulcer treatment. *Wound Repair and Regeneration, 23*(6), 891–900.

Eisenberg, M., & Llewelyn, D. (1998). Surgical management of hands in children with recessive dystrophic epidermolysis bullosa: Use of allogeneic composite cultured skin grafts. *British Journal of Plastic Surgery, 51,* 608–613.

Falanga, V., Margolis, D., Alvarez, O., et al. (1998). Rapid healing of venous ulcers and lack of clinical rejection with an allogeneic cultured human skin equivalent. *Archives of Dermatology, 134,* 293–300.

Falanga, V., & Sabolinski, M. (1999). A bilayered living skin construct (Apligraf) accelerates complete closure of hard-to-heal venous ulcers. *Wound Repair and Regeneration, 7,* 201–207.

Forbes, J., & Fetterolf, D. (2012). Dehydrated amniotic membrane allografts for the treatment of chronic wounds: A case series. *Journal of Wound Care, 21*(6), 290–296.

Gilbert, T. W., Nieponice, A., Spievack, A. R., et al. (2008). Repair of the thoracic wall with an extracellular matrix scaffold in a canine model. *The Journal of Surgical Research, 147,* 61–67.

Gravante, G., Delogu, D., Giordan, N., et al. (2007). The use of Hyalomatrix PA in the treatment of deep partial-thickness burns. *Journal of Burn Care & Research, 28,* 269–274.

Greaves, N., Iqbal, S. A., Baguneid, M., et al. (2013). The role of skin substitutes in the management of chronic cutaneous wounds. *Wound Repair and Regeneration, 21,* 194–210.

Greenwood, J. E., Schmitt, B. J., & Wagstaff, M. J. (2018). Experience with a synthetic bilayer biodegradable temporising matrix in significant burn injury. *Burns Open, 2*(1), 17–34.

Griffiths, M., Ojeh, N., Livingstone, R., et al. (2004). Survival of Apligraf in acute human wounds. *Tissue Engineering, 10,* 1180–1195.

Gurtner, G. C., Garcia, A. D., Bakewell, K., & Alarcon, J. B. (2019). A retrospective matched-cohort study of 3994 lower extremity wounds of multiple etiologies across 644 institutions comparing a bioactive human skin allograft, TheraSkin, plus standard of care, to standard of care alone. *International Wound Journal, 17*(1), 55–64.

Harding, K., Sumner, M., & Cardinal, M. (2013). A prospective, multicentre, randomised controlled study of human fibroblast-derived dermal substitute (Dermagraft) in patients with venous leg ulcers. *International Wound Journal, 10*(2), 132–137. https://doi.org/10.1111/iwj.12053.

Hashimoto, K. (2000). Regulation of keratinocyte function by growth factors. *Journal of Dermatological Science, 24,* S46–S50.

Hodde, J. P., Ernst, D. M., & Hiles, M. C. (2005). An investigation of the long-term bioactivity of endogenous growth factor in OASIS Wound Matrix. *Journal of Wound Care, 14,* 23–25.

Humphries, L. K., & Mansavage, V. L. (2006). Quality control in tissue banking-ensuring the safety of allograft tissues. *AORN Journal, 84,* 385–398.

Jang, J. C., Choi, R. J., Han, S. K., et al. (2015). Effect of fibroblast-seeded artificial dermis on wound healing. *Annals of Plastic Surgery, 74*(4), 501–507.

Kagan, R. J., Robb, E. C., & Plessinger, R. T. (2005). Human skin banking. *Clinics in Laboratory Medicine, 25,* 587–605.

Kahn, S., Beers, R. J., & Lentz, C. W. (2011). Use of acellular dermal replacement in reconstruction of nonhealing lower extremity wounds. *Journal of Burn Care & Research, 32*(1), 124–128.

Kavros, S. J., Dutra, T., Gonzalez-Cruz, R., Liden, B., Marcus, B., Mcguire, J., et al. (2014). The use of PriMatrix, a fetal bovine acellular dermal matrix, in healing chronic diabetic foot ulcers. *Advances in Skin & Wound Care, 27*(8), 356–362.

Lantis, J. C., & Polanco, T. O. (2016). Tissue generation with acellular dermal collagen matrices: Clinical comparison of human and fetal bovine matrices. In *9th Symposium on biologic scaffolds for regenerative medicine, Napa, California, April 28–30.*

Lavery, L. A., Davis, K. E., Berriman, S. J., Braun, L., Nichols, A., Kim, P. J., et al. (2016). WHS guidelines update: Diabetic foot ulcer treatment guidelines. *Wound Repair and Regeneration, 24*(1), 112–126. https://doi.org/10.1111/wrr.12391. PMID: 26663430.

Límová, M. (2010). Active wound coverings: Bioengineered skin and dermal substitutes. *The Surgical Clinics of North America, 90,* 1237–1255.

Malhotra, C., & Jain, A. K. (2014). Human amniotic membrane transplantation: Different modalities of its use in ophthalmology. *World Journal of Transplantation, 4*(2), 111.

Mandal, A. (2007). Paediatric partial-thickness scald burns—Is Biobrane the best treatment available? *International Wound Journal, 4,* 15–19.

Marston, W. A., Hanft, J., Norwood, P., et al. (2003). The efficacy and safety of Dermagraft in improving the healing of chronic diabetic foot ulcers: Results of a prospective randomized trial. *Diabetes Care, 26,* 1701–1705.

Metcalfe, A. D., & Ferguson, M. W. J. (2007). Tissue engineering of replacement skin: The crossroads of biomaterials, wound healing, embryonic development, stem cells and regeneration. *Journal of the Royal Society Interface, 4,* 413–437.

Michael, S., Winters, C., & Khan, M. (2019). Acellular fish skin graft use for diabetic lower extremity wound healing: A retrospective study of 58 ulcerations and a literature review. *Wounds, 31*(10), 262–268.

Mostow, E. N., Haraway, G. D., Dalsing, M., et al. (2005). Effectiveness of an extracellular matrix graft (OASIS Wound Matrix) in the treatment of chronic leg ulcers: A randomized clinical trial. *Journal of Vascular Surgery, 41,* 837–843.

Nieponice, A., Gilbert, T. W., & Badylak, S. F. (2006). Reinforcement of esophageal anastomoses with an extracellular matrix scaffold in a canine model. *The Annals of Thoracic Surgery, 82,* 2050–2058.

Price, R. D., Das-Gupta, V., Leigh, I. M., et al. (2006). A comparison of tissue-engineered hyaluronic acid dermal matrices in a human wound model. *Tissue Engineering, 12,* 2985–2995.

Reyzelman, A. M., & Bazarov, I. (2015). Human acellular dermal wound matrix for treatment of DFU: Literature review and analysis. *Journal of Wound Care, 24*(3), 128, 129–134.

Reyzelman, A., Crews, R. T., Moore, J. C., et al. (2009). Clinical effectiveness of a acellular dermal regenerative tissue matrix compared to standard wound management in healing diabetic foot ulcers: A prospective, randomized multicentre study. *International Wound Journal, 6,* 196–208.

Roberts, C., & Mansbridge, J. (2002). The scientific basis and differentiating features of Dermagraft. *Canadian Journal of Plastic Surgery, 10*(Suppl. A), 6A–13A.

Robson, M. C., Cooper, D. M., Aslam, R., et al. (2006). Guidelines for the treatment of venous ulcers. *Wound Repair and Regeneration, 14,* 649–662.

Rommer, E. A., Peric, M., & Wong, A. (2013). Urinary bladder matrix for the treatment of recalcitrant nonhealing radiation wounds. *Advances in Skin & Wound Care, 26*(10), 450–455.

Rosales, M. A., Bruntz, M., & Armstrong, D. G. (2004). Gamma-irradiated human skin allograft: A potential treatment modality for lower extremity ulcers. *International Wound Journal, 1,* 201–206.

Ryssel, H., Gazyakan, E., Germann, G., et al. (2008). The use of MatriDerm in early excision and simultaneous autologous skin grafting in burns—A pilot study. *Burns, 34,* 93–97.

Ryssel, H., Germann, G., Czermak, C., et al. (2010). Matriderm® in depth-adjusted reconstruction of necrotising fasciitis defects. *Burns, 36*(7), 1107–1111.

Schaum, K. D. (2014). More 2014 code changes and medicare payment changes for wound care providers. *Advances in Skin & Wound Care, 27*(3), 108–110.

Shevchenko, R., James, S. L., & James, S. E. (2009). A review of tissue-engineered skin bioconstructs available for skin reconstruction. *Journal of the Royal Society Interface, 7,* 229–258.

Shores, J. T., Gabriel, A., & Gupta, S. (2007). Skin substitutes and alternatives: A review. *Advances in Skin & Wound Care, 20,* 493–508.

Still, J., Glat, P., Silverstein, P., et al. (2003). The use of a collagen sponge/living cell composite material to treat donor sites in burn patients. *Burns, 29,* 837–841.

Ter Horst, B., Chouhan, G., Moiemen, N. S., & Grover, L. M. (2018). Advances in keratinocyte delivery in burn wound care. *Advanced Drug Delivery Reviews, 123,* 18–32. https://doi.org/10.1016/j.addr.2017.06.012.

Towler, M. A., Rush, E. W., Richardson, M. K., & Williams, C. L. (2018). Randomized, prospective, blinded-enrollment, head-to-head venous leg ulcer healing trial comparing living, bioengineered skin graft substitute (Apligraf) with living, cryopreserved, human skin allograft (TheraSkin). *Clinics in Podiatric Medicine and Surgery, 35*(3), 357–365.

Troy, J., et al. (2013). The use of EZ Derm® in partial-thickness burns: An institutional review of 157 patients. *Eplasty, 13,* e14.

van Winterswijk, P. J., & Nout, E. (2007). Tissue engineering and wound healing: An overview of the past, present, and future. *Wounds, 19,* 277–284.

Veves, A., Falanga, V., Armstrong, D. G., et al. (2001). Graftskin, a human skin equivalent, is effective in the management of noninfected neuropathic diabetic foot ulcers: A prospective randomized multicenter clinical trial. *Diabetes Care, 24,* 290–295.

Wagstaff, M. J., Schmitt, B. J., Coghlan, P., Finkelmeyer, J. P., Caplash, Y., & Greenwood, J. E. (2015). A biodegradable polyurethane dermal matrix in reconstruction of free flap donor sites: A pilot study. *Eplasty, 15,* e13.

Whitaker, I. S., Prowse, S., & Potokar, T. S. (2008). A critical evaluation of the use of Biobrane as a biologic skin substitute: A versatile tool for the plastic and reconstructive surgeon. *Annals of Plastic Surgery, 60,* 333–337.

Williams, M. L., & Holewinski, J. E. (2015). Use of a human acellular dermal wound matrix in patients with complex wounds and comorbidities. *Journal of Wound Care, 24*(6), 261–262. 264–267.

Yang, C. K., Polanco, T. O., & Lantis, J. C. (2016). A prospective, postmarket, compassionate clinical evaluation of a novel acellular fish-skin graft which contains omega-3 fatty acids for the closure of hard-to-heal lower extremity chronic ulcers. *Wounds, 28*(4), 112–118. 27071138.

FURTHER READING

Brockmann, I., Ehrenpfordt, J., Sturmheit, T., Brandenburger, M., Kruse, C., Zille, M., et al. (2018). Skin-derived stem cells for wound treatment using cultured epidermal autografts: Clinical applications and challenges. *Stem Cells International, 2018,* 4623615. https://doi.org/10.1155/2018/4623615.

Campitiello, F., Mancone, M., Corte, A. D., Guerniero, R., & Canonico, S. (2018). Acellular flowable matrix in the treatment of tunneled or cavity ulcers in diabetic feet. *Advances in Skin & Wound Care, 31*(6), 270–275.

Caputo, W. J., Vaquero, C., Monterosa, A., Monterosa, P., Johnson, E., Beggs, D., et al. (2016). A retrospective study of cryopreserved umbilical cord as an adjunctive therapy to promote the healing of chronic, complex foot ulcers with underlying osteomyelitis. *Wound Repair and Regeneration, 24*(5), 885–893.

Caravaggi, C., De Giglio, R., Pritelli, C., et al. (2003). Hyaff 11-based autologous dermal and epidermal grafts in the treatment of noninfected diabetic plantar and dorsal foot ulcers: A prospective, multicenter, controlled, randomized clinical trial. *Diabetes Care, 26,* 2853–2859.

Ehrenreich, M., & Ruszczak, Z. (2006). Update on tissue-engineered biological dressings. *Tissue Engineering, 12,* 2407–2424.

Hrabchak, C., Flynn, L., & Woodhouse, K. A. (2006). Biological skin substitutes for wound cover and closure. *Expert Review of Medical Devices, 3,* 373–385.

Kamolz, L. P., Lumenta, D. B., Kitzinger, H. B., et al. (2008). Tissue engineering for cutaneous wounds: An overview of current standards and possibilities. *European Surgery, 40,* 19–26.

Kulkarni, M., O'Loughlin, A., Vazquez, R., et al. (2014). Use of a fibrin-based system for enhancing angiogenesis and modulating inflammation in the treatment of hyperglycemic wounds. *Biomaterials, 36,* 2001–2010.

Mulder, G., & Lee, D. (2009a). Case presentation: Xenograft resistance to protease degradation in a vasculitic ulcer. *The International Journal of Lower Extremity Wounds, 8,* 157–161.

Mulder, G., & Lee, D. (2009b). A retrospective clinical review of extracellular matrices for tissue reconstruction: Equine pericardium as a biological covering to assist with wound closure. *Wounds, 19,* 254–261.

Mulder, G., & Lee, D. (2009c). Use of equine derived pericardium as a biological cover to promote closure of a complicated wound with associated scleroderma and Raynaud's disease. *Wounds, 21,* 297–301.

Prystowsky, J. H., Nowygrod, R., Marboe, C. C., Benvenisty, A. I., Ascherman, J. A., & Todd, G. J. (2000). Artificial skin (Integra dermal regeneration template) for closure of lower extremity wounds. *Vascular Surgery, 34*(6), 557–567.

Raphael, A. (2016). A single-centre, retrospective study of cryopreserved umbilical cord/amniotic membrane tissue for the treatment of diabetic foot ulcers. *Journal of Wound Care, 25* (Sup7), S10–S17.

Reyzelman, A. M. (2015). Human acellular dermal wound matrix for treatment of DFU: Literature review and analysis. *Journal of Wound Care, 24*(3), 128–134.

Schurr, M. J., Foster, K. N., Centanni, J. M., et al. (2009). Phase I/II clinical evaluation of StrataGraft: A consistent pathogen-free human skin substitute. *The Journal of Trauma, 66,* 866–874.

Wilkins, L. M., Watson, S. R., Prosky, S. J., Meunier, S. F., & Parenteau, N. L. (1994). Development of a bilayered living skin construct for clinical applications. *Biotechnology and Bioengineering, 43*(8), 747–756.

Williams, M. L., & Holewinski, J. (2013). Experience using a flowable soft tissue scaffold in conjunction with a human dermal matrix in lower extremity wounds. *Journal of Diabetic Foot Complications, 5*(3), 55–61.

Woodley, D. T., Peterson, H. D., Herzog, S. R., et al. (1998). Burn wounds resurfaced by cultured epidermal autografts show abnormal reconstitution of anchoring fibrils. *Journal of the American Medical Association, 259,* 2566–2571.

23

Molecular and Cellular Regulators

Gregory S. Schultz

OBJECTIVES

1. Describe the importance of adhesion and migration of leukocytes in inflammation.
2. Distinguish between growth factors and cytokines.
3. Identify important processes in wound healing that are regulated by growth factors, cytokines, proteases, or hormones.
4. Describe the molecular environment that growth factors need to promote wound healing.
5. For each growth factor family, list one member, a key target cell, one main action, and one therapeutic use.
6. Describe the molecular differences between acute, healing wounds and chronic, nonhealing wounds.
7. Review two key updated points for wound bed preparation, biofilms, and point-of-care diagnostics and their application for the removal of barriers to wound healing.

At the cellular level, the complex process of the healing of skin wounds involves platelets, leukocytes, epidermal cells, fibroblasts, and vascular endothelial cells. At the molecular level, many growth factors, cytokines, proteases, and hormones regulate most of the key actions of cells during wound healing, such as the directed movement of cells into a wound (chemotactic migration), replacement of damaged epidermal and dermal cells (mitosis), growth of new blood vessels (neovascularization), formation of scar tissue (synthesis of extracellular matrix proteins), and remodeling of scar tissue (proteolytic turnover of extracellular matrix proteins) (Bennett & Schultz, 1993a, 1993b). Any condition that disrupts the normal actions of these molecular regulators in wounds will directly disrupt healing and promote the establishment and maintenance of chronic wounds (Mast & Schultz, 1996; Tarnuzzer & Schultz, 1996). By identifying abnormalities in the actions of molecular regulators in chronic wounds, therapies can be designed that will reestablish an environment that permits molecular regulators to function normally and achieve healing.

BIOLOGIC ROLES OF CYTOKINES AND GROWTH FACTORS

Growth factors are polypeptide proteins produced by the body to regulate proliferation, migration, and differentiation of target cells (e.g., expression of specialized genes) by binding to receptors on the cell surface. Specifically, proliferation and differentiation of nonimmune system cells are regulated primarily by growth factors. In contrast, cytokines are protein molecules that primarily regulate the interactions between cells that participate in the immune response (Frenette & Wagner, 1996a, 1996b; Springer, 1990).

Cytokines are a unique family of growth factors that are small signaling proteins that mediate and regulate immunity, inflammation, and hematopoiesis. Produced in response to an immune stimulus, cytokines are secreted primarily from leukocytes, although other wound cells can also secrete cytokines. Cytokines function at very low concentration and act over short distances. After the cytokines bind to specific membrane receptors, secondary messengers are triggered that signal the cell to alter its behavior by increasing or decreasing membrane proteins, proliferation, and secretion of molecules. The same cytokine may be secreted by different types of cells, and the same cytokine may act on several different cell types.

General Phases of Wound Healing

The four phases of acute wound healing are hemostasis, inflammation, repair, and remodeling. There is considerable temporal overlap of these phases of healing, and the entire process lasts for several months. Immediately after injury, the process of blood clotting is initiated by activation of a proteolytic cascade, which ultimately converts fibrinogen into fibrin. As the fibrin molecules self-associate into a weblike net, red blood cells (RBCs) and platelets become entrapped. The aggregate of fibrin, RBCs, and platelets quickly grows large enough to form a stable clot that acts as a tamponade to physically block an injured capillary and stop the flow of blood.

The process of blood clotting also induces platelet degranulation, which releases a burst of preformed growth factors stored in platelet granules. These include platelet-derived growth factor (PDGF), transforming growth factor-β (TGF-β), epidermal growth factor (EGF), and insulin-like growth factor-1 (IGF-1). In addition, platelets release tumor necrosis factor-alpha (TNF-α) and mRNA for interleukin-1β (IL-1β), which provides a mechanism for rapid synthesis by wound cells. Platelet activation induces rapid and sustained synthesis of pro-IL-1β protein, a response that is abolished by translational inhibitors. A portion of the IL-1β is shed in its mature form in membrane microvesicles and induces adhesiveness of human endothelial cells for neutrophils (Lindemann et al., 2001). Thus, platelet activation initiates two major processes: inflammation and tissue repair. The growth factors released from platelets quickly diffuse from the wound into the surrounding tissues and attract leukocytes into the injured area (Bennett & Schultz, 1993a, 1993b). Neutrophils, which are the first major inflammatory cell type that is chemotactically drawn into an acute skin wound, enter within 12 h after injury and are followed by macrophages that begin to enter an acute wound within 24 h. Importantly, macrophages initially activate into the M1 type of macrophages that are predominately proinflammatory in their actions, secreting more proinflammatory cytokines, engulfing and killing contaminating bacteria, and releasing proteases that help to remove denatured proteins in the extracellular matrix (Ley, 2017). As the bacterial bioburden is reduced and levels of proinflammatory molecules such as interferon-gamma (INF-γ) and lipopolysaccharides decrease, macrophages entering a wound bed can be stimulated by cytokines and growth factors to differentiate into the M2 phenotype, which synthesize and secrete antiinflammatory cytokines (IL-4 and IL-10) and prohealing growth factors (VEGF, EGF, TGF-β) that promote angiogenesis, wound cell proliferation, and migration and synthesis of ECM, as described in more detail in the following sections.

Adhesion Molecules and Adhesion Receptors in Inflammation

The chemotactic attraction of leukocytes to a wound and the movement of leukocytes from the blood into wounded tissue (extravasation) involve expression and activation of adhesion molecules and adhesion receptors on leukocytes, platelets, and vascular endothelial cells. Cytokines and growth factors play key roles in these processes (Arai, Lee, Miyajima, et al., 1990; Frenette & Wagner, 1996a, 1996b; Springer, 1990). Among the many types of adhesion molecules and receptors on the cell surface, four major families of transmembrane proteins stand out in the process of inflammation: integrins, selectins, cell adhesion molecules (CAMs), and cadherins (Fig. 23.1).

Integrins are glycoproteins composed of two different types of subunits, designated α and β. In simple terms, integrins are cellular receptors for extracellular matrix proteins, as shown with $\alpha_5\beta_1$, which is a receptor for fibronectin. A short amino acid sequence, such as arginine-glycine-aspartate, is often the site of recognition by the integrin receptor. Integrins are important because they are capable of generating signals inside cells when the integrin receptor binds to a specific extracellular matrix protein, in much the same way the insulin receptor generates intracellular signals, which regulate glucose transport into a cell when insulin binds to its cellular receptor. Expression of β_2 integrins is limited to leukocytes, whereas β_1 integrins are expressed on most cell types. β_1 Integrins primarily bind to extracellular matrix components such as fibronectin, laminin, and collagens. (These substances are discussed in more detail in Chapter 8.)

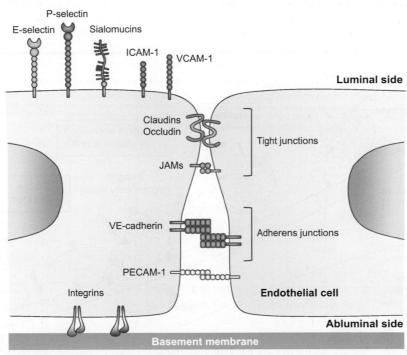

Fig. 23.1 Four major classes of adhesion proteins and adhesion receptors embedded in a theoretic plasma membrane: integrins, selectins, cell adhesion molecules (platelet–endothelial cell adhesion molecule [PECAM-1] and vascular cell adhesion molecule [VCAM-1]), and cadherins. (From Ratcliffe, M. J. H. (2016). Encyclopedia of immunobiology. London: Elsevier Ltd.)

Selectins are proteins that have a unique structure called a *lectin domain* at the distal end, which can bind specific carbohydrate groups of glycoproteins or mucins on adjacent cells. Thus, unlike other adhesion proteins, which recognize specific protein structures, selectins recognize and bind to carbohydrate ligands on leukocytes and vascular endothelial cells. E-selectin appears on endothelial cells after they have been activated by inflammatory cytokines, and P-selectin is stored in the α-granules of platelets and the storage granules of endothelial cells (Weibel–Palade bodies).

CAMs are members of the immunoglobulin superfamily of proteins. CAMs can bind to other CAMs or to integrins on cells. CAMs that are important in inflammation include the platelet–endothelial cell adhesion molecule (PECAM), vascular cell adhesion molecule (VCAM), and intercellular adhesion molecule-1 (ICAM-1).

Cadherins are important in establishing molecular links between adjacent cells, especially during embryonic development. They form zipper-like structures of dimers at specialized regions of contact between neighboring cells called *adherens junctions.* Cadherins are linked to the cytoskeleton through molecules called *catenins,* which associate with actin microfilaments.

During the process of extravasation of inflammatory cells into a wound, important interactions occur between blood vessels and blood cells (Arai et al., 1990; Frenette & Wagner, 1996a, 1996b; Springer, 1990). Initially, circulating leukocytes begin rolling on endothelial cells through the binding of glycoproteins expressed on their cell surface to selectins, transiently expressed by activated endothelial cells of venules (Fig. 23.2). The binding affinity of selectins is relatively low, but is enough to serve as a biologic brake, making leukocytes quickly decelerate by rolling on endothelial cells. While rolling, leukocytes can become activated by chemoattractants (cytokines, growth factors, or bacterial products). After activation, leukocytes firmly adhere to endothelial cells as a result of the binding between their β_2 class of integrins and ligands, such as VCAM and ICAM expressed on activated endothelial cells. Chemotactic signals present outside the venule induce leukocytes to squeeze between endothelial cells of the venule and migrate into the inflammatory center by using their β_1 class of integrins to recognize and bind to extracellular matrix components.

Adhesion and degranulation of platelets at sites of vascular injury also use a system of adhesion molecules and adhesion receptor proteins. Vascular injury immediately induces endothelial cells to release the contents of their storage granules (Weibel–Palade bodies), including the proteins P-selectin and von Willebrand factor. P-selectin promptly moves to the plasma membrane of endothelial cells, where it induces rolling of platelets on endothelial cells, and von Willebrand factor is quickly deposited on the exposed extracellular matrix, where it plays a crucial role in the adhesion of platelets to the damaged site.

Inflammatory Cell Proteases

When the inflammatory cascade is activated, neutrophils enter the wound initially, followed by macrophages. Neutrophils and macrophages become activated and engulf and destroy bacteria through their production of reactive oxygen species (ROS) (hydrogen peroxide hypochlorous acid). Activated neutrophils and macrophages also release several proteases, including neutrophil elastase (a serine type of protease), neutrophil collagenase (a matrix metalloproteinase [MMP] type of protease designated MMP-8), and macrophage metalloelastase (MMP-12). These

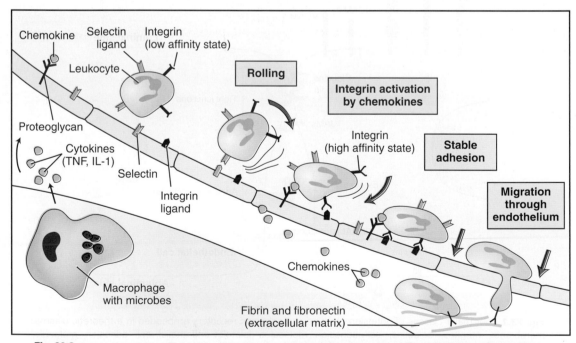

Fig. 23.2 Interactions between blood cells and a stimulated or injured venule. *vWF,* von Willebrand factor. (From Banasik, J. (2022). *Pathophysiology* (6th ed.). St. Louis: Elsevier)

proteases play important, beneficial roles in initiating normal wound healing by removing proteolytically degraded and, damaged extracellular matrix components, which must be replaced by new, intact extracellular matrix molecules for wound healing to proceed. These proteases also are important for enabling inflammatory cells to move through the basement membrane that surrounds capillaries.

Inflammatory Cell Cytokines and Growth Factors in Proliferation and Repair

The growth factors released by platelets diffuse away from a wound within a few hours, but they are replaced by growth factors and cytokines that are produced by neutrophils, macrophages, activated fibroblasts, vascular endothelial cells, and epidermal cells that are drawn into the wound area. For example, activated macrophages secrete several important cytokines, including TNF-α and IL-1β, which have a variety of actions on different cells. TNF-α and IL-1β are potent inflammatory cytokines, which further stimulate inflammation. TNF-α also induces macrophages to produce IL-1β, which is mitogenic for fibroblasts and upregulates expression of MMPs. Both TNF-α and IL-1β directly influence deposition of collagen in the wound by inducing synthesis of collagen by fibroblasts and by upregulating expression of MMPs. In addition, these cytokines downregulate expression of the tissue inhibitors of metalloproteinases (TIMPs), which are the natural inhibitors of MMPs. IFN-γ, produced by lymphocytes attracted into the wound, inhibits fibroblast migration and downregulates collagen synthesis (Table 23.1).

TABLE 23.1 Growth Factor Families

Growth Factor Family	Cell Source	Actions	Relevant Research
Transforming growth factor-β (TGF-β_1, TGF-β_2, TGF-β_3)	Platelets Fibroblasts Macrophages	Fibroblast chemotaxis and activation ECM deposition Collagen synthesis TIMP synthesis MMP synthesis Reduces scarring Collagen synthesis Fibronectin synthesis	Chronic skin ulcers (Robson, Abdullah, Burns, et al., 1994)
Platelet-derived growth factor (PDGF-AA, PDGF-BB, vascular endothelial growth factor)	Platelets Macrophages Keratinocytes Fibroblasts	Activation of immune cells and fibroblasts ECM deposition Collagen synthesis TIMP synthesis MMP synthesis Angiogenesis	Pressure injuries (Robson, Phillips, Lawrence, et al., 1992) Diabetic ulcers (Steed, 1995)
Fibroblast growth factor (acidic FGF, basic FGF, keratinocyte growth factor)	Macrophages Endothelial cells Fibroblasts	Angiogenesis Endothelial cell activation Keratinocyte proliferation and migration ECM deposition	Pressure injuries (Robson, Phillips, Thomason, et al., 1992) Second-degree burns (Fu, Shen, Chen, et al., 1998)
Insulin-like growth factor (IGF-1, IGF-2, insulin)	Liver Skeletal muscle Fibroblasts Macrophages Neutrophils	Keratinocyte proliferation Fibroblast proliferation Endothelial cell activation Angiogenesis Collagen synthesis ECM deposition Cell metabolism	No published reports evaluating IGF-1 for treatment of wounds
Epidermal growth factor (EGF, heparin-binding epidermal growth factor, transforming growth factor-α, amphiregulin, betacellulin)	Keratinocytes Macrophages	Keratinocyte proliferation and migration ECM deposition	Burns, donor sites (Brown, Curtsinger, Brightwell, et al., 1986; Brown, Nanney, Griffen, et al., 1989) Venous ulcers (Falanga, Eaglstein, Bucalo, et al., 1992)
Connective tissue growth factor (CTGF)	Fibroblasts Endothelial cells Epithelial cells	Mediates action of TGF-βs on collagen synthesis, cell proliferation and migration	No published reports evaluating CTGF for treatment of wounds

ECM, extracellular matrix; *MMP*, matrix metalloproteinase; *TIMP*, tissue inhibitor of metalloproteinase.

Inflammatory cells secrete other growth factors, including TGF-β, TGF-α, heparin-binding epidermal growth factor (HB-EGF), and basic fibroblast growth factor (bFGF). The growth factors secreted by macrophages continue to stimulate migration of fibroblasts, epithelial cells, and vascular endothelial cells into the wound. As the fibroblasts, epithelial cells, and vascular endothelial cells migrate into the site of injury, they begin to proliferate, and the cellularity of the wound increases. This begins the proliferative and repair phase, which often lasts several weeks. If the wound is not infected, the number of inflammatory cells in a wound begins to decrease after a few days. Other types of cells, such as fibroblasts, endothelial cells, and keratinocytes, are drawn into the wound and begin to synthesize growth factors. Fibroblasts secrete IGF-1, bFGF, TGF-β, PDGF, and keratinocyte growth factor (KGF). Endothelial cells produce vascular endothelial growth factor (VEGF), bFGF, and PDGF. Keratinocytes synthesize TGF-α, TGF-β, and IL-1β. These growth factors continue to stimulate cell proliferation and synthesis of extracellular matrix proteins and to promote formation of new capillaries.

A recent meta-analysis of multiple publications that characterized the bioburden of chronic wounds determined that most chronic wounds (~80%) have bacteria present in the biofilm phenotype as well as the well-known planktonic phenotype that are single, proliferating bacteria (Malone et al., 2017). Bacteria in biofilm communities are typically encased in a self-produced exopolymeric matrix (EPM) that typically consists of unique polysaccharides (e.g., polyalginate, poly-N-acetylglucosamine) and extracellular bacteria DNA that help to firmly attach the biofilm community to the surface and into the superficial levels of the wound bed tissues (Phillips, Wolcott, Fletcher, & Schultz, 2010). Many of the EPM components are highly inflammatory to both the innate immune system (Toll-like receptors) and the adaptive immune system (antibodies and induced killer T cells). Importantly, a substantial percentage of bacteria in biofilm communities develop high tolerance to antibodies and phagocytic cells (neutrophiles and macrophages) of patients and also to most antibiotics and many antiseptics that effectively kill planktonic bacteria. Thus, bacterial biofilms in chronic wounds make important contributions to stimulating the chronic inflammatory state that characterizes most chronic wounds (Omar, Wright, Schultz, Burrell, & Nadworny, 2017). This leads to highly elevated levels of proteases (matrix metalloproteases, MMPs, and neutrophil elastase NE) and ROS that degrade proteins (growth factors, receptors, ECM) that are essential to healing (World Union of Wound Healing Societies [WUWHS], 2016). This better understanding of the critical roles that bacterial biofilms play in impairing healing has led to the clinical principles of "Biofilm-Based Wound Care" that emphasize "step-down then step-up" treatment. This clinical concept specifies beginning treatment with effective debridement of biofilms combined with dressings and treatments that effectively prevent reformation of biofilms, which can reform in less than 3 days (Schultz et al., 2017).

As the levels of biofilm and planktonic bacteria are reduced to levels that reduce the levels of inflammatory proteases and ROS, endogenous healing factors can resume proper functioning and traditional wound care practices can resume (step-down). In patients who need extra exogenous therapies to stimulate healing, advanced wound care products can be used because the wound bed has been properly prepared to enable advanced therapies to function effectively (step-up) and accelerate healing (International Wound Infection Institute, 2022; Eriksson et al., 2022).

Remodeling Phase

After the initial scar forms, proliferation and neovascularization cease and the wound enters the remodeling phase, which can last for many months. During this last phase, a new balance is reached between the synthesis of extracellular matrix components in the scar and their degradation by metalloproteinases such as collagenase, gelatinase, and stromelysin. Fibroblasts synthesize a majority of the collagen, elastin, and proteoglycans that compose the dermal scar matrix. Fibroblasts also are a major source of the MMPs that degrade the scar matrix, as well as their inhibitors, the TIMPs. They also secrete lysyl oxidase, an enzyme that covalently cross-links components of the extracellular matrix, such as collagen and elastin molecules, producing a stable extracellular matrix. Keratinocytes secrete much of the type IV collagen that re-forms the basement membrane, which separates the epidermal and dermal layers and forms the surface on which keratinocytes prefer to migrate. Angiogenesis ceases and the density of capillaries decreases in the wound site as a result of programmed cell death (apoptosis) of the vascular endothelial cells. Eventually, remodeling of the scar tissue reaches equilibrium, although the mature scar is never as strong as uninjured skin.

CYTOKINES

Cytokines are produced extensively by activated T cells and macrophages, although nonimmune system cells such as keratinocytes and vascular endothelial cells also produce some cytokines. Studies have revealed that cytokines generally induce multiple biologic activities (pleiotropic) and that a single cytokine can act as both a positive signal and a negative signal, depending on the type of the target cell. Cytokines such as IL-1, IL-2, IL-3, IL-4, IL-5, IL-6, and IL-10; granulocyte–macrophage colony-stimulating factor; granulocyte colony-stimulating factor; IFN-γ; and TNF-α are key mediators of immune and inflammatory responses. A cytokine is also referred to as a *lymphokine* (cytokine made by lymphocytes), *monokine* (cytokine made by monocytes), *chemokine* (cytokine with chemotactic action), and *interleukin* (cytokines made by one leukocyte and acting on other leukocytes). Two cytokines in particular, TNF-α and IL-1β, have activities that substantially influence skin wound healing through their ability to increase production of MMPs and suppress production of TIMPs. Table 23.2 lists the cytokines

TABLE 23.2 Cytokines Involved in Wound Healing

Cytokine	Cell Source	Biologic Activity
Proinflammatory Cytokines		
TNF-α	Macrophages	PMN margination and cytotoxicity; collagen synthesis; provides metabolic substrate
IL-1	Macrophages Keratinocytes	Fibroblast and keratinocyte chemotaxis; collagen synthesis
IL-2	T lymphocytes	Increases fibroblast infiltration and metabolism
IL-6	Macrophages PMNs Fibroblasts	Fibroblast proliferation; hepatic acute-phase protein synthesis
IL-8	Macrophages Fibroblasts	Macrophage and PMN chemotaxis; keratinocyte maturation
IFN-γ	T lymphocytes Macrophages	Macrophage and PMN activation; retards collagen synthesis and cross-linking; stimulates collagenase activity
Antiinflammatory Cytokines		
IL-4	T lymphocytes Basophils Mast cells	Inhibition of TNF, IL-1, IL-6 production; fibroblast proliferation; collagen synthesis
IL-10	T lymphocytes Macrophages Keratinocytes	Inhibition of TNF, IL-1, IL-6 production; inhibits macrophage and PMN activation

IFN, interferon; *IL*, interleukin; *PMN*, polymorphonuclear leukocyte; *TNF*, tumor necrosis factor.

involved in wound healing, along with cell source, biologic activity, and their subclassification as proinflammatory or antiinflammatory.

Cytokines have not been investigated extensively in human wound-healing studies. IL-1β was evaluated in a prospective, randomized, double-blind, placebo-controlled trial performed on 26 patients with stage 3 and 4 pressure injuries (Robson, et al., 1994). No statistically significant differences were seen in the percentage decrease in wound volumes between the treatment groups.

GROWTH FACTORS

Discovery, Purification, and Cloning of Growth Factors

Protein growth factors were discovered as a consequence of their ability to stimulate multiple cycles of cell growth (mitosis) when added to cultures of normal, quiescent cells. This process distinguishes growth factors from essential nutrients such as vitamins, cofactors, and trace minerals (e.g., selenium), which are required for metabolic processes but are not sufficient to initiate cell division by themselves. Both nutrients and growth factors are necessary for mitosis, but only growth factors can initiate mitosis of quiescent cells.

Based on the ability of growth factors to stimulate continuous mitosis of cells in culture, it is not surprising that many growth factors initially were isolated from medium conditioned by tumor cells. Other sources of growth factors included platelets, macrophages, and normal tissues that can proliferate rapidly, such as ovarian follicles and placenta. Although growth factors were present in minute quantities from these natural sources, tiny amounts eventually were purified using traditional biochemical methods. The amino acid sequences of the proteins were determined, which permitted cloning and sequencing of the growth factor genes. With the development of recombinant DNA technology, large amounts of synthetic human growth factors were produced from cultures of bacteria, yeast, or human cells that carried the gene for the growth factor. The availability of large amounts of the synthetic growth factors enabled research that led to a better understanding of the biologic roles of growth factors in wound healing and other physiologic processes, such as fetal development, aging, and cancer. Ultimately, this led to experiments that evaluated the effects of synthetic growth factors in animal wound-healing models and eventually to clinical trials in patients.

Autocrine and Paracrine Action of Growth Factors

Growth factors are synthesized and secreted by many types of cells involved in wound healing, including platelets, inflammatory cells, fibroblasts, epithelial cells, and vascular endothelial cells. Moreover, growth factors usually act either on the producer cell (autocrine stimulation) or on adjacent cells (paracrine stimulation). In contrast to classic endocrine hormones, growth factors generally do not enter the bloodstream and act on cells at a great distance (Fig. 23.3) (Barrientos, Brem, Stojadinovic, et al., 2008).

Receptors

All peptide growth factors initiate their effects on target cells by binding to specific, high-affinity receptor proteins located in the plasma membrane of target cells (Fantl, Johnson, & Williams, 1993). Only cells that express the specific receptor protein can respond to the growth factor. Binding of the growth factor to its receptor activates a region of the receptor protein called a *kinase domain*, which is located inside the cell

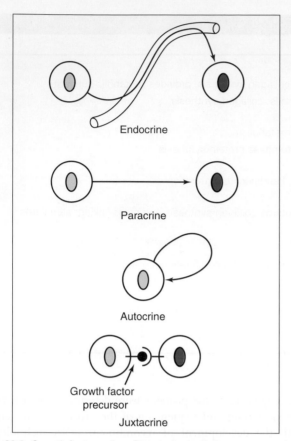

Fig. 23.3 Growth factor action. Secreted growth factors act predominately by an autocrine (self-stimulation) or a paracrine (adjacent cells) pathway and usually not by classic endocrine pathways. Membrane-bound growth factors may also interact with adjacent cells by juxtacrine stimulation. (From Bennett, N. T., & Schultz, G. S. (1993). Growth factors and wound healing: Biochemical properties of growth factors and their receptors. *American Journal of Surgery, 165,* 728.)

(Fig. 23.4). Kinase domains have the enzymatic ability to covalently transfer a phosphate group from the high-energy adenosine triphosphate molecule to an amino acid, such as tyrosine, serine, or threonine, in a protein. The activated receptor protein is the "first messenger" in the response system of a cell to a growth factor.

The activated receptor kinase domain then phosphorylates amino acids on a small number of specific cytoplasmic proteins. These cytoplasmic proteins become activated when phosphorylated and are the first in a series of "second messenger" proteins that eventually generate a response in the cell to the growth factor. Second messenger proteins also typically contain kinase domains that are activated when the proteins are phosphorylated. The activated cytoplasmic kinase proteins in turn phosphorylate other cytoplasmic proteins in a sequential cascade of phosphorylations and activations that eventually leads to activation of special proteins called *RNA transcription factors.* Activated RNA transcription factors bind with selected regions of the DNA to help initiate transcription of genes into messenger RNAs (mRNAs), which are translated into proteins that ultimately alter the functions of the target cell.

Another system of cytoplasmic proteins acts to turn off the transcription of genes that are turned on by growth factors. These proteins are called *phosphatases.* They remove the phosphate groups that were added to the amino acids of the second messenger kinase proteins and to the RNA transcription factors. Removal of the phosphate groups inactivates the second messenger proteins and the transcription factors. Thus, the effects of growth factors on target cells require an integrated balance among receptor proteins, second messenger kinase proteins, RNA transcription factors, and phosphatases.

MAJOR FAMILIES OF GROWTH FACTORS

The first attempt to use growth factors to promote healing of human wounds was based on the concept that platelets contained numerous growth factors that were released at the time of injury. Furthermore, substantial amounts of activated platelet supernatant could be obtained from individual patients with chronic skin ulcers or from apheresis donors. This would permit patients to be treated with their own activated platelet supernatant or from carefully screened platelet donors. To test this concept, a U.S. Food and Drug Administration (FDA)-approved, randomized, controlled, multicenter, dose–response trial of topically applied activated platelet supernatant in 97 patients with a chronic, nonhealing diabetic wound was conducted (David, Goslen, Holloway, et al., 1992; Holloway, Steed, DeMarco, et al., 1993).

The use of placebo treatment, combined with good basic wound care, reduced wound area 77% and reduced wound volume 83% from baseline to final visit, although only 29% of the placebo group healed completely compared with 63% of the patients treated with platelet releasate. All healing parameters were significantly improved in the patients who were treated with all doses of platelet releasate. These results demonstrated the benefit of treatment of chronic diabetic wounds with a mixture of growth factors and proteins released from platelets. Table 23.1 presents an overview of the major families of growth factors, including those growth factors that have been shown to play roles in wound healing in animals or humans (not all known growth factors are included).

Epidermal Growth Factor Family

EGF was the first growth factor to be purified and biochemically characterized (Carpenter & Cohen, 1990). Other members of the EGF family that influence wound healing are TGF-α (Massague, 1990) and HB-EGF (Higashiyama et al., 1992). Members of the EGF family are small single-chain proteins that bind to a common receptor protein (EGF receptor) that has tyrosine kinase activity and is expressed on almost all types of cells. Members of the EGF family have similar, but not identical, biologic effects on target cells. They are chemoattractants and mitogens for epidermal cells, fibroblasts, and vascular endothelial cells but are most effective for epidermal cells.

EGF and TGF-α are synthesized as membrane-bound precursors that are released by proteolysis in a wide range of

Fig. 23.4 Growth factor receptor signal generation. Growth factors typically affect cells by binding to specific, high-affinity receptor proteins located in the plasma membrane of target cells, which then dimerize and activate tyrosine or serine/threonine kinase domains located in the cytoplasmic region of the receptor. The activated receptor then phosphorylates second messenger proteins, which frequently also are kinases that participate in a cascade of phosphorylation/activation steps that ultimately activate an RNA transcription factor, which selectively initiates synthesis of proteins that alter the behavior of the target cell. The second messenger system is turned off by enzymes called phosphatases that remove phosphate groups from proteins.

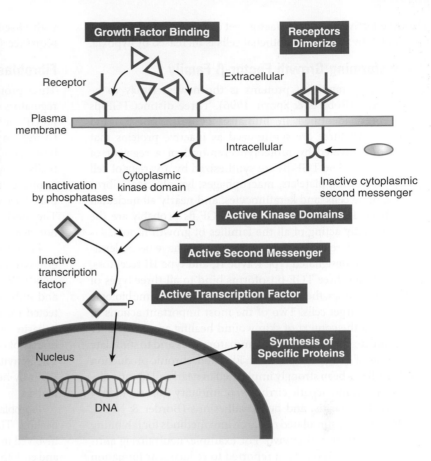

cells, including cells of the lacrimal and salivary glands. EGF and TGF-α are present in saliva and tears, and data from many different types of experiments strongly suggest that EGF and TGF-α play important roles in both the normal turnover of epithelial cells of the gut and cornea and in the healing of wounds in these tissues. Specifically, in the skin, epidermal cells synthesize large amounts of TGF-α. Mice that lack TGF-α or EGF receptors have abnormal hair and skin architecture. Levels of EGF receptor are elevated in the leading edge of epidermal cells in burn wounds (Nanney & King, 1996). Specific inhibition of the EGF receptor delays healing of partial-thickness skin injuries in animals. HB-EGF is produced by macrophages and presumably is retained in a wound for longer periods than EGF or TGF-α because of reversible binding to heparin.

Current models of skin wound healing propose that TGF-α is the growth factor that is primarily responsible for the normal maintenance and turnover of epidermal cells of the skin. When a skin injury occurs, epidermal cell proliferation and migration are stimulated by TGF-α produced by epidermal cells; EGF produced by epithelial cells lining the hair follicles, sweat glands, and sebaceous glands; and HB-EGF produced by macrophages that enter the wound. In addition, fibroblasts surrounding the wound secrete KGF, a member of the fibroblast growth factor system, which exclusively promotes migration and mitosis of keratinocytes.

Injections of recombinant human EGF into the dermal tissue at the edge of chronic diabetic foot ulcers promoted healing and reduced amputations compared with standard care of wet-to-dry gauze dressings (Acosta, Savigne, Valdez, et al., 2006).

Platelet-Derived Growth Factor Family

The PDGF family comprises two major proteins, PDGF and VEGF, which influence wound healing (Heldin & Westermark, 1996). PDGF and VEGF share about 25% of the amino acid sequence homology, and both are composed of two subunits that are covalently linked by disulfide bonds. PDGF has two different subunits (designated types A and B). Human platelets contain high levels of PDGF, and many types of human cells important in skin wound healing can secrete PDGF, including fibroblasts, vascular smooth muscle cells, and vascular endothelial cells.

PDGF and VEGF bind to different receptor proteins (both are tyrosine kinases) and stimulate different biologic actions. Two distinct PDGF receptors have been characterized. The PDGF-α receptor recognizes both α and β subunits of PDGF, whereas the PDGF-β receptor only recognizes the β subunit of PDGF.

PDGF is a chemoattractant and mitogen primarily for fibroblasts, whereas VEGF is a chemoattractant and mitogen primarily for vascular endothelial cells. VEGF is one of the most effective angiogenic factors yet discovered, and synthesis of VEGF by vascular endothelial cells is increased by hypoxia.

Transforming Growth Factor-β Family

The TGF-β family of proteins is the newest family to be discovered (Roberts & Sporn, 1996). Three distinct TGF-βs have been identified in humans: TGF-$β_1$, TGF-$β_2$, and TGF-$β_3$. All three are synthesized as inactive proteins that must be activated by proteolytic removal of a segment of the proteins. The TGF-βs are synthesized by a variety of cell types, including platelets, macrophages, lymphocytes, fibroblasts, bone cells, and keratinocytes, and nearly all nucleated cells have TGF-β receptors. Thus, TGF-βs probably are the most broadly acting of all the families of growth factors.

Three different TGF-β receptor proteins have been identified and are designated type I, type II, and type III receptors. Although all three TGF-β isoforms bind to all three types of TGF-β receptors, they do not appear to have the same biologic effects on target cells. Two of the most important actions of TGF-βs in the context of skin wound healing are their ability to stimulate chemotaxis of inflammatory cells and to stimulate synthesis of extracellular matrix. Elevated, chronic production of TGF-β has been strongly implicated in nearly all fibrotic diseases, including hepatic cirrhosis, pulmonary fibrosis, kidney glomerulonephritis, and pelvic adhesions (Border & Noble, 1994). This has stimulated research into methods for inhibiting the action of TGF-β in vivo. For example, neutralizing antibodies to TGF-βs has been reported to reduce scar formation in rat skin incisions (Shah, Foreman, & Ferguson, 1992, 1994; Stromberg, Collins, Gordon, et al., 1992).

Connective Tissue Growth Factor

TGF-β has been shown to induce synthesis of another important protein, connective tissue growth factor (CTGF) (Bradham, Igarashi, Potter, et al., 1991; Frazier, Williams, Kothapalli, et al., 1996). CTGF is a potent inducer of extracellular matrix synthesis, and much of the increase in extracellular matrix that occurs in the skin after treatment with TGF-β probably is due to the action of CTGF. Many human fibrotic diseases have been reported to contain elevated levels of CTGF protein (Ito, Aten, Bende, et al., 1998; Kucich, Rosenbloom, Herrick, et al., 2001). Macrophages, fibroblasts, and epithelial cells all secrete CTGF. The receptor for CTGF has not been conclusively identified. No clinical studies of CTGF have been performed, but adding exogenous CTGF to stimulate healing of chronic wounds is logical. Conversely, inhibiting CTGF action by adding neutralizing antibodies or antisense oligonucleotides (ASO) to wounds should reduce fibrosis.

Recent animal studies reported that injections of ASO targeting CTGF mRNA dramatically reduced hypertrophic scarring of full-thickness skin excisions that extended to the cartilage layer in rabbit ears (Sisco, Kryger, O'Shaughnessy, et al., 2008). More importantly, phase II clinical studies assessing the effect of injections of ASO CTGF into the edges of surgically excised hypertrophic scars reported significant reduction of the visible appearance of the new incisional scars compared with no treatment or treatment with negative-control ASO with scrambled nucleotide sequence (R. Galiano, personal communication).

Fibroblast Growth Factor Family

Three proteins of the FGF family are thought to be important regulators of wound healing: acidic fibroblast growth factor (aFGF or FGF-1), bFGF (or FGF-2), and KGF (FGF-7) (Abraham & Klagsbrun, 1996). More than 30 synonyms have been reported in the literature describing proteins that eventually were shown to be either aFGF or bFGF. As their names imply, aFGF and bFGF are potent mitogens for fibroblasts that share many similar biochemical and biologic properties. The mechanism of release for aFGF and bFGF from cells is not clear.

Fibroblast growth factors have the ability to bind the glycosaminoglycan heparin and the proteoglycan heparan sulfate. When FGF is associated in the extracellular matrix and in basement membranes with heparan sulfate, it is protected from proteolytic degradation. The binding of FGF to heparin or to heparan sulfate proteoglycans in the membranes of cells results in a substantial increase in cell division. The activity of FGF appears to be regulated by the binding FGFs by heparin-containing components of the extracellular matrix.

Fibroblast growth factors appear to play major roles in wound healing. They stimulate proliferation of the major cell types involved in wound healing, including fibroblasts, keratinocytes, and endothelial cells. Fibroblast growth factors and VEGF probably are the major angiogenic factors in wound healing. Many of the cells that respond to FGF also synthesize the peptide, including fibroblasts, endothelial cells, and smooth muscle cells.

KGF shares the ability to bind to heparin. In contrast to aFGF and bFGF, synthesis of KGF is restricted to fibroblasts, and KGF expression is rapidly upregulated in fibroblasts after an injury (Werner, Peters, Longaker, et al., 1992). More importantly, KGF only stimulates mitosis of keratinocytes and not fibroblasts, as the receptor for KGF is not expressed by fibroblasts. This has led to the concept that KGF is a paracrine effector of epithelial cell growth. Palifermin, a recombinant derivative of human KGF, is the first active agent approved by the FDA for the prevention of severe oral mucositis in patients undergoing hematopoietic stem cell transplantation (Vadhan-Raj, Goldberg, Perales, et al., 2013).

Four FGF receptors have been identified: FGFR-1, FGFR-2, FGFR-3, and FGFR-4. However, the receptors differ in their ability to bind bFGF and KGF. Expression of different FGF receptor variants by cells may provide another method for regulating the response of cells to FGFs.

Insulin-Like Growth Factor Family

IGF-1 and IGF-2 have substantial amino acid sequence homology to proinsulin, and both are synthesized as precursor molecules that are proteolytically cleaved to generate active monomeric proteins of approximately 7000 molecular weight. IGF-2 is synthesized more prominently during fetal development, whereas IGF-1 synthesis persists at high levels in many adult tissues, especially in the liver in response to stimulation by pituitary-derived growth hormone. Many of the biologic actions originally attributed to growth hormone, such as cartilage and bone growth, are mediated in part by IGF-1. However, combinations of growth hormone and IGF-1 are more effective than either hormone alone.

Unlike other growth factors, IGF-1 is present in substantial levels in plasma, which primarily reflects hepatic synthesis. High-affinity IGF-binding proteins reversibly bind almost all the IGF-1 in plasma. Because the IGFs are inactive while bound to their binding proteins, the dynamic balance between free and bound IGFs has a substantial influence on the effects of IGF-1 in wound healing. IGF-1 is also found in high levels in platelets and is released during platelet degranulation. It is a potent chemotactic agent for vascular endothelial cells, and IGF-1 released from platelets or produced by fibroblasts may promote migration of vascular endothelial cells into the wound area, resulting in increased neovascularization. IGF-1 stimulates mitosis of fibroblasts and may act synergistically with PDGF to enhance epidermal and dermal regeneration.

IGF-1 and -2 each has distinct receptor proteins. The IGF-1 receptor is similar in structure to the insulin receptor. It consists of two α subunits that contain the IGF-1 binding site linked by disulfide bonds to the two β subunits that contain the transmembrane and cytoplasmic regions with the tyrosine kinase domain. The IGF-1 receptor binds IGF-1 with high affinity, binds IGF-2 with lower affinity, and binds insulin weakly. The IGF-2 receptor is a monomeric protein that has no kinase activity but binds proteins that contain the sugar mannose-6-phosphate. The IGF-2 receptor binds IGF-2 with high affinity, binds IGF-1 with low affinity, and does not bind insulin.

There are no published reports of clinical studies evaluating IGF-1 treatment of wounds. However, IGF-1 and growth hormone may act synergistically to promote wound healing. Two small double-blind, placebo-controlled studies showed improved healing with topical application of growth hormone to leg ulcers and systemic administration of growth hormone to severely burned pediatric patients (Gilpin, Barrow, Rutan, et al., 1994; Rasmussen, Karlsmark, Avnstorp, et al., 1991).

INTEGRATING GROWTH FACTORS INTO CLINICAL PRACTICE

Recombinant human PDGF-BB protein (becaplermin or Regranex) has been approved by the FDA for treatment of chronic diabetic foot ulcers but concerns about an increased rate of mortality secondary to malignancy that was observed in patients treated with three or more tubes of Regranex gel in a postmarketing retrospective cohort study led to a black box warning on the product label. However, a more extensive postmarketing retrospective cohort study did not find this association.

Although no growth factor has received approval for pressure injuries treatment, the Wound Healing Society guidelines for pressure injuries suggest considering PDGF use for pressure injuries that are not responsive to comprehensive therapy or before surgical repair (Whitney, Phillips, Aslam,

et al., 2006). International guidelines for prevention and treatment of pressure ulcers/injuries recommend considering the application of platelet-rich plasma (an autologous source of PDGF) for promoting healing in stage 3 and 4 pressure injuries (European Pressure Ulcer Advisory Panel, National Pressure Injury Advisory Panel, Pan Pacific Pressure Injury Alliance [EPUAP, NPIAP, PPPIA], 2019).

From a practical clinical perspective, whether manipulating the wound topically with growth factors or with semiocclusive dressings (as discussed in Chapter 21), the three principles of wound management remain the same and must be followed:

1. The underlying condition that caused the wound must be controlled or alleviated.
2. Cofactors that impair healing must be corrected. Similar to the concept of "barren soil," the cells in or adjacent to the wound must be properly prepared so that they can respond to stimulation by growth factors. For example, the cells must have adequate levels of oxygen, nutrients, and intact extracellular matrix components to be able to support cell mitosis, migration, and attachment.
3. A physiologic wound environment (both cellular and molecular) must be created for topical growth factors to be effective, also referred to as *wound bed preparation* (Schultz, Sibbald, Falanga, et al., 2003).

To create a physiologic wound environment, molecular imbalances that are common to chronic wounds (Box 23.1) and detrimental to healing must be corrected. The level of protease activities has emerged as one of the most important factors preventing chronic wounds from healing because the protease will degrade proteins that are essential for healing, such as growth factors, their receptors, and extracellular matrix proteins. Growth factors added to chronic wound fluids are quickly degraded by the proteases (MMPs and serine proteases such as neutrophil elastase) present in the fluid. Fortunately, levels of protease activity decrease in chronic wounds as they begin to heal (Figs. 23.5 and 23.6).

BOX 23.1 Molecular Imbalances in Chronic Wounds

- Chronic wound fluid does not consistently stimulate growth (mitosis) of skin fibroblasts (Alper, Tibbetts, & Sarazen, 1985; Bucalo, Eaglstein, & Falanga, 1993; Katz, Alvarez, Kirsner, et al., 1991).
- Ratios of proinflammatory cytokines (tumor necrosis factor-α and interleukin-1β) and natural receptors are significantly increased (Harris, Yee, Walters, et al., 1995; Mast & Schultz, 1996).
- Protease activity is significantly elevated (Bullen, Longaker, Updike, et al., 1995; Harris et al., 1995; Mast & Schultz, 1996; Nwomeh, Liang, Diegelmann, et al., 1998; Rogers, Burnett, Moore, et al., 1995; Tarnuzzer & Schultz, 1996; Yager, Zhang, Liang, et al., 1996).
- Cells may be unable to respond or may be senescent (Hopf, Ueno, Aslam, et al., 2006; Robson, Cooper, Aslam, et al., 2006; Steed, Attinger, Colaizzi, et al., 2006; Whitney et al., 2006).

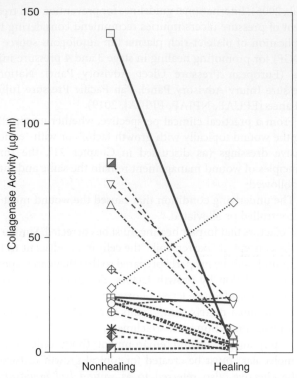

Fig. 23.5 Protease levels in fluids from chronic venous ulcers before and after initiating healing. Protease activity was measured in fluids collected from nonhealing venous leg ulcers of 15 patients at the start of hospitalization and 2 weeks later, after the ulcers had clinical evidence of healing. *Lines* connecting the protease levels measured in the two samples from each patient (nonhealing and healing) indicate that protease activity tends to decrease as ulcers begin to heal. (From Schultz, G. S., & Mast, B. A. (1998). Molecular analysis of the environment of healing and chronic wounds: Cytokines, proteases, and growth factors. *Wounds, 10*, 1f–9f.)

Numerous interventions are available to facilitate wound bed preparation and the creation of a physiologic wound environment. The acronym "TIME," as described in Chapter 21 identifies clinical interventions that should be used. For example, sharp debridement to remove nonviable tissue may be necessary to convert the detrimental chronic wound environment into a pseudoacute wound environment in which growth factors can function more effectively. Topical dressings that contain collagen (e.g., Promogran or Endoform) are designed as "sacrificial substrates" for wound proteases (MMPs and elastase) and thereby "spare" proteolytic destruction of the proteins in the wound bed that is essential for healing, such as growth factors, receptors, and extracellular matrix proteins. An added benefit to sharp debridement is that it will help to remove bacterial biofilms, which have been reported to be present in over 60% of chronic wounds (James, Swogger, Wolcott, et al., 2008). Biofilm is discussed in Chapter 19. Specific aspects of wound bed preparation were updated in 2012 to include new information that was generated in the 10 years since the original publication on wound bed preparation (Leaper, Schultz, Carville, et al., 2012). Biophysical and biologic agents can be used to alter the wound environment and correct senescent cells. These agents are described in detail in Chapters 24–27.

MOLECULAR ENVIRONMENT OF WOUNDS

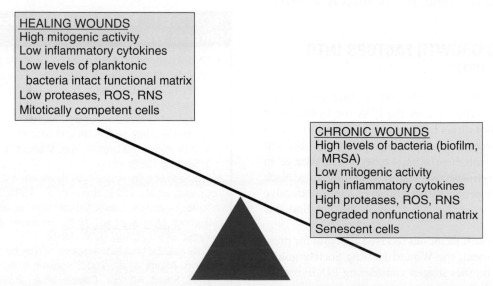

HEALING WOUNDS
High mitogenic activity
Low inflammatory cytokines
Low levels of planktonic
  bacteria intact functional matrix
Low proteases, ROS, RNS
Mitotically competent cells

CHRONIC WOUNDS
High levels of bacteria (biofilm, MRSA)
Low mitogenic activity
High inflammatory cytokines
High proteases, ROS, RNS
Degraded nonfunctional matrix
Senescent cells

Fig. 23.6 Imbalanced molecular environments of healing and chronic wounds. *MRSA,* methicillin-resistant *Staphylococcus aureus*; *RNS,* reactive nitrogen species; *ROS,* reactive oxygen species.

CLINICAL CONSULT

A: A 50-year-old female with a lower right extremity leg ulcer referred to wound clinic by friend. Patient wants growth factors because they worked so well on her friend's diabetic foot wound. Pitting edema and hemosiderin staining present on right lower leg gaiter area. Ulcer is irregular-shaped 2 × 1 × 0.4 cm with clean, red, viable wound base. No history of diabetes. ABI and foot sensation within normal limits, no signs of neuropathy. Ulcer has been present for 9 months, and patient indicates she is "tired of it being there." Uses several layers of gauze over ulcer and has to change twice daily to prevent soaking through to socks.
D: Venous ulceration.

P: Graduated compression, absorptive topical dressings, collagen wound dressing to reduce breakdown of desirable wound proteins and growth factors.
I: (1) Provide education related to venous insufficiency and need for compression. (2) Recommend collagen wound dressing to attract MMPs and preserve growth factors. (3) Alginate followed by foam cover dressing over collagen to absorb exudate. (4) Wrap with two-layer compression. (5) Change dressing and apply compression dressing twice weekly in clinic.
E: Patient verbalizes understanding and rationale for plan of care. Return to clinic in 4 days to evaluate effectiveness of compression and local wound care.

SUMMARY

- Increased knowledge of the molecular regulation of normal wound healing has led to a better understanding of the molecular imbalances that occur frequently in chronic wounds and that impair healing.
- The presence of bacterial biofilms in a high percentage of chronic wounds stimulates chronic inflammation, which leads to elevated levels of proteases that destroy proteins essential for healing.
- Dressings that contain collagen help to reduce elevated levels of destructive proteases, improve effectiveness of endogenous growth factors and exogenously applied recombinant growth factors (PDGF, EGF), as well as other advanced therapies, including biologically active, engineered, artificial skin substitutes.
- Advanced therapies only function optimally when they are applied to wound beds that are properly prepared and contain cells that are able to respond to them.

SELF-ASSESSMENT QUESTIONS

1. Small signaling proteins that mediate and regulate immunity, inflammation, and hematopoiesis are called:
   a. Cytokines
   b. Growth factors
   c. Proteases
   d. a and b
2. Sources of growth factors include:
   a. Platelets
   b. Macrophages
   c. Placenta
   d. All of the above

3. Which of the following statements about chronic wounds is false?
   a. Chronic wound fluid does not consistently stimulate growth of skin fibroblasts
   b. Ratios of proinflammatory cytokines decrease
   c. Protease activity is elevated
   d. Cells may be senescent
4. Which of the following statements about collagen dressings is true?
   a. They reduce elevated levels of destructive proteases
   b. They should not be used with topical growth factors
   c. Both a and b
   d. None of the above

REFERENCES

Abraham, J., & Klagsbrun, M. (1996). Modulation of wound repair by members of the fibroblast growth factor family. In R. A. F. Clark (Ed.), *The molecular and cellular biology of wound repair.* New York: Plenum Press.

Acosta, J., Savigne, W., Valdez, C., et al. (2006). Epidermal growth factor intralesional infiltrations can prevent amputation in patients with advanced diabetic foot wounds. *International Wound Journal, 3,* 232.

Alper, J. C., Tibbetts, L. L., & Sarazen, A. A., Jr. (1985). The in vitro response of fibroblasts to the fluid that accumulates under a vapor-permeable membrane. *The Journal of Investigative Dermatology, 84*, 513.

Arai, K., Lee, F., Miyajima, A., et al. (1990). Cytokines: Coordinators of immune and inflammatory responses. *Annual Review of Biochemistry, 59*, 783.

Barrientos, S., Brem, H., Stojadinovic, O., et al. (2008). Growth factors and cytokines in wound healing. *Wound Repair and Regeneration, 16*, 585.

Bennett, N. T., & Schultz, G. S. (1993a). Growth factors and wound healing: Biochemical properties of growth factors and their receptors. *American Journal of Surgery, 165*, 728.

Bennett, N. T., & Schultz, G. S. (1993b). Growth factors and wound healing. II. Role in normal and chronic wound healing. *American Journal of Surgery, 166*, 74.

Border, W. A., & Noble, N. A. (1994). Transforming growth factor-β in tissue fibrosis. *The New England Journal of Medicine, 10*, 1286.

Bradham, D. M., Igarashi, A., Potter, R. L., et al. (1991). Connective tissue growth factor: A cysteine-rich mitogen secreted by human vascular endothelial cells is related to the SRC-induced immediate early gene product CEF-10. *The Journal of Cell Biology, 114*(6), 1285.

Brown, G. B., Curtsinger, L., 3rd, Brightwell, J. R., et al. (1986). Enhancement of epidermal regeneration by biosynthetic epidermal growth factor. *The Journal of Experimental Medicine, 163*, 1319.

Brown, G. L., Nanney, L. B., Griffen, J., et al. (1989). Enhancement of wound healing by topical treatment with epidermal growth factor. *The New England Journal of Medicine, 321*, 76.

Bucalo, B., Eaglstein, W. H., & Falanga, V. (1993). Inhibition of cell proliferation by chronic wound fluid. *Wound Repair and Regeneration, 1*, 181.

Bullen, E. C., Longaker, M. T., Updike, D. L., et al. (1995). Tissue inhibitor of metalloproteinases-1 is decreased, and activated gelatinases are increased in chronic wounds. *The Journal of Investigative Dermatology, 104*, 236.

Carpenter, G., & Cohen, S. (1990). Epidermal growth factor. *The Journal of Biological Chemistry, 265*, 7709.

David, L. S., Goslen, J. B., Holloway, G. A., et al. (1992). Randomized prospective double-blind trial in healing chronic diabetic foot ulcers. *Diabetes Care, 11*, 1598.

Eriksson, E., Liu, P. Y., Schultz, G. S., Martins-Green, M., Tanaka, R., Weir, D., et al. (2022). Chronic wounds—Treatment consensus. *Wound Repair and Regeneration, 30*, 156. https://www.ncbi.nlm.nih.gov/pubmed/35130362.

European Pressure Ulcer Advisory Panel, National Pressure Injury Advisory Panel, Pan Pacific Pressure Injury Alliance (EPUAP, NPIAP, PPPIA). (2019). In E. Haesler (Ed.), *Prevention and treatment of pressure ulcers/injuries*. Osborne Park: Cambridge Media.

Falanga, V., Eaglstein, W. H., Bucalo, B., et al. (1992). Topical use of human recombinant epidermal growth factor (h-EGF) in venous ulcers. *Phlebology, 18*, 604.

Fantl, W. J., Johnson, D. E., & Williams, L. T. (1993). Signaling by receptor tyrosine kinases. *Annual Review of Biochemistry, 62*, 453.

Frazier, K., Williams, S., Kothapalli, D., et al. (1996). Stimulation of fibroblast cell growth, matrix production, and granulation tissue formation by connective tissue growth factor. *The Journal of Investigative Dermatology, 107*, 404.

Frenette, P. S., & Wagner, D. D. (1996a). Adhesion molecules—Part II: Blood vessels and blood cells. *The New England Journal of Medicine, 335*, 43.

Frenette, P. S., & Wagner, D. D. (1996b). Molecular medicine: Adhesion molecules—Part I. *The New England Journal of Medicine, 334*, 1526.

Fu, X., Shen, Z., Chen, Y., et al. (1998). Randomised placebo-controlled trial of use of topical recombinant bovine basic fibroblast growth factor for second-degree burns. *Lancet, 352*, 1661.

Gilpin, D. A., Barrow, R. E., Rutan, R. L., et al. (1994). Recombinant human growth hormone accelerates wound healing in children with large cutaneous burns. *Annals of Surgery, 220*, 19.

Harris, I. R., Yee, K. C., Walters, C. E., et al. (1995). Cytokine and protease levels in healing and non-healing chronic venous leg ulcers. *Experimental Dermatology, 4*, 342.

Heldin, C., & Westermark, B. (1996). Role of platelet derived growth factor in vivo. In R. A. F. Clark (Ed.), *The molecular and cellular biology of wound repair*. New York: Plenum Press.

Higashiyama, S., et al. (1992). Structure of heparin-binding EGF-like growth factor. *The Journal of Biological Chemistry, 267*, 6205.

Holloway, G. A., Steed, D., DeMarco, M., et al. (1993). A randomized, controlled, multicenter, dose response trial of activated platelet supernatant, topical CT-102 in chronic, nonhealing, diabetic wounds. *Wounds, 5*, 198.

Hopf, H. W., Ueno, C., Aslam, R., et al. (2006). Guidelines for the treatment of arterial insufficiency ulcers. *Wound Repair and Regeneration, 14*(6), 693.

International Wound Infection Institute (IWII). (2022). Wound infection in clinical practice. *Wounds International*.

Ito, Y., Aten, J., Bende, R. J., et al. (1998). Expression of connective tissue growth factor in human renal fibrosis. *Kidney International, 53*, 853.

James, G., Swogger, E., Wolcott, R., et al. (2008). Biofilms in chronic wounds. *Wound Repair and Regeneration, 16*, 37.

Katz, M. H., Alvarez, A. F., Kirsner, R. S., et al. (1991). Human wound fluid from acute wounds stimulates fibroblast and endothelial cell growth. *Journal of the American Academy of Dermatology, 25*, 1054.

Kucich, U., Rosenbloom, J. C., Herrick, D. J., et al. (2001). Signaling events required for transforming growth factor–beta stimulation of connective tissue growth factor expression by cultured human lung fibroblasts. *Archives of Biochemistry and Biophysics, 395*, 103.

Leaper, D., Schultz, G., Carville, K., et al. (2012). Extending the TIME concept: What have we learned in the past 10 years? *International Wound Journal, 9*(Suppl. 2), S1.

Ley, K. (2017). M1 means kill; M2 means heal. *Journal of Immunology, 199*(7), 2191–2193. https://doi.org/10.4049/jimmunol.1701135. 28923980.

Lindemann, S., Tolley, N. D., Dixon, D. A., McIntyre, T. M., Prescott, S. M., Zimmerman, G. A., et al. (2001). Activated platelets mediate inflammatory signaling by regulated interleukin 1beta synthesis. *The Journal of Cell Biology, 154*(3), 485–490. https://doi.org/10.1083/jcb.200105058.

Malone, M., Bjarnsholt, T., McBain, A. J., James, G. A., Stoodley, P., Leaper, D., et al. (2017). The prevalence of biofilms in chronic wounds: A systematic review and meta-analysis of published data. *Journal of Wound Care, 26*, 20–25.

Massague, J. (1990). Transforming growth factor-alpha. A model for membrane-anchored growth factors. *The Journal of Biological Chemistry, 265*(35), 21393.

Mast, B. A., & Schultz, G. S. (1996). Interactions of cytokines, growth factors, and proteases in acute and chronic wounds. *Wound Repair and Regeneration, 4,* 411.

Nanney, L. B., & King, L. E. (1996). Epidermal growth factor and transforming growth factor-α. In R. A. F. Clark (Ed.), *The molecular and cellular biology of wound repair.* New York: Plenum Press.

Nwomeh, B. C., Liang, H. X., Diegelmann, R. F., et al. (1998). Dynamics of the matrix metalloproteinases MMP-1 and MMP-8 in acute open human dermal wounds. *Wound Repair and Regeneration, 6,* 127.

Omar, A., Wright, J. B., Schultz, G., Burrell, R., & Nadworny, P. (2017). Microbial biofilms and chronic wounds. *Microorganisms, 5*(1), 9. https://doi.org/10.3390/microorganisms5010009. 28272369. PMCID: PMC5374386.

Phillips, P. L., Wolcott, R. D., Fletcher, J., & Schultz, G. S. (2010). Biofilms made easy. *Wounds International, 1*(3). Retrieved 3/21/2021, from https://www.woundsinternational.com.

Rasmussen, L. H., Karlsmark, T., Avnstorp, C., et al. (1991). Topical human growth hormone treatment of chronic leg ulcers. *Phlebology, 6,* 23.

Roberts, A. B., & Sporn, M. B. (1996). Transforming growth factor-beta. In R. A. F. Clark (Ed.), *The molecular and cellular biology of wound repair.* New York: Plenum Press.

Robson, M. C., Abdullah, A., Burns, B. F., et al. (1994). Safety and effect of topical recombinant human interleukin-1β in the management of pressure sores. *Wound Repair and Regeneration, 2,* 177.

Robson, M. C., Cooper, D. M., Aslam, R., et al. (2006). Guidelines for the treatment of venous ulcers. *Wound Repair and Regeneration, 14*(6), 649.

Robson, M. C., Phillips, L. G., Lawrence, W. T., et al. (1992). The safety and effect of topically applied recombinant basic fibroblast growth factor on the healing of chronic pressure sores. *Annals of Surgery, 216,* 401.

Robson, M. C., Phillips, L. G., Thomason, A., et al. (1992). Recombinant human platelet-derived growth factor-BB for the treatment of chronic pressure ulcers. *Annals of Plastic Surgery, 29,* 193.

Rogers, A. A., Burnett, S., Moore, J. C., et al. (1995). Involvement of proteolytic enzymes—Plasminogen activators and matrix metalloproteinases—In the pathophysiology of pressure ulcers. *Wound Repair and Regeneration, 3,* 273.

Schultz, G., Bjarnsholt, T., James, G. A., Leaper, D. J., McBain, A. J., Malone, M., et al. (2017). Consensus guidelines for the identification and treatment of biofilms in chronic nonhealing wounds. *Wound Repair and Regeneration, 25*(5), 744–757. https://doi.org/10.1111/wrr.12590. 28960634.

Schultz, G., Sibbald, R., Falanga, V., et al. (2003). Wound bed preparation, a systemic approach to wound bed management. *Wound Repair and Regeneration, 11*(Suppl. 1), S1.

Shah, M., Foreman, D. M., & Ferguson, M. W. (1992). Control of scarring in adult wounds by neutralising antibody to transforming growth factor beta. *Lancet, 339,* 213.

Shah, M., Foreman, D. M., & Ferguson, M. W. (1994). Neutralising antibody to TGF-beta 1,2 reduces cutaneous scarring in adult rodents. *Journal of Cell Science, 107,* 1137.

Sisco, M., Kryger, Z., O'Shaughnessy, K., et al. (2008). Antisense inhibition of connective tissue growth factor (CTGF/CCN2) mRNA limits hypertrophic scarring without affecting wound healing in vivo. *Wound Repair and Regeneration, 16,* 661.

Springer, T. A. (1990). Adhesion receptors of the immune system. *Nature, 346,* 425.

Steed, D. L. (1995). Clinical evaluation of recombinant human platelet-derived growth factor for the treatment of lower extremity diabetic ulcers. Diabetic Ulcer Study Group. *Journal of Vascular Surgery, 21,* 71.

Steed, D. L., Attinger, C., Colaizzi, T., et al. (2006). Guidelines for the treatment of diabetic ulcers. *Wound Repair and Regeneration, 14*(6), 680.

Stromberg, S., Collins, T. J., Gordon, A. Q., et al. (1992). Transforming growth factor-alpha acts as an autocrine growth factor in ovarian carcinoma cell lines. *Cancer Research, 52,* 341.

Tarnuzzer, R. W., & Schultz, G. S. (1996). Biochemical analysis of acute and chronic wound environments. *Wound Repair and Regeneration, 4,* 321.

Vadhan-Raj, S., Goldberg, J., Perales, M., et al. (2013). Clinical applications of palifermin: Amelioration of oral mucositis and other potential indications. *Journal of Cellular and Molecular Medicine, 17,* 1371.

Werner, S., Peters, K. G., Longaker, M. T., et al. (1992). Large induction of keratinocyte growth factor expression in the dermis during wound healing. *Proceedings of the National Academy of Sciences of the United States of America, 89,* 6896.

Whitney, J., Phillips, L., Aslam, R., et al. (2006). Guidelines for the treatment of pressure ulcers. *Wound Repair and Regeneration, 14*(6), 663.

World Union of Wound Healing Societies (WUWHS). (2016). Florence congress, position document. Management of biofilm. *Wounds International.*

Yager, D. R., Zhang, L. Y., Liang, H. X., et al. (1996). Wound fluids from human pressure ulcers contain elevated matrix metalloproteinase levels and activity compared to surgical wound fluid. *The Journal of Investigative Dermatology, 107,* 743.

24

Negative Pressure Wound Therapy

Debra S. Netsch and Denise P. Nix

OBJECTIVES

1. Compare and contrast two different types of negative pressure wound therapy (NPWT).
2. Discuss three mechanisms for the effects of NPWT on wound healing.
3. Describe three indications, contraindications, and precautions for NPWT.
4. Describe the application of NPWT, including undermined or sinus areas.

Negative pressure wound therapy (NPWT) is the application of subatmospheric (negative) pressure to a wound through suction to facilitate healing and collect wound fluid (Campbell, Smith, & Smith, 2008; Vikatmaa, Juutilainen, Kuukasjärvi, et al., 2008). NPWT has become a common modality for the temporary management of a wide variety of acute and chronic wounds. Numerous NPWT systems are commercially available, each consisting of the following components: a wound filler dressing, a negative pressure device (disposable or reusable), a cover dressing or drape, a source for negative pressure (e.g., pump), and a fluid containment mechanism (i.e., a container or absorbent dressing). As shown in Table 24.1, components vary by manufacturer and product. For example, wound fillers range from open cell foam, silicone tubing wrapped with gauze (either plain or antimicrobial), honeycomb configured nonadherent matrix, nonwoven superabsorbent polymer, hydrocolloid, to gauze. Table 24.1 lists NPWT features and options. Available combinations of features and options are contingent on the manufacturer and device. Due to considerable variability, specific brand names are not listed.

MECHANISM OF ACTION

NPWT facilitates wound healing through the use of controlled subatmospheric pressure to trigger and enhance the body's wound-healing response at a cellular level (Ubbink, Westerbos, Evans, et al., 2008). Primary effects include (1) edema reduction and fluid removal, (2) macrodeformation and wound contraction, and (3) microdeformation and mechanical stretch perfusion (Saxena, Hwang, Huang, et al., 2004). Secondary effects include increased angiogenesis, granulation tissue formation, and reduction in bacterial bioburden (Orgill, Manders, Sumpio, et al., 2009).

Edema Reduction and Removal of Wound Fluid

Removal of exudate containing toxic cytokines, bacteria, and matrix metalloproteinases and reduction of interstitial edema is a primary benefit of NPWT (Ubbink et al., 2008). By reducing tissue edema, the compressive effects of edema upon the periwound vasculature are decreased, thereby improving tissue perfusion, delivery of nutrients, and uptake of oxygen, culminating in the wound's ability to resist bacterial proliferation and microbial penetration (Orgill et al., 2009). A decrease in wound bacterial load was first described in the porcine model by Morykwas, Argenta, Shelton-Brown, et al. (1997) and is attributed to: (1) removal of stagnant wound fluid, (2) direct removal of bacteria from the wound bed, (3) removal of third-space fluid, and (4) increased blood flow and thus increased immunity and oxygenation (Orgill et al., 2009). A significant decrease in nonfermentative, gram-negative bacilli has been reported with the use of NPWT compared with moist saline dressings (Mouës, Vos, van den Bemd, et al., 2004). NPWT was found to decrease bacteria counts, including both virulence and biofilm of *Pseudomonas aeruginosa* more than dry sterile gauze in vivo (Wang, Zhirui, Tongtong, Wang, et al., 2018). However, it is important to note that an increase in *Staphylococcus aureus* compared with the wounds managed with moist saline dressings was also reported, suggesting close monitoring is warranted. Removal and collection of wound exudate via a closed containment system may also facilitate bioburden reduction by decreasing the frequency of dressing changes and exposure to potential external contaminants (Hinck, Franke, & Gatzka, 2010; Pham, Middleton, & Maddern, 2006).

Macrodeformation and Wound Contraction

Intact skin and soft tissue have a natural tension that, when disrupted, causes skin and soft tissues to typically pull apart

TABLE 24.1   NPWT Features and Options[a]

Wound filler	Green foam
	Nonadherent gauze
	Oil emulsion nonadherent gauze
	Polyurethane black foam
	Polyvinyl alcohol white foam
	Proprietary hydrocolloid dressing over antimicrobial gauze or foam interface dressing
	Silver-impregnated polyurethane foam
Canister volume (mL)	45
	60 mL cartridge
	No canister; absorb up to 140 mL
	250
	500
	1200
Setting variability	Continuous
	Continuous and dynamic/variable
	Continuous and intermittent
	Continuous, dynamic/variable, and instill irrigant
	Continuous, intermittent, and instills irrigant
Pump weight (lb)	<0.5
	1.9
	2.4
	3.2
	4.5
	5.5 lb
	7.4 lb
	12.3 lb
	14.5 lb
Settings (mmHg)	10–200
	40–125
	50–100
	60–200
	70, 120 or 150
	75, 100 or 125
Battery life (h)	4
	6
	9
	12
	14
	24
	8 days
	3 weeks alkaline batteries
	No battery proprietary spring mechanism

NPWT, negative pressure wound therapy.
[a]Examples only, list not inclusive. Available combinations of features and options are contingent on the manufacturer and device.

(separate). Distractive tissue forces may act to keep a wound open, with vectors that oppose contraction, thereby delaying healing. NPWT provides a mechanism to oppose these distractive soft tissue vectors (Franz, Robson, Steed, et al., 2008). The application of negative pressure facilitates contraction, or pulling together, of the wound edges, simulating the application of an abdominal binder. The pulling together of the wound edges (contraction) promotes earlier wound healing by delayed primary or secondary intention. This contraction process occurs three dimensionally through mechanical forces, thus allowing decreased wound volume symmetrically and facilitating faster wound closure (Orgill et al., 2009; Ubbink et al., 2008).

Microdeformation and Mechanical Stretch

Histologic wound sections have demonstrated microdeformations of the wound surface present with NPWT that is not present underneath occlusive dressings alone (Saxena et al., 2004). Mechanically, deformation results in fluid flow within the matrix and strain where the matrix cells are anchored. Thus cells are subjected to both mechanical stretch mediated by their attachments to the matrix and shear stresses due to fluid flow. Fluid shear stresses are known to regulate cellular proliferation (Ubbink et al., 2008).

Wound surface microdeformations also stimulate increased vascular growth. The stretching of the wound surface stimulates cell division, proliferation, and angiogenesis (Orgill, Austen, Butler, et al., 2004). In vivo models have demonstrated that cells respond to tension with directional growth and specific gene release (vascular endothelial growth factor) when mechanical tension has been applied (Orgill et al., 2004; Saxena et al., 2004). The application of mechanical force also initiates a cellular response, inducing a cascade of cellular proliferation, angiogenesis, and promotion of wound healing. The term *mechanotransduction* has been adopted to denote this cellular and physiologic response to mechanical strain (Orgill et al., 2009). An in vivo porcine study has found the degree of microdeformation and macrodeformation to be similar between gauze- and foam-based NPWT (Borgquist, Gustafsson, Ingemansson, et al., 2010). In terms of the effect of NPWT on surrounding skin perfusion, it is hypothesized that increased perfusion occurs with the treatment, although the testing mechanism (laser Doppler) was criticized as being an indirect measure of blood flow (Morykwas, Simpson, Punger, et al., 2006; Orgill et al., 2009).

Morykwas et al. (1997) reported an increase of more than 60% in granulation tissue formation using NPWT in comparison to moist gauze in porcine wounds. Numerous human studies have found increased and/or faster closure rates of wounds when treated with NPWT versus standard practice (Vuerstaek, Vainas, Wuite, et al., 2006). Comparison of NPWT to standard compression therapy in primarily venous lower leg ulcerations revealed faster wound bed preparation (7 vs 17 days) and faster healing rates (29 vs 45 days) (Vuerstaek et al., 2006). Faster granulation tissue coverage over diabetic foot wounds resulted in accelerated wound closure when NPWT was used (Blume, Walters, Payne, et al., 2008).

INDICATIONS AND USES

NPWT is approved by the Food and Drug Administration (FDA) for use with chronic, acute, traumatic, subacute, and dehisced wounds; partial-thickness burns; ulcers (e.g., diabetic or pressure); flaps and grafts once nonviable tissue is removed; and select high-risk postoperative surgical incisions (e.g., orthopedic, sternal). The modality is used clinically with wounds of all sizes and depths, but most favorably in complicated deep wounds. NPWT can be used in wounds with tunnels, undermining, or sinus tracts when the foam is used as a wound filler to fill the dead space and can be easily retrieved (Andros, Armstrong, Attinger, et al., 2006).

Acute Wounds

The use of NPWT has been reported in acute wounds, including the intact postoperative surgical incision, open surgical wounds, contaminated surgical wounds, and burns.

Incisional NPWT

The prophylactic application of incisional NPWT (iNPWT) in the operating room over a sterile incision is used on "at-risk" incisions to bolster the incision by keeping the cutaneous, dermal, and subcutaneous wound edges approximated and reducing horizontal and vertical shear forces. Physiologically, iNPWT reduces lateral stresses on the wound up to 50%. The macrodeformation created by iNPWT mimics intact skin elasticity forces. Although findings are inconsistent, the reported benefits of iNPWT in high-risk surgical patients include reduced incidence of surgical site infection and reduced seroma and hematoma formation and dehiscence (Ingargiola, Daniali, & Lee, 2013; Kubec, Badeau, Materazzi, et al., 2013).

Metaanalysis conducted by other researchers suggested the use of iNPWT of closed incisions compared with traditional dressing concluded iNPWT usage demonstrated a statistically significant decrease in surgical site infection ($P < 0.05$) (Li et al., 2019; Singh et al., 2019). NICE guidelines (2019) recommend use of iNPWT noting clinical evidence shows fewer surgical site infections for closed surgical incisions with iNPWT as well as a reduction in the rate of seromas compared with standard wound dressings. In contrast, a Cochrane review (Webster et al., 2019) noted numerous study design limitations with iNPWT research.

Infected and Complex Surgical Wounds

NPWT can be used with clean or contaminated surgical wounds and with use of dense foam or contact layer over orthopedic hardware, tendons, bone, and Gor-Tex sheets. It can also be used in the presence of wound infection or osteomyelitis *after* appropriate debridement and antibiotics have been initiated (Andros et al., 2006; Shweiki & Gallagher, 2013). A review of NPWT for prevention and treatment of surgical-site infections after vascular surgery (Acosta, Björck, & Wanhainen, 2017) found improved healing rates with low risk of NPWT-related bleeding from underlying vessels and the high rate of graft preservation.

National Institute for Health and Care Excellence (NICE) guidelines (2013) recommend NPWT as a viable option for the management of the open abdominal wound. The open abdominal wound is often used as a "bridge" until the patient is stabilized, and the wound is amenable to closure. In addition to providing stabilization of the wound edges, containment of exudate, and a moist wound environment and promoting granulation tissue formation, NPWT has been reported to improve wound closure rates in the repair of hernias with infected mesh (Baharestani & Gabriel, 2011; DeFranzo, Argenta, Marks, et al., 2001). Evidence also suggests that NPWT increases the chance of successful delayed primary fascial closure and reduced negative clinical outcomes (e.g., ventral hernias and prolonged hospitalization), compared with select alternative temporary abdominal closure (TAC) methods (Moües, Heule, & Hovius, 2011; Roberts, Zygun, Grendar, et al., 2012; Stevens, 2009).

The use of NPWT in burn management has been minimally investigated. One NPWT has received FDA approval for partial-thickness burns, although a Cochrane review found only one randomized controlled trial (RCT) addressing this indication (Dumville & Munson, 2012). The physiologic advantages to using NPWT are similar as in other wounds; however, the reduced edema mediated capillary stasis and improved blood flow, particularly within the first 12–24 h postburn, and has been noted to reduce the progression to full-thickness burns. In addition, with the removal of wound fluid containing proteolytic enzymes, acute-phase protein, and metalloproteinases, a reduced systemic inflammatory response has been observed (Bovill, Banwell, Teot, et al., 2008). The use of NPWT for full-thickness burns is unclear and should be explored within the scope of the specialist burn center following a rigorous study protocol.

Chronic Wounds

Multiple studies have found efficacious and safe use of NPWT with treatment of chronic wounds. Among national evidence-based guidelines for chronic wounds, NPWT is recommended for the treatment of nonhealing venous ulcers and diabetic wounds when conventional therapies have failed (Dowsett, 2012; Moües et al., 2011; Steed, Attinger, Colaizzi, et al., 2006; Whitney, Phillips, Aslam, et al., 2006; WOCN®, 2019). NPWT may have an adjunct role in the management of arterial ulcers when there is adequate perfusion for healing (Hopf, Ueno, Aslam, et al., 2006; Moües et al., 2011). International pressure injury guidelines recommend NPWT as an early adjuvant for the treatment of deep Stage 3 and 4 pressure injuries (EPIUAP, NPIAP, & PPPIA, 2019). Adequate wound debridement remains an important precursor to the implementation of NPWT with chronic wounds.

The use of NPWT for the management of diabetic foot ulcers after debridement is increasingly prevalent. Armstrong, Lavery, Abu-Rumman, et al. (2002) reported that in patients with refractory diabetic foot ulcers, 90.3% ($n = 28$) of wounds healed after debridement and NPWT within a mean of 8.1 weeks (± 5.5 weeks). The remaining three patients required a transmetatarsal amputation or below-the-knee amputation. Enhanced wound healing, reduced time to healing, and fewer amputations have been reported (Armstrong, Lavery, & Boulton, 2007; Blume et al., 2008). NPWT is recognized in national guidelines as a recommended treatment of diabetic foot ulcers with and without partial foot amputations (Crawford &

Fields-Varnado, 2013; Game, Almqvist, Attinger, et al., 2016; Steed et al., 2006; WOCN®, 2019).

Flaps and Grafts

NPWT has also been used to prepare a granular wound bed to receive a graft and to manage the donor, graft, and flap site postoperatively (Gray & Peirce, 2004; Murphy & Evan, 2012; Robson, Cooper, Aslam, et al., 2006). Stimulation of angiogenesis, granulation formation, and reduction of edema all prepare the wound and improve the success for surgical repair. Additionally, NPWT provides the opportunity of scheduling the elective surgical procedure at a time that is optimal for the patient and does not jeopardize outcomes (Dowsett, 2012; Murphy & Evan, 2012; Robson et al., 2006). Staged use of different types of NPWT has been utilized to help manage cardiac sternal wounds that failed to close following a previous procedure. In this study (Chowdhry & Wilhelmi, 2019), NPWTi-d was used as an adjunct therapy along with debridement and systemic antibiotics with a significantly shorter time to primary wound closure when compared with the standard care group ($P < 0.0001$). The mean time to primary wound closure for the NPWTi-d group was 7.9 ± 2.3 days with a median of 8 days, whereas patients in the standard care group required 13.9 ± 3.2 days to primary wound closure with a median of 15 days. The NPWTi-d group utilized iNPWT after muscle flap reconstruction and closure. The iNPWT group had a significantly shorter drain duration when compared with patients in the standard care group ($P = 0.0001$). The mean drain duration for the iNPWT group was 15.0 ± 2.0 days with a median of 14 days, whereas the mean drain duration for the standard care group was 21.7 ± 3.9 days with a median of 22 days. Thus, the use of different types of NPWT at appropriate stages was found to be statistically significant over the standard care group.

Enteric Fistulas

Chapter 39 provides a comprehensive review of the assessment and management of fistulas. NPWT is one management strategy that may be used with a fistula that has been explored and evaluated and the following criteria is confirmed:

- the fistula exhibits the potential for spontaneous closure (i.e., no evidence of pseudostoma formation),
- lack of exposed bowel in the wound base, and
- lack of abscess or distal obstruction.

Typically, when managing an enterocutaneous fistula, the actual fistula orifice is separated from the wound (see Plate 69) and the fistula effluent is contained by a pouching system. The remainder of the wound is then managed with NPWT (Bruhin, Ferreira, Chariker, et al., 2014; Heineman, Garcia, Obst, et al., 2015; Reider, 2017). Plate 70 provides a pictorial step-by-step procedure for isolating and pouching a fistula. Additional pictorial step-by-step procedures for isolating fistulas with and without the use of commercially available devices and can be accessed at the Nurses Specialized in Wound, Ostomy and Continence Canada (NSWOCC) Nursing Best Practice Recommendations: Enterocutaneous Fistula

and Enteroatmospheric Fistula website http://nswoc.ca/ecf-best-practices/ (Brooke, El-Ghaname, Napier, & Sommerey, 2018).

To minimize trauma to the fascia in the bed of an open abdominal wound and potential fistula formation, NPWT should be used cautiously by applying a lower amount of pressure (i.e., 75 to 90 mmHg), utilizing a nonadherent wound liner between the wound bed and filler dressing, and/or positioning the catheter so that it does not contact the wound bed (Mouës et al., 2011; Stevens, 2009).

Although containment of fistula effluent is neither a recommended nor intended use of the commercial vacuum-assisted closure (VAC), it is an appropriate indication for most NPWT systems using gauze wound-filler dressings (Mouës et al., 2011; Stevens, 2009).

SAFETY, CONTRAINDICATIONS, AND PRECAUTIONS

NPWT is generally considered to be a safe advanced-practice wound dressing, with rare serious adverse events (Peinemann & Sauerland, 2011; Sullivan, Snyder, Tipton, et al., 2009; Ubbink et al., 2008; Vikatmaa et al., 2008). Between the years 2007 and 2011, however, the FDA received reports of 12 deaths and 174 injuries related to NPWT. Most adverse events and deaths occurred either at home or in a long-term care facility. Bleeding was the most serious complication, with reports of bleeding associated with nine of the overall deaths. According to these reports, extensive bleeding has occurred in patients

- with blood vessel grafts in the leg,
- with breastbone or groin wounds,
- receiving medication for blood clots, and
- during removal of dressings attached to the tissues.

Patients with bleeding required emergency room visits and/or hospitalization and were treated with surgery and blood transfusions. Wound infection occurred in many of the additional cases, the majority of which were related to the retention of foam dressing pieces in the wounds. Most of these patients required surgery, additional hospitalization, and antibiotics (Wallis, 2010).

Contraindications and precautions for NPWT listed by the FDA can be found in Checklist 24.1. NPWT is contraindicated in the presence of untreated osteomyelitis, necrotic tissue, exposed blood vessels, exposed organs, nonenteric or unexplored fistulas, and malignancy in the wound (select manufacturers). Precautions and close monitoring are indicated with the use of NPWT in the presence of treated infection, treated osteomyelitis, potential for hemorrhage, anticoagulation therapy, postsurgical malignancy excision, and patients who have poor adherence to follow-up for monitoring of wound progress by the care provider (Andros et al., 2006; Wallis, 2010).

Debridement and appropriate antibiotics should be implemented before using NPWT in an infected wound or when osteomyelitis is present. It is essential that all infected and nonviable tissue or bone be debrided in conjunction with

CHECKLIST 24.1 Negative Pressure Wound Therapy: Contraindications and Precautions

Contraindications to NPWT
✓ Necrotic tissue with eschar present
✓ Untreated osteomyelitis
✓ Nonenteric and unexplored fistulas
✓ Malignancy in the wound
✓ Exposed vasculature
✓ Exposed nerves
✓ Exposed anastomotic site
✓ Exposed organs

Patient Risk Factors/Characteristics to Consider Before NPWT Use
✓ Patients at high risk for bleeding and hemorrhage, including immediately postoperatively
✓ Patients on anticoagulants or platelet aggregation inhibitors
✓ Patients with:
  • Friable vessels and infected blood vessels
  • Vascular anastomosis
  • Treated infected wounds
  • Treated osteomyelitis
  • Exposed organs, vessels, nerves, tendons, and ligaments
  • Sharp edges in the wound (i.e., bone fragments)
  • Spinal cord injury (stimulation of sympathetic nervous system)
  • Enteric fistulas
✓ Patients requiring:
  • Magnetic resonance imaging
  • Hyperbaric chamber
  • Defibrillation
✓ Patient size and weight
✓ Use near vagus nerve (bradycardia)
✓ Circumferential dressing application
✓ Mode of therapy (intermittent vs continuous negative pressure)

appropriate antibiotic coverage before NPWT placement. To help minimize the risk of retained dressing pieces, keep track of the number of dressing pieces placed in the wound, and do not cut the dressing directly over the wound to avoid dressing fragments or debris falling into the wound area while cutting (Wallis, 2010).

As shown in Table 24.2, when the potential for hemorrhage exists, NPWT can be used, but cautiously. If the patient's coagulation tests cannot be maintained within a therapeutic range, ecchymosis develops in the wound or periwound area or wound drainage becomes bloody, the pressure setting of the NPWT should be reduced. A nonadherent contact layer or a less adherent, higher-density, moist NPWT foam may be indicated (Andros et al., 2006).

Manufacturers' instructions state that NPWT dressing must be removed if defibrillation is required in the area of dressing placement because it may inhibit transmission of electrical energy and/or patient resuscitation. Some NPWT electrical units and silver dressings are not designed or compatible with hyperbaric oxygen therapy (HBO) or magnetic resonance imaging (MRI) environments. Typically, dressings can remain in place if they are not silver, but the electrical NPWT unit should not be taken into the area.

After surgical excision of the malignancy, all NPWT systems can be implemented in the acute surgical wound to aid in closure. NPWT has been used for palliative care purposes (e.g., reduced frequency of painful dressing changes, containment of exudate and odor); however, it is important to again check the manufacturer's guidelines for that device (Ford-Dunn, 2006). In addition, the insurance provider may not approve use of NPWT for palliative outcomes (as opposed to healing outcomes), and the wound care specialist may need to advocate strongly on the behalf of the patient and family for this type of intervention.

TABLE 24.2 Examples of Wound Characteristics Matched With Wound Filler

Wound Characteristic	NPWT Open-Cell Foam	NPWT Higher-Density, Moist, Open-Cell Foam	Gauze-Based Filler	Contact Layer (Under Filler)	Antibacterial Layer Under Filler or Silver-Coated Cell Foam	Irrigation With Open-Cell Foam
Deep but visible wound cavity	x		x			
Wound cavity with tunnels or deep undermining		x	x			
Infected wound					x	X
Wound with exposed structures		x		x		
Skin graft bolster	x			x		
Fragile wounds (bleeding potential, friable tissue)		x		x		

Birke-Sorensen et al. (2011); Dowsett (2012); Glass and Nanchahal (2012); Vig, Dowsett, Berg, et al. (2011).
NPWT, negative pressure wound therapy.

CLINICAL APPLICATION

Clinical application considerations for NPWT include the patient's need for and access to assistance and supplies, pain management, product selection, and amount of negative pressure.

Pain Management

Pain during dressing change removal and application of negative pressure has been frequently noted and is cited as a common cause for NPWT discontinuation (Malmsjö, Gustafsson, Lindstedt, et al., 2012; Sullivan et al., 2009). Pain has been associated with the type of wound filler used and may be more pronounced in the acute wound such as the fasciotomy and explant pacer sites. Multiple studies, including one systemic review, confirmed that there is less pain with gauze-based NPWT (Hurd, Chadwick, Cote, et al., 2010; Malmsjö et al., 2012; Upton & Andrews, 2015). Malmsjö, Ingemansson, Martin, et al. (2009) reported significantly higher levels of neuropeptides (calcitonin gene-related peptide [CGRP] and substance P) with the use of foam-based NPWT; both are known to cause inflammation and signal pain when tissue trauma occurs. Instillation of 2% lidocaine solution diluted 50/50 with normal saline can be instilled into the NPWT tubing with dressing changes or directly into the foam which will reduce pain during the dressing change procedure (Franczyk, Lohman, Agarwal, et al., 2009). The solution should be allowed to dwell in the wound bed for at least 15 min to attain the desired effect. Often simply instilling normal saline into the foam will facilitate easier lifting of the wound filler from the wound bed. Conscious sedation may be warranted for the pediatric patient to minimize emotional and physical trauma of the dressing change. Premedication before the dressing change should also be considered. Box 24.1 offers additional interventions for reducing pain upon dressing removal (EPIUAP, NPIAP, & PPPIA, 2019; Franczyk et al., 2009; Gupta, Baharestani, Baranoski, et al., 2004; Pham et al., 2006; Sullivan et al., 2009).

BOX 24.1   Reducing Pain Upon Dressing Removal

- Instill normal saline to moisten wound-filler dressing and allow it to loosen the wound-filler dressing from granulation tissue (either with or without adherent cover dressing in place).
- Decrease pressure setting.
- Change from intermittent to continuous cycling.
- Use nonadherent contact layers (e.g., silicone mesh dressing, impregnated wide-mesh dressings).
- Instill topical diluted lidocaine without epinephrine into wound-filler dressing and/or use systemic analgesics per prescriber's directions.
- Change wound-filler dressing to one less likely to allow granulation growth into dressing.
- Change type of NPWT system.

NPWT, negative pressure wound therapy.

Product Selection

Each system uses the same basic principles of negative pressure despite wound-filler dressing differences. Although each company denotes the nuances of their product, more research is needed to compare effectiveness between different products and wound-filler dressings. One in vivo study found that the pressure delivered with gauze and foam was similar and concluded that the overall NPWT impact should be the same (Malmsjö et al., 2009). Wall suction-based gauze NPWT compared with standard foam NPWT were found to have no statistical significance in healing (Hu, Zhang, Zhou, et al., 2009). Therefore, until research suggests otherwise, NPWT product selection should be based on features, availability, reimbursement, and cost (Campbell et al., 2008; Glass & Nanchahal, 2012; Long & Blevins, 2009). Systematic reviews of NPWT correlating with different wound types have been performed (Birke-Sorensen et al., 2011; Glass & Nanchahal, 2012; Krug et al., 2011; Sullivan et al., 2009; Vig et al., 2011). The recommendations for NPWT selection based on wound characteristics are summarized in Table 24.2. This table is based on the summarization of multiple systematic reviews and not from anecdotal experience or case studies (Birke-Sorensen et al., 2011; Dowsett, 2012; Glass and Nanchahal, 2012; Vig et al., 2011).

Adjunctive Interventions for NPWT

Adjunct wound dressings (e.g., antimicrobial dressings, enzymatic debridement agents, impregnated wide-mesh gauze, silicone mesh dressings, collagen wound dressings, skin substitutes, and skin grafts) may be used in conjunction with NPWT, although research regarding their combined use is limited. Instillation of fluids, including topical or antiseptic solutions, can be used with the NPWT tubing clamped for short periods of time to hold the fluids at the wound site.

In addition, the use of topical or antimicrobial or silver dressings, including silver-coated polyurethane foam, also may provide improved bioburden reduction than NPWT alone (Glass & Nanchahal, 2012; Orgill et al., 2009). As such, the combined use of NPWT with antimicrobial products (e.g., silver and impregnated gauze) may provide a mechanism for reducing the bioburden of the wound (Orgill et al., 2009). The adjunct use of nonsilver bacterial binding dressings is also becoming commonplace.

Negative Pressure Wound Therapy Instillation and Dwell Time (NPWTi-d)

NPWT has been used successfully in the management of acute and chronic wounds since 1997. As clinical applications and product use have advanced, the benefits of routine wound cleansing between dressing changes have become more apparent to address healing impediments. Thus, the incorporation of instillation of a topical solution with dwell time alternating with removal via negative pressure cycles is an important evolution of NPWT therapy which has been shown to facilitate regular wound cleansing and wound bed preparation to help promote wound healing in certain complex wounds. Best practices for NPWTi-d use, based on a growing body of evidence, have shifted from being last resort therapy to increasingly being used to impact the wound-healing process by combining the mechanisms of action of NPWT with cyclic cleansing as a means to dilute and solubilize wound debris. In addition, a new reticulated open cell foam dressing with "through" holes expands the use of NPWTi-d therapy to include wounds that contain devitalized tissue. Clinical goals of NPWTi-d therapy include preparation for reconstructive surgery; stabilization, decontamination, and restoration of wound bed integrity; or stimulation of granulation tissue. Goals of therapy should be determined during routine serial assessments at each dressing change. Discontinuation of the therapy is recommended if the wound is not progressing within 7 days, even after therapy adjustments are made (Kim, Attinger, Constatine, et al., 2020).

Comparison of NPWTi-d use with NPWT in a retrospective, historical, cohort-control study (Kim, Attinger, Steinberg, et al., 2014) concluded that NPWTi-d group had statistically significant better outcomes than the NPWT group in the following areas: less operative visits for the 6- and 20-min dwell time (2.4 + 0.9 and 2.6 + 0.9, respectively) compared with the standard NPWT (3.0 + 0.9) ($P < 0.05$); Shorter hospital stay for the 20 min dwell time NPWTi-d group (11.4 + 5.1 days) compared with the no instillation group (14.92 + 9.23 days) ($P < 0.05$); percentage of wounds healed before discharge for the 6 min dwell NPWTi-d group (94%) compared with the no instillation group (62%) ($P < 0.05$); and culture improvement for Gram-positive bacterial in the 6-min dwell NPWTi-d group being significantly higher (90%) compared with the no instillation group (63%) ($P < 0.05$) (Kim et al., 2014).

International consensus guidelines (2019) do not recommend NPWTi-d use: (a) in wounds with exposed, unprotected organs and vessels; (b) in wounds with undrained abscess(es); (c) over split-thickness skin grafts; (d) over dermal substitutes; and (e) in acutely ischemic wounds.

These guidelines recommend for wounds with clinical signs of infection, an antiseptic solution such as hypochlorous acid solution or sodium hypochlorite solution, as the topical solution for the initial 24–48 h, followed by saline instillation. This recommendation incorporates the wound benefits from the antiseptic effects without cytotoxic effects of long-term use. It should be noted that the achievement of bioburden reduction with instilled antiseptic solutions can have various effects on wound healing depending not only on the solution type but also on the host, wound type. Use of instilled antibiotic solutions is not recommended due to the potential development of local resistance and contact sensitization. Appropriate systemic antibiotic therapy use, and the change to instilled saline are recommended based on serial patient and wound assessments. More research is needed to understand the effects of different solutions as it is possible that the cleansing effects of an instilled topical wound solution may have a greater impact on NPWTi-d outcomes more than the solution type itself (Kim et al., 2020).

Intermittent vs Continuous Pressure

Negative pressure can be delivered intermittently or continuously, most often continuously. Review of evidence by national guidelines have concluded that there is improved microvascular blood flow and granulation tissue formation with intermittent therapy compared with continuous therapy delivered at 125 mmHg (WOCN®, 2016). However, the potential loss of seal and subsequent backflow of wound fluid onto the wound, as well as the increased caregiver supervision required to monitor the intermittent therapy, increase the "work" of providing intermittent therapy and consequently outweigh its benefits. Studies have shown that after pressures fall, reexpansion of sponge fillers can lead to tissue disruption and increased pain (Ahearn, 2009). Variable/dynamic pressure is instrumental to intermittent pressure. Variable/dynamic pressure cycles between a higher pressure and a lower pressure but does not allow the pressure to drop to zero. The premise is that this allows for the aforementioned benefits without the problems of intermittent pressure. In vivo studies of variable/dynamic pressure compared with intermittent and continuous pressures found similar results in efficacy between the variable/dynamic pressure and intermittent pressure for both gauze- and foam-based NPWT (Diehm et al., 2020; Glass & Nanchahal, 2012; Malmsjö et al., 2012). Continuous therapy delivered at 125 mmHg is most routinely used; however, variable/dynamic pressure is currently becoming more popular (Glass and Nanchahal, 2012). In addition to the interventions listed in Box 24.1, lower levels of pressure (75–80 mmHg) can be used to reduce pain without compromising effectiveness (Isago, Nozaki, Kikuchi, et al., 2003; EPIUAP, NPIAP, & PPPIA, 2019).

Procedure Components

Once it has been determined that NPWT is appropriate, principles and procedures for application of most brands are similar. However, it is important to follow the specific manufacturer's instructions. Box 24.2 contains general considerations for application and use of NPWT devices (Gupta et al., 2004).

Prepare the Skin

The cover dressing requires an airtight seal to allow NPWT to function properly (Fig. 24.1). Most air leaks can be prevented by (1) drying the periwound skin; (2) framing the periwound area with skin sealant, skin barrier, hydrocolloid, or transparent film dressing; and (3) filling uneven skin surfaces (e.g., creases, scars, and folds) with a skin barrier product (paste, strip, etc.) or hydrocolloid. Contact dermatitis may result if negative pressure is applied directly to the skin (see Plate 71). This can be prevented by protecting intact periwound skin under the foam with a hydrocolloid or transparent film dressing (Kim et al., 2020; Gupta et al., 2004).

Fill Wound Depth, Undermining, Tunneling, or Sinus Tracts

Nonviable tissue should be removed and exposed structures (e.g., bone, surgical mesh, tendon) protected with a contact layer before applying the wound-filler dressing. The brand of NPWT or specific wound-filler dressing may need to be adjusted based on undermining, tunneling, or sinus tracts present. Infections from retained pieces of foam filler that

BOX 24.2 NPWT Application and Use

Preparation

1. Assessment of wound and periwound is the initial step to NPWT application.
2. Debridement of eschar or slough, if present, should be performed for removal of devitalized tissue as a step in wound bed preparation.
3. Measurement of wound is necessary as a key assessment of wound-healing progression in addition for justification of continuation of NPWT with third-party payers.

Dressing Application

1. Cover exposed structures (e.g., bone, surgical mesh, tendon) with a nonadherent contact dressing (e.g., silicone or impregnated mesh).
2. Fill wound with wound-filler dressing.
3. Cover with adherent dressing.
4. Mark on adherent dressing the number of wound-filler pieces used.
5. Typically change entire dressing, including wound filler, every 48 hours or three times per week.

Negative Pressure Activation

1. Apply negative pressure device per manufacturer's recommendations.

2. Secure all tubing connections.
3. Ensure that all clamps are open.
4. Activate negative pressure with settings ordered according to patient tolerance, type of wound, and underlying structures.
5. Verify negative pressure settings and maintenance of seal.
6. Change canister weekly unless wound drainage collection necessitates earlier changes.
7. Ensure therapy for at least 20 hours of every 24 hours with disruption no more than 2 hours at a time.
8. Disconnect negative pressure tubing from the NPWT before defibrillation, magnetic resonance imaging, or hyperbaric oxygen therapy.

Documentation

1. Removal process: Ease of removal, wound-filler dressing type, and number of wound-filler dressing pieces removed
2. Assessment process: Assessment of periwound skin, wound, exudate
3. Application process: Nonadherent dressing type and number of pieces, if used; wound-filler dressing type and number of wound-filler dressing pieces used; negative pressure settings; patient's tolerance of procedure

NPWT, negative pressure wound therapy.

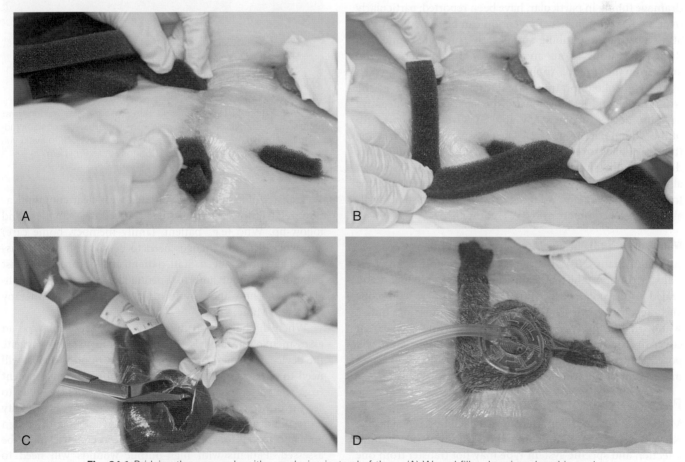

Fig. 24.1 Bridging three wounds with one device instead of three. (A) Wound filler dressing placed in each wound. Transparent dressing applied to protect intact skin under the intended bridge from negative pressure. (B) Wound filler strips applied to touch each other and connect/bridge the wounds. (C) Transparent drape is applied over the entire configuration. An opening is made to accommodate the negative pressure. Note foam is bubbled up above skin level because negative pressure and vacuum has not yet been applied. (D) Dressing attached to negative pressure; airtight seal achieved. Courtesy Debra S. Netsch.

subsequently required surgery and antibiotics have been reported by MedWatch (Wallis, 2010). Therefore, it is imperative that products are selected, prepared, and used to ensure retrieval of the wound-filler dressing. Undermining, tunneling, or sinus tracts should *not* be packed tightly. Rather, the wound-filler dressing should be gently placed all the way into the undermined, tunneled, or sinus area. Then 1–2 cm of the wound filler dressing should be withdrawn from the opening of the undermined, tunneled, or sinus area. The higher pressures will collapse the undermined portion together and promote granulation of the undermined area from the innermost aspect of the wound toward the exterior surface. Progressively smaller amounts of wound filler dressing should be used to allow for contraction and decrease in wound volume over time.

Bridge Multiple Wounds/Areas

If more than one wound/area requires NPWT, these areas can be Y-connected together to the same NPWT device. If a Y-connector is not feasible or available, these multiple areas can be "bridged together" (see Fig. 24.1).

Prevent Pressure from Device/Tubes

Pressure injuries associated with the device, and with the drainage tubing in particular, have been reported, particularly over a bony prominence. Prevention can be achieved by creating a path for the tubing and negative pressure connection device that leads to an area without pressure points and away from the wound. Apply a thin dressing to the skin (such as a hydrocolloid or transparent dressing) starting at the wound edge and leading toward the site where the negative pressure device can be safely applied. Over this lay a strip of the wound filler (Fig. 24.2). The transparent cover dressing then is applied over the wound itself and the wound-filler dressing path. This transparent cover dressing or drape can also be applied in two sections, one to the wound and one to the path separately. Bridging dressings may also be available with the commercial NPWT company.

Maintain a Seal

Although many NPWT systems compensate for small air leaks, it is important that significant air leaks are found and sealed. Air leaks can be identified with the use of a stethoscope and repaired with the transparent dressing or drape. Although one or two additional layers of the transparent cover dressing will repair large air leaks, multiple layers will potentially reduce moisture vapor transmission and cause maceration of the wound and periwound area.

Patient Discharge or Transfer of Care

Most hospitals and long-term care facilities rent specific NPWT systems based on contracts and formularies. Vendor selection and specific system type may not transfer from one facility to another or to the home care venue. Having access to vendor-supported education for both staff and physicians with annual competencies may be necessary for safe NPWT practice.

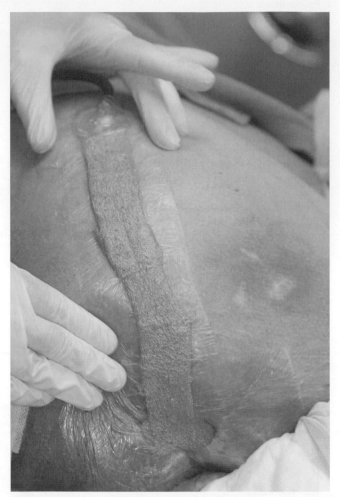

Fig. 24.2 Patient laying on left side with pressure ulcer evident over right ischial tuberosity. Bridge created from ischial ulcer to position tubing and negative pressure device on right lateral buttock to avoid vulnerable pressure points near ulcer. Courtesy Julie Freyberg.

Transfer of care must be initiated with clear communication related to vendor, system, procedure, supplies, and follow-up. Who (e.g., patient, family member, home care) and when dressing changes need to be done should be discussed and prearranged. Staff, patient, and/or caregivers must be educated about how to operate the device, respond to alarms, and how and why to turn off or disconnect therapy (Ousey & Milne, 2014).

When discharging to the community, there must be an assessment of the family's or patient's ability to safely navigate the device in the new environment. The wound specialist will need to obtain information about the physical environment (e.g., stairways, electrical outlets) and the patient's ability to see the device controls and hear the alarms. Cognitive ability to respond appropriately to the alarms and identify when and who to call for complications and emergencies must be assessed. Patients with high-output wounds will need to change or have immediate access to having their canister changed before filling so the dressing seal is not compromised. In the absence of constant supervision by trained staff or caregivers, NPWT may not be an appropriate option for the patient who is unable to cooperate with keeping the system intact (e.g., dementia, agitation). Checklist 24.2 provides a list of questions and factors to consider during discharge planning for the patient with NPWT (Ousey & Milne, 2014).

Checklist 24.3 provides questions for patients and/or their caregivers to ask health care providers before transitioning from receiving NPWT in a health care facility to using it at home (Birke-Sorensen et al., 2011).

CHECKLIST 24.2 NPWT Factors to Consider Before Discharge

✓ Patient mobility—does the patient use a walking aid?
✓ Is the patient able to carry the device and manage the weight and tubing?
✓ Is the patient at risk of falling because of the device?
✓ Is the patient/caregiver cognitively able to manage the therapy?
✓ Does the patient have sufficient hearing/vision to manage the system and to hear alarms and read the controls?
✓ Is the patient in a psychological and social situation appropriate for NPWT?
✓ Is the patient's home electricity supply safe?
✓ Are there stairs or other obstacles that the patient will need to negotiate with the device?
✓ Does the patient know who to contact in an emergency and what would constitute an emergency?
✓ Is there a risk of potential loss of equipment?
✓ Does community staff have access to the equipment with or without funding?

NPWT, negative pressure wound therapy.
Adapted from Ousey, K.J., Milne, J. (2014). Exploring portable negative pressure wound therapy devices in the community. *British Journal of Community Nursing, 19*(Suppl. 1), S14–S20.

CHECKLIST 24.3 NPWT: Transitioning From Inpatient to Home

✓ Am I using the NPWT device correctly?
✓ How long should I expect to use the NPWT device?
✓ What serious complications might occur in my situation?
✓ What should I do if any of those complications occur?
  • Whom do I contact?
  • How do I recognize bleeding?
  • How do I recognize serious infection?
  • How do I recognize if my wound condition is worsening?
✓ Do I need to stop taking aspirin or any other medicines that affect my bleeding system or platelet function? What's the risk associated with stopping or avoiding such medicines?
✓ Can you provide me with patient instructions or tell me where I can find them?

NPWT, negative pressure wound therapy.
Source: (Birke-Sorensen et al. (2011). Evidence-based recommendations for negative pressure wound therapy: Treatment variables (pressure levels, wound filler and contact layer)—Steps towards an international consensus. *Journal of Plastic, Reconstructive & Aesthetic Surgery, 64*(Suppl. 1), S1–S16).

CLINICAL CONSULT

A: Wound care referral received for a 43-year-old male with diabetic neuropathic ulceration of the left dorsal foot. Patient reports that the ulcer developed due to swelling in his foot and rubbing on his shoe. The wound was surgically debrided 24 hours ago following arterial blood flow testing. Ulcer is 3 cm × 2 cm × 2 cm; 90% red vascular tissue, 10% slough; no tunneling, undermining, periwound erythema, induration, or crepitus.
D: Diabetic neuropathic ulceration, left dorsal foot.

P: Optimize nutrition and management of blood glucose, offload pressure and repetitive stress, initiate NPWT for rapid wound contraction and containment.
I: (1) Dietician referral. (2) Continue with the postoperative offloading shoe. (3) Elevate left foot when sitting. (4) Noninvasive peripheral arterial testing. (5) Home care referral for 3× weekly dressing changes.
E: Patient verbalizes understanding and agreed to the plan once he learned we could use a smaller device than the one he saw in the hospital. Return to clinic in 2 weeks to reevaluate.

SUMMARY

• As with other topical therapies, the efficacy of NPWT is contingent upon correcting host cofactors (e.g., nutritional status, oxygenation, perfusion, and pressure redistribution).
• NPWT has become an interim adjunctive intervention to prepare the acute wound for definitive closure, such as the fasciotomy, dehisced sternal or abdominal surgical wounds, and donor sites.

• iNPWT has been found to reduce SSIs.
• NPWTi-d has been shown to be efficacious with faster healing rates than NPWT or standard of care.
• Additional well-designed comparative studies with standardized protocols are needed to further explore clinical outcomes, the patient's experience, and effectiveness of alternative NPWT systems.

SELF-ASSESSMENT QUESTIONS

1. Which of the following is *not a primary* mechanism of action of negative pressure wound therapy (NPWT)?
   a. Wound edge contraction
   b. Wound environment stabilization
   c. Reduction of bioburden
   d. Wound surface microdeformations

2. Bioburden reduction with use of NPWT is believed to occur through which of the following?
   a. Removal of growth factors
   b. Increased perfusion
   c. Irrigation daily with normal saline
   d. Creation of hypoxic environment for bacteria with negative pressure

3. Which of the following describes appropriate use of NPWT in the care of enteric fistulas?
   a. It can only be used after exploration of the enteric fistula.
   b. It is only used to contain effluent.
   c. It is never indicated with enteric fistulas.
   d. The wound should be covered with a wound liner instead of porous foam filler dressing.

4. Serious complications associated with NPWT, including death, are related to which of the following?
   a. Hemorrhage
   b. Retrograde migration of bacteria from canister to wound surface
   c. Fluid and electrolyte depletion
   d. Excess wound moisture

5. Contraindications to NPWT include which of the following?
   a. Patient taking anticoagulants
   b. Treated osteomyelitis
   c. Nonenteric or unexplored fistulas
   d. Postsurgical dehiscence

REFERENCES

Acosta, S., Björck, M., & Wanhainen, A. (2017). Negative-pressure wound therapy for prevention and treatment of surgical-site infections after vascular surgery. *BJS, 104*, e75–e84.

Ahearn, C. (2009). Intermittent negative pressure wound therapy and lower negative pressures—Exploring the disparity between science and current practice: A review of the literature. *Ostomy/Wound Management, 55*(6), 22–28.

Andros, G., Armstrong, D. G., Attinger, C. E., et al. (2006). Consensus statement on negative pressure wound therapy (VAC therapy) for the management of diabetic foot wounds. *Ostomy/Wound Management, 52*(Suppl), S1–S32.

Armstrong, D. G., Lavery, L. A., Abu-Rumman, P., et al. (2002). Outcomes of subatmospheric pressure dressing therapy on wounds of the diabetic foot. *Ostomy/Wound Management, 48*(4), 64–68.

Armstrong, D. G., Lavery, L. A., & Boulton, A. J. (2007). Negative pressure wound therapy via vacuum-assisted closure following partial foot amputation: What is the role of wound chronicity? *International Wound Journal, 4*, 79–86.

Baharestani, M. M., & Gabriel, A. (2011). Use of negative pressure wound therapy in the management of infected abdominal wounds containing mesh: An analysis of outcomes. *International Wound Journal, 8*, 118–125.

Birke-Sorensen, et al. (2011). Evidence-based recommendations for negative pressure wound therapy: Treatment variables (pressure levels, wound filler and contact layer)—Steps towards an international consensus. *Journal of Plastic, Reconstructive & Aesthetic Surgery, 64*(Suppl. 1), S1–S16.

Blume, P. A., Walters, J., Payne, W., et al. (2008). Comparison of negative pressure wound therapy using vacuum-assisted closure with advanced moist wound therapy in the treatment of diabetic foot ulcers: A multicenter randomized controlled trial. *Diabetes Care, 31*(4), 631–636.

Borgquist, O., Gustafsson, L., Ingemansson, R., et al. (2010). Micro- and macromechanical effects on the wound bed of negative pressure wound therapy using gauze and foam. *Annals of Plastic Surgery, 64*(6), 789–793.

Bovill, E., Banwell, P. E., Teot, L., et al. (2008). Topical negative pressure wound therapy: A review of its role and guidelines for its use in the management of acute wounds. *International Wound Journal, 5*(4), 511–529.

Brooke, J., El-Ghaname, A., Napier, K., & Sommerey, L. (2018). Executive summary: Nurses Specialized in Wound, Ostomy and Continence Canada (NSWOCC) nursing best practice recommendations: Enterocutaneous Fistula and enteroatmospheric fistula. *Journal of Wound, Ostomy, and Continence Nursing.* Jul/Aug;46(4).

Bruhin, A., Ferreira, F., Chariker, M., et al. (2014). Systematic review and evidence-based recommendations for the use of negative pressure wound therapy in the open abdomen. *International Journal of Surgery, 12*(10), 1105–1114.

Campbell, P., Smith, G., & Smith, J. (2008). Retrospective clinical evaluation of gauze-based negative pressure wound therapy. *International Wound Journal, 5*(2), 280–286.

Chowdhry, S., & Wilhelmi, B. (2019). Comparing negative pressure wound therapy with instillation and conventional dressings for sternal wound reconstructions. *Plastic and Reconstructive Surgery. Global Open, 7*, e2087.

Crawford, P. E., & Fields-Varnado, M. (2013). Guideline for the management of wounds in patients with lower-extremity neuropathic disease. *Journal of Wound, Ostomy, and Continence Nursing, 40*(1), 34–45.

DeFranzo, A. J., Argenta, L. C., Marks, M. W., et al. (2001). The use of vacuum-assisted closure therapy for the treatment of lower-extremity wounds with exposed bone. *Plastic and Reconstructive Surgery, 108*(5), 1184–1191.

Diehm, Y. F., Loew, J., Will, P. A., Fischer, S., Hundeshagen, G., Ziegler, B., Gazyakan, E., Kneser, U., & Hirche, C. (2020). Negative pressure wound therapy with instillation and dwell time (NPWTi-d) with V. A. C. VeraFlo in traumatic, surgical, and chronic wounds-A helpful tool for decontamination and to prepare successful reconstruction. *International Wound Journal, 17*(6), 1740–1749. https://doi.org/10.1111/iwj.13462.

Dowsett, C. (2012). Clinical research/audit: Recommendations for the use of negative pressure wound therapy. *Wounds UK, 8*(2), 48–59.

Dumville, J. C., & Munson, C. (2012). Negative pressure wound therapy for partial-thickness burns. *Cochrane Database of Systematic Reviews, 12*, CD006215.

European Pressure Ulcer Advisory Panel, National Pressure Injury Advisory Panel, & Pan Pacific Pressure Injury Alliance (EPIUAP, NPIAP, & PPPIA). (2019). In E. Haesler (Ed.), *Prevention and treatment of pressure ulcers/injuries*. Osborne Park: Cambridge Media.

Ford-Dunn, S. (2006). Use of vacuum assisted closure therapy in the palliation of a malignant wound. *Palliative Medicine, 20*(4), 477–478.

Franczyk, M., Lohman, R. F., Agarwal, J. P., et al. (2009). The impact of topical lidocaine on pain level assessment during and after vacuum-assisted closure dressing changes: A double-blind, prospective, randomized study. *Plastic and Reconstructive Surgery, 124*(3), 854–861.

Franz, M. G., Robson, M. C., Steed, D. L., et al. (2008). Guidelines to aid healing of acute wounds by decreasing impediments of healing. *Wound Repair and Regeneration, 16*(6), 723–748.

Game, F., Almqvist, J., Attinger, C., et al. (2016). IWGDF guidance on use of interventions to enhance the healing of chronic ulcers of the foot in diabetes. *Diabetes/Metabolism Research and Reviews, 32*(Suppl. 1), 75–83.

Glass, G., & Nanchahal, J. (2012). The methodology of negative pressure wound therapy: Separating fact from fiction. *Journal of Plastic, Reconstructive & Aesthetic Surgery, 65*, 989–1001.

Gray, M., & Peirce, B. (2004). Is negative pressure wound therapy effective for the management of chronic wounds? *Journal of Wound, Ostomy, and Continence Nursing, 31*(3), 101–105.

Gupta, S., Baharestani, M., Baranoski, S., et al. (2004). Guidelines for managing pressure ulcers with negative pressure wound therapy. *Advances in Skin & Wound Care, 17*(Suppl. 2), 1–16.

Heineman, J. T., Garcia, L. J., Obst, M. A., et al. (2015). Collapsible enteroatmospheric fistula isolation device: A novel, simple solution to a complex problem. *Journal of the American College of Surgeons, 221*, e7–e14.

Hinck, D., Franke, A., & Gatzka, F. (2010). Use of vacuum-assisted closure negative pressure wound therapy in combat-related injuries—Literature review. *Military Medicine, 175*(3), 173–181.

Hopf, H., Ueno, C., Aslam, R., et al. (2006). Guidelines for the treatment of arterial insufficiency ulcers. *Wound Repair and Regeneration, 14*(6), 693–710.

Hu, K. X., Zhang, H. W., Zhou, F., et al. (2009). A comparative study of the clinical effects between two kinds of negative pressure wound therapy. *Zhonghua Shao Shang Za Zhi, 25*(4), 253–257.

Hurd, T., Chadwick, P., Cote, J., et al. (2010). Impact of gauze based NPWT on the patient and nursing experience in the treatment of challenging wounds. *International Wound Journal, 7*(6), 448–455.

Ingargiola, M. J., Daniali, L. N., & Lee, E. S. (2013). Does the application of incisional negative pressure therapy to high-risk wounds prevent surgical site complications? A systematic review. *Eplasty, 13*, e49.

Isago, T., Nozaki, M., Kikuchi, Y., et al. (2003). Effects of different negative pressures on reduction of wounds in negative pressure dressings. *The Journal of Dermatology, 30*(8), 596–601.

Kim, P., Attinger, C., Constantine, T., et al. (2020). Negative pressure wound therapy with instillation: International consensus guidelines update. *International Wound Journal, 17*, 174–186.

Kim, P., Attinger, C., Steinberg, J., et al. (2014). The impact of negative-pressure wound therapy with instillation compared with standard negative-pressure wound therapy: A retrospective, historical, cohort, controlled study. *Plastic and Reconstructive Surgery, 133*(3), 709–716.

Krug, E., et al. (2011). Evidence-based recommendations for the use of negative pressure wound therapy in traumatic wounds and reconstructive surgery: Steps towards an international consensus. *Injury, 42*(Suppl. 1), S1–S12.

Kubec, E., Badeau, A., Materazzi, S., et al. (2013). Negative pressure wound therapy and the emerging role of incisional negative pressure wound therapy as prophylaxis against surgical site infections. In A. Méndez-Vilas (Ed.), *Microbial pathogens and strategies for combating them: science, technology, and education*. Badajoz: Formatex.

Li, H. Z., Xu, X. H., Wang, D. W., Lin, Y. M., Lin, N., & Lu, H. D. (2019). Negative pressure wound therapy for surgical site infections: A systematic review and meta-analysis of randomized controlled trials. *Clinical Microbiology and Infection, 25*(11), 1328–1338.

Long, M. A., & Blevins, A. (2009). Challenges in practice: options in negative pressure wound therapy. Five case studies. *Journal of Wound, Ostomy, and Continence Nursing, 36*(2), 202–211.

Malmsjö, M., Gustafsson, L., Lindstedt, S., et al. (2012). The effects of variable, intermittent, and continuous negative pressure wound therapy, using foam or gauze, on wound contraction, granulation tissue formation, and ingrowth into the wound filler. *Eplasty, 12*, e5.

Malmsjö, M., Ingemansson, R., Martin, R., et al. (2009). The physical properties of gauze and polyurethane open cell foam in negative pressure wound therapy. *Wound Repair and Regeneration, 17*(2), 200–205.

Morykwas, M., Argenta, L. C., Shelton-Brown, E. I., et al. (1997). Vacuum-assisted closure: A new method for wound control and treatment: Animal studies and basic foundation. *Annals of Plastic Surgery, 38*(6), 553–562.

Morykwas, M., Simpson, J., Punger, K., et al. (2006). Vacuum-assisted closure: State of basic research and physiologic foundation. *Plastic and Reconstructive Surgery, 117*(Suppl. 7), S121–S126.

Mouës, C. M., Heule, F., & Hovius, S. E. R. (2011). A review of topical negative pressure therapy in wound healing: sufficient evidence? *American Journal of Surgery, 201*(4), 544–556.

Mouës, C. M., Vos, M. C., van den Bemd, G. J., et al. (2004). Bacterial load in relation to vacuum-assisted closure wound therapy: A prospective randomized trial. *Wound Repair and Regeneration, 12*(1), 11–17.

Murphy, P., & Evan, G. (2012). Advances in wound healing: A review of current wound healing products. *Plastic Surgery International.* http://www.ncbi.nlm.nih.gov/pmc/articles/PMC3335515/ accessed August 28, 2021.

National Institute for Health and Care Excellence (NICE). (2013). *Negative pressure wound therapy for the open abdomen (NICE interventional procedure guidance no 467).* November 2013. https://www.nice.org.uk/guidance/ipg467 accessed August 28, 2021.

NICE. (2019). *PICO negative pressure wound dressings for closed surgical incisions.* Medical technologies guidance MTG43. May 2019. www.nice.org.uk/guidance/mtg43 accessed August 28, 2021.

Orgill, D. P., Austen, W. G., Butler, C. E., et al. (2004). Guidelines for treatment of complex chest wounds with negative pressure wound therapy. *Wounds, 16*(Suppl. B), 1–23.

Orgill, D. P., Manders, E. K., Sumpio, B. E., et al. (2009). The mechanisms of action of vacuum assisted closure: More to learn. *Surgery, 146*(1), 40–51.

Ousey, K., & Milne, J. (2014). Exploring portable negative pressure wound therapy devices in the community. *British Journal of Community Nursing, 19*(Suppl. 1), S14–S20.

Peinemann, F., & Sauerland, S. (2011). Negative-pressure wound therapy: Systematic review of randomized controlled trials. *Deutsches Ärzteblatt International, 108*(22), 381–389.

Pham, C., Middleton, P., & Maddern, G. (2006). The safety and efficacy of topical negative pressure in non-healing wounds: A systematic review. *Journal of Wound Care, 15*(6), 240–250.

Reider, K. (2017). Fistula isolation and the use of negative pressure to promote wound healing. a case study. *Journal of Wound, Ostomy, and Continence Nursing, 44*(3), 293–298.

Roberts, D. J., Zygun, D. A., Grendar, J., et al. (2012). Negative-pressure wound therapy for critically ill adults with open abdominal wounds: A systematic review. *Journal of Trauma and Acute Care Surgery, 73*, 629–639.

Robson, M., Cooper, D. M., Aslam, R., et al. (2006). Guidelines for the treatment of venous ulcers. *Wound Repair and Regeneration, 14*(6), 649–662.

Saxena, V., Hwang, C. W., Huang, S., et al. (2004). Vacuum-assisted closure: Microdeformations of wounds and cell proliferation. *Plastic and Reconstructive Surgery, 114*(5), 1086–1096.

Shweiki, E., & Gallagher, K. E. (2013). Negative pressure wound therapy in acute, contaminated wounds: Documenting its safety and efficacy to support current global practice. *International Wound Journal, 10*, 13–43.

Singh, D., Gabriel, A., Parvizi, J., Kim, P., Attinger, C., et al. (2019). Meta-analysis of comparative trials evaluating a single-use closed-incision negative-pressure therapy system. *Plastic and Reconstructive Surgery, 143*(1S), 41S–46S.

Steed, D., Attinger, C., Colaizzi, T., et al. (2006). Guidelines for the treatment of diabetic ulcers. *Wound Repair and Regeneration, 14*(6), 680–692.

Stevens, P. (2009). Vacuum-assisted closure of laparostomy wounds: a critical review of the literature. *International Wound Journal, 6*(4), 259–266.

Sullivan, N., Snyder, D. L., Tipton, K., et al. (2009). *Negative pressure wound therapy devices technology assessment report (Project ID: WNDT1108).* Rockville: Agency for Healthcare and Research Quality.

Ubbink, D. T., Westerbos, S. J., Evans, D., et al. (2008). Topical negative pressure for treating chronic wounds. *Cochrane Database of Systematic Reviews, 3*, CD001898.

Upton, D., & Andrews, A. (2015). Pain and trauma in negative pressure wound therapy: A review. *International Wound Journal, 12*(1), 100–105.

Vig, S., Dowsett, C., Berg, L., et al. (2011). Evidence-based recommendations for the use of negative pressure wound therapy in chronic wounds: Steps towards an international consensus. *Journal of Tissue Viability, 20*(Suppl. 1), S1–S18.

Vikatmaa, P., Juutilainen, V., Kuukasjärvi, P., et al. (2008). Negative pressure wound therapy: A systematic review on effectiveness and safety. *European Journal of Vascular and Endovascular Surgery, 36*(4), 438–448.

Vuerstaek, J., Vainas, T., Wuite, J., et al. (2006). State of the art treatment of chronic leg ulcers: A randomized controlled trial comparing vacuum-assisted closure (V.A.C.) with modern wound dressings. *Journal of Vascular Surgery, 44*(5), 1029–1038.

Wallis, L. (2010). Food and Drug Administration (FDA) warning about negative pressure wound therapy (NPWT). *The American Journal of Nursing, 110*(3).

Wang, G., Zhirui, L., Tongtong, L., Wang, S., et al. (2018). Negative-pressure wound therapy in a *Pseudomonas aeruginosa* infection model. *BioMed Research International, 9496183.* 11 pages.

Webster, J., Liu, Z., Norman, G., Dumville, J. C., Chiverton, L., Scuffham, P., et al. (2019). Negative pressure wound therapy for surgical wounds healing by primary closure. *The Cochrane Database of Systematic Reviews, 3*(3).

Whitney, J., Phillips, L., Aslam, R., et al. (2006). Guidelines for the treatment of pressure ulcers. *Wound Repair and Regeneration, 14*(6), 663–679.

Wound, Ostomy and Continence Nurses Society™ (WOCN®). (2016). *Guideline for prevention and management of pressure ulcers (WOCN® clinical practice guideline series no. 2).* Glenview: WOCN®.

Wound, Ostomy and Continence Nurses Society™ (WOCN®). (2019). *Venous, arterial, and neuropathic lower-extremity wounds: clinical resource guide.* Mt. Laurel: WOCN®.

FURTHER READING

Chariker, M. E., Jeter, K. F., Tintle, T. E., et al. (1989). Effective management of incisional and cutaneous fistulae with closed suction wound drainage. *Contemporary Surgery, 34*, 59–63.

Irrgang, S., & Bryant, R. (1984). Management of the enterocutaneous fistula. *Journal of Enterostomal Therapy, 11*(6), 211–228.

Lessing, C. M., James, R. B., & Ingram, S. C. (2013). Comparison of the effects of different negative pressure wound therapy modes—Continuous, noncontinuous, and with instillation—On porcine excisional wounds. *Eplasty, 13*(1), 443–454.

Orringer, J. S., Mendeloff, E. N., & Eckhauser, F. E. (1987). Management of wounds in patients with complex enterocutaneous fistulas. *Surgery, Gynecology & Obstetrics, 165*(1), 79–80.

25

Hyperbaric Oxygenation

William H. Tettelbach, Geness Koumandakis, and Brenda Freymiller

OBJECTIVES

1. List at least two indications for hyperbaric oxygen therapy.
2. List at least two contraindications for hyperbaric oxygen therapy.

3. Explain the physiologic effects of hyperbaric oxygen therapy.

Hyperbaric oxygen (HBO_2) therapy entails the systemic intermittent administration of oxygen delivered under pressure. A hyperbaric environment exists when atmospheric pressure is greater than 1 atmosphere absolute (ATA) (Hammarlund, 1995). For clinical purposes HBO_2 therapy is defined as an intervention in which an individual breathes near 100% oxygen while inside a hyperbaric chamber at a pressure equal to or greater than 1.4 ATA (Bird, 2018). HBO_2 therapy targeting skin, soft tissue or bone typically range from pressures of 2.0–2.5 ATA, or 14.7–22.0 pounds per square inch gauge (PSIG). Presently most outpatient wound clinics offering HBO_2 therapy have migrated to treating patients using 2.0 ATA with no air breaks for 90 min due to its preferred safety profile and simple standardized approach.

Although often viewed as being complementary to each other, wound care is not a formal subspecialty of hyperbaric medicine, neither is hyperbaric medicine a subspecialty of wound care. In certain situations, HBO_2 therapy represents the primary treatment modality while in other circumstances it is an adjunct to surgical and pharmacologic interventions. Beyond skin and soft tissue-related management, HBO_2 is indicated for many other conditions, such as carbon monoxide poisoning, chronic refractory osteomyelitis, air/gas embolism and decompression sickness. Oxygen under pressure can be thought of as a pharmacologic agent in that it has a therapeutic dose, a toxic dose, side effects, contraindications, interactions with other drugs, and incompatibilities with other drugs (Heimbach, 1998).

HISTORY

Much of what is known about the effects of hyperbaric treatment comes from observations and studies of caisson workers and divers. The first description of a pressurization vessel dates to 1662, when Henshaw used bellows to increase and decrease pressures to treat respiratory problems. The nineteenth century saw the advent of caisson workers for bridge construction and the subsequent description of caisson's disease (or decompression sickness), bubble theory, and oxygen toxicity by Paul Bert in 1878 (Elliott, 1995). A little more than a decade later, Moir used recompression to treat decompression sickness in caisson workers building the Hudson River tunnel. During the 20th century, the military supported research and developed applications of HBO_2 therapy for decompression sickness. The potential benefits of HBO_2 continue to expand with current research being conducted in areas that include ischemic stroke, posttraumatic stress disorder symptoms and mild traumatic brain injuries (Weaver et al., 2018).

Modern use of HBO_2 to potentiate the effects of radiation in cancer patients began in 1955 (Kindwall, 1995). The National Academy of Science–National Research Council appointed a committee to review the physiologic basis for HBO_2 in 1962. In 1966, this group published *Fundamentals of Hyperbaric Medicine,* which describes the physical and physiologic effects of HBO_2. However, it did not address clinical conditions treated with hyperbaric treatment. The Undersea Medical Society (UMS) was founded in 1967 and was primarily devoted to diving and undersea medicine. The UMS became the Undersea and Hyperbaric Medical Society (UHMS) in 1986. The UHMS is the primary, worldwide source of information on hyperbaric and diving medicine. Part of the mission of the UHMS is "to develop and promote educational activities and other programs, which improve the scientific knowledge of matters related to undersea and hyperbaric environments" and "to promote cooperation between the life sciences and other disciplines concerned with undersea activity, hyperbaric medicine, and wound care" (UHMS, 2015).

PHYSIOLOGIC EFFECTS

The mechanical effect of HBO$_2$ follows the physical law described by Boyle, which states that as pressure increases, volume decreases. Therefore, in the case of decompression sickness or air/gas embolism, hyperbaric treatment is used to decrease the size of the air bubble or embolism. Physiologic effects of HBO$_2$ use the physical law described by Henry's law, which states that the amount of gas dissolved in a liquid is directly proportional to the partial pressure of the dissolved gas. As a result, oxygen tensions can be raised 10–13 times higher than oxygen breathed at ambient pressure (Hammarlund, 1995). A pressure of 3 ATA results in 6 mL of O$_2$ being dissolved per 100 mL of plasma, thus rendering as much O$_2$ delivery as by hemoglobin bound O$_2$. With these increases in oxygen tension, oxygen acts as a drug and has several effects on wound healing (Table 25.1).

As previously noted, the delivery of oxygen under pressure increases the capacity of the blood plasma to carry and deliver oxygen to tissues systemically. Consequently, HBO$_2$ can significantly augment oxygen delivery by increasing the oxygen gradient into hypoxic tissues while concurrently stimulating angiogenesis, thus enhancing perfusion to compromised areas. HBO$_2$ has been shown to upregulate the expression of a whole host of growth factors and receptors including vascular endothelial growth factor (Sheikh, 2000), transforming growth factor (Lin, Wang, & Lee, 2002), matrix metalloproteinase-2 (MMP-2), matrix metalloproteinase-9 (MMP-9), tissue inhibitor of metalloproteinase-1 (TIMP-1)

TABLE 25.1 Effects and Mechanisms of Hyperbaric Oxygen Therapy on Wound Healing

Effect	Mechanism
Hyperoxygenation	Improved oxygen-carrying capacity Increased distance of diffusion Improved local tissue oxygenation Vasoconstriction and decreased local tissue edema Improved cellular energy metabolism
Improved growth factor expression	Upregulation of platelet-derived growth factor receptor Increased angiogenesis Increased extracellular matrix formation and granulation tissue (may see clinical signs of granulation tissue within 2 weeks of treatment) Enhanced epithelial cell proliferation and migration
Fibroblast proliferation	Increased collagen deposition Improved collagen cross-linking Increased production of fibronectin
Increased nitric oxide production	Enhanced neutrophil activity Enhanced macrophage activity Increased leukocyte-killing ability Enhanced effectiveness of antibiotics

(Sander et al., 2009), basic fibroblast growth factor (bFGF) (Kang, Gorti, Quan, Ho, & Koch, 2004) and platelet-derived growth factor (PDGF) receptors (Bonomo et al., 1998). There are statements that HBO$_2$ is able to accelerate epithelialization by approximately 30% (Winter & Perrins, 1970), while wound contraction seems to be independent of ambient oxygen tensions (Pai & Hunt, 1972).

Oxygen is a powerful vasoconstrictor and can be helpful in managing edema related to traumatic wounding or crush injuries. Although HBO$_2$ may seem injurious in that it decreases blood supply to an injured area, the increase in blood plasma oxygen tension and in diffusion of oxygen more than compensates for the decrease in circulation associated with vasoconstriction. An additional favorable effect of HBO$_2$ includes its capacity to mitigate the effects of ischemic-reperfusion (IR) injury caused by adherence of circulating neutrophils to the vascular endothelium. HBO$_2$ in both animal and human models has demonstrated the ability of circulating neutrophils to bind to the vascular endothelium by means of the B$_2$ integrin adhesion molecule, reducing IR-related inflammation and edema (Thom, 1993) (Thom et al., 1997). Leukocytes have an impaired ability to generate reactive oxygen species in a hypoxic environment, so the delivery of increased tissue oxygenation also enhances leukocyte function and the penetration of concomitant antibiotic therapy (Dauwe, Pulikkottil, Lavery, Stuzin, & Rohrich, 2014). It is worth noting HBO$_2$ does not impede the antimicrobial functions of neutrophils, for instance, degranulation, phagocytosis or the oxidative burst (Juttner et al., 2003). The effect of HBO$_2$ in blood is instantaneous, with a subsequent plateau in soft tissues approximately 1 h after exposure. The effect of HBO$_2$ declines steadily over 2–4 h after exposure (Hammarlund, 1995).

INDICATIONS

The UHMS continuously reviews scientific data regarding the therapeutic benefit of HBO$_2$. It currently has designated the conditions or disease processes listed in Box 25.1 as indications for hyperbaric therapy (Moon, 2019). Hyperbaric oxygenation is the primary therapy for air or gas embolism, carbon monoxide poisoning, and decompression sickness. When used for any other indication, hyperbaric therapy must be incorporated as part of the plan of care that includes appropriate medical and surgical treatments (Cianci & Sato, 1994; FDA, 2021; Federman et al., 2016; Marx, 1995). The effects of HBO$_2$ on wound healing and the mechanisms for those effects are listed in (Table 25.1). Patient selection should focus on the origin and hypoxic nature of the wound. For example, a pressure injury is best treated with pressure redistribution; an ischemic wound is best treated by, whenever possible, optimizing perfusion to the affected region. Indications specific to wound management recommended by national organizations and guidelines are listed in (Table 25.2).

Hyperbaric oxygenation may be considered for the treatment of patients with limb-threatening diabetic and vascular

BOX 25.1 Indications for Hyperbaric Oxygen Therapy

1. Air or gas embolism[a]
2. a. Carbon monoxide poisoning[a]
   b. Carbon monoxide poisoning complicated by cyanide poisoning
3. Clostridial myositis and myonecrosis (gas gangrene)
4. Crush injury, compartment syndrome, and other acute traumatic ischemias
5. Decompression sickness[a]
6. Arterial inefficiencies:
   a. Central retinal artery occlusion
   b. Arterial inefficiencies: enhancement of healing in selected problem wounds
7. Severe anemia
8. Intracranial abscess
9. Necrotizing soft tissue infections
10. Osteomyelitis (refractory)
11. Delayed radiation injury (soft tissue and bony necrosis)
12. Compromised grafts and flaps
13. Acute thermal burn injury
14. Idiopathic sudden sensorineural hearing loss

[a]Primary therapy.
Adapted from Undersea and Hyperbaric Medical Society (UHMS). *Indications for hyperbaric oxygen therapy*, https://www.uhms.org/resources/hbo-indications.html?highlight=WyJpbmRpY2F0aW9ucyJd. Accessed March 23, 2020.

TABLE 25.2 Wound-Related Indications for Hyperbaric Oxygen Therapy

Indication	Source
Adjunctive HBO$_2$ therapy in the treatment of thermal burns	Moon (2020)
Acute arterial ischemias	Moon (2020)
Necrotizing soft tissue infections	Moon (2020)
Osteomyelitis (refractory)	Moon (2020)
Delayed radiation injury (soft tissue and bony necrosis)	Moon (2020)
Compromised grafts and flaps	Moon (2020)
Selected problem wounds that fail to respond to established medical and surgical management	Moon (2020)
Diabetic Wagner grade 3 or higher lower extremity wounds not responsive to established medical and surgical management	CMS (2002)
Diabetic limb-threatening lower extremity wound	Crawford and Fields-Varnado (2013); Lavery et al. (2016)
Arterial limb-threatening lower extremity wound	Bonham et al. (2016); Federman et al. (2016); Norgren et al. (2007)

insufficiency wounds of the lower extremity (Bonham et al., 2016; Federman et al., 2016; Lavery et al., (2016); Moon, 2019; Norgren et al., 2007). Löndahl (2012) also recommended HBO$_2$ as an adjunctive therapy in a selected group of patients with diabetic foot ulcers, such as those complicated with a deep tissue infection (e.g., chronic osteomyelitis, infectious tenosynovitis, joint capsule infection) not responding to optimal treatment within a multidisciplinary approach. A 2015 Cochrane review analyzed 12 trials (577 participants), of which 10 trials (531 participants) enrolled candidates with a diabetic foot ulcer (DFU). Pooled data from five trials with 205 participants showed an increase in the rate of DFU healing (risk ratio [RR] 2.35, 95% confidence interval [CI] 1.19–4.62; $P = 0.01$) with HBO$_2$ therapy at 6 weeks reported there was some evidence that in patients with DFUs, the use of HBO$_2$ in conjunction with appropriate wound care resulted in meaningful healing by 6 weeks (Kranke et al., 2015). Unfortunately, this effect did not appear to be sustained at 1 year or greater follow-up and further research is needed. In 2018, a retrospective observational study using a real-world data set was published, reporting on the modified-intent-to-treat outcomes of HBO$_2$ therapy on diabetic ulcers limited to the foot and specifically only the more complex Wagner grades 3 and 4 diabetic foot ulcers. During the study time frame, a total of 2,651,878 wounds were evaluated. The analysis demonstrated that adjunctive HBO$_2$ therapy can be effective for hard-to-heal Wagner grades 3 and 4 diabetic foot ulcers. Furthermore, the results underscore the importance of treatment adherence when analyzing the effectiveness of HBO$_2$ therapy (Ennis, Huang, & Gordon, 2018).

To meet Centers for Medicare and Medicaid Services (CMS) criteria, the lower extremity diabetic wound must be Wagner grade 3 or higher and not responsive to standard wound care, including assessment and correction of vascular insufficiency, maximization of nutritional status, optimization of glycemic control, debridement of nonvital tissue, and maintenance of moist wound healing with the use of topical dressings. Whereas other classification systems are recommended for use with diabetic foot ulcers, for reimbursement purposes, the National Coverage Determination (NCD) continues to insist that the Wagner Classification System be used (CMS, 2017a, 2017b). Active infections should receive appropriate targeted antimicrobial therapy when possible, and the wound must be suitably offloaded. Transcutaneous oximetry (TcPO$_2$) values of <100 mmHg during HBO$_2$ exposure were correlated with a low probability of healing, while an in-chamber TcPO$_2$ > 200 mmHg provided the best single discriminator (reliability of 74% and positive predictive value [PPV] of 58%) for healing (Fife et al., 2002). Alternatively, combining 1 ATA air TcPO$_2$ < 15 mmHg and in-chamber TcPO$_2$ <400 mmHg predicts wound healing failure with a reliability of 75.8% and PPV of 73.3% (Fife et al., 2002). Wounds associated with a TcPO$_2$ reading of <20 mmHg on room air demonstrated a significantly decreased probability of healing compared with those associated with a TcPO$_2$ of >40 mmHg ($P = 0.008$) (Ladurner et al., 2010). Although it is understood that not all wounds heal, consideration for hyperbaric treatment should be considered for those patients with refractory lower extremity wounds meeting guidance criteria. Hyperbaric treatment could mean the difference between limb salvage and a trans metatarsal, below-the-knee or above-the-knee amputation if appropriate circulatory assessment, intervention, and preamputation preparation are part of the comprehensive workup.

Crush injury, compartment syndrome, and acute traumatic ischemia benefit from HBO_2 therapy because of the improved oxygen tension in tissue that is inadequately perfused because of a disruption of blood supply and edema associated with injury. Hyperbaric oxygenation helps to decrease edema through its vasoconstrictive action. In addition, it helps to decrease reperfusion injury. The use of HBO_2 therapy in these cases is emergent, and patients should be treated as early as possible (within 4–6 h after injury or surgery) for the best outcome (Latham, 2020). It is recommended that treatment (2–2.5 ATA for 60–90 min) be repeated three times daily for 2–3 days, then twice daily for 2–3 days, and then daily for 2–3 days. However, a recent Cochrane review reported there was insufficient evidence to support or refute the effectiveness of HBO_2 therapy for acute wounds, and further quality randomized controlled trials are needed (Eskes, Ubbink, Lubbers, Lucas, & Vermeulen, 2010).

Clostridial myonecrosis and necrotizing fasciitis are emergent conditions treated with surgical excision and HBO_2 therapy. Clostridial myonecrosis is caused by the toxin-producing organism *Clostridium perfringens*. The most prevalent toxin is the O_2-stable lecithinase-C, alpha-toxin, which is hemolytic and tissue-necrotizing. It destroys platelets and polymorphonuclear leukocytes and causes widespread capillary damage and is often lethal (Heimbach, 1994). A tissue PO_2 of 250 mmHg is necessary to stop alpha-toxin production which concurrently can inhibit bacterial growth, thus enabling the body to more effectively use its own host defense mechanisms (Van, 1965). The only way to achieve this is to start HBO_2 therapy as soon as possible. A minimum of 3–4 HBO_2 treatments are necessary for this response. Necrotizing fasciitis is an acute bacterial infectious process that may include both anaerobic and aerobic bacteria that act synergistically to cause rapid tissue destruction. Using HBO_2 therapy as an adjunct to surgical intervention improves oxygenation and may have a direct effect on the culprit bacteria, as well as improving neutrophil activity.

Chronic osteomyelitis occurs when extended or repeated attempts of standard interventions have failed. It is thought that HBO_2 improves available oxygen at the bone site to improve leukocyte killing ability through oxidative mechanisms. In addition, antibiotic activity may be enhanced. It is also thought that osteoclastic activity and osteogenesis are improved with the use of HBO_2.

Delayed radiation injury results from endarteritis and subsequent tissue hypoxia. There typically is a latent period of at least 6 months before the effects of delayed injury become apparent. Injury that was not apparent for many years can be precipitated by injury or surgical procedures. Hyperbaric oxygenation is used prophylactically for decades before

---

BOX 25.2   Situations for Hyperbaric Oxygen Therapy Under Investigation

- Acute myocardial infarction
- Acute cerebrovascular accident
- Mild traumatic brain injury
- Spinal cord injury
- Sickle cell crisis
- Rheumatic diseases
- Migraine/cluster headache
- Multiple sclerosis
- Radiation cystitis/proctitis
- Human immunodeficiency virus/acquired immunodeficiency syndrome
- Cerebral palsy
- Autism
- Bell palsy
- Fibromyalgia
- Traumatic brain injury
- Posttraumatic stress disorder
- Insulin resistance
- Near-drowning/anoxic brain injury
- Crohn's disease
- Ulcerative colitis
- Preconditioning before vascular surgery (diabetics)

---

oromaxillary surgical procedures to mitigate the potential postprocedure progression to osteoradionecrosis. However, a recent Cochrane review noted that more well-designed RCTs with larger samples are required to make conclusive statements regarding the efficacy of this prophylactic intervention (El-Rabbany et al., 2019).

Soft tissue radiation injuries, including proctitis and cystitis, can be treated with HBO_2. The rationale for the use of HBO_2 therapy is induction of neovascularization in the irradiated area.

Compromised grafts and flaps benefit from HBO_2 by facilitating increased distance of oxygen diffusion, thereby supporting the ischemic graft or flap. In addition, it now is believed that graft and flap failure may have a component of reperfusion injury that is overcome with the administration of HBO_2. Of note, HBO_2 therapy is not indicated in uncomplicated grafts or flaps, nor is it indicated in bioengineered tissues or human-derived allograft.

Hyperbaric oxygenation has been and is being used for many other disease processes and conditions, as outlined in Box 25.2. However, these are currently not recognized by the UHMS as indications for HBO_2 therapy. In a systematic review of the literature, the WOCN® Society (2016) concluded there is insufficient evidence to support the use of HBO_2 in the treatment of pressure injuries.

CONTRAINDICATIONS

Rigorous assessment of the patient must be completed to rule out contraindications to hyperbaric therapy (Tables 25.3 and 25.4). Any air-filled cavity must be assessed. The gas law described by Boyle states that as pressure increases, volume decreases, and vice

TABLE 25.3 Absolute Contraindications to Hyperbaric Oxygen Therapy

	Rationale for Contraindication	Corrective Interventions Necessary Prior to HBO_2
Untreated pneumothorax	• Gas emboli • Tension pneumothorax • Pneumomediastinum	Thoracostomy
Bleomycin	Interstitial pneumonitis	Elective treatment with HBO_2 is contraindicated in patients with even a remote history of bleomycin administration. However, in emergency, life-threatening situations, the benefits of HBO_2 might outweigh the possibility of bleomycin toxicity
Cisplatin	Impaired wound healing	In animals, concurrent administration of HBO_2 and cis-platinum was associated with an increase in wound breakdown. HBO_2 should be held until cis-platinum therapy is finished, if possible
Doxorubicin	Cardiotoxicity	In animals, administering HBO_2 concurrently with doxorubicin was associated with cardiac toxicity. It is advisable to wait (at a minimum of 72 h from last dose) until the drug has been cleared from the body before initiating HBO_2 therapy
Mafenide acetate (sulfamylin)	Impaired wound healing	Discontinue and remove medication
Disulfiram	Potentiates oxygen toxicity	Blocks the production of superoxide dismutase, which could lead to decreased free radical scavenging in hyperbaric environments

TABLE 25.4 Examples of Relative Contraindications to Evaluate Prior to Initiating Hyperbaric Oxygen Therapy

Relative Contraindications	Rationale for Contraindication	Corrective Interventions Necessary Prior to HBO_2
Asthma	Increased risk of air trapping leading to barotrauma during decompression	Must be well controlled with medications
Chronic obstructive pulmonary disease (COPD)	Increased risk of air trapping leading to barotrauma during decompression Loss of hypoxic drive to breathe	Assess for possible bullous lung disease and risk for air trapping prior to HBO_2. May not be appropriate to treat Monitor closely
Claustrophobia	Anxiety	Treat with benzodiazepines
Congenital spherocytosis	Severe hemolysis	None; HBO_2 for emergencies only
Congestive heart failure with ejection fraction <35%	HBO_2 therapy can potentially exacerbate congestive heart failure and/or flash pulmonary edema	Consult with cardiologist
Contact lenses	Needs to be gas permeable, no hard contact lenses	Include in pretreatment check list and ask patient to remove if hard contact lenses present
Eustachian tube dysfunction	Barotrauma to tympanic membrane	Training, PE tubes
High fever	Higher risk of seizures	Provide antipyretic
Pacemakers or epidural pain pump	Malfunction or deformation of device under pressure	Ensure company has pressure-tested device at the appropriate depth
Pregnancy	Unknown effect on fetus (previous studies from Russia suggest HBO_2 is safe)	None, but HBO_2 may be warranted in emergencies
Recent eye/retinal/cataract surgery or optic neuritis	Buckle procedure can have air trapped; other procedures can leave bubbles inside	Usually requires a few months waiting period before initiation of treatment
Recent thoracic surgery	Possible persisting pneumothorax	Recommend imaging to rule out pneumothorax
Seizures	May have lower seizure threshold	Should be stable on medications; may be treated with benzodiazepines

Continued

TABLE 25.4   Examples of Relative Contraindications to Evaluate Prior to Initiating Hyperbaric Oxygen Therapy—cont'd

Relative Contraindications	Rationale for Contraindication	Corrective Interventions Necessary Prior to HBO$_2$
Uncontrolled hypertension	Blood pressure can increase during treatment	Patient should be on appropriate medication(s). Document blood pressure before and after treatment session
Upper respiratory infection (URI/chronic sinus condition)	Risk for barotrauma	Evaluate for ability to equalize on the descent. Risk of reverse sinus block on the ascent. May need to wait for resolution of symptoms or use decongestants

versa. This guides the practitioner to assess air-filled body cavities, such as ears and sinus cavities, and the patient's ability to equalize pressure to prevent barotrauma. A chest X-ray examination will rule out trapping of air in the lungs. Patients with a history of seizure activity should be assessed for seizure control. Hyperbaric treatment is absolutely contraindicated for patients who have a history of receiving bleomycin because of its lifelong increased risk for oxygen toxicity. Hyperbaric treatment also is contraindicated for patients receiving *cis*-platinum, mafenide acetate (Sulfamylon), or disulfiram. Chemotherapeutic medications that generate oxygen-free radicals, such as cyclophosphamide and the anthracyclines daunorubicin and doxorubicin, are contraindicated with hyperbaric oxygen therapy (Dougherty, 2013). Clinicians need to understand the following pharmacotherapy interactions with hyperbaric oxygen treatments. Bleomycin can lead to interstitial pneumonitis (recent exposure, usually within a 12-month period), pulmonary fibrosis. Sulfamylon and cisplatin impair wound healing. Disulfiram blocks superoxide dismutase, which is protective against oxygen toxicity, and doxorubicin can cause cardiotoxicity (must wait a minimum of 72 h from the last dose) (Howell, Criscitelli, Woods, Gillette, & Gorenstein, 2018). Another absolute contraindication is an untreated pneumothorax (see Table 25.3).

Relative contraindications to hyperbaric treatment include pregnancy, known malignancy, emphysema, pneumonia, bronchitis, and hyperthermia (see Table 25.4) (Foster, 1992; Heimbach, 1998). Congestive heart failure (CHF) may be a relative contraindication to HBO$_2$ therapy depending on severity and current management. There are a number of recognized risks and side effects of HBO$_2$ therapy most of which are either uncommon or of minimal consequence. One such complication is an exacerbation of CHF. When pulmonary edema occurs, it is typically observed in the latter half of a 90-min treatment and, though infrequent, this complication can be substantial. Patients may respond favorably to simple decompression. Others may require a diuresis while some may require hospitalization and cardio-respiratory support in the Intensive Care Unit. Some deaths have been reported in the literature from exacerbations of pulmonary edema during HBO$_2$ therapy (Weaver & Churchill, 2001).

PROTOCOLS AND CLINICAL APPLICATION

Hyperbaric treatment protocols depend on the specific disease process. The UHMS has outlined acceptable protocols for hyperbaric exposure. However, this does not preclude provider preference and individualization to meet the patient's needs. Typically, a patient will receive a daily hyperbaric exposure five to seven times per week. The treatment will last for 90 min at 2.0–2.5 ATA. The number of total treatments is generally tailored to the patient response to HBO$_2$ and adjunctive indication to ongoing concomitant therapies. Therefore, continuous assessment of the patient's progress is required to determine when the maximum benefit from HBO$_2$ therapy has been reached (FDA, 2021).

Staff Education and Certification

The American Board of Medical Specialties offers a board examination for undersea and hyperbaric medicine that requires completion of a fellowship in undersea and hyperbaric medicine. The Undersea and Hyperbaric Medical Society (UHMS) offers a Program for Advanced Training in Hyperbarics (PATH) (UHMS, 2020). The PATH does not replace fellowship training or board certification in undersea and hyperbaric medicine, which is considered the gold standard for hyperbaric training. The PATH program is intended to demonstrate that a candidate has completed a formal education program covering advanced topics in undersea and hyperbaric medicine, as well as having submitted clinical cases for formal review. The PATH program is intended to take between 6 and 12 months to complete and represents approximately 100 h of continuing education credits.

The Baromedical Nurses Association (BNA) provides guidance for providing nursing care in the hyperbaric environment. Nurses may obtain national certification in hyperbaric nursing through the Baromedical Nurses Association Certification Board (BNACB), an association that promotes the status and standards of baromedical nursing practice. Three levels of certification are available, depending on practice participation and educational background (BNA, 2020). Physician assistants, respiratory therapists, paramedics, and EMT's can also obtain national certification in hyperbaric. Certification for hyperbaric technologists is available through the National Board of Diving and Hyperbaric Medicine after completion of an approved 40 h primary training course and 480 h internship (NBDHMT, 2019). The National Fire Protection Association requires each hyperbaric facility to designate an on-site hyperbaric safety director. This individual is responsible to oversee operational safety and maintenance of all hyperbaric equipment. There are additional educational opportunities available for those interested in becoming a hyperbaric safety director.

Methods and Chambers

To achieve a hyperbaric state, the patient is placed into either a monoplace or multiplace chamber. The American Society of Mechanical Engineers (ASME) provides standards for pressure vessels for human occupancy (PVHO-2). The National Fire Protection Association sets forth construction requirements for the physical structure containing the chamber (NFPA, 2018). The monoplace chamber (Fig. 25.1) has rapidly become the predominant chamber in outpatient settings. A monoplace chamber typically is compressed with oxygen. These chambers are rated for a maximum clinical pressurization of 44 pounds per square inch absolute (psia), or three atmospheres absolute (ATA). The major advantages of using monoplace chambers is that they are relatively inexpensive, have less space requirements and are much easier to install. Another advantage is that the monoplace chamber can be staffed by either a nurse or technician and a provider. Current reimbursement guidelines dictate that a provider must be immediately available for the duration of a hyperbaric treatment.

Disadvantages of the monoplace chamber include the lack of direct patient contact and the difficulty involved in monitoring the patient other than visually. Methods are available to monitor electrocardiogram, arterial blood pressure, pulmonary artery pressure, wedge pressure, central venous pressure, cuff blood pressure, temperature, and transcutaneous partial pressure of oxygen ($TcPO_2$) monitoring. It also is possible to ventilate a patient in the monoplace chamber; however, most hyperbaric chambers that are integrated within an outpatient wound care clinic do not have the ability to provide support to the critically ill patient.

The multiplace chamber (Fig. 25.2) allows a caregiver to enter the chamber with the patient. The caregiver, or *tender,* may be a technician, nurse, or provider. The multiplace chamber can accommodate multiple patients in a single treatment. The number of patients who can be treated simultaneously depends on the size of the chamber and whether the patients are ambulatory, chair bound, or bed bound. The multiplace chamber is compressed with air. Oxygen is delivered to the patient through either a mask or a hood. The multiplace chamber can easily be equipped to handle the critically ill.

The major disadvantages of the multiplace chamber are the cost and housing requirements for the chamber. Another disadvantage of the multiplace chamber, if the chamber is not a multilock design, a multioccupant treatment will need to be aborted if a patient is unable to equalize pressure during pressurization or is unable to complete the treatment. A final consideration of the multiplace chamber is staffing. The multiplace chamber requires a greater expenditure for staff than does the monoplace chamber. The multiplace chamber is typically staffed with a chamber operator, inside attendant, outside attendant, and attending provider. There are also additional risks to staff members who work as inside attendants, especially at higher treatment pressures and longer treatment profiles.

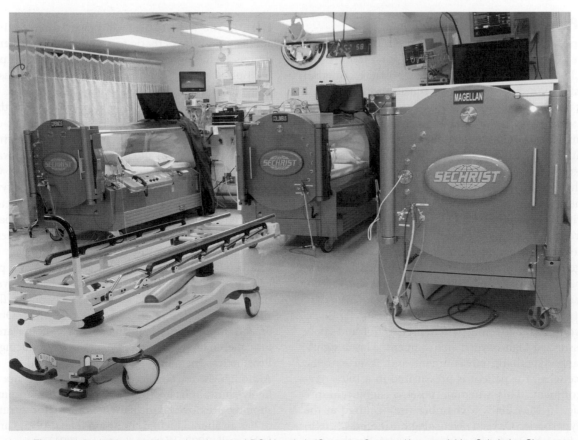

Fig. 25.1 Sechrist monoplace chambers at LDS Hospital. (Courtesy Geness Koumandakis, Salt Lake City, UT, USA.)

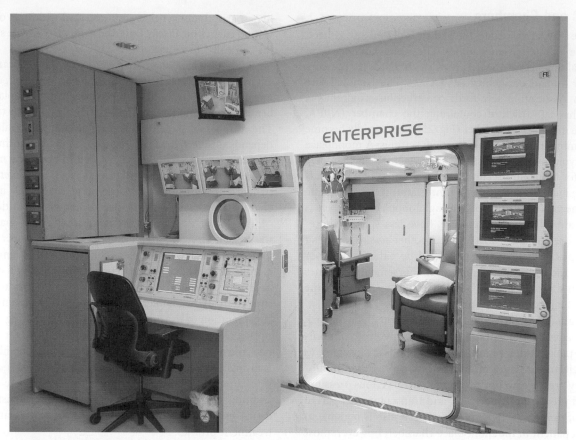

Fig. 25.2 Fink multiplace chamber at Intermountain Medical Center. (Courtesy Geness Koumandakis, Salt Lake City, UT, USA.)

Patient Preparation and Safety

Two factors dictate the need to follow rigorous procedures for patient preparation and patient safety. The first factor is the nature of hyperbarics (e.g., atmospheric pressure changes). Patient instruction should include air equalization techniques to prevent aural or sinus barotrauma. The patient should be instructed not to hold his or her breath during ascent to prevent pneumothorax. The caregiver responsible for assessing the patient before treatment should assess breath sounds to prevent exposing the patient with compromised pulmonary status to the hyperbaric environment. A random blood sugar measurement before treatment should be obtained for all patients with diabetes because HBO_2 therapy has the potential to significantly lower blood sugar levels. Vital signs are obtained to assess for hypertension and hyperthermia. Hyperbaric oxygenation is a potent vasoconstrictor and can predispose the patient to a hypertensive crisis; an oral temperature greater than 102°F (38.9°C) predisposes the patient to an oxygen toxicity seizure.

The second factor affecting patient preparation and safety is the pressurized high-oxygen environment. This is significant in any hyperbaric environment and is of extreme importance when the patient is pressurized in a 100% oxygen environment. This situation poses a significant fire safety issue. In May 2009, a chamber fire occurred at the Ocean Hyperbaric Oxygen Neurologic Center, a freestanding hyperbaric facility in Lauderdale-by-the Sea,

Florida. The hyperbaric facility specialized in neurologic applications of hyperbaric oxygen for the treatment of conditions including stroke, brain injury, cerebral palsy, and multiple sclerosis. The fire resulted in the deaths of a 62-year-old woman and her 4-year-old grandson who was receiving treatment for cerebral palsy. Neither the grandmother nor the grandchild died in the fire but died later as a result of burn injuries received due to a spark from static electricity; the patient and the grandmother who was accompanying the grandson in the chamber were not wearing a grounding bracelet to dissipate static electricity (Ortega, 2009; Roustan, 2012). Patients should be instructed not to use products that have a petroleum or alcohol base before they go into the chamber. Checklist 25.1 provides a list of materials banned in the hyperbaric chamber. Cosmetic products such as hair spray, hair creams, lotions, petroleum jelly, deodorants, and perfumes must be removed before treatment. Almost all skin care products pose a flammable risk and should be removed before treatment. Only cotton or cotton/polyester blend linens and clothing are allowed into the chamber to decrease risk for producing a spark. Prosthetics, including hearing aids, should be removed. Although glasses, contact lenses, and dentures are not absolutely contraindicated in the hyperbaric environment, they should be removed if the patient is at risk for seizure activity or has an altered mental condition (Hart, 1995; Larson-Lohr & Norvell, 2002; Weaver & Straas, 1991).

CHECKLIST 25.1 Materials Banned From the Hyperbaric Chamber

✓ Cosmetic products, including the following:
- Hair spray
- Hair cream
- Skin care products, including lotions and barrier ointments
- Deodorant
- Perfume
- Lipstick
- Fingernail polish

✓ Petrolatum and products containing petrolatum and paraffin
✓ Mineral oil and products containing mineral oil
✓ Dressing products containing synthetic fibers (e.g., nylon)
✓ Elastic products (e.g., compression wraps)
✓ Any device with a battery (e.g., hearing aid, cell phone)
✓ Dentures if patient at risk for seizure activity
✓ All jewelry
✓ Magnesium eyeglass frames

Side Effects

The most common side effect or complication of HBO_2 is middle ear barotrauma. Aural barotrauma, referred to as an *ear squeeze*, will manifest as ear pain and may result in a hematoma to the tympanic membrane, hemorrhage in the middle ear, or tympanic rupture. If a patient experiences an ear squeeze, placement of pressure equalization tubes or a myringotomy may be necessary. Sinus barotrauma, or sinus squeeze, results in extreme sinus pain and may lead to hemorrhage of the sinus. The patient who comes for a hyperbaric treatment and has a congested nasal passage may benefit from nasal decongestant sprays before the treatment. However, the possibility of a reverse sinus squeeze on decompression should be considered. Oral decongestants may be indicated for a more long-term approach (Capes & Tomaszewski, 1996; Kidder, 1995; Vrabec, Clements, & Mader, 1998).

Another common side effect is claustrophobia. This can occur in either the monoplace or multiplace chamber. Patients who experience claustrophobia should be reassured, and a tender should be present and in contact with the patient at all times. In the multiplace chamber, the tender can offer direct physical comfort. In the monoplace chamber, the tender should maintain both visual and verbal contact with the patient. Benzodiazepines offer relief of claustrophobia in most cases. Occasionally, a treatment is aborted, and subsequent hyperbaric therapy is discontinued as a result of claustrophobia.

Visual acuity changes during hyperbaric therapy are not rare. Myopia may worsen after 20 or more hyperbaric exposures. Frequently, a patient who uses glasses to correct presbyopia will find that he or she is able to read without corrective lenses. The exact mechanism behind these visual changes is not fully understood. The patient who experiences a visual change should be instructed not to change prescription eyewear for 2–3 months after hyperbaric treatment because the visual change usually is temporary (Maki, 1996).

A physiologic anomaly, breath holding, or cessation of respiration can cause air to be trapped in the lungs. This trapped air can lead to a tension pneumothorax. Should this occur in a multiplace chamber, the patient can be recompressed and the pneumothorax corrected within the chamber before decompression of the chamber. In a monoplace environment, the patient should be recompressed to treatment depth until supplies, equipment, and personnel are available. Once the team and supplies are assembled, the patient should be decompressed and treated immediately upon removal from the chamber.

Seizure activity from oxygen toxicity, although ominous in appearance, is self-limiting and benign. The patient in the monoplace environment should be maintained at pressure until seizure activity has stopped. If the patient is breathing oxygen by mask or hood, the oxygen should be stopped, and the patient placed on air. Once the seizure has stopped, the patient can be removed from the chamber. Generally, no further precautions or anticonvulsant medications are necessary for subsequent treatments. Patients with a known history of seizure or who are predisposed to seizure activity would benefit from periodic, scheduled discontinuation of oxygen breathing (air breaks) during the treatment (Clark, 1995).

TOPICAL OXYGEN IS NOT HBO₂

Various methods for providing topical oxygen have been created, including plastic chambers over a limb; continuous oxygen flow through a battery-operated system or a reservoir within a bandage; and gas dissolved or saturated within saline, gel, or foam (Federman et al., 2016). Topical oxygen therapy has been in clinical use for over 50 years with promising but preclinical and clinical studies that have shown improved closure rates when compared to standard care (Frykberg, 2021). However, until recently there has been insufficient rigorous level one evidence to recommend topical oxygen therapy for the treatment of wounds. In 2020 a multinational, multicenter, randomized, double blinded, placebo-controlled trial was published that evaluated the efficacy of topical wound oxygen therapy in the treatment of chronic diabetic foot ulcers with 220 patients completing the 12-week treatment phase. The study results demonstrated that topical oxygen therapy was superior in healing chronic DFUs at 12 weeks and reduced recidivism at 12 months compared to optimal SOC alone (Federman et al., (2016); Frykberg, Franks, Edmonds, et al., 2020; Marston, Tang, Kirsner, & Ennis, 2016; NPUAP, EPUAP, and PPPIA, 2019; WOCN, 2016).

Published information related to topical oxygen can be confusing when the modality is inaccurately labeled topical hyperbaric oxygen (THBO). Topical therapy literature can further confuse the consumer by using by using HBO^2 to demonstrate its value. In fact, topical oxygen therapy is not HBO_2; the route of delivery and the mode of action are different. It is important to distinguish between the two modalities in order to clarify the discussion of efficacy (Federman et al., 2016). In 2017, CMS announced that decisions related to reimbursement for topical hyperbaric therapy DME equipment for treatment of chronic wounds would be left to the individual MACs. It is important to understand that CMS will not cover physician or professional services with this treatment (Center for Medicare and Medicaid Services, 2017a, 2017b). Information from the Noridian and Cigna MACs currently indicates that the HCPCS codes for topical hyperbaric oxygen therapy are considered investigational and not covered DME services (DME Non Covered Items, 2019; Medical Coverage Policy Hyperbaric and Topical Oxygen Therapies, 2019). These types of coverage barriers will hopefully be addressed over time. In fact as of 2022 topical oxygen therapy is covered by NY Medicaid with expected adoption by other medicaid payers in 2023. Remember, it is important to check with your local MAC or payer's policies for coverage information in your area.

Topical oxygen may produce transient, slight elevations in ambient pressure applied to the wound (as high as 1.03 ATA). In contrast, HBO_2 therapy (systemic) is defined medically as the application of pressures greater than atmospheric to a patient who is entirely enclosed within the pressurized chamber, at pressures that equal or exceed 1.4 ATA while breathing near 100% oxygen. The United States Pharmacopoeia (USP) and Compressed Gas Association (CGA) Grade A specify medical grade oxygen to be not less than 99.0% by volume, and the National Fire Protection Association specifies USP medical grade oxygen.

SUMMARY

- Oxygen is a powerful and versatile agent used in many aspects of medicine.
- The therapeutic use of oxygen under pressure has been used for many years for multiple medical conditions, including wound healing.
- Hyperoxygenation of tissue, vasoconstriction, downregulation of inflammatory cytokines, upregulation of growth factors, and antibacterial effects of HBO_2 can benefit patients with specific wound types.
- As with other biophysical modalities used in wound care today, more research is needed before expanding the list of indications.

SELF-ASSESSMENT QUESTIONS

1. Which of the following statements about hyperoxygenation that occurs with hyperbaric treatment is *true*?
   a. Hyperoxygenation occurs because the hemoglobin molecule is saturated with oxygen molecules.
   b. Hyperoxygenation results from increasing the oxygen-carrying capacity of the plasma.
   c. Several treatments are needed to achieve hyperoxygenation.
   d. Hyperoxygenation may be sustained for 8–10 h after exposure.

2. All of the following personal care items are contraindicated during hyperbaric treatment *except*:
   a. Hairspray
   b. Hearing aids
   c. Gas permeable contact lenses
   d. Perfume

3. True or False: Wound care dressings with a petrolatum base should be removed prior to hyperbaric oxygen treatment.

4. True or False: Hyperbaric oxygen is a definitive treatment of hard-to-heal wounds.

5. HBO_2 benefits wound healing through the following mechanism(s):
   a. Tissue oxygen tension restored to >30 mmHg
   b. Augments transport of certain antibiotics across bacterial cell walls
   c. Promotes capillary angiogenesis
   d. Prevents polymorphonuclear leukocytes from adhering to damaged blood vessel linings
   e. All of the above

REFERENCES

Baromedical Nurses Association (BNA) Certification. (2020). Retrieved August 19, 2020, from http://hyperbaricnurses.org/certification.

Bird, N. (2018). *Undersea and hyperbaric medical society position statement: Low-pressure fabric hyperbaric chambers.* Retrieved August 19, 2020, from https://www.uhms.org/images/Position-Statements/UHMS_Position_Statement_LP_chambers_revised.pdf.

Bonham, P. A., Flemister, B. G., Droste, L. R., Johnson, J. J., Kelechi, T., Ratliff, C. R., et al. (2016). 2014 Guideline for management of wounds in patients with lower-extremity arterial disease (LEAD). *Journal of Wound, Ostomy and Continence Nursing, 43*(1), 23–31. https://doi.org/10.1097/won.0000000000000193.

Bonomo, S. R., Davidson, J. D., Yu, Y., Xia, Y., Lin, X., & Mustoe, T. A. (1998). Hyperbaric oxygen as a signal transducer: Upregulation of platelet derived growth factor-beta receptor in the presence of HBO2 and PDGF. *Undersea & Hyperbaric Medicine, 25*(4), 211–216.

Capes, J. P., & Tomaszewski, C. (1996). Prophylaxis against middle ear barotrauma in US hyperbaric oxygen therapy centers. *The American Journal of Emergency Medicine, 14*(7), 645–648. https://doi.org/10.1016/s0735-6757(96)90079-0.

Centers for Medicare and Medicaid Services (CMS). (2002). *Coverage of hyperbaric oxygen (HBO) therapy for the treatment of diabetic wounds of the lower extremities (Program memorandum in-termediaries/carriers, Transmittal AB-02-183)*. Washington, DC: Department of Health and Human Services. Retrieved August 19, 2020 from http://www.cms.gov/transmittals/downloads/AB02183.pdf.

Centers for Medicare and Medicaid Services (CMS). (2017a). *Medicare learning network*. Retrieved August 19, 2020 from https://www.cms.gov/Outreach-and-Education/Medicare-Learning-Network-MLN/MLNMattersArticles/Downloads/MM10220.pdf.

Centers for Medicare and Medicaid Services (CMS). (2017b). *National coverage determination (NCD) for hyperbaric oxygen therapy (20.29) (Publication no. 100-3), Manual section no. 20.29, Vol. 4*. Retrieved April 11, 2020, from https://www.cms.gov/medicare-coverage-database/details/ncd-details.aspx?NCDId=12.

Cianci, P., & Sato, R. (1994). Adjunctive hyperbaric oxygen therapy in the treatment of thermal burns: A review. *Burns, 20*(1), 5–14. https://doi.org/10.1016/0305-4179(94)90099-x.

Clark, J. M. (1995). Oxygen toxicity. In E. P. Kindwall (Ed.), *Hyperbaric medicine practice*. Flagstaff: Best.

Crawford, P. E., & Fields-Varnado, M. (2013). Guideline for the management of wounds in patients with lower-extremity neuropathic disease. *Journal of Wound, Ostomy and Continence Nursing, 40*(1), 34–45. https://doi.org/10.1097/won.0b013e3182750161.

Dauwe, P. B., Pulikkottil, B. J., Lavery, L., Stuzin, J. M., & Rohrich, R. J. (2014). Does hyperbaric oxygen therapy work in facilitating acute wound healing. *Plastic and Reconstructive Surgery, 133*(2). https://doi.org/10.1097/01.

DME Non Covered Items. (2019). *Noridian Healthcare Solutions*. Retrieved August 19, 2020 from https://med.noridianmedicare.com/web/jddme/topics/noncovered-items.

Dougherty, J. E. (2013). The role of hyperbaric oxygen therapy in crush injuries. *Critical Care Nursing Quarterly, 36*(3), 299–309. https://doi.org/10.1097/cnq.0b013e318294ea41.

El-Rabbany, M., Duchnay, M., Raziee, H. R., Maria, Z. M., Tenenbaum, H., Shah, P. S., et al. (2019). Interventions for preventing osteoradionecrosis of the jaws in adults receiving head and neck radiotherapy. The Cochrane Database of Systematic Reviews, 2019(11), CD011559. https://doi.org/10.1002/14651858.CD011559.pub2.

Elliott, D. H. (1995). Decompression sickness. In E. P. Kindwall (Ed.), *Hyperbaric medicine practice*. Flagstaff: Best.

Ennis, W. J., Huang, E. T., & Gordon, H. (2018). Impact of hyperbaric oxygen on more advanced Wagner Grades 3 and 4 diabetic foot ulcers: Matching therapy to specific wound conditions. *Advances in Wound Care, 7*(12), 397–407. https://doi.org/10.1089/wound.2018.0855.

Eskes, A., Ubbink, D. T., Lubbers, M., Lucas, C., & Vermeulen, H. (2010). Hyperbaric oxygen therapy for treating acute surgical and traumatic wounds. *The Cochrane Database of Systematic Reviews*. https://doi.org/10.1002/14651858.cd008059.pub2.

FDA (U.S. Food & Drug Administration). (2021). Hyperbaric oxygen therapy: Get the facts. Retrieved November 14, 2022 from https://www.fda.gov/consumers/consumer-updates/hyperbaric-oxygen-therapy-get-facts.

Federman, D. G., Ladiiznski, B., Dardik, A., Kelly, M., Shapshak, D., Ueno, C. M., et al. (2016). Wound Healing Society 2014 update on guidelines for arterial ulcers. *Wound Repair and Regeneration, 24*(1), 127–135. https://doi.org/10.1111/wrr.12395. PMID: 26663663.

Fife, C. E., Buyukcakir, C., Otto, G. H., Sheffield, P. J., Warriner, R. A., Love, T. L., et al. (2002). The predictive value of transcutaneous oxygen tension measurement in diabetic lower extremity ulcers treated with hyperbaric oxygen therapy: A retrospective analysis of 1144 patients. *Wound Repair and Regeneration, 10*(4), 198–207. https://doi.org/10.1046/j.1524-475x.2002. 10402.x.

Foster, J. H. (1992). Hyperbaric oxygen therapy: Contraindications and complications. *Journal of Oral and Maxillofacial Surgery, 50*(10), 1081–1086. https://doi.org/10.1016/0278-2391(92)90495-l.

Frykberg, R. G. (2021). Topical wound oxygen therapy in the treatment of chronic diabetic foot ulcers. *Medicina (Kaunas), 57*(9), 917. https://doi.org/10.3390/medicina57090917.

Frykberg, R. G., Franks, P. J., Edmonds, M., et al. (2020). A multinational, multicenter, randomized, double-blinded, placebo-controlled trial to evaluate the efficacy of cyclical topical wound oxygen (TWO2) therapy in the treatment of chronic diabetic foot ulcers: The TWO2 study. *Diabetes Care, 43*(3), 616–624. https://doi.org/10.2337/dc19-0476.

Hammarlund, C. (1995). The physiologic effects of hyperbaric oxygen. In E. P. Kindwall (Ed.), *Hyperbaric medicine practice*. Flagstaff: Best.

Hart, G. B. (1995). The monoplace chamber. In E. P. Kindwall (Ed.), *Hyperbaric medicine practice*. Flagstaff: Best.

Heimbach, R. D. (1994). Gas gangrene. In E. P. Kindwall (Ed.), *Hyperbaric medicine practice* (pp. 373–394). Flagstaff: Best Publishing Co.

Heimbach, R. D. (1998). Physiology and pharmacology of HBO_2. In C. Jefferson (Ed.), *Davis wound care and hyperbaric medicine center (Course)*. San Antonio: Hyperbaric Medicine Team Training, Southwest Texas Methodist Hospital and Nix Medical Center.

Howell, R. S., Criscitelli, T., Woods, J. S., Gillette, B. M., & Gorenstein, S. (2018). Hyperbaric oxygen therapy: Indications, contraindications, and use at a tertiary care center. *AORN Journal, 107*(4), 442–453. https://doi.org/10.1002/aorn.12097.

Juttner, B., Scheinichen, D., Bartsch, S., Heine, J., Ruschulte, H., Elsner, H. A., et al. (2003). Lack of toxic side effects in neutrophils following hyperbaric oxygen. *Undersea & Hyperbaric Medicine, 30*(4), 305–311.

Kang, T. S., Gorti, G. K., Quan, S. Y., Ho, M., & Koch, R. J. (2004). Effect of hyperbaric oxygen on the growth factor profile of fibroblasts. *Archives of Facial Plastic Surgery, 6*(1), 31. https://doi.org/10.1001/archfaci.6.1.31.

Kidder, T. M. (1995). Myringotomy. In E. P. Kindwall (Ed.), *Hyperbaric medicine practice*. Flagstaff: Best.

Kindwall, E. P. (1995). A history of hyperbaric medicine. In E. P. Kindwall (Ed.), *Hyperbaric medicine practice*. Flagstaff: Best.

Kranke, P., Bennett, M. H., James, M. M.-S., Schnabel, A., Debus, S. E., & Weibel, S. (2015). Hyperbaric oxygen therapy for chronic wounds. *The Cochrane Database of Systematic Reviews*. https://doi.org/10.1002/14651858.cd004123.pub4.

Ladurner, R., Küper, M., Königsrainer, I., Löb, S., Wichmann, D., Königsrainer, A., et al. (2010). Predictive value of routine transcutaneous tissue oxygen tension (tcpO2) measurement for the risk of non-healing and amputation in diabetic foot ulcer patients with non-palpable pedal pulses. *Medical Science Monitor, 16*(6), CR273–277.

Larson-Lohr, V., & Norvell, H. (Eds.). (2002). *Hyperbaric nursing*. Flagstaff: Best.

Latham, E. (2020). *Hyperbaric oxygen therapy*. Retrieved April 11, 2020, from http://emedicine.medscape.com/article/1464149-overview#a2.

Lavery, L. A., Davis, K. E., Berriman, S. J., Braun, L., Nichols, A., Kim, P. J., et al. (2016). WHS guidelines update: Diabetic foot ulcer treatment guidelines. *Wound Repair and Regeneration, 24*(1), 112–126. https://doi.org/10.1111/wrr.12391. PMID: 26663430.

Lin, C.-M., Wang, F.-H., & Lee, P.-K. (2002). Activated human CD4⁺ T cells induced by dendritic cell stimulation are most sensitive to transforming growth factor-B: Implications for dendritic cell immunization against cancer. *Clinical Immunology, 102*(1), 96–105.

Löndahl, M. (2012). Hyperbaric oxygen therapy as treatment of diabetic foot ulcers. *Diabetes/Metabolism Research and Reviews, 28*(Suppl. 1), 78–84.

Maki, R. D. (1996). Ophthalmic side effects of hyperbaric oxygen therapy. *Insight, 21*(4), 114–117.

Marston, W., Tang, J., Kirsner, R. S., Ennis, W. (2016). Wound Healing Society 2015 update on guidelines for venous ulcers. *Wound Repair and Regeneration, 24*(1), 136–144. https://doi.org/10.1111/wrr.12394. PMID: 26663616.

Marx, R. E. (1995). Radiation injury to tissue. In E. P. Kindwall (Ed.), *Hyperbaric medicine practice*. Flagstaff: Best.

Medical Coverage Policy Hyperbaric and Topical Oxygen Therapies. (2019). *Cigna Corporation*. Retrieved August 19, 2020 from https://cignaforhcp.cigna.com/public/content/pdf/coveragePolicies/medical/mm_0053_coveragepositioncriteria_hyperbaric_oxygen.pdf.

Moon, R. E. (2019). *Undersea and Hyperbaric Medical Society (UHMS): Indications for hyperbaric oxygen therapy*. Retrieved April 12, 2020, from https://www.uhms.org/resources/hbo-indications.html?highlight=WyJpbmRpY2F0aW9ucyJd.

Moon, R. E. (2020). *Undersea and Hyperbaric Medical Society: Indications for hyperbaric oxygen therapy*. Retrieved April 12, 2020, from https://www.uhms.org/resources/hbo-indications.html?highlight=WyJpbmRpY2F0aW9ucyJd.

National Board of Diving and Hyperbaric Medical Technology (NBDHMT). (2019). *Certified hyperbaric technologic resource manual*. Retrieved April 11, 2020, from http://www.nbdhmt.org/forms/CHT_Resource_Manual.pdf.

National Fire Protection Association. (2018). *NFPA 99: Standard for health care facilities*. Retrieved April 11, 2020, from https://www.nfpa.org/codes-and-standards/all-codes-and-standards/list-of-codes-and-standards/detail?code=99.

National Pressure Ulcer Advisory Panel (NPUAP), European Pressure Ulcer Advisory Panel (EPUAP) and Pan Pacific Pressure Injury Alliance (PPPIA). (2019). *Prevention and treatment of pressure ulcers: Clinical practice guideline*. Retrieved April 11, 2020, from https://guidelinesales.com.

Norgren, L., Hiatt, W., Dormandy, J., Nehler, M., Harris, K., & Fowkes, F. (2007). Inter-society consensus for the management of peripheral arterial disease (TASC II). *Journal of Vascular Surgery, 45*(Suppl. S), S5–S67. https://doi.org/10.1016/j.jvs.2006.12.037.

Ortega, J. (2009). *Child in blast dies from injuries*. Retrieved April 11, 2020 from http://articles.sun-sentinel.com/2009-06-12/news/0906110581_1_hyperbaric-italian-boy-boy-s-family.

Pai, M. P., & Hunt, T. K. (1972). Effect of varying oxygen tensions on healing of open wounds. *Surgery, Gynecology & Obstetrics, 135*(5), 756–758.

Roustan, W. K. (2012). *Two charged in deadly 2009 hyperbaric chamber fire*. Retrieved April 11, 2020 from http://articles.sun-sentinel.com/2012-04-25/news/fl-hyperbaric-chamber-deaths-0426-20120425_1_francesco-martinisi-hyperbaric-clinic-pure-oxygen.

Sander, A. L., Henrich, D., Muth, C. M., Marzi, I., Barker, J. H., & Frank, J. M. (2009). In vivo effect of hyperbaric oxygen on wound angiogenesis and epithelialization. *Wound Repair and Regeneration, 17*(2), 179–184. https://doi.org/10.1111/j.1524-475x.2009.00455.x.

Sheikh, A. Y. (2000). Effect of hyperoxia on vascular endothelial growth factor levels in a wound model. *Archives of Surgery, 135*(11), 1293–1297. https://doi.org/10.1001/archsurg.135.11.1293.

Thom, S. R. (1993). Functional inhibition of leukocyte B2 integrins by hyperbaric oxygen in carbon monoxide-mediated brain injury in rats. *Toxicology and Applied Pharmacology, 123*(2), 248–256. https://doi.org/10.1006/taap.1993.1243.

Thom, S. R., Mendiguren, I., Hardy, K., Bolotin, T., Fisher, D., Nebolon, M., et al. (1997). Inhibition of human neutrophil beta2-integrin-dependent adherence by hyperbaric O_2. *American Journal of Physiology, 272*(3 Pt. 1), C770–C777. https://doi.org/10.1152/ajpcell.1997.272.3.C770.

Undersea and Hyperbaric Medical Society (UHMS). (2015). *About the UHMS*. Retrieved April 12, 2020, from https://www.uhms.org/about-the-uhms.html.

Undersea and Hyperbaric Medical Society (UHMS) Program for Advanced Training in Hyperbarics (PATH). (2020). Retrieved April 12, 2020, from https://www.uhms.org/education/credentialing/caq-hyperbaric-physician-certification.html2020.

Van, U. (1965). Inhibition of toxin production in Clostridium perfringens in vitro by hyperbaric oxygen. *Antonie Van Leeuwenhoek, 31*, 181–186.

Vrabec, J. T., Clements, K. S., & Mader, J. T. (1998). Short-term tympanostomy in conjunction with hyperbaric oxygen therapy. *Laryngoscope, 108*(8), 1124–1128. https://doi.org/10.1097/00005537-199808000-00004.

Weaver, L. K., & Churchill, S. (2001). Pulmonary edema associated with hyperbaric oxygen therapy. *Chest, 120*(4), 1407–1409. https://doi.org/10.1378/chest.120.4.1407.

Weaver, L. K., & Straas, M. B. (1991). *Monoplace hyperbaric chamber safety guidelines: Report to the Hyperbaric Chamber Safety Committee of the Undersea and Hyperbaric Medical Society*. Retrieved April 12, 2020, from https://www.uhms.org/images/Safety-Articles/Monoplace_Hyperbaric_Chamber_Guidlelines.pdf.

Weaver, L. K., Wilson, S. H., Lindblad, A. S., Churchill, S., Deru, K., Price, R. C., et al. (2018). Hyperbaric oxygen for post-concussive symptoms in United States military service members: A randomized clinical trial. *Undersea & Hyperbaric Medicine, 45*(2), 129–156.

Winter, G., & Perrins, D. (1970). In *Effects of hyperbaric oxygen treatment on epidermal regeneration Paper Presented at: Fourth International Congress on Hyperbaric Medicine, Tokyo*.

Wound, Ostomy and Continence Nurses Society. (2016). *Guideline for management of patients with pressure ulcers (injuries), WOCN clinical practice guideline series #2*, Mt. Laurel, Author.

FURTHER READING

Fries, R. B., Wallace, W. A., Roy, S., Kuppusamy, P., Bergdall, V., Gordillo, G., et al. (2005). Dermal excisional wound healing in pigs following treatment with topically applied pure oxygen. *Mutation Research/Fundamental and Molecular Mechanisms of Mutagenesis, 579*(1–2), 172–181. https://doi.org/https://doi.org/10.1016/j.mrfmmm.2005.02.023.

Edsberg, L. E., Brogan, M. S., Jaynes, C. D., & Fries, K. (2002). Topical hyperbaric oxygen and electrical stimulation: Exploring potential synergy. *Ostomy Wound Manage, 48*(11), 42–50.

Gordillo, G. M., & Sen, C. K. (2003). Revisiting the essential role of oxygen in wound healing. *The American Journal of Surgery, 186*(3), 259–263. https://doi.org/https://doi.org/10.1016/s0002-9610(03)00211-3.

Heng, M. C., Harker, J., Bardakjian, V. B., & Ayvazian, H. (2000). Enhanced healing and cost effectiveness of low-pressure oxygen therapy in healing necrotic wounds: A feasibility

study of technology transfer. *Ostomy Wound Manage, 46*(3), 52–60, 62.

Kalliainen, L. K., Gordillo, G. M., Schlanger, R., & Sen, C. K. (2003). Topical oxygen as an adjunct to wound healing: A clinical case series. *Pathophysiology, 9*(2), 81–87. https://doi.org/https://doi.org/10.1016/s0928-4680(02)00079-2.

Undersea & Hyperbaric Medicine Society. (2019). Hyperbaric oxygen therapy indications (14th ed.). Best Publishing Company.

Whelan, H. T., Kindwall, E., et al. (2017). Hyperbaric medicine practice (4th ed.). Best Publishing Company.

26

Electrical Stimulation

Frank Aviles

OBJECTIVES

1. Explain the physiologic effects of electrical stimulation.
2. List at least two indications for electrical stimulation.
3. List at least two contraindications for electrical stimulation.

4. Describe electrode placements when treating wounds with electrical stimulation.

Wound healing occurs through an overlapping cascade of events that are characterized by specific cellular and biomechanical processes. These processes transpire in response to chemical signals as well as bioelectrical currents. When the wound-healing process is disrupted, the wound shifts to a chronic state. Electrical stimulation is a valuable and effective (Thakral et al., 2013) adjunctive modality that can impact the human body's bioelectric system and accelerate wound healing. Considered as a biophysical energy, electrical stimulation has been noted to increase capillary density and perfusion, improve wound oxygenation, encourage granulation, and fibroblast activity (Kloth, 2002), and provide an antibacterial effect (Barnes, Shahin, Gohil, & Chetter, 2014). Various electrical stimulation devices exist. Their ability to promote chronic wound healing is based on their galvanotaxic effect and how they mimic the natural current of injury. Furthermore, ES has been demonstrated to be effective in the care of various wound etiologies including recalcitrant wounds and pressure injuries (Hunckler & de Mel, 2017; Kloth, 2005; Thakral et al., 2013).

Devices used for wound healing applications consist of a source of electrical current, a minimum of two wires or leads, and their corresponding electrodes (Fig. 26.1). One lead is connected to the negative output of the device and is the source of negatively charged electrons in an electrical circuit; this is referred to as the cathode. The other lead is connected to a positive output on the device that serves as an electron

depository for the flow of electrons in the electrical circuit; this is called the anode. Electrodes are attached to the patient end of the wires and placed on either the patient's wound bed or the adjacent skin. A unidirectional current flows through this circuit when the device is operating, causing positively charged ions (Na^+, K^+, H^+) in the tissues and positively charged cells (activated neutrophils and fibroblasts) to migrate toward the cathode; negatively charged ions (Cl^-, HCO_3^- P^-) and negatively charged cells (epidermal, neutrophils, and macrophages) migrate toward the anode. To understand the basis of electrical stimulation as an adjunctive therapy for wounds, it is important to understand several terms. Table 26.1 provides definitions of relevant terms.

EFFECTS OF ELECTRICAL STIMULATION

In an effort to examine the entire body of evidence on electrical stimulation and chronic wound healing, Gardner, Frantz, and Schmidt (1999) conducted a meta-analysis of 15 studies that assessed efficacy. Studies included in the meta-analysis were limited to randomized controlled trials ($n = 9$) and nonrandomized controlled trials ($n = 6$). Meta-analysis procedures were applied to 24 electrical stimulation samples ($n = 591$ wounds) and 15 control wound samples ($n = 212$). The calculated average rate of healing for the electrical stimulation samples was 22% per week compared with 9% for the control samples. The net effect of electrical stimulation therapy was 13% per week, a 144% increase over the control rate. These data provide an abundance of evidence that electrical stimulation can produce substantial improvement in the healing of chronic wounds. The physiologic effects of electrical stimulation that contribute to its wound healing efficacy include galvanotaxis, stimulatory, antibacterial, blood flow, and tissue oxygenation (Polak, Kloth, Blaszczak, Taradaj, & Nawrat-Szoltysik, 2016). In a 2014 meta-analysis, Barnes et al. (2014) examined the impact of

---

☆The editors gratefully acknowledge Dr. Rita Frantz for her pioneering work creating this chapter in the first edition (1992) of Acute and Chronic Wounds: Current Concepts and providing updates in each subsequent edition. Her scientific and scholarly framework to advance our understanding of electrical stimulation and its application to wound healing is unmatched. Many of the components and concepts she put forth are reflected in this chapter and we are appreciative of her significant contribution.

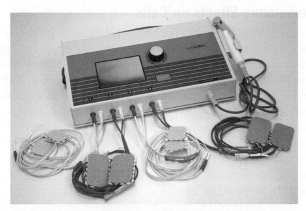

Fig. 26.1 Example of a high-voltage pulsed current electrical stimulation device. (Courtesy Rich-Mar Corporation, Inola, OK, USA.)

electrical stimulation on chronic wound healing irrespective of the wound etiology when compared with standard of care and/or sham stimulation. There findings included a mean percentage change in ulcer size of 24%–62% and a decrease in ulcer size by 2.42 cm^2. While daily and weekly changes in ulcer size did not reach statistical significance, which may be attributable to small sample size and small number of studies, these findings are clinically significant.

The underlying physiologic effects of electrical stimulation are mediated by the endogenous bioelectric system in the human body and its response to positive and negative polarity. Several investigators have demonstrated the existence of transepithelial potential on the skin surface (Barker, Jaffe, & Vanable, 1982; Hunckler & de Mel, 2017; Illingsworth &

Barker, 1980). Transepithelial electric potential, also known as "skin battery," occurs through the movement of ions (Zhao et al., 2006). The transepithelial potential arises from Na$^+$ channels on the mucosal surface of the skin that allow Na$^+$ to diffuse from the area surrounding epidermal cells to the inside of the cells. As a result of the movement of Na$^+$ from the skin surface to the interior of epidermal cells, the exterior of the skin maintains a variable level of negative electrical charge (Foulds & Barker, 1983; Viera, Reid, Mannis, Schwab, & Zhao, 2011). Jaffe and Vanable (1984) demonstrated that when the epidermis is injured, current flows as ions are transmitted through the tissue fluid between the damaged regions of the epidermis (Eltinge, Cragoe, & Vanable, 1986). This "current of injury" has a positive polarity, whereas the adjacent intact skin retains its negative polarity (Reid, Song, McCaig, & Zhao, 2005; Zhao et al., 2006), producing a unidirectional force sufficient to attract reparative cells to the wound bed during the inflammatory and proliferative phases of healing (Vanable, 1989). When this natural conductive electrical process is disturbed, such as in chronic wounds, healing may be halted. Electrical stimulation can be used to jumpstart this natural process, attracting the correct cells to the wound. Once reepithelialization has closed the wound, the current of injury disappears, suggesting that it does not play a role in the remodeling phase of healing. However, studies demonstrate that an advanced remodeling phase is achieved by utilizing delivery of an exogenous current, cathodal, and anodal actually triggers an advanced remodeling phase by attracting critical cells that expedite the inflammatory response (Hunckler & de Mel, 2017) and stimulate

TABLE 26.1　Terms and Definitions for Electrical Stimulation

Terms	Definitions
Alternating current	Uninterrupted, bidirectional current flow
Amperage	Measure of rate of flow of current; expressed as amperes (A), milliamperes (mA), or microamperes (μA)
Amplitude	Maximum (peak) excursion of voltage or current pulse
Charge	Property of matter determined by proportion of electrons (negatively charged particles) contained by the matter; substance may be neutral, positively charged, or negatively charged; measured in units of coulombs (C) or microcoulombs (μC)
Current	Rate of flow of charged particles (ions or electrons); measured in units of amperes (A) or milliamperes (mA)
Direct current	Uninterrupted, unidirectional current flow
Frequency	Number of pulses delivered per unit of time; also termed pulse rate; frequency is the reciprocal of cycle time; usually measured as pulses per second or hertz (Hz); 0.1 Hz is on for 10 s, and a pulse of 1000 Hz is on for 1 ms
Interpulse interval	Time between pulses when no voltage is applied and no current is flowing
Polarity	Property of possessing two oppositely charged electrodes in an electrical circuit (positive and negative); negative electrode (cathode) provides electrons in a circuit; positive electrode (anode) serves as depository to which electrons flow
Pulse duration	Time during which current is flowing
Voltage	Measure of force of flow of electrons through a conductor (wound tissue) between two or more electrodes; created by difference of charges between two electrodes (one with excess in relation to the other); electrodes are polarized in comparison to each other (negative electrode and positive electrode)
Waveform	Graphic representation of current flow; may be monophasic (current that deviates from isoelectric zero line in one direction and then returns to baseline) or biphasic (current that deviates above and below isoelectric zero line); may be symmetric or asymmetric

collagen synthesis, thus increasing the tensile strength of the healing tissue (Sussman & Bates-Jensen, 2012). Importantly, the flow of current from the wound is blocked if the wound bed is allowed to desiccate and form a scab (Alvarez, Mertz, Smerback, et al., 1983), underscoring the significance of the moist environment.

Galvanotaxic Effects

Positively and negatively charged cells are attracted toward an electric field of opposite polarity, a process termed galvanotaxis. Using an exogenous electrical current on wounded tissue can improve the endogenous natural bioelectric current, thus improving the galvanotaxic effect (Kloth, 2005) to provide cellular migration. Multiple in vitro studies have established that cells essential to tissue repair will migrate toward the anode or cathode created by an electric field within a tissue culture (Bourguignon & Bourguignon, 1987; Eberhardt, Szczypiorski, & Korytowski, 1986; Orida & Feldman, 1982; Stromberg, 1988). Preliminary evidence from in vivo studies has demonstrated that electrical stimulation creates a similar galvanotaxic response. Studies have demonstrated that positive (anode) currents have an antibacterial effect as well as fibroblast and macrophage attraction, while negative (cathode) currents attract keratinocytes, epidermal cells, and neutrophils, and increase fibroblast proliferation (Khouri et al., 2017). In reviewing the literature, some studies report that using the cathode electrode stimulates granulation tissue by increasing the vascular endothelial growth factor (VEGF), while the anode electrode stimulates epithelialization of wounds. Eberhardt et al. (1986) showed that treating wounds with electrical stimulation for 30 min increased the relative number of neutrophils in the wound exudate compared with control wounds. Using a pig model, Mertz, Davis, Cazzaniga, et al. (1993) treated experimentally induced wounds with two 30-min sessions of monophasic pulsed current (PC) using varying polarity and found that wounds initially treated with negative polarity (day 0) followed by positive polarity (on days 1–7) showed 20% greater epithelialization compared with wounds that received only one type of polarity. In the wounds treated daily by alternating polarity (alternating daily between negative and positive), epithelialization was limited by 45%. Although the influence of polarity on cell migration in human wounds remains to be elucidated more completely, these findings suggest that bioelectric signals play a role in facilitating the phases of healing. Polarity appears to enhance the cellular needs during the inflammatory and proliferative phases of healing (Kloth & Zhao, 2010; Polak et al., 2016). Specifically, anodal electrical stimulation facilitates cells involved in the inflammatory phase of wound healing and cathodal promotes cellular proliferations (European Pressure Ulcer Advisory Panel, National Pressure Injury Advisory Panel, and Pan Pacific Pressure Injury Alliance, 2019; Polak et al., 2016, 2017) while both positive and negative polarity stimulate cellular processes that enhance the growth of blood vessels (European Pressure Ulcer Advisory Panel, National Pressure Injury Advisory Panel, and Pan Pacific Pressure Injury Alliance, 2019).

Stimulatory Effects on Cells

Electrical stimulation has been reported to influence the electrical activity of the cell membrane, inducing various cellular responses including migration of macrophages, granulocytes, fibroblasts, and epithelial cells (Orida & Feldman, 1982; Taskan et al., 1997; Zhao et al., 2006). Several laboratories and in vivo studies have demonstrated electrical current has a stimulatory effect on fibroblasts. The stimulatory effect of electrical current on fibroblasts, reported by Bourguignon and Bourguignon (1987), was observed when fibroblasts in culture increased DNA and protein (including collagen) synthesis in response to electrical stimulation. This effect was most noticeable near the negative electrode. Using a pig model, Cruz, Bayron, and Suarez (1989) demonstrated the presence of significantly more fibroblasts in burn wounds treated with electrical stimulation as opposed to in controls. Increased collagen density with burn wounds were also reported in the rat model by Castillo, Sumano, Fortoul, et al. (1995). More fibroblasts and increased collagen synthesis has also been reported in partial-thickness wounds using a pig model (Alvarez et al., 1983). More recent in vivo studies also report, enhanced fibroblast activity resulting in an increased fibroblast number (Bayat et al., 2006; Taskan et al., 1997), collagen synthesis, and tensile strength (Bayat et al., 2006).

Blood Flow and Tissue Oxygen Effects

Accumulating evidence indicates that electrical stimulation exerts a positive influence on blood flow and localized tissue oxygen. Hecker, Carron, and Schwartz (1985) showed that negative polarity increased blood flow in the upper extremity, as measured by plethysmography. In a sample of patients diagnosed with Raynaud disease and diabetic polyneuropathy, Kaada (1982) demonstrated that application of distant, low-frequency, transcutaneous electrical stimulation (TENS) produced pronounced and prolonged cutaneous vasodilation. Using skin temperature as a measurement of peripheral vasodilation, Kaada found a rise in the temperature of ischemic extremities from 71.6–75.2°F (22–24°C) to 87.8–93.2°F (31–34°C). The latency from stimulus onset to the abrupt rise in temperature averaged 15–30 min, with a duration of response ranging from 4 to 6 h. Kaada (1983) subsequently reported successful treatment of 10 patients with 19 leg ulcers that were previously resistant to treatment by applying a TENS device to the web space between the first and second metacarpals of the ipsilateral wrist. Using the burst mode, Kaada delivered 15–30 mA of pulsed direct current by the cathode for 30–34 min three times per day. He proposed that the remote application of electrical stimulation enhanced microcirculation in the tissues of the ipsilateral lower extremity, as demonstrated by the increase in toe temperature and ulcer healing. Based on the findings from subsequent basic research, Kaada suggested that the improvement in tissue microcirculation was the result of activation of a central serotonergic link that inhibits sympathetic vasoconstriction (Kaada, Hegland, Okteldalen, et al., 1984; Kaada & Helle, 1984).

Additional evidence of increased blood flow in wounds treated with electrical stimulation is provided by reports of increasing capillary density after implementation of this therapy. Fifteen venous leg ulcers, previously resistant to healing, were treated for 30 min daily for an average of 38 days (Jünger, Zuder, Steins, et al., 1997). Using light microscopy to measure capillary density, researchers found densities increased from a prestimulation baseline of 8.05–11.55 capillaries/mm^2 after stimulation ($P < 0.039$). Transcutaneous oxygen in the periwound skin was noted to increase from 13.5 to 24.7 mmHg. Increased periwound transcutaneous oxygen has also been reported in patients with arterial insufficiency and lower extremity wounds following high-voltage PC (HVPC) (Ashrafi, Alonso-Rasgado, Baguneid, & Bayat, 2017). At 1 year, the rate of healing in a retrospective study of 11 patients was 90% compared with 29% for the standard-of-care group (Goldman, Brewley, Zhou, et al., 2003).

Further support for the effect on blood flow by ES includes increased VEGF in patients with and without diabetes (Bevilacqua, Dominguez, Barrella, & Barbagallo, 2007), increased plasma levels of VEGF and nitric oxide in patients with diabetic ulcers (Mohajeri-Tehrani et al., 2014), and the release of VEGF by a direct effect on endothelial cells (Zhao, Bai, Wang, Forrester, & McCaig, 2004). Increases in VEGF can help increase local tissue oxygenation.

Antibacterial Effects

Electrical stimulation has bacteriostatic (Asadi & Torkaman, 2014) and bactericidal effects on microorganisms that are known to infect chronic wounds (Daeschlein, 2007). In a study of 20 patients with burn wounds that had been unresponsive to conventional therapy for 3 months to 2 years, Fakhri and Amin (1987) showed a quantitatively lower level of organisms after treatment for 10-min intervals twice weekly. This decrease in bacterial count was accompanied by epithelialization of the wound margins within 3 days of beginning electrical stimulation. Although the mechanism underlying the bactericidal or bacteriostatic effects remains unclear, the galvanotaxic effect on macrophages and neutrophils has been implicated (Eberhardt et al., 1986; Orida & Feldman, 1982). These studies suggest that the anodal attraction of neutrophils to tissue with high bacterial levels may be a primary mode of action, rather than destruction of pathogens by electrolysis or elevation of tissue pH. However, these studies used direct current, which is not as commonly used in wound management as the PC type (see Section "Types of Electrical Stimulation"). It appears that the voltage required to produce an antibacterial effect with PC would create profound muscle contractions and therefore would not be applicable in clinical practice (Guffey & Asmussen, 1989; Kincaid & Lavoie, 1989; Szuminsky, Albers, Unger, et al., 1994). However, recent studies have shown where PC along with direct current (DC) decreases and kills *Staphylococcus aureus*, *Escherichia coli*, and *Pseudomonas aeruginosa* (Gomez et al., 2015; Merriman et al., 2004).

INDICATIONS AND CONTRAINDICATIONS

The US Food and Drug Administration (FDA) has not yet approved any type of electrical stimulation device for wound healing. Consequently, devices cannot be marketed for this indication, although they can be marketed for other already approved indications, such as edema and pain, and subsequently used as an off-label treatment of wound healing.

Among national guidelines disseminated by professional societies dedicated to wound care, recommendations related to electrical stimulation as therapy for chronic wounds vary. International pressure injury guidelines (European Pressure Ulcer Advisory Panel, National Pressure Injury Advisory Panel, and Pan Pacific Pressure Injury Alliance, 2019), the Wound Healing Society (Gould et al., 2016) as well as the Wound, Ostomy and Continence Nurses Society™ (WOCN®) (2016) report electrical stimulation may be useful in the treatment of pressure injuries that have not healed with conventional therapy. Guideline #7.2.3: Electrical stimulation is recommended to accelerate wound closure. (Level I) Principle: Application of electric current to diabetic foot wounds increases local tissue perfusion and may affect protein synthesis, cell migration, and bacterial growth to improve wound healing. The Wound Healing Society guidelines recommend electrical stimulation for the treatment of diabetic foot wounds to increase local tissue perfusion and accelerate wound closure (Lavery et al, 2016) and state it may be useful in reducing the size of venous leg ulcers (Marston, Tang, Kirsner, & Ennis, 2016). Based on existing data at the time, the authors were unable to determine which voltage, type, or current may be superior (Gould et al., 2016; Lavery et al., 2016; Marston et al., 2016). A study analyzed 15 randomized controlled studies showing that electrical stimulation provided an additional 27.7% reduction in pressure injury size (Koel & Houghton, 2014) while another study demonstrated a reduction in pressure injury area by 43% using high-voltage electrical stimulation (Karsli, Gurcay, Karaahmet, & Cakci, 2017). Recio, Felter, Schneider, and McDonald (2012) demonstrated that by using high-voltage electrical stimulation, recalcitrant pressure injuries (8–14 months duration) were completely healed after 7–22 weeks of treatments performed three times per week.

As is the case with most therapies, certain contraindications apply to the use of electrical stimulation (Checklist 26.1). It should not be used when basal or squamous cell carcinoma is suspected in the wound or surrounding tissue or when osteomyelitis is present. Patients with electronic implants, such as pacemakers, should not be treated with electrical stimulation. Electrical stimulation is also

---

CHECKLIST 26.1 Contraindications for Electrical Stimulation

- ✓ Placement of electrodes tangential to the heart
- ✓ Presence of cardiac pacemaker
- ✓ Placement of electrodes along regions of phrenic nerve
- ✓ Presence of malignancy
- ✓ Placement of electrodes over carotid sinus
- ✓ Placement of electrodes over laryngeal musculature
- ✓ Placement of electrodes over topical substances containing metal ions, exogenous iodine, povidone–iodine, or mercurochrome
- ✓ Placement of electrodes over osteomyelitis

contraindicated for use over the heart or when iodine or silver ion residues are present in the wound.

TYPES OF ELECTRICAL STIMULATION

Although several electrotherapy modalities are cited in the literature, the three basic types of electrical current are DC, PC, and alternating current (Fraccalvieri, Salomone, Zingarelli, Rivarossa, & Bruschi, 2014). In general, alternating current is not used for wound treatment and is not described in this chapter. DC is characterized as continuous and monophasic (unidirectional) in which the voltage does not vary with time. DC can irritate the wound (Kloth, 2014), therefore, low-intensity DC (LIDC) is typically used. DC can be subdivided into LIDC and microcurrent, providing a subsensory stimulation (Ashrafi et al., 2017). The parameters used to stimulate wound healing typically are 200–300 µA at a low voltage (<100 V). The polarity that is selected determines the direction of current flow delivered to the wound tissue, with positively charged ions migrating toward the cathode and negatively charged ions migrating toward the anode. Small, older clinical trials have demonstrated benefits from the use of DC with chronic wounds (Carley & Wainapel, 1985; Gault & Gatens, 1976). However, charged ions of Na^+ and Cl^- in the wound tissue move toward the cathode and anode, respectively, producing a chemical reaction with caustic end-products at the interface of the electrode and tissue. In the case of the cathode, Na^+ reacts with H_2O to form $NaOH$ and H_2, whereas the anode reacts with Cl^- and H_2O to form HCl and O_2. Even when DC is delivered at therapeutic doses, these products form at the electrode tissue interface, creating acid–base changes. If the dosage of DC is delivered at high amplitude over an extended period, the acid–base changes lead to tissue irritation that varies in intensity from erythema to blistering due to electrochemical burning. This side effect can be diminished to some extent by using current amplitudes in the microamperage (µA) range.

Pulsed Current Electrical Stimulation

Devices used to deliver the DC are also capable of delivering PC, a pattern or flow that has become the predominant type of electrical stimulation used for wound healing. PC can be unidirectional or bidirectional and can have a monophasic or biphasic waveform. Monophasic PC can describe an HVPC or low-voltage PC. The biphasic PC can be asymmetric or symmetric (Ashrafi et al., 2017). Electrodes placed on the tissues deliver the PC as a series of pulses, with each pulse separated by a period in which no current is flowing. PC can be visually constructed as a waveform that plots amplitude and time.

Waveform Patterns (Monophasic and Biphasic)

Two waveform patterns are available as PC (Fig. 26.2). Monophasic (unidirectional) PC is the movement of current in one direction away from the isoelectric zero line. Monophasic (bidirectional) PC has been applied to clinical treatment of wounds using a rectangular waveform (Feedar, Kloth, &

Gentzkow, 1991; Gentzkow, Alon, Taler, et al., 1993; Gentzkow, Pollack, Kloth, et al., 1991; Jünger et al., 1997) and twin-peak waveform of high voltage (Fitzgerald & Newsome, 1993; Griffin, Tooms, Mendius, et al., 1991; Kloth & Feedar, 1988). Biphasic PC is the movement of current in two directions on either side of the isoelectric zero line. Biphasic PC is configured as charged particles moving above and below the isoelectric zero line in brief succession. The biphasic waveform may be symmetric or asymmetric with respect to the isoelectric zero line. The biphasic symmetric waveform is characterized by amplitude, duration, and rate of rise and decays of current that are identical in relation to the isoelectric zero line. This creates a balanced electrical charge. In contrast, with the biphasic asymmetric waveform, one or more of these elements of the current are unequal in relation to the isoelectric zero line. This produces waveforms that may be electrically balanced or unbalanced. Both biphasic symmetric (Baker, Chambers, DeMuth, et al., 1996, 1997; Baker, Rubayi, Villar, et al., 1996; Debreceni, Gyulai, Debreceni, et al., 1995) and asymmetric (Baker et al., 1996, 1997) waveforms have been studied as a modality for promoting wound healing.

Application and Administration Methods

Regardless of the waveform of PC selected for treatment, the electrodes are applied using one of two methods (Baker et al., 1996; Kloth & Feedar, 1988). The first method involves placing one electrode in direct contact with a clean, electrically conductive material (commonly a saline-moistened gauze dressing) that is positioned in the wound; then the second electrode is placed on intact skin approximately 15–30 cm from the wound edge. With the second method, the electrodes are positioned on the skin at the wound edges on opposite sides of the wound. The treatment protocol is similar whether the device is a low-voltage or a high-voltage stimulator. The pulse frequency is set to 100 pulses per second, with a current or voltage sufficient to produce a comfortable tingling sensation or, in insensate skin, at a level just below the motor threshold (Feedar et al., 1991; Gentzkow et al., 1991, 1993; Griffin et al., 1991; Kloth & Feedar, 1988; Kloth & McCulloch, 1996). As summarized in Box 26.1, polarity is determined by the status of the wound and the specific cells that are to be targeted for migration into the wound (Bourguignon & Bourguignon, 1987). The treatment electrode is placed over the wound and the polarity may be selected as follows: positive electrode for autolysis, epithelialization or negative electrode for infection/inflammation, and granulation (Kloth & McCulloch, 1996). Treatments are administered for 1 h, 5–7 days per week, and are continued as long as the wound is progressing toward closure.

Research identifies a range of electrical charge that has supported positive wound healing outcomes. This dosage of current, defined in microcoulombs (µC), is between 250 and 500 µC/s (Feedar et al., 1991; Gentzkow et al., 1991, 1993; Griffin et al., 1991; Jünger et al., 1997; Kloth & Feedar, 1988). The evolution of electrical stimulation devices led to the evaluation of two different types of PC for the

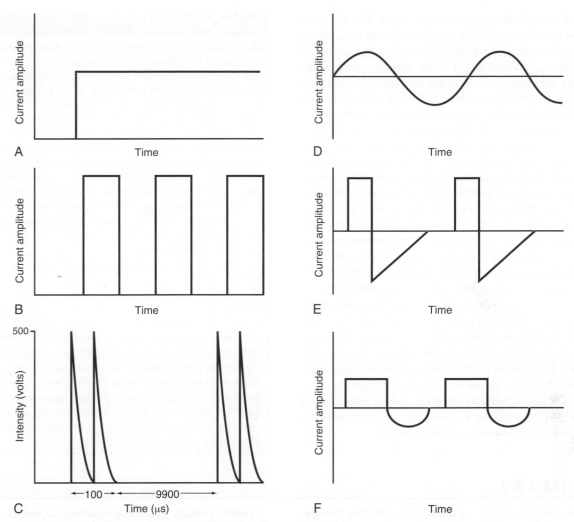

Fig. 26.2 Waveforms used in electrical stimulation. (A) Direct current. (B) Monophasic pulsed current. (C) Monophasic high-voltage pulsed current. (D) Symmetric biphasic pulsed current (balanced). (E) Asymmetric biphasic pulsed current (balanced). (F) Asymmetric biphasic pulsed current (unbalanced). (Modified from Dyson, M. (2004). Adjuvant therapies: Ultrasound, laser therapy, electrical stimulation, hyperbaric oxygen and negative pressure therapy. In M. J. Morison & L. G. Ovington (Eds.), *Chronic wound care: A problem-based learning approach*. Edinburgh: Mosby.)

BOX 26.1   Cellular Response to Polarity

Anode (+)

Assists: cells involved in the inflammatory phase

Stimulation of epithelialization

Attracts: neutrophils, macrophages, and fibroblasts

Cathode (−)

Assists: stimulation of granulation tissue

Cell proliferation

Attracts: keratinocytes and epidermal cells

* Polarity differed between studies.
* Some studies alternate polarity.
* Bacteriostatic effect noted on both, anode and cathode but stronger at cathode electrode.

---

treatment of chronic wounds: low-voltage amplitude and high-voltage amplitude. Low-voltage amplitude devices deliver PC with either a monophasic or a biphasic waveform. Their pulse durations are relatively long, so low-driving voltages (<150 V) are adequate. High-voltage amplitude devices provide only monophasic PC. Their pulses are of short duration (10–20 μs), so these devices must have a high-driving voltage (>150 V). Each voltage type of electrical stimulation devices has been examined in clinical studies of wound healing.

PAYMENT COVERAGE

Policies related to payment coverage for the treatment of chronic wounds with electrical stimulation differ dramatically among third-party payers. In 2002, the Centers for Medicare & Medicaid Services (CMS) approved payment for electrical stimulation when used for the treatment of chronic Stage 3 or Stage 4 pressure injuries and for wounds of the lower extremity caused by arterial and venous insufficiency and diabetes, if no measurable improvement is evidenced after at least 30 days of standard wound therapy. CMS also states that electrical stimulation must be used with standard wound care, which includes optimization of nutritional status, debridement of nonviable tissue, maintaining a moist wound environment with proper dressing, and resolving any possible infection. Interventions to correct or reduce the effect of those factors associated with the underlying wound etiology are essential, such as support surface, offloading, glucose control, optimizing blood flow, adequate graduated compression, etc. After the start of electrical stimulation, 30-day reassessments are required, and, if no measurable progress is noted, coverage or this modality will not continue. National coverage determinations became effective in July 2004 (CMS, 2004). Generally, electrical stimulation is only reimbursed when the treatment is performed by a physical therapist, although local coverage determinations vary in defining practice parameters that will be reimbursed. In contrast to CMS policies, a health technology assessment of electrical stimulation as an adjuvant treatment of chronic wounds conducted by Blue Cross Blue Shield Association (Lefevre & Samson, 2005) in April 2005 concluded that the available evidence does not demonstrate convincingly that electrical stimulation results in clinically significant improvement in the most relevant outcome—the percentage of patients whose wounds heal completely. Blue Cross Blue Shield Corporate medical policy review as of November 2019 continues to consider electrostimulation for the treatment of wounds as investigational.

CLINICAL CONSULT

A: Consulted for unresponsive left trochanter pressure injury. 70-Year-old Caucasian female bedridden with Parkinson's disease. History and physical reveals hypertension managed with diuretics; negative for cardiac, renal, or metabolic disorder. Wound has been unresponsive to standard therapy for more than 1 month, including low air loss, repositioning to avoid left trochanter, optimal nutrition per dietitian and tube feedings, and bioburden management with debridement and antimicrobial dressings. Medical history includes Parkinson's disease. Wound dimensions remain 4.8 × 8.2 × 1 cm Stage 3, wound bed clean and smooth, absent of granulation. Wound edges attached, periwound skin intact, scant serous exudate, and no local signs of infection. Current local wound care includes daily hydrogel impregnated gauze and covered with nonadherent border cover dressing.

D: Stage 3 pressure injury resistant to healing despite conventional therapy.

P: Initiate daily high-voltage pulsed current electrical stimulation.

I: (1) Continue all current interventions, including daily hydrogel dressings to maintain a continuously moist environment. (2) Set voltage between 75 and 200 V to create a tingling paresthesia at a frequency of 100 pulses per second.

E: Benefits and risks explained to family and they want to proceed. Family understands that therapy can be administered by qualified wound clinic staff only while nurses will continue to manage dressings as indicated. If healing progress ceases, the polarity will be switched daily.

SUMMARY

- Many wound specialists are unfamiliar with this therapy. The transfer of electrical stimulation to mainstream wound care practice continues to be variable and inconsistent.
- Many clinical settings do not have personnel with the necessary expertise to administer electrical stimulation.
- The FDA has not approved any electrical stimulation device for wound healing (it is an off-label use).
- Emerging data reports that the electrical stimulation has multiple benefits for treating chronic wounds or wounds that do not respond to conventional treatment.
- PC has demonstrated wound-healing effects at the cellular level.
- Studies also recommend electrical stimulation therapy for treating wounds of various etiologies. International

pressure injury guidelines recommend electrical stimulation to facilitate healing in recalcitrant pressure injuries.
- Literature has demonstrated electrical stimulation to be an adjunctive modality to treat ulcers with the following benefits:
  - improve ulcer size,
  - restart the body's endogenous electrical field when current of injury exists,
  - attract and stimulate cells using a galvanotaxic effect,
  - promote the release of VEGF,
  - provide an antibacterial effect, and
  - improve collagen synthesis.

SELF-ASSESSMENT QUESTIONS

1. Cathode polarity attracts:
   a. epidermal cells
   b. macrophages
   c. fibroblasts
   d. All of the above
2. Anode polarity attracts and increases:
   a. macrophages and fibroblast proliferation
   b. epidermal cells and macrophages

   c. both a and b
   d. none of the above
3. True/False: The epidermis possesses a natural endogenous "skin battery" that generates an electric current when wounded.
4. Electrical stimulation benefits the wound by:
   a. promote the release of VEGF
   b. improve collagen synthesis

c. promote a galvanotaxic effect

d. all of the above

5. When using electrical stimulation as an adjunctive modality for wound healing, the electrodes can be placed as follows:

a. One electrode over the wound and saline dressing and the other electrode on intact skin

b. Both electrodes on the opposite nonwounded extremity

c. Electrodes on opposite sides of the wound on intact skin

d. a and c

e. All of the above

6. The following are considered contraindications for electrical stimulation except:

a. wounds with osteomyelitis

b. wounds in the inflammatory phase

c. areas near/over a pacemaker

d. wounds with malignancy

REFERENCES

Alvarez, O. M., Mertz, P. M., Smerback, R. V., et al. (1983). The healing of superficial skin wounds is stimulated by external electrical current. *The Journal of Investigative Dermatology*, *81*(2), 144.

Asadi, M. R., & Torkaman, G. (2014). Bacterial inhibition by electrical stimulation. *Advances in Wound Care*, *3*(2), 91–97.

Ashrafi, M., Alonso-Rasgado, T., Baguneid, M., & Bayat, A. (2017). The efficacy of electrical stimulation in lower extremity cutaneous wound healing: A systematic review. *Experimental Dermatology*, *26*, 171–178.

Baker, L., Chambers, R., DeMuth, S. K., et al. (1997). Effects of electrical stimulation on wound healing in patients with diabetic ulcers. *Diabetes Care*, *20*(3), 405.

Baker, L., Rubayi, S., Villar, F., et al. (1996). Effect of electrical stimulation waveform on healing of ulcers in human beings with spinal cord injury. *Wound Repair and Regeneration*, *4*(1), 21.

Barker, A., Jaffe, L. F., & Vanable, J. W., Jr. (1982). The glabrous epidermis of cavies contains a powerful battery. *The American Journal of Physiology*, *11*, R358.

Barnes, R., Shahin, Y., Gohil, R., & Chetter, I. (2014). Electrical stimulation vs. standard of care for chronic ulcer healing: A systematic review and meta-analysis of randomized controlled trials. *European Journal of Clinical Investigation*, *44*(4), 429–440.

Bayat, M., Asgari-Moghadam, Z., Maroufi, M., Rezaie, F. S., Bayat, M., & Rakhshan, M. (2006). Experimental wound healing using microamperage electrical stimulation in rabbits. *Journal of Rehabilitation Research and Development*, *43*, 219–226.

Bevilacqua, M., Dominguez, L. J., Barrella, M., & Barbagallo, M. (2007). Induction of vascular endothelial growth factor release by transcutaneous frequency modulated neural stimulation in diabetic polyneuropathy. *Journal of Endocrinological Investigation*, *30*, 944–947.

Bourguignon, G., & Bourguignon, L. (1987). Electric stimulation of protein and DNA synthesis in human fibroblasts. *The FASEB Journal*, *1*(5), 398.

Carley, P. J., & Wainapel, S. F. (1985). Electrotherapy for acceleration of wound healing: Low intensity direct current. *Archives of Physical Medicine and Rehabilitation*, *66*(7), 443.

Castillo, E., Sumano, H., Fortoul, T. I., et al. (1995). The influence of pulsed electrical stimulation on the wound healing of burned rat skin. *Archives of Medical Research*, *26*(2), 185.

Centers for Medicare & Medicaid Services (CMS). (2004). *National coverage determination (NCD) for electrical stimulation (ES) and electromagnetic therapy for the treatment of wounds (270.1)*. Publication Number 100-3, Manual Section Number 270.1.

Retrieved 8/10/2020 from: https://www.cms.gov/medicare-coverage-database/details/ncd-details.aspx?NCDId=131.

Cruz, N., Bayron, F., & Suarez, A. (1989). Accelerated healing of full-thickness burns by the use of high-voltage pulsed galvanic stimulation in the pig. *Annals of Plastic Surgery*, *23*(1), 49.

Daeschlein, G. (2007). Antibacterial activity of positive and negative polarity low-voltage pulsed current (LVPC) on six typical Gram-positive and Gram-negative bacterial pathogens of chronic wounds. *Wound Repair and Regeneration*, *15*(3), 399.

Debreceni, L., Gyulai, M., Debreceni, A., et al. (1995). Results of transcutaneous electrical stimulation (TNS) in cure of lower extremity arterial disease. *Angiology*, *46*(7), 613.

Eberhardt, A., Szczypiorski, P., & Korytowski, G. (1986). Effect of transcutaneous electrostimulation on the cell composition of skin exudate. *Acta Physiologica Polonica*, *37*(1), 41.

Eltinge, E. M., Cragoe, E. J., Jr., & Vanable, J. W., Jr. (1986). Effects of amiloride analogues on adult *Notophthalmus viridescens* limb stump currents. *Comparative Biochemistry and Physiology. A, Comparative Physiology*, *84*(1), 39–44.

European Pressure Ulcer Advisory Panel, National Pressure Injury Advisory Panel, and Pan Pacific Pressure Injury Alliance. (2019). In E. Haesler (Ed.), *Prevention and treatment of pressure ulcers/injuries: Clinical practice guideline. The international guideline* EPUAP/NPIAP/PPPIA.

Fakhri, O., & Amin, M. (1987). The effect of low-voltage electric therapy on the healing of resistant skin burns. *Journal of Burn Care & Research*, *8*(1), 15.

Feedar, J., Kloth, L. C., & Gentzkow, G. D. (1991). Chronic dermal ulcer healing enhanced with monophasic pulsed electrical stimulation. *Physical Therapy*, *71*(9), 639.

Fitzgerald, G. K., & Newsome, D. (1993). Treatment of a large infected thoracic spine wound using high voltage pulsed monophasic current. *Physical Therapy*, *73*(6), 355.

Foulds, I., & Barker, A. (1983). Human skin battery potentials and their possible role in wound healing. *The British Journal of Dermatology*, *109*, 515.

Fraccalvieri, M., Salomone, M., Zingarelli, E., Rivarossa, F., & Bruschi, S. (2014). Electrical stimulation for difficult wounds: Only an alternative procedure? *International Wound Journal*, *12*(6), 669–673.

Gardner, S., Frantz, R. A., & Schmidt, F. L. (1999). The effect of electrical stimulation on chronic wound healing: A meta-analysis. *Wound Repair and Regeneration*, *7*(6), 495.

Gault, W., & Gatens, P. (1976). Use of low intensity direct current in management of ischemic skin ulcers. *Physical Therapy*, *56*(3), 265.

Gentzkow, G. D., Alon, G., Taler, G. A., et al. (1993). Healing of refractory stage III and IV pressure ulcers by a new electrical stimulation device. *Wounds, 5*(3), 160.

Gentzkow, G. D., Pollack, S. V., Kloth, L. C., et al. (1991). Improved healing of pressure ulcers using Dermapulse®, a new electrical stimulation device. *Wounds, 3*(5), 158.

Goldman, R., Brewley, B., Zhou, L., et al. (2003). Electrotherapy reverses inframalleolar ischemia: A retrospective, observational study. *Advances in Skin & Wound Care, 16*, 79–89.

Gomez, R. C., Brandino, H. E., de Sousa, N. T., Santos, M. F., Martinez, R., & Guirro, R. R. (2015). Polarized currents inhibit in vitro growth of bacteria colonizing cutaneous ulcers. *Wound Repair and Regeneration, 23*(3), 403–411.

Gould, L., Stuntz, M., Giovannelli, M., Ahmad, A., Aslam, R., Mullen-Fortino, M., et al. (2016). Wound Healing Society 2015 update on guidelines for pressure ulcers. *Wound Repair and Regeneration, 24*(1), 145–162. https://doi.org/10.1111/wrr.12396. Epub 2016 Mar 4. PMID: 26683529.

Griffin, J. W., Tooms, R. E., Mendius, R. A., et al. (1991). Efficacy of high voltage pulsed current for healing of pressure ulcers in patients with spinal cord injury. *Physical Therapy, 71*(6), 433.

Guffey, J. S., & Asmussen, M. D. (1989). In vitro bactericidal effects of high voltage pulsed current versus direct current against *Staphylococcus aureus. Journal of Clinical Electrophysiology, 1*(1), 5.

Hecker, B., Carron, H., & Schwartz, D. P. (1985). Pulsed galvanic stimulation: Effects of current frequency and polarity on blood flow in healthy subjects. *Archives of Physical Medicine and Rehabilitation, 66*(6), 369.

Hunckler, J., & de Mel, A. (2017). A current affair: Electrotherapy in wound healing. *Journal of Multidisciplinary Healthcare, 10*, 179–194.

Illingsworth, C. M., & Barker, A. T. (1980). Measurement of electrical currents emerging during the regeneration of amputated fingertips in children. *Clinical Physics and Physiological Measurement, 1*, 87.

Jaffe, L., & Vanable, J. (1984). Electric fields and wound healing. *Clinics in Dermatology, 2*(3), 34.

Jünger, M., Zuder, D., Steins, A., et al. (1997). Treatment of venous ulcers with low frequency pulsed current (Dermapulse): Effect on cutaneous microcirculation. *Hautarzt, 48*(12), 879.

Kaada, B. (1982). Vasodilation induced by transcutaneous nerve stimulation in peripheral ischemia (Raynaud's phenomenon and diabetic polyneuropathy). *European Heart Journal, 3*(4), 303.

Kaada, B. (1983). Promoted healing of chronic ulceration by transcutaneous nerve stimulation (TNS). *VASA, 12*(3), 262.

Kaada, B., Hegland, O., Okteldalen, O., et al. (1984). Failure to influence the VIP level in the cerebrospinal fluid by transcutaneous nerve stimulation in humans. *General Pharmacology, 15*(6), 563.

Kaada, B., & Helle, K. (1984). In search of mediators of skin vasodilation induced by transcutaneous nerve stimulation: IV. In vitro bioassay of the vasoinhibitory activity of sera from patients suffering from peripheral ischaemia. *General Pharmacology, 15*(2), 115.

Karsli, P. B., Gurcay, E., Karaahmet, O. Z., & Cakci, A. (2017). High-voltage electrical stimulation versus ultrasound in the treatment of pressure ulcers. *Advances in Skin and Wound Care, 30*(12), 565–570.

Khouri, C., Kotzki, S., Roustit, M., Blaise, S., Gueyffier, F., & Cracowski, J. (2017). Hierarchical evaluation of electrical

stimulation protocols for chronic wound healing: An effect size meta-analysis. *Wound Repair and Regeneration, 25*, 883–891.

Kincaid, C., & Lavoie, K. (1989). Inhibition of bacterial growth in vitro following stimulation with high voltage, monophasic, pulsed current. *Physical Therapy, 69*(8), 651.

Kloth, L. C. (2002). How to use electrical stimulation for wound healing. *Nursing, 32*(12), 17. https://doi.org/10.1097/00152193-200212000-00009.

Kloth, L. C. (2005). Electrical stimulation for wound healing: A review of evidence from in vitro studies, animal experiments, and clinical trials. *The International Journal of Lower Extremity Wounds, 4*, 23–44.

Kloth, L. C. (2014). Electrical stimulation technologies for wound healing. *Advances in Wound Care, 3*, 81–90.

Kloth, L., & Feedar, J. (1988). Acceleration of wound healing with high voltage, monophasic, pulsed current. *Physical Therapy, 68*(4), 503.

Kloth, L. C., & McCulloch, J. (1996). Promotion of wound healing with electrical stimulation. *Advances in Wound Care, 9*(5), 42–45.

Kloth, L. C., & Zhao, M. (2010). Endogenous and exogenous electrical fields for wound healing. In J. M. McCulloch, & L. C. Kloth (Eds.), *Wound healing. Evidence-based management* (4th ed., pp. 450–513). Philadelphia: FA Davis Company.

Koel, G., & Houghton, P. E. (2014). Electrostimulation: Current status, strength of evidence guidelines, and meta-analysis. *Advances in Wound Care, 3*(2), 118–126.

Lavery, L. A., Davis, K. E., Berriman, S. J., Braun, L., Nichols, A., Kim, P. J., et al. (2016). WHS guidelines update: Diabetic foot ulcer treatment guidelines. *Wound Repair and Regeneration, 24*(1), 112–126. https://doi.org/10.1111/wrr.12391. PMID: 26663430.

Lefevre, F., & Samson, D. (2005). *Electrical stimulation or electromagnetic therapy as adjunctive treatments for chronic skin wounds.* Chicago: Blue Cross and Blue Shield Association.

Marston, W., Tang, J., Kirsner, R. S., Ennis, W. (2016). Wound Healing Society 2015 update on guidelines for venous ulcers. *Wound Repair and Regeneration, 24*(1), 136–144. https://doi.org/10.1111/wrr.12394. PMID: 26663616.

Merriman, H. L., Hegyi, C. A., Albright-Overton, C. R., Carlos, J. J. R., Putnam, R. W., & Mulcare, J. A. (2004). A comparison of four electrical stimulation types on *Staphylococcus aureus* growth in vitro. *Journal of Rehabilitation Research and Development, 41*(2), 139–146.

Mertz, P. M., Davis, S., Cazzaniga, A., et al. (1993). Electrical stimulation: Acceleration of soft tissue repair by varying the polarity. *Wounds, 5*(3), 153.

Mohajeri-Tehrani, M. R., Nasiripoor, F., Torkaman, G., Hedayati, M., Annabestani, Z., & Asadi, M. R. (2014). Effect of low-intensity direct current on expression of vascular endothelial growth factor and nitric oxide in diabetic foot ulcer. *Journal of Rehabilitation Research and Development, 51*, 815–824.

Orida, N., & Feldman, J. (1982). Directional protrusive pseudopodial activity and motility in macrophages induced by extracellular electric fields. *Cell Motility, 2*, 243.

Polak, A., Kloth, L. C., Blaszczak, E., Taradaj, J., & Nawrat-Szoltysik, A. (2016). Evaluation of the healing progress of pressure ulcers treated with cathodal high-voltage monophasic pulsed current: Results of a prospective, double-blind, randomized clinical trial. *Advances in Skin & Wound Care, 29* (10), 447–459.

Polak, A., Kloth, L. C., Blaszczak, E., Taradaj, J., Nawrat-Szoltysik, A., Ickowicz, T., et al. (2017). The efficacy of pressure ulcer treatment with cathodal and cathodal-anodal high-voltage monophasic pulsed current: A prospective, randomized, controlled clinical trial. *Physical Therapy, 97*(8), 777–789.

Recio, A., Felter, C., Schneider, A. C., & McDonald, J. (2012). High-voltage electrical stimulation for the management of stage III and IV pressure ulcers among adults with spinal cord injury: Demonstration of its utility for recalcitrant wounds below the level of injury. *Journal of Spinal Cord Medicine, 35*, 58–63.

Reid, B., Song, B., McCaig, C. D., & Zhao, M. (2005). Wound healing in rat cornea: The role of electric currents. *The FASEB Journal, 19*, 379–386. https://doi.org/10.1096/fj.04-2325com.

Stromberg, B. V. (1988). Effects of electrical currents on wound contraction. *Annals of Plastic Surgery, 21*(2), 121.

Sussman, C., & Bates-Jensen, B. (2012). *Wound care: A collaborative practice for manual health professionals*. Philadelphia: Wolters Kluwer.

Szuminsky, N. J., Albers, A. C., Unger, P., et al. (1994). Effect of narrow, pulsed high voltages on bacterial viability. *Physical Therapy, 74*(7), 660.

Taskan, I., Ozyazgan, I., Tercan, M., Kardas, H. Y., Balkanli, S., Sarayment, R., et al. (1997). A comparative study of the effect of ultrasound and electrostimulation on wound healing in rats. *Plastic and Reconstructive Surgery, 100*, 966–972.

Thakral, G., LaFontaine, J., Najafi, B., Talal, T., Kim, P., & Lavery, L. (2013). Electrical stimulation to accelerate wound healing. *Diabetic Foot & Ankle, 4*, 1. https://doi.org/10.3402/dfa.v4i0.22081.

Vanable, J. W., Jr. (1989). Integumentary potentials and wound healing. In R. B. Borgan, et al. (Eds.), *Electric fields in vertebrate repair*. New York: Liss.

Viera, A. C., Reid, B., Mannis, M. J., Schwab, I. R., & Zhao, M. (2011). Ionic components of electric current at rat corneal wounds. *PLoS One, 6*(2), e17411.

Wound, Ostomy and Continence Nurses Society™ (WOCN®). (2016). *Guideline for the management of patients with pressure ulcers/injuries. (WOCN® clinical practice guideline series no. 2)*. Mt. Laurel: WOCN®.

Zhao, M., Bai, H., Wang, E., Forrester, J. V., & McCaig, C. D. (2004). Electrical stimulation directly induces pre-angiogenic responses in vascular endothelial cells by signaling through VEGF receptors. *Journal of Cell Science, 117*, 397–405.

Zhao, M., Song, B., Pu, J., Wada, T., Reid, B., Tai, G., et al. (2006). Electrical signals control wound healing through phosphatidylinositol-3-OH kinasegamma and PTEN. *Nature, 442*, 457–460.

27

Ultraviolet Light and Ultrasound

Renee Cordrey

OBJECTIVES

1. List at least one indication each for ultraviolet-C, high-frequency ultrasound, and low-frequency ultrasound use.

2. List at least one contraindication for each modality.
3. Explain the mechanism of action for each modality.

The use of physical agents can support wound healing through mechanical action or by their effect on tissue function. Common modalities include ultraviolet (UV) light and ultrasound. Each of these tools offer parameter options with different effects. Selective use of these devices may reduce wound bioburden, facilitate wound debridement, or speed granulation and reepithelialization.

ULTRAVIOLET LIGHT

Ultraviolet (UV) light consists of the portion of the electromagnetic spectrum that is at a higher frequency than visible light. There are three types of UV light which are classified by their wavelength and differ in their biological activity and extent to which they penetrate the skin. UV-A is a long wavelength and ranges from 320 to 400 nm. The vast majority of UV radiation reaching the Earth is UVA. UV-B is the medium wavelength, 290–320 nm, and is mostly filtered by the atmosphere. The short wavelength, UV-C, is 185–290 nm and is completely filtered by the atmosphere therefore does not reach the earth's surface.

Ultraviolet light has long been used for the treatment of many skin conditions, including psoriasis (Kirke et al., 2007; Lapidoth, Adatto, & David, 2007) and acne vulgaris. In recent decades, usage for those conditions has declined due to the advent of more topical and systemic treatments and the increased awareness of the potential damage from UV radiation. However, UV-C has seen a resurgence in chronic wound management.

Ultraviolet light is a simple-to-use modality that may be a valuable tool in addressing wound bioburden, especially in this era of resistant organisms. Specialized lamps generate UV light; hot quartz mercury vapor lamps produce UV-A and UV-B light, while cold quartz lamps create UV-C light. These lamps are generally easy to use, and, because they do not require a warm-up or cool-down period, treatment may be started immediately (Fig. 27.1).

Physiologic Effects

Ultraviolet light is hypothesized to alter several aspects of cellular function: (1) increased cell wall permeability through altering the shape of proteins, (2) increased stimulation of the production of various chemicals such as prostaglandins and arachidonic acid, and (3) increased production of adenosine triphosphate (ATP) (Camp, Greaves, Hensby, Plummer, & Warin, 1978). UV light does not heat tissue. While erythema at the site may be observed, it is a result of the increased local vasodilation, tissue oxygenation, and histamine release.

Each form of UV light has different effects on tissue. UV-A penetrates most deeply into the skin (several millimeters) and is responsible for immediate tanning; it is also recognized as contributing to skin aging, wrinkling, and skin cancers. UV-A. is known to produce a mild erythema. The impact of UV-A can be increased with the use of oral psoralens, a photosensitizing agent, before treatment. In contrast, UV-B elicits a stronger erythematous response; it is responsible for delayed tanning and burning and significantly increases the risk of skin cancer. UV-B produces hyperplasia of the dermis and stratum corneum 3 days after treatment and has been used to toughen scars (Parrish, Zaynoun, & Anderson, 1981).

UV-C is ionizing and mutagenic but is not linked to skin cancers for several reasons: (1) UV-C only penetrates the most superficial layers of the epidermis; (2) the superficial layers of the epidermis are sloughed often enough to prevent development of neoplasms; and (3) naturally occurring UV-C is blocked by the atmosphere before it reaches the earth's surface. However, as wound treatment exposes the more permanent healing tissue, not the epidermis, to UV-C radiation, the long-term cancer risk is unknown. Mouse studies by Dai et al. (Dai, Vrahas, Murray, & Hamblin, 2012) suggests that most of the DNA damage is repaired by the body within 48 h.

UV-C is recognized to be germicidal, which has come to be the primary use for UV treatment. Other evidence suggests that UV-C can increase epithelialization, epithelial cell turnover (Freytes, Fernandez, & Fleming, 1965), granulation

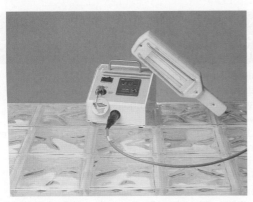

Fig. 27.1 Ultraviolet light. (Courtesy National Biological Corporation, Twinsburg, Ohio, USA.)

tissue growth and tissue perfusion at lower doses (Ramsay & Challoner, 1976), basic fibroblast growth factor and transforming growth factor-β release (Gupta, Avci, Dai, Huant, & Hamblin, 2013; James et al., 1991), fibronectin release (Morykwas & Marks, 1998) transforming growth factor-beta expression (Suo, Wang, & Wang, 2002), autolysis (Kloth, 1995; Spielholz & Kloth, 2000), and speed wound contraction (Morykwas & Marks, 1998). However, caution is advised in interpreting these studies because a different standard of care was used in older studies than the standard of care today.

Ultraviolet-C treatment has been used for decades, in formal and informal ways (such as "sunlight treatments" for infectious diseases), to reduce bioburden. Early research on this modality was promising, though limited to in vitro and animal models. Over time, as newer, more advanced interventions became available, interest in ultraviolet waned in favor of the higher tech and newer options. As a result, there is limited research on chronic wounds in humans. In recent years, there has been a resurgence of interest in this inexpensive tool, especially in an era of multiple drug-resistant organisms, antibacterial stewardship, and cost-effective care.

The bacteriocidal effects of UV light have been recognized for more than a century (Gates, 1928). The mechanism of action is theorized to be inhibition of DNA synthesis (Hall & Mount, 1981). Another in vitro study (Sheldon, Kokjohn, & Martin, 2005) found MRSA eradication with use of UV-C, with an even greater impact on *Pseudomonas*. A case series (Thai, Houghton, Campbell, & Woodbury, 2002) reported reduced bacterial counts and more wound rapid healing with UV-C use, although treatment was not standardized and there was no control group. Thao, Keast, Campbell, Woodbury, and Houghton (2005) later studied the effect of one 180-s UV-C treatment session on semiquantitative swab culture results in 22 patients with a variety of chronic wounds (pressure, venous, diabetic and arterial) each with high levels of bacteria and signs of infection. Results showed a statistically significant reduction of the predominant bacteria, including *Pseudomonas*, MRSA, and *Staphylococcus aureus*. *Aspergillus* was also successfully eradicated after one 15- to 30-s treatment, and prokaryotic organisms such as *Pseudomonas aeruginosa* and *Mycobacterium abscessus*

demonstrated eradication with only 3–5 s of exposure (Sullivan & Conner-Kerr, 2000). *Acinetobacter baumannii* was also shown to be susceptible to UV-C in a mouse study (Dai et al., 2012). Other work shows multiple-drug resistant organisms needed less exposure time than susceptible ones, as little as 5–15 s (Rao, Kumar, Rao, & Gurung, 2011). In a study with mice, UV-C demonstrated nearly complete inactivation of *Candida albicans* after one 15- to 30-s treatment, performing better than the antifungal drug nystatin (Dai et al., 2011); however, fungi often require a higher dose than do bacteria (Yin et al., 2013). The dose needed to damage pathogens has been shown to be nondamaging or minimally damaging to keratinocytes and other mammalian cells, with 6–19% destruction of keratinocytes and no damage to corneal epithelial cells (Buonanno et al., 2013; Rao et al., 2011; Yin et al., 2013). Platelets may be mildly damaged; however, that damage can lead to increased platelet activity, which can also reduce pH further, inhibiting bacterial growth (Yin et al., 2013).

Evidence suggests that a higher dose of UV-C may be needed when treating biofilms to overcome the innate resistance of biofilms and because the biofilm matrix may block some of the UV light penetration (Dai et al., 2011; Dai, Vrahas, et al., 2012). Treatment of *P. aeruginosa* biofilms on urinary catheters achieved full disinfection in 30–300 min, depending on the catheter material, but shorter times were not assessed (Bak, Ladefoged, Tvede, Begovic, & Gregersen, 2010). Resistance to UV-C has not been observed but is theoretically possible. Evidence regarding the use of UV-C and its effects on antibiotic utilization in a clinical setting is nonexistent at this time.

A recent placebo-controlled randomized trial compared UVC as a generalized wound modality to promote healing of pressure ulcers/injuries. Forty-three patients with paralysis with a total of 58 pressure injuries ranging in severity from superficial to eschar-covered were randomized to either UV-C or visible white light while also receiving standard of care for topical management (Nussbaum et al., 2013). Wounds were irradiated for 15 s to the periwound, at a one-inch distance from the wound, then from 15 to 360 s based on wound presentation, three times per week until wound closure or hospital discharge. Although significant results were reported in Stage 2 pressure injuries, overall results were inconclusive due to small sample size and methodological design (e.g., lack of homogeneity of wound severity, wound management, treatment setting). Furthermore, the study design did not match the optimum use of UV-C.

Indications and Use

Because of its antimicrobial effects, UV-C is sometimes used in hospital patient rooms and operating rooms to reduce surgical infections (Buonanno et al., 2013; Curtis et al., 2018; Lindblad, Tano, Lindahl, & Huss, 2019; Ritter, Olberding, & Malinzak, 2007). UV-C devices have even been marketed to the consumer to sterilize everything from toothbrushes to drinking water to personal protective equipment that is reused. Yamada, Yamada, Ueda, and Sakurai (2014) found that UV-C treatment of titanium hardware reduced biofilm adhesion. The UV-C irradiated discs showed significantly less biofilm formation on them than the control discs did, after soaking in an incubating bath for up to 8 h. The treated titanium showed increased hydrophilicity and a reduction of surface hydrocarbon, which are two mechanisms that could inhibit bacterial adhesion via increasing wettability of the surface. However, the UV-exposure in this study was 48 h, far longer than would be used in a clinical situation. Interestingly, the UV-C irradiation also appears to improve bony adherence to an implant due to these changes to the titanium surface, a result confirmed by Park, Koak, Kim, Han, and Heo (2013).

Following a systemic review, Reddy et al. (2008) did not recommend UV treatment of pressure injuries. International pressure ulcer/injury guideline (EPUAP, NPIAP, PPPIA, 2019) does not comment on ultraviolet, though there was a recommendation for it in the preceding edition. New evidence has been published in recent years, though the quantity of clinical research is still limited., and the next updates to these guidelines and reviews may reach different conclusions. A retrospective study including 224 wounds treated with UV-C noted no adverse effects from the intervention (Yarboro, Millar, & Smith, 2019).

There is no standardized way to apply UV-C light to a wound. A common protocol involves protecting the peri-wound skin from UB exposure with petrolatum, a towel, aluminum foil, or sheet drape. UV treatment to unprotected periwound skin has been used to promote wound closure and stimulate cellular activity, however, evidence of efficacy is quite limited (Yarboro et al., 2019).

The UV lamp is positioned 1 inch above the wound and parallel with the skin, so the light waves are perpendicular to the wound. Treatment is applied directly over the wound, for 90–120 s, although recent research indicates a shorter time may be effective, without any materials between the wound bed and the light. Plastic transparent films have been shown to block transmission of the UV-C light; therefore, any material between the wound bed and the light must be removed (Rao et al., 2011). Treatment is discontinued when the bioburden is adequately reduced. UV-C does not penetrate deeply into the tissue and therefore is reserved for superficial infections (Yin et al., 2013).

Both the patient and the clinician must wear UV-blocking eye protection. Even if a person does not look directly at the light, the waves may bounce off surfaces and reflect into the eye, causing damage. UV-C is most commonly performed by physical therapists and physical therapist assistants, as ultraviolet therapy is covered in their curriculum, but it may be administered by other trained clinicians.

Contraindications and Precautions

Safe and effective dosage of UV-C may vary based on the distance from the light source, the intensity of the light source, and the size of the treated area. UV-C has a very low risk of causing burns. Contraindications, precautions, and conditions that can be exacerbated by UV treatment (especially with UV-A or UV-B over large areas of the body) can be

---

> **BOX 27.1 Contraindications and Conditions Exacerbated by Ultraviolet (UV) Light Therapy**
>
> **Absolute Contraindications**
> - History of skin cancer
> - Systemic lupus erythematosus
> - Fever
> - Radiation therapy anywhere on body within previous 3 months
> - Sarcoidosis
> - Treatment over eye
> - Presence of erythema from last UV treatment
>
> **Conditions That Can Be Exacerbated by UV Treatment (Especially UV-A or UV-B Over Large Areas of Body)**
> - Pulmonary tuberculosis
> - Cardiac disease
> - Renal disease
> - Hepatic disease
> - Human immunodeficiency virus/acquired immunodeficiency syndrome
> - Hyperthyroidism
> - Diabetes
> - Herpes simplex infection

> **BOX 27.2 Precautions for Ultraviolet (UV) Light Therapy**
>
> - Acute eczema or dermatitis
> - Radiation therapy more than 3 months earlier
> - Photosensitivity
> - Human immunodeficiency virus/acquired immunodeficiency syndrome
> - Use of photosensitizing medication (may shorten treatment time or preclude treatment altogether)
>   - Psoralens (intentionally given to increase susceptibility to UV-A)
>   - Tetracycline
>   - Sulfonamides
>   - Quinolones
>   - Gold medications for rheumatoid arthritis
>   - Thiazide diuretics
>   - Diphenhydramine
>   - Oral contraceptives
>   - Phenothiazines

found in Box 27.1. Conditions and medications requiring caution with UV, usually UV-A and UV-B treatment are listed in Box 27.2 (Cameron, 2017).

ULTRASOUND

Ultrasound is a term used to describe sound waves greater than 20,000 Hz, the upper limit of human hearing. Three forms of ultrasound are commonly used: 1–3.3 MHz, 40 Hz, and 22–35 kHz. Each has distinct uses.

Traditional High-Frequency Ultrasound (1.0–3.3 MHz)

Traditional clinical therapeutic applications use a frequency of 1 or 3.3 MHz. Most users may elect to use a duty cycle. This parameter results in pulsing of the current, with periods of wave production followed by quiet periods. A 20% duty cycle is most commonly used, in which the sound waves are on for 1 ms and then off for 4 ms. Heat is produced but is dispersed so quickly when good perfusion is present that no temperature change occurs in the tissue. Ultrasound has been used to promote soft tissue healing for more than six decades, primarily for orthopedic conditions. More recently, that use has extended to wound healing.

An ultrasound device consists of the control unit and the handheld sound head, or *transducer* (Fig. 27.2). The user is able to control the intensity (amount of power used), whether the waves are continuous or pulsed, the duration of treatment, and, on some units, the wavelength. The device runs electricity through a crystal in the sound head, causing the crystal to vibrate through a reverse piezoelectric effect. These vibrations create sound waves that pass through the sound head membrane and into the tissue. These waves elicit both thermal and nonthermal effects.

Physiologic Effects. Nonthermal effects are attributed to cavitation and acoustic microstreaming. Stable cavitation is the vibration of tiny bubbles within the interstitial spaces. With microstreaming, current eddies form around gas bubbles that are near vibrating particles. In addition, streaming stimulates the movement of fluid within and between cells. Some investigators believe that using ultrasound in a water bath stimulates mechanical wound debridement through acoustic streaming of the water itself. These nonthermal effects occur with both pulsed and continuous ultrasound. The resulting forces stimulate an inflammatory response in wounds (Young & Dyson, 1990a), with an increase in histamine release (Demir, Yaray, Kirnap, & Yaray, 2004; Fyfe & Chahl, 1984). Pulsed ultrasound has been shown to stimulate fibroblast proliferation and macrophage phagocytic activity in vitro (Young & Dyson, 1990b; Zhou et al., 2004, 2008). However, peak benefit occurred after 20 min of treatment, which is longer than is usually acceptable by the clinician providing the treatment. Other effects of ultrasound include leukocyte adhesion and increased fibrinolysis, permeability of cell membranes and skin, mast cell degranulation, and production of growth factors and nitric oxide (Ennis, Lee, & Meneses, 2007; Stanisic, Provo, Larson, & Kloth, 2005; Young & Dyson, 1990b).

The thermal effects of continuous ultrasound stimulate an increase in local circulation that disperses heat and increases cell metabolism (Taskan et al., 1997). Increases in macrophage activity, protein synthesis by fibroblasts, and angiogenesis occur (Young & Dyson, 1990a). As a result, wounds may progress through the inflammatory phase more quickly (Demir et al., 2004) or acute inflammation may be reinitiated if healing has stalled. Additional effects reported include increased tensile strength and collagen deposition after ultrasound treatments (Byl, McKenzie, Wong, West, & Hunt, 1993; Demir et al., 2004).

Protocol and Clinical Application. Based on the theory and in vitro research, high-frequency ultrasound should have a significant impact on wound healing. However, in the more complex in vivo environment, this expectation has not borne out consistently. A common limit of the available research is that treatment time and sound head movement patterns have not always been modified appropriately to accommodate wound size and the effective radiating area of the transducer. Ultrasound treatment is commonly combined with other modalities, which also may influence study results. Robertson and Baker (2001) identified eight randomized clinical trials addressing ultrasound. Seven of the studies were rejected because of inadequate controls, inadequate analysis, inadequate treatment details, insufficient sample size, or the use of multiple interventions. More current studies continue

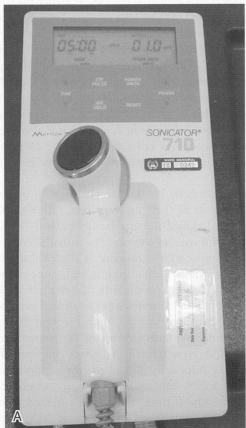
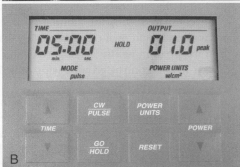

Fig. 27.2 (A) Ultrasound device. (B) Close-up of ultrasound parameter settings. (Courtesy Renee Cordrey.)

to omit full descriptions of parameters and technique. Seven of the nine high-frequency US trials included in the most recent Cochrane review of US for venous leg ulcers delivered the soundwaves through water (Cullum & Liu, 2017). As venous insufficiency is exacerbated by placing a leg in a dependent position in warm water, this method of treatment could worsen the condition, or mask any benefit of the ultrasound. Therefore, no standard protocol for high frequency ultrasound exists and its application to clinical practice is difficult.

In general, low-intensity, high-frequency ultrasound has ranged from 0.1 to 0.3 W/cm^2, medium-intensity ultrasound from 0.3 to 1.2 W/cm^2, and high-intensity ultrasound from 1.2 to 3.0 W/cm^2. Time of treatment varies from 1 to 10 min, and transducer frequency has run between 0.3 and 3 MHz. Frequency of treatment has ranged between 1 and 5 days per week, and treatment duration has ranged from 2 weeks through wound closure. Most of these studies used periwound techniques, although Peschen, Weichenthal, Schopf, and Vanscheidt (1997) used a water immersion technique. Most studies used pulsed ultrasound, possibly because of the risks of thermal heating in a person with sensory, vascular, or cognitive compromise, common comorbidities in people with chronic wounds.

Evidence for Clinical Use. Pressure injury research on high-frequency ultrasound points to a lack of benefit. Two older randomized controlled trials demonstrated no difference in healing rates (McDiarmid, Burns, Lewith, & Machin, 1985; ter Reit, Kessels, & Knipschild, 1996). A meta-analysis combining the two studies strengthened that conclusion with a stronger sample size (Flemming & Cullum, 2001). Although some trials did show a small improvement in the ultrasound group, the sample sizes were too small to reach statistical significance. Selkowitz, Cameron, Mainzer, and Wolfe (2002) conducted a single-subject baseline–ultrasound–sham trial on a Stage 3 coccyx pressure injury using low-intensity pulsed ultrasound. The baseline period had the greatest healing rate and the sham the poorest, although this result may be attributed to natural variation as a wound heals.

A Cochrane review of ultrasound for pressure injuries concluded that there was no evidence supporting the efficacy of high-frequency ultrasound (Baba-Akbari Sari, Flemming, Cullum, & Wollina, 2006). The WOCN® Society (2016) concurs that there is a lack of evidence about high-frequency ultrasound and pressure ulcers/injuries. However, international pressure ulcer/injuries guidelines recommend considering the use of high-frequency ultrasound as an adjunct for the treatment of stage 3 and 4 pressure injuries and deep tissue pressure injuries (DTPI), at a 1 MHz setting (EPUAP, NPIAP, PPPIA, 2019). The strength of evidence in that guideline is B1, moderate quality evidence, including evidence generated since those prior works.

Research has been more promising, with less severe stage 2 ulcers. A 2014 randomized controlled trial included 43 patients, living in long-term care facilities in Poland, with stage 2–3 trunk or pelvic pressure ulcers/injuries (Polak

et al., 2014). The wounds in the experimental group were treated with 1 MHz ultrasound 5 days per week, with variable times based on wound area and week of the study, in addition to standard care. Stage 2 ulcers did show significant improvements in area decrease weekly (2.6 cm^2 vs 1.52) and overall (68.8% vs 37.2%), and the proportion which closed (50.0% vs 16.7%). Stage 3 pressure injuries had no significant differences between groups.

Limitations in this study were that it did not consider that stage 2 and 3 pressure injuries are quite different clinically and physiologically. There were standard care dressing options—including nonadherent pads, saline gauze, hydrogel, and plant extracts—without information on how those treatments were distributed. It also excluded necrotic, deep, or tunneling wounds, which are the ones potentially most likely in need of energy therapies. While the authors did include information on the device specifications and treatment parameters, they used a 2- to 8-min 20% duty cycle, rather the very brief pulses usually used. As a result, the wound may have received only active treatment, or a brief treatment with a long period of inactivity, treating only part of the wound bed or periwound. Additionally, this long on-time would likely result in thermal heating, while the pulsed setting is typically used to eliminate tissue heating by allowing rapid heat dispersal. Therefore, the heat, not the nonthermal effects of ultrasound, may be the beneficial factor in this study. It is also interesting that 1 MHz penetrates more deeply than 3 MHz, yet, the more superficial ulcers appeared to be more responsive to ultrasound.

A second study by Polak et al. (2016), with many of the same limitations as their previous one, followed 90 long-term care and skilled nursing facility patients with stages 2–4 pressure injuries for 6 weeks. The patients received standard care alone or with ultrasound or electrical stimulation. As in their previous study, necrotic and tunneling wounds were excluded, as were people with diabetes, venous insufficiency, and lymphatic insufficiency. Standard care included appropriate measures, but the topical wound therapy was highly variable. Wounds, including the wound bed and the periwound, were treated five times per week. The US protocol was minimally described; the authors reported 1 MHz and a 20% duty cycle were used, but not the time frame of that on-off time. The wounds treated with ultrasound did show a significant improvement in area reduction (77% vs 49%) and the proportion of wounds that closed (46% vs 23%), compared with the standard care control group. There was no breakdown of outcomes by stage, but the wounds were predominantly stage 2 (64% in the US group, and 74% in the control group), with only 7% and 3% as stage 4 pressure injuries.

Outcome trials using high-intensity and low-intensity pulsed ultrasound on patients with venous ulcers are inconclusive; offering low quality evidence, potential bias and lack of statistical significance (Cullum & Liu, 2017; WOCN Society, 2017). Taradaj et al. (2008) found that patients with venous ulcers healed equally with compression alone verses compression with venous surgery, pulsed ultrasound, or both. However, findings may have been influenced by the patients self-selecting into the surgery or nonsurgery group and ultrasound delivered in warm water with the leg in a dependent position. Ericksson, Lundeberg, and Malm (1991) found no significant difference in the percentage of wounds that closed using low-intensity pulsed or ultrasound treatment versus sham treatment. Studies showing improvement with use of ultrasound lacked baseline data and control of variables such as wound size and follow-up (Cullum & Liu, 2017; Johannsen, Gam, & Karlsmark, 1998; Peschen et al., 1997). Both of these factors could alter the findings.

Newer research has addressed some of these study design concerns, but limitations remain. Dolibog et al. (2018) examined a 1 MHz US, 0.5 W/cm², 20% duty cycle protocol on venous ulcers, treating the wound bed directly, compared with shockwave therapy and standard of care. All patients received saline moistened gauze under elastic wraps, changed daily. This plan cannot manage the exudate volume of a typical venous ulcer, and is not the standard of care, but the care was consistent between groups. The treatment time was 1 min per square centimeter. However, the size of the transducer, or its ERA was not described, so it cannot be determined whether the dosage was appropriate. The US group had newer ulcers (mean 5.3 months compared with 8.1 and 8.8 months), and the control group wounds were larger (mean 11.8 cm² vs 9.8 and 9.2 cm²). After 4 weeks of five times weekly treatments, the US group reduced area by 67.6%, the shockwave group 38.2%, and the control group 15.8%. Polak et al. (2016) compared US with electrical stimulation and standard of care groups in a randomized clinical trial with 77 participants who had Stage 2–4 pressure injuries over a 6-week time period. The US protocol involved treating the wound and periwound 5 days per week with 1 MHz and 20% duty cycle. Treatment times for the US were 1 min per square centimeter in the 1st week, 2 min/cm² in the 2nd week, and 3 min/cm² from the 3rd week onward. They weaned patients onto the treatment to monitor for adverse effects; the authors did not report on actual adverse effects. The transducer had an ERA of 4 cm². At 6 weeks, the wound surface area reduced by 77.48% in the US group, and 48.97% in the control group. ES performed similarly to US with a 76.19% reduction in area.

Contraindications and Precautions. With high-frequency ultrasound, the sound head must be kept in constant motion. If the sound head stays in place for even 0.1 ms, standing waves and banding may occur. A *standing wave* occurs when the sound wave reflects off tissue back onto itself. The resulting interference wave is twice as strong as the original wave, which increases tissue heating and potentially leads to burning. *Banding* is the separation of cells and plasma within the blood vessels. This action causes irreversible damage to the endothelial linings of the vessel walls.

Contraindications are related to the thermal and nonthermal effects of ultrasound (Cameron, 2017). Ultrasound must not be used over the eyes, the heart, the carotid sinuses, a pregnant uterus, or the exposed central nervous system (e.g., over a laminectomy site). The inflammatory, cavitation, and metabolic effects of ultrasound contraindicate its use in situations where it would be harmful, such as areas of active bleeding, active infection, over saline or silicone-filled

implants, over malignancies, and in the presence of thrombophlebitis. Ultrasound should not be used over pacemakers, active epiphyseal plates, the reproductive organs, or orthopedic cement or plastic components because the increased reflection of sound waves overheats local tissue. The VenUS III trial with 337 participants with venous leg ulcers found more adverse events in the ultrasound group compared with standard of care group, but at a rate similar to the rate from other trials (Cullum & Liu, 2017; Watson et al., 2011). The risk ratio for nonserious adverse events was 1.29 (95% CI 1.02–1.64). There may have been a higher occurrence of serious adverse events as well, with a risk ratio of 1.21 (0.78–1.89). However, the serious events count included situations such as the new diagnosis of diabetes, which cannot be attributed to ultrasound treatment. Serious adverse effects were also associated with larger and longer duration wounds, but there was no association for nonserious adverse effects.

Due to insufficient evidence, the WOCN Society (2014) does not recommend the used of ultrasound for the treatment of arterial ulcers until larger, robust studies that focus on patients with arterial wounds show safety and effectiveness

In summary the use of traditional high frequency ultrasound for wound care is off label use. If used, it should be performed by a therapist with appropriate credentials and training. The clinician must exercise good judgment when deciding whether to use ultrasound. Ultrasound may be used in the presence of a contraindication only when the treatment location is remote to the site of contraindication. For example, ultrasound may be used on a foot wound despite the presence of a cardiac pacemaker, total hip replacement, or pregnancy because of the localized effects of ultrasound. Caution should be used around superficial bones because periosteum heats and burns easily from reflection off the bone. The clinician should be especially vigilant when thermal ultrasound is used in a person with sensory or cognitive deficits who is unable to provide feedback relating to tissue heating. Ultrasound may be used with caution in an area of acute inflammation if the benefits outweigh the risks of increasing inflammation.

Noncontact Low-Frequency Ultrasound (40 kHz)

Noncontact low-frequency ultrasound (NCLFU) is a noncontact method benefiting from the nonthermal effects of ultrasound. At this time, there is one commercially available NCLFU device (UltraMIST, Sanuwave) (Fig. 27.3).

This intervention may be performed by any licensed trained practitioner. The device vaporizes saline into microdroplets (60 μm), which are then propelled to the wound bed via 40-kHz ultrasonic waves, with an intensity of 1.5 W/cm². A handset is held close to the wound and is moved in a zigzag pattern across the wound in each direction, taking care to maintain cavitation at the wound surface while spraying a fine mist of saline, though other substances may be used, such as antimicrobial agents. The duration of treatment is based upon wound size, from 3 to 20 min.

Noncontact low-frequency ultrasound has been found to have two primary benefits: wound size reduction and bioburden reduction (Ennis et al., 2007; Kavros & Schenck, 2007; Lai & Pittelkow, 2007). Microstreaming and cavitation, which are

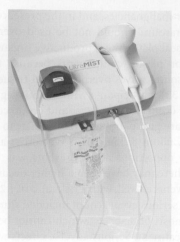

Fig. 27.3 UltraMIST® control unit. (Copyright Sanuwave Wound Care Technologies, Suwanee, Georgia.)

thought to be the primary sources of any healing effect from ultrasound, are more common with kilohertz ultrasound than with megahertz (high frequency) ultrasound (Ennis et al., 2007; Kavros & Schenck, 2007). Those mechanisms lead to DNA synthesis diminishing for 4 h after treatment, but then increasing for a 2-day period, stimulating tissue growth (Lai & Pittelkow, 2007). Additionally, a mouse study found that treated wounds had a greater concentration of collagen and blood vessels in the new tissue (Thawer & Houghton, 2004). A mechanism for this effect may be the morphologic changes in fibroblasts treated with 35 kHz ultrasound in vitro (Conner-Kerr, Malpass, Steele, & Howlett, 2015). Further, over time, the fibroblasts that entered the scratch wound on the petri dish became more perpendicular to the wound when treated with US compared with the control dishes. The treated fibroblasts also presented as more elongated and were more evenly spaced with less bunching across the scratch.

With 12 weeks of NCLFU therapy, increased closure rates have been reported with venous insufficiency and Wagner grade 1 and 2 diabetic foot ulcers compared with conventional wound care (Peschen et al., 1997; Weichenthal, Mohr, Stegman, & Breitbart, 1997). In addition, studies noted a reduction in wound size in patients with critical limb ischemia (Kavros et al., 2008; Kavros, Miller, & Hanna, 2007). A systematic review showed that NCLFU, low-frequency, and high-intensity contact ultrasound improved healing in patients with chronic wounds (venous ulcers and diabetic ulcers), although the authors note that the quality of the data may be threatened by researcher biases (Voigt, Wendelken, Driver, & Alvarez, 2011).

More recent research by White, Ivins, Wilkes, Carolan-Rees, and Harding (2016) examined the effect of adding NCLFU thrice weekly to the standard of care in an RCT for venous leg ulcers. The 36 participants, 8-week trial found no significant differences between groups in area reduction (46.6% vs 39.2%), infection rates, and quality of life scores. Pain was reduced by 14.4 points on visual analog scale compared with 5.3 points; that difference was not statistically significant ($P = 0.078$) but may be clinically relevant. Positive trends were noted in the NCLFU group, but the study was likely too

underpowered due to high variance to provide conclusive evidence. The ultrasound-treated wounds were on average 15 months older, with the longest duration ulcer being 14 years older than the oldest ulcer in the control group. Wound duration is known to be a risk factor for poor healing of venous ulcers. No adverse effects from the US were noted. Gibbons et al. (2015) conducted an RCT with 81 participants with venous leg ulcers. After 4 weeks of treatment, the NCLFU group showed greater reductions in wound area reduction (61.6% vs 45%), actual area reduction (9.0 cm^2 vs 4.1 cm^2), and pain (0.6 vs 2.4, both with a starting score of 3). The area reduction was more pronounced when evaluating the newer ulcers, those under 6-months duration. In these wounds, the treatment group reduced 79.4% compared with 49.2% in the standard care group. Quality of life scores were similar between groups. NCLFU treatment was delivered three times per week, in addition to the standard care both groups received, with time based on wound size. The investigator could provide a standard care participant NCLFU in the follow-up period if desired or provide other nonstandard interventions to all participants. Few participants had any energy modalities (pulse electromagnetic induction, electrical stimulation, NCLFU) prior to the trial enrollment, though 10% of the standard group and 5% of the test group did receive NCLFU treatment previously for the study ulcers. The standard care group did have significantly more cellular-based tissue products used prior to this trial (5.1 mean compared with 2.0).

Additional studies with NCLFU have been observed to include increased granulation tissue, decreased periwound maceration, and decreased volume of exudate (Bell & Cavorsi, 2008). Conversely, the following adverse events were reported with patients with diabetic foot ulcers: pain, erythema, blisters, edema, and ulcer enlargement (Ennis et al., 2005). A study with chronic venous ulcers (Wiegand, Bittenger, Galiano, Driver, & Gibbons, 2017) included 36 people, randomized to an NCLFU or control group after showing <30% size change in the 2-week run in period. NCLFU was performed three times per week. The NCLFU group reduced area 67% within 4 weeks, while the standard of care group reduced 41.6%. Those in the treatment group, especially those who responded to care, saw lower IL-6 and higher IL-10 levels, as well as a greater reduction in fibrinogen levels, though most of their analysis was between responders and nonresponders, not the treatment group and the SOC control group. The variables they studied did not appear to relate to the improvement seen with NCLFU treatment.

According to the WOCN Society clinical practice guidelines, the benefit of ultrasound for treating pressure injuries and lower extremity venous, arterial, and diabetic wounds is uncertain due to limited evidence or inconsistent study findings. Continued research is recommended (WOCN, 2014, 2016, 2017, 2021).

International pressure ulcer/injury guidelines recommend considering the use of NCLFU (40 kHz) for the treatment of stage 3 and 4 pressure injuries and DTPIs. These recommendations are based on level B2 evidence (EPUAP, NPIAP, PPPIA, 2019). An observational study with historical controls using a validated DTPI severity scale (Honaker, Brockopp, &

Moe, 2014a) reported that more wounds resolved spontaneously (18% vs 2% of control) and those that did open were less severe when treated with NCLFU (Honaker, Brockopp, & Moe, 2014b). The effect of this treatment on DTPI remains a hypothesis that needs further investigation.

Other wound etiologies may benefit from NCLFU. An RCT with split thickness skin graft donor sites (Prather, Tummel, Patel, Smith, & Gould, 2015) treated 27 participants with daily sessions for 5 days. Most of the participants were being treated for burns (84%). The treatment group closed faster, 12.1 vs 21.3 days. It also demonstrated a distinct improvement in maintained closure, with 8% of the NCLFU treatment group reopening within the 6-week follow-up period, and 45% of the standard care group opening, though the result was not statistically significant ($P = 0.06$). In weeks five and six, the participants reported significantly reduced pruritis within the treatment group.

There is limited evidence that NCLFU may reduce bioburden. In a study by Serena et al. (Serena et al., 2009), NCLFU was applied to in vitro bacterial samples and to people with pressure ulcers. In this study, one treatment of ultrasound reduced *Pseudomonas* by 33%, *Escherichia coli* by 40%, and *Enterococcus faecalis* by 27%. However, MRSA and *S. aureus* were not affected. When treating 11 people with Stage III pressure ulcers for 2 weeks, bioburden reduced from 4×10^7 to 2×10^7 overall, although beta-hemolytic streptococcus G was stable and beta-hemolytic streptococcus group A increased. A study with venous ulcers found reductions in *peptoniphilus* after the ultrasound treatment period, but other bacteria were consistent between groups (Wiegand et al., 2017).

Some preliminary research suggests that low-frequency ultrasound can work synergistically with antibiotics, improving the effectiveness of both interventions (Cai, Wang, Liu, Wang, & Xia, 2017). Pitt, McBride, Lunceford, Roper, and Sagers (1994) tested subtherapeutic levels of gentamycin with and without 67 kHz continuous ultrasound in an in vitro study. The US was used at an intensity lower than antimicrobial levels. The pseudomonas and *E. coli* cultures showed the bacteria reduced by several orders of magnitude when the ultrasound was added, and the minimum inhibitory concentration of the antibiotic reduced from 4 to 3 µg/mL with the pseudomonas, and from 6 to 3 µg/mL with the *E. coli*. Older cultures, presumably with more biofilm, showed greater susceptibility to the gentamycin with ultrasound. The gram-positive bacteria tested did not show a similar effect. Other studies have achieved similar results involving several antibiotics and 40–80 kHz ultrasound on planktonic cultures, including some Gram-positive strains (Cai et al., 2017). Studies looking at low-frequency US against biofilms have found that higher intensities (10 W/cm^2 vs 1), and longer treatment times, from 2 to 6 h, which is not practical in a clinical setting, are needed in order to reduce bacterial viability (Cai et al., 2017). Komrakov and Antipov (1990) did use this combination in patients with wound infections. They found that the rate of purulent-septic complications was lower in the group combining the ultrasound and gentamycin, decreasing from 35.7% to 5.9%.

A systematic review and meta-analysis by Michailidis, Bergin, Haines, and Williams (2018) compared healing outcomes of diabetic foot ulcers with debrided with ultrasound compared to nonsurgical sharp debridement. Researchers noted similar outcomes with use of NCLFU and non surgical sharp debridement.

The clinician should consider NCLFU as an option when developing a plan of care for a person with a wound. While the material costs may be higher than for a sharp debridement, there are few risks of complications and it is often less painful for the patient.

Ultrasonic Low-Frequency Debridement (22.5–35 kHz)

The third form of ultrasound is ultrasonic debridement. Ultrasonic kilohertz frequencies have been effective at fibrinolysis of the wound surface without causing damage to underlying granulation tissue. Softer fibrinous slough is more responsive to ultrasonic debridement than drier, tougher fibrinous tissue (Stanisic et al., 2005; Tan, Abisi, Smith, & Burnand, 2007).

The limited number of controlled clinical trials on human chronic ulcers led Ramundo and Gray (2008) to conclude that low-frequency ultrasound may be beneficial for removing necrotic tissue, but the evidence was inconclusive. Amini et al. (2013) compared the standard care for diabetic foot ulcers with diagnosed osteomyelitis with and without ultrasonic debridement. They found a small but significant improvement in healing rate in months two and three, but not at month six. However, there were some notable differences between groups, such as the ultrasound group having much higher rates of peripheral arterial disease, ischemic heart disease, and anemia, and the study was underpowered. Further, it is not clear if sharp or surgical debridement was included in the standard care of wound. Off-loading, antibiotics, and an unspecified daily dressing comprised the standard plan of care.

Ultrasonic debridement at 35 kHz may also be effective in reducing bioburden by damaging cell walls. After 30 s of treatment, MRSA was reduced from 1 million colony-forming units (CFUs) to 6 CFUs, and MRSA's susceptibility to methicillin improved (Conner-Kerr et al., 2010). More recently, Attinger and Wolcott (2012) reported that ultrasound is a useful adjunct for debriding biofilm (see Chapter 19).

Saline is used as the transfer media, and the air bubbles in the fluid expand and collapse, causing shockwave formation, cavitation, and erosion and fragmentation of the dead tissue (Wendelken, Alvarez, Markowitz, Comfort, & Waltrous, 2006). A variety of probes are available and selected according to the wound surface to be treated. Ultrasound intensity can be adjusted. The treatment is often painless or minimally pain inducing; some patients may benefit from a topical anesthetic or pain medication before treatment. Ultrasonic debridement may take more time to complete than sharp debridement. Contraindications and precautions are similar to those for sharp debridement. Therefore, it should be performed only by practitioners who are qualified for wound debridement.

CLINICAL CONSULT

A: Referral received to consult on a 64-year-old woman with a right lateral leg wound that developed after falling and scraping her leg on a car door 5 months ago. Comorbidities include type 2 diabetes, venous insufficiency in right leg with edema. She is a manager and sits most of the day at work. She walks independently without an assistive device but does not engage in any exercise program. Past treatment includes dressings, surgical debridement, multilayer compression wraps, negative pressure wound therapy, oral antibiotics, and a cellular-tissue-derived product graft, which failed. Current wound presentation is a full-thickness lesion on right lateral calf, 11.7 × 6.2 × 0.4 cm. Wound base is covered with thick biofilm layer; after debridement, the base is fibrogranular. The copious wound exudate is yellow-green with a sweet odor. Periwound is macerated. Ankle-brachial index (ABI) right leg was 1.05 at the dorsalis pedis and 0.96 at the posterior tibialis. 2+ palpable pulses at both. Right leg with circumferential hemosiderin staining. Hemoglobin A1c from 1 month ago was 6.4. Her reported diet should be adequate, including protein, fruits, and vegetables.

D: Wound presentation is consistent with a traumatic wound, complicated by an edematous limb with venous insufficiency and a history of diabetes under adequate control. The high level of bioburden with biofilm will impair healing, and many past treatments have been unsuccessful.

P: Reduce bioburden in the wound, provide compression and moist wound healing. Consult physical therapy for UV-C to further stimulate cellular activity to promote healing.

I: (1) Routine weekly sharp debridement by wound care as needed to reduce bioburden. Topical cadexomer iodine to manage/treat bioburden. (2) Ultraviolet-C treatments to the right leg wound three times per week initially. Several treatments may be necessary. (3) Consider noncontact, low-frequency ultrasound two to three times per week if wound fails to respond to the UV-C after 2 weeks. (4) Multilayer compression wraps. (5) Teach patient to elevate leg above heart twice daily for 30 min. (6) Therapeutic exercise to improve ankle range of motion and calf muscle pump strength; instruct patient on a home exercise program and a walking program. She should be encouraged to get up frequently while at work and walk.

E: Weekly wound measurements/assessments by PT and notify wound care team if dimensions unchanged after 2 weeks of UV-C. Will modify plan as needed.

SUMMARY

- Ultraviolet C light has been used for decades to reduce bioburden but is under-utilized at this time.
- UV-C can also stimulate wound healing at the cellular level.
- Megahertz frequency ultrasound may benefit pressure ulcer/injury and venous ulcer healing.

- Kilohertz frequency ultrasound may support healing in multiple wound types through reducing bioburden and stimulating cellular activity.
- Well-designed clinical trials and bench science have increased in recent years, but more evidence is desirable.
- UV-C and US can be useful adjuncts for wound healing.

SELF-ASSESSMENT QUESTIONS

1. Which of the following conditions would contraindicate UV-C as a viable treatment option for a sacral ulcer?
   a. A history of sunburns as a child
   b. Radiation therapy for breast cancer last month
   c. Unable to stay in position for 20 min
   d. Use of levothyroxine for hypothyroidism

2. Low-frequency ultrasound generates which of the following beneficial effects on tissue?
   a. Heating
   b. Standing waves
   c. Banding
   d. Cavitation

3. Ultrasound wound be contraindicated in which of the following conditions?
   a. A dehisced Cesarian section surgical wound
   b. A person in a hypercoagulable state
   c. Fournier's gangrene in a man
   d. A neuropathic ulcer in a patient with a pacemaker

4. Which of the following modalities is effective at debriding nonviable tissue?
   a. Ultraviolet-C
   b. 1 MHz ultrasound
   c. 3 MHz ultrasound
   d. 25 kHz ultrasound

5. Which category of microorganisms appear to be most easily destroyed by ultraviolet-C?
   a. Multiple drug-resistant bacteria
   b. Yeast
   c. Biofilm
   d. Viruses

REFERENCES

Amini, S., ShojaeeFard, A., Annabestani, Z., Hammami, M. R., Shaiganmehr, Z., Larijani, B., et al. (2013). Low-frequency ultrasound debridement in patients with diabetic foot ulcers and osteomyelitis. *Wounds, 25*(7), 193–198.

Attinger, C., & Wolcott, R. (2012). Clinically addressing biofilm in chronic wounds. *Advances in Wound Care (New Rochelle), 1*(3), 127–132.

Baba-Akbari Sari, A., Flemming, K., Cullum, N. A., & Wollina, U. (2006). Therapeutic ultrasound for pressure ulcers. *Cochrane Database of Systematic Reviews, 3*, CD001275.

Bak, J., Ladefoged, S., Tvede, M., Begovic, T., & Gregersen, A. (2010). Disinfection of *Pseudomonas aeruginosa* biofilm contaminated tube lumens with ultraviolet C light emitting diodes. *Biofouling, 26*(1).

Bell, A. L., & Cavorsi, J. (2008). Noncontact ultrasound therapy for adjunctive treatment of nonhealing wounds: Retrospective analysis. *Physical Therapy, 88*(12), 1517–1524.

Buonanno, M., Randers-Pehrson, G., Bigelow, A. W., Trivedi, S., Lowy, F. D., Spotnitz, H. M., et al. (2013). 207-nm UV light—A promising tool for safe low-cost reduction of surgical site infections. I: In vitro studies. *PLoS One, 8*(10).

Byl, N. N., McKenzie, A., Wong, T., West, J., & Hunt, T. K. (1993). Incisional wound healing: A controlled study of low and high dose ultrasound. *The Journal of Orthopaedic and Sports Physical Therapy, 18*(5), 619–628.

Cai, Y., Wang, J., Liu, X., Wang, R., & Xia, L. (2017). A review of the combination therapy of low frequency ultrasound with antibiotics. *BioMed Research International, 2017.*

Cameron, M. H. (2017). *Physical agents in rehabilitation: An evidence-based approach to practice* (5th ed.). Elsevier.

Camp, R. D., Greaves, M. W., Hensby, C. N., Plummer, N. A., & Warin, A. P. (1978). Irradiation of human skin by short wavelength ultraviolet radiation (100–290 nm) (u.v.C): Increased concentrations of arachidonic acid and prostaglandines E2 and F2alpha. *British Journal of Clinical Pharmacology, 6*(2), 145–148.

Conner-Kerr, T., Alston, G., Stovall, A., Vernon, T., Winter, D., Meixner, J., et al. (2010). The effects of low-frequency ultrasound (35 kHz) on methicillin-resistant *Staphylococcus aureus* (MRSA) in vitro. *Ostomy/Wound Management, 56*(5), 32–43.

Conner-Kerr, T., Malpass, G., Steele, A., & Howlett, A. (2015). Effects of 35 kHz, low-frequency ultrasound application in vitro on human fibroblast morphology and migration patterns. *Ostomy/Wound Management, 61*(3), 34–41.

Cullum, N., & Liu, Z. (2017). Therapeutic ultrasound for venous leg ulcers. *Cochrane Database of Systematic Reviews,* (5), CD001180. https://doi.org/10.1002/14651858.CD001180.pub4.

Curtis, G. L., Faour, M., Jawad, M., Klika, A. K., Barsoum, W. K., & Higuera, C. A. (2018). Reduction of particles in the operating room using ultraviolet air disinfection and recirculation units. *The Journal of Arthroplasty, 33*(7S), S196–S200.

Dai, T., Kharkwal, G. B., Zhao, J., St Denis, T. G., Wu, Q., Xia, Y., et al. (2011). Ultraviolet-C light for treatment of *Candida albicans* burn infection in mice (Research Support, N.I.H., Extramural Research Support, Non-U.S. Gov't Research Support, U.S. Gov't, Non-P.H.S). *Photochemistry and Photobiology, 87*(2), 342–349.

Dai, T., Murray, C. K., Vrahas, M. S., Baer, D. G., Tegos, G. P., & Hamblin, M. R. (2012). Ultraviolet C light for Acinetobacter baumannii wound infections in mice: Potential use for battlefield wound decontamination? (Comparative Study Research Support, N.I.H., Extramural Research Support, Non-U.S. Gov't). *Journal of Trauma and Acute Care Surgery, 73*(3), 661–667.

Dai, T., Vrahas, M. S., Murray, C. K., & Hamblin, M. R. (2012, Feb). Ultraviolet C irradiation: An alternative antimicrobial approach to localized infections? (Research Support, N.I.H., Extramural Research Support, U.S. Gov't, Non-P.H.S. Review). *Expert Review of Anti-Infective Therapy, 10*(2), 185–195.

Demir, H., Yaray, S., Kirnap, M., & Yaray, K. (2004). Comparison of the effects of laser and ultrasound treatments on experimental wound healing in rats. *Journal of Rehabilitation Research and Development, 41*(5), 721–728.

Dolibog, P., Dolibog, P. T., Franek, A., Brzezińska-Wcisło, L., Wróbel, B., Arasiewicz, H., et al. (2018). Comparison of ultrasound therapy and radial shock wave therapy in the treatment of venous leg ulcers—Clinical, pilot study. *Postepy Dermatologii i Alergologii, 35*(5), 454–461. https://doi.org/10.5114/ada.2018.79191.

Ennis, W. J., Foremann, P., Mozen, N., Massey, J., Conner-Kerr, T., & Meneses, P. (2005). Ultrasound therapy for recalcitrant diabetic foot ulcers: results of a randomized, double-blind, controlled, multicenter study. *Ostomy/Wound Management, 51*(8), 24–39.

Ennis, W. J., Lee, C., & Meneses, P. (2007). A biochemical approach to wound healing through the use of modalities. *Clinics in Dermatology, 25*(1), 63–72. https://doi.org/10.1016/j.clindermatol.2006.09.008.

Ericksson, S., Lundeberg, T., & Malm, M. (1991). A placebo controlled trial of ultrasound therapy in chronic leg ulceration. *Scandinavian Journal of Rehabilitation Medicine, 23*(4), 211–213.

European Pressure Ulcer Advisory Panel, National Pressure Injury Advisory Panel, and Pan Pacific Pressure Injury Alliance. (2019). In E. Haesler (Ed.), *Prevention and Treatment of Pressure Ulcers/Injuries: Quick Reference Guide.*

Flemming, K., & Cullum, N. (2001). Systematic reviews of wound care management: (5) beds; (6) compression; (7) laser therapy, therapeutic ultrasound, electrotherapy and electromagnetic therapy. *Health Technology Assessment, 5*(9), 1–221.

Freytes, H. A., Fernandez, B., & Fleming, W. C. (1965). Ultraviolet light in the treatment of indolent ulcers. *Southern Medical Journal, 58*, 223–226.

Fyfe, M., & Chahl, L. (1984). Mast cell degranulation and increased vascular permeability induced by "therapeutic" ultrasound in the rat ankle joint. *British Journal of Experimental Pathology, 65*, 671–676.

Gates, F. (1928). Discussion and correspondence on nuclear derivatives and the lethal action of ultraviolet light. *Science, 68*, 479.

Gibbons, G. W., Orgill, D. P., Serena, T. E., Novoung, A., O'Connell, J. B., Li, W. W., et al. (2015). A prospective, randomized, controlled trial comparing the effects of noncontact, low-frequency ultrasound to standard care in healing venous leg ulcers. *Ostomy/Wound Management, 61*(1), 16–29.

Gupta, A., Avci, P., Dai, T., Huant, Y., & Hamblin, M. (2013). Ultraviolet radiation in wound care: Sterilization and stimulation. *Advances in Wound Care, 2*(8), 422–437.

Hall, J. D., & Mount, D. W. (1981). Mechanisms of DNA replication and mutagenesis in ultraviolet-irradiated bacteria and mammalian cells. *Progress in Nucleic Acid Research and Molecular Biology, 25*, 53–126.

Honaker, J., Brockopp, D., & Moe, K. (2014a). Development and psychometric testing of the honaker suspected deep tissue injury severity scale. *Journal of Wound, Ostomy, and Continence Nursing, 41*(3), 238–241.

Honaker, J., Brockopp, D., & Moe, K. (2014b). Suspected deep tissue injury profile: A pilot study. *Advances in Skin & Wound Care, 27* (3), 133–140. quiz 141–132.

James, L. C., Moore, A. M., Wheeler, L. A., Murphy, G. M., Dowd, P. M., & Greaves, M. W. (1991). Transforming growth factor alpha: In vivo release by normal human skin following UV irradiation and abrasion. *Skin Pharmacology, 4*(2), 61–64.

Johannsen, F., Gam, A. N., & Karlsmark, T. (1998). Ultrasound therapy in chronic leg ulceration: A meta-analysis. *Wound Repair and Regeneration, 6*(2), 121–126.

Kavros, S. J., Liedl, D. A., Boon, A. J., Miller, J. L., Hobbs, J. A., & Andrews, K. L. (2008). Expedited wound healing with noncontact, low-frequency ultrasound therapy in chronic wounds: A retrospective analysis. *Advances in Skin & Wound Care, 21*(9), 416–423.

Kavros, S. J., Miller, J. L., & Hanna, S. W. (2007). Treatment of ischemic wounds with noncontact, low-frequency ultrasound: The Mayo Clinic experience, 2004–2006. *Advances in Skin & Wound Care, 20*(4), 221–226.

Kavros, S. J., & Schenck, E. C. (2007). Use of noncontact low-frequency ultrasound in the treatment of chronic foot and leg ulcerations: A 51-patient analysis. *Journal of the American Podiatric Medical Association, 97*(2), 95–101.

Kirke, S. M., Lowder, S., Lloyd, J. J., Diffey, B. L., Matthews, J. N., & Farr, P. M. (2007). A randomized comparison of selective broadband UVB and narrowband UVB in the treatment of psoriasis. *The Journal of Investigative Dermatology, 127*(7), 1641–1646.

Kloth, L. C. (1995). Physical modalities in wound management: UVC, therapeutic heating and electrical stimulation. *Ostomy/ Wound Management, 41*(5), 18–20. 22-14, 26-17.

Komrakov, V. E., & Antipov, S. V. (1990). Use of ultrasonics and antibiotics in the treatment of wounds in patients with high risk of infection of vascular transplants. *Klin Khir*, (7), 10–11.

Lai, J., & Pittelkow, M. R. (2007). Physiological effects of ultrasound mist on fibroblasts. *International Journal of Dermatology, 46*(6), 587–593.

Lapidoth, M., Adatto, M., & David, M. (2007). Targeted UVB phototherapy for psoriasis: A preliminary study. *Clinical and Experimental Dermatology, 32*(6), 642–645.

Lindblad, M., Tano, E., Lindahl, C., & Huss, F. (2019). Ultraviolet-C decontamination of a hospital room: Amount of UV light needed. *Burns: Journal of the International Society for Burn Injuries,* S0305-4179(0319). 30092-30090.

McDiarmid, T., Burns, P., Lewith, G., & Machin, D. (1985). Ultrasound in the treatment of pressure sores. *Physiotherapy, 71,* 66–70.

Michailidis, L., Bergin, S. M., Haines, T. P., & Williams, C. M. (2018). A systematic review to compare the effect of low-frequency ultrasonic versus nonsurgical sharp debridement on the healing rate of chronic diabetes-related foot ulcers. *Ostomy/ Wound Management, 64*(9), 39–46.

Morykwas, M., & Marks, M. W. (1998). Effects of ultraviolet light on fibroblast fibronectin production and lattice contraction. *Wounds, 10*(4), 111–117.

Nussbaum, E. L., Flett, H., Hitzig, S. L., McGillivray, C., Leber, D., Morris, H., et al. (2013). Ultraviolet-C irradiation in the management of pressure ulcers in people with spinal cord injury: a randomized, placebo-controlled trial. *Archives of Physical Medicine and Rehabilitation, 94*(4), 650–659.

Park, K.-H., Koak, J.-Y., Kim, S.-K., Han, C.-H., & Heo, S.-J. (2013). The effect of ultraviolet-C irradiation via a bactericidal ultraviolet sterilizer on an anodized titanium implant: A study in rabbits.

The International Journal of Oral & Maxillofacial Implants, 28(1), 57–66.

Parrish, J. A., Zaynoun, S., & Anderson, R. R. (1981). Cumulative effects of repeated subthreshold doses of ultraviolet radiation. *The Journal of Investigative Dermatology, 76*(5), 356–358.

Peschen, M., Weichenthal, M., Schopf, E., & Vanscheidt, W. (1997). Low-frequency ultrasound treatment of chronic venous leg ulcers in an outpatient therapy. *Acta Dermato-Venereologica, 77*(4), 311–314.

Pitt, W. G., McBride, M. O., Lunceford, J. K., Roper, R. J., & Sagers, R. D. (1994). Ultrasonic enhancement of antibiotic action on gram-negative bacteria. *Antimicrobial Agents and Chemotherapy, 38*(11), 2577–2582.

Polak, A., Franek, A., Blaszczak, E., Nawrat-Szoltysik, A., Taradaj, J., Wiercigroch, L., et al. (2014). A prospective, randomized, controlled, clinical study to evaluate the efficacy of high-frequency ultrasound in the treatment of Stage II and Stage III pressure ulcers in geriatric patients. *Ostomy/Wound Management, 60*(8), 16–28.

Polak, A., Taradaj, J., Nawrat-Szoltysik, A., Stania, M., Dolibog, P., Blaszczak, E., et al. (2016). Reduction of pressure ulcer size with high-voltage pulsed current and high-frequency ultrasound: A randomised trial. *Journal of Wound Care, 25*(12), 742–754.

Prather, J. L., Tummel, E. K., Patel, A. B., Smith, D. J., & Gould, L. J. (2015). Prospective randomized controlled trial comparing the effects of noncontact low-frequency ultrasound with standard care in healing split-thickness donor sites. *Journal of the American College of Surgeons, 221*(2), 309–318.

Ramsay, C. A., & Challoner, A. V. (1976). Vascular changes in human skin after ultraviolet irradiation. *The British Journal of Dermatology, 94*(5), 487–493.

Ramundo, J., & Gray, M. (2008). Is ultrasonic mist therapy effective for debriding chronic wounds? *Journal of Wound, Ostomy, and Continence Nursing, 35*(6), 579–583.

Rao, B. K., Kumar, P., Rao, S., & Gurung, B. (2011). Bactericidal effect of ultraviolet C (UVC), direct and filtered through transparent plastic, on gram-positive cocci: An in vitro study [In Vitro]. *Ostomy/Wound Management, 57*(7), 46–52.

Reddy, M., Gill, S. S., Kalkar, S. R., Wu, W., Anderson, P. J., & Rochon, P. A. (2008). Treatment of pressure ulcers: A systematic review. *JAMA, 300*(22), 2647–2662.

Ritter, M. A., Olberding, E. M., & Malinzak, R. A. (2007). Ultraviolet lighting during orthopaedic surgery and the rate of infection. *The Journal of Bone and Joint Surgery. American Volume, 89*(9), 1935–1940.

Robertson, V. J., & Baker, K. G. (2001). A review of therapeutic ultrasound: Effectiveness studies. *Physical Therapy, 81*(7), 1339.

Selkowitz, D. M., Cameron, M. H., Mainzer, A., & Wolfe, R. (2002). Efficacy of pulsed low-intensity ultrasound in wound healing: A single-case design. *Ostomy/Wound Management, 48*(4), 40–44, 46–50.

Serena, T., Lee, S. K., Lam, K., Attar, P., Meneses, P., & Ennis, W. (2009). The impact of noncontact, nonthermal, low-frequency ultrasound on bacterial counts in experimental and chronic wounds. *Ostomy/Wound Management, 55*(1), 22–30.

Sheldon, J. L., Kokjohn, T. A., & Martin, E. L. (2005). The effects of salt concentration and growth phase on MRSA solar and germicidal ultraviolet radiation resistance. *Ostomy/Wound Management, 51*(1), 36–38, 42–34, 46 passim.

Spielholz, N. I., & Kloth, L. C. (2000). Electrical stimulation and pulsed electromagnetic energy: Differences in opinion. *Ostomy/ Wound Management, 46*(5), 8, 10, 12.

Stanisic, M. M., Provo, B. J., Larson, D. L., & Kloth, L. C. (2005). Wound debridement with 25 kHz ultrasound. *Advances in Skin & Wound Care, 18*(9), 484–490.

Sullivan, P. K., & Conner-Kerr, T. A. (2000). A comparative study of the effects of UVC irradiation on select procaryotic and eucaryotic wound pathogens. *Ostomy/Wound Management, 46* (10), 28–34.

Suo, W., Wang, X., & Wang, D. (2002). Effect of Ultraviolet C irradiation on expression of transforming growth factor-beta in wound. *Chinese Journal of Rehabilitation Theory Practices, 8*(5).

Tan, J., Abisi, S., Smith, A., & Burnand, K. G. (2007). A painless method of ultrasonically assisted debridement of chronic leg ulcers: A pilot study. *European Journal of Vascular and Endovascular Surgery, 33*(2), 234–238.

Taradaj, J., Franek, A., Brzezinska-Wcislo, L., Cierpka, L., Dolibog, P., Chmielewska, D., et al. (2008). The use of therapeutic ultrasound in venous leg ulcers: A randomized, controlled clinical trial. *Phlebology, 23*(4), 178–183.

Taskan, I., Ozyazgan, I., Tercan, M., Kardas, H. Y., Balkanli, S., Saraymen, R., et al. (1997). A comparative study of the effect of ultrasound and electrostimulation on wound healing in rats. *Plastic and Reconstructive Surgery, 100*(4), 966–972.

ter Reit, G., Kessels, A. G., & Knipschild, P. (1996). A randomized clinical trial of ultrasound in the treatment of pressure ulcers. *Physical Therapy, 76*(12), 1301–1312.

Thai, T. P., Houghton, P. E., Campbell, K. E., & Woodbury, M. G. (2002). Ultraviolet light C in the treatment of chronic wounds with MRSA: A case study. *Ostomy/Wound Management, 48*(11), 52–60.

Thao, T. P., Keast, D. H., Campbell, K. E., Woodbury, M. G., & Houghton, P. E. (2005). Effect of ultraviolet light C on bacterial colonization in chronic wounds. *Ostomy/Wound Management, 51*(10), 32–45.

Thawer, H. A., & Houghton, P. E. (2004). Effects of ultrasound delivered through a mist of saline to wounds in mice with diabetes mellitus. *Journal of Wound Care, 13*(5), 171–176.

Voigt, J., Wendelken, M., Driver, V., & Alvarez, O. M. (2011). Low-frequency ultrasound (20–40 kHz) as an adjunctive therapy for chronic wound healing: A systematic review of the literature and meta-analysis of eight randomized controlled trials. *The International Journal of Lower Extremity Wounds, 10*(4), 190–199.

Watson, J. M., Kang'ombe, A. R., Soares, M. O., Chuang, L. H., Worthy, G., Bland, J. M., et al. (2011). Use of weekly, low dose, high frequency ultrasound for hard to heal venous leg ulcers: The VenUS III randomised controlled trial. *BMJ, 342*, d1092.

Weichenthal, M., Mohr, P., Stegman, W., & Breitbart, E. (1997). Low-frequency ultrasound treatment of chronic venous ulcers. *Wound Repair and Regeneration, 5*(1), 18–22.

Wendelken, M., Alvarez, O., Markowitz, L., Comfort, C., & Waltrous, L. (2006). Key insights on mapping wounds with ultrasound. *Podiatry Today, 19*(7), 70–74.

White, J., Ivins, N., Wilkes, A., Carolan-Rees, G., & Harding, K. G. (2016). Non-contact low-frequency ultrasound therapy compared with UK standard of care for venous leg ulcers: A single-centre, assessor-blinded, randomised controlled trial. *International Wound Journal, 13*(5), 833–842.

Wiegand, C., Bittenger, K., Galiano, R. D., Driver, V. R., & Gibbons, G. W. (2017). Does noncontact low-frequency ultrasound therapy contribute to wound healing at the molecular level? *Wound Repair and Regeneration, 25*(5), 871–882.

Wound, Ostomy and Continence Nurses Society. (2014). *Guideline for management of wounds in patients with lower-extremity arterial disease.* WOCN Clinical Practice Guideline Series 1. Mt. Laurel, NJ: Author.

Wound, Ostomy and Continence Nurses Society. (2016). *Guideline for management of patients with pressure ulcers (injuries).* WOCN Clinical Practice Guideline Series #2. Mt. Laurel, Author.

Wound, Ostomy and Continence Nurses Society. (2017). *Guideline for management of wounds in patients with lower-extremity venous disease.* WOCN Clinical Practice Guideline Series 4. Mt. Laurel, NJ: Author.

Wound, Ostomy and Continence Nurses Society. (2021). *Guideline for management of patients with lower extremity wounds due to diabetes mellitus and/or neuropathic disease.* WOCN Clinical Practice Guideline Series 3. Mt. Laurel, NJ: Author.

Yamada, Y., Yamada, M., Ueda, T., & Sakurai, K. (2014). Reduction of biofilm formation on titanium surface with ultraviolet-C pre-irradiation. *Journal of Biomaterials Applications, 29*(2), 161–171.

Yarboro, D., Millar, A., & Smith, R. (2019). The effects of ultraviolet c irradiation in the treatment of chronic wounds: A retrospective, descriptive study. *Wound Management & Prevention, 65*(7), 16–22.

Yin, R., Dai, T., Avci, P., Jorge, A. E. S., de Melo, W. C. M. A., Vecchio, D., et al. (2013). Light based anti-infectives: Ultraviolet C irradiation, photodynamic therapy, blue light, and beyond. *Current Opinion in Pharmacology, 13*(5), 731–762.

Young, S., & Dyson, M. (1990a). Effect of therapeutic ultrasound on the healing of full-thickness excised lesions. *Ultrasonics, 28*, 175–180.

Young, S., & Dyson, M. (1990b). Macrophage repsonsiveness to therapeutic ultrasound. *Ultrasound in Medicine & Biology, 16*, 809–816.

Zhou, S., Bachem, M. G., Seufferlein, T., Li, Y., Gross, H. J., & Schmelz, A. (2008). Low intensity pulsed ultrasound accelerates macrophage phagocytosis by a pathway that requires actin polymerization, Rho, and Src/MAPKs activity. *Cellular Signalling, 20*(4), 695–704.

Zhou, S., Schmelz, A., Seufferlein, T., Li, Y., Zhao, J., & Bachem, M. G. (2004). Molecular mechanisms of low intensity pulsed ultrasound in human skin fibroblasts. *The Journal of Biological Chemistry, 279*(52), 54463–54469.

28

Wound Pain

Alisha Oropallo and Waqaas Quraishi

OBJECTIVES

1. List 5 parameters for wound pain assessment.
2. Distinguish between manifestations of wound pain at rest and wound pain during dressing change procedure.
3. Identify key nonpharmacologic interventions for wound pain.
4. Describe three strategies for managing procedural wound pain and managing nonprocedural wound pain.

5. Describe the pharmacologic options for treating wound pain.
6. Describe appropriate indications for and application of topical analgesics.
7. Identify the principles that guide chronic wound pain management.

Although not all wounds are painful, in general, most acute and chronic wounds cause moderate to severe pain. Consequences of wound pain range from self-care deficit and declination of care to loss of income and poor quality of life (see Chapter 4). Management of this pain can be challenging. Given a thoughtful approach and modern pharmacologic and nonpharmacologic interventions, most patients can achieve an acceptable level of pain control. This chapter presents approaches to preventing and managing acute and chronic wound pain.

PAIN ASSESSMENT

Pain related to wounds is complex involving physiological and psychological components and often underreported. Physiologic components may involve both nociceptive and neuropathic elements depending on the tissue damage or neuronal dysfunction (Bechert & Abraham, 2009). Wound pain may also be affected by the personal, familial, and cultural backgrounds creating different patient's experiences and expression of pain (Smith, 2020).

The World Union of Wound Healing Society's consensus document categorizes wound pain as: (1) background pain or basal or baseline pain felt at rest including pain associated with an infection; (2) incident pain or breakthrough pain occurring during the patient's activities of daily living; (3) procedural pain during routine dressing changes; and (4) operative pain associated with wound debridement and wound biopsy (Smith, 2020).

Assessment of wound pain is not only critical to determine management strategies, the US Joint Commission mandates regular and ongoing assessment of pain in hospitalized patients (Joint Commission, 2000). Wound pain assessments should be conducted before, during, and after wound procedures such as dressing changes and debridement (see Checklist 28.1). Experts advocate the use of a valid and reliable self-reported pain assessment tools as one component of a comprehensive wound pain assessment. To be effective, however, the pain scale must be compatible with the patient's age and cognitive ability (Ahn, Stechmiller, Fillingim, Lyon, & Garvan, 2015; European Pressure Ulcer Advisory Panel, National Pressure Injury Advisory Panel, Pan Pacific Pressure Injury Alliance (EPIAP, NPIAP, PPPIA), 2019; Gunes, 2008; Reddy, Kohr, Queen, Keast, & Sibbald, 2003; World Union of Wound Healing Societies (WUWHS), 2004; Wound, Ostomy and Continence Nurses Society, 2014, 2016, 2017). Various pain scales are available for use. Table 28.1 lists the examples of pain assessment tools and their intended populations. Appendix A provides several illustrations of pain assessment scales and wound pain models available. Chapter 13, Table 13.2, provides the typical assessment findings for venous, arterial, and neuropathic leg ulcer pain.

NONPHARMACOLOGIC PAIN CONTROL

Many nonpharmacologic pain control measures are essential when caring for a patient with a wound. A simple and effective intervention is acknowledging a patient's pain and making a commitment to the patient to address it. Explaining the

CHECKLIST 28.1 Wound Pain Assessments Before, During, and After Wound Procedures

Wound Pain at Rest
- ✓ Description (e.g., aching, throbbing, sharp, burning, tingling)
- ✓ Location (e.g., wound only, surrounding area, both)
- ✓ Triggers (e.g., touch, pressure, movement, positioning, day vs night)
- ✓ Pain reducers (e.g., analgesia, bathing, repositioning)
- ✓ Pain intensity (e.g., pain scale)

Wound Pain During Dressing-Related Procedures
- ✓ Description (e.g., aching, throbbing, sharp, burning, tingling)
- ✓ Location (e.g., wound only, surrounding area, both)
- ✓ Triggers (e.g., dressing removal, exposure to air, cleansing, dressing application)
- ✓ Pain reducers (e.g., time-out, slow or self-removal of dressing)
- ✓ Pain intensity (e.g., pain scale)

Wound Pain After Dressing-Related Procedures
- ✓ Time it to for pain to return to baseline
- ✓ Pain intensity (e.g., pain scale)

TABLE 28.1 Examples of Self-Reported Pain Assessment Tools and Intended Population

Pain Assessment Tool	Intended Population
FLACC (Face, Leg, Activity Cry and Consolability) Pain Scale	Children 2 months to 7 years
CRIES Pain Scale	Neonates (0–6 months)
COMFORT Scale	Children, adults, adults with cognitive impairment or inability to communicate
Wong-Baker FACES Pain Rating Scale	Children, adults, adults with cognitive impairment or inability to communicate
Visual Analog Scale	Adults
Numerical Rating Scales (NRS)	Adults
McGill Pain Index or Questionnaire	Adults
Abbey Pain Scale	Adults with cognitive impairment
PAINAD Pain Assessment in Advanced Dementia	Adults with advanced dementia

BOX 28.1 Nonpharmacologic Interventions for Pain Reduction During Dressing Changes

- Minimize degree of sensory stimulus (e.g., drafts from open windows, prodding, and poking).
- Allow patient to perform own dressing changes.
- Allow "time-outs" during painful procedures.
- Schedule dressing changes when patient is feeling best.
- Give an analgesic and then schedule dressing change during time of drug's peak effect.
- Moisten dried dressings before removal.
- Avoid use of cytotoxic cleansers.
- Avoid excessive packing.
- Minimize number of dressing changes.
- Prevent periwound trauma.
- Position and support wounded area for comfort.
- Consider using low-adhesive or nonadhesive dressings.
- Offer and use distraction techniques/alternative therapies (e.g., headphones, TV, music, warm blanket, visualization, acupuncture, and music therapy).

potential harmful effects of pain on healing, along with a careful explanation of how to manage pain, will help to shape the patient's expectations and increase the individual's sense of control. Both of these strategies may reduce the pain experienced (Acute Pain Management Panel (APMP), 1992). Additional interventions related to pain control begin with controlling and reducing procedural pain or cyclic acute pain through appropriate and conscientious topical care. Active nonpharmacologic pain control measures can include

acupuncture, music therapy, a fleece warming boot or a warm blanket, and visualization. Such measures are listed in Box 28.1. Emerging technologies such as virtual reality may have a role in acutely painful procedures (Chan, Foster, Sambell, & Leong, 2018).

Wound Cleansing

Avoiding cytotoxic topical agents including antiseptics and antimicrobials, harsh chemicals, and highly concentrated agents for wound cleansing can significantly reduce wound pain. In general, judicious use of these agents should be utilized. Additionally, clinicians should take into consideration efficacy, adverse reactions, dosing, and systemic absorption (Tong et al., 2018).

Periwound Skin Care

Eroded or denuded wound margins can contribute significantly to the pain experienced by the patient. Use of nonsting skin protectants, silicone adhesive, and self-adhesive polyurethane foam on intact skin can prevent painful denuding of skin or skin stripping of the stratum corneum (Matsumura et al., 2014). Use of moisture barrier ointments, protective barrier films, or skin barriers on open areas can prevent and/or minimize the pain secondary to damaged wound margins especially in the aging population (Holloway & Mahoney, 2021). Chapter 10 provides a detailed description and formulary of products useful for prevention and management of moisture, chemical, and adhesive-related skin damage.

Debridement

Although many factors are considered when a method of debridement is selected, pain is a frequently neglected consideration. Regardless of the method of debridement selected, pain assessment and management must be considered. Nonselective wet-to-dry dressing changes for mechanical debridement should be used sparingly secondary to increased pain levels (Wongkietkachorn, Surakunprapha, Titapun, Wongkietkachorn, & Wongkietkachorn, 2019). Using autolysis for debridement, when feasible and appropriate, can significantly reduce the pain associated with this procedure. Recent debridement methods include hydrosurgery, low-frequency ultrasonic, and enzymatic collagenase debridement may be less painful. However, these newer types of debridement demonstrate inconclusive findings in a recent review with patient safety not clearly defined (Thomas et al., 2021).

Conservative or surgical sharp debridement provokes acute noncyclical pain, which leads patients to ask the clinician to stop the debridement unless they are given additional analgesia or anesthesia (Evans & Gray, 2005). When sharp debridement is indicated, properly timed pharmacologic interventions are an important consideration and are described in detail later in this chapter (Cazander et al., 2020).

Inflammation and Edema

Inflammation and edema contribute to wound pain, so measures that reduce them will provide pain relief. Such measures include elevation of edematous extremities, appropriate edema-reducing dressings, devices such as compression bandaging and sequential compression pumps, and systemic medications (O'Donnell et al., 2014). Application of ice may be effective if edema is largely related to inflammation from traumatic injury (Sugasawa et al., 2020). Local cryotherapy in a normothermic individual may reduce inflammation both at the gene and the protein levels. IL-6, IL-17A, and IL-1β gene expression levels were significantly downregulated in animal models (Guillot et al., 2017).

Support and Positioning

Binders, splints, body positioners, and other devices that stabilize a wound can significantly reduce pain, especially pain related to mobilization. Care must be taken to fit these devices properly so that the wound dressing is appropriately accommodated and increased pressure on the wound is not created. However, certain medical devices, such as immobilizers and negative pressure therapy devices, can become a source of pain. Various methods can be used to reduce pain and include pressure redistribution mattress for pressure injury and use of nonadherent foam dressings at the device–wound interface.

Positioning patients for comfort and offloading their wound can reduce pain at the wound site and improve healing. Recommendations of the National Pressure Injury Advisory Panel suggest that offloading support surfaces can offer pain relief to bed-bound or chair-bound patients. Individuals should be encouraged to request a "time-out" during any procedure that causes pain. Patients should be premedicated, if needed, before activities that cause or trigger pain. Using lift sheets (to lift and move) instead of draw sheets (that drag) to move patients in bed prevents friction and shear, which can cause painful injuries to the skin and deeper tissues (Kottner et al., 2019).

Wound Dressings

Many commercially available moisture-retentive dressings are designed to manage the wound. The main analgesic efficacy of these products appears to stem from their ability to keep the wound moist, maintain a consistent wound microenvironment that is protected from the external environment, reduce inflammation, and stimulate healing. Moisture-retentive dressings have at least some capacity to reduce pain associated with wounds (Kottner et al., 2019). Thus, dressings can be selected with the aim of reducing pain in a particular patient. The most effective dressing will depend on patient factors such as volume of exudate, condition of surrounding skin, wound depth, and necrotic tissue. Dry, wet-to-dry, or wet-to-damp dressings are not moisture retentive and consequently are the most painful. As the gauze dehydrates, it tends to adhere to the wound surface and, along with damaging new granulation tissue, is painful to remove (Kottner et al., 2019). The psychological impact of pain can in turn physiologically impact wound healing by stressors increasing cortisol levels and the subsequent repercussions (Matsumura et al., 2014). Dressings should be selected that will, upon removal, minimize the degree of sensory stimulus to the wound area (Kottner et al., 2019).

Box 28.1 lists several interventions for nonpharmacologic pain control during dressing changes.

PHARMACOLOGIC INTERVENTIONS

The World Health Organization's (WHO) Pain Clinical Ladder, a three-step analgesic ladder approach initially for the treatment of cancer pain, has also been used to guide the treatment of nonmalignant pain (Boxes 28.2 and 28.3 and Fig. 28.1). This approach uses a combination of pain control medications based on assessment of pain intensity. If pain persists after reassessment, the ladder guides the clinician in adding a medication or combination of medications to effectively control pain (Anekar & Cascella, 2021). However, in light of the national opioid crisis, "WHO Pain Ladder" protocol initially developed in 1986 has been challenged with modifications providing a wide range of safe alternatives before resorting to potent opioids and invasive interventions (Pergolizzi & Raffa, 2014). New approaches to pain control include neuromodulation, nerve blocks, intrathecal drug administration, peripheral nerve blockade, and neurolysis (Pergolizzi & Raffa, 2014). Pharmacologic interventions can be topical, subcutaneous or perineural injectable, or systemic.

Topical Medications

Topical analgesics are commonly used before debridement or before manipulation inside the wound margins, which includes wound packing or application of materials that contact the wound. These medications usually are in the form of a jelly, cream, or ointment, although liquid forms, sprays, and patches are available. They generally include lidocaine or another local anesthetic with sodium channel receptor blockade activity. Topical anesthetics require at least 15–30 minutes to reach optimal analgesic states. Although lidocaine

---

BOX 28.2 World Health Organization Analgesic Ladder*

Step 1

Patients with mild to moderate pain should be treated with a nonopioid analgesic, which should be combined with an adjuvant drug if an indication for one exists.

For example: Nonsteroidal antiinflammatory drugs, acetylsalicylic acid, and acetaminophen.

Step 2

Patients who have limited opioid exposure and moderate to severe pain or who fail to achieve adequate relief after a trial of a nonopioid analgesic should be treated with an opioid conventionally used for moderate pain.

For example: Step 1 medications plus codeine, tramadol, and hydrocodone.

Step 3

Patients who have severe pain or who fail to achieve adequate relief after appropriate administration of drugs in step 2 of the analgesic ladder should receive an opioid conventionally used for severe pain.

For example: Step 1 medications and morphine (discontinue step 2 medications).

Note: Unrelieved pain should raise a red flag that attracts the clinician's attention.

Data from Anekar, A. A., & Cascella, M. (2022). WHO analgesic ladder. In *StatPearls*. Treasure Island, FL: StatPearls Publishing. Available from: https://www.ncbi.nlm.nih.gov/books/NBK554435/.
*See Fig. 28.1.

BOX 28.3 Examples of Opioid, Nonopioid, and Adjuvant Medications

Opioids
- Codeine
- Dolophine (Methadone)
- Fentanyl
- Hydromorphone (Dilaudid)
- Levorphanol
- Morphine
- Oxycodone
- Tramadol

Combination Medications
- Percocet (oxycodone/acetaminophen)
- Lortab, Vicodin, Norco (hydrocodone/acetaminophen)

Nonopioids
- Aspirin
- Acetaminophen
- Nonsteroidal antiinflammatory drugs (NSAIDs)

Adjuvant Medications
- Tricyclic antidepressants
- Anticonvulsants
- Systemic local anesthetics
- Topical anesthetics

Note that many of these medications should be avoided or given at an adjusted dose in the elderly.

---

preparations have been widely available and safely used for years, topical use of these preparations in open wounds is considered off-label in the United States. Topical lidocaine products should be used with caution, taking into consideration toxic doses and levels, especially with large wounds, where systemic absorption of very large doses could potentially lead to neurologic and/or cardiovascular toxicity.

The most commonly used topical analgesics include 2% and 4% lidocaine jelly, which act on only the superficial layer of tissue and can inactivate exposed wound pain receptors.

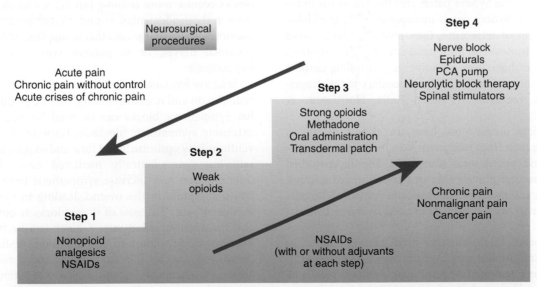

Fig. 28.1 Transition from the original WHO three-step analgesic ladder to the revised WHO fourth-step form. The additional step 4 is an "interventional" step and includes invasive and minimally invasive techniques. This updated WHO ladder provides a bidirectional approach.

BOX 28.4 Application of Eutectic Mixture of Local Anesthetics (EMLA) Cream

- 10 g EMLA can safely cover a surface area of approximately 100 cm².
- Apply directly to wound.
- Cover with plastic or transparent wrap for 20 min.
- If pain is not managed after 20 min, increase time to 45–60 min.

Note that this is an off-label use of EMLA cream. The product insert directions state to apply to intact skin; however, extensive experience with topical use on open wounds suggests this is safe. The recommendation is to limit to 10 g of EMLA per use.

Data from Evans, E., & Gray, M. (2005). Do topical analgesics reduce pain associated with wound dressing changes? *Journal of Wound Ostomy & Continence Nursing, 32*(5), 287–290.

The strongest evidence base for the effectiveness of topical analgesics in wound care is associated with eutectic mixture of local anesthetics (EMLA) cream, which contains 2.5% lidocaine and 2.5% prilocaine. Although manufacturer's instructions indicate EMLA should only be used on intact skin, there is no evidence of harm from application to open wounds, and it is widely used. It is applied 30–60 minutes before debridement under occlusion with a film dressing (Navarro-Rodriguez, Suarez-Serrano, Martin-Valero, Marcen-Roman, & de-la-Casa-Almeida, 2021). Instructions for use of EMLA cream are given in Box 28.4 (Evans & Gray, 2005). A Cochrane review found statistically significant reduction in debridement pain scores with EMLA cream (Briggs et al., 2012). A recent randomized controlled trial demonstrated EMLA cream as the primary dressing for relieving wound-related pain for patients with painful chronic leg ulcers (Purcell, Buckley, King, Moyle, & Marshall, 2018).

Topical transdermal anesthetic patches also may be useful. Examples include the Synera patch and the Lidoderm (lidocaine) patch. The Synera patch incorporates 70 mg of lidocaine and 70 mg of tetracaine, thus providing fairly rapid onset (20–30 minutes) and prolonged duration (up to hours). Fentanyl patches have been effective in controlling chronic pain but are to be used with caution secondary to their capricious systemic regulation (Pastore, Kalia, Horstmann, & Roberts, 2015).

Topical opioid preparations have also shown efficacy in the controlling pain from malignant skin infiltration, cutaneous ulcers, and severe oral mucositis. The most-studied preparations use morphine either in a compounded solution or gel form. A recent study demonstrates improved wound-related pain relief with morphine-loaded hydrogel (Mateus et al., 2019).

Cannabis-based therapies have been gaining traction in medical use. Preliminary studies using topical cannabis with venous leg ulcers demonstrate promising results in pain control (Maida, Shi, Fazzari, & Zomparelli, 2021). More vigorous clinical trials are needed before adoption into clinical practice guidelines.

Subcutaneous or Perineural Injectable Medications

Injectable medications (subcutaneous or perineural) frequently contain the same type of active drug that is found in the topical analgesic formulations (local anesthetics such as lidocaine). However, these medications are in solution and are designed to be injected into the soft tissue. These medications include lidocaine or longer-acting agents (e.g., bupivacaine and tetracaine). Epinephrine can be added to these medications to cause vasoconstriction, increasing the duration of action, as well as decreasing bleeding. Epinephrine is contraindicated for use in distal areas such as hands and feet because of the risk of necrosis from interruption of blood supply. Epinephrine is generally avoided in wounds due to concern of impairing blood supply, although it may be useful in extremely vascular wounds. Injectable local anesthetics can be used for either field or regional blockade.

A *field blockade* is accomplished by injecting local anesthetic adjacent to or directly into the wound margins, encircling the entire area (Robards & Hadzic, 2007). It blocks transmission of pain signals that are carried in the superficial cutaneous nerves that supply the wound area. At times, injection within the wound edges is less painful. If tolerated, however, the block is generally more effective when the injection is made outside the wound margins. Inflammation in the wound may inactivate or reduce the activity of the local anesthetic.

A *regional* or *nerve block* is accomplished by injecting local anesthetic into an often singular, proximal location where the larger nerve bundles are contained. Examples of regional blocks include not only digital, wrist, and ankle blocks but also other larger, more proximal nerves. Brachial plexus blockade and blockade of lower extremity nerves in the popliteal fossa may provide larger areas of coverage. Regional blocks require more training but are useful in the management and debridement of wounds that either cross many dermatomes, cover a large area that is supplied by many separate proximal nerves, or in patients with severe periwound hyperalgesia.

Selective blockade of the sympathetic nervous system may reduce pain and improve healing. Stellate ganglion and lumbar sympathetic blocks can be used for upper and lower extremity sympathetic blockade, respectively. These interventions may optimize blood flow and oxygen delivery while relieving sympathetically mediated pain. Trauma and inflammation may increase sympathetic tone and upregulate α-receptors in the wound, leading to sympathetically mediated pain. The goal of these blocks is both diagnostic and therapeutic. Oftentimes a block can be followed with a neurolytic procedure to provide longer-lasting analgesia. Neurolysis can be thermal (cryoablation, radiofrequency ablation), chemical (alcohol-based), or even mechanical (surgical resection). Dorsal column stimulation is another method for effective long-term sympathetic blockade (Wu et al., 2008).

Use of Regional and General Anesthesia for Debridement

Sharp surgical debridement in patients without complete neuropathy requires anesthesia to protect the patient from the stress response initiated by the painful stimulus (O'Neill et al., 2012). Sodium channel blockade with "local anesthetics" such as lidocaine, bupivacaine, or mepivacaine defines the basis of regional anesthesia, which in turn protects the central nervous system (CNS) from assault of action potentials associated with afferent information. The neuroanatomy and the dermatomal distribution of the surgical stimulus form the basis of selection of the mode for drug disposition: locally (field block), peripherally (nerve bundle), or centrally (neuroaxial: epidural, intrathecal). In the absence of sodium channel blockade, some reasonable combination of intravenous and/or inhalational anesthetics in the form of general anesthesia would be required to prevent autonomic or musculoskeletal reflexes. Standard real-time physiologic monitoring as recommended by the American Society of Anesthesiologists (ASA) would be utilized by a qualified anesthesia personnel to support homeostasis (ASA, 2020).

Systemic Medications

The goal of systemic medication administration as a pain control strategy is not to stop pain signal transmission from the wound but to modulate the response of the CNS to that pain signal. Whether given intravenously, subcutaneously, transcutaneously, or orally, many pain management choices are available when utilizing systemic pain control (Tables 28.2–28.4). These include nonsteroidal antiinflammatory drugs (NSAIDs), opioids (e.g., morphine, methadone), oral lidocaine, acetaminophen, partial μ-receptor agonists (e.g., tramadol), anticonvulsants (e.g., gabapentin [Neurontin]), antidepressants (e.g., Cymbalta, Elavil), and clonidine (central α2-adrenergic agonist that reduces sympathetic outflow) (Giovannitti, Thoms, & Crawford, 2015). These

TABLE 28.2 Recommended Starting Doses (and Equivalence) for Opioid Treatment of Intrinsic Wound Pain

PO/PR (mg)	Analgesic	IV or IM (mg)
30	Morphine	1–5 IV or 5–10 IM
6	Hydromorphone (Dilaudid)	0.2–0.6 or 1.5
20	Methadone	10–20
Not recommended	Meperidine (Demerol)	10–30 or 100[a]
60	Codeine	30–60
5–10	Oxycodone (Percocet)	N/A

IM, intramuscular; *IV*, intravenous; *PO*, by mouth; *PR*, per rectum.
[a]Meperidine should not be used for analgesia because normeperidine, a metabolite, may accumulate. Seizures are common when high doses (1000 mg in 1 day or 600 mg/day for several days) are given. Meperidine is more likely to cause dependence than other clinically used opioids. Note that many of these medications should be avoided or given at an adjusted dose in the elderly (American Geriatrics Society, 2019).

TABLE 28.3 Agents Appropriate for Sedation/Analgesia for Procedures in Adults

Agent	Dose (IV)	Frequency
Diazepam	1–2 mg	Every 3–10 min
Lorazepam	0.05 mg/kg (max 4 mg)	One time
Midazolam	0.25–1 mg	Every 1–5 min
Fentanyl	Loading dose up 1 μg/kg, then 12.5–50 μg	Every 5–10 min
Meperidine	12.5–25 mg	Every 2–15 min
Morphine	1–3 mg	Every 2–15 min
Droperidol	0.625–1.25 mg	Every 5–10 min

Note that many of these medications should be avoided or given at an adjusted dose in the elderly (American Geriatrics Society, 2019).

TABLE 28.4 Pharmacologic Interventions for Neuropathic Pain

Type of Pain	Medication
Dysesthesia	Capsaicin cream topically applied three to four times a day; may take 3 weeks for effect to be seen Gabapentin or pregabalin Selective serotonin reuptake inhibitor (e.g., fluoxetine, paroxetine) Serotonin and noradrenergic reuptake inhibitors (e.g., venlafaxine) Dextromethorphan syrup Tricyclic antidepressant (e.g., imipramine, amitriptyline)
Paresthesia	Anticonvulsant (e.g., carbamazepine [Tegretol], and phenytoin) Analgesic (e.g., Tramadol)
Muscular pain	Muscle relaxant (e.g., metaxalone, baclofen [Lioresal], tizanidine by mouth)
General neuropathic pain	Analgesics (e.g., lidocaine [Lidoderm] patch or lidocaine and tetracaine patch [Synera]) Gabapentin or pregabalin Hemorheologic agent (e.g., pentoxifylline [Trental]) Diuretic (e.g., furosemide, metolazone, bumetanide); may diminish pain with reduction in vasodilation Platelet inhibitor, cilostazol (Pletal) Bisphosphonate (e.g., pamidronate) Aldose reductase inhibitor (e.g., fidarestat, sorbinil) Antithromboembolitic therapy (e.g., heparin, warfarin, acetylsalicylic acid, antiinflammatory drugs) Clopidogrel (Plavix)

medications act on different target locations to combat the perception of pain. One of the actions of opioids is stimulation of receptors in the central and peripheral nervous system that downregulate both the afferent response to pain and central pain perception. For example, predominantly neuropathic pain is more responsive to antidepressants and anticonvulsants than to NSAIDs and opioids (Wound,

Ostomy and Continence Nurses Society, 2021). Some medications (e.g., NSAIDs) can also act by secondary means to reduce pain; that is, besides their direct analgesic properties, they reduce inflammation in the wound area, leading to a decrease in pain.

Combining several analgesic agents as part of a multifaceted approach is often more successful than using a single agent. Drugs may act additively or synergistically, allowing a reduction in the required dose of each agent, thus potentially reducing side effects while providing equal or even superior analgesia (Hopf & Weitz, 1994). For example, patients with mixed nociceptive and neuropathic pain respond better to a combination of an opioid and an adjunct medication such as pregabalin, gabapentin, duloxetine, or amitriptyline.

Further research is necessary to confirm which strategies or groups of strategies optimize pain relief and for which type of pain. For example, will applying a topical anesthetic compress before sharp debridement be more effective for this type of acute noncyclical pain than taking an oral pain medication? Around-the-clock medications might be most effective for chronic wound pain. Applying pain-reducing dressings or selecting pressure-reducing devices may prove to reduce acute cyclic pressure ulcer pain more effectively than pharmacologic measures.

Potential Complications of Medical Pain Management

Medications are rarely benign. Almost every drug has an associated set of potential side effects that can be inconvenient or harmful to the patient. The *Physician's Desk Reference* lists every reported side effect for each medication, but certain sets of complications are commonly encountered in the setting of analgesic control. The most powerful systemic analgesic agents are opioids; they have the most deleterious side effects, including sedation and respiratory depression. Elderly patients may be at greater risk of complications due to comorbid conditions and changes in pharmacokinetics and pharmacodynamics. On the other hand, pain may also be undertreated in the elderly due to underreporting and barriers to pain assessment (Kaye et al., 2020). Careful assessment and management are therefore critical.

Whenever opioids are administered, attention must be given to avoid excess sedation and respiratory depression (O'Neill et al., 2012). This is particularly true when opioids are given to manage procedural pain. Most health care facilities recognize five categories of sedation (Table 28.5). However, these categories are artificially drawn because sedation is a continuum. Sedation is different from simple pain control; sedation implies that the medications are given to specifically facilitate the ability to perform a painful procedure. The use of analgesics or sedatives solely to provide analgesia and/or allay anxiety (as occurs during dressing changes) but with no intention of performing a procedure is not considered sedation. Nonetheless, such drugs must be used with caution because respiratory depression and sedation can be induced whenever these drugs are used. Box 28.5 lists prescribing principles developed by the American Geriatrics Society Panel on

TABLE 28.5   Categories of Sedation

Level	Category	Definition
1	No sedation	
2	Minimal or light sedation	Patient responds normally to verbal commands
		Patient's ventilatory and cardiac functions are unaffected
3	Moderate or conscious sedation	Patient responds purposefully to verbal commands
		Patient's spontaneous ventilation is adequate
4	Deep sedation	Patient cannot be easily aroused
		Patient can respond purposefully following repeated or painful stimulation
		Patient has increased probability of respiratory or hemodynamic compromise
5	Anesthesia	Most often performed in operating room
		Patient is not arousable by painful stimulation

BOX 28.5   Principles That Guide Chronic Wound Pain Management

1. Manage intrinsic (background) pain with medications provided on a routine schedule.
2. Manage breakthrough pain with fast-acting medications as required (PRN).
3. Consider the following regarding route of administration:
   a. Use the least invasive route first (i.e., administer medications orally, when feasible).
   b. Use topical patches or creams when oral medications are insufficient.
4. Analgesic dose should be titrated to an effective level, starting with a low dose and advancing slowly.
5. Reassessment of background pain, as well as procedural or incident pain, should be ongoing and treatment individualized per patient need.
6. Monitor elderly patients closely for undesirable effects

American Geriatrics Society Panel on Persistent Pain in Older Persons (2002). The management of persistent pain in older persons. *Journal of the American Geriatrics Society, 50*(S6), S205–S224.

Pharmacological Management of Persistent Pain in Older Persons (2009) for chronic pain management in the long-term care setting.

A patient receiving sedation requires constant monitoring, which includes, at a minimum, cardiac monitoring, pulse oximetry, and direct supervision by a provider not involved in performing the procedure (Practice Guidelines for Moderate Procedural Sedation and Analgesia 2018, 2018). When a patient is being managed using sedation, the most serious common complication is respiratory depression. Therefore, the sedation should be performed only in a setting where a medical practitioner is available who can provide a definitive airway and handle the complications of ventilatory and/or circulatory collapse. Whenever patients are given analgesics for procedural pain, consideration should be given to monitoring, and facility guidelines should always be followed.

Potential side effects of opioid medications should be discussed at the initiation of therapy. High-dose and/or long-term opioid therapy may place patients at higher risk for hormonal disturbances (decreased testosterone) or sleep disorders. Respiratory depression is the most serious side effect. Other less serious but common side effects include nausea, vomiting, constipation, urinary retention, and pruritus. All patients receiving opioids should be given stool softeners and counseled on ways to prevent constipation, including increased fluid and fiber intake. Antiemetic medications, changing to a different opioid, or limiting opioid dose by using nonopioid analgesics (e.g., NSAIDs) can manage nausea and vomiting. Pruritus can be managed with diphenhydramine or other antihistamines.

Side effects of NSAIDs include stomach pain, ulcers, gastrointestinal bleeding, renal impairment, allergies, and platelet inhibition (Sostres, Gargallo, & Lanas, 2013). Side effects of acetaminophen are few, but overdoses (>4–6 g/day) can result in acute fulminant liver failure. Care should be exercised when using opioid–acetaminophen combinations, especially those with relatively low-potency opioids and high-dose acetaminophen (500 mg per tablet), such as Vicodin (hydrocodone–acetaminophen). Acetaminophen is a powerful adjunct, so it should be used when possible. For tolerant patients, it should be given separately as an around-the-clock drug to reduce the risk of liver injury. More potent opioids (e.g., oxycodone, hydromorphone [Dilaudid], morphine, and methadone) should be selected as well to reduce the number of doses required daily.

Side effects of antiepileptics and antidepressants include sedation, which usually resolves with continued use. These drugs can be started as a bedtime dose for several days to allow acclimatization.

Side effects of clonidine include sedation and dry mouth (acclimatization is rapid). It can decrease blood pressure and heart rate, but the low doses used to treat wound pain (lower than those commonly used to treat hypertension) rarely causes hypotension or bradycardia. Clonidine is available as a transdermal patch, which allows constant plasma levels and improved compliance. Usually the lowest dose (no. 1 or 2 patch) is sufficient. Clonidine should be used with caution and at the lowest possible dose in the elderly, as side effects are more common. American Geriatrics Society Panel on Pharmacological Management of Persistent Pain in Older Persons (2009) recommends against routine use of clonidine for treatment of hypertension in the elderly due to the potential for orthostatic hypotension and bradycardia (quality of evidence is low), but lower-dose clonidine has been used safely in the elderly for treatment of wound pain. Dexmedetomidine may reduce opioid requirements in tolerant patients (Kaye et al., 2020). It often increases perfusion and oxygenation in patients with hypoxic wounds because of their excess sympathetic tone or peripheral vascular disease, which may also reduce pain (Hopf & Weitz, 1994).

Addiction Concerns

The degree of pain that a patient experiences and reports often is influenced by the patient's fear of addiction. A common social and medical problem is substance abuse and treating painful wounds can be especially difficult in this population. Because patients who are addicted to alcohol or drugs can exhibit tolerance to CNS depressants and opioids, higher dosages of analgesic medications may be required. In addition, liver and kidney disease associated with alcohol or other drug abuse may alter the metabolism and excretion of opioids and other analgesics. Tolerance and altered metabolism, along with variability in recent drug use by the patient and attitudes among health care providers toward addicted patients, are factors that make designing an effective analgesic regimen for these patients difficult (Smith, 2020).

Furthermore, opioid-addicted patients may exhibit a tendency for hyperalgesia, in which patients experience a greater intensity of pain than expected for a given wound. When treating these individuals, the fundamental principle of pain management is the same as it is for other patients: complaints of pain should be taken seriously and treated aggressively (Cohen et al., 2004). Intravenous drug abusers may require higher doses of analgesics to obtain similar degrees of pain relief because of the development of opioid cross-tolerance. Careful consideration of adjunctive medications or interventions may be useful in this patient population.

The history of opioid prescribing has been particularly variable. Patients have commonly been undertreated with opioid pain medications when opioids were indicated (Owen et al., 1990). However, recent data show some alarming trends in prescription drug misuse and abuse over the past 10 years. In 2009, the American Pain Society detailed the guidelines for opioid prescribing. Most recently, the culture of opioid prescription has shifted once again. Prescribing of opioids for nonmalignant pain has decreased by nearly 40% over the past decade. The risks and benefits of opioid therapy should be carefully weighed and continually assessed in each patient (Manchikanti et al., 2017). Medication contracts between patient and prescriber, urine drug screenings, and periodic monitoring of prescriptions filled are instrumental in maintaining adherence to medical management.

Because patients frequently take inadequate doses of opioids because of their fear of addiction, they should be counseled as to proper and safe use of their medication. When doses are inadequate due to untoward side effects, different opioids should be tried and adjunct agents added to reduce the required opioid dose. Referral to a pain medicine specialist may be warranted if pain is poorly controlled or is refractory to appropriate dose escalation; interventions are needed; or comprehensive, multidisciplinary treatment is needed. Pain relief, safety, and active monitoring for medication misuse should be the cornerstones of opioid therapy (Smith, 2020).

Use of opioids for the treatment of chronic pain has come under recent scrutiny because of long-term consequences of opioid use (Dowell, Ragan, Jones, Baldwin, & Chou, 2022). An important consideration in the treatment of wound pain is the distinction between treating acute and chronic pain. Opioids are appropriate for management of severe acute interventional pain, for example, for debridement. A short course of opioids is appropriate for treatment of chronic wound pain, particularly at the start of treatment, when more procedures and lack of healing lead to more severe wound pain. The responsibility of the provider to exercise opioid stewardship is essential. The goal of therapy should be to transition to nonopioid wound management when feasible and not to routinely continue opioids long term.

CLINICAL CONSULT

A: Consult requested for an 82-year-old woman who bumped her shin on the dishwasher a month ago, causing a small wound that has increased in size and pain. The wound measures 4.5 × 2.5 × 0.2 cm is highly exudative with yellow slough. No periwound erythema. Polyurethane foam dressing in place and is changed daily. Both legs are edematous to the knee. Comorbidities include well-controlled hypertension and mild renal insufficiency (creatinine of 1.2 mg/dL). Formerly quite active; now resides in a skilled nursing facility due to leg ulcer. Has taken metoprolol 25 mg PO daily for many years. Recently began furosemide for leg edema and hydromorphone with acetaminophen as needed for pain. Patient states the pain score has remained 8 out of 10 for the past week.

D: Trauma-induced leg ulcer with severe pain and untreated edema.
P: Improve pain management, edema control, and removal of nonviable wound tissue.
I: (1) Apply topical anesthetic. (2) Debridement. (3) Begin modified compression (25% stretch) initially to accommodate pain. (4) Music therapy or visualization distraction. (5) May apply ice pack over the dressing if it provides relief.
E: Reassessment in 1 week. Patient understands that she will require compression therapy.

SUMMARY

- Managing pain associated with the presence of a wound enhances the cellular and molecular activities of wound healing.
- Pain management increases the patient's ability to participate in activities essential to healing.

- Pharmacologic agents need to be selected and titrated to the type and severity of pain.
- Nonpharmacologic interventions are also important to prevent exacerbation of pain.

SELF-ASSESSMENT QUESTIONS

1. True or False. Pain control for wound care involves a holistic individualized approach to the patient.
2. In a patient with edema, pain control can be managed by:
   a. Compression therapy
   b. Ambulation
   c. Position and support
   d. All of the above
3. True or False. A step-wise ladder of pharmacological agents is used when addressing patients with pain.

4. Pharmacologic interventions include:
   a. Topical analgesics
   b. Transdermal patches
   c. Injectable medications
   d. Field, selective, regional blocks
   e. All of the above

REFERENCES

Acute Pain Management Panel (APMP). (1992). Acute pain management: Operative or medical procedures and trauma. In *Clinical practice guideline. AHCPR publication no. 92-0032.* Rockville, MD: US Department of Health and Human Services, Public Health Service.

Ahn, H., Stechmiller, J., Fillingim, R., Lyon, D., & Garvan, C. (2015). Bodily pain intensity in nursing home residents with pressure ulcers: Analysis of national minimum data set 3.0. *Research in Nursing & Health, 38*(3), 207–212.

American Society of Anesthesiologists (ASA). (2020). *Standards for basic anesthetic monitoring.* Retrieved 3/13/2023 from:

https://www.openanesthesia.org/keywords/asa_standards_for_monitoring/.

American Geriatrics Society Panel on Pharmacological Management of Persistent Pain in Older Persons. (2009). Pharmacological management of persistent pain in older persons. *Journal of the American Geriatrics Society, 57*(8), 1331–1346. https://doi.org/10.1111/j.1532-5415.2009.02376.x. Epub 2009 Jul 2. PMID: 19573219.

American Geriatrics Society. (2019). Updated AGS Beers Criteria® for Potentially Inappropriate Medication Use in Older Adults. *Journal of the American Geriatrics Society, 67*(4), 674–694. https://doi.org/10.1111/jgs.15767.

Anekar, A. A., & Cascella, M. (2021). WHO analgesic ladder. In *StatPearls* StatPearls Publishing. http://www.ncbi.nlm.nih.gov/books/NBK554435/.

Bechert, K., & Abraham, S. E. (2009). Pain management and wound care. *The Journal of the American College of Certified Wound Specialists, 1*(2), 65–71. https://doi.org/10.1016/j.jcws.2008.12.001.

Briggs, M., Nelson, E. A., & Martyn-St James, M. (2012). Topical agents or dressings for pain in venous leg ulcers. *Cochrane Database of Systematic Reviews, 11*(11), Art. No.: CD001177. https://doi.org/10.1002/14651858.CD001177.pub3. Accessed 10 March 2023.

Cazander, G., Ottelander, B. K., Kamga, S., Doomen, M. C. H. A., Damen, T. H. C., & Well, A. M. E. (2020). Importance of debriding and wound cleansing agents in wound healing. In *Therapeutic dressings and wound healing applications* (pp. 59–89). New York: Wiley. https://doi.org/10.1002/9781119433316.ch4.

Chan, E., Foster, S., Sambell, R., & Leong, P. (2018). Clinical efficacy of virtual reality for acute procedural pain management: A systematic review and meta-analysis. *PLoS One, 13*(7), e0200987. https://doi.org/10.1371/journal.pone.0200987.

Cohen, S. P., Christo, P. J., & Moroz, L. (2004). Pain management in trauma patients. *American Journal of Physical Medicine and Rehabilitation, 83*(2), 142–161. https://doi.org/10.1097/01.PHM.0000107499.24698.CA. PMID: 14758300.

Dowell, D., Ragan, K. R., Jones, C. M., Baldwin, G. T., & Chou, R. (2022). CDC Clinical Practice Guideline for Prescribing Opioids for Pain—United States, 2022. *MMWR. Recommendations and Reports: Morbidity and Mortality Weekly Report. Recommendations and Reports, 71*(3), 1–95. https://doi.org/10.15585/mmwr.rr7103a1.

European Pressure Ulcer Advisory Panel, National Pressure Injury Advisory Panel, Pan Pacific Pressure Injury Alliance (EPIAP, NPIAP, PPPIA). (2019). In E. Haesler (Ed.), *Prevention and treatment of pressure ulcers/injuries*. Osborne Park, Western Australia: Cambridge Media.

Evans, E., & Gray, M. (2005). Do topical analgesics reduce pain associated with wound dressing changes or debridement of chronic wounds? *Journal of Wound, Ostomy, and Continence Nursing, 32*(5), 287–290. https://doi.org/10.1097/00152192-200509000-00002.

Giovannitti, J. A., Jr., Thoms, S. M., & Crawford, J. J. (2015). Alpha-2 adrenergic receptor agonists: A review of current clinical applications. *Anesthesia Progress, 62*(1), 31–39. https://doi.org/10.2344/0003-3006-62.1.31. PMID: 25849473; PMCID: PMC4389556.

Guillot, X., Martin, H., Seguin-Py, S., Maguin-Gaté, K., Moretto, J., Totoson, P., et al. (2017). Local cryotherapy improves adjuvant-induced arthritis through down-regulation of IL-6/IL-17 pathway but independently of TNFα. *PLoS One, 12*(7), e0178668. https://doi.org/10.1371/journal.pone.0178668.

Gunes, U. Y. (2008). A descriptive study of pressure ulcer pain. *Ostomy Wound Management, 54*(2), 56.

Holloway, S., & Mahoney, K. (2021). Periwound skin care considerations for older adults. *British Journal of Community Nursing, 26*(Suppl. 6), S26–S33. https://doi.org/10.12968/bjcn.2021.26.Sup6.S26.

Hopf, H. W., & Weitz, S. (1994). Postoperative pain management. *Archives of Surgery, 129*(2), 128–132. https://doi.org/10.1001/archsurg.1994.01420260014002. PMID: 8304824.

Joint Commission. (2000). *Pain assessment and management: An organizational approach.* Oakbrook Terrace, IL: The Joint Commission.

Kaye, A. D., Chernobylsky, D. J., Thakur, P., Siddaiah, H., Kaye, R. J., Eng, L. K., et al. (2020). Dexmedetomidine in enhanced recovery after surgery (ERAS) protocols for postoperative pain. *Current Pain and Headache Reports, 24*(5), 21. https://doi.org/10.1007/s11916-020-00853-z.

Kottner, J., Cuddigan, J., Carville, K., Balzer, K., Berlowitz, D., Law, S., et al. (2019). Prevention and treatment of pressure ulcers/injuries: The protocol for the second update of the international Clinical Practice Guideline 2019. *Journal of Tissue Viability, 28*(2), 51–58. https://doi.org/10.1016/j.jtv.2019.01.001.

Maida, V., Shi, R. B., Fazzari, F. G. T., & Zomparelli, L. (2021). Topical cannabis-based medicines—A novel adjuvant treatment for venous leg ulcers: An open-label trial. *Experimental Dermatology, 30*(9), 1258–1267. https://doi.org/10.1111/exd.14395.

Manchikanti, L., Kaye, A. M., Knezevic, N. N., McAnally, H., Slavin, K., Trescot, A. M., et al. (2017). Responsible, safe, and effective prescription of opioids for chronic non-cancer pain: American Society of Interventional Pain Physicians (ASIPP) Guidelines. *Pain Physician, 20*(2S), S3–S92.

Mateus, D., Marto, J., Trindade, P., Gonçalves, H., Salgado, A., Machado, P., et al. (2019). Improved morphine-loaded hydrogels for wound-related pain relief. *Pharmaceutics, 11*(2), E76. https://doi.org/10.3390/pharmaceutics11020076.

Matsumura, H., Imai, R., Ahmatjan, N., Ida, Y., Gondo, M., Shibata, D., et al. (2014). Removal of adhesive wound dressing and its effects on the stratum corneum of the skin: Comparison of eight different adhesive wound dressings. *International Wound Journal, 11*(1), 50–54. https://doi.org/10.1111/j.1742-481X.2012.01061.x.

Navarro-Rodriguez, J. M., Suarez-Serrano, C., Martin-Valero, R., Marcen-Roman, Y., & de-la-Casa-Almeida, M. (2021). Effectiveness of topical anesthetics in pain management for dermal injuries: A systematic review. *Journal of Clinical Medicine, 10*(11), 2522. https://doi.org/10.3390/jcm10112522.

O'Donnell, T. F., Passman, M. A., Marston, W. A., Ennis, W. J., Dalsing, M., Kistner, R. L., et al. (2014). Management of venous leg ulcers: Clinical practice guidelines of the Society for Vascular Surgery® and the American Venous Forum. *Journal of Vascular Surgery, 60*(2 Suppl), 3S–59S. https://doi.org/10.1016/j.jvs.2014.04.049.

O'Neill, D. K., Robins, B., Ayello, E. A., Cuff, G., Linton, P., & Brem, H. (2012). Regional anaesthesia with sedation protocol to safely debride sacral pressure ulcers. *International Wound Journal, 9*(5), 525–543. https://doi.org/10.1111/j.1742-481X.2011.00912.x.

Owen, H., McMillan, V., & Rogowski, D. (1990). Postoperative pain therapy: A survey of patients' expectations and their experiences. *Pain, 41*(3), 303–307. https://doi.org/10.1016/0304-3959(90)90007-Z.

Pastore, M. N., Kalia, Y. N., Horstmann, M., & Roberts, M. S. (2015). Transdermal patches: History, development and pharmacology. *British Journal of Pharmacology, 172*(9), 2179–2209. https://doi.org/10.1111/bph.13059.

Pergolizzi, J. V., & Raffa, R. B. (2014). The WHO pain ladder: Do we need another step? *Practical Pain Management, 14*(1). Retrieved 3/13/2023 from https://www.practicalpainmanagement.com/resources/who-pain-ladder-do-we-need-another-step.

Practice Guidelines for Moderate Procedural Sedation and Analgesia. (2018). A Report by the American Society of Anesthesiologists Task Force on Moderate Procedural Sedation and Analgesia, the American Association of Oral and Maxillofacial Surgeons, American College of Radiology, American Dental Association, American Society of Dentist Anesthesiologists, and Society of Interventional Radiology (2018). *Anesthesiology, 128*(3), 437–479. https://doi.org/10.1097/ALN.0000000000002043.

Purcell, A., Buckley, T., King, J., Moyle, W., & Marshall, A. P. (2018). Eutectic mixture of local anaesthetics (EMLA®) as a primary dressing on painful chronic leg ulcers: A pilot randomised controlled trial. *Pilot and Feasibility Studies, 4*, 123. https://doi.org/10.1186/s40814-018-0312-6.

Reddy, M., Kohr, R., Queen, D., Keast, D., & Sibbald, R. G. (2003). Practical treatment of wound pain and trauma: A patient-centered approach. An overview. *Ostomy Wound Management, 49*(4 Suppl), 2–15.

Robards, C., & Hadzic, A. (2007). Chapter 33. Lumbar plexus block. In A. Hadzic (Ed.), *NYSORA textbook of regional anesthesia and acute pain management* McGraw Hill. https://accessanesthesiology.mhmedical.com/Content.aspx?bookid=413&sectionid=39828184.

Smith, R. G. (2020). Mitigating the opioid crisis for wound care providers using opioid stewardship. *Wounds, 32*(6), 146–151.

Sostres, C., Gargallo, C. J., & Lanas, A. (2013). Nonsteroidal anti-inflammatory drugs and upper and lower gastrointestinal mucosal damage. *Arthritis Research & Therapy, 15*(Suppl. 3), S3. https://doi.org/10.1186/ar4175.

Sugasawa, T., Tome, Y., Takeuchi, Y., Yoshida, Y., Yahagi, N., Sharma, R., et al. (2020). Influence of intermittent cold stimulations on CREB and its targeting genes in muscle: Investigations into molecular mechanisms of local cryotherapy. *International Journal of Molecular Sciences, 21*(13), 4588. https://doi.org/10.3390/ijms21134588.

Thomas, D. C., Tsu, C. L., Nain, R. A., Arsat, N., Fun, S. S., & Sahid Nik Lah, N. A. (2021). The role of debridement in wound bed preparation in chronic wound: A narrative review. *Annals of Medicine and Surgery, 71*, 102876. https://doi.org/10.1016/j.amsu.2021.102876.

Tong, Q.-J., Hammer, K. D., Johnson, E. M., Zegarra, M., Goto, M., & Lo, T. S. (2018). A systematic review and meta-analysis on the use of prophylactic topical antibiotics for the prevention of uncomplicated wound infections. *Infection and Drug Resistance, 11*, 417–425. https://doi.org/10.2147/IDR.S151293.

Wongkietkachorn, A., Surakunprapha, P., Titapun, A., Wongkietkachorn, N., & Wongkietkachorn, S. (2019). Periwound challenges improve patient satisfaction in wound care. *Plastic and Reconstructive Surgery. Global Open, 7*(3), e2134. https://doi.org/10.1097/GOX.0000000000002134.

World Union of Wound Healing Societies (WUWHS). (2004). *Principles of best practice: Minimising pain at wound dressing-related procedures. A consensus document.* Accessed 11/13/2021 from https://www.woundsinternational.com/resources/details/minimising-pain-wound-dressing-related-procedures-wuwhs-consensus-document.

Wound, Ostomy and Continence Nurses Society. (2014). Guideline for management of wounds in patients with lower-extremity arterial disease. In *WOCN Clinical Practice Guideline Series 1*. Mt. Laurel, NJ: Author.

Wound, Ostomy and Continence Nurses Society. (2016). Guideline for management of pressure ulcers. In *WOCN clinical practice guideline series 2*. Mt. Laurel, NJ: Author.

Wound, Ostomy and Continence Nurses Society. (2017). Guideline for management of wounds in patients with lower-extremity venous disease. In *WOCN clinical practice guideline series 4*. Mt. Laurel, NJ: Author.

Wound, Ostomy and Continence Nurses Society. (2021). Guideline for management of wounds in patients with lower-extremity neuropathic disease. In *WOCN clinical practice guideline series 3*. Mt. Laurel, NJ: Author.

Wu, M., Linderoth, B., & Foreman, R. D. (2008). Putative mechanisms behind effects of spinal cord stimulation on vascular diseases: A review of experimental studies. *Autonomic Neuroscience: Basic & Clinical, 138*(1–2), 9–23. https://doi.org/10.1016/j.autneu.2007.11.001.

29

Nutritional Assessment and Support[*]

Joshua R. Dilley, Lucian G. Vlad, and Joseph A. Molnar

OBJECTIVES

1. Compare and contrast the etiology of starvation-related malnutrition, disease-related malnutrition, and acute disease- or injury-related malnutrition.
2. Distinguish between nutrition screening and nutrition assessment, as well as who performs each.
3. Compare and contrast the criteria for malnutrition in the context of starvation, chronic disease, and acute injury.

4. List at least one role for each of the following nutrients in wound healing: protein; carbohydrate; fat; vitamins A, B, C, D, and E; and minerals zinc, copper, and magnesium.
5. Identify the required daily dose for the patient with a wound for calories, protein, zinc, vitamin C, and fluid.

Nutrition is fundamental to normal cellular integrity, as well as tissue repair and regeneration. Carbohydrates, proteins, fat, minerals, vitamins, and fluids are required in sufficient amounts to meet nutritional requirements for these basic processes. Individual needs vary depending on the underlying nutritional status, metabolic rate, and concomitant biologic demands (e.g., diabetes, heart failure, pneumonia, and kidney disease).

Wound healing is an anabolic process that requires specific nutrients to fuel the biochemical processes in healing (e.g., vitamin C and iron are required for hydroxylation of proline in collagen formation) (Arnold & Barbul, 2006; Demling, 2009; Stechmiller, 2010). Although adequate nutrition is important for all patients, it is of particular importance for the patient with a wound to prevent severe or prolonged depletion of nutrients that can affect healing. A patient with a wound may lose as much as 100 g of protein per day through wound exudate (Pompeo, 2007). Furthermore, once malnourished, the tube-fed patient may require 4 weeks or longer before protein stores normalize. This is even more difficult to correct in the outpatient population where it is more difficult to control and monitor dietary intake.

MALNUTRITION

Nationwide, the prevalence of malnutrition in hospitals is a significant and underappreciated problem. It was recognized as the "The Skeleton in the Hospital Closet" by Harvard

Surgeon C. Butterworth in 1974 (Butterworth, 1974). The incidence is estimated at between 30% and 50% (Jensen et al., 2013), but it is recognized as a clinical diagnosis in only 5% of hospitalized patients according to a large study that looked at 6 million patients across 110 institutions (Tobert et al., 2018). Some patients are admitted malnourished, and others experience deterioration of nutritional status during their hospitalization. This high prevalence of malnutrition is particularly alarming because malnutrition is associated with increased morbidity, mortality and decreased quality of life in patients with acute or chronic disease, as well as longer hospitalization and higher treatment costs, compared with patients without malnutrition (Corkins et al., 2014; Correia, 2018). Pediatric inpatient undernutrition has been estimated between 2.5% and 51% and is increasing (McCarthy et al., 2019). Nutrition assessment within 24 h of hospital admission has been mandated by the Joint Commission since 1995 for the hospitalized patient, but there was not a commonly accepted assessment tool.

This issue has a completely different magnitude and is even harder to assess in the outpatient setting where incidence is between 7.2% and 30% (Graham et al., 2017). Approximately 15% of US households face food insecurity placing them at high risk for malnutrition (Gundersen & Ziliak, 2015). This problem is even greater in the geriatric patients with a fixed income, immobility, and physiologic loss of appetite (Molnar et al., 2014). Risk factors for malnutrition are listed in Table 29.1.

Malnutrition is a state in which an imbalance between nutrient intake and nutrient demands causes measurable adverse effects on tissue, body structure, and body functions. It is apparent from this definition that the metabolic state of

[*]The editors acknowledge and appreciate the contributions of Nancy Stotts RN, EdD, FAAN for her work on previous editions of this chapter.

TABLE 29.1   Risk Factors for Malnutrition Divided Into Categories Under Mode of Influence

Physiological or Anatomic	Social Causes	Increased Demands
Dental disease	Poverty	Hypermetabolism
Dementia, altered mental status	Social isolation/depression	Trauma
Alterations in swallowing, ingestion, digestion, or absorption	Inability to buy or prepare food	Sepsis
Decreased appetite	Inability to feed self	Surgery
Weight loss	Therapeutic dietary restriction	Chronic wound
Medication side effect (i.e., chemotherapy)	Poor patient choices	

the individual creating metabolic demands is as important as the intake. Malnutrition is also classified as undernutrition or overnutrition and is caused by a deficit or excess of nutrients in the diet, respectively. Historically, the focus of malnutrition has been on the individual's intake, because of the potential for the development of protein malnutrition, or protein–calorie malnutrition. Appreciation of the role of inflammation in malnutrition has turned our thinking about malnutrition upside down (White et al., 2012).

The inflammatory response elevates energy requirements and nitrogen excretion increasing both energy and protein demands (Jensen et al., 2010). The inflammatory response to injury consists of three phases: the ebb phase of decreased metabolism, the flow or catabolic phase, and the anabolic phase (Şimşek et al., 2014; Sobotka & Soeters, 2009). The ebb phase occurs during the first hours after injury and is characterized by a decreased metabolic rate with increased catecholamine release. In the phase flow, hypermetabolism occurs and there is significant increase in substrate to meet the body's increasing metabolic demands. During severe injury, food intake is generally stopped, and the organism depends on consuming its own energy to cover its metabolic needs. Peripheral tissues such as adipose tissue, skin and muscle are catabolized. The body increases the production of glucose and frees amino acids from muscle tissue to support synthesis of acute phase proteins, inflammatory cells, and collagen to heal the wound (Şimşek et al., 2014; Sobotka & Soeters, 2009). If the stress or injury is prolonged, eventually the visceral organs will begin to catabolize as well. The anabolic phase occurs days to weeks after the injury depending on the severity of injury. This phase begins with a positive nitrogen balance that increases protein synthesis with associated gains in weight and muscle (Şimşek et al., 2014).

Classic parameters of malnutrition have included weight loss, inadequate intake, and the proteins albumin, prealbumin, and transferrin. Shifts in body water, inaccuracies in intake measurement and recording, and inflammatory processes that lower serum protein levels lead to inaccurate diagnoses (Jensen et al., 2009). This metabolic response to infection or trauma results in reduction of protein levels within 24 h—even for patients who are not malnourished (Jensen et al., 2012; Zhang et al., 2017).

Inflammation is an important mediator for nutrition as seen in the etiologic classifications of malnutrition provided by the International Guideline Committee of the American Society for Parenteral and Enteral Nutrition and the European Society for Clinical Nutrition and Metabolism. The three etiologic categories of malnutrition are starvation-related malnutrition, disease-related malnutrition, and acute disease- or injury-related malnutrition (Jensen & Wheeler, 2012) (Table 29.2). These categories incorporate both undernutrition and overnutrition. Patients can be assigned to more than one of these classifications and may move among them as their situation changes (Jensen et al., 2009, 2013). Diagnostic criteria accompany these etiologic classifications (White et al., 2012).

Starvation-Related Malnutrition

Starvation occurs when caloric intake is inadequate to meet metabolic needs over time. Famine often is the cause in underdeveloped countries, and inadequate intake due to insufficient income or conditions such as depression or anorexia nervosa are seen in developed countries (Jensen & Wheeler, 2012; White et al., 2012). The classic picture of starvation-related malnutrition is the individual with inadequate intake who is in an unstressed state and is hypometabolic (Heimburger, 2008). Initially, with inadequate intake, compensatory processes meet the glucose needs of essential tissues (e.g., brain, white blood cells). Glycogen that is stored in the liver is mobilized for energy; however, stores are small and are exhausted in less than 24 h. Subsequently, glucose needed for cellular activities is formed by the catabolism of protein in muscle and tissues. Protein is not stored in the body. When protein is used for gluconeogenesis, tissues containing protein, especially the carcass tissues of muscle and skin, are broken down to support this process. Weight loss occurs from both the breakdown of protein and the osmotic diuresis that allows for excretion of the byproducts of protein metabolism in urine.

If inadequate intake persists, compensatory processes allow fat to become the primary energy source and for protein to be used at a much slower rate (Heimburger, 2008). The brain adapts and uses ketones from fat metabolism for energy, the muscle releases less protein, and the kidneys recycle the end products of protein metabolism for glucose. Over time, the basal metabolic rate decreases, and weight loss is slowed. Gluconeogenesis continues for use by only a few tissues that are unable to adapt to use of other nutrients for energy (e.g., red blood cells, fibroblasts, and renal medulla) (Berg et al.,

TABLE 29.2 Criteria for Malnutrition
Starvation-Related, Chronic Disease-Related, and Acute or Injury-Related[a]

	STARVATION-RELATED MALNUTRITION		CHRONIC DISEASE-RELATED MALNUTRITION[B]		ACUTE OR INJURY-RELATED MALNUTRITION	
	Nonsevere	Severe	Nonsevere	Severe	Nonsevere	Severe
Estimated energy intake	<75% for ≥3 months	<50% for >1 month	<75% for ≤1 month		<75% for >7 days	≤50% for >5 days
Weight loss	5% in 1 month	>5% in 1 month	5% in 1 month	>5% in 1 month	1%–2% in 1 week	>2% in 1 week
	7.5% in 3 months	>7.5% in 3 months	7.5% in 3 months	>7.5% in 3 months	5% in 1 month	>5% in 1 month
	10% in 6 months	>10% in 6 months	10% in 6 months	>10% in 6 months	7.5% in 3 months	>7.5% in 3 months
	20% in 1 year	>20% in 1 year	20% in 1 year	>20% in 1 year		
Body fat reduction	Mild	Severe	Mild	Severe	Mild	Moderate
Muscle mass reduction	Mild	Severe	Mild	Severe	Mild	Moderate
Fluid accumulation	Mild	Severe	Mild	Severe	Mild	Moderate to severe
Hand-grip strength reduction	Not applicable	Measurably	Not applicable	Measurably	Not applicable	Measurably

[a]Two or more characteristics must be present for malnutrition to be diagnosed.
[b]Adapted from Table. White, J. V., Guenter, P., Jensen, G., et al. (2012). Consensus statement: Academy of Nutrition and Dietetics and American Society for Parenteral and Enteral Nutrition: Characteristics recommended for the identification and documentation of adult malnutrition (undernutrition). *Journal of Parenteral and Enteral Nutrition, 36*(3), 275–283.

2002). Serum protein measures decline gradually (Glasgow & Herrmann, 2006).

When fat stores are depleted, protein again becomes the primary energy source and is rapidly depleted. The carcass is also broken down to support visceral protein synthetic processes but eventually when this resource is exhausted the visceral organs suffer as well (Sobotka & Soeters, 2009). Skeletal muscle size rapidly decreases, and serum protein levels fall. If treatment is not prompt, death will ensue.

Disease-Related Malnutrition

This category of malnutrition is seen in persons with chronic diseases where inflammation is chronic and often mild to moderate. Examples include organ failure, rheumatoid arthritis, pancreatic cancer, and sarcopenic obesity (Jensen et al., 2012; White et al., 2012). Here the underlying disease (e.g., end-stage renal disease, asthma, or rheumatoid arthritis) is characterized by a chronic inflammatory response that contributes to the effects of the disease (Gupta et al., 2012; Murdoch & Lloyd, 2010; Wong & Lord, 2004). Obesity is characterized by a chronic inflammatory component that increases activation of kinases, resulting in upregulation of proinflammatory cytokines and weight loss in these individuals leads to a reduction in the inflammatory state (Ferrucci & Fabbri, 2018).

It is important to recognize that the excess weight of an obese patient does not necessarily reflect adequate nutritional health. Protein deficiency and deficiencies of vitamins and minerals are increasingly common in the obese patient due to the highly refined western diet (Kaidar-Person et al., 2008). The combination of obesity and malnutrition has been termed the "obesity paradox" (Tanumihardjo et al., 2007). Unfortunately, nutritional evaluation of the obese person is often incorrectly deferred simply because the individual's weight is so much more than normal (Gallagher & Gates, 2003).

Acute Disease- or Injury-Related Malnutrition

Classically, this type of malnutrition is seen with trauma, surgery, or rapid severe infection (Jensen & Wheeler, 2012; White et al., 2012). Injury causes stress, catecholamine release, and increased resting energy expenditure. The degree of hypermetabolism is directly related to the severity of injury. For example, severe burns cause a greater increase in metabolic rate than uncomplicated surgery (Demling, 2009). The inflammatory response is elicited concomitantly. Cortisol released from the adrenal cortex enhances protein catabolism, amino acid mobilization, and hepatic glucose production (Heimburger, 2008). Cytokines, including tumor necrosis factor, transforming growth factor-β, and interleukin-1 and interleukin-6, contribute to the stress response. While insulin levels are elevated, insulin resistance prevents anabolism. Positive acute phase proteins increase (e.g., C-reactive protein). Less albumin is synthesized, catabolism increases, and fluids leak into the interstitium and create edema. The low albumin level (<3.5 g/dL) with the elevation of C-reactive protein is an indicator of inflammation (Jensen, 2006). During hypermetabolic periods, caloric needs increase and protein requirements increase disproportionately. Hypermetabolic demands decrease gradually, and, if no additional insult occurs, metabolic needs return to baseline within 10–14 days of the acute injury.

In the injured but healthy person, inadequate intake for 5–7 days usually is not a problem. Surgical patients are an excellent example. A combination of hypermetabolism and starvation occurs due to inadequate intake. The hypermetabolic response is a physiologic response to injury and results in increased energy needs. At the same time, patients initially are provided with intravenous fluids containing 5% glucose (about 200 calories per liter). The glucose administered spares protein but is not able to meet metabolic needs. As oral intake resumes, caloric intake is less than normal, and autocatabolism occurs to meet metabolic needs. These patients usually have a brief but rapid decrease in weight. When they return to adequate caloric intake, they regain the lost weight (Heimburger, 2008). If the cause of the stress is not resolved, additional stresses occur (e.g., infection), or the individual's intake does not meet metabolic needs, the patient is set up for a downward spiral.

SCREENING AND ASSESSMENT

Healthy people ingest sufficient carbohydrates, protein, fat, vitamins, minerals, and fluids to meet nutritional needs and maintain a positive nitrogen balance. Wound healing requires additional nutrients, mostly commonly increased protein demand, and it is important to evaluate patients with wounds early and at regular intervals.

Screening for Possible Malnutrition

Nutrition *screening* identifies patients who are at risk for malnutrition while assessment determines the specific nutritional diagnosis or deficiency. Anyone who screens positive indicates the need for a nutritional *assessment* by a registered dietitian (Anthony, 2008; European Pressure Ulcer Advisory Panel, National Pressure Injury Advisory Panel, and Pan Pacific Pressure Injury Alliance, 2019). Professional guidelines recommend routine nutrition screening within 24 h of admission for hospitalized patient (Green & Watson, 2006; Munoz et al., 2020). No outpatient nutrition screening guidelines have been established. Malnutrition can contribute to development of chronic wounds so screening the outpatient wound patient would be prudent (Ord, 2007). The nutritional screening tool used should be validated, reliable, relevant to the desired patient group, applicable to different health care settings, able to detect undernutrition and overnutrition, cost effective and quick and easy to use (Charney, 2008; European Pressure Ulcer Advisory Panel, National Pressure Injury Advisory Panel, and Pan Pacific Pressure Injury Alliance, 2019).

The most common nutrition screening tools include the Malnutrition Universal Screening Tool (MUST), the Short Nutritional Assessment Questionnaire (SNAQ), and the Mini Nutritional Assessment (MNA). The MUST, SNAQ, and MNA are all recommended by the International Pressure Injury Guidelines for screening (European Pressure Ulcer Advisory Panel, National Pressure Injury Advisory Panel, and Pan Pacific Pressure Injury Alliance, 2019). The MNA is used to provide information on nutritional status in elderly adults. The MUST and SNAQ are applicable to all health care settings (inpatient, outpatient, nursing homes) and both consist of three items (Reber et al., 2019; Yaxley et al., 2015). Composed of questions that are most predictive of malnutrition, these tools are easy to implement. Most screening tools have two common questions: unintentional recent weight loss (5%–10%) and inadequate intake for the previous 1 or 2 weeks. A positive answer to either of these should lead to a more in-depth nutritional assessment (Correia, 2018). Each health care setting should have a policy on nutritional screening that acknowledges the need to refer those at risk to a registered dietitian or nutritional support team for a nutritional assessment.

The MNA is an instrument designed for use in older patients that combines screening with assessment. It is a reliable and valid 18-item tool that consists of anthropometric, general, dietary, and subjective assessments. Furthermore, it has been used in a variety of health care settings and has been shown to detect malnutrition before changes in weight or serum protein levels, especially in an elderly population (Bauer et al., 2008). From a cross-sectional study of elderly patients with pressure injuries, Langkamp-Henken et al. (2005) concluded that use of the MNA was advantageous over serum protein levels for screening or assessment. Additional studies have demonstrated that the MNA can accurately predict pressure injury formation (Yatabe et al., 2013).

Recently the new MNA-Short Form has been validated as a standalone screening tool consisting of six items; requiring less time to complete and being more user friendly, the MNA-Short Form has become the preferred form for clinical practice (DiMaria-Ghalili, 2014; Kaiser et al., 2009). Furthermore, it has been demonstrated that when body mass index (BMI) is not available, the calf circumference is a valid alternative.

Assessment of Nutritional Status

A nutritional assessment is indicated for the patient who has a wound, is obese, or is screened as being at potential risk for malnutrition using any of the approved screening methods. Nutrition assessment is a more in-depth nutrition focused examination to determine if there is a nutritional deficiency and indicate the severity of the problem (Correia, 2018). Although the nurse may be instrumental in gathering the data used in a nutritional assessment, assimilation of the data into an assessment requires a referral to a dietitian or a multidisciplinary nutrition support team (dietitians, nurses, pharmacists, and providers). With the implementation of interventions, the patient's response should be monitored closely. Reassessments are recommended every week, with changes in the patient's condition, and with any significant weight loss. For individuals in home care, it is important to be vigilant to changes in patient status and weight. Although no consensus definition currently exists, significant weight loss is commonly defined as weight loss of 5% within 6–12 months (Wong, 2014).

The nutritional assessment is multifactorial and includes several different components as no individual parameter can identify malnutrition. A systematic approach to nutritional assessment is recommended and includes:

- History and clinical diagnosis.
- Clinical signs and physical examination (fever/hypothermia, nonspecific signs of inflammation; e.g., tachycardia).
- Anthropometric data (weight, height, and skinfolds).
- Laboratory data.
- Dietary information (diet history, 24-h recall).
- Functional assessment (strength and physical performance) (Jensen et al., 2012).

History and Clinical Diagnosis

No single parameter is a reliable marker of nutritional status. Instead, one must look at the aggregate of the information together to determine the status of the patient. Furthermore, many assessment parameters commonly used are affected by other conditions (e.g., kidney disease, dehydration, cancer, and pregnancy). Research is ongoing to determine which parameters provide the most reliable and accurate representation of the malnourished state.

Nutritional status is sometimes evaluated based entirely on data from the patient's history and physical. In these situations, the initial assessment should sequence the history taking so that significant dimensions reflective of nutritional status are clustered. This information can be used to direct the physical examination, laboratory work, and referrals.

Clinical Signs and Physical Examination

The physical examination is performed after the history is taken. Although no single physical finding is diagnostic of malnutrition, many different signs and symptoms are associated with specific nutritional alterations, such as corkscrew hair or neuropathy. Signs and symptoms associated with nutritional alterations are listed in Table 29.3. However, these findings correlate with other conditions, such as disease process, medication side effects, metabolic alterations, and age-related changes (Reber et al., 2019). Often the physical assessment findings can be used to confirm concerns or suspicions derived from the data obtained from the patient's history or the laboratory work. For patients at risk of or with early malnutrition, the physical findings for malnutrition may be subtle or absent because many signs do not appear until the malnutrition becomes advanced. With overt malnutrition, anthropometric changes often are key findings. Obese patients are especially difficult to evaluate because their weight may mask the skeletal muscle wasting of malnutrition (Johnson Stoklossa et al., 2017).

Anthropometric Measures

Anthropometric measures are easy to perform and are pivotal in the evaluation of nutritional status. The most used anthropometric parameters are height, weight, and head

TABLE 29.3 Physical Findings Associated With Nutritional Deficiencies

Site	Signs and Symptoms	Nutritional Deficit
Skin	Cracking	Protein
	Edema	Protein, vitamin B1
	Pallor	Folic acid, iron, vitamin B12
	Petechiae	Vitamin A, C
	Purpura	Vitamin C, K
	Scaling	Vitamin A
Hair	Corkscrew hairs	Vitamin C
	Easily pluckable hair	Protein
	Alopecia or thin/sparse	Zinc, biotin, or protein
Nails	Transverse ridging/banding	Protein
	Clubbing, spoon shaped	Iron
Nervous system	Peripheral neuropathy	Vitamins B2, B6, B12
	Ataxia	Vitamin B12
	Muscle cramps	Calcium, magnesium
Muscles	Weakness	Protein, calories
Mouth	Bleeding	Vitamins C, K
	Atrophic tongue	Niacin iron
	Cheilosis	Niacin, vitamins B2, B6

circumference (children only). Less frequently used are midarm muscle circumference and skinfold measurements (Table 29.4). Body composition scans such as computed tomography, ultrasound, or dual X-ray absorptiometry can identify losses of muscle mass, subcutaneous tissue, and the presence of intermuscular adipose tissue. These methods are rarely used clinically due to cost and potential radiation exposure (Correia, 2018).

Weight is the cornerstone in the diagnosis of malnutrition and can be used alone or in relation to height or frame size. Weight is often considered in relation to height. Recent tables for interpretation of these parameters are based on the National Research Council data on weight and height,

TABLE 29.4 Anthropometric Measures

	Measures	Condition Measure Reflects
Common measures	Height and weight (body mass index)	Overnutrition, undernutrition
	Head circumference in children	Undernutrition
Less frequently used measures[a]	Midarm circumference	Muscle stores
	Skinfold measurements	Fat stores
	Hand-grip strength	Muscle strength Undernutrition

[a]Measures performed by dietitian or occupational therapist.

the dietary guidelines, and BMI. The BMI is calculated by dividing weight (in kilograms) by height (in meters) squared and most often is used to determine whether people are underweight or overweight. BMI is a predictor of morbidity and mortality (Abdelaal et al., 2017; Aune et al., 2016). BMI does not evaluate body composition or fat distribution; therefore, it should be considered in conjunction with other assessment findings (Evans, 2005). Also, the Centers for Disease Control and Prevention advise that age and gender can affect the relationship between BMI and body fat, as women and older persons have a greater proportion of fat than do men and younger persons.

Head circumference is used in children to evaluate their growth. Measurements are compared with tables of norms, allowing head size to be classified in percentiles. Chronic undernutrition impacts weight first, then length and finally head growth, and its identification and treatment are important so that permanent neurological damage does not occur (Homan, 2016; Jeong, 2011).

Although the test measures are performed primarily by dietitians, it is important to understand what the test measures mean in order to appreciate the relevance of the findings. Arm muscle circumference and skinfold measures initially were used in underdeveloped countries to evaluate the nutritional status of the population (Jelliffe and World Health Organization, 1966). Standards exist in the United States for specific age groups, gender, and ethnicity (McDowell et al., 2008). Both are impacted by obesity and edema and used more for research purposes than in daily clinical practice (Correia, 2018; Reber et al., 2019). Mid-upper arm circumference is a measure of muscle mass, bones, and skin. It is used to calculate midarm muscle circumference as a measure of lean body mass (Heimburger, 2008). A decrease in arm muscle mass occurs with protein and calorie deficiencies.

Fat stores are measured with a skinfold caliper. The triceps site is most frequently used; other sites include the scapula and waist. Fat stores do not change rapidly, so skinfold thickness is not a sensitive measure of malnutrition. Dietitians and the nutritional support team may perform arm muscle circumference and skinfold measures. There is high interindividual variability with measurement (Reber et al., 2019).

Laboratory Data

There is no laboratory test that is pathognomonic or diagnostic of malnutrition. Instead, laboratory assessment should be used in conjunction with clinical assessment. Serum proteins include albumin, prealbumin, transferrin, retinol-binding protein (RBP) (Table 29.5). Serum proteins are synthesized primarily by the liver and are commonly used to help assess nutritional status.

Serum proteins are negative acute phase proteins or reactants during the inflammatory response. Inflammatory processes such as acute or chronic infection, surgery, trauma, and burns trigger a systemic response referred to as the *acute phase response.* The serum levels of most proteins either increase or decrease during the acute phase response. Serum proteins that decrease levels during inflammation are called

TABLE 29.5   Laboratory Measures of Adequate Hydration

Laboratory Test	Underhydration	Normal Values
Serum sodium	>150 mEq/L	130–150 mEq/L
Osmolality	>295 mOsm/L	285–295 mOsm/L
Blood urea nitrogen (BUN)	Elevated	7–23 mg/dL
BUN–creatinine ratio	>25:1	10:1
Urine-specific gravity	>1.028	1.003–1.028

negative acute phase reactants (e.g., albumin and prealbumin) and are expected to return to normal as the inflammatory process resolves. Positive acute phase reactants are proteins that increase levels during times of stress because they are essential for the immune response. C-reactive protein, fibrinogen, protein S, and fibronectin are examples of positive acute phase reactants. C-reactive protein can be utilized to monitor acute changes in inflammation because of its short half-life (4–7 h) (Litao & Kamat, 2014).

Historically, albumin has commonly been used as a marker of nutritional status. It is a carrier protein and primarily helps to maintain oncotic pressure. Albumin has a long half-life (17–21 days) and is not sensitive to rapid changes in nutritional status. Previous studies have demonstrated that restriction of protein or caloric intake does not consistently decrease albumin levels (Afolabi et al., 2004; Scalfi et al., 1990). Albumin levels fall only late during the course of prolonged and premorbid starvation (Demling, 2009). Additionally, increasing caloric or protein intake does not reliably increase albumin levels if there is an ongoing inflammatory condition (Banh, 2006; Friedman & Fadem, 2010; Marcason, 2017). As a negative acute phase protein influenced by many factors, serum albumin by itself is not an appropriate measure of malnutrition but can help identify patients at risk for malnutrition due to an underlying inflammatory state. In summary, a low albumin level may be the result of malnutrition or an inflammatory response and further workup is necessary. A normal albumin is still helpful as it suggests a better metabolic situation than a low albumin and because it is a slow turnover protein it is more useful for looking at the chronic condition rather than acute changes.

Prealbumin, also known as *thyroxin-binding prealbumin* or *transthyretin,* is a transport protein for thyroxine and vitamin A (Evans, 2005). It is affected by many of the same factors that affect albumin. Prealbumin is degraded by the kidneys so any renal dysfunction will increase serum levels (Bharadwaj et al., 2016). Because of its short half-life (2 days), prealbumin is believed to reflect changes in nutrient intake more rapidly but the acute phase response limits its clinical utility (Bharadwaj et al., 2016).

Transferrin, also an acute phase protein, has a shorter half-life than albumin (8–10 days) and a smaller body pool. Its major function is iron transport. Usually, about one-third of the body's transferrin is bound to iron. In iron-deficiency states, transferrin is increased due to higher amounts of iron absorption and in iron-overload states transferrin is decreased. Transferrin level is not sufficiently sensitive or specific to be a meaningful measurement of nutritional status unless one is using it to look at iron status (Roza et al., 1984; Sergi et al., 2006).

Less commonly measured is RBP, a plasma protein with a very short half-life (12 h) and very low serum levels. It participates in the transport of vitamin A, and its response follows that of prealbumin. Similar to prealbumin, renal dysfunction increases serum levels of RBP. Although it has a theoretical advantage over other plasma proteins by virtue of its short half-life, its low normal values and the technical difficulties associated with its measurement limit its usefulness compared with other measures of nutrient status (Evans, 2005).

It should be noted that hydration status affects serum protein levels. When the patient is dehydrated, serum albumin and prealbumin levels will be falsely elevated. Conversely, when the patient is overhydrated, serum protein levels will be falsely low. Serum proteins are also affected by a number of other factors (Table 29.6) (Banh, 2006).

One commonly available and inexpensive laboratory test that provides nutritional information is often overlooked. The complete blood count has several nutritional indicators. Microcytic or hypochromic indices may represent iron deficiency (although there are other causes such as anemia of chronic disease). Megaloblastic indices may represent folate or B12 deficiency (Cascio & DeLoughery, 2017). A decreased total lymphocyte count may also be and index of protein–calorie malnutrition (Omran & Morley, 2000).

Creatinine levels have been used for years to evaluate lean body mass. Creatinine is breakdown product of muscle that is metabolized and released as a constant rate allowing it to serve as a surrogate marker of muscle mass or skeletal muscle (Datta et al., 2018). Creatinine assessment is complex in the general population because it is affected by hydration status, activity level, recent high-protein diet and requires a 24-h

urine collection. In hemodialysis patients, there is increasing evidence that creatinine is strongly associated with lean body mass and higher creatinine correlates with improved longevity (Patel et al., 2013).

Nutritional status also can be evaluated using a 24-h urine creatinine excretion divided by normal creatinine for height, producing a creatinine height index. An index of 80% or more is normal. An index of 40%–60% reflects moderate protein depletion, whereas an index less than 40% indicates severe nutrition depletion (Medhat et al., 2016). Age-specific tables are used to interpret the findings.

Nitrogen balance measures whether sufficient protein is being ingested, absorbed, and metabolized. Nitrogen intake and loss from the body are carefully regulated and, under normal nutritional circumstances, closely approximate each other so that nitrogen turnover is in balance. Anabolism and repair require positive nitrogen balance. Negative nitrogen balance reflects catabolism or inadequate ingestion of protein. Measuring nitrogen balance is difficult in clinical practice because it requires accurate determination of protein intake and nitrogen loss (Dickerson, 2016; Kondrup, 2008).

Dietary Intake

A diet history and a 24-h recall help the dietitian evaluate recent intake although studies demonstrate individuals tend to underreport their intake and their recall may not represent their usual diet because eating behaviors can vary day to day. In order to limit these biases, collecting 24-h diet recalls on multiple days may improve accuracy (Tucker, 2007). When patients are unable to provide this information due to cognitive status or severity of illness, family members will be called upon to provide recent data.

Functional Assessment

Evaluation of functional ability with hand-grip strength is recommended. Using a simple dynamometer, this evaluation is quick and easy to use and can provide information about function but cannot be used as a surrogate for muscle

TABLE 29.6 Acute Phase Response to Inflammation

Acute Phase Reactants[a] (Normal Values)	Factors Affecting Reliability (Direction of Response)	Effect of Inflammation	Effect of Recovery From Inflammation
Albumin (3.5–5.0 g/dL)	Overhydration (↓) Bed rest (↓) Zinc deficiency (↓)	Negative	Positive (return to normal)
Prealbumin (18–45 mg/dL)	Steroid use (↑) Hyperglycemia (↓) Kidney disease (↑)	Negative	Positive (return to normal)
Transferrin (188–341 mg/dL)	Iron deficiency (↑) Zinc deficiency (↓) Old age (↓)	Negative	Positive (return to normal)
C-reactive protein (<0.8 mg/L)	Heart disease (↑) Leukemia (no change) Ulcerative colitis (no change)	Positive	Negative (return to normal)

[a]Values decrease by 25%.
Banh, L. (2006). Serum proteins as markers of nutrition: What are we treating? *Practical Gastroenterology, 30*(10), 46.

function in the lower limb (Russell, 2015). Other potential usable measures of physical function include the stair climb test, timed get up go, 6-min walk test, and 30-s chair stand (Russell, 2015). Unfortunately, as the variability of absolute numbers in a population is quite large due to body habitus, amount of exercise, neuropathy, and various disease states, such functional assessments cannot be used as isolated information but must be interpreted in light of the complete clinical evaluation. These measures are very useful when used as repeated measures during treatment of a patient to determine response to treatment.

Diagnosis of malnutrition. The diagnosis of malnutrition is made in the context of the patient's overall situation. Six characteristics from the history and physical are evaluated: (1) decreased energy intake; (2) weight loss; (3) fat loss; (4) muscle loss; (5) fluid accumulation; and (6) diminished grip strength (Jensen et al., 2012; White et al., 2012). The criteria for malnutrition in the context of starvation, chronic disease (chronic defined as at least 3 months), and acute illness are listed in Table 29.2. At least two characteristics must be present in order to diagnose either severe or nonsevere malnutrition. The duration of reduced estimated energy intake is an important criterion for severity. Also, the timeframe of weight loss can guide the clinician. White et al, (2012) recommend that weight and height should be measured, rather than estimated. Clinical judgment is needed in evaluating fat and muscle loss, as well as fluid accumulation. Hand-grip strength measures function as mentioned previously. Registered dietitians and occupational therapists usually have a dynamometer as part of their equipment and are qualified to perform this measure. Absent from the list are the serum proteins (albumin, prealbumin, etc.) that historically have been an integral part of nutritional assessment due to their variability with an inflammatory response (White et al., 2012).

NUTRIENT NEEDS FOR HEALING

Body composition is conceptualized as having two components: fat mass and fat-free mass (Demling, 2009). Fat is a calorie-dense substrate that acts as a calorie reservoir, with 9 calories per gram of fat. When the body's intake of calories is greater than expenditure, fat deposits form and weight increases. In times of need or caloric deficit, fat is catabolized, and weight loss occurs.

In contrast, the fat-free compartment, or lean body mass, is composed primarily of protein and water. The protein portion is located predominantly in muscles, red blood cells, connective tissues, and organs, including the skin, which is the largest of the body's organs. Healing requires protein synthesis (Demling, 2009). When energy requirements exceed intake, even for short periods, body protein is broken down to meet metabolic need. The protein in this situation is used for energy rather than for anabolism. Protein has less than half the calories of fat (4 calories per gram) when it is catabolized, weight loss is rapid. Catabolism of protein results in loss of functional tissue (muscle and organs), which is referred to as *muscle wasting*.

Normal healing requires adequate protein, fat, and carbohydrates, as well as vitamins and minerals (Stechmiller, 2010). When intake, absorption, or metabolism of nutrients does not meet metabolic requirements, biochemical changes occur that have implications for healing (e.g., impaired fibroplasia). However, these changes often occur without clinical manifestations and severe changes must occur before signs and symptoms of impaired healing due to malnutrition are manifest (e.g., dehiscence). In part, the wound receives the biologic priority of muscle catabolism, which provides substrates that preferentially allow repair of injured tissues. This protection is tightly tied to the percentage of lean body mass. When more than 15% of lean body mass is lost, impaired healing and increased risk of infection are seen (Barchitta et al., 2019). At 30% loss of lean body mass, more severe alterations in healing occur and predisposes the patient to new wound formation (e.g., dehiscence). With 40% loss of lean body mass, death occurs, often due to pneumonia (Molnar et al., 2014).

The best data about nutritional requirements for healing come from the surgical and pressure injury literature (Demling, 2009; European Pressure Ulcer Advisory Panel, National Pressure Injury Advisory Panel, and Pan Pacific Pressure Injury Alliance, 2019; Posthauer, 2006a, 2006b). Energy needs usually are based on a modification of the Harris–Benedict equation, which takes into account the person's age, gender, height, and weight. The equation also considers the individual's stress from the injury or wound and activity. This equation provides a good starting point for determining energy requirements but is inaccurate in overweight or obese individuals (Douglas et al., 2007). The most accurate way to assess energy needs is indirect calorimetry. This approach usually is reserved for the inpatient setting in patients who are hypermetabolic from sepsis or trauma where it is particularly easy to employ in intubated patients (Haugen et al., 2007). Once caloric needs are determined, protein, fat, carbohydrate, and vitamin and mineral distributions are planned.

Calories

The range of normal calories administered is broad and is based on a multitude of factors. Usual caloric needs are 20–35 calories per kilogram of body weight. Lower estimates are used for patients with chronic illness who are chronically starved, whereas higher estimates are used for those who are hypermetabolic and have significant injuries (Bistrian & Driscoll, 2008; Posthauer, 2006b). Caloric demand is increased for healing in individuals with wounds. About 50%–60% of an individual's caloric needs are met through carbohydrates, 20%–25% through protein, and the remainder from fat (Posthauer, 2006b).

Protein

Protein needs are disproportionally increased after injury, and a protein deficiency can prolong a person's healing time (Arnold & Barbul, 2006). In adults, 15% of lean body weight is composed of protein, of which 3% (approximately 300 mg) is turned over daily during normal protein metabolism. Most of this protein is reused in the synthesis of new proteins, and some is lost through excretion. The recommended daily allowance (RDA) of protein for a healthy person is 0.8 g of protein per kilogram per 24 h. Protein needs with injury may increase to 1.25–1.5 g per kilogram per day (European Pressure Ulcer Advisory Panel, National Pressure Injury Advisory Panel, and Pan Pacific Pressure Injury Alliance, 2019). Protein intake goals can be modified to be higher for those with preexisting deficiencies or obesity to a safe goal of 2 g per kilogram per day in those without liver or renal disease (Dickerson et al., 2017; Wu, 2016). Older adults are at higher risk of protein malnutrition due to increased rates of protein catabolism and higher protein requirements compared with younger adults. Older adults have higher protein needs because they generate a smaller anabolic response to amino acids than younger adults. Higher protein intake in older adults can lead to increased anabolic response similar to young adults (Baum et al., 2016). Inadequate protein intake in older adults is common and places them at further risk of malnutrition (Baum et al., 2016). The inadequate intake in the geriatric population is influenced by physiological changes (changes in smell, taste, appetite) and financial restraints due to fixed income (Molnar et al., 2016).

Proteins are made of amino acids, which are necessary to generate acute phase proteins, including collagen and proteoglycans, and are essential for wound healing, hormonal and immune balance, and muscle health. Under metabolic stress, the amino acids arginine and glutamine become conditional essential amino acids because the body cannot produce these amino acids at a rate adequate to meet the increased need (Posthauer, 2006b).

Arginine

Arginine is converted to ornithine, a precursor to proline and subsequent collagen formation. In animal models, arginine decreases nitrogen loss, chance of infection and stimulates immune function, wound-breaking strength, nitric oxide and collagen formation. It also facilitates wound healing by augmenting the release of the anabolic hormones insulin, insulin-like growth factors, glucagon, prolactin, and various growth factors (Posthauer, 2006b; Stechmiller, 2010; Stechmiller et al., 2005). Small clinical studies show the value of arginine in wound healing (Brewer et al., 2010; De Luis et al., 2009; Desneves et al., 2005; Evans et al., 2014; Leigh et al., 2012). Enteral feeding solutions contain arginine (Stechmiller, 2010) and arginine supplementation is commercially available for clinical use. Of important note, energy and protein requirements must be met before supplementation can be effective (Alexander & Supp, 2014).

Glutamine

As the most abundant amino acid in the body, glutamine preserves the intestinal brush border, synthesizes nonessential fatty acids and the nucleotide units of RNA and DNA. Additionally, glutamine is the principle fuel source for rapidly dividing epithelial cells during healing and helps stimulate lymphocyte proliferation (Demling, 2009). With stress, glutamine levels diminish (400 μmol/L), thereby compromising the integrity of the immune system. Replacement is important to reduce infectious complications by upregulating heat shock proteins and by stimulating growth hormone (Wischmeyer, 2002). Normal glutamine levels of 600 μmol/L or higher facilitate intact immunologic function. The patient with a major wound has a glutamine requirement of 0.3–0.5 g per kilogram per day. Supplementation has showed mixed results in regard to wound healing (Chow & Barbul, 2014; Demling, 2009; Ellinger, 2014).

Carbohydrates

Carbohydrates provide a significant portion of nutrients. Carbohydrate is turned into glucose, which is available immediately for adenosine triphosphate formation and provides the energy for phagocytosis and collagen development. Carbohydrates play an important role in enzymatic functions and hormonal functions that regulate wound healing. Glucose levels must be kept within normal limits to facilitate healing. Excessive hyperglycemia results in impaired healing and immune system dysfunction. Provision of adequate glucose is useful to inhibit gluconeogenesis from amino acid precursors, thus allowing amino acids to be used for anabolic processes.

Fats

Fats are important for development and stability of cell membranes (both intracellular and cell wall) and serve as precursors for signaling molecules such as leukotrienes and prostaglandins (Chow & Barbul, 2014). Fats also participate actively in various aspects of the inflammatory response to injury and thus in healing. Omega-3 fatty acids have antiinflammatory and vasodilatory properties that may provide benefit during the inflammatory phase of wound healing. Omega-6 fatty acids contribute to the inflammatory response, vasospasm, platelet aggregation and vasoconstriction (Molnar et al., 2014; Simopoulos, 2016). Evidence is mixed on whether omega fatty acid supplementation benefits wound healing and further studies are needed (Barchitta et al., 2019; Chow & Barbul, 2014; Theilla et al., 2012).

Vitamins

All of the vitamins are needed for tissue repair and regeneration because of their various functions in normal cellular metabolism. Table 29.7 lists the role of various nutrients in healing. Vitamins A and C are especially critical for healing. Vitamin A is an essential fat-soluble molecule that must be obtained through the diet and is important in various steps of collagen deposition. Collagen is the most important component in scar formation and in maintaining wound closure. Diets low in fresh vegetables and meat are subject to vitamin A deficiency, which slows epithelial growth and wound healing (Polcz & Barbul, 2019). In persons treated with corticosteroids, vitamin A is an important antagonist as it reverses the negative effects of corticosteroids. A short course of 15,000–25,000 IU/day of vitamin A orally for 14–21 days based on the size and overall nutritional status of the patient can help counter the deleterious effects of steroids on wound healing (Polcz & Barbul, 2019; Zinder et al., 2019).

TABLE 29.7	Role of Nutrients in Wound Healing
Nutrient	**Role in Healing**
Protein	Angiogenesis
	Collagen synthesis/remodeling
	Wound contraction
	Immune function
	Precursor to nitric oxide
Carbohydrate	Energy source
	Protein sparing
	Angiogenesis
Fat	Cell walls
	Intracellular structures
	Inflammation
Vitamin A[a]	Epithelialization
	Angiogenesis
	Fibroblast stimulation
B vitamins	Cofactor in enzymes
	Immune response
	Macronutrient metabolism
Vitamin C	Collagen synthesis
	Capillary wall integrity
	Fibroblast function
	Immune function
	Antioxidant
Vitamin D[a]	Calcium metabolism
	Immune function
Vitamin E[a]	Antioxidant
Vitamin K[a]	Coagulation
Copper	Cross-linking collagen
Iron	Collagen formation
	Immune function
	Oxygen transport
Zinc	Collagen formation
	Protein synthesis
	Cell membrane stability
	Immune function

[a]Fat soluble.

Caution should be taken when prescribing vitamin A in situations of decreased RBP due to malnutrition or liver disease.

Vitamin C is a water-soluble vitamin, a cofactor in collagen formation, and is important to fibroplasia. Vitamin C influences the activity of the immune system and works synergistically with vitamin E to prevent oxidative cell damage (Moores, 2013). When vitamin C intake ceases, the stores become depleted within 2–3 months (Arnold & Barbul, 2006). Vitamin C deficiency results in poor collagen formation, subcutaneous bleeding due to loss of connective tissue and thickening of the stratum corneum (Pullar et al., 2017). There are recommendations for supplementing 500 mg to 2 g of vitamin C daily depending on the severity of the wound although there is no consensus guideline (Molnar et al., 2014). The benefit of vitamin C supplementation may only have a beneficial effect in pressure injury patients when combined with arginine and zinc (Ellinger & Stehle, 2009). Evidence remains mixed on vitamin C supplementation (Chow & Barbul, 2014; Ellinger & Stehle, 2009; Moores, 2013).

Minerals

Among the minerals, zinc, copper, and iron have received the most attention in the context of wound healing. Zinc is important because of its role in protein synthesis, DNA synthesis, enzyme systems, immune competence, and collagen formation (Lin et al., 2018). During the remodeling phase of wound healing, zinc plays a key role in fibroblast proliferation and epithelialization (Barchitta et al., 2019). Zinc supplementation enhances collagen formation in patients with zinc deficiency. In persons with normal zinc levels, oral supplementation has not been shown to alter healing, but topical zinc oxide has evidence showing improvement in wound healing regardless of the patient's zinc status (Kogan et al., 2017). Oral supplementation should be based on serum deficits, and treatment should be limited to 10–14 days (220 mg of zinc sulfate daily). Supplementation in those who are not in need may result in disruption of normal phagocyte, neutrophil, and lymphocyte function and cause copper or calcium deficiency (Saghaleini et al., 2018).

Copper is key for collagen cross-linking and connective tissue production. Copper deficiency may result in weaker scar tissue and decreased tensile strength, predisposing the person to dehiscence and poor wound healing (Kornblatt et al., 2016). Iron is important in hemoglobin for oxygen transport and consequently tissue perfusion. Persons with anemia may experience impaired collagen formation and ineffective phagocytic activity slowing wound healing, but evidence is limited (Ferris & Harding, 2019). To date, there is no evidence that iron supplementation benefits wound healing unless the patient is iron deficient (Wright et al., 2014).

Electrolytes

Water and balanced electrolytes are the sea in which the various nutrients function. Adequate hydration and electrolytes provide the physiologic space in which nutrients and oxygen are transported to the site of injury so that healing can occur. The usual rule for fluid is at least 1500 mL per 24 h, with most individuals receiving fluids based on the equation 30 mL per kilogram body weight (Dwyer, 2008). The exception to this rule is people with heart or kidney disease, for whom the recommendation is 25 mL/kg or replacement of fluid losses. High levels of wound exudate or treatment with an air-fluidized bed may increase the patient's fluid requirement needs (Posthauer, 2006a, 2006b). Evaluation of hydration status is an integral part of nutritional assessment (Posthauer, 2006a). Table 29.5 lists laboratory measures of hydration.

NUTRITIONAL SUPPORT

Depending on the health care system, the appropriate action to take when a patient is screened as being malnourished or at risk for malnutrition is referring the patient to a dietitian, notifying the provider of the findings, or calling the nutritional support team. A sequence of events for providing nutritional support is summarized in Box 29.1.

Nutritional needs are dependent on many variables, including age, gender, height, weight, presence of severe wasting or obesity, comorbidities, and severity of illness. Additional nutrient needs are present when the patient has a wound due to loss of protein and fluid from the wound, as well as the increased demands required to support the wound-healing process. When the patient is at risk for pressure injuries as identified by the nutrition subscale of the Braden scale, supplementation has been shown to reduce incidence of pressure injuries by 25% (Saghaleini et al., 2018).

Most diets are a combination of protein, carbohydrate, fat, vitamins, and minerals, so deficiencies of individual nutrients are uncommon. Increased intake or supplementation is needed if the patient is undernourished or at risk for impaired healing (Stechmiller, 2010). Protein intake should be sufficient to support growth of granulation tissue and to place in a state of anabolism (Baum et al., 2016; Stechmiller, 2010; Whitney et al., 2006). Goals of nutritional support for the patient who is at risk or who has an existing wound are to provide a minimum of 30–35 kcal per kilogram of body weight per day, with 1.25–2.0 g per kilogram per day of protein and 1 mL per kilocalorie per day of fluid intake (Dickerson et al., 2017; European Pressure Ulcer Advisory

BOX 29.1 Sequence of Events for Nutritional Support

1. Screen nutritional status of all patients upon admission to hospital and initial visit to outpatient wound care center
2. Nutritional assessment performed on patients who screen positive, have a wound, or are obese
3. Estimate nutritional requirements
4. Compare nutrient intake with estimated requirements
5. Provide appropriate nutrition intervention based on nutritional requirements
6. Provide sufficient nutrients
   - 30–35 kcal per kilogram of body weight per day
   - 1.25–2.0 g of protein per kilogram per day
   - 1 mL of fluid intake per kcal per day
   - 1600–2000 retinol equivalents of vitamin A
   - 100–1000 mg of vitamin C
   - 15–30 mg of zinc
   - 200% of recommended dietary allowance of the B vitamins
   - 20–30 mg of iron
   - 0.3–0.4 g of glutamine per kilogram per day
   - Daily multivitamin and mineral supplement
7. Monitor intake to ensure patient is meeting nutritional requirements
8. Monitor and evaluate nutritional outcomes, with reassessment of nutritional status at frequent intervals

Panel, National Pressure Injury Advisory Panel, and Pan Pacific Pressure Injury Alliance, 2019; Whitney et al., 2006; Wu, 2016). In patients who are chronically or acutely ill, they may be unable to eat a balanced diet that provides the required vitamins and minerals. In that case, a daily multivitamin is recommended, as well as treatment of any detected or suspected deficiencies (European Pressure Ulcer Advisory Panel, National Pressure Injury Advisory Panel, and Pan Pacific Pressure Injury Alliance, 2019). Daily vitamin and mineral needs are increased to 1600–2000 retinol equivalents of vitamin A, 100–1000 mg of vitamin C, 15–30 mg of zinc, 200% of the RDA of the B vitamins, and 20–30 mg of iron. Most of these needs can be met with a daily multivitamin and mineral supplement (Bistrian & Driscoll, 2008; Posthauer, 2006b). Evidence demonstrates supplemental vitamin A may combat the negative side effects of chronic steroids on wound healing. Oral zinc has only been shown to be beneficial in those with documented deficiency. Arginine, glutamine, and vitamin C supplementation have not been shown conclusively to accelerate wound healing as much of the data is mixed.

Anabolic steroids have been recommended and demonstrated to be useful in supporting healing in some populations by stimulating protein synthesis, new tissue formation, weight gain and decreasing protein degradation (Demling, 2009). Approved by the US Food and Drug Administration in the 1960s for treatment of severe weight loss due to chronic infections, severe trauma, or failure to thrive anabolic steroids have been used to treat severe malnourishment and wasting syndrome typical with human immunodeficiency virus and burns. The anabolic steroid oxandrolone (Oxandrin), a testosterone analog, has been shown to decrease catabolism and significantly attenuate lost lean mass with severe wounds. Androgens influence wound healing by increasing collagen deposition and facilitating leukocyte migration and monocyte adhesion to enhance the inflammatory response (Levine, 2017). Shortened healing times have also been reported with human growth hormone, another anabolic steroid (Oh & Phillips, 2006). A recent Cochrane review concluded there is no strong evidence to support the use of anabolic steroids in pressure injuries (Naing & Whittaker, 2017).

Estrogen has been reported to have antiinflammatory properties, decreasing elastase activity so that fibronectin degradation is decreased, and collagen content deposition is increased. Estrogen deficiency increases the inflammatory process and delays angiogenesis. Exogenous estrogen supplementation increases the risk of endometrial hyperplasia, blood clots, and cancer and has been observed to adversely affect the quality of scar formation (Oh & Phillips, 2006). The selective estrogen receptor modulators may offer promise to promote wound healing, but their effects have yet to be studied (Levine, 2017).

The preferred route of nutritional support is oral, and, whenever possible, the gastrointestinal tract should be used for feeding. The benefits of enteral (gastrointestinal) over parenteral nutrition are numerous and include fewer infectious complications, earlier return of gut function, reduced cost, and reduced length of stay in hospitalized patients (Seres et al., 2013). A person who is feeding orally should be counseled to select foods that contain protein. Foods high in protein, including milk, eggs, cheese, tuna, lentils, and meat, should be encouraged. Supplemental snacks, including shakes, peanut butter, protein bars, and protein-enriched ice cream, are other sources of protein.

If the patient's intake is inadequate with oral feeding, then tube feedings should be considered to supplement or supplant the oral feeding. As with other patient populations, use of specialized nutritional support (tube feeding or parenteral nutrition) is based on the likelihood that prevention or treatment of protein–calorie malnutrition will increase the possibility of recovery, mitigate infection, improve healing, or shorten hospital stay (Bistrian & Driscoll, 2008). For a portion of those who are malnourished, weight loss and debilitation are inevitable consequences.

Historically, research on nutrition and wound healing focused on the acutely ill trauma patient in the hospital. The evidence from these patients were then extrapolated to patients with chronic wounds. While both patients may have wounds, their underlying nutritional status and characteristics are drastically different. The acute wound patient is typically younger (<35 years old), healthier with few comorbidities and well nourished. The acute wound patient has an appropriate hypermetabolic response to injury and is unlikely to have repeated injury. The acute wound will progress through the normal stages of healing in an orderly fashion (Molnar et al., 2016).

The chronic wound patient is usually older, unhealthier with multiple comorbidities, and malnourished. These patients typically have a blunted response to injury given their underlying comorbidities. Additionally, they are likely to have repeated injury. The chronic wound is stalled in the healing stage due to prolonged inflammation, which prevents the wound from healing. Clearly, the patient population and wounds are fundamentally distinct between acute and chronic wound patients. As a result, their underlying nutritional and metabolic needs are different (Molnar et al., 2016).

For the outpatient chronic wound patient with multiple comorbidities, a high-protein diet is still recommended. The focus of the nutritional recommendations should be on high protein and concentrate less on specific calorie intake goal. Obviously, patients with diabetes should try to ingest a low-carbohydrate diet to improve glycemic control and wound healing (Xiang et al., 2019). Additionally, supplementation with a multivitamin including vitamin C and zinc could be beneficial as they likely have deficiencies. Since these patients are outpatients, it takes more individualization and troubleshooting to ensure adherence. A dietician can be an excellent resource to help improve a patient's diet.

CLINICAL CONSULT

A: 84-year-old Latina woman with a history of glaucoma and dementia is admitted from a nursing home after a fall that resulted in a fractured hip. She has an abdominal wound from surgery 5 weeks ago for a perforated bowel managed with NPWT. Documentation indicates wound size has not decreased in 2 weeks. She is able to follow directions, has a body mass index (BMI) of 30 (height 5 ft 5 in, weight 180 lbs). Discussion with the nursing home staff facilitated completion of a Mini Nutritional Assessment, which indicates a decreased appetite, recent 8 lbs weight loss, and minimal ability to feed herself. Her complete blood count is normal. Her albumin is 2.2 g/dL.

D: Starvation-related malnutrition; not compatible with wound healing. At risk for pressure injury related to hip fracture and decreased mobility.

P: Control wound bioburden until nutrition improves enough to support wound healing. Prevent further skin breakdown.

I: (1) Immediate referral to dietitian. (2) Assist patient with eating and offer protein-rich fluid at each visit to the room. (3) C-reactive protein to rule out coexisting inflammation. (4) Continue with NPWT to abdominal wound and silver-impregnated hydrocolloid island dressing over hip incision. (5) Reposition every 2 h and as needed while in bed; use offloading mattress. (6) Continuous passive motion machine on while patient is in bed. (7) Consult with physical therapy for strengthening exercises and ambulation twice daily.

E: Family understands that wound healing cannot be expected until nutrition improves. Plan to revisit in 1 week to review recommendations from dietitian and physical therapy and adjust local wound care as indicated.

SUMMARY

- Adequate nutrition is fundamental to wound healing.
- All patients with a wound should undergo a nutritional assessment. The nutritional assessment will determine if malnutrition and any micronutrient deficiencies are present.
- After nutritional assessment, an individualized nutrition plan should be established to correct any deficiencies.

Correcting underlying malnutrition is crucial to wound healing.
- The patient's nutritional status should be regularly reevaluated to determine the effectiveness of the plan.

SELF-ASSESSMENT QUESTIONS

1. Supplementing which of the following is key to wound healing?
   a. Carbohydrates
   b. Fat
   c. Protein
   d. Vitamin C
2. Which of the following is not an acute phase reactant?
   a. Albumin
   b. Prealbumin
   c. Transferrin
   d. Magnesium
3. Which of the following is a nutritional screening tool valid ONLY for screening elderly adults?
   a. Mini Nutritional Assessment (MNA)
   b. Malnutrition Universal Screening Tool (MUST)
   c. Short Nutritional Assessment Questionnaire (SNAQ)
   d. Obesity Nutritional Screen (ONS)

REFERENCES

Abdelaal, M., le Roux, C. W., & Docherty, N. G. (2017). Morbidity and mortality associated with obesity. *Annals of Translational Medicine*, 5(7).

Afolabi, P. R., Jahoor, F., Gibson, N. R., & Jackson, A. A. (2004). Response of hepatic proteins to the lowering of habitual dietary protein to the recommended safe level of intake. *American Journal of Physiology. Endocrinology and Metabolism*, 287(2), E327–E330.

Alexander, J. W., & Supp, D. M. (2014). Role of arginine and omega-3 fatty acids in wound healing and infection. *Advances in Wound Care*, 3(11), 682–690.

Anthony, P. S. (2008). Nutrition screening tools for hospitalized patients. *Nutrition in Clinical Practice*, 23(4), 373–382.

Arnold, M., & Barbul, A. (2006). Nutrition and wound healing. *Plastic and Reconstructive Surgery*, 117(7S), 42S–58S.

Aune, D., Sen, A., Prasad, M., Norat, T., Janszky, I., Tonstad, S., et al. (2016). BMI and all cause mortality: Systematic review and non-linear dose-response meta-analysis of 230 cohort studies with 3.74 million deaths among 30.3 million participants. *British Medical Journal*, 353.

Banh, L. (2006). Serum proteins as markers of nutrition: What are we treating? *Practical Gastroenterology*, 30(10), 46.

Barchitta, M., Maugeri, A., Favara, G., Lio, R. M. S., Evola, G., Agodi, A., et al. (2019). Nutrition and wound healing: An overview focusing on the beneficial effects of curcumin. *International Journal of Molecular Sciences*, 20(5), 1119.

Bauer, J. M., Kaiser, M. J., Anthony, P., Guigoz, Y., & Sieber, C. C. (2008). The Mini Nutritional Assessment®—Its history, today's practice, and future perspectives. *Nutrition in Clinical Practice*, 23(4), 388–396.

Baum, J. I., Kim, I. Y., & Wolfe, R. R. (2016). Protein consumption and the elderly: What is the optimal level of intake? *Nutrients*, 8(6), 359.

Berg, J. M., Tymoczko, J. L., & Stryer, L. (2002). Food intake and starvation induce metabolic changes. Biochemistry W H Freeman: New York.

Bharadwaj, S., Ginoya, S., Tandon, P., Gohel, T. D., Guirguis, J., Vallabh, H., et al. (2016). Malnutrition: Laboratory markers vs nutritional assessment. *Gastroenterology Report*, 4(4), 272–280.

Bistrian, B. R., & Driscoll, D. F. (2008). Enteral and parenteral nutrition therapy. In *Vol. 18. Harrison's principles of internal medicine* (pp. 612–621).

Brewer, S., Desneves, K., Pearce, L., Mills, K., Dunn, L., Brown, D., et al. (2010). Effect of an arginine-containing nutritional supplement on pressure ulcer healing in community spinal patients. *Journal of Wound Care*, 19(7), 311–316.

Butterworth, C. E., Jr. (1974). The skeleton in the hospital closet. *Nutrition Today*, 9(2), 4–8.

Cascio, M. J., & DeLoughery, T. G. (2017). Anemia: Evaluation and diagnostic tests. *Medical Clinics*, 101(2), 263–284.

Charney, P. (2008). Nutrition screening vs nutrition assessment: How do they differ? *Nutrition in Clinical Practice*, 23(4), 366–372.

Chow, O., & Barbul, A. (2014). Immunonutrition: Role in wound healing and tissue regeneration. *Advances in Wound Care*, 3(1), 46–53.

Corkins, M. R., Guenter, P., DiMaria-Ghalili, R. A., Jensen, G. L., Malone, A., Miller, S., et al. (2014). Malnutrition diagnoses in hospitalized patients: United States, 2010. *Journal of Parenteral and Enteral Nutrition*, 38(2), 186–195.

Correia, M. I. T. D. (2018). Nutrition screening vs nutrition assessment: What's the difference? *Nutrition in Clinical Practice*, 33(1), 62–72.

Datta, D., Foley, R., Wu, R., Grady, J., & Scalise, P. (2018). Can creatinine height index predict weaning and survival outcomes in patients on prolonged mechanical ventilation after critical illness? *Journal of Intensive Care Medicine*, 33(2), 104–110.

De Luis, D. A., Izaola, O., Cuellar, L., Terroba, M. C., Martin, T., & Aller, R. (2009). High dose of arginine enhanced enteral nutrition in postsurgical head and neck cancer patients. A randomized clinical trial. *European Review for Medical and Pharmacological Sciences*, 13(4), 279–283.

Demling, R. H. (2009). Nutrition, anabolism, and the wound healing process: An overview. *Eplasty*, 9.

Desneves, K. J., Todorovic, B. E., Cassar, A., & Crowe, T. C. (2005). Treatment with supplementary arginine, vitamin C and zinc in patients with pressure ulcers: A randomised controlled trial. *Clinical Nutrition*, 24(6), 979–987.

Dickerson, R. N. (2016). Nitrogen balance and protein requirements for critically ill older patients. *Nutrients*, 8(4), 226.

Dickerson, R. N., Patel, J. J., & McClain, C. J. (2017). Protein and calorie requirements associated with the presence of obesity. *Nutrition in Clinical Practice*, 32, 86S–93S.

DiMaria-Ghalili, R. A. (2014). Integrating nutrition in the comprehensive geriatric assessment. *Nutrition in Clinical Practice*, 29(4), 420–427.

Douglas, C. C., Lawrence, J. C., Bush, N. C., Oster, R. A., Gower, B. A., & Darnell, B. E. (2007). Ability of the Harris-Benedict formula to predict energy requirements differs with weight history and ethnicity. *Nutrition Research*, 27(4), 194–199.

Dwyer, D. J. (2008). Nutritional requirements and dietary assessment. In *Vol. 17. Harrison's principles of internal medicine*.

Ellinger, S. (2014). Micronutrients, arginine, and glutamine: Does supplementation provide an efficient tool for prevention and treatment of different kinds of wounds? *Advances in Wound Care, 3*(11), 691–707.

Ellinger, S., & Stehle, P. (2009). Efficacy of vitamin supplementation in situations with wound healing disorders: Results from clinical intervention studies. *Current Opinion in Clinical Nutrition & Metabolic Care, 12*(6), 588–595.

European Pressure Ulcer Advisory Panel, National Pressure Injury Advisory Panel, and Pan Pacific Pressure Injury Alliance. (2019). In E. Haesler (Ed.), *Prevention and treatment of pressure ulcers/ injuries: Clinical practice guideline. The international guideline.* Osborne Park: Cambridge Media.

Evans, E. (2005). Nutritional assessment in chronic wound care. *Journal of Wound Ostomy & Continence Nursing, 32*(5), 317–320.

Evans, D. C., Martindale, R. G., Kiraly, L. N., & Jones, C. M. (2014). Nutrition optimization prior to surgery. *Nutrition in Clinical Practice, 29*(1), 10–21.

Ferris, A. E., & Harding, K. G. (2019). An overview of the relationship between anaemia, iron, and venous leg ulcers. *International Wound Journal, 16*(6), 1323–1329.

Ferrucci, L., & Fabbri, E. (2018). Inflammageing: Chronic inflammation in ageing, cardiovascular disease, and frailty. *Nature Reviews. Cardiology, 15*(9), 505–522.

Friedman, A. N., & Fadem, S. Z. (2010). Reassessment of albumin as a nutritional marker in kidney disease. *Journal of the American Society of Nephrology, 21*(2), 223–230.

Gallagher, S., & Gates, J. L. (2003). Obesity, panniculitis, panniculectomy, and wound care: Understanding the challenges. *Journal of Wound, Ostomy, and Continence Nursing, 30*(6), 334–341.

Glasgow, S., & Herrmann, V. (2006). Surgical metabolism and nutrition. *Current Surgical Diagnosis and Treatment,* 140–169.

Graham, J., Fan, L., Meadows, E. S., Hang, L., Partridge, J., & Goates, S. (2017). Addressing malnutrition across the continuum of care: Which patients are likely to receive oral nutritional supplements. *Journal of Ageing Research and Healthcare, 1,* 9.

Green, S. M., & Watson, R. (2006). Nutritional screening and assessment tools for older adults: Literature review. *Journal of advanced Nursing, 54*(4), 477–490.

Gundersen, C., & Ziliak, J. P. (2015). Food insecurity and health outcomes. *Health Affairs, 34*(11), 1830–1839.

Gupta, J., Mitra, N., Kanetsky, P. A., Devaney, J., Wing, M. R., Reilly, M., et al. (2012). Association between albuminuria, kidney function, and inflammatory biomarker profile in CKD in CRIC. *Clinical Journal of the American Society of Nephrology, 7*(12), 1938–1946.

Haugen, H. A., Chan, L. N., & Li, F. (2007). Indirect calorimetry: A practical guide for clinicians. *Nutrition in Clinical Practice, 22*(4), 377–388.

Heimburger, D. C. (2008). Malnutrition and nutritional assessment. In *Harrison's principles of internal medicine* (18th ed., pp. 605–611). New York: McGraw-Hill.

Homan, G. J. (2016). Failure to thrive: A practical guide. *American Family Physician, 94*(4), 295–299.

Jelliffe, D. B., & World Health Organization. (1966). *The assessment of the nutritional status of the community (with special reference to field surveys in developing regions of the world).* World Health Organization.

Jensen, G. L. (2006). Inflammation as the key interface of the medical and nutrition universes: A provocative examination of the future of clinical nutrition and medicine. *Journal of Parenteral and Enteral Nutrition, 30*(5), 453–463.

Jensen, G. L., Bistrian, B., Roubenoff, R., & Heimburger, D. C. (2009). Malnutrition syndromes: A conundrum vs continuum. *Journal of Parenteral and Enteral Nutrition, 33*(6), 710–716.

Jensen, G. L., Compher, C., Sullivan, D. H., & Mullin, G. E. (2013). Recognizing malnutrition in adults: Definitions and characteristics, screening, assessment, and team approach. *Journal of Parenteral and Enteral Nutrition, 37*(6), 802–807.

Jensen, G. L., Hsiao, P. Y., & Wheeler, D. (2012). Adult nutrition assessment tutorial. *Journal of Parenteral and Enteral Nutrition, 36*(3), 267–274.

Jensen, G. L., Mirtallo, J., Compher, C., Dhaliwal, R., Forbes, A., Grijalba, R. F., et al. (2010). Adult starvation and disease-related malnutrition: A proposal for etiology-based diagnosis in the clinical practice setting from the International Consensus Guideline Committee. *Journal of Parenteral and Enteral Nutrition, 34*(2), 156–159.

Jensen, G. L., & Wheeler, D. (2012). A new approach to defining and diagnosing malnutrition in adult critical illness. *Current Opinion in Critical Care, 18*(2), 206–211.

Jeong, S. J. (2011). Nutritional approach to failure to thrive. *Korean Journal of Pediatrics, 54*(7), 277.

Johnson Stoklossa, C. A., Sharma, A. M., Forhan, M., Siervo, M., Padwal, R. S., & Prado, C. M. (2017). Prevalence of sarcopenic obesity in adults with class II/III obesity using different diagnostic criteria. *Journal of Nutrition and Metabolism, 2017,* 7307618.

Kaidar-Person, O., Person, B., Szomstein, S., & Rosenthal, R. J. (2008). Nutritional deficiencies in morbidly obese patients: A new form of malnutrition? *Obesity Surgery, 18*(7), 870–876.

Kaiser, M. J., Bauer, J. M., Ramsch, C., Uter, W., Guigoz, Y., Cederholm, T., et al. (2009). Validation of the Mini Nutritional Assessment Short-Form (MNA®-SF): A practical tool for identification of nutritional status. *The Journal of Nutrition, Health and Aging, 13*(9), 782.

Kogan, S., Sood, A., & Garnick, M. (2017). Zinc and wound healing: A review of zinc physiology and clinical applications. *Wounds: A Compendium of Clinical Research and Practice, 29*(4), 102–106.

Kondrup, J. (2008). Basic concepts in nutrition: Energy and protein balance. *e-SPEN, the European e-Journal of Clinical Nutrition and Metabolism, 3*(3).

Kornblatt, A. P., Nicoletti, V. G., & Travaglia, A. (2016). The neglected role of copper ions in wound healing. *Journal of Inorganic Biochemistry, 161,* 1–8.

Langkamp-Henken, B., Hudgens, J., Stechmiller, J. K., & Herrlinger-Garcia, K. A. (2005). Mini nutritional assessment and screening scores are associated with nutritional indicators in elderly people with pressure ulcers. *Journal of the American Dietetic Association, 105*(10), 1590–1596.

Leigh, B., Desneves, K., Rafferty, J., Pearce, L., King, S., Woodward, M. C., et al. (2012). The effect of different doses of an arginine-containing supplement on the healing of pressure ulcers. *Journal of Wound Care, 21*(3), 150–156.

Levine, J. M. (2017). The effect of oral medication on wound healing. *Advances in Skin & Wound Care, 30*(3), 137–142.

Lin, P. H., Sermersheim, M., Li, H., Lee, P. H., Steinberg, S. M., & Ma, J. (2018). Zinc in wound healing modulation. *Nutrients, 10*(1), 16.

Litao, M. K. S., & Kamat, D. (2014). Erythrocyte sedimentation rate and C-reactive protein: How best to use them in clinical practice. *Pediatric Annals, 43*(10), 417–420.

Marcason, W. (2017). Should albumin and prealbumin be used as indicators for malnutrition? *Journal of the Academy of Nutrition and Dietetics, 117*(7), 1144.

McCarthy, A., Delvin, E., Marcil, V., Belanger, V., Marchand, V., Boctor, D., et al. (2019). Prevalence of malnutrition in pediatric hospitals in developed and in-transition countries: The impact of hospital practices. *Nutrients, 11*(2), 236.

McDowell, M. A., Fryar, C. D., Ogden, C. L., & Flegal, K. M. (2008). Anthropometric reference data for children and adults: United States, 2003–2006. *National Health Statistics Reports, 10*(1–45), 5.

Medhat, A. S., Ahmed, A. O., Thabet, A. F., & Amal, M. (2016). Creatinine height index as a predictor of nutritional status among patients with liver cirrhosis. *Journal of Public Health and Epidemiology, 8*, 220–228.

Molnar, J. A., Underdown, M. J., & Clark, W. A. (2014). Nutrition and chronic wounds. *Advances in Wound Care, 3*(11), 663–681.

Molnar, J. A., Vlad, L. G., & Gumus, T. (2016). Nutrition and chronic wounds: Improving clinical outcomes. *Plastic and Reconstructive Surgery, 138*(3S), 71S–81S.

Moores, J. (2013). Vitamin C: A wound healing perspective. *British Journal of Community Nursing, 18*(Suppl. 12), S6–S11.

Munoz, N., Posthauer, M. E., Cereda, E., Schols, J. M., & Haesler, E. (2020). The role of nutrition for pressure injury prevention and healing: The 2019 International Clinical Practice Guideline recommendations. *Advances in Skin & Wound Care, 33*(3), 123–136.

Murdoch, J. R., & Lloyd, C. M. (2010). Chronic inflammation and asthma. *Mutation Research. Fundamental and Molecular Mechanisms of Mutagenesis, 690*(1–2), 24–39.

Naing, C., & Whittaker, M. A. (2017). Anabolic steroids for treating pressure ulcers. *Cochrane Database of Systematic Reviews, 2017*(6), CD011375.

Oh, D. M., & Phillips, T. J. (2006). Sex hormones and wound healing. *Wounds: A Compendium of Clinical Research and Practice, 18*(1), 8–18.

Omran, M. L., & Morley, J. E. (2000). Assessment of protein energy malnutrition in older persons. Part II: Laboratory evaluation. *Nutrition, 16*(2), 131–140.

Ord, H. (2007). Nutritional support for patients with infected wounds. *British Journal of Nursing, 16*(21), 1346–1352.

Patel, S. S., Molnar, M. Z., Tayek, J. A., Ix, J. H., Noori, N., Benner, D., et al. (2013). Serum creatinine as a marker of muscle mass in chronic kidney disease: Results of a cross-sectional study and review of literature. *Journal of Cachexia, Sarcopenia and Muscle, 4*(1), 19–29.

Polcz, M. E., & Barbul, A. (2019). The role of vitamin A in wound healing. *Nutrition in Clinical Practice, 34*(5), 695–700.

Pompeo, M. (2007). Misconceptions about protein requirements for wound healing: Results of a prospective study. *Ostomy/Wound Management, 53*(8), 30–32.

Posthauer, M. E. (2006a). Hydration: Does it play a role in wound healing? *Advances in Skin & Wound Care, 19*(2), 97–102.

Posthauer, M. E. (2006b). The role of nutrition in wound care. *Advances in Skin & Wound Care, 19*(1), 43–52.

Pullar, J. M., Carr, A. C., & Vissers, M. (2017). The roles of vitamin C in skin health. *Nutrients, 9*(8), 866.

Reber, E., Gomes, F., Vasiloglou, M. F., Schuetz, P., & Stanga, Z. (2019). Nutritional risk screening and assessment. *Journal of Clinical Medicine, 8*(7), 1065.

Roza, A. M., Tuitt, D., & Shizgal, H. M. (1984). Transferrin—A poor measure of nutritional status. *Journal of Parenteral and Enteral Nutrition, 8*(5), 523–528.

Russell, M. K. (2015). Functional assessment of nutrition status. *Nutrition in Clinical Practice, 30*(2), 211–218.

Saghaleini, S. H., Dehghan, K., Shadvar, K., Sanaie, S., Mahmoodpoor, A., & Ostadi, Z. (2018). Pressure ulcer and nutrition. *Indian Journal of Critical Care Medicine: Peer-Reviewed, Official Publication of Indian Society of Critical Care Medicine, 22*(4), 283.

Scalfi, L., Laviano, A., Reed, L., Borrelli, R., & Contaldo, F. (1990). Albumin and labile-protein serum concentrations during very-low-calorie diets with different compositions. *The American Journal of Clinical Nutrition, 51*(3), 338–342.

Seres, D. S., Valcarcel, M., & Guillaume, A. (2013). Advantages of enteral nutrition over parenteral nutrition. *Therapeutic Advances in Gastroenterology, 6*(2), 157–167.

Sergi, G., Coin, A., Enzi, G., Volpato, S., Inelmen, E. M., Buttarello, M., et al. (2006). Role of visceral proteins in detecting malnutrition in the elderly. *European Journal of Clinical Nutrition, 60*(2), 203–209.

Simopoulos, A. P. (2016). An increase in the omega-6/omega-3 fatty acid ratio increases the risk for obesity. *Nutrients, 8*(3), 128.

Şimşek, T., Şimşek, H. U., & Cantürk, N. Z. (2014). Response to trauma and metabolic changes: Posttraumatic metabolism. *Turkish Journal of Surgery/Ulusal cerrahi dergisi, 30*(3), 153.

Sobotka, L., & Soeters, P. B. (2009). Basics in clinical nutrition: Metabolic response to injury and sepsis. *e-SPEN, the European e-Journal of Clinical Nutrition and Metabolism, 1*(4), e1–e3.

Stechmiller, J. K. (2010). Understanding the role of nutrition and wound healing. *Nutrition in Clinical Practice, 25*(1), 61–68.

Stechmiller, J. K., Childress, B., & Cowan, L. (2005). Arginine supplementation and wound healing. *Nutrition in Clinical Practice, 20*(1), 52–61.

Tanumihardjo, S. A., Anderson, C., Kaufer-Horwitz, M., Bode, L., Emenaker, N. J., Haqq, A. M., et al. (2007). Poverty, obesity, and malnutrition: An international perspective recognizing the paradox. *Journal of the American Dietetic Association, 107*(11), 1966–1972.

Theilla, M., Schwartz, B., Cohen, J., Shapiro, H., Anbar, R., & Singer, P. (2012). Impact of a nutritional formula enriched in fish oil and micronutrients on pressure ulcers in critical care patients. *American Journal of Critical Care, 21*(4), e102–e109.

Tobert, C. M., Mott, S. L., & Nepple, K. G. (2018). Malnutrition diagnosis during adult inpatient hospitalizations: Analysis of a multi-institutional collaborative database of academic medical centers. *Journal of the Academy of Nutrition and Dietetics, 118*(1), 125–131.

Tucker, K. L. (2007). Assessment of usual dietary intake in population studies of gene–diet interaction. *Nutrition, Metabolism and Cardiovascular Diseases, 17*(2), 74–81.

White, J. V., Guenter, P., Jensen, G., Malone, A., Schofield, M., Academy Malnutrition Work Group, et al. (2012). Consensus statement: Academy of Nutrition and Dietetics and American Society for Parenteral and Enteral Nutrition: Characteristics recommended for the identification and documentation of adult malnutrition (undernutrition). *Journal of Parenteral and Enteral Nutrition, 36*(3), 275–283.

Whitney, J., Phillips, L., Aslam, R., Barbul, A., Gottrup, F., Gould, L., et al. (2006). Guidelines for the treatment of pressure ulcers. *Wound Repair and Regeneration, 14*(6), 663–679.

Wischmeyer, P. E. (2002). Glutamine and heat shock protein expression. *Nutrition, 18*(3), 225–228.

Wong, C. J. (2014). Involuntary weight loss. *The Medical Clinics of North America, 98*(3), 625–643.

Wong, S. H., & Lord, J. M. (2004). Factors underlying chronic inflammation in rheumatoid arthritis. *Archivum Immunologiae et Therapiae Experimentalis, 52*(6), 379–388.

Wright, J. A., Richards, T., & Srai, S. K. (2014). The role of iron in the skin and cutaneous wound healing. *Frontiers in Pharmacology, 5,* 156.

Wu, G. (2016). Dietary protein intake and human health. *Food & Function, 7*(3), 1251–1265.

Xiang, J., Wang, S., He, Y., Xu, L., Zhang, S., & Tang, Z. (2019). Reasonable glycemic control would help wound healing during the treatment of diabetic foot ulcers. *Diabetes Therapy, 10*(1), 95–105.

Yatabe, M. S., Taguchi, F., Ishida, I., Sato, A., Kameda, T., Ueno, S., et al. (2013). Mini nutritional assessment as a useful method of predicting the development of pressure ulcers in elderly inpatients. *Journal of the American Geriatrics Society, 61*(10), 1698–1704.

Yaxley, A., Crotty, M., & Miller, M. (2015). Identifying malnutrition in an elderly ambulatory rehabilitation population: Agreement between mini nutritional assessment and validated screening tools. In *Vol. 3. Healthcare* (pp. 822–829). Multidisciplinary Digital Publishing Institute.

Zhang, Z., Pereira, S. L., Luo, M., & Matheson, E. M. (2017). Evaluation of blood biomarkers associated with risk of malnutrition in older adults: A systematic review and meta-analysis. *Nutrients, 9*(8), 829.

Zinder, R., Cooley, R., Vlad, L. G., & Molnar, J. A. (2019). Vitamin A and wound healing. *Nutrition in Clinical Practice, 34*(6), 839–849.

FURTHER READING

Abbott Nutrition. (n.d.) Malnutrition Screening Tool (MST). Retrieved 8/5/2020 from: http://static.abbottnutrition.com/cms-prod/abbottnutrition.com/img/Malnutrition%20Screening%20Tool_FINAL.pdf.

Dutch Malnutrition Steering Group. (n.d.) Short Nutritional Assessment Questionnaire (SNAQ). Retrieved 8/5/2020 from: https://www.fightmalnutrition.eu/toolkits/summary-screening-tools.

Nestlé Nutrition Institute. (n.d.) MNA® elderly—Overview. Retrieved 8/5/2020 from: http://mna-elderly.com/.

30

Medications and Phytotherapy: Impact on Wounds

Janice M. Beitz

OBJECTIVES

1. Describe phases of wound healing and how they may be affected by traditional and alternative medications.
2. Analyze classes of traditional medications noted to affect wound healing.
3. Describe how medications can cause skin reactions and wounds.
4. Describe how the off-label application of prescription medications may affect wound healing.
5. Discuss selected oral or topical alternative therapies (phytotherapy) that can affect wound healing.
6. Describe clinical practices that can help mitigate the negative impact of medication therapy on wound healing.

INTRODUCTION

Medications have the potential to affect any phase of wound healing and impair one or more of the essential processes. Additionally, use of medications is quite prevalent in society for prevention and management of chronic diseases. In the United States, nearly 32% of Americans over 65 years have one chronic medical condition for which they take one prescription medication monthly. Twenty-two percent have four to five chronic conditions for which they take related medications monthly. Over 17% of Americans have six or more chronic diseases for which they take prescription medications monthly (Centers for Medicare and Medicaid Service, 2020). When both Medicare and Medicaid beneficiaries are considered, the prevalence of chronic disease percentages goes even higher (Centers for Medicare and Medicaid Service, 2020). In addition, millions of Americans (four out of five) take herbal and/or dietary supplements as well (Council for Responsible Nutrition, 2019). The collective impact of prescribed, over-the-counter (OTC) and alternative medicines on the American population is evident. When one considers the factors promoting delayed wound healing (Armstrong & Meyr, 2020a, 2020b, 2020c; Azevedo, Lisboa, Cobrado, Pina-Vaz, & Rodrigues, 2020; Sharma, Schaper, & Rayman, 2019), the surge of chronic illness in America, the aging of Americans, and the occurrence of chronic illnesses in younger persons, medication therapy impact on wound care practice is progressively, relentlessly enlarging.

MEDICATIONS INHIBITING WOUND HEALING

Medications reported to delay wound healing incorporate several categories of agents including: anticoagulants, antimicrobials (select antibiotic classes), antiangiogenesis agents (e.g., bevacizumab), antineoplastics, antirheumatoids drugs (e.g., methotrexate), bisphosphonates (e.g., Zoledronate), nonsteroidal antiinflammatories (NSAIDs) (e.g., aspirin, ibuprofen), colchicine, nicotine, steroids (e.g., glucocorticoids like prednisone), and vasoconstrictors (Ahn et al., 2019; Berry et al., 2018; Cevirme et al., 2020; Cheng, Nayernama, Jones, Casey, & Waldren, 2019; Gaucher, Nicholas, Piveteau, Phillippe, & Blanche, 2017; Ginestal et al., 2019; Hull, Garcia, & Vasquez, 2021; Soundia et al., 2018; Young, 2019). A literature synthesis is organized in Table 30.1 with supporting references.

Because of their ubiquity of usage, two categories deserve special focus: steroids and NSAIDs. Multiple literature reviews support that short-term use of both categories has limited impact on wound healing (Assante, Collins, & Hewer, 2015; Chen & Dragoo, 2013; Treadwell, 2013; Wang, Armstrong, & Armstrong, 2013). Conversely, long-term use, especially at higher doses, can substantively interfere with wound healing and generate metabolic/physiologic changes such as osteoporosis and renal impairment.

Steroids impair normal wound healing while generating systemic effects (e.g., hyperglycemia, mood alterations, osteoporosis). Narrative literature reviews explain how steroids

TABLE 30.1 Medication Effects on Wound Healing

Class	Medications	Mechanism of Action/Category	Reported Effects on Wound Healing
Anabolic Steroids	Oxandrolone	Anabolism related to hormonal effect	Theorized to help decrease weight loss
		Anabolic effect; derivative of dihydrotestosterone	Promote weight gain and tissue growth
Antibiotics		Antiinfective	Removal of inflammation caused by infection
	Doxycycline	Antiinfective–antiinflammatory	Accelerates healing via MMP-9 and VEGF activation
	Tetracycline	Antiinfective–antiinflammatory	Inhibition leukocyte chemotaxis
	Erythromycin	Antiinfective–antiinflammatory	Inhibition leukocyte chemotaxis
	Neomycin	Antiinfective–Gram positive	Reepithelialization promoted
	Polymyxin-B	Antiinfective–Gram negative	Reepithelialization promoted
	Bacitracin	Antiinfective–Gram positive	Reepithelialization promoted
	Gentamicin	Antiinfective–Gram negative	Contraction inhibited
	Mupirocin	Antiinfective–Gram negative	Reepithelialization delayed
	Silver sulfadiazine	Antiinfective–Gram positive	Contraction inhibited
		Antiinfective–Gram negative	
		Candida, fungi, herpes simplex	
Anticoagulants		Inhibit coagulation cascade intrinsic and extrinsic pathways	Prevent fibrin deposition avoids injury and inflammation
Anticonvulsants		Decrease electrical activity of neuronal cell membranes limiting seizures	Can affect balance of tissue growth and cessation
	Phenytoin	Affects collagen remodeling	Decreased collagenase reduction; increases granulation tissue and angiogenesis
Antihypertensive Drugs		Decrease blood pressure via inhibition of angiotensin-converting enzyme (ACE)	
	ACE-I	Inhibit deposition of collagen I in wounds	Inhibit collagen deposition in wounds; decreased granulation
Antiinflammatory Drugs		Decrease inflammatory response	
	Dapsone	Sulfone antibiotic with antiinflammatory effects; inhibits polymorphonuclear neutrophil leukocytes	Limits PMN-mediated injury and inflammatory response
Antiplatelet/ Anticoagulant Drugs		Inhibit platelet aggregation	Inhibition of inflammation mediated by arachidonic acid metabolites
		Inhibit arachidonic acid pathway	
	Coumadin	Interferes with vitamin K pathways	Can cause unexpected skin damage/ necrosis
	Heparin	Interferes with clotting pathways	Can cause skin necrosis and damage
Antitumor Angiogenesis Inhibitors		Humanized monoclonal antibody	Affects growth of new blood vessels
	Bevacizumab	Blocks VEGF (vascular endothelial growth factor) and impairs angiogenesis	Increased wound dehiscence
			Infection
			Not within 28–30 days of elective surgery
	Sorafenib	Tyrosine kinase inhibitor; antiangiogenesis effect	Can cause hand foot skin reaction; not to be used within 1 week of surgery
Chemotherapeutic Agents for Cancer (General)		Suppress immune response; affect both normal cells and target tumor cells	Reduced inflammatory response
			Suppression of protein synthesis
			Inhibition of cell reproduction
			Increased risk of wound infection
			Decreased fibrin deposition
Agents for Cancer	Hydroxyurea	Classified as antineoplastic agent; used in sickle cell anemia and as antitumor agent/ myeloproliferative disorder	May hinder perfusion via megaloblastic erythrocytes: cutaneous, atrophy, via keratinocyte, cytotoxicity

TABLE 30.1	**Medication Effects on Wound Healing—cont'd**		
Class	**Medications**	**Mechanism of Action/Category**	**Reported Effects on Wound Healing**
Corticosteroids		Inhibition of gene expression Long-term use more deleterious Affect all phases of wound healing	Decreased inflammatory mediators Decreased platelet adhesion Decreased WBC recruitment and phagocytosis Decreased tissue formation Decreased tissue remodeling Note: Local topical use of steroids may *help* wound healing
Antigout Agent	Colchicine	Inhibition of microtubule formation	Decreased cytokine release Decreased granulocyte migration Decreased blood supply from vasoconstriction Decreased fibroblast activity Interrupted extracellular transport of procollagen Increased collagenase synthesis
Hemorheological Agents	Pentoxifylline	Enhanced tissue perfusion Phosphodiesterase inhibitor; acts to improve perfusion due to decreased blood viscosity; may also inhibit TNF	Increased blood supply Enhance wound healing and flap survival
Hormones	Estrogen (Topical)	Enhances collagen formation	Faster wound healing; stronger wound matrix
Hormone-Like Drugs (Prostaglandins)	Misoprostol (Synthetic PGE1) (Topical)	Prostaglandins are locally acting vasodilators	Facilitates collagen synthesis Inhibit TNF and IL-1
Immunosuppressants		Suppress immune system function	Decreased inflammatory response
	mTOR Inhibitors Rapamycin (now called Sirolimus)	mTOR (mammalian target of rapamycin) pathway plays key role in cellular proteins important for angiogenesis, metabolism, and cell proliferation; mTOR suppression causes immune suppression	Inhibits angiogenesis Inhibits fibroblast and matrix deposition (antimitotic)
	T Cell Inhibitors	Decreased T cell activity	Decreased inflammatory response
	Cyclosporine Tacrolimus	Calcineurin inhibition Decreased T cell activity	Inhibit fibroplasia and decreased wound strength
	TNF-α Inhibitors	TNF regulates fibroblast proliferation, prostaglandin production and angiogenesis; blockade decreases activity	Inhibit fibroplasia and decreased wound strength
	Infliximab Adalimumab	Monoclonal antibody (chimeric) Humanized monoclonal antibody	Potential for impaired surgical healing within 1–2 weeks before/after surgery (range 2–8 weeks)
Nonsteroidal Agents (NSAIDs)		Affect cyclooxygenase and lipoxygenase creating antiinflammatory effect	Retard inflammatory response
	Ibuprofen Diclofenac	Longer-term use more deleterious	Reduced wound tensile strength; reduced proliferation; increased bleeding risk
	Indomethacin		Detrimental effect on bone healing
Vasoconstrictors	Cocaine-epinephrine	Impaired microcirculation	Increased ulcer necrosis Lidocaine with epinephrine may have antibacterial effect
Smoking[a]	Nicotine	Agonist at nicotinic cholinergic receptors; nicotine constricts blood vessels	Decreases RBCs, fibroblasts Increased scarring Increased platelet adhesion

TABLE 30.1	Medication Effects on Wound Healing—cont'd		
Class	**Medications**	**Mechanism of Action/Category**	**Reported Effects on Wound Healing**
Ascorbic Acid (Deficiency)	(Deficiency)	Essential cofactor for hydroxylation of proline and lysine	Poor wound healing due to impaired collagen synthesis Decreased tensile strength Increased capillary fragility

Note: Nicotine replacement therapy does **not** impair healing.
aDisclaimer: Please note that medications may have different trade and generic names in Canada and other foreign countries. Sources for this table are listed in Further Reading.

alter gene expression once they cross the cell membrane and thereby alter almost every phase of wound healing. Steroids impair the inflammatory response, decrease fibroblast activity, slow epithelial regeneration and, with long-term use, thin epidermis. Wound contraction is also hampered (Anderson & Hamm, 2012; Poetker & Reh, 2010). Similarly, NSAIDs can impair wound healing when used long-term or at higher doses. The wound healing effects of NSAIDs include inhibition of inflammation, delayed bone healing, impaired ligament health, and adverse skin reactions (Barry, 2010; Levine, 2018; Ward, Archambault, & Mersfelder, 2010). Fibroblast inhibition has been observed specifically with diclofenac (an NSAID) in animal tests (Krischak, Augat, Claes, Kinzl, & Beck, 2007). Preliminary evidence suggests that SSRIs (selected serotonin reuptake inhibitors) and PPIs (proton pump inhibitors) *may* have a negative effect on implant integration (Aghaloo et al., 2019). With over 120 million Americans missing at least one tooth, the relationship of medications to boney healing needs more research (American College of Prosthodontists, 2020).

MEDICATIONS FACILITATING WOUND HEALING

Selected drugs/drug categories can *promote* wound repair. These include hemorrheologic (e.g., pentoxifylline) agents, hormones (e.g., estrogen), phenytoin, prostaglandins, vitamins A and C, and zinc (Afzali et al., 2019; Amaya, 2015; Levine, 2017, 2018; Mii, Guntani, Kawakubo, Tanaka, & Kyuragi, 2018; Zinder, Cooley, Vlad, & Molnar, 2019). Appetite stimulants (orexigenic drugs) like megestrol, dronabinol (a synthetic active ingredient of marijuana), and other agents such as SSRIs, can help with wound healing by increasing intake of nutrients (Levine, 2018). Notably, synthetic testosterone (oxandrolone), previously used to assist with weight gain, is associated with complications including hepatitis and liver cell tumors (Levine, 2018). Anabolic steroids (e.g., oxandrolone) lack quality evidence to support their use in wound healing (Bauman et al., 2013; Naing & Whitaker, 2017).

Probiotics (either systemic or topical) have been studied to examine their antagonistic activity against pathogens associated with wound infections (Fijan et al., 2019). The use of various well-known strains of live lactobacillus (e.g., casei, acidophilus) has been reported efficacious in reducing wound infections and presents an intriguing opportunity for future wound management.

Prescription medications have been used off-label, both orally or systemically, to potentially enhance wound healing. For example, β-blockers, most known for their usage in cardiac arrythmias, angina, migraine, and hypertension via blockade of β-adrenergic receptors, have been described as effective for dermatologic conditions of vascular origin (Chen & Tsai, 2018). The authors noted several diseases (e.g., pyoderma gangrenosum) wherein topical β-blocker (0.5% topical timolol) promoted wound healing.

Similarly, vitamin A (a retinoid) is commonly used to reverse the negative wound-healing effects of prolonged glucocorticoids, specifically in restoring the inflammatory response and epithelialization. For selected populations, however, vitamin A usage poses a problem. Vitamin A in large doses can markedly increase intracranial pressure with catastrophic results for the neurosurgical patient. Therefore, large-dose vitamin A is contraindicated in neurosurgical patients (Berry et al., 2018).

MEDICATIONS *CAUSING* SKIN DAMAGE AND WOUNDS

Cutaneous drug reactions are reported to be some of the most common manifestations of adverse drug effects (ADEs) (Kuklik, Stausberg, Amiri, & Jockel, 2019; Zhu & Weingart, 2020). Almost any medication can cause or induce skin reactions with possible subsequent wound development. Selected patient factors increase the risk for skin ADEs including a history of ectopy, older age, past drug allergies, and organ dysfunction (e.g., renal insufficiency) (Mendes, Alves, Loureiro, Fonte, & Batel-Marques, 2019). Almost 1 in 1000 hospitalized patients has a serious cutaneous drug reaction (Kuklik et al., 2019; Samel & Chu, 2020). Two recent retrospective reviews of electronic medical records for patients with skin ADEs in Portugal and the United States, respectively, noted that the number one category of drugs causing skin ADEs is antibiotics/antibacterials (Mendes et al., 2019; Zhang, Van, Hieu, & Craig, 2019). Of the antibiotics, β-lactams (penicillin/cephalosporin) and sulfonamide agents are most commonly implicated (Kuklik et al., 2019; Samel & Chu, 2020).

BOX 30.1 Categories of Immunologic or Hypersensitivity Reactions

Type I—Immediate in onset and mediated by IgE, mast cells and basophils; associated with rash, wheeling angioedema and, most severely, anaphylaxis.

Type II—Delayed in onset and caused by antibody-mediated cell destruction; associated with hemolytic anemia, thrombocytopenia and neutropenia.

Type III—Delayed in onset and caused by IgG: Drug immune complex deposition and complement activation; can be associated with serum sickness (fever, rash), vasculitis.

Type IV—Delayed in onset and mediated by T-cells; can be associated with contact dermatitis, maculopapular rashes, drug fever, Stevens-Johnson syndrome and TENS (toxic epidermal necrolysis syndrome).

Adverse skin reactions are commonly categorized according to predictability or immunologic pathomechanism. Regarding predictability, Type A (predictable) ADEs include gastritis (due to NSAID use) or diarrhea (due to antibiotics) and are related to the pharmacologic properties of the drug. Type B (unexpected, idiosyncratic) ADEs represent hypersensitivity reactions such as developing ringing in the ears (tinnitus) from a single dose of aspirin (Dykewicz & Lam, 2020; Kuklik et al., 2019; Mendes et al., 2019; Pichler, 2020a, 2020b; Warrington, Silvio-Dan, & Wong, 2018). Immunologic or severe hypersensitivity reactions are classified into one of four categories as described in Box 30.1 (Kaniwa & Saito, 2013; Pichler, 2020a, 2020b). Medications usually cause one type of response; Type I and Type IV forms occur most commonly. Penicillin, however, can cause all four types (Koh et al., 2019; Pichler, 2020a, 2020b; Trommell, Hofland, Van Komen, Dokter, & Van Baar, 2019; Zhang et al., 2020).

Skin eruptions can also occur and are associated with ADEs. These range from erythema (redness) to morbilliform (resembling measles), or maculopapular lesions. Reactions can be widespread or localized (occurring in one location, often referred to as a "fixed" drug reaction). Lesions may also be a blister or resemble psoriasis (psoriasiform) or may be a plaque, ulcer, or as severe as necrosis, depending on the underlying etiology (Beitz, 2017; Dykewicz & Lam, 2020; Pichler, 2020a, 2020b; Samel & Chu, 2020; Zhang et al., 2019). Chapter 32 provides an indepth discussion of atypical wounds including those precipitated by medications.

OFF-LABEL USE OF TRADITIONAL MEDICATIONS

While "natural" (i.e., nonprescription or alternative therapy) medications have been used for centuries across the planet to promote wound healing, more recently, prescription pharmacologic agents have been used off-label as topical therapy to facilitate wound healing. These medications include calcium channel blockers, regular insulin, nitroglycerine, opioid-related drugs, phenytoin (e.g., Dilantin), retinoids, sildenafil, and sucralfate (Table 30.2). Available studies range from animal models, in vitro approaches, and clinical testing. Please note that the following description of off-label use of prescription medications is NOT an endorsement of their usage. The explanation is to make readers aware of what research testing is occurring.

Subcutaneous injection of low molecular weight heparin (LMWH) had a positive effect on Achilles tendon healing in rats ($N = 36$) (Eren et al., 2018). In a clinical trial with burn patients, researchers reported faster healing and lower pain when given LMWH topical antibiotics (Manzoor et al., 2019).

Other scientists are testing topical formulations of drugs usually used orally/systemically. For example, a case study analyzed the stability of topical doxycycline in vitro and in a clinical application for diabetic foot ulcers (DFUs) (Gabriele et al., 2019). Two formulations of 2% doxycycline were stable for 70 days and promoted faster wound healing when clinically tested. Further testing is needed for full assessment of efficacy.

Another study investigated the use of topical hyaluronic acid and silver on the healing of pressure injuries or vascular wounds (e.g., arterial, venous) (Gazzabin, Serantoni, Palumbo, & Giordan, 2019). Although limited to only 25 patients, the topical combination (a spray form) of these two components applied once daily was reported to reduce wound area and keep bacterial growth "under control."

Topical phenytoin has been utilized in a variety of chronic wounds. A recent Cochrane Review (Hao et al., 2017) systematically analyzed three randomized control trials on phenytoin vs hydrocolloid dressings, triple antibiotic ointment, and simple dressings in 148 participants. The topical application of phenytoin to the wound bed was reported as "uncertain evidence" for use with grade (Stage) 1 and 2 pressure injuries and further research warranted prior to clinical application.

Another convulsant (topiramate) was used off-label topically in an animal study with diabetic mice. The researchers reported faster healing, better quality collagen deposition, and enhanced scar formation (wound strength) in the mice who received topiramate cream daily (Jara et al., 2019). The researchers noted that topiramate affected the insulin pathway in wound healing and could potentially be a therapeutic agent in patients with diabetes who have a chronic wound.

An interesting off-label topical use of corticosteroids was reported (Pearson, Prentice, Sinclair, Lim, & Carville, 2019). In a case series of seven patients with peristomal pyoderma gangrenosum (PPG) done in Australia, a crushed prednisolone tablet was combined with barrier powder and sprinkled on the PPG wounds. In six of the seven patients, the wounds healed, and pain was relieved. An earlier study done in the United States using crushed prednisone tablets had similar success (DeMartyn, Faller, & Miller, 2014).

TABLE 30.2   Off-Label Topical Medications and Wound Healing[a]

Off-Label Topical Agents (Level of Evidence)	Mechanism of Action/Category	Reported Effect on Wound Healing	References
Calcium Channel Blockers Nifedipine (Literature Review)	Affects calcium channels in blood vessels	Increased vascular perfusion and wound healing	Helmke, 2004a, 2004b; Jacobs, 2014
Insulin Topical (Regular) (Human Clinical Trials)	Antidiabetic agent with growth factor effect	Accelerates wound healing process	Attia, Belal, Samahy, & El Hamamsy, 2014; Rezvani et al., 2009; Singh & Pawar, 2020; Smith, 2010
Morphine and Morphine Blockers (Animal Studies)	Opioid narcotic and opioid narcotic blocker	Affect wound healing processes via opioid receptor impact; decreases inflammation	Rook, Hasan, & McCarson, 2008; Zaslansky, Schramm, Stein, Guthoff, & Schmidt-Westhausen, 2018
Naltrexone (Topical) (Animal Studies)	Antagonizes opioid receptors from opioid receptors	Assists with wound contraction	McLaughlin, Potering, Immonen, & Zagon, 2011
Nitroglycerine (glyceryl trinitrate) (Topical) (Animal Studies and Human Clinical Trials)	Organic nitrate; increases vasodilation	Accelerates wound healing	Hotkar, Avachat, Bhosale, & Oswal, 2015; Miles, Lord, Williams, & Fulbrook, 2019
Phenytoin Topical (Animal Studies and Systematic Review of Human Testing)	Anticonvulsant	Promotes granulation tissue formation; stimulates collagen, protein and hydroxyproline synthesis	Firmino et al., 2014; Hao et al., 2017; Smith, 2010
Retinoids (tretinoin) (Literature Review of Human Clinical Trials)	Antiacne agent	Increases granulation tissue; increases angiogenesis	Abdelmalek & Spencer, 2006; Helmke, 2004b
Sildenafil Topical and oral (Animal Studies and Human Clinical Trials)	Phosphodiesterase type 5 inhibitor; increases nitric oxide release	Accelerates wound healing and tissue perfusion; increases granulation	Derici et al., 2010; Farsaei, Khalil, Farboud, & Khazaeipour, 2015; Gursoy et al., 2014
Sucralfate (Topical)	Antiulcer (agent); coats gastric mucosa	Inhibits inflammatory cytokines; stimulates angiogenesis	Gupta, Heda, Shrirao, & Kalaskar, 2011; Helmke, 2004b

[a]Disclaimer: Please note that medications may have different trade and generic names in Canada and other foreign countries. Additional sources for this table are listed in Further Reading.

Topical insulin (10 units per 1 mL of saline) has also been trialed in patients with leprosy and chronic foot ulcers (Singh & Pawar, 2020). When compared with topical saline only, patients with topical insulin experienced statistically significantly faster wound healing ($P < 0.0001$) and reduced number of days to healing (average of 13 days less) ($P = 0.02$). The researchers concluded topical insulin therapy is a safe, efficacious, cheap, and easily available option for persons with chronic trophic ulcers.

The topical application of glyceryl trinitrate 2% ointment has been used in patients with chronic venous leg ulcers in an attempt to accelerate healing by capitalizing on the donation of the drug's nitrous oxide (Miles et al., 2019). Thus far, results are inconclusive.

Topical metformin hydrochloride hydrogel has also been studied in the animal model and in humans to explore wound healing (Tawfeek, Abou-Taleb, Badary, Ibrahim, & Abdellatif, 2020). The animal model demonstrated faster wound contraction; the clinical trial revealed topical metformin gel was well tolerated, reduced pain and edema as well as complete healing of the traumatic extremity and cutaneous extremity ulcers after 21 and 30 days, respectively. Researchers suggested that the wound healing effects were due to metformin's antiinflammatory effect, promotion of angiogenesis, and regulation of cell proliferation.

Another animal model study (with rats) demonstrated the local application of metformin accelerated wound healing (Zhao et al., 2017). The researchers identified accelerated collagen deposition and improved hair follicles and epidermis in the young rodents. A similar positive effect was noted in aged rodents wherein topical metformin promoted improved cell viability in wound beds.

In some instances, off-label topical use of a traditional drug is not effective. Topical application of morphine (0.2 or 0.4 mg of morphine dissolved in glycerine three times daily) in patients with erosive or ulcerative oral Lichen Planus (a chronic inflammation of oral mucosa) did not enhance wound healing, although all wounds eventually healed (Zaslansky et al., 2018). Impact on wound pain could not be assessed as patients experienced only mild levels of pain.

Gentamicin, an aminoglycoside antibiotic, is commonly used systemically to treat infections (including wound infections) caused by multiresistant bacteria. A major concern with systemic use is its intrinsic toxicity when given intravenously or by deep intramuscular injection. Therefore, topical application of gentamicin has been tested more frequently. In a systematic review and meta-analysis of the efficacy of topical gentamicin for patients with local wound infection or infection risk, researchers reported topical gentamycin application had significantly stronger clinical efficacy rates (OR = 3.57; 95% CI 2.52–5.07) and shorter time to healing (OR = −4.94; 95% CI 8.37–1.51) than other routes (Wang et al., 2019). The researchers concluded that topical gentamicin was significantly stronger for clinical efficacy and decreased duration of wound healing outcomes. Given the challenge of healing refractory chronic wounds, unique use of prescription medications in topical application warrants further research with full human subject protections. Future testing may identify safer uses of these approaches and generate approved topical usage.

SPECIAL CASE OF TOPICAL ANTIMICROBIALS

Though not always considered off-label usage, for persons with chronic wounds, utilization of topical antimicrobials (antibiotics and antiseptics) is a common part of therapy from pressure injuries to DFUs (Block & Wu, 2019). Topical antimicrobials act to impede bacterial growth of pathogens without harming the patient significantly. Antimicrobials can be divided into two groups: antibiotics and antiseptics. Antibiotics are chemicals that kill or inhibit microbial activity/growth. Antibiotics belong to various classes of drugs (penicillins, quinolones, sulfa agents) and generally are specifically focused on a narrow spectrum of activity. Topical antibiotics are not the first-line choice in wound infection as systemic therapy works better for deeper wound infections (Stevens et al., 2014). Conversely topical agents (e.g., metronidazole) may be used off-label very effectively to control wound odor (Akhmetova et al., 2016; Ousey, 2018).

Antiseptics are broad-spectrum disinfectants including substances like chlorhexidine, iodine (Betadine), hydrogen peroxide, sodium hypochlorite (e.g., Dakin's Solution), acetic acid, octenidine, and biguanide. Certain antiseptics are associated with wound healing delays by damaging fibroblasts, keratinocytes, and inflammation mediators (Block & Wu, 2019; Nikolic et al., 2019).

Antiseptics are designed to reduce microbial content within a wound. However, dilution level and length of use play a *pivotal* role in minimizing deleterious effects to the wound. Formulation also plays a role. Iodine inherent in cadexomer iodine is safer in wound care than povidone-iodine, and iodine scrub formulations should not be used in wounds as the detergent component has increased cytotoxic effects on exposed tissues (Leise, 2018). Sodium hypochlorite (e.g., Dakin's Solution) is safe only when used in dilute concentrations (0.0125%). But hypochlorous acid (a similar but different agent) is much more effective in inactivating bacteria and is associated with low or no cytotoxicity (Leise, 2018; Pure and Clean Wound Management Technology, 2020). For example, hypochlorous acid can kill *Acinetobacter baumannii*, *Enterococcus faecalis* (VRE), *Staphylococcus aureus* (MRSA), and *Candida albicans* in as little as 60 s (Pure and Clean Wound Management Technology, 2020; info@pureandclean.us). See Chapter 19 and Table 19-2 for an extensive review of topical antimicrobials in wound care.

PLANT AND HERBACEOUS ANIMAL SOURCES

Multiple narrative literature reviews support that selected plant based interventions, topical or oral, can augment wound healing. Many have been used for centuries, and are currently utilized in a variety of countries and cultures (India, Iran, Iraq, Turkey, Chinese, Islamic, Ayurveda, Unani) (Dorai, 2012; Gouveia et al., 2015; Gupta & Nautiyal, 2016; Majumdar & Sangole, 2016; Medellin-Luna, Castaneda-Delgao, Martinez-Balderas, & Cervantes-Villagrana, 2019; Shedoeva, Leavesly, Upton, & Fan, 2019; Siddique et al., 2019) to assist wound healing. When used outside of Western Society medical therapies, cultural "traditional" medicine (based on plant, animal, and mineral-based medicines) is often called Complementary and Alternative Medicine (Dorai, 2012).

Notably, between 25% and 50% of approved medical therapeutic prescription drugs are derivatives of natural products (Singh, Fisher, Shagalou, Varma, & Siegel, 2018). Not all plants used to promote wound healing or other positive outcomes are positive. Some plant and mushroom species have been used for inebriation and/or intoxication. Such substances include cannabis, euphorbia, ricinus, podophyllum, veratrum, and nightshades. The reader is referred to other sources for further reading but should recognize that some traditional plants are dangerous and, if used at all, must be used for specified purposes with full understanding of side effects and possible toxicities (Singh et al., 2018).

Complementary approaches do offer intriguing opportunities to improve clinical care. These "traditional" cultural therapies can potentially promote wound healing because of their simplicity, affordability, and increasing trial-based support for clinical efficacy. Notably, these traditional substances (e.g., aloe) can be combined with modern clinical therapies, biomaterials, and selected drugs to substantively improve care (Pereira & Bartoo, 2016). Living organisms (maggots and leeches) and metals (e.g., silver, copper) can augment wound healing and are discussed in Chapters 19 and 20. Herbal-derived compounds (e.g., aloe, vinca, marigold, curcumin, etc.) and selected animal-derived substances (e.g., honey, propolis, and sea cucumber) will be discussed primarily with a focus on topical therapy use. Table 30.3 lists a variety of topical therapies and their impact on healing. Hundreds of compounds are used across the planet in a variety of cultures. The focus here is those with some animal model and/or human clinical trial evidence. The reader is referred to the references list for further reading on the larger variety of available topical products used for wound healing globally.

Aloe vera has been used for skin and wound healing since at least 1500 BC and possibly for over 5000 years (Shakib, Shahraki, Razavi, & Hosseinzadeh, 2019). It belongs to the Liliaceae family and is similar to a cactus. Topical aloe has achieved positive results in patients with skin ulcers, burns, postoperative wounds, cracked nipples, genital herpes, and chronic wounds like pressure injuries (Hekmatpou et al., 2019). Researchers report the positive effects of aloe vera to include antibacterial, antiviral, antiinflammatory effects, and moisture retention. Active ingredients of aloe vera

include vitamins (C, E, B1, 2, 6, 12), anthraquinones, salicylic acid, amino acids, sterols, and other sugars. The oral administration of aloe vera has also been investigated. A systematic literature review reported the oral intake of aloe vera reversed impaired glucose tolerance, and lowered blood glucose, low-density lipoprotein (sometimes called "bad" cholesterol), and blood pressure. Researchers have subsequently suggested testing aloe vera for its impact on metabolic syndrome (Shakib et al., 2019).

Calendula officinalis, a garden plant of the Asteraceae family, commonly called marigold, is used worldwide both orally and topically for treating herpes, wounds, and scars. *C. officinalis* contains many compounds with positive biologic effects (e.g., flavonoids, triterpenoids, and polyphenols). Although inconsistent, positive effects include an antiinflammatory response, increased production of granulation tissue, and an antioxidant effect. Researchers suggest continued study of *C. officinalis* for wound healing as warranted (Givol et al., 2019; Leach, 2008).

Curcuma mangga is one of the zingiberaceous plants that has been used traditionally in elixir form for a variety of conditions including skin/wound issues. Srirod and Tewtrakul (2019) studied the effect of *C. mangga* extract in a cream formulation in an in vitro study of wound healing cells (murine type). They found that the cream was stable over time and

TABLE 30.3 Phytotherapy Effects on Wound Healing

Product (Oral and/or Topical)	Description	Purported Effects	References
Aloe vera	Topical gel derived from succulent aloe plant	Soothing; improves collagen production; antimicrobial; assists collagen formation antiinflammatory	Eshghi et al., 2010; Hashemi, Madani, & Abediankenari, 2015; Hekmatpou, Mehrabi, Rahzani, & Aminiyan, 2019; Helmke, 2004a, 2004b; Topman, Lin, & Gefen, 2013
Cayenne pepper	Extracted from Capsicum annuum, frutescens, red pepper	Relieves pain with short-term topical use; formulations available over the counter and by prescription; enhances blood circulation, helps vascular integrity	Beitz, 2017
Curcumin (*Zingiberaceae*)	From turmeric shrub	Antiinflammatory; analgesic activities; antimicrobial	Majumdar & Sangole, 2016; Shedoeva et al., 2019; Srirod & Tewtrakul, 2019; Topman et al., 2013
Ginger	Produced from rhizome of zingiber officinale plant	Antiinflammatory and antimicrobial	Topman et al., 2013
Goldenseal	Dry root herb in the buttercup family	Increases granulation; antimicrobial effects	Beitz, 2017
Plantain	From the banana plant genus Musa	Antioxidant	Beitz, 2017; Majumdar & Sangole, 2016

TABLE 30.3   Phytotherapy Effects on Wound Healing—cont'd

Product (Oral and/or Topical)	Description	Purported Effects	References
Tea Tree Oil (Topical)	Also known as melaleuca oil, an essential that comes from leaves of a tea tree; toxic if swallowed	Antiinflammatory; antimicrobial effects; may be active with MRSA	Beitz, 2017; Labib et al., 2019
Camellia sinensis	Contains flavonoids, tannins, caffeine, and amino acids.	Reduces wound healing time; topical ointment stimulates wound healing	Pereira & Bartoo, 2016; Shedoeva et al., 2019
Rosmarinus officinalis L. (Rosemary)	Contains terpenoids, and polyphenols enhances angiogenesis (topical-extract and essential oil)	Reduces inflammation; enhances collagen deposition	Labib et al., 2019; Pereira & Bartoo, 2016
Hippophae rhamnoides (Sea Buckthorn)	Contains flavonoids, carotenoids, tannins, amino acids (available in topical and oral use such as gels, and solutions)	Antioxidant antiinflammatory stimulates healing process and improves epithelialization; increase protein content in wounds; enhance wound contraction	Pereira & Bartoo, 2016
Catharanthus rosea (Vinca rosea)	Contains alkaloids and tannins (topical)	Antimicrobial improves epithelialization; enhances wound contraction and wound strength	Al-Shmgani, Mohammed, Sulaiman, & Saadoon, 2017; Pereira & Bartoo, 2016; Singh, Singh, & Singh, 2014
Calendula officinalis (Marigold)	Contains triterpenoids and flavonoids (available as topical gels and extracts)	Enhances collagen production antiinflammatory, antibacterial; stimulates proliferation/migration of fibroblasts; stimulate angiogenesis	Givol et al., 2019: Leach, 2008; Pereira & Bartoo, 2016; Shedoeva et al., 2019
Morinda citrifolia (Noni)	Contains acids, phenols, flavonoids, triterpenoid, etc. (extract-oral)	Reduces wound area and enhances epithelialization	Pereira & Bartoo, 2016
Achille millefolium (Asteraceae Family Herb Family)	Contains Azulen (oral and topical; tonic and essential oil)	Antiinflammatory antioxidant accelerates wound closure; assists fibroblast proliferation; accelerates collagen production, inhibits MMPs	Medellin-Luna et al., 2019
Opuntia ficus-indica L. (Prickly Pear)	Contains flavonoids, alkaloids, fatty acids, phytosterols, tocopherus (essential oil, topical)	Antibacterial; accelerates wound closure and contraction	Khemiri, Hedi, Zouaoui, Gdara, & Bitri, 2019
Grape seed	Contains phenolic compounds like catechins, epilatechins, and proanthocyanidins; and vitamins (E) and tannins (extract ointment)	Antioxidant, antiinflammatory	Izadpanah, Sourgi, Geraminejad, & Hosseini, 2019; Majumdar & Sangole, 2016
Propolis (Honey Bee—*Apis mellifera*)	Contains polyphenols caffeic acid, flavonoids. Increases migration and proliferation of fibroblasts	Antibacterial; antiinflammatory; induces wound contraction; accelerates wound healing; increases migration and proliferation of fibroblasts	Afkhamizadeh et al., 2018; Elkhenany, El-Badri, & Dhar, 2019; Martinotti, Pellavio, Laforenza, & Ranzato, 2019; Moon, Lee, Chung, Rhee, & Lee, 2018

Phytotherapy is not regulated by the Federal Drug and Administration (FDA). Phytotherapy can cause side affects ranging from mild to severe, and interact with other medications, potentially making them less effective.
Additional sources for this table are listed in Further Reading.

that *C. mangga* ointment increased cell viability, served as an antioxidant, and increase cell proliferation. The researchers suggested that in its cream formulation, *C. mangga* could be used as a wound-healing agent.

In an in vitro study of traditionally used Nepalese plants, researchers analyzed the effects of nine plant extracts on cells necessary for wound healing (Zimmerman-Klemd et al., 2019). Two plants, *Bassia longifolia* (tree bark from Sapotaceae family) and *Gmelina arborea* (tree bark from Verbenaceae family), formulated in an ethyl acetate extract decreased inflammation (reducing activation and proliferation of T-cells) and augmented keratinocyte and fibroblast cells activity in cell-based assays. Both substances also are suggested to assist epithelialization and promote granulation tissue growth.

Clinical trial testing of a phytotherapy (betulin or birch bark) linked with an oleogel (Episalvan) has also been reported (Schleffler, 2019). The active ingredient, triterpene dry extract (betulin) of the now approved drug, Episalvan, has been purported to affect all phases of wound healing. Faster wound closure and reduced pain was reported in Phase II and III trials of burn wounds and split-thickness skin graft donor sites. Betulin was noted to upregulate inflammatory cells, promote autolysis, and promote fibroblast and keratinocyte cell migration resulting in new tissue growth and faster epithelialization.

Opuntia ficus-indica inermis (OFI), an oil extracted from the seeds of mature prickly pears fruits, has been studied in full-thickness skin wounds (Khemiri et al., 2019). When tested in animal models against bacteria, yeast, and fungi, OFI oil was demonstrated to inhibit bacteria (e.g., *Enterobacter*), *Candida* species of yeast, *Aspergillus*, and other fungi. Statistically significant faster wound healing within 5 days ($P < 0.001$) was also reported in the rat model.

Herbs such as henna, pomegranate, and myrrh have been widely used in traditional cultural systems of medicine because of their purported antiseptic and antiinflammatory effects. Known for centuries and mentioned in both the Bible and Koran, these herbs are currently under investigation for their effect on wound healing. Elzayat, Auda, Alanazi, and Al-Agamy (2018) studied the effect of an herbal ointment blend on full-thickness wounds in rats compared with gentamicin. Natural extracts of all three herbs were used in ointments either singly or in combination. The blended formulation showed the highest percentage of wound contraction and decrease in time for epithelialization compared with the control group. The blended ointment was somewhat comparable to gentamicin ointment in the animal testing of antibacterial activity; it also had antifungal activity. The authors suggest that the positive wound healing effects are due to faster collagen deposition, formation of stronger connective tissue, and antibacterial activity.

Topical vinca (*Catharanthus roseus*), also called annual vinca or periwinkle, has been tested in both animal models and human clinical studies. It is theorized to promote increased tensile strength, granulation tissue, and wound contraction. Methanolic extract of *C. roseus* dried leaves has been applied topically on full-thickness wounds in mice (Singh et al., 2014). A statistically significant increase in collagen fibers ($P < 0.001$) and rate of wound contraction was reported. An intriguing use of vinca plant is the phytochemicals. These are theorized to generate silver nanoparticles (AgNP) from the plant (i.e., green synthesis) with strong in vitro antioxidant and antimicrobial effects against pathogens (Al-Shmgani et al., 2017). In the laboratory setting with animal models, the AgNP-treated mice has faster healing activity by day 12 (98%) when compared with the control groups (85%).

An extract of the Gamat or Sea Cucumber, an animal that thrives on the seabed, especially in Southeast Asia, has been used in topical ointments, oils, or gels. The extract contains essential amino acids, and fatty acids. In a study of patients ($N = 25$) who underwent split-thickness skin grafts, the topical application of the animal substance was compared with a hydrogel (Wen, Halim, Saad, Nor, & Sulaiman, 2018). After 10 days, there was no difference in epithelialization, pain level, or pruritus scores between the two products. However, the Gamat gel was less expensive, raising its possible use in resource-limited situations.

Topical application of propolis, the resin in bee glue, has been studied in a variety of settings and models to explore its impact on wound healing. In patients with a DFU, propolis, theorized to be both antiinflammatory and antimicrobial, significantly faster ulcer size reduction in 4 weeks ($P = 0.001$) when compared with conventional therapies was reported (Afkhamizadeh et al., 2018). The researchers suggested that the outcome may be due to antimicrobial effects of propolis. Green propolis, theorized to also recruit and stimulate stem cells, has been studied for its effect on proliferation, differentiation, and migration of bone marrow stromal cells (Elkhenany et al., 2019). Over 3 days, the propolis extract was applied to tissue cultures of bone marrow cells. The researchers found that propolis in concentrations of <400 mcg/mL were not cytotoxic to bone marrow stem cells. Higher concentrations inhibited proliferation and were cytotoxic. Propolis has also been studied in posttonsillectomy patients. When applied topically via gargling, postoperative pain was significantly better in the propolis group by day 3 and days 7–10. Postoperative hemorrhage was significantly less ($P < 0.05$) and wound healing significantly better ($P = 0.002$) than the control group who gargled with plain fluid. Finally, the effect of topical propolis has been studied on human keratinocytes (Martinotti et al., 2019). Using an in vitro scratch wound healing model (confluent layers of human keratinocytes were scratch wounded), propolis induced a pronounced increase in wound repair abilities of keratinocytes. A cell migration assay showed propolis stimulated keratinocytes to close the wound.

Medicinal or medical-grade honey has gained wide acceptance in recent decades. Notably, medicinal honey is dissimilar to honey used in cooking in terms of strength and safe preparation. Medicinal honey has become well established in the topical management of wounds and is presented in Chapter 20.

CLINICAL PRACTICES MITIGATING DRUG EFFECTS ON WOUND HEALING

Since chronic wounds are an expensive, compelling clinical challenge, knowledgeable clinicians of all disciplines and specialties need to be cognizant of the potential for medications to impair wound healing. A thorough intake of medication history by the provider and/or pharmacist is critical when managing a patient with a wound, particularly a nonhealing wound (Demidova-Rice, Hamblin, & Herman, 2012; Kaufman, 2015; Rutecki, 2012; Sen et al., 2009; Shirin, 2015).

Critical components of the medication history intake include the following items:

1. Medication dosage, frequency, start date, etc.
2. Past medication reactions, connective tissue disease, or previous wound healing delays, and use of OTC medications.
3. Use of "natural" medications (e.g., herbals), specifically:
   a. What product(s) do you use?
   b. What form is the product in? (tea, liquids)
   c. Do you space product use away from prescription or OTC medications?
   d. Do you use any topical natural or herbal substance on year wound or skin?
4. "Red Flag" prescription medications with possible drug interactions (e.g., cyclosporine, digoxin, lithium, protease inhibitors, warfarin).
5. Recent use or exposure to vaccines or contrast dye.
6. An analysis of medical history/history of present problem for other hidden factors potentially affecting drug therapy and/or wound healing in patients with refractory wounds.

7. A consideration of chronic disease comorbidities and pertinent drug therapy for elders with or at risk for chronic wounds.

Multiple underlying factors can occur that impact how drugs affect wound healing. Malnutrition (often present in elders and the chronically ill) can affect blood protein levels (e.g., albumin) which will alter drug-binding processes (e.g., phenytoin) and increase circulating drug levels. Patients may also have mouth ulcers, bad teeth or chronic pain affecting oral intake (Harris & Fraser, 2004).

Aging and chronic disease will also alter body physiology. Both liver and kidney function decrease with age, therefore renal function needs to be monitored (e.g., use creatinine clearance in the elderly rather than creatinine to assess renal function), and drugs noted in the Beers criteria (e.g., antipsychotics like Haldol, hypnotics [e.g., diazepam]) need to be avoided as possible. Additionally, DMARDs (disease-modifying antirheumatic drugs), such as methotrexate and sulfasalazine, need to be noted as they can impair wound healing.

Polypharmacy, the use of many drugs for multiple conditions when possibly not all are needed is a notable problem in U.S. elders. Wound patients often experience polypharmacy related to underlying chronic medical conditions (multimorbidity overlaid with need for treating wound care situations [e.g., an infected wound]). Polypharmacy is associated with adverse outcomes including mortality, falls, adverse drug reactions, and potentially, delayed wound healing (Masnoon, Shakib, Kalisch-Ellett, & Caughey, 2017). A helpful mnemonic, "ARMOR," can assist clinicians:

Assess (check Beers criteria, use of other "Red Flag" drugs)
Review (review drug–drug and drug–disease interactions)
Minimize (minimize number of medications pertinent to patient's status)
Optimize (optimize for renal/hepatic function), and
Reassess (reassess functional/cognitive status periodically and after drug changes; Haque, 2009).

CLINICAL CONSULT

A: Received referral for wound consult on multiple skin changes (all called pressure injuries) on an 80-year-old bedfast white female with a history of frailty, malnutrition, Alzheimer's dementia (newer diagnosis), hypertension, previous CVA, and renal insufficiency. Physical assessment shows that likely pressure injuries are on bilateral trochanters, sacrum. Multiple small wounds (scabs) are also on sternum and both arms. Patient is on a pressure redistribution support surface, the dietitian is on consult for poor albumin, low prealbumin, and weight loss (>10%). The pressure injuries on trochanters and sacrum are round in shape, Stage 4, and with the following measurements: right hip 4 × 4 × 2 cm, left hip 3 × 5 × 1.5 cm and sacrum 5 × 3 × 2 cm, respectively. All wound bases are 20% slough and 80% pale pink tissue. Surrounding skin intact. No local signs of infection.

Sternal "pressure injuries" are multiple thin scabs. Both arms have multiple thin scabs; both arms also showing intact skin with erythematous rash. Medication review shows following medications: Lisinopril (10 mg), multivitamin one daily, Iron (Ferrous Sulfate), and Aricept (donepezil) (10 mg daily). The Aricept is newly ordered for the last 5 days.

D: Assessment of sternal wounds and arm lesions is not consistent with pressure injury (not over a bony prominence with long weight loading). Risk factors and patient history are consistent with pressure injuries on hips and sacrum but not for other skin lesions. Patient has not been lying face down in bed (e.g., prone) at any time; had not had any recent surgery or procedures.

P: Provide appropriate care for pressure-related wounds on trochanters and sacrum. Investigate potential integumentary adverse drug event (ADE) related to Aricept use.

Continued

CLINICAL CONSULT—cont'd

I: Nurse consultant discusses situation with attending provider pointing out skin changes on arms and sternum are *not* pressure-related injuries. Given renal status and new use of Aricept, consultant suggests that Aricept (donepezil) is causing integumentary adverse drug event (review of drug literature shows that Aricept can cause integumentary ADEs).
Provider agreed to following plan of care:
1. Discontinue Aricept, monitor neurologic state
2. Apply moisturizing lotion to arms and sternum daily
3. Consider future use of Benadryl and/or topical steroid if sternum and extremity wounds worsen

4. Institute pressure injury treatment protocol (turn and reposition, elevate heels off bed, manage urinary incontinence with external female device [e.g., Purewick])
5. Upgrade support surface to low air loss system
6. Topical therapy for pressure injuries: hydrogel daily with fluffed 4 × 4 dressings
E: Follow-up at next assessment to evaluate sternum and arms for ADE; monitor pressure injury.
Note: This is a real-life case—The "pressure injuries" on sternum and arms were an ADE and resolved when the drug was discontinued.

SUMMARY

This chapter examined the following critical concepts:
- Medications can assist or impair wound healing affecting some or all of the four phases.
- Selected medications notoriously impairing wound healing include steroids, NSAIDs, anticancer chemotherapy, antiangiogenesis agents and selected antirheumatoid and antigout agents.
- Selected traditional prescription medications (topical insulin, phenytoin, nitroglycerine, sildenafil) are being used off-label in clinical testing of wound healing effects.

- Antibiotics and antiseptics are both used topically in wounds; their spectrum of efficacy and safety parameters for cytotoxicity differ significantly.
- Phytotherapy (use of plants and natural substances) used in cultural practices globally can alter wound healing and skin integrity.
- Polypharmacy is a substantial problem especially affecting the elderly; mitigating strategies can be used to minimize adverse effects.

SELF-ASSESSMENT QUESTIONS

1. A healthcare student is asking questions about drugs impairing wound healing. Which of the following drugs/drug categories would the wound clinician be *unlikely* to include:
   a. Steroids (e.g., prednisone)
   b. Hormones (estrogen)
   c. Antiangiogenesis drugs (e.g., bevacizumab)
   d. Antirheumatoid drugs (e.g., methotrexate)
2. Which wound healing phase would likely be *most* impaired when a patient is receiving oral prednisone?
   a. Maturation
   b. Proliferation
   c. Inflammation
   d. Hemostasis
3. Medications purported to support tissue regeneration in wound healing include the following:
   a. Megestrol
   b. Phenytoin
   c. Estrogen
   d. Pentoxifylline
   e. All of the above
4. Vitamin A in large doses would be an *inappropriate* medication in which patient care situation:
   a. Patient receiving oral steroids
   b. Patient with retinol insufficiency

   c. Patient with age-related macular degeneration
   d. Patient who has had recent neurosurgery
5. Risk factors for adverse drug events (ADEs) would be *unlikely* to include the following characteristic/situation:
   a. Creatinine level of 3.0
   b. Family history of skin allergies
   c. Middle age group
   d. Personal history of drug allergy
6. A patient is given penicillin for the first time and develops a Type I drug reaction. Which of the following responses is typical of this form of reaction:
   a. Decrease in platelet levels
   b. Angioedema and wheezing
   c. Vasculitic skin reaction
   d. Delayed onset of allergic reaction for 24 h
7. Case series research in the United States and Australia examined off-label topical therapy for patients with peristomal pyoderma gangrenosum (PPG). Which class of drug therapy was used in the form of crushed tablets applied to the PPG wounds?
   a. Hormones
   b. Calcium channel blockers
   c. Antiangiogenesis agents
   d. Steroids

8. Topical antiseptics have a broad spectrum of antimicrobial activity but can be cytotoxic as well. Which of the following agents is associated with good antimicrobial activity with low cytotoxicity in wounds?
   a. Povidone-iodine
   b. Hypochlorous acid
   c. Hydrogen peroxide
   d. Sodium hypochlorite

9. Aloe vera, a form of phytotherapy, has been used for centuries for skin and wound healing to achieve: debridement, balanced MMP-TIMP levels, increased collagen synthesis, reduce bacterial load. Its effects include:
   a. Antimicrobial
   b. Antiviral
   c. Moisture retention
   d. Antiinflammatory
   e. All of the above

10. A wound care clinician is caring for an elderly patient with multiple comorbidities and polypharmacy. Which of the following actions would assist with mitigating adverse drug events?
   a. Identifying "Red Flag" prescription drugs like Digoxin or Lithium
   b. Completing a thorough family and personal history for drug-related skin reactions
   c. Questioning with regard to use of OTC and herbal agents
   d. All of the above

REFERENCES

Abdelmalek, M., & Spencer, J. M. (2006). Retinoids and wound healing. *Dermatologic Surgery, 32*(10), 1219–1230. https://doi.org/10.1111/j.1524-4725.20086.32280.x.

Afkhamizadeh, M., Aboutorabi, R., Davari, H., Najafi, M., Azimi, S., Langaroudi, A., et al. (2018). Topical propolis improves wound healing in patients with diabetic foot ulcer: A randomized controlled trial. *Natural Product Research, 32*(17), 2096–2099. https://doi.org/10.1080/14786419.2017.1363755.

Afzali, H., Kashi, A., Momen-Heravi, M., Razzaghi, R., Amirani, E., Bahmani, F., et al. (2019). The effects of magnesium and vitamin E co-supplementation on wound healing and metabolic status in patients with diabetic foot ulcer: A randomized, double blind, placebo-controlled trial. *Wound Repair and Regeneration, 27*, 277–284. https://doi.org/10.1111/wrr.12701.

Aghaloo, T., Pi-Anfrons, J., Moshaverina, A., Sim, D., Grogan, T., & Hadaya, D. (2019). The effects of systemic diseases and medications on implant osseointegration: A systematic review. *International Journal of Oral & Maxillofacial Implants, 34*(Suppl), S35–S49. https://doi.org/10.11607/jomi.19suppl.g3.

Ahn, J. W., Shalabi, D., Correa-Selm, L., Dasgeb, B., Nikbakht, N., & Cha, J. (2019). Impaired wound healing secondary to bevacizumab. *International Wound Journal, 16*, 1009–1012. https://doi.org/10.1111/iwj.13139.

Akhmetova, A., Saliev, T., Allan, I., Illsley, M., Nurgozhin, T., & Mikhalovsky, S. (2016). A comprehensive review of topical odor-controlling treatment options for chronic wounds. *Journal of Wound, Ostomy, and Continence Nursing, 43*(6), 98–607. https://doi.org/10.1097/WON.0000000000000273.

Al-Shmgani, H., Mohammed, W. H., Sulaiman, G. M., & Saadoon, A. H. (2017). Biosynthesis of silver nanoparticles from Catharanthus roseus leaf extract an assessing their antioxidant, antimicrobial, and wound healing activities. *Artificial Cells, Nanomedicine, and Biotechnology, 45*(6), 1234–1240. https://doi.org/10.1080/21691401.2016.1220950.

Amaya, R. (2015). Safety and efficacy of active Leptospermum honey in neonatal and pediatric wound debridement. *Journal of Wound Care, 24*(3), 95–103. https://doi.org/10.12968/jowc.2015.24.3.95.

American College of Prosthodontists. (2020). *Facts and figures: Tooth loss.* Retrieved 6/5/2020 from www.gotoapro.org.

Anderson, K., & Hamm, R. L. (2012). Factors that impair wound healing. *Journal of American College of Clinical Wound Specialists, 4*(4), 84–91. https://doi.org/10.1016/j.jccw.2014.03.001.

Armstrong, D. G., & Meyr, A. (2020a). Basic principles of wound healing. In *UptoDate.* Retrieved 4/2/2020 from www.uptodate.com.

Armstrong, D. G., & Meyr, A. (2020b). Risk factors for impaired wound healing and wound complications. In *UptoDate.* Retrieved 4/2/2020 from www.uptodate.com.

Armstrong, D. G., & Meyr, A. (2020c). Basic principles of wound management. In *UptoDate.* Retrieved 4/2/2020 from www.uptodate.com.

Assante, J., Collins, S., & Hewer, I. (2015). Infection associated with single-dose dexamethasone for prevention of postoperative nausea and vomiting: A literature review. *AANA Journal, 83*(4), 281–288.

Attia, E. A., Belal, D. M., Samahy, M. H., & El Hamamsy, M. H. (2014). A pilot trial using topical regular crystalline insulin vs. aqueous zinc solution for uncomplicated cutaneous wound healing: Impact on quality of life. *Wound Repair and Regeneration, 22*, 52–57. https://doi.org/10.1111/wrr.12122.

Azevedo, M., Lisboa, C., Cobrado, L., Pina-Vaz, C., & Rodrigues, A. (2020). Hard-to-heal wounds, biofilm, and wound healing: An intricate relationship. *British Journal of Nursing, 29*(5), S6–S13. https://doi.org/10.12968/bjon.2020.29.5.s6.

Barry, S. (2010). Non-steroidal anti-inflammatory drugs inhibit bone healing: A review. *Veterinary and Comparative Orthopaedics and Traumatology, 23*(6), 385–392. https://doi.org/10.3415/VCOT-10-01-0017.

Bauman, W. A., Spungen, A. M., Collins, J. F., Raisch, D. W., Ho, C., Deitrick, G. A., et al. (2013). The effect of oxandrolone on the healing of chronic pressure ulcers in persons with spinal cord injury: A randomized trial. *Annals of Internal Medicine, 158*(10), 718–726. https://doi.org/10.7326/0003-4819-158-10-201305210-00006.

Beitz, J. (2017). Pharmacologic impact (AKA "breaking bad") of medications on wound healing and wound development: A literature-based overview. *Ostomy Wound Management*, 63(3), 18–35.

Berry, J. D., Miulli, D., Lam, B., Elia, C., Minasian, J., Podkovik, S., et al. (2018). The neurosurgical wound and factors that can affect cosmetic functional, and neurological outcomes. *International Wound Journal*, 16, 71–78. https://doi.org/10.1111/iwj.12993.

Block, A., & Wu, S. (2019). Topical antibiotic use in diabetic wound healing. *Podiatry Management, November*, 73–79.

Centers for Medicare and Medicaid Service. (2020). *Chronic illness chart book and charts 2017*. Retrieved 3/26/2020 from https://www.cms.gov/research.statistics-data-and-systems/statistics-trends-and-reports/chronic-conditions/chartbook_charts.

Cevirme, D., Savluk, O., Basaran, E., Aksoy, R., Elibol, A., Bas, T., et al. (2020). Effects of anticoagulant drugs on wound healing process in a rat model: A comparative study. *Journal of Wound Care*, 29(1), 44–50.

Chen, L., & Tsai, T. F. (2018). The role of B-blockers in dermatological treatment: A review. *Journal of the European Academy of Dermatology & Venereology*, 32(3), 363–371.

Cheng, C., Nayernama, A., Jones, S. C., Casey, D., & Waldren, P. E. (2019). Wound healing complications with lenvatinib identified in a pharmacovigilance database. *Journal of Oncology Pharmacy Practice*, 25(8), 1817–1822. https://doi.org/10.1177/1078155218817109.

Council for Responsible Nutrition. (2019). Dietary supplement use reaches all time high. In *CRN*. Retrieved 6/5/2020 from https://www.crnusa.org/newsroom/dietary-supplement-use-reaches-all-time-high.

DeMartyn, L., Faller, N., & Miller, L. (2014). Treating pyoderma gangrenosum with topical crushed prednisone: A report of three cases. *Ostomy Wound Management*, 60(6), 50–54.

Demidova-Rice, T. N., Hamblin, M. R., & Herman, I. M. (2012). Acute and impaired wound healing: Pathophysiology and current methods for drug delivery, part I: Normal and chronic wounds: Biology, causes, and approaches to care. *Advances in Skin & Wound Care*, 25(7), 304–314.

Derici, H., Kamer, E., Unalp, H., Diniz, G., Bozdag, A., Tansug, T., et al. (2010). Effect of sildenafil on wound healing: An experimental study. *Langenbeck's Archives of Surgery*, 395(6), 713–718.

Dorai, A. A. (2012). Wound care with traditional, complementary, and alternative medicine. *Indian Journal of Plastic Surgery*, 45(2), 418–424.

Dykewicz, M. S., & Lam, J. K. (2020). Drug hypersensitivity reactions. *Medical Clinics of North America*, 104, 109–128. https://doi.org/10.1016/j.mcna.2019.09.003.

Elkhenany, H., El-Badri, N., & Dhar, M. (2019). Green propolis extract promotes in vitro proliferation, differentiation, and migration of bone marrow stromal cells. *Biomedicine & Pharmacotherapy*, 115, 108861. https://doi.org/10.1016/j.biopha.2019.108861.

Elzayat, E. M., Auda, S. H., Alanazi, F. K., & Al-Agamy, M. (2018). Evaluation of wound healing activity of henna, pomegranate and myrrh herbal ointment blend. *Saudi Pharmaceutical Journal*, 26, 733–738.

Eren, Y., Adenir, O., Dincel, Y., Genc, E., Arslan, Y., & Caglar, A. (2018). Effects of low molecular weight heparin and rivaroxaban on rat Achilles tendon healing. *Joint Diseases and Related Surgery*, 29(1), 13–19.

Eshghi, F., Jalal Hosseinmehr, S., Rahmani, N., Khademloo, M., Norozi, M. S., & Hojati, O. (2010). Effects of aloe vera cream on posthemorrhoidectomy pain and wound healing: Results of a randomized, blind, placebo-control study. *The Journal of Alternative and Complementary Medicine*, 16(6), 647–650.

Farsaei, S., Khalil, H., Farboud, E., & Khazaeipour, Z. (2015). Sildenafil in the treatment of pressure ulcer: A randomized clinical trial. *International Wound Journal*, 12(1), 111–117.

Fijan, S., Frauwallaner, A., Langerhole, T., Krebs, B., Ter Harr, J. A., Heschl, A., et al. (2019). Efficacy of using probiotics with antagonistic activity against pathogens of wound infections: An integrative review of the literature. *BioMed Research International*, 219, 7585486. https://doi.org/10.1155/2019/7585486.

Firmino, F., Pereira de Almeida, A., Griijo e Silva, R., Da Silva Alves, G., Da Silva Granadiero, D., & Garcia Penna, L. (2014). Scientific production on the application of phenytoin in wound healing. *Revista da Escola de Enfermagem da U S P*, 48(1), 162–169.

Gabriele, S., Buchanan, B., Kundu, A., Dwyer, H., Gabriele, J., Mayer, P., et al. (2019). Stability, activity, an application of topical doxycycline formulation in a diabetic wound case study. *Wounds*, 31(2), 49–54.

Gaucher, S., Nicholas, C., Piveteau, O., Phillippe, H. J., & Blanche, P. (2017). Sarcoidosis and wound healing after cellulitis of the lower limb. Is methotrexate responsible for skin graft failure? *Wounds*, 29(8), 229–230.

Gazzabin, L., Serantoni, S., Palumbo, F., & Giordan, N. (2019). Hyaluronic acid and metallic silver treatment of chronic wounds: Healing rate and bacterial load control. *Journal of Wound Care*, 28(7), 482–490.

Ginestal, R., Perez-Kohler, B., Perez-Lopez, P., Rodriguez, M., Pascual, G., Cebrian, D., et al. (2019). Comparing the influence of two immunosuppressants (fingolimod, azathioprine) on wound healing in a rat model of primary and secondary intention wound closure. *Wound Repair and Regeneration*, 27, 59–68.

Givol, O., Kornhaber, R., Visentin, D., Cleary, M., Haik, J., & Harats, M. (2019). A systematic review of Calendula officinalis extract for wound healing. *Wound Repair and Regeneration*, 27, 548–561.

Gouveia, B., Albuquerque, A., Dos Santos, S., Da Silva, A., De Oliviera, L., & Costa, M. (2015). Wound management: Empirical practices under the cultural and religious point of view. *Revista de Enfermagem UFPE On line*, 9(3), 7046–7054.

Gupta, P., Heda, P., Shrirao, S., & Kalaskar, S. (2011). Topical sucralfate treatment of anal fistulotomy wounds: A randomized placebo-controlled trial. *Diseases of the Colon and Rectum*, 54(6), 699–704. https://doi.org/10.1007/dcr.0b013e31820fcd89.

Gupta, D., & Nautiyal, U. (2016). Ayurvedic remedies for the healing of wounds: A review. *International Journal of Pharmaceutical and Medicinal Research*, 4(4), 342–349.

Gursoy, K., Oruc, M., Kankaya, Y., Ulusoy, M., Kocer, U., Kankaya, D., et al. (2014). Effect of topically applied sildenafil citrate on wound healing: An experimental study. *Bosnian Journal of Basic Medical Sciences*, 14(3), 125–131.

Hao, X., Li, H., Su, H., Cai, H., Guo, T., Liu, R., et al. (2017). Topical phenytoin for treating pressure ulcers. *Cochrane Database of Systematic Reviews*. https://doi.org/10.1002/14651858.CD008251.pub2.

Haque, R. (2009). ARMOR: A tool to evaluate polypharmacy in elderly persons. *Annals of Long-Term Care*, 17, 26–30.

Harris, C. L., & Fraser, C. (2004). Malnutrition in the institutionalized elderly. *Ostomy Wound Management, 50*(10), 54–63.

Hashemi, S. A., Madani, S. A., & Abediankenari, S. (2015). The review on properties of aloe-vera in healing of cutaneous wounds. *BioMED Research International, 2015,* 714216.

Hekmatpou, D., Mehrabi, F., Rahzani, K., & Aminiyan, A. (2019). The effect of aloe vera clinical trials on prevention and healing of skin wound: A systematic review. *Iranian Journal of Medical Sciences, 44*(1), 1–9.

Helmke, C. D. (2004a). Current topical treatments in wound healing, part I. *International Journal of Pharmaceutical Compounding, 8*(4), 269–273.

Helmke, C. D. (2004b). Current topical treatments in wound healing, part II. *International Journal of Pharmaceutical Compounding, 8*(5), 354–357.

Hotkar, M., Avachat, A., Bhosale, S., & Oswal, Y. (2015). Preliminary investigation of topical nitroglycerin formulations containing natural wound healing agent in diabetes-induced foot ulcer. *International Wound Journal, 12*(2), 210–217.

Hull, R. D., Garcia, D. A., & Vasquez, S. (2021). Warfarin and other vitamin K antagonists: Dosing and adverse effects. In *UptoDate.* Retrieved 3/23/2023. https://www.uptodate.com/contents/warfarin-and-other-vkas-dosing-and-adverse-effects.

Izadpanah, A., Sourgi, S., Geraminejad, N., & Hosseini, M. (2019). Effect of grapeseed extract ointment on cesarean section wound healing: A double-blind, randomized, controlled clinical trial. *Complementary Therapies in Clinical Practice, 35,* 323–328.

Jacobs, A. (2014). Using topical compounded medications to modulate wound healing. *Podiatry Today, 27*(8). Retrieved 8/19/2020 from https://www.podiatrytoday.com/utilizing-topical-compounded-medications-modulatewoundhealing.

Jara, C. P., Do Prado, T., Bobbo, V. C. P., Ramalho, A., Lima, M., Velloso, L., et al. (2019). Topical topiramate improves wound healing in an animal model of hyperglycemia. *Biological Research for Nursing, 21*(4), 420–430.

Kaniwa, N., & Saito, Y. (2013). Pharmacogenomics of severe cutaneous adverse reactions and drug-induced liver injury. *Journal of Human Genetics, 58,* 317–326.

Kaufman, G. (2015). Multiple medicines: The issues surrounding polypharmacy. *Nursing and Residential Care, 17*(4), 198–203.

Khemiri, I., Hedi, B., Zouaoui, N., Gdara, N., & Bitri, L. (2019). The antimicrobial and wound healing potential of Opuntia ficus indica L. inermis extracted oil from Tunisia. *Evidence-Based Complementary and Alternative Medicine, 2019,* 9148762. https://doi.org/10.1155/2019/9148782.

Koh, H., Chai, Z., Tay, H., Fook-Chong, S., Choo, K. J., Oh, C., et al. (2019). Risk factors and diagnostic markers of bacteremia in Stevens-Johnson syndrome and toxic epidermal necrolysis: A cohort of 176 patients. *Journal of the American Academy of Dermatology, 81*(3), 686–693. https://doi.org/10.1016/j.jaad.2019.05.096.

Krischak, G. D., Augat, P., Claes, L., Kinzl, L., & Beck, A. (2007). The effects of non-steroidal anti-inflammatory drug application on incisional wound healing in rats. *Journal of Wound Care, 16*(2), 76–78.

Kuklik, N., Stausberg, J., Amiri, M., & Jockel, K. (2019). Improving drug safety in hospitals: A retrospective study on the potential adverse drug events coded in routine data. *BMC Health Services Research, 19,* 555. https://doi.org/10.1186/s12913-019-4381-x.

Labib, R. M., Ayoub, I. M., Michel, H. E., Mehanny, M., Kamil, V., Hany, M., et al. (2019). Appraisal on the wound healing potential of *Melaleuca alternifolia* and *Rosmarinus officinalis* L. essential oil-loaded chitosan topical preparations. *PLoS One, 14*(9), e0219561. https://doi.org/10.1371/journal.pone.0219561.

Leach, M. J. (2008). Calendula officinalis and wound healing: A systematic review. *Wounds: A Compendium of Clinical Research and Practice, 20,* 236–243.

Leise, B. S. (2018). Topical wound medications. *Veterinary Clinics of North America. Equine Practice, 34*(3), 485–498.

Levine, J. (2017). The effect of oral medications on wound healing. *Advances in Skin & Wound Care, 30*(3), 137–142.

Levine, J. (2018). How oral medications affect wound healing. *Nursing, 48*(3), 35–40.

Majumdar, A., & Sangole, P. (2016). Alternative approaches in wound healing. In *Wound healing—New insights into ancient challenges* (pp. 459–482). Intech. https://doi.org/10.5772/63636.

Manzoor, S., Khan, F., Muhammads, S., Qayyam, R., Muhammad, I., Nazir, V., et al. (2019). Comparative study of conventional and topical heparin treatment in second degree burn patients for burn analgesia and wound healing. *Burns, 45,* 379–386.

Martinotti, S., Pellavio, G., Laforenza, U., & Ranzato, E. (2019). Propolis induces AQP3 expression: A possible way of action in wound healing. *Molecules, 25,* 1544. https://doi.org/10.3390/molecules24081544.

Masnoon, N., Shakib, S., Kalisch-Ellett, L., & Caughey, G. E. (2017). What is polypharmacy? A systematic review of definitions. *BMC Geriatrics, 17,* 230. https://doi.org/10.1186/S12877-017-0621-2.

McLaughlin, P. J., Potering, C. A., Immonen, J. A., & Zagon, I. S. (2011). Topical treatment with the opioid antagonist naltrexone facilitates closure of full-thickness wounds in diabetic rats. *Experimental Biology and Medicine, 236,* 1122–1132.

Medellin-Luna, M. F., Castaneda-Delgao, J. E., Martinez-Balderas, V. Y., & Cervantes-Villagrana, A. R. (2019). Medicinal plant extracts and their use as wound closure inducing agents. *Journal of Medicinal Food, 22*(5), 435–443.

Mendes, D., Alves, C., Loureiro, M., Fonte, A., & Batel-Marques, F. (2019). Drug-induced hypersensitivity: A 5-year retrospective study in a hospital electronic health records database. *Journal of Clinical Pharmacy and Therapeutics, 44,* 54–61.

Mii, S., Guntani, A., Kawakubo, E., Tanaka, K., & Kyuragi, R. (2018). Cilostazol improves wound healing in patients undergoing open bypass for ischemic tissue loss: A propensity score matching analysis. *Annals of Vascular Surgery, 49,* 30–38.

Miles, S. J., Lord, R., Williams, P., & Fulbrook, P. (2019). Study protocol: A pilot clinical trial of topical glyceryl trinitrate for chronic venous leg ulcer healing. *Wound Practice and Research, 27*(3), 131–134.

Moon, J., Lee, M., Chung, Y., Rhee, C., & Lee, S. (2018). Effect of topical propolis on wound healing process after tonsillectomy: Randomized controlled study. *Clinical and Experimental Otorhinolaryngology, 11*(2), 146–150.

Naing, C., & Whitaker, M. A. (2017). Anabolic steroids for treating pressure ulcers (review). *Cochrane Database of Systematic Reviews,* (6), CD011375. https://doi.org/10.1002/14651858.CD011375.PUB2.

Nikolic, N., Kienzl, P., Tajpara, P., Vierhapper, M., Matiasek, J., & Elbe-Burger, A. (2019). The antiseptic octenidine inhibits Langerhans cells activation and modulates cytokine expression upon superficial wounding with tape stripping. *Journal of Immunology Research, 2019,* 5143635. https://doi.org/10.1155/2019/5143635.

Ousey, K. (2018). The role of topical metronidazole in the management of infected wounds. *Wounds UK, 14*(5), 78–83.

Pearson, W. A., Prentice, D. A., Sinclair, D. L., Lim, L. Y., & Carville, K. J. (2019). A novel topical therapy for resistant and early peristomal pyoderma gangrenosum. *International Wound Journal, 16*, 1136–1143.

Pereira, R. E., & Bartoo, P. J. (2016). Traditional therapies for skin wound healing. *Advances in Wound Care, 5*(5), 208–229.

Pichler, W. J. (2020a). Drug allergy: Pathogenesis. In *UptoDate*. Retrieved 4/2/2020 from www.uptodate.com.

Pichler, W. J. (2020b). Drug hypersensitivity: Classification and clinical features. In *UptoDate*. Retrieved 4/2/2020 from www.uptodate.com.

Poetker, D., & Reh, D. (2010). A comprehensive review of the adverse effects of systemic corticosteroids. *Otolaryngologic Clinics of North America, 43*(4), 753–768.

Pure and Clean Wound Management Technology. (2020). *Hypochlorous acid*. Retrieved 8/19/2020 from https://pureandclean.us.

Rezvani, O., Shabbak, E., Aslani, A., Bidar, R., Jafari, M., & Safarnezhad, S. (2009). A randomized, double-blind, placebo-controlled trial to determine the effects of topical insulin on wound healing. *Ostomy Wound Management, 55*(8), 22–28.

Rook, J. M., Hasan, W., & McCarson, K. E. (2008). Temporal effects of topical morphine application on cutaneous wound healing. *Anesthesiology, 109*(1), 130–136.

Rutecki, G. W. (2012). Polypharmacy. What can we do to curtail harmful polypharmacy? Consultant, 360, 52(2). Retrieved 2/16/2023 from: https://www.consultant360.com/article/what-can-we-do-curtail-harmful-polypharmacy.

Ryan, T. (2003). Use of herbal medicines in wound healing. *International Journal of Lower Extremity Wounds, 2*(1), 22–24.

Samel, A. D., & Chu, C. (2020). Drug eruptions. In *UpToDate*. Retrieved 2/29/2020 from www.uptodate.com.

Schleffler, A. (2019). The wound healing properties of betulin from birch bark from bench to bedside. *Planta Medica, 85*, 524–527.

Sen, C. K., Gordillo, G. M., Roy, S., Kirsner, R., Lambert, L., Hunt, T. K., et al. (2009). Human skin wounds: A major and snowballing threat to public health and the economy. *Wound Repair and Regeneration, 17*, 763–771.

Shakib, Z., Shahraki, N., Razavi, B. M., & Hosseinzadeh, H. (2019). Aloe vera as an herbal medicine in the treatment of metabolic syndrome: A review. *Phytotherapy Research, 33*(10), 2649–2660. https://doi.org/10.1002/ptr.6465.

Sharma, S., Schaper, N., & Rayman, G. (2019). Microangiopathy: Is it relevant to wound healing in diabetic foot disease. *Diabetes Metabolism Research and Reviews, 36*(Suppl. 1), e3244. https://doi.org/10.1002/dmrr.3244.

Shedoeva, A., Leavesly, D., Upton, Z., & Fan, C. (2019). Wound healing and the use of medicinal plants. *Evidence-Based Complementary and Alternative Medicine, 2019*, 2684108. https://doi.org/10.1155/2019/2684108.

Shirin, J. (2015). Polypharmacy, the elderly, and deprescribing. *Consultant Pharmacist, 30*(9), 527–532.

Siddique, Z., Shah, G., Ahmed, A., Nisa, S., Khan, A., Idrees, M., et al. (2019). Ethnophytotherapy practices for wound healing among populations of district Haripur, KPK, Pakistan. *Evidence-Based Complementary and Alternative Medicine, 2019*, 4591675. https://doi.org/10.1155/2019/4591675.

Singh, D., Fisher, J., Shagalou, D., Varma, A., & Siegel, D. M. (2018). Dangerous plants in dermatology: Legal and controlled. *Clinics in Dermatology, 36*(3), 399–419.

Singh, M., & Pawar, M. (2020). Effects of topical insulin therapy for chronic trophic ulcers in patients with leprosy: A randomized intervention pilot study. *Advances in Skin & Wound Care, 33*(2), 1–6. https://doi.org/10.1097/01.asw.0000617856.84426.9f.

Singh, A., Singh, P., & Singh, R. (2014). Antidiabetic and wound healing activity of *Catharanthus roseus* L. in streptozotocin-induced diabetic mice. *American Journal of Phytomedicine and Clinical Therapeutics, 2*(6), 686–692.

Smith, R. G. (2010). Off-label use of prescription medication: A literature review. *Wounds, 22*(4), 78–86.

Soundia, A., Hadaya, D., Esfandi, N., Gkooveris, I., Christensen, R., Dry, S. M., et al. (2018). Zoledronate impairs socket healing after extraction of teeth with experimental periodontitis. *Journal of Dental Research, 97*(3), 312–326.

Srirod, S., & Tewtrakul, S. (2019). Anti-inflammatory and wound healing effects of cream containing Curcuma mangga extract. *Journal of Ethnopharmacology, 238*, 111828. https://doi.org/10.1016/j.jep.2019.111828.

Stevens, D. L., Bisno, A. L., Chambers, H. F., Delinger, E. P., Goldstein, E. J., Gorbach, S. L., et al. (2014). Practice guidelines for the diagnosis and management of skin and soft tissue infections: 2014 update by the Infectious Diseases Society of America. *Clinical Infectious Diseases, 59*(2), e10–e52. https://doi.org/10.1093/CID/CIU296.

Tawfeek, H. M., Abou-Taleb, D., Badary, D. M., Ibrahim, M., & Abdellatif, A. A. (2020). Pharmaceutical, clinical, and immunohistochemical studies of metformin hydrochloride topical hydrogel for wound healing application. *Archives of Dermatological Research, 312*, 113–121.

Topman, G., Lin, F., & Gefen, A. (2013). The natural medications for wound healing-curcumin, aloe-vera, and ginger—Do not induce a significant effect on the migration kinematics of cultured fibroblasts. *Journal of Biomechanics, 46*, 170–174.

Treadwell, T. (2013). Editorial message: Corticosteroids and wound healing. *Wounds, 25*(10). Retrieved 2/29/2020 from www.wounds.research.com.

Trommell, N., Hofland, H. W., Van Komen, R. S., Dokter, J., & Van Baar, M. E. (2019). Nursing problems in patients with toxic epidermal necrolysis and Stevens-Johnson syndrome in a Dutch burn center: A 30-year retrospective review. *Burns, 45*, 1625–1633. https://doi.org/10.1016/j.burns.2019.07.004.

Wang, A., Armstrong, E. J., & Armstrong, A. W. (2013). Corticosteroids and wound healing: Clinical considerations in the perioperative period. *American Journal of Surgery, 206*(3), 410–417.

Wang, P., Long, Z., Yu, Z., Liu, P., Wei, D., Fang, Q., et al. (2019). The efficacy of topical gentamicin wound infection: A systematic review and meta-analysis. *International Journal of Clinical Practice, 73*, e13334. https://doi.org/10.1111/ifcp.13334.

Ward, K. E., Archambault, R., & Mersfelder, T. L. (2010). Severe adverse skin reactions to nonsteroidal anti-inflammatory drugs: A review of the literature. *American Journal of Health-System Pharmacy, 67*, 206–213.

Warrington, R., Silvio-Dan, F., & Wong, T. (2018). Drug allergy. *Allergy, Asthma, & Clinical Immunology, 14*(Suppl. 2), 60. https://doi.org/10.1186/s13223-018-0289-y.

Wen, A., Halim, A., Saad, A., Nor, F., & Sulaiman, W. (2018). A prospective study evaluating wound healing with sea cucumber gel compared with hydrogel in treatment of skin graft donor sites. *Complementary Therapies in Medicine, 41*, 261–266. https://doi.org/10.1016/j.ctim.2018.10.006.

Young, T. (2019). Rheumatoid arthritis and its impact on ulceration and haling. *Wounds UK, 15*(4), 40–43.

Zaslansky, R., Schramm, C., Stein, C., Guthoff, C., & Schmidt-Westhausen, A. (2018). Topical application of morphine for wound healing and analgesia in patients with oral lichen planus: A randomized double-blind placebo-controlled trial. *Clinical Oral Investigations, 22*(1), 305–311. https://doi.org/10.1007/500784-017-2112-4.

Zhang, Z., Li, S., Zhang, Z., Yu, K., Duan, X., Long, L., et al. (2020). Clinical features, risk factors, and prognostic markers of drug-induced liver injury in patients with Stevens-Johnson syndrome/toxic epidermal necrolysis. *Indian Journal of Dermatology, 65*(4), 274–278. https://doi.org/10.4103/ijd.IJD_217_19.

Zhang, C., Van, D. N., Hieu, C., & Craig, T. (2019). Drug-induced severe cutaneous adverse reactions. *Annals of Allergy, Asthma, and Immunology, 123*, 483–487.

Zhao, P., Sui, B., Liu, N., Lv, Y., Zheng, C., Lu, Y., et al. (2017). Anti-aging pharmacology in cutaneous wound healing: Effects of metformin, resveratrol, and rapamycin by local application. *Aging, 16*, 1083–1093.

Zhu, J., & Weingart, S. N. (2020). Prevention of adverse drug events in hospitals. In *UptoDate*. Retrieved 5/29/2020 from www.uptodate.com.

Zimmerman-Klemd, A. M., Konradi, V., Steinborn, C., Ucker, A., Falanga, C., Woelfe, U., et al. (2019). Influence of traditionally used Nepalese plants on wound healing and immunological properties using human cells in vitro. *Journal of Ethnopharmacology, 235*, 415–423.

Zinder, R., Cooley, R., Vlad, L., & Molnar, J. A. (2019). Vitamin A and wound healing. *Nutrition in Clinical Practice, 34*(6), 839–849.

FURTHER READING

Adler, B. L., & Friedman, A. J. (2014). News, views, & reviews. Repurposing of drugs for dermatologic applications: Five key medications. *Journal of Drugs in Dermatology, 13*(11). Retrieved 2/29/2020 from http://jddonline.com/articles/dermatology/S1545961614P1413X.

Atkin, L. (2019). Chronic wounds: The challenges of appropriate management. *British Journal of Community Nursing, 24*(Suppl. 9), S26–S32.

Bassas, P., Bartralot, R., & Garcia-Patos, V. (2009). Anticoagulation an antiplatelet therapy in dermatology. *Actas Dermo-Sifiliográficas, 100*(1), 7–16.

Bauer, K. A. (2020). Protein C deficiency. In *UptoDate*. Retrieved 5/29/2020 from www.uptodate.com.

Benhadou, F., & Del Marmol, V. (2013). The mTOR inhibitors and the skin wound healing. *EWMA Journal, 13*(1), 20–22.

Biswas, T. K., & Mukherjee, B. (2003). Plant medicines of Indian origin for wound healing activity: A review. *International Journal of Lower Extremity Wounds, 2*(1), 25–39. https://doi.org/10.1177/1534734603002001006.

Buscemi, C. P., & Romeo, C. A. (2014). Wound healing, angiotensin-converting enzyme inhibition, and collagen-containing products. *Journal of Wound, Ostomy, and Continence Nursing, 41*(6), 611–614.

Butcher, M. (2012). PHMB: An effective antimicrobial in wound bioburden management. *British Journal of Nursing, 21*(12), S16–S21.

Cakmak, E., Yesilada, A., Sevim, K., Sumer, O., Tatildede, H., & Sakiz, D. (2014). Effects of sildenafil citrate on secondary healing in full thickness skin defects in experiment. *Bratisl Leklisty, 115*(6), 267–271.

Chen, M. R., & Dragoo, J. L. (2013). The effect of nonsteroidal anti-inflammatory drugs on tissue healing. *Knee Surgery, Sports Traumatology, Arthroscopy, 21*, 540–549.

Choueiri, T. K., & Sonpavde, G. (2020). Toxicity of molecularly targeted antiangiogenic agents: Non-cardiovascular effects. In *UptoDate*. Retrieved 5/29/2020 from www.uptodate.com.

Cotti, E., Mezzena, S., Schirru, E., Ottonello, O., Mura, M., Ideo, F., et al. (2018). Healing of apical periodontitis in patients with inflammatory bowel diseases and under anti-tumor necrosis factor alpha therapy. *Journal of Endodontics, 44*, 1777–1782.

Coutre, S., & Crowther, M. (2020). Clinical presentation and diagnosis of heparin-induced thrombocytopenia. In *UptoDate*. Retrieved 5/29/2020 from www.uptodate.com.

Dinarvand, P., & Moser, K. A. (2019). Protein C deficiency. *Archives of Pathology and Laboratory Medicine, 143*, 1281–1285.

Duarte, B., Cabete, J., Formiga, A., & Neves, J. (2017). Dakin's solution: Is there a place for it in the 21st century? *International Wound Journal, 14*, 918–920.

Elsass, F. (2017). A sweet solution: The use of medical-grade honey on oral mucositis in the pediatric oncology patient. *Journal of Wound, Ostomy, and Continence Nursing, 44*(Suppl. 3), S9.

Evans, K., & Kim, P. J. (2020). Overview of treatment of chronic wounds. In *UptoDate*. Retrieved 5/29/2020 from www.uptodate.com.

Goodman, S. M., & Paget, S. (2012). Perioperative drug safety in patients with rheumatoid arthritis. *Rheumatic Diseases Clinics of North America, 38*, 747–759.

Hermanns, R., & Rodriguez, B. (2019). A case report: Pilonidal sinus management with medical-grade honey. *Journal of European Wound Management Association, 20*(1), 73–78.

High, W. A. (2020). Stevens-Johnson syndrome and toxic epidermal necrolysis: Pathogenesis, clinical manifestations, and diagnosis. In *UptoDate*. Retrieved 5/29/2020 from www.uptodate.com.

High, W. A., & Nirken, M. H. (2020). Stevens-Johnson syndrome and toxic epidermal necrolysis: Management, prognosis, and long-term sequelae. In *UpToDate*. Retrieved 2/29/2020 from www.uptodate.com.

Jafari, M., Tessier, W., Hajbi, F., Mirabel, X., & Decanter, G. (2016). Delayed anastomotic leakage following bevacizumab administration in colorectal cancer patients. *Acta Oncologica, 55*(9–10), 1250–1252. https://doi.org/10.3109/0284186x.2016.1171393.

Jung, K., Woo, J., & Park, C. (2019). Effects of aqueous suppressants and prostaglandin analogues on early wound healing after glaucoma implant surgery. *Scientific Reports, 9*(1), 525.

Kadota, Y., Nishida, K., Hashizome, K., Nasu, Y., Nakahara, R., Kanazawa, T., et al. (2016). Risk factors for surgical site infections and delayed wound healing after orthopedic surgery in rheumatoid arthritis patients. *Modern Rheumatology, 26*(1), 68–74.

Karukonda, S. R. K., Flynn, T. C., Boh, E. E., McBurney, E. I., Russo, G. G., & Millikan, L. E. (2000a). The effects of drugs on wound healing: Part I. *International Journal of Dermatology, 39*(4), 250–257.

Karukonda, S. R. K., Flynn, T. C., Boh, E. E., McBurney, E. I., Russo, G. G., & Millikan, L. E. (2000b). The effects of drugs on wound healing: Part II. *International Journal of Dermatology, 39*(5), 321–333.

Keating, G. (2014). Bevacizumab: A review of its use in advanced cancer. *Drugs, 74*, 1891–1925.

Kesici, S., Demirci, M., & Kesici, V. (2019). Antibacterial effects of lidocaine and adrenaline. *International Wound Journal, 16,* 1190–1194.

Kotagal, M., Hakkarainen, T. W., Simianu, V., Beck, S. J., Alfonso-Cristancho, R., & Flum, D. R. (2016). Ketorolac use and postoperative complications in gastrointestinal surgery. *Annals of Surgery, 263*(1), 71–75.

Kotian, S., Bhat, K., Pai, S., Nayak, J., Souza, A., Gourisheti, K., et al. (2018). The role of natural medicines on wound healing: A biomechanical, histological, biochemical, and molecular study. *Ethiopian Journal of Science, 28*(6), 459. https://doi.org/10.4314/ejhs.v28i6.

Kyllo, R. L., & Anadkat, J. J. (2014). Dermatologic adverse events to chemotherapeutic agents. Part I: Cytotoxic agents, epidermal growth factor inhibitors, multikinase inhibitors, and proteosome inhibitors. *Seminars in Cutaneous Medicine and Surgery, 33,* 28–39.

Leach, M. J. (2014). Horse-chestnut (*aesculus hippocastanum*) seed extract for venous leg ulceration: A comparative multiple case study of healers and non-healers. *Focus on Alternative and Complementary Therapies, 19*(4), 184–190.

Levine, J. (2013). Dakin's solution: Past, present, and future. *Advances in Skin & Wound Care, 26*(9), 410–414.

Moores, J. (2013). Vitamin C: A wound healing perspective. *Wound Care, December,* S6–S11.

Mufti, A., Maliyar, K., Syed, M., Pagnoux, C., & Alavi, A. (2020). Approaches to microthrombotic wounds: A review of pathogenesis and clinical features. *Advances in Skin & Wound Care, 33,* 68–75. https://doi.org/10.1097/01.ASW.0000617860.92050.9e.

Murdoch, R., & Lagan, K. M. (2013). The role of povidone and cadexomer iodine in the management of acute and chronic wounds. *Physical Therapy Reviews, 18*(3), 207–216.

Nedorost, S. T., & Stevens, S. R. (2011). Diagnosis and treatment of allergic skin disorders in the elderly. *Drugs & Aging, 18*(11), 827–835.

Nijhuis, W., Houwing, R., Van der Zwet, W., & Jansman, F. (2012). A randomized trial of honey barrier cream versus zinc oxide ointment. *British Journal of Nursing, 21*(20), S10–S13.

Pichler, W. J. (2020c). Drug allergy: Classification and clinical features. In *UptoDate.* Retrieved 2/29/2020 from www.uptodate.com.

Polachek, A., Caspi, D., & Elkayam, O. (2012). The perioperative use of biologic agents in patients with rheumatoid arthritis. *Autoimmunity Reviews, 12,* 164–168.

Quattrone, F., Dini, V., Barbanera, S., Zerbinati, N., & Romanelli, M. (2013). Cutaneous ulcers associated with hydroxyurea therapy. *Journal of Tissue Viability, 22,* 112–121.

Ranade, D., & Collins, N. (2014). Nutrition 411: An introduction to herbs for wound healing professionals. *Ostomy Wound Management, 60*(6). Retrieved 2/29/2020 from www.o-wm.com.

Rothenberger, J., Krause, S., & Tschumi, C. (2016). The effect of polyhexanide octenidine hydrochloride and tea tree oil as topical antiseptic agents on in vivo microcirculation of the human skin: A noninvasive quantitative analysis. *Wounds, 28*(10), 341–346.

Serra, R., Gallelli, L., Buffone, G., Molinari, V., Stilitano, D. M., Palmieri, C., et al. (2015). Doxycycline speeds up healing of chronic venous ulcers. *International Wound Journal, 12,* 179–184.

Sharpe, A., Neves, J., Formica, A., Silva, C., Serfino, E., & Machado, M. (2018). Case studies: Octenidine in the management of diabetic foot ulcers. *Diabetic Foot Journal, 21*(3), 192–197.

Shaw, J., Hughes, C. M., Lagan, K. M., Stevenson, M. R., Irwin, C. R., & Bell, P. M. (2011). Short report: Treatment—The effect of topical phenytoin on healing in diabetic foot ulcers: A randomized controlled clinical trial. Diabetic Medicine, *28,* 1154–1157.

Shukla, S., Sharma, A., Gupta, V., & Yashavarddhan, M. H. (2019). Pharmacological control of inflammation in wound healing. *Journal of Tissue Viability, 28,* 218–222.

Singh, S., & Pardi, D. S. (2014). Update on anti-tumor necrosis factors agents in Crohn's disease. *Gastroenterology Clinics of North America, 43,* 457–478.

Smith, R. G. (2008). The effects of medications in wound healing. *Podiatry Management,* 195–202. Accessed 3/23/2023 from https://www.podiatrym.com/cme/cmeaug08.pdf.

Smith, R. G. (2009). Nanopharmaceuticals and gene therapy applied to wound care. *Podiatry Management,* 187–194. Accessed 3/23/2023 from https://www.podiatrym.com/cme/aug09cme.pdf.

Sussman, G. (2007). The impact of medicines on wound healing. *Pharmacists, 26*(11), 874–876.

Vallejo, A., Wallis, M., Horton, E., & McMillan, D. (2018). Low-frequency ultrasonic debridement and topical antimicrobial solution polyhexamethylene biguanide for use in chronic wounds: A case series. *Wound Practice and Research, 26*(1), 4–13.

Wang, C., Guo, M., Zhang, N., & Wang, P. (2019). Effectiveness of honey dressings in the treatment of diabetic foot ulcers: A systematic review and meta-analysis. *Complementary Therapies in Clinical Practice, 34,* 123–131.

Warkentin, T. E. (2006). Think of HIT. *American Society of Hematology, 2006*(1), 408–414. https://doi.org/10.1182/asheducation-2006.1.408.

Warkentin, T. E., & Greinacher, A. (2016). Management of heparin-induced thrombocytopenia. *Current Opinion in Hematology, 23*(5), 462–470. https://doi.org/10.1097/coh.0000000000000273.

Wigston, C., Hassan, S., Turvey, S., Baosanquet, D., Richards, A., Holloway, S., et al. (2013). Impact of medications and lifestyle factors on wound healing: A pilot study. *Wounds, 9*(1), 22–28.

Zelenikova, R., & Vyhlidalove, D. (2019). Applying honey dressings to non-healing wounds in elderly persons receiving home care. *Journal of Tissue Viability, 28,* 139–143.

Zhu, G., Wang, Q., Lu, S., & Niu, Y. (2017). Hydrogen peroxide: A potential wound therapeutic target. *Medical Principles and Practice, 26,* 301–308. https://doi.org/10.1159/000475501.

31

Perfusion, Oxygenation, and Incision Care

Alisha Oropallo

OBJECTIVES

1. Identify factors that impair perfusion and related wound repair processes.
2. Describe interventions to increase tissue oxygen or improve wound healing.
3. Discuss current issues related to surgical wound infection and recommendations made by national collaboratives or

evidence-based guidelines to address these problems and improve outcomes.
4. Identify evidence-based measures for surgical wounds, including dressings; topical treatment; and care of sutures, staples, and tissue adhesives.

A great deal has been learned over several decades about tissue repair and the importance of perfusion and oxygenation to healing, although much of that information has not been applied widely in daily clinical practice. Recognition is growing that inadequate wound healing and complications of acute wounds including infections such as surgical site infection, likely have their origins early in the initial inflammatory response and early in the healing process (Yip, 2015).

Classic and recent evidence serves as a guide to understanding the importance of adequate blood flow to peripheral tissues with an adequate oxygen supply so that optimal healing and resistance to infection for acute and chronic wounds may occur. This chapter addresses factors that influence perfusion and local wound oxygenation during wound repair, including autonomic nervous system activation, fluids, supplemental oxygen, pain, stress, hypothermia, obesity, and tobacco use. The efficacy of interventions for modifying these factors to achieve better wound tissue perfusion and healing responses is discussed in light of current evidence.

EFFECT OF OXYGEN AND PERFUSION IN WOUND HEALING

The critical roles of oxygen in healing are summarized in Table 31.1 (Dunnill et al., 2017; Yip, 2015). Oxygen fuels the cellular functions essential to the repair process; therefore, the ability to perfuse the tissues and the availability of oxygen (partial pressure of oxygen [Po_2]) to the local wound area are critical to wound healing. The processes of tissue repair that require oxygen include oxidative bacterial killing and resistance to infection, collagen synthesis and fibroplasia, angiogenesis, and epithelialization. Evidence has suggested the

radical derivatives of oxygen such as reactive oxygen species (ROS) are involved in each phase of wound healing (Dunnill et al., 2017; Oropallo, Serena, Armstrong, & Niederauer, 2021).

Tissue oxygen levels are dependent on both perfusion status and oxygen content of the blood. However, because wounds remove only 1 mL of oxygen per each 100 mL of blood perfusing the tissues, compromised perfusion is more likely to jeopardize wound healing than is compromised oxygenation secondary to pulmonary conditions (Waldorf & Fewkes, 1995). Tissues that are adequately perfused are often able to heal even if the blood is poorly oxygenated or the patient is anemic. In fact, anemia usually does not significantly affect repair unless the hematocrit drops below 20% (Stotts & Wipke-Tevis, 1996). Arterial oxygen levels are not necessarily reflective of tissue oxygen delivery. Although PaO_2 of 90 mmHg in a healthy volunteer breathing room air maintains a wound Po_2 of 50 mmHg or greater, the postoperative patient experiencing autonomic nervous system activation or periodic desaturation will exhibit predictably low oxygen levels within the wound. This observation led to an approach of adrenergic activation as an etiology for wound hypoxia (West, 1990). Thus, even when the wound has areas of hypoxia, the goal is to reestablish normoxia via oxygen sensing in the areas of hypoxia without exposing the wound to high levels of oxygen which might cause oxygen toxicity (Kimmel, Grant, & Ditata, 2016).

Wound Tissue Hypoxia

Wound tissue hypoxia occurs to some extent at the time of injury in everyone, regardless of their age or state of health (Silver, 1980). Incisions closed during elective surgery under

TABLE 31.1   Important Roles of Oxygen in Wound Healing

Event in Wound Healing	Specific Role of Oxygen
Inflammation: Bacteria control	Oxygen is substrate for enzymatic step for leukocyte production of reactive oxygen species (superoxide and other oxidants) during phagocytosis
Proliferation: Angiogenesis	Local tissue hypoxia and oxidants induce release of growth factors that stimulate angiogenesis
Proliferation: Collagen synthesis and cellular export	Oxygen with adequate vitamin C is required for enzymatic hydroxylation of procollagen to form triple helical, mature collagen structure for export from fibroblasts Production and release of collagen are necessary for tissue strength
Remodeling: Epithelialization	Oxygen and growth factors are needed for generation of new epithelium

the best of aseptic conditions appear to have the fewest reparative obstacles to healing. However, any tissue injury disrupts vascular and therefore oxygen supply. All wounds are relatively hypoxic at the center, in the range from 0 to 5 mmHg (Niinikoski, Heughan, & Hunt, 1972; Silver, 1969). After oxygen leaves the red blood cells in the capillaries, it diffuses into the wound space. The driving force of diffusion is partial pressure. In wounds, damage to the microvasculature, vasoconstriction, and intravascular fluid overload markedly increase intercapillary distances (Hunt & Hopf, 1997).

Local oxygen tension influences wound healing and bacterial control in several ways. Initial injured tissue is hypoxic, a state that acts as a stimulus for repair. The one potentially beneficial effect of moderate hypoxia is enhanced stimulus to neoangiogenesis (Wilson & Clark, 2003; Zamboni, Browder, & Martinez, 2003). However, prolonged and decreased local wound oxygen (tissue hypoxia) is a major contributor to wound complications (Goodson, Andrews, Thakrai, et al., 1979; Jönsson, Hunt, & Mathes, 1988; Knighton, Halliday, & Hunt, 1984). Prolonged effects of hypoxia can lead to changes in gene expression (D'Alessandro et al., 2019). A main role of oxygen during repair is that of controlling bacteria within the wound site. During repair, production of reactive oxygen species by leukocytes for phagocytosis is needed before rebuilding tissue (Dunnill et al., 2017; Oropallo et al., 2021). Oxidant production by leukocytes requires molecular oxygen and the presence of tissue oxygen levels of 45–80 mmHg up to 300 mmHg (Allen, Maguire, Mahdavian, et al., 1997). In addition to their role in controlling bacteria, reactive oxygen species serve other roles in healing, which include acting as chemical signals

and mitogens for fibroblasts and other cells, inducing cellular adhesion in neutrophils and macrophages, hemostasis, and cellular expression of growth factors that are critical for repair (Dunnill et al., 2017). Low levels of ROS are cytostatic and excessive ROS activates cell destruction. Maintaining the balance of ROS in a basal state can maintain normal cell functioning (Dunnill et al., 2017). In response to ROS, mesenchymal extracellular vesicles can protect the keratinocytes from oxidative stress-induced apoptosis (Bray, Oropallo, Grande, Kirsner, & Badiavas, 2021).

Many factors are stimulated by wound hypoxia including vascular endothelial growth factor (VEGF-A and Angiopoietin Like 4 (ANGPTLY), known to stimulate angiogenesis including anastomotic integrity (D'Alessandro et al., 2019; Giannis, Geropoulos, Ziogas, Gitlin, & Oropallo, 2021) Transforming growth factor beta one (TGF-B1) is involved in the collagen synthesis (Kimmel et al., 2016) In response to hypoxia, cells undergo a metabolic change by hypoxia-inducible factors (HIFs) targeting genes. Upregulated genes such as MMP-9 and TIMP1 proteins are involved with the glycolytic metabolism, cellular proliferation and apoptosis, as well as transcription and signaling (Kimmel et al., 2016). In hypoxia, low level expression of the leptin gene (LEP) is found in the adipocytes. The transcription of this protein is involved in all of the phases of wound healing including bone formation (Francisco et al., 2018). Endothelial-expressed genes such as CDH5 encoding VE-cadherin are involved in vessel organization. NOS3 associated with endothelial nitric oxide synthetase is upregulated in hypoxia (D'Alessandro et al., 2019). Hypoxia also creates both pro- and antiapoptotic factors inducing cell proliferation (D'Alessandro et al., 2019). The complexity of wound healing involves the maintenance of the balance of these mechanisms.

FACTORS THAT ALTER PERFUSION AND OXYGENATION

Pain and Stress

Cannon (1970) revealed the mechanisms that activate the autonomic nervous system to respond to stress. He directly observed the constriction of blood vessels in peripheral tissues during stress in animals. The mediators of the sympathetic and adrenal response to stress (epinephrine and norepinephrine) induced profound vasoconstriction in subcutaneous and skin blood vessels supplying peripheral tissues (Katlein and Mohammad, 2017). Sympathetic activation in the postoperative period is a function of the severing of afferent nerves, hypovolemia, fear, pain, and cold rather than anesthesia (Halter, Pflug, & Porte, 1977). Catecholamine levels may remain elevated for days after surgery (Derbyshire & Smith, 1984; Halter et al., 1977), and concentrations vary with the length and severity of surgery (Chernow, Alexander, Smallridge, et al., 1987). Norepinephrine is increased threefold in the early postoperative hours (Derbyshire & Smith, 1984), peaking with the patient's first expression of pain (Niinikoski et al., 1972). Increased levels of circulating catecholamines, including epinephrine, triggered by pain and stress, lead to peripheral vasoconstriction, decreased perfusion of blood to the skin and extremities, and, consequently, reduced oxygen availability in the tissues (Jensen, Jönsson, Goodson, et al., 1985). Evidence of how stress and pain limit perfusion has been demonstrated by infusion of exogenous epinephrine in healthy subjects. In a study designed to mimic the body's response to stress, increasing levels of epinephrine decreased the level of subcutaneous tissue oxygen 45%, whereas heart rate and arterial Po_2 did not markedly change (Jensen et al., 1985). The stress response is complex with multiple mechanisms involving glucocorticoid hormones affecting the immune system including interleukin 1 (IL-1). Increased stress has been demonstrated to increase the glucocorticoids levels which negatively affects the production of wound healing cytokines (IL1α, IL1β, and TNFα) (Charalambous et al., 2018). More specifically, stress before a procedure is a significant predictor of low IL-1 and MMP 9 levels in wound fluids, followed by increased pain (Woo, 2012). Overproduction of cortisol and catecholamines as a result of the stress response can have a significant impact on wound healing due to alteration in the immune system and tissue hypoxia. Stress and pain often lead to stress activation and delayed wound healing (Brown, 2016).

Hypothermia

Adverse consequences of perioperative body heat loss are significant and include prolonged hypothermia and postanesthesia recovery, longer postoperative warming time, shivering and thermal discomfort, reduced antibody and cell-mediated responses, reduced tissue oxygen peripherally, and increased incidence of wound infections, as well as poorer wound healing (Reynolds, Beckmann, & Kurz, 2008; Xu et al., 2021). The effects of temperature on the amount of vasomotor tone primarily determine cutaneous capillary blood flow. Cooling increases norepinephrine affinity to alpha-adrenergic receptors on vascular smooth muscle. This augments the response of cutaneous vessels to autonomic activation, which increases constrictive vessel tensions up to fivefold (Vanhoutte, Verbeuren, & Webb, 1981).

Hypothermia-induced vasoconstriction has decreased subcutaneous oxygen tension in anesthetized volunteers (Fio_2 0.6 mmHg) to a mean of 50 mmHg (Sheffield, Hopf, Sessler, et al., 1992). Furthermore, a lower blood temperature shifts the oxyhemoglobin curve to the left, thereby increasing the amount of oxygen carried in the blood but decreasing the amount of oxygen released (Severinghaus, 1958). This effect may exacerbate tissue hypoxia induced by peripheral vasoconstriction.

Virtually all anesthetic agents are vasodilators and may cause a rapid initial decrease in core temperature (1–2°C) during the first hour after induction of anesthesia (Sessler, 1993). Internal redistribution of body heat from core to periphery is exacerbated by conductive and evaporative losses as a result of visceral exposure in a cold environment (Roe, 1971). Rapid initial body heat loss can be limited by heating the operating room and aggressive preoperative warming

(Morris, 1971). Preinduction warming may nearly prevent rapid initial body heat loss (Hynson & Sessler, 1992).

Perioperative shivering in the elderly, although rare, is dangerous because oxygen demand may increase by 400%–500% (Bay, Nunn, & Prys-Roberts, 1968). This drastic increase in oxygen demand increases cardiac workload. Increased oxygen consumption has been shown to coincide with core decrements of 0.3–1.2°C (Roe, Goldberg, Blair, et al., 1966). Prolonged postoperative hypothermia is associated with increased mortality (Slotman, Jed, & Burchard, 1985) and myocardial ischemia (Frank, Beattie, Christopherson, et al., 1993).

Tobacco

Smoking is associated with poor wound outcomes in part through the catecholamine-mediated vasoconstrictive effects of nicotine, increases in carbon monoxide that reduce blood oxygen content, and effects on immune and proliferative cell function that reduce repair (Gottrup, 2004; Warner, 2005). Vasoconstrictive effects resulting in significant decreases in tissue oxygen tension occur after a single cigarette is smoked, and tissue oxygen requires an hour to return to baseline levels (Jensen, Goodson, Hopf, et al., 1991). Reductions in tissue oxygen translate clinically into lower amounts of collagen production and reduced wound strength (Jorgensen, Kallehave, Christensen, et al., 1998). A recent systematic review of studies evaluating wound outcomes for smokers and nonsmokers documented increased risk for wound necrosis, healing delay, dehiscence, and complications, including infections associated with smoking (Sørensen, 2012). Based on multiple studies and reviews demonstrating an association between smoking and wound-related problems, including infection and poor wound healing, all patients with wounds should be advised to abstain from smoking.

Smoking is the single most predictive factor of wound complications in patients undergoing elective hip or knee replacement (Møller, Pedersen, Villebro, et al., 2003). Forty-seven percent of patients undergoing abdominoplasty who smoked had wound complications compared with 14.7% of those who did not smoke (Manassa, Hertl, & Olbrisch, 2003). Due to the reductions in tissue oxygen supply when a person smokes, a substantial amount of time is needed for levels to recover. At least one study has shown that 2 weeks of abstinence is inadequate to limit wound-related problems, whereas a minimum of 3–4 weeks of abstinence has been associated with reduced incisional wound infection and improved wound healing (Kuri, Nakagawa, Tanaka, et al., 2005; Sørensen, Karlsmark, & Gottrup, 2003). In an analysis of 18 meta-analyses and systematic reviews, current smoking increases in-hospital mortality by about 20% and major postoperative complications including infection by 40%. Current smoking increases all specific surgical complications (Pierre et al., 2017). Smoking cessation over 8 weeks before the intervention reduced respiratory complications by close to 50%. In terms of impaired wound healing, the benefits of quitting were apparent after 3–4 weeks of smoking cessation. Education regarding the risks of smoking is imperative before elective surgical intervention (Pierre et al., 2017).

Abstaining from smoking before surgery decreases surgical wound infections, but has not been shown to reduce other wound-healing problems (Sørensen, 2012). In recent years, the use of new forms of tobacco products is increasing in popularity without significant knowledge of their effects.

With over 10,000 e-liquids available from online, restaurants, and retail vape shops, the delivery methods for electronic cigarettes are continuously changing. With the different nicotine concentrations and other chemicals, aerosolization methods, or entirely new devices (JUUL), the proper testing mechanism has not been validated for its overall impact in chronic diseases, including wound healing. Thus, the major knowledge gaps exist in the use of these products and the impact in wound healing and disease (Aghaloo, Kim, Gordon, & Behrsing, 2019).

Obesity

Wound-healing problems are more likely to occur in patients who are overweight, which is a growing national problem. The US obesity prevalence was 42.4% in 2017–2018. The obesity prevalence was 40.0% among adults aged 20–39 years, 44.8% among adults aged 40–59 years, and 42.8% among adults aged 60 and older. From 1999–2000 through 2017–2018, US obesity prevalence increased from 30.5% to 42.4% (Centers for Disease Control and Prevention, 2022). Individuals who are severely obese often suffer from a number of related health problems that potentially affect healing: type 2 diabetes, hypertension, coronary artery disease, sleep apnea, venous stasis disease, lower extremity ulcers, osteoarthritis, urinary incontinence, gastroesophageal reflux disease, fatty liver, cholelithiasis, and depression (Mun, Blackburn, & Matthews, 2001).

Obesity as a single factor is an independent predictor of surgical site infection (Harrington et al., 2004). Regardless of the surgical procedure, the incidence of postsurgical wound complications, such as infection and wound dehiscence, are higher in patients with obesity compared with those of normal weight. Postsurgical wound complication rates of patients with obesity have been reported to be as high as 15%–22% (Fried, Peskova, & Kasalicky, 1997; Israelsson and Jonsson, 1997; Myles, Gooch, & Santolaya, 2002; Vastine et al., 1999; Winiarsky, Barth, & Lotke, 1998).

Several studies document low oxygen levels associated with obesity. Abdominal tissue oxygen tension is reported to be negatively associated with the percentage of fat as measured by body composition dual-energy X-ray absorptiometry, with obese subjects found to have lower adipose tissue capillary density (Pasarica, Sereda, Redman, et al., 2009). In surgical populations, patients with BMI greater than 30 kg/m^2 who had undergone abdominal surgery had significantly lower tissue oxygen readings compared with those with BMI less than 30 kg/m^2 (Fleischmann, Kurz, Niedermayr, et al., 2005; Kabon, Nagele, Reddy, et al., 2004). Tissue oxygen levels measured in patients with obesity fell below normal, even with administration of supplemental oxygen, and were within a range associated with increased surgical site infection risk. Prolonged administration of supplemental oxygen postoperatively (80% oxygen for 12–18 h) is reported to significantly increase both wound and upper arm tissue oxygen (Kabon, Rozum, Marschalek, et al., 2010).

Because of the increased vulnerability to wound complications, extra vigilance and measures to ensure peripheral perfusion must be taken with patients who are obese, including maintenance of normothermia and adequate fluid resuscitation. Higher doses of preoperative prophylactic antibiotic regiment, most commonly cefazolin, are administered to obese patients to reduce infection. There is general paucity of data regarding the pharmacokinetics of antimicrobials active against MRSA in obese patients, especially for the target tissue (Grupper & Nicolau, 2017). Obesity is addressed in greater detail in Chapter 35.

INTERVENTIONS TO IMPROVE PERFUSION AND OXYGEN

Wound tissue oxygen delivery may be impaired unless conditions of diminished peripheral perfusion are anticipated and corrected. Factors most likely to adversely affect perfusion to the wound bed include hypovolemia, hypotension, factors producing vasoconstriction (e.g., cold, sympathetic stimulation), vascular disease, and edema. Correction of adrenergic vasoconstrictive stimuli, particularly cold, pain, and volume loss, elevates tissue Po$_2$ and leads to fewer postoperative infections (Hopf, Hunt, West, et al., 1997; Kurz, Sessler, & Lenhardt, 1996). The degree of regional tissue perfusion regulates the supply of oxygen and therefore is the prime determinant of the competency of wound healing. Strategies for optimizing perfusion by addressing specific sympathetic nervous system activators are described in this section and listed in Table 31.2. As previously described, pain management is a critical strategy for improving perfusion and oxygenation. Techniques for pain control are described in Chapter 26.

Warming

Aggressive intraoperative warming and rapid postoperative warming are effective modalities for minimizing the risks of prolonged hypothermia (Hynson & Sessler, 1992). Sympathetic vasoconstriction can be overcome by warmth to provide uncomplicated healing. In a large study combining intraoperative and postoperative warming, wound infection rates were reduced by 60% (Kurz et al., 1996). Maintenance of normothermia during surgery and in the immediate recovery period is defined as sustaining a minimum core temperature of 36.5°C. In patients undergoing colorectal surgery, a temperature higher than 36°C immediately after surgery is recommended as one of the metrics for documenting optimal care for prevention of surgical infection (Bratzler and Hunt, 2006). Warming before and after surgery may also provide benefit and should be considered. Fewer wound infections (13% vs 27%) were observed within 8 weeks of elective abdominal surgery in patients who were warmed for 2 h before and after surgery in addition to the standard warming of all patients during the operation (Wong, Kumar, Bohra, et al., 2007).

TABLE 31.2   Interventions to Reduce Factors That Impair Perfusion and Oxygenation

Factor	Examples of Interventions
Hypothermia	Provide active warming to maintain perioperative normothermia Provide postoperative warming and warm blankets Prevent heat loss and shivering Apply socks, slippers, sweaters, blankets
Pain	Provide analgesia and nonpharmacologic measures (e.g., repositioning, relaxation for pain control) (see Chapter 26)
Fear/stress	Provide patient teaching to reduce fear related to procedures or knowledge deficits Administer medications as needed to reduce anxiety and fear
Pharmacologic	If possible, avoid medications that activate the sympathetic nervous system (e.g., beta blockers) Avoid high-dose alpha-adrenergic agonists
Smoking	Encourage minimum of 4 weeks' abstinence before surgery until incision is healed Refer to tobacco cessation program and encourage successful completion
Obesity	Increase FiO_2 perioperatively unless contraindicated Maintain normothermia and fluid balance Realize larger doses of prophylactic antibiotics may be needed

Local Warming

Local wound temperature modification using controlled warming improves blood flow directly to sites of injury and may benefit healing. Multiple small clinical studies examining local warming with chronic wounds (pressure, venous, diabetic, arterial) suggest benefits that include increased transcutaneous wound oxygen, less pain, and fewer infections (Puzziferri, West, Hunt, et al., 2001; Whitney & Wickline, 2003). Surgical sites with local warming have shown significantly higher tissue oxygen in the immediate recovery period and on the first postoperative day (Plattner, Akça, Herbst, et al., 2000) and fewer wound-related complications compared with systemic warming or no warming (Melling, Ali, Scott, et al., 2001; Whitney, Dellinger, & Wickline, 2004). Although these studies suggest benefits of local warming, more rigorous research is needed to confirm these benefits, as well as the best methodology (i.e., temperature, duration, frequency) and method of delivery for maximizing them. Enhanced Recovery After Surgery (ERAS) is a global interdisciplinary approach to the care of the surgical patient. Enhanced Recovery After Surgery process implementation involves a team consisting of surgeons, anesthetists, an ERAS coordinator (often a nurse or a physician assistant), and staff from units that care for the surgical patient. The ERAS Society, an international nonprofit professional society, establishes guidelines based on evidence-based medicine. ERAS Society supports preservation of normal body temperature which reduces wound infections, cardiac complications, bleeding, and transfusion requirements. Recommendations include forced air heating of the upper body, intravenous fluids given with extending heating to 2 h before and after surgery for additional benefits (Pędziwiatr et al., 2018).

Supplemental Oxygen

A growing number of researchers have suggested that increased fraction of inspired oxygen (FiO_2) be routinely prescribed for postoperative patients to increase oxygen delivery to the reparative site. However, it is important to recognize that correcting tissue hypoxia requires more than simply providing increased FiO_2 to increase arterial saturation (SaO_2) and arterial PO_2. Wound PO_2 may remain unchanged even while the patient is breathing additional oxygen if other important clinical factors are not also addressed. In a study of patients who underwent general surgery, approximately 30% had reduced tissue oxygen tension levels despite adequate urine output and arterial oxygen levels (Chang, Goodson, Gottrup, et al., 1983). This is a result of early postoperative compartmental fluid shifts, in which kidney perfusion is restored at the expense of peripheral vasculature vasoconstriction. A Cochrane metaanalysis evaluating the effect of increased FiO_2 provided intraoperatively demonstrated no beneficial effect of a fraction of inspired oxygen of 60% or higher on surgical site infection; thus, suggesting insufficient evidence to support the routine use of a high fraction of inspired oxygen during anesthesia and surgery (Wetterslev et al., 2015).

To increase the perfusion, hyperbaric oxygenation (HBO) is recommended for specific clinical conditions and wound types. More specifically, HBO therapy saturates the plasma via pressurized oxygen, thus, directly addressing the impairment oxygen at the microcirculatory system level such as with diabetic foot ulcers, radiation necrosis, and compromised skin flaps. Recent ongoing evidence of newer devices has challenged prior reports regarding the efficacy of topical oxygen on wound healing (Oropallo & Andersen, 2021). Topical oxygen at the wound surface and HBO are discussed in Chapter 22.

Volume Support

Jönsson, Jensen, Goodson, et al. (1987) demonstrated that low tissue oxygen levels in general surgery patients could be raised with infusion of fluids and that a fluid bolus of 250 mL of normal saline was sufficient in most cases. In well-perfused patients, tissue oxygen pressure continues to rise as PaO_2 rises. Findings of subsequent clinical studies in which supplemental fluids were provided perioperatively have produced mixed results of tissue PO_2 change and wound infection related to increasing fluids. In patients undergoing abdominal and colon surgeries, those who received aggressive fluid repletion (defined as maintenance levels of 16–18 mL/kg/h during surgery and 1 h postoperatively, or for the first 24 postsurgical hours, for an average 1.1-L increase above standard fluids) showed significantly higher wound P_{O_2} than did patients who received standard fluids (Arkiliç, Taguchi, Sharma, et al., 2003). Higher levels of collagen deposition were associated with the increased fluids and improved wound oxygen status. Testing of fluid supplementation in randomized clinical trials has not shown benefit in terms of reducing surgical site infection. Fewer postsurgical complications, including wound dehiscence, were reported in a randomized clinical trial of 152 cases of elective intraabdominal surgeries in patients randomized to restricted versus liberal fluid repletion protocols (Nisanevich, Felsenstein, Almogy, et al., 2005). The fluid protocols in each study are not directly comparable, and neither study documented tissue oxygen levels in response to fluid, so interpretation of these differing findings is difficult. Similar lack of benefit associated with higher intraoperative fluids was also shown in a study using a surgical porcine model that measured perianastomotic and anastomotic colon tissue oxygen levels (Kimberger, Fleischmann, Brandt, et al., 2007). At present, data suggest that fluid supplementation as a single intervention is not sufficient to reduce wound infections or improve clinical healing outcomes. For most surgical procedures, proper dosing of IV fluids that outweighed the losses during surgery is recommended by ERAS guidelines (Pędziwiatr et al., 2018).

Combining More Than Two Interventions

Combining the interventions of fluid repletion, oxygen support and warming, and pain control seems warranted, given the existing evidence. Hypovolemia is a powerful physiologic vasoconstrictor. Therefore, volume replacement and oxygen therapy must coincide with postoperative warming to benefit peripheral perfusion and tissue oxygen supply. Core temperature is not a clinically useful indicator in this equation. Skin surface temperatures do correlate with fingertip blood flow; a forearm-minus-fingertip difference of 4°C defines a state of peripheral vasoconstriction. However, this method is not commonly used in practice (Rubinstein & Sessler, 1990).

The concept of combined interventions received early testing many years ago. In a prospective randomized trial that combined interventions, aggressive postoperative warming and pain control increased the wound P_{O_2} to 70 mmHg within 4–6 h, a level nearly equal to that found in normal volunteers (West, 1994). In addition, the actively rewarmed patients who had undergone lengthy abdominal surgeries were given a 1-L fluid bolus to replace fluids lost as urine during the diuresis, which commonly accompanies hypothermia and vasoconstriction. These same interventions have been applied to trauma patients who have demonstrated improved regional perfusion, but only after warming and adequate fluid resuscitation (Knudson, Bermudez, Doyle, et al., 1997). Patients who are warm, well perfused, and oxygenated rarely develop wound infections (Hopf & Holm, 2008; Hopf et al., 1997). In order to test future combined interventions pragmatically, there is need for clinically feasible, reliable, and valid methods to measure the effect of combined interventions on tissue oxygenation (Schreml et al., 2010).

To predict fluid responsiveness, most studies have focused on validating new tests and the limitations of each test. Obtaining pulse pressure/stroke volume variations are numerous, but recent efforts have been made to overcome these limitations, such as with low tidal volume ventilation. Following pulse pressure/stroke volume variations, new tests have emerged which assess preload responsiveness. Given the risk of fluid overload that is inherent to the "classical" fluid challenge, a "mini" fluid challenge, made of 100 mL of fluid only, has been utilized.

Passive leg raising creates a reversible increase in venous return allowing for the prediction of fluid responsiveness. However, the amount of venous return may vary in various clinical settings potentially affecting the diagnostic performance of passive leg raising (Cherpanath et al., 2016). The reliability of the passive leg-raising test is now well established and the development of defining several noninvasive estimates of cardiac output is ongoing. By establishing indices of fluid responsiveness, excessive fluid balance may be avoided (Monnet & Teboul, 2018).

Other methods of evaluating resuscitation goals are lactate normalization (≤ 2 mmol/L) or a 20% decrease every 2 h. Other forms of multimodal perfusion monitoring include sublingual microcirculatory assessment; plasma-disappearance rate of indocyanine green; muscle oxygen saturation; central venous-arterial pCO_2 gradient/arterial-venous O_2 content difference ratio; and lactate/pyruvate ratio. Additional research on end resuscitative measures using capillary refill targeted fluid resuscitation suggests comparable effects on regional and microcirculatory flow parameters and hypoxia surrogates, and a faster achievement of the predefined resuscitation target. Fluid cessation in patients with capillary refill time ≤ 3 s appears as reliable method to assess tissue perfusion (Castro et al., 2020).

Patient Education

The knowledgeable provider uses theory-based assessment and a coordinated therapeutic plan to optimize wound care within the context of a larger plan, including patient teaching and necessary follow-up. Patients in acute care settings require instruction on wound care, fluid replacement, avoidance of dehydration, cessation of tobacco use, and practical ways to conserve body heat. Unfortunately, this instruction frequently occurs at a time when the patient is fatigued and somewhat overwhelmed by the entire surgical experience. In this case, teaching is best done succinctly and should be reinforced by providing the patient or family member with written guidelines. Follow-up of the patient's understanding and emphasis on healthy postoperative behaviors at clinic appointments reinforce initial teaching.

Cigarette smoking and obesity are particularly deleterious to wound repair because of their effects on both perfusion and oxygenation. Studies indicate a higher incidence of wound infection, dehiscence, and delayed healing among smokers and obese individuals compared with nonsmokers and nonobese individuals. Therefore, patients should be counseled regarding the negative effect of smoking and obesity on wound-healing outcomes and should be offered programs and resources as needed to address these lifestyle choices or addictions (Fleischmann et al., 2005; Kabon et al., 2004; Manassa et al., 2003; Sørensen, 2012; Sørensen et al., 2003; Stotts & Wipke-Tevis, 1996). Lifestyle modifications present challenges and may require specialized, targeted interventions that include techniques such as motivational interviewing or other methods to encourage individual willingness and commitment to adopt new behaviors.

MEASURING THE RESPONSE

Although low periwound oxygen is an initial feature of most wounds, continued and unexplained hypoxia is of particular importance. Wound healing is proportional to local oxygen tension. Transcutaneous oxygen tension is a useful, noninvasive way to assess the adequacy of tissue oxygenation near a wound or suture line in relationship to Fio_2 (Fig. 31.1). Defining the contribution of hypoxia in the context of the recent history of the patient and time from wounding clarifies the reason for low wound Po_2. Tests can be conducted to reveal the responsiveness of the wound to factors such as local warming, vasodilating drugs, oxygen therapies, sympathetic blockade, positioning, pain, and anxiety management. For example, during an oxygen challenge (e.g., breathing increased, controlled oxygen via face mask) in the absence of vasoconstriction, significant oxygen diffusion into the capillary-perfused wound edge will occur. Simple, effective, and conservative corrective therapy then can be initiated. Because improved wound Po_2 is a real measure of wound-healing progress, serial measurements of damaged tissue can be obtained during the course of healing. Traditional methods to evaluate for ischemia and perfusion such as ankle-brachial and toe-brachial indices and pressures have advantages of use in a noninvasive way of measuring perfusion. However, emerging technology may address some of the pitfalls of traditional methods. Color photo and blood flow images provided by a camera and illumination system uses the laser speckle contrast technique to deliver real-time,

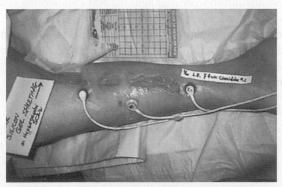

Fig. 31.1 Recording transcutaneous oxygen tension near a lower leg wound.

high-resolution blood flow images, providing a wide range of preclinical and clinical research applications. The images are recorded where the average speed and concentration of moving red blood cells in the living tissue sample volume can be analyzed (Sarojini et al., 2021). Thermal imaging using near-infrared light has improved in technology and translation to the bedside to help assist in determining areas of ischemia (Koerner, Adams, Harper, Black, & Langemo, 2019).

INCISION CARE

Sutures and Staples

Multiple techniques and suture materials are available for closing an incision. National guidelines state that the type of suture material used does not matter in terms of SSI or postsurgical wound complications, as long as the primary repair is anatomic and perfused (Hemming, Pinkney, Futaba, et al., 2013). The choice of suture technique depends on the type and anatomic location of the wound, the thickness of the skin, the degree of tension, and the desired cosmetic result. For example, absorbable sutures are used to close tissues deeper than the epidermis and to provide tissue support, relieve skin tension, and reduce wound dead space (Hollander et al., 2003). Continuous sutures are recommended for closure of laparotomy fascial incisions; however, the type of suture does not affect healing. Surgical site infection in wounds after saphenous vein graft harvesting is problematic, but current evidence does not favor staples or sutures in terms of infection risk. There is a lack of evidence to suggest that sutures are better than staples in terms of wound infection, readmission rate, adverse events, and postoperative pain. Yet with low quality of evidence, sutures reduce postoperative pain and improve grade of satisfaction with the cosmetic outcome (Cochetti et al., 2020).

Sutures should be removed within 1–2 weeks of their placement, depending on the anatomic location: 3 to 5 days for the face; 7–10 days for scalp, chest, fingers, hand, and lower extremity; and 10–14 days for the back, forearm, and foot (Hollander et al., 2003; Wu, 2006). Sutures left in too long can lead to suture marks, local tissue reaction, and scarring. Premature suture removal places the wound at risk for reopening (Hollander, 2003; Wu, 2006). With the appropriate equipment, suture and staple removal is not difficult. The suture should be gently grasped by the knot and elevated slightly with forceps. One side of the suture is cut at skin level. With the forceps still grasping the knot, the suture is gently pulled toward the wound or suture line until the suture material is completely removed (Wilson, Kocurek, & Doty, 2000).

Skin Adhesives

Tissue adhesives and derivatives of cyanoacrylate and other materials that add strength and flexibility have been used for several years for lacerations and other types of wound closure. An updated Cochrane review compared adhesives to sutures (10 trials) or adhesives to staples used for incision closure. The review identified a difference in rate of dehiscence between adhesives and sutures, favoring the use of sutures to reduce dehiscence; faster time to closure was found for staples in comparison to adhesives, but this was based on a single trial (Coulthard, Esposito, Worthington, et al., 2010). The overall conclusion was that there is no evidence that SSI rates differ based on wound closure with tissue adhesives, sutures, tapes, or staples or between types of tissue adhesives. The authors also noted that evaluation of adhesives in patients with healing risk factors and for wounds with high tension requires additional study because these subpopulations were excluded from the trials that were reviewed; therefore, the comparative effectiveness is not known. Skin adhesives are not recommended for use with complex lacerations with wound edges that are difficult to approximate (Hollander, 2003). However, a prospective, double-blind randomized controlled trial performed in 51 patients undergoing total knee arthroplasty completion with a subcuticular stitch versus 2-octyl cyanoacrylate topical adhesive with flexible self-adhesive polyester mesh demonstrated improvement (Choi et al., 2021). The primary and secondary outcome measures were compared between groups provided quicker wound closure, shorter stitch out time, and better wound margin coaptation in the early postoperative period but similar cosmetic efficacy compared with subcuticular suture (Choi et al., 2021). No removal is required for adhesives, although some cannot be exposed to water. Ointments should be avoided because they may loosen the adhesive and cause wound dehiscence (Hollander, 2003). Tissue adhesives slough off 5 to 10 days after they are applied.

Steri-Strip™ S Wound closure tapes, or Steri-Strips™, are reinforced microporous surgical adhesive tape. Steri-Strip™ are used to provide extra support to a suture line when running subcuticular sutures are used or after sutures are removed. Wound closure tapes may reduce spreading of the scar if they are kept in place for several weeks after suture removal. Often they are used with a tissue adhesive. These tapes are rarely used for primary wound closure (Wilson et al., 2000). There is very little evidence of use for primary closure. Even recent Steri-Strip™ S demonstrated no significant differences in wound healing of median sternotomy incisions in children closed with either a subcuticular suture or Steri-Strip™ S using the Patient and Observer Scar Assessment Scale (POSAS) which measures the pliability, thickness, and surface area. Additionally, significant differences regarding scar formation and final cosmetic results of the scars favored subcuticular closure (van de Kar, Koolbergen, van Avendonk, & van der Horst, 2019).

SURGICAL WOUND ASSESSMENT

Clinically, there is no single, standard, widely accepted method for assessing healing of acute wounds. Additional issues arise because assessment parameters that are documented and descriptions of surgical incision healing by care providers vary and in some cases are not recorded. This concern is illustrated by a retrospective chart audit of surgical cases that documented 59.6% (89/152) did not have complete wound assessments (Gillespie, Chaboyer, Kang, et al., 2014).

Physiologically, deposition of collagen in the wound begins immediately in the inflammatory phase and peaks during the proliferative phase, approximately 4–21 days after wounding. Sufficient synthesis of collagen early during the healing process is critical to successful repair. Wound dehiscence is most likely to occur fairly early after surgery (by postoperative day 5–8) in patients in whom normal physiologic healing responses, such as collagen synthesis, lag. However, a method for direct observation of collagen production in acute wounds has been evaluated on a molecular level confirming collagen production even from macrocytic involvement (Sarojini et al., 2021).

Scoring Tools

Acute wound complications can be evaluated on the basis of specific parameters using the a variety of scoring tools; most commonly, the CDC criterion, Southampton and ASEPSIS (shown in Appendix B) The CDC has issued an SSI criterion that distinguishes superficial incisional SSI, deep incisional SSI, and organ/space SSI (Berríos-Torres, Umscheid, & Bratzler, 2017). The Southampton score was originally designed to assess hernia wounds. Wounds are graded according to any complications and their extent (Campwala, Unsell, & Gupta, 2019). The ASEPSIS method (acronym for Additional treatment, Serous discharge, Erythema, Purulent exudate, Separation of deep tissues, Isolation of bacteria, and prolonged inpatient Stay) was originally developed in cardiac surgery patients to evaluate characteristics of the surgical incision associated with infection (Wilson, Treasure, Sturridge, et al., 1986). In a validation study, ASEPSIS was reported to be as sensitive and significantly more specific compared with other clinical indicators of wound problems or to wound assessments made using standard definitions of wound infections (Wilson, Weavill, Burridge, et al., 1990). Interrater reliability of 0.96 has been reported in patients undergoing general surgery (Byrne, Malek, Davey, et al., 1989). Similar reliability has been shown for sternal and leg wounds of patients after cardiac surgery (Wilson, Webster, Gruneberg, et al., 1986). Topaloglu, Akin, Avsar, et al. (2008) noted statistically significant correlations between preoperative wound infection risk indices and ASEPSIS scores. A systematic review in 2012 demonstrated the potential for its efficacy; however, caution regarding its validation (Siah & Childs, 2012). However, comparative studies between the CDC criterion, ASEPSIS score, and Southampton score highlight the ASEPSIS scoring system showing substantial predictive value of outcomes in the setting of breast reconstruction (Campwala et al., 2019). Other pitfalls with the CDC criterion is its reliance on subjective physician diagnosis; thus, allowing for varying rates of infection diagnosis (Campwala et al., 2019).

Impediments to Surgical Wound Healing

Although ongoing assessment of the surgical wound is critical, identifying impediments to healing is important so that they may be minimized or eliminated when possible. Box 31.1 lists impediments to surgical wound healing. Most of these (perfusion and smoking, nonviable tissue, infection, mechanical factors, obesity, diabetes, malnutrition, and burn

BOX 31.1 Impediments to Surgical Wound Healing

- Inadequate wound perfusion
- Presence of nonviable tissue
- Wound hematoma or seroma
- Infection or increased tissue bioburden
- Mechanical factors during wound repair
- Systemic immunodeficiencies
- Cancer and cancer treatment factors
- Systemic conditions, uncontrolled diabetes mellitus, obesity, malnutrition
- Burn injuries
- External agents (e.g., tobacco, drugs)
- Excessive scar formation

TABLE 31.3 CDC Criteria for Incisional, Deep, and Organ/Space Infection

Superficial SSI	Deep Incisional SSI	Organ/Space SSI
Purulent damage	Purulent damage	Purulent damage
Positive wound culture	Incision dehisces or is opened by physician when patient has one of the following: fever, local pain, tenderness (unless site is culture negative)	Positive wound culture
At least one of the following: signs or symptoms of infection: pain, or tenderness; local swelling; redness; heat	Abscess or other evidence of infection found on examination, X-ray study, histopathology	Abscess or other evidence of infection found on examination, X-ray study, histopathology
Superficial incision is deliberately opened by a surgeon unless incision culture is negative		
Diagnosis by surgeon or attending physician	Diagnosis by surgeon or attending physician	Diagnosis by surgeon or attending physician

CDC, Centers for Disease Control and Prevention; SSI, surgical site infection. Berríos-Torres et al. (2017).

injuries) are discussed in greater detail in chapters throughout this text.

Hematoma or Seroma

The occurrence of hematoma or seroma in surgical wounds has increased because of greater clinical use of anticoagulants and prophylactic treatments now recommended and implemented for deep vein thrombosis. When detected, hematoma or seroma requires intervention for removal by needle aspiration or prophylactic drainage. The presence of fluid collections, seromas, or hematomas delays healing in acute wounds through mechanisms of pressure and ischemia to the wound edges and adjacent tissues.

Surgical Wound Infection

Centers for Disease Control and Prevention criteria for diagnosing various types of SSIs are widely accepted; the criteria are listed in Table 31.3 (Berríos-Torres et al., 2017). Infections of episiotomies, newborn circumcision sites, burns, and stitch abscesses are not classified as SSIs.

Box 31.2 lists both intrinsic and extrinsic risk factors for SSI that have been identified in many studies. However, the risk factors most commonly reported amongst most surgical procedures include length of preoperative hospital stay more than 24 h; duration of surgery in hours; wound class clean-contaminated, contaminated and dirty/infected; ASA index classified into ASA II, III, and IV/V, and if *Staphylococcus aureus* and *Escherichia coli* were identified (de Carvalho, Campos, de Castro Franco, Rocha, & Ercole, 2017). Although there are global variations around the definition of an SSI, an SSI is defined typically as infections occurring within 30 days after surgery and affecting either the incision or organ. Infectious complications are the predominate reason for unplanned 30-day readmissions in vascular surgery patients. Expected patient risk factors, such as diabetes, obesity, renal insufficiency, and cigarette smoking, were less important in predicting infectious complications compared with operative time, presence of a preoperative open wound, and inpatient operation. Recent findings suggest that careful operative planning and expeditious operations may be the most effective approaches to reducing infections (Hicks et al., 2016). In

many regions, SSIs are part of reportable hospital acquired conditions that have potential for decreased reimbursement (Alverdy, Hyman, & Gilbert, 2020). Among other risk factors (e.g., advanced age, frailty, diabetes mellitus, and surgery complexity), the review reported that increased duration of surgery was found consistently to be associated with SSI. 87% of reported studies demonstrated a statistically significant association between longer operative time and SSI (Cheng et al., 2017). Risk factors can vary due operative procedure and etiology. Recent reports of conflicting results regarding intraoperative contamination, cultures, and use of antibiotics lead to other opportunities (Alverdy et al., 2020).

A number of risk factors are irreversible, but several may be modified through patient advisement and modification of aspects of perioperative care. Understanding who is at risk for SSI provides an opportunity for both preventive measures and to increase surveillance so that early detection can occur, and timely intervention can be initiated. ERAS updated guidelines for many operations include changes from overnight fasting to carbohydrate drinks 2 h before surgery (Box 31.3).

BOX 31.2 Risk Factors for Surgical Site Infection

Intrinsic

Existing Disease
- Chronic obstructive pulmonary disease
- Congestive cardiac failure
- Diabetes
- Peripheral vascular disease
- Skin disease in surgical area

Additional Factors
- Age
- Ascites
- Chronic inflammation
- Excessive alcohol use
- Hypercholesterolemia
- Hyperglycemia
- Hypoxemia
- Low albumin
- Low hemoglobin or hematocrit
- Malnutrition

- Nicotine use
- Prior surgical site radiation
- Remote infection
- Skin carrier of staphylococcus
- Steroid or other immunosuppressive medications

Extrinsic

Presurgical Factors
- Current surgery through previous incision
- Emergency surgery
- Previous surgery
- Hair removal

Perioperative Factors
- Estimated blood loss $\geq$500 mL
- Hypothermia
- Blood products
- Surgery $\geq$2 h

BOX 31.3 ERAS Guidelines

Preoperative
- Counseling
- Fluid and Carbohydrate loading
- No prolonged fasting
- No selective bowel prep
- Antibiotic prophylaxis
- Thromboprophylaxis
- No premedication

Intraoperative
- Short-acting anesthesia
- Epidural anesthesia
- No salt and water overload
- Normothermia

Postoperative
- Epidural anesthesia
- No nasogastric tubes
- Nausea and vomiting prevention
- No salt and water overload
- Early mobilization, nutrition
- Removal of catheters
- NSAIDs, avoid opioids

Data from Pędziwiatr, M., Mavrikis, J., Witowski, J., et al. (2018). Current status of enhanced recovery after surgery (ERAS) protocol in gastrointestinal surgery. *Medical Oncology, 35*, 95.

Minimally invasive approaches instead of large incisions are encouraged. The management of fluids seek balance rather than large volumes of intravenous fluids. Avoidance of or early removal of drains and tubes is recommended as well as early mobilization and serving of drinks and food the day of the operation. These protocols have resulted in shorter length of hospital stay and, reduced complications, while readmissions

and costs are reduced. Stress of the operation to retain anabolic homeostasis. has been shown to improve outcomes in almost all major surgical specialties (Ljungqvist, Scott, & Fearon, 2017).

Yet in the past 10 years, oral antibiotics before colon surgery have made a major comeback and are now considered to be standard of care (Rollins, Javanmard-Emamghissi, Acheson, & Lobo, 2019). Approximately 50% of the microbes causing SSI today have been shown to be resistant to the antibiotics used for prophylaxis (Teillant, Gandra, Barter, Morgan, & Laxminarayan, 2015). With the use of sequencing technology, exact sequence variants can be tracked from their original site of colonization to the surgical wound and to the actual clinical infection site. Targeted therapies include application of mouth hygiene, personalized diets and bowel preparations, and fecal transplants to eliminate multidrug-resistant pathogens to enhance the microbiome rather than nonselectively eliminating it (Alverdy et al., 2020).

TOPICAL INCISION CARE

Regardless of their origin, wounds progress through the same phases of the reparative process in order to heal: inflammation, angiogenesis, fibroplasia and matrix deposition, and epithelialization. Knowledgeable assessment of the patient's surgical incision site includes evaluation of the primary dressing, epithelial resurfacing, wound closure, and local changes at the wound site that may signal infection. All healing incisions should be protected from sun exposure to prevent permanent hyperpigmentation (Ship & Weiss, 1985). General components of topical incision care are listed in Box 31.4 and described in this section.

Dressings provide initial protection, exudate absorption, and thermal insulation for acute wounds. Studies evaluating

BOX 31.4 Topical Incision Care

1. Keep incisions dry without prolonged exposure to moisture.
2. Maintain original postoperative dressing for 48–72 h (cleanse incision with sterile saline and use aseptic technique for changing dressings if needed in first 48 h).
3. After 48–72 h, patient may shower if suture line is closed with no drainage.
4. Timing of suture or staple removal depends on wound location:
   - 3–5 days face
   - 7–10 days for scalp, chest, fingers, hand, lower extremity
   - 10–14 days for the back
5. Protect surgical wound incision from exposure to sun.

dressings that provide a moist, occlusive, or semiocclusive environment compared with standard dry absorbent gauze postsurgical dressings find no difference in the incidence of SSI for wounds after cardiac, vascular, or gastrointestinal surgeries; in patient comfort; or in cost (Shinohara, Yamashita, Satoh, et al., 2008; Vogt, Uhlyarik, & Schroeder, 2007; Wynne, Botti, Stedman, et al., 2004). A recent systematic review and metaanalysis of 16 randomized controlled trials (RCTs) ($n = 2594$ patients) (Dumville, Walter, Sharp, et al., 2011; Walter, Dumville, Sharp, et al., 2012) included comparisons of basic contact dressings with no dressing; different types of basic contact dressings; or basic contact dressings with film, hydrocolloid/matrix hydrocolloid, or hydrofiber. The 16 studies in the review included children or adults with surgical incisions healing by primary intention, wounds of all contamination levels (clean, clean-contaminated, contaminated), and dressings applied immediately after surgery. The metaanalysis found no statistically significant differences in rates of SSI for any of the comparisons, and the authors concluded there is insufficient evidence to suggest the type of surgical wound dressing reduces SSI (Aduba & Yang, 2017).

Additional outcomes relevant to surgical incision beyond SSI include patient satisfaction, comfort, pain, convenience, and cost. In terms of the outcome of cost, the data are mixed. Dry absorbent dressings are reported to be less expensive (Vogt et al., 2007; Wynne et al., 2004), although Shinohara et al. (2008) found hydrocolloid dressings were less costly. None of the studies or the metaanalysis found differences in comfort between dressing types, and it is noted that meaningful data on pain are lacking (Walter et al., 2012). Further research on the impact of various dressings on meaningful outcomes with quality measurement methods is needed. Multiple systematic reviews and metaanalyses have supported the use of negative pressure over primary incision site in different types of surgeries (Sahebally et al., 2018; Yin et al., 2018). A recent Cochrane report people experiencing primary **wound** closure of their surgical **wound** and treated prophylactically with NPWT

following surgery probably experience fewer SSI than people treated with standard dressings (moderate-certainty evidence (Webster et al., 2019)).

More detailed information on NPWT is presented in Chapter 21.

Of interest, some data suggest that dressings that provide some level of pressure or compression may actually impede local tissue perfusion (Plattner et al., 2000). This finding was based on the observation that wounds covered with dressings that provide some level of pressure had tissue oxygen levels 12 mmHg lower than wounds with less constrictive covers. In the interest of supporting oxygen delivery to acute wounds, avoiding extra pressure over the wound seems prudent unless required for hemostasis.

Surgical dressings usually are removed 48–72 h after injury, which is consistent with CDC guidelines for prevention of SSIs (Berríos-Torres et al., 2017). Aseptic technique for dressing changes and use of sterile saline if needed for cleansing are recommended within the 48-h timeframe (Leaper, Burman-Roy, Palanca, et al., 2008). If the wound is closed and dry after 48 h, patients may shower.

Use of topical antibiotics on closed surgical incisions is not supported by current evidence and is not recommended by recent guidelines (Leaper et al., 2008). A trial comparing no ointment, paraffin, and mupirocin ointment on excised and sutured skin lesions ($n = 562$ wounds) reported no differences in wound infection rate and, interestingly, significantly fewer scar complications in patients treated without any ointment (Dixon, Dixon, & Dixon, 2006).

Resurfacing of the wound closed by primary intention occurs within 2–3 days after wounding because of the presence of intact epithelial appendages, such as hair follicles, and the relatively short distance that cells in the interrupted epithelial tissue must traverse. Although the incisional wound does not have the structural integrity (tensile strength) to withstand force at this time, by postoperative day 2 or 3, the incision is "sealed" and impenetrable to bacteria. However, many patients prefer that the wound remain covered. As healing evolves, some incisions begin to itch as a result of wound contraction or simply dry skin. Wound dressings manage and encourage the wound healing procedure for proper recovery. To compare with excisional wounds, there have been few studies exploring dressing effect on wound healing strength without consistent results to prevent surgical site dehiscence. Malnutrition, sepsis, anemia, uremia, liver failure, diabetes, obesity, malignancy, use of steroids, and many other diseases can all contribute to surgical wound dehiscence (Aduba & Yang, 2017). Studies cited in the Cochrane review conclude that it is "low or very low certainty for all outcomes" (Webster et al., 2019). One direct effect of ischemia is a reduction of tissue high-energy phosphate reserve. Preliminary results using intracellular delivery of Mg-ATP (ATP-vesicles) to enhance excisional skin wound healing process in nonischemic and ischemic wounds both in nondiabetic and diabetic animals is promising to help assist in incisional wound healing (Mo et al., 2019).

CLINICAL CONSULT

A: This 66-year-old woman presents for a preoperative clinic appointment prior to a scheduled colon surgery in 3 weeks for the treatment of stage II colorectal cancer. The patient lives in a rural part of the state, 3 h from the medical center. The patient is under treatment for hypertension (controlled) and also type 2 diabetes (controlled, Hb A_{1c} 5%). She smokes ¼ pack per day and has a body mass index of 33. She is anxious about the upcoming procedure and particularly concerned about postprocedure pain and complications, including wound infection.

D: Patient presents with multiple factors placing her at high risk for postoperative wound-healing problems. Her diabetes is controlled, but of particular concern are the use of tobacco and obesity making her vulnerable to low tissue oxygen levels and risk for wound-healing complications. Her anxiety is also a factor that may contribute to and exacerbate procedure-related pain, thus influencing tissue perfusion to the surgical wound.

P: Selected interventions will be discussed with both the patient and the interdisciplinary operative team preoperatively.

I: (1) Wound-related risks of smoking reviewed with patient and plan for smoking cessation for 2 weeks prior to surgery agreed on. (2) Prescription for nicotine patch obtained and provided to patient. (3) Discuss patient interest in smoking cessation as a personal goal and refer to cessation program as indicated. (4) Discuss with surgical/anesthesia team intraoperative management, including systemic warming, pain management, and fluid replacement.

E: Follow postoperatively for wound healing and early detection of problems (wound dehiscence and/or infection) in hospital, with telecheck in at-home and at postoperative clinic visits. Follow up postoperatively on smoking cessation plans and needed support.

SUMMARY

- Emerging technology continues to address intravascular fluid shifts.
- Adequate oxygen delivery to the tissues is necessary for wound fibroblasts, collagen formation, and wound tensile strength.
- ERAS-based intervention can enhance tissue perfusion include measures to prevent hypothermia and hypovolemia, reduce pain and anxiety including edema.

- Postoperative wound assessment is essential to detect SSI and dehiscence.
- National safety initiatives, quality reporting measures, and evidence-based guidelines for acute wounds offer new insights into risk and strategies to decrease wound-healing failure after surgery.

SELF-ASSESSMENT QUESTIONS

1. Ways to improve oxygenation to the wound bed include is to address patient:
   a. Pain and stress
   b. Hypothermia
   c. Obesity
   d. Tobacco use
   e. All of the above

2. True or False. SSI is defined typically as infections occurring within 30 days after surgery and affecting either the incision or organ and reportable leading to decreased hospital reimbursement.

3. Postoperative recovery involves:
   a. Epidural anesthesia
   b. Prevention of nausea and vomiting
   c. No nasogastric tubes
   d. Early removal of catheters
   e. All of the above

4. The most commonly used acute wound complication scoring tool includes:
   a. CDC criterion
   b. ASEPSIS
   c. Southampton
   d. None of the above

5. True or False. Routine use of topical antibiotics should be used when dressing wounds.

REFERENCES

Aduba, D. C., & Yang, H. (2017). Polysaccharide fabrication platforms and biocompatibility assessment as candidate wound dressing materials. *Bioengineering (Basel, Switzerland), 4*(1), E1. https://doi.org/10.3390/bioengineering4010001.

Aghaloo, T., Kim, J. J., Gordon, T., & Behrsing, H. P. (2019). In vitro models, standards, and experimental methods for tobacco products. *Advances in Dental Research, 30*(1), 16–21. https://doi.org/10.1177/0022034519872474.

Allen, D. B., Maguire, J. J., Mahdavian, M., et al. (1997). Wound hypoxia and acidosis limit neutrophil bacterial killing mechanisms. *Archives of Surgery, 132*(9), 991–996.

Alverdy, J. C., Hyman, N., & Gilbert, J. (2020). Re-examining causes of surgical site infections following elective surgery in the era of asepsis. *The Lancet Infectious Diseases, 20*(3), e38–e43. https://doi.org/10.1016/S1473-3099(19)30756-X.

Arkiliç, C. F., Taguchi, A., Sharma, N., et al. (2003). Supplemental perioperative fluid administration increases tissue oxygen pressure. *Surgery, 133*(1), 49–55.

Bay, J., Nunn, J. F., & Prys-Roberts, C. (1968). Factors influencing arterial PO2 during recovery from anaesthesia. *British Journal of Anaesthesia*, 40(6), 398–407.

Berríos-Torres, S. I., Umscheid, C. A., & Bratzler, D. W. (2017). Centers for Disease Control and Prevention Guideline for the Prevention of Surgical Site Infection, 2017. *JAMA Surgery*, 152(8), 784–791. https://doi.org/10.1001/jamasurg.2017.0904.

Bratzler, D. W., & Hunt, D. R. (2006). The surgical infection prevention and surgical care improvement projects: National initiatives to improve outcomes for patients having surgery. *Clinical Infectious Diseases*, 43(3), 322–330.

Bray, E. R., Oropallo, A. R., Grande, D. A., Kirsner, R. S., & Badiavas, E. V. (2021). Extracellular vesicles as therapeutic tools for the treatment of chronic wounds. *Pharmaceutics*, 13(10), 1543. https://doi.org/10.3390/pharmaceutics13101543.

Brown, J. (2016). The impact of stress on acute wound healing. *British Journal of Community Nursing*, 21(Sup12), S16–S22. https://doi.org/10.12968/bjcn.2016.21.Sup12.S16.

Byrne, D., Malek, M. M., Davey, P. G., et al. (1989). Postoperative wound scoring. *Biomedicine & Pharmacotherapy*, 43, 669–673.

Campwala, I., Unsell, K., & Gupta, S. (2019). A comparative analysis of surgical wound infection methods: Predictive values of the CDC, ASEPSIS, and Southampton scoring systems in evaluating breast reconstruction surgical site infections. *Plastic Surgery (Oakville, ON)*, 27(2), 93–99. https://doi.org/10.1177/2292550319826095.

Cannon, W. B. (1970). *Bodily changes in pain, hunger, fear and rage: An account of recent researches into the function of emotional excitement.* College Park: McGrath.

Castro, R., Kattan, E., Ferri, G., Pairumani, R., Valenzuela, E. D., Alegría, L., et al. (2020). Effects of capillary refill time-vs. lactate-targeted fluid resuscitation on regional, microcirculatory and hypoxia-related perfusion parameters in septic shock: A randomized controlled trial. *Annals of Intensive Care*, 10(1), 150. https://doi.org/10.1186/s13613-020-00767-4.

Centers for Disease Control and Prevention. (2022). Adult obesity facts. *Obesity is a common, serious, and costly disease.* Centers for Disease Control and Prevention. Retrieved December 27, 2022 from https://www.cdc.gov/obesity/data/adult.html.

Chang, N., Goodson, W. H., 3rd, Gottrup, F., et al. (1983). Direct measurement of wound and tissue oxygen tension in postoperative patients. *Annals of Surgery*, 197(4), 470–478.

Charalambous, C., Vassilopoulos, A., Koulouri, A., Eleni, S., Popi, S., Antonis, F., et al. (2018). The impact of stress on pressure ulcer wound healing process and on the psychophysiological environment of the individual suffering from them. *Medical Archives (Sarajevo, Bosnia and Herzegovina)*, 72(5), 362–366. https://doi.org/10.5455/medarh.2018.72.362-366.

Cheng, H., Chen, B. P.-H., Soleas, I. M., Ferko, N. C., Cameron, C. G., & Hinoul, P. (2017). Prolonged operative duration increases risk of surgical site infections: A systematic review. *Surgical Infections*, 18(6), 722–735. https://doi.org/10.1089/sur.2017.089.

Chernow, B., Alexander, H. R., Smallridge, R. C., et al. (1987). Hormonal responses to graded surgical stress. *Archives of Internal Medicine*, 147(7), 1273–1278.

Cherpanath, T. G. V., Hirsch, A., Geerts, B. F., Lagrand, W. K., Leeflang, M. M., Schultz, M. J., et al. (2016). Predicting fluid responsiveness by passive leg raising: A systematic review and meta-analysis of 23 clinical trials. *Critical Care Medicine*, 44(5), 981–991. https://doi.org/10.1097/CCM.0000000000001556.

Choi, K. Y., Koh, I. J., Kim, M. S., Park, D. C., Sung, Y. G., & In, Y. (2021). 2-Octyl cyanoacrylate topical adhesive as an alternative to subcuticular suture for skin closure after total knee arthroplasty: A randomized controlled trial in the same patient. *The Journal of Arthroplasty*, 36(9), 3141–3147. https://doi.org/10.1016/j.arth.2021.04.033.

Cochetti, G., Abraha, I., Randolph, J., Montedori, A., Boni, A., Arezzo, A., et al. (2020). Surgical wound closure by staples or sutures?: Systematic review. *Medicine*, 99(25), e20573. https://doi.org/10.1097/MD.0000000000020573.

Coulthard, P., Esposito, M., Worthington, H. V., et al. (2010). Tissue adhesive for closure of surgical incisions. *The Cochrane Database of Systematic Reviews*, 5, CD004287.

D'Alessandro, S., Magnavacca, A., Perego, F., Fumagalli, M., Sangiovanni, E., Prato, M., et al. (2019). Effect of hypoxia on gene expression in cell populations involved in wound healing. *BioMed Research International*, 2019. https://doi.org/10.1155/2019/2626374. 2626374–20.

de Carvalho, R. L. R., Campos, C. C., de Castro Franco, L. M., Rocha, A. D. M., & Ercole, F. F. (2017). Incidence and risk factors for surgical site infection in general surgeries. *Revista Latino-Americana De Enfermagem*, 25, e2848. https://doi.org/10.1590/1518-8345.1502.2848.

Derbyshire, D., & Smith, G. (1984). Sympathoadrenal responses to anaesthesia and surgery. *British Journal of Anaesthesia*, 56, 725–739.

Dixon, A. J., Dixon, M. P., & Dixon, J. B. (2006). Randomized clinical trial of the effect of applying ointment to surgical wounds before occlusive dressing. *The British Journal of Surgery*, 93, 937–943.

Dumville, J. C., Walter, C. J., Sharp, C. A., et al. (2011). Dressings for the prevention of surgical site infection. *Cochrane Database of Systematic Reviews*, 7, CD003091.

Dunnill, C., Patton, T., Brennan, J., Barrett, J., Dryden, M., Cooke, J., et al. (2017). Reactive oxygen species (ROS) and wound healing: The functional role of ROS and emerging ROS-modulating technologies for augmentation of the healing process. *International Wound Journal*, 14(1), 89–96. https://doi.org/10.1111/iwj.12557.

Fleischmann, E., Kurz, A., Niedermayr, M., et al. (2005). Tissue oxygenation in obese and non-obese patients during laparoscopy. *Obesity Surgery*, 15, 813–819.

Francisco, V., Pino, J., Campos-Cabaleiro, V., Ruiz-Fernández, C., Mera, A., Gonzalez-Gay, M. A., et al. (2018). Obesity, fat mass and immune system: Role for leptin. *Frontiers in Physiology*, 9, 640. https://doi.org/10.3389/fphys.2018.00640.

Frank, S. M., Beattie, C., Christopherson, R., et al. (1993). Unintentional hypothermia is associated with postoperative myocardial ischemia: The Perioperative Ischemia Randomized Anesthesia Trial Study Group. *Anesthesiology*, 78, 468–476.

Fried, M., Peskova, M., & Kasalicky, M. (1997). Bariatric surgery at the 1st surgical department in Prague: History and some technical aspects. *Obesity Surgery*, 7, 22–25.

Giannis, D., Geropoulos, G., Ziogas, I. A., Gitlin, J., & Oropallo, A. (2021). The anti-adhesive effect of anti-VEGF agents in experimental models: A systematic review. *Wound Repair and Regeneration: Official Publication of the Wound Healing Society [and] the European Tissue Repair Society*, 29(1), 168–182. https://doi.org/10.1111/wrr.12879.

Gillespie, B. M., Chaboyer, W., Kang, E., et al. (2014). Postsurgery wound assessment and management practices: A chart audit. *Journal of Clinical Nursing*, 8. https://doi.org/10.1111/jocn.

Goodson, W. H., 3rd, Andrews, W. S., Thakrai, K. K., et al. (1979). Wound oxygen tension of large vs small wounds in man. *Surg Forum, 30*, 92–95.

Gottrup, F. (2004). Oxygen in wound healing and infection. *World Journal of Surgery, 28*, 312–315.

Grupper, M., & Nicolau, D. P. (2017). Obesity and skin and soft tissue infections: How to optimize antimicrobial usage for prevention and treatment? *Current Opinion in Infectious Diseases, 30*(2), 180–191. https://doi.org/10.1097/QCO.0000000000000356.

Halter, J. B., Pflug, A. E., & Porte, D., Jr. (1977). Mechanism of plasma catecholamine increases during surgical stress in man. *The Journal of Clinical Endocrinology and Metabolism, 45*(5), 936–944.

Harrington, G., Russo, P., Spelman, D., Borrell, S., Watson, K., Barr, W., et al. (2004). Surgical-site infection rates and risk factor analysis in coronary artery bypass graft surgery. *Infection Control & Hospital Epidemiology, 25*(6), 472–476.

Hemming, K., Pinkney, T., Futaba, K., et al. (2013). A systematic review of systematic reviews and panoramic meta-analysis: Staples versus sutures for surgical procedures. *PLoS One, 8*(10), e75132.

Hicks, C. W., Bronsert, M., Hammermeister, K. E., Henderson, W. G., Gibula, D. R., Black, J. H., et al. (2016). Operative variables are better predictors of postdischarge infections and unplanned readmissions in vascular surgery patients than patient characteristics. *Journal of Vascular Surgery, 65*(4), 1130–1141. e9. https://doi.org/10.1016/j.jvs.2016.10.086.

Hollander, D. A., Erli, H. J., Theisen, A., Falk, S., Kreck, T., & Müller, S. (2003). Standardized qualitative evaluation of scar tissue properties in an animal wound healing model. *Wound Repair and Regeneration, 11*(2), 150–157.

Hopf, H. W., & Holm, J. (2008). Hyperoxia and infection. *Best Practice & Research Clinical Anaesthesiology, 22*(3), 553–569.

Hopf, H. W., Hunt, T. K., West, J. M., et al. (1997). Wound tissue oxygen tension predicts the risk of wound infection in surgical patients. *Archives of Surgery, 132*, 997–1004.

Hunt, T. K., & Hopf, H. (1997). Wound healing and wound infection: what surgeons and anesthesiologists can do. *The Surgical Clinics of North America, 77*, 587–606.

Hynson, J. M., & Sessler, D. I. (1992). Intraoperative warming therapies: A comparison of three devices. *Journal of Clinical Anesthesia, 4*, 194–199.

Israelsson, L. A., & Jonsson, T. (1997). Overweight and healing of midline incisions: the importance of suture technique. *European Journal of Surgery = Acta Chirurgica, 163*(3), 175–180.

Jensen, J. A., Goodson, W. H., Hopf, H. W., et al. (1991). Cigarette smoking decreases tissue oxygen. *Archives of Surgery, 126*, 1131–1134.

Jensen, J. A., Jönsson, K., Goodson, W. H., 3rd, et al. (1985). Epinephrine lowers subcutaneous wound oxygen tension. *Current Surgery, 42*(6), 472–474.

Jönsson, K., Hunt, T. K., & Mathes, S. J. (1988). Oxygen as an isolated variable influences resistance to infection. *Annals of Surgery, 208*, 783–787.

Jönsson, K., Jensen, J. A., Goodson, W. H., 3rd, et al. (1987). Assessment of perfusion in postoperative patients using tissue oxygen measurements. *British Journal of Surgery, 74*, 263–267.

Jorgensen, L. N., Kallehave, F., Christensen, E., et al. (1998). Less collagen production in smokers. *Surgery, 123*, 450–455.

Kabon, B., Nagele, A., Reddy, D., et al. (2004). Obesity decreases perioperative tissue oxygenation. *Anesthesiology, 100*(2), 274–280.

Kabon, B., Rozum, R., Marschalek, C., et al. (2010). Supplemental postoperative oxygen and tissue oxygen tension in morbidly obese patients. *Obesity Surgery, 20*, 885–894.

Katlein, F., & Mohammad, J. (2017). In K. França, & M. Jafferany (Eds.), *Stress and Skin Disorders Basic and Clinical Aspects* (1st ed.). Springer International Publishing. https://doi.org/10.1007/978-3-319-46352-0.

Kimberger, O., Fleischmann, E., Brandt, S., et al. (2007). Supplemental oxygen, but not supplemental crystalloid fluid, increases tissue oxygen tension in healthy and anastomotic colon in pigs. *Anesthesia Analgesia, 105*, 773–779.

Kimmel, H. M., Grant, A., & Ditata, J. (2016). The presence of oxygen in wound healing. *Wounds: A Compendium of Clinical Research and Practice, 28*(8), 264–270.

Knighton, D. R., Halliday, B., & Hunt, T. K. (1984). Oxygen as an antibiotic: The effect of inspired oxygen on infection. *Archives of Surgery, 119*, 199–204.

Knudson, M. M., Bermudez, K. M., Doyle, C. A., et al. (1997). Use of tissue oxygen tension measurements during resuscitation from hemorrhagic shock. *The Journal of Trauma, 42*, 608–614.

Koerner, S., Adams, D., Harper, S. L., Black, J. M., & Langemo, D. K. (2019). Use of thermal imaging to identify deep-tissue pressure injury on admission reduces clinical and financial burdens of hospital-acquired pressure injuries. *Advances in Skin & Wound Care, 32*(7), 312–320. https://doi.org/10.1097/01.ASW.0000559613.83195.f9.

Kuri, M., Nakagawa, M., Tanaka, H., et al. (2005). Determination of the duration of preoperative smoking cessation to improve wound healing after head and neck surgery. *Anesthesiology, 102*, 892–896.

Kurz, A., Sessler, D. I., & Lenhardt, R. (1996). Perioperative normothermia to reduce the incidence of surgical-wound infection and shorten hospitalization. *New England Journal of Medicine, 334*, 1209–1215.

Leaper, D., Burman-Roy, S., Palanca, A., et al. (2008). Prevention and treatment of surgical site infection: Summary of NICE guidance. *British Medical Journal, 337*, a1924.

Ljungqvist, O., Scott, M., & Fearon, K. C. (2017). Enhanced recovery after surgery: A review. *JAMA Surgery, 152*(3), 292–298. https://doi.org/10.1001/jamasurg.2016.4952.

Manassa, E. H., Hertl, C. H., & Olbrisch, R. (2003). Wound healing problems in smokers and nonsmokers after 132 abdominoplasties. *Plastic and Reconstructive Surgery, 111*, 2082–2087.

Melling, A. C., Ali, B., Scott, E. M., et al. (2001). Effects of preoperative warming on the incidence of wound infection after clean surgery: A randomized controlled trial. *Lancet, 358*, 876–880.

Mo, Y., Sarojini, H., Wan, R., Zhang, Q., Wang, J., Eichenberger, S., et al. (2019). Intracellular ATP delivery causes rapid tissue regeneration via upregulation of cytokines, chemokines, and stem cells. *Frontiers in Pharmacology, 10*, 1502. https://doi.org/10.3389/fphar.2019.01502.

Møller, A. M., Pedersen, T., Villebro, N., et al. (2003). Effect of smoking on early complications after elective orthopaedic surgery. *The Journal of Bone and Joint Surgery. British Volume, 85*, 178–181.

Monnet, X., & Teboul, J.-L. (2018). Assessment of fluid responsiveness: Recent advances. *Current Opinion in Critical Care, 24*(3), 190–195. https://doi.org/10.1097/MCC.0000000000000501.

Morris, R. H. (1971). Influence of ambient temperature on patient temperature during intraabdominal surgery. *Annals of Surgery, 173*, 230–233.

Mun, E. C., Blackburn, G. L., & Matthews, J. B. (2001). Current status of medical and surgical therapy for obesity. *Gastroenterology, 120*, 660–681.

Myles, T. D., Gooch, J., & Santolaya, J. (2002). Obesity as an independent risk factor for infectious morbidity in patients who undergo cesarean delivery. *Obstetrics & Gynecology, 100*(5), 959–964.

Niinikoski, J., Heughan, C., & Hunt, T. K. (1972). Oxygen tensions in human wounds. *Journal of Surgical Research, 12*, 77–82.

Nisanevich, V., Felsenstein, I., Almogy, G., et al. (2005). Effect of intraoperative fluid management on outcome after intraabdominal surgery. *Anesthesiology, 103*, 25–32.

Oropallo, A., & Andersen, C. A. (2021). Topical oxygen. In *StatPearls*. StatPearls Publishing. http://www.ncbi.nlm.nih.gov/books/NBK574579/.

Oropallo, A. R., Serena, T. E., Armstrong, D. G., & Niederauer, M. Q. (2021). Molecular biomarkers of oxygen therapy in patients with diabetic foot ulcers. *Biomolecules, 11*(7), 925. https://doi.org/10.3390/biom11070925.

Pasarica, M., Sereda, O. R., Redman, L. M., et al. (2009). Reduced adipose tissue oxygenation in human obesity: Evidence for rarefaction, macrophage chemotaxis, and inflammation without an angiogenic response. *Diabetes, 58*(3), 718–725.

Pędziwiatr, M., Mavrikis, J., Witowski, J., Adamos, A., Major, P., Nowakowski, M., et al. (2018). Current status of enhanced recovery after surgery (ERAS) protocol in gastrointestinal surgery. *Medical Oncology (Northwood, London, England), 35*(6), 95. https://doi.org/10.1007/s12032-018-1153-0.

Pierre, S., Rivera, C., Le Maître, B., Ruppert, A.-M., Bouaziz, H., Wirth, N., et al. (2017). Guidelines on smoking management during the perioperative period. *Anaesthesia, Critical Care & Pain Medicine, 36*(3), 195–200. https://doi.org/10.1016/j.accpm.2017.02.002.

Plattner, O., Akça, O., Herbst, F., et al. (2000). The influence of two surgical bandage systems on wound tissue oxygen tension. *Archives of Surgery, 135*(7), 818–822.

Puzziferri, N., West, J. M., Hunt, T. K., et al. (2001). Local warming increases oxygenation and decreases pain in ischemic ulcers. *Wound Repair and Regeneration, 9*(2), 146–147.

Reynolds, L., Beckmann, J., & Kurz, A. (2008). Perioperative complications of hypothermia. *Best Practice & Research Clinical Anaesthesiology, 22*, 645–657.

Roe, C. F. (1971). Effect of bowel exposure on body temperature during surgical operations. *American Journal of Surgery, 122*, 13–15.

Roe, C. F., Goldberg, M. J., Blair, C. S., et al. (1966). The influence of body temperature on early postoperative oxygen consumption. *Surgery, 60*, 85.

Rollins, K. E., Javanmard-Emamghissi, H., Acheson, A. G., & Lobo, D. N. (2019). the role of oral antibiotic preparation in elective colorectal surgery: A meta-analysis. *Annals of Surgery, 270*(1), 43–58. https://doi.org/10.1097/SLA.0000000000003145.

Rubinstein, E. H., & Sessler, D. I. (1990). Skin-surface temperature gradients correlate with fingertip blood flow in humans. *Anesthesiology, 73*, 541–545.

Sahebally, S. M., McKevitt, K., Stephens, I., Fitzpatrick, F., Deasy, J., Burke, J. P., et al. (2018). Negative pressure wound therapy for closed laparotomy incisions in general and colorectal surgery: A systematic review and meta-analysis. *JAMA Surgery, 153*(11), e183467. https://doi.org/10.1001/jamasurg.2018.3467.

Sarojini, H., Bajorek, A., Wan, R., Wang, J., Zhang, Q., Billeter, A. T., et al. (2021). Enhanced skin incisional wound healing with intracellular ATP delivery via macrophage proliferation and direct collagen production. *Frontiers in Pharmacology, 12*, 594586. https://doi.org/10.3389/fphar.2021.594586.

Schreml, S., Szeimies, R. M., Prantl, L., Karrer, S., Landthaler, M., & Babilas, P. (2010). Oxygen in acute and chronic wound healing. *British Journal of Dermatology, 163*(2), 257–268.

Sessler, D. I. (1993). Perianesthetic thermoregulation and heat balance in humans. *FASEB Journal, 7*(8), 638–644.

Severinghaus, J. (1958). Oxyhaemoglobin dissociation curve correction for temperature and pH variation in human blood. *Journal of Applied Physiology, 12*, 485–486.

Sheffield, C. W., Hopf, H. W., Sessler, D. I., et al. (1992). Thermoregulatory vasoconstriction decreases subcutaneous oxygen tension in anesthetized volunteers. *Anesthesiology, 77*, A96.

Shinohara, T., Yamashita, Y., Satoh, K., et al. (2008). Prospective evaluation of occlusive hydrocolloid dressing versus conventional gauze dressing regarding the healing effect after abdominal operations: Randomized controlled trial. *Asian Journal of Surgery, 31*(1), 1–5.

Ship, A. G., & Weiss, P. R. (1985). Pigmentation after dermabrasion: An avoidable complication. *Plastic and Reconstructive Surgery, 75*, 528–532.

Siah, C. J., & Childs, C. (2012). A systematic review of the ASEPSIS scoring system used in non-cardiac-related surgery. *Journal of Wound Care, 21*(3), 124–130. https://doi.org/10.12968/jowc.2012.21.3.124.

Silver, I. A. (1969). The measurement of oxygen tension in healing tissue. *Progress in Respiratory Research, 3*, 124.

Silver, I. A. (1980). The physiology of wound healing. In T. Hunt (Ed.), *Wound healing and wound infection: Theory and surgical practice*. New York: Appleton-Century-Crofts.

Slotman, G. J., Jed, E. H., & Burchard, K. W. (1985). Adverse effects of hypothermia in postoperative patients. *American Journal of Surgery, 49*, 495–501.

Sørensen, L. T. (2012). Wound healing and infection in surgery. *Archives in Surgery, 147*, 373–383.

Sørensen, L. T., Karlsmark, T., & Gottrup, F. (2003). Abstinence from smoking reduces incisional wound infection: A randomized controlled trial. *Annals of Surgery, 238*, 1–5.

Stotts, N. A., & Wipke-Tevis, D. (1996). Co-factors in impaired wound healing. *Ostomy Wound Manage, 42*(2). 44–46, 48, 50–54.

Teillant, A., Gandra, S., Barter, D., Morgan, D. J., & Laxminarayan, R. (2015). Potential burden of antibiotic resistance on surgery and cancer chemotherapy antibiotic prophylaxis in the USA: A literature review and modelling study. *The Lancet. Infectious Diseases, 15*(12), 1429–1437. https://doi.org/10.1016/S1473-3099(15)00270-4.

Topaloglu, S., Akin, M., Avsar, F. M., et al. (2008). Correlation of risk and postoperative assessment methods in wound surveillance. *Journal of Surgical Research, 146*, 211–217.

van de Kar, A. L., Koolbergen, D. R., van Avendonk, J. P. H., & van der Horst, C. M. A. M. (2019). Comparison of wound closure techniques in median sternotomy scars in children: Subcuticular suture versus Steri-Strip™ S. *Journal of Plastic Surgery and Hand Surgery, 53*(3), 161–166. https://doi.org/10.1080/2000656X.2019.1566737.

Vanhoutte, P. M., Verbeuren, T. J., & Webb, R. C. (1981). Local modulation of adrenergic neuroeffector interaction in the blood vessel well. *Physiological Reviews, 61,* 151–247.

Vastine, V. L., Morgan, R. F., Williams, G. S., Gampper, T. J., Drake, D. B., Knox, L. K., et al. (1999). Wound complications of abdominoplasty in obese patients. *Annals of Plastic Surgery, 42*(1), 34–39.

Vogt, D. C., Uhlyarik, M., & Schroeder, T. V. (2007). Moist wound healing compared with standard care of treatment of primary closed vascular surgical wound: A prospective randomized controlled study. *Wound Repair and Regeneration, 15,* 624–627.

Waldorf, H., & Fewkes, J. (1995). Wound healing. *Advances in Dermatology, 10,* 77–96.

Walter, C. J., Dumville, J. C., Sharp, C. A., et al. (2012). Systematic review and meta-analysis of wound dressings in the prevention of surgical-site infections in surgical wounds healing by primary intention. *British Journal of Surgery, 99,* 1185–1194.

Warner, D. O. (2005). Preoperative smoking cessation. How long is long enough? *Anesthesiology, 102,* 883–884.

Webster, J., Liu, Z., Norman, G., Dumville, J. C., Chiverton, L., Scuffham, P., et al. (2019). Negative pressure wound therapy for surgical wounds healing by primary closure. *The Cochrane Database of Systematic Reviews, 3,* CD009261. https://doi.org/10.1002/14651858.CD009261.pub4.

West, J. M. (1990). Wound healing in the surgical patient: influence of the perioperative stress response on perfusion. *AACN Clinical Issues in Critical Care Nursing, 1*(3), 595–601.

West, J. M. (1994). *The effect of postoperative forced-air rewarming on subcutaneous tissue oxygen tension and wound healing in hypothermic abdominal surgery patients, San Francisco.* San Francisco: University of California.

Wetterslev, J., Meyhoff, C. S., Jørgensen, L. N., Gluud, C., Lindschou, J., & Rasmussen, L. S. (2015). The effects of high perioperative inspiratory oxygen fraction for adult surgical patients. *The Cochrane Database of Systematic Reviews, 6,* CD008884. https://doi.org/10.1002/14651858.CD008884.pub2.

Whitney, J. D., Dellinger, E. P., & Wickline, M. (2004). Warming surgical wounds: Effects on healing and wound complications. *Wound Repair and Regeneration, 12,* A8.

Whitney, J. D., & Wickline, M. M. (2003). Treating chronic and acute wounds with warming: Review of the science and practice implications. *Journal of Wound, Ostomy, and Continence Nursing, 30*(4), 199–209.

Wilson, J. A., & Clark, J. J. (2003). Obesity: Impediment to wound healing. *Critical Care Nursing Quarterly, 26*(2), 119–132.

Wilson, J. L., Kocurek, K., & Doty, B. J. (2000). A systematic approach to laceration repair. Tricks to ensure the desired cosmetic result. *Postgraduate Medicine, 107*(4). 77–83, 87–88.

Wilson, A. P. R., Treasure, T., Sturridge, M. F., et al. (1986). A scoring method (ASEPSIS) for postoperative wound infections for use in clinical trials of antibiotic prophylaxis. *Lancet, 1*(8476), 311–313.

Wilson, A. P. R., Weavill, C., Burridge, J., et al. (1990). The use of the wound scoring method "ASEPSIS" in postoperative wound surveillance. *The Journal of Hospital Infection, 16*(4), 297–309.

Wilson, A. P. R., Webster, A., Gruneberg, R. N., et al. (1986). Repeatability of ASEPSIS wound scoring method. *Lancet, 849,* 1208–1209.

Winiarsky, R., Barth, P., & Lotke, P. (1998). Total knee arthroplasty in morbidly obese patients. *Journal of Bone and Joint Surgery, 80*(12), 1770–1774.

Wong, P. F., Kumar, S., Bohra, A., et al. (2007). Randomized clinical trial of perioperative systemic warming in major elective abdominal surgery. *British Journal of Surgery, 94,* 421–426.

Woo, K. Y. (2012). Exploring the effects of pain and stress on wound healing. *Advances in Skin & Wound Care, 25*(1), 38–44. https://doi.org/10.1097/01.ASW.0000410689.60105.7d.

Wu, T. L. (2006). Plastic surgery made easy. Simple techniques for closing skin defects and improving cosmetic results. *Australian Family Physician, 35,* 492–496.

Wynne, R., Botti, M., Stedman, H., et al. (2004). Effect of three wound dressings on infection, healing comfort, and cost in patients with sternotomy wounds: A randomized trial. *Chest, 125*(1), 43–49.

Xu, H., Tian, Y., Zhang, J., Sun, L., Yang, T., Ma, T., et al. (2021). Clinical outcomes of venous self-expanding stent placement for iliofemoral venous outflow obstruction. *Journal of Vascular Surgery. Venous and Lymphatic Disorders.* https://doi.org/10.1016/j.jvsv.2021.01.016. S2213-333X(21)00076-7.

Yin, Y., Zhang, R., Li, S., Guo, J., Hou, Z., & Zhang, Y. (2018). Negative-pressure therapy versus conventional therapy on split-thickness skin graft: A systematic review and meta-analysis. *International Journal of Surgery (London, England), 50,* 43–48. https://doi.org/10.1016/j.ijsu.2017.12.020.

Yip, W. L. (2015). Influence of oxygen on wound healing. *International Wound Journal, 12*(6), 620–624. https://doi.org/10.1111/iwj.12324.

Zamboni, W. A., Browder, L. K., & Martinez, J. (2003). Hyperbaric oxygen and wound healing. *Clinics in Plastic Surgery, 30,* 67–75.

Uncommon Wounds and Manifestations of Intrinsic Disease

Ruth A. Bryant

OBJECTIVES

1. Differentiate between staphylococcal scalded skin syndrome and toxic epidermal necrolysis (TEN) and between graft-vs-host disease (GVHD) and pyoderma gangrenosum in terms of manifestations and etiology.
2. Describe the process of tissue damage and treatment options for vasculitis, calciphylaxis, epidermolysis bullosa (EB), GVHD, frostbite, and TEN.
3. Discriminate among the patient populations at risk for calciphylaxis, frostbite, TEN, and extravasation.

4. Compare and contrast the role of debridement in necrotizing fasciitis, TEN, extravasation, and frostbite.
5. Describe the distinguishing features of a chronic wound with malignant transformation.
6. Identify four conditions that require a tissue biopsy for diagnosis.
7. Describe cutaneous manifestations associated with COVID-19 infection.

Wounds commonly referred to as atypical are actually typical manifestations of uncommon conditions. This chapter discusses less common skin pathologies that often are intrinsic to another disease such as infection, inflammatory processes, metabolic disorders, and neoplasms. Although some may be rare, they are often associated with significant morbidity and mortality. When the patient's clinical history or wound progression is inconsistent with common skin lesions or the wound is unresponsive to appropriate treatment, uncommon cutaneous wounds should be considered. The wound specialist should be familiar with the clinical manifestations of these less common conditions to facilitate early detection and prompt referral for appropriate medical management. In many situations, early detection is essential to arrest the underlying pathology and to prevent progression of ulcerations, infection, sepsis, and death.

INFECTIOUS ETIOLOGY

Staphylococcal Scalded Skin Syndrome

Staphylococcal scalded skin syndrome (SSSS) is a superficial blistering skin disorder caused by the exfoliative toxins of some strains of *Staphylococcus aureus*. Initially an infection is present most commonly in the oral or nasal cavities, neck, axillae, groin, or umbilicus (King, Carone, & de Saint Victor, 2019). The toxins produced by the infecting organism are transferred through the bloodstream to a site remote from the original infection, where

significant erythema will develop, followed by separation of the superficial epidermis (i.e., desquamation). Initially a diffuse tender erythema appears and the skin may have a sandpaper texture. Within 1–2 days, superficial bullae develop, and the skin wrinkles and peels off in large sheets revealing a superficial loss of epidermis that is moist and red. Gentle touching of the skin can induce skin separation, known as Nikolsky sign. Significant pain is unusual for SSSS and, if present, suggests another diagnosis, such as toxic epidermal necrolysis (TEN), a drug-induced necrosis of the epidermis.

Although SSSS has been reported in adults, it most commonly occurs in healthy children 6 years or younger and in neonates (Dinulos, 2021; King et al., 2019). The absence of antibodies to these toxins and an impaired ability to excrete the toxin due to immature renal function are contributing factors to this condition (Dinulos, 2021; Jeyakumari, Eswaran, et al., 2009). Mortality in children is very low (1%–5%) unless SSSS is associated with sepsis or a coexisting serious medical condition. SSSS, when it develops in adults, occurs in adults who are chronically ill, immunocompromised, or with renal failure. The mortality rate in adults is substantial (50%–60%), although this may be attributable to the overall health status of the adults rather than the SSSS (King et al., 2019).

Suspicious sites (nose, eyes, ears, throat, and vagina) should be swabbed for microbial cultures to confirm the diagnosis. Bullae from the primary lesion usually yield cultures that are negative for bacteria. A frozen section of sloughing skin is needed to differentiate SSSS from a drug-induced skin reaction (TEN). Full-thickness epidermal necrosis is inconsistent with SSSS and suggests a drug-induced process. Bullous impetigo is a localized form of SSSS in which the endotoxin can be obtained from the bullae (Dinulos, 2021). Important distinctive features of SSSS include involvement of the face around the mouth, chin, eyes, and nose and absence of mucosal involvement (Jeyakumari et al., 2009).

Once SSSS is diagnosed, treatment consists of supportive care and elimination of the primary infection. Debridement and antibiotics (e.g., B-lactamase-resistant penicillin, clindamycin, or, for limited disease, dicloxacillin or a cephalosporin) are essential to managing the infection (Dinulos, 2021). Topical management of the desquamated skin should address exudate management, pain control, and maintenance of a moist environment. Foam dressings, superabsorbent dressings, sheet hydrogels, and alginates are preferred dressing options; adhesives should be avoided. Steroids may worsen immune function, and nonsteroidal antiinflammatory drugs (NSAIDs) should be avoided because they potentially can reduce renal function (King et al., 2019). When massive tissue loss is apparent, the wound should be managed according to the principles for burn therapy as outlined in Chapter 34.

Toxic Shock Syndrome

Toxic shock syndrome (TSS) is caused by the production of superantigens by *S. aureus* or group A streptococci. Superantigens are polypeptide proteins manufactured by bacteria and viruses that activate T cells which then trigger extreme production of proinflammatory cytokines. Staphylococcal TSS can be caused by any staphylococcal infection including very minor infections (Dinulos, 2021). In contrast, streptococcal TSS (STSS) is most often associated with severe necrotizing soft tissue infection, cellulitis, myonecrosis, and bacteremia (Dinulos, 2021). While both types of TSS are severe and result in multisystem failure, the mortality for STSS is 30% when compared with 5% for staphylococcal TSS.

Acute onset consists of a widespread macular erythematous eruption that extends to include the soles of the feet and the palms of the hands. Desquamation of the skin is highly characteristic of TSS occurring 10 days to 3 weeks after onset and primarily including the fingertips and plantar surfaces of the palms and feet (Habif, Campbell, Chapman, et al., 2005).

The CDC diagnosis of TSS requires a constellation of symptoms: fever (>38.9°C), hypotension with systolic blood pressure less than 90 mmHg, diffuse macular rash progressing to desquamation 1–2 weeks after onset of rash, evidence of multiple organ system involvement and exclusion of other reasonable pathogens (Dinulos, 2021). Multisystem involvement can be evidenced by impaired functioning of at least three of the following organ systems: muscular, gastrointestinal, mucous membrane, central nervous system, renal, hepatic, hematologic, and cardiopulmonary (Dinulos, 2021; Vyas, 2020). A skin biopsy may be helpful in the early stages.

The goal of treatment of TSS is preventing organ damage through supportive care (hydration and vasopressors), incision and drainage of abscesses, and aggressive antibiotic therapy. Extensive debridement is warranted for necrotizing soft tissue infection. Local wound management is based on wound needs (e.g., exudate absorption with topical antimicrobial dressings). Topical dressings should be nonocclusive and nonadhesive.

Necrotizing Fasciitis

Necrotizing fasciitis is an uncommon but serious subcutaneous tissue infection that spreads rapidly along the superficial fascial plane destroying fascia and fat. The overall mortality rate from this very rapidly spreading condition is variable: 20% in pediatric cases and anywhere from 6% to 73% in adults (Anaya & Dellinger, 2007). Necrotizing fasciitis is characterized by widespread necrosis of the fascia and deep subcutaneous tissue, with thrombosis of nutrient vessels and sloughing of overlying tissue (see Plate 73). Although it can occur anywhere in the body, such as the abdomen, perianal area, or inguinal area, it usually occurs in the extremities after a minor operation or injury (Park, Choi, Song, et al., 2014).

The clinical markers of necrotizing fasciitis are a rapidly spreading erythema in the skin around the wound and subcutaneous crepitus that may be visible on radiograph. Initial signs of necrotizing fasciitis are pain (considered to be out of proportion for the extent of the skin damage), erythema, swelling, cellulitis, and a fever. The skin may initially appear normal over the cellulitis, but as the infectious process compromises blood supply, the skin becomes erythematous, edematous, and reddish-purple to patchy blue-gray. Bullae form within 3–5 days from onset and progress to necrosis of the skin, sloughing, and frank cutaneous gangrene (Anaya & Dellinger, 2007). Tendon sheaths and muscle will liquefy when infected; in the operating room, "dishwater fluid" is the hallmark of liquefactive necrosis. Death occurs in 25% due to septic shock and organ failure (Dinulos, 2021).

Necrotizing fasciitis can be detected by its dramatic clinical presentation and by probing the wound. When the affected area is probed with a hemostat through a limited incision, the instrument passes easily along a plane of superficial to deep fascia. This examination helps to distinguish necrotizing fasciitis from cellulitis. This infection is most often polymicrobial with group A streptococci or *S. aureus* predominating. A subset of necrotizing soft tissue infections are monomicrobial, which are associated with a significantly worse prognosis (50%–70% mortality in patient with hypotension and organ failure) (Dinulos, 2021).

The presence of necrotizing fasciitis requires aggressive surgical debridement; any nonviable or questionably viable tissue must be removed. Because the infection spreads subcutaneously, a wound may need to be extended to allow access to and debridement of all necrotic tissue (Attinger, Janis, Steinberg, et al., 2006). Despite aggressive local control, necrotizing fasciitis has a 24%–50% mortality rate secondary to persistent wound sepsis or systemic sepsis (Martin, Nanci, Marlowe, et al., 2008). Local wound care consists of close monitoring for further dissection, which indicates progression of the infection. Topical dressing recommendations are largely based on expert opinion or preference. Dressings should be used that meet the needs of the wound (e.g., fill dead space, and absorb exudate), allow for frequent monitoring of the wound, deliver topical antimicrobial activity, and are non-adhesive and nonocclusive. Negative pressure wound therapy (NPWT) is an appropriate option for managing the open wound after debridement. Surgical reconstruction of large tissue defects can be achieved with NPWT, skin grafts, and tissue-based products (Mazzone & Schiestl, 2013).

CORONAVIRUS DISEASE 2019 (COVID-19)

Numerous skin manifestations have been associated with the severe acute respiratory syndrome coronavirus 2 (COVID-19). While the array of conditions is broad, six major morphologies have emerged that can be categorized as an immune response to the virus or thrombotic vasculopathy based on the pathologic process (Klejtman, 2020). Immune response-based COVID-19 cutaneous manifestations are nonischemic in nature and comprise the following manifestations: (1) maculopapular, (2) urticarial, and (3) vesicular (Freeman et al., 2020). The immune response and inflammatory-based manifestations are theorized to be an indication of the "cytokine storm" occurring in the skin (Criado et al., 2020). Lesions classified as thrombotic vasculopathy demonstrate noninflammatory thrombi in the skin and manifestations include (1) chilblain-like (also referred to as pernio-like), (2) petechiae/purpura, and (3) livedoid (ischemic microangiopathy) (Freeman et al., 2020; Rahimi & Tehranchinia, 2020; Singh, Kaur, Singh, & Sem, 2021). Patients may have more than one type of lesion. Lesions are further described as acral (occurring distally such as on the feet) or reticular (with a net-like or lacey type of distribution). The vast majority of cutaneous manifestations occur after COVID-19 symptoms; from 5% to 18% have been reported before COVID-19 symptoms (Freeman et al., 2020). The predominant symptom with all cutaneous manifestations is pruritus; pain and burning occurs much less frequently.

Among the inflammatory-based skin manifestations, a maculopapular rash (Plate 74A) is the most common in COVID-19 and occurs predominantly on the trunk of the body (Rahimi & Tehranchinia, 2020; Singh et al., 2021). This is often described as morbilliform in that it resembles measles and is widespread (described as exanthem). Lesions may occur simultaneously with COVID-19 symptoms or 3 weeks later. Urticarial lesions (Plate 75), often presenting as hives or angioedema, are an erythematous slightly raised papular rash accompanied by pruritis. Outside of COVID-19, urticaria occurs in the general population as an allergic reaction and is typically self-limited. Urticaria has also been observed as an adverse drug reaction with many medications used to treat COVID-19 (e.g., lopinavir/ritonavir, nitazoxanide, corticosteroids, baricitinib, and IVIG treatments). Therefore, urticaria cannot be assumed to be a COVID-19-related manifestation.

Vesicular lesions (Plate 75) associated with COVID-19 are clear fluid-filled lesions that develop in the epidermal layer, often described as blisters, and tend to be less than 1 cm in diameter. Vesicular lesions are not as common as other immune-based cutaneous manifestations. Much like urticaria and maculopapular rash, vesicles also are associated with non-COVID-19-related conditions (Plate 6H) such as heat

contact dermatitis, medications, or bacterial or viral infections (e.g., varicella-zoster, herpes simplex) (Singh et al., 2021). However, unlike urticaria and maculopapular eruptions, vesicular lesions are not related to the medications used to treat COVID-19 including the antiviral drugs. Therefore, the onset of vesicular lesions may be interpreted as a specific cutaneous manifestation of COVID-19, unlike maculopapular and urticarial lesions (Singh et al., 2021).

Several COVID-19 skin manifestations have been reported with COVID-19 and are associated with the vascular or thrombotic vasculopathy abnormalities that occur with the COVID-19 disease process. For example, combined nonblanching lesions less than 2 mm in diameter (petechiae) (Plate 43) and greater than 2 mm in diameter (purpura) (Plate 42) have been reported (Singh et al., 2021). These less common cutaneous manifestations tend to be diffuse, acral, or on distal extremities. Petechiae reflect subdermal hemorrhages with many possible pathophysiological causes including thrombocytopenia, platelet dysfunction, disorders of coagulation, and loss of vascular integrity. As with urticarial manifestations, petechial rashes occur with other viral conditions and are not unique to COVID-19; petechiae may also develop as an adverse reaction to COVID-19 drugs or high-dose IVIG treatments. In COVID-19, petechial lesions are not common and are hypothesized to result from thrombogenic vasculopathy. Retiform purpuria has also been observed (Plate 74B) (McBride et al., 2020; Caldeira et al., 2021) and may include necrosis (Plates 74C and D). A biopsy at the periphery of the wound edge is essential to establish a diagnosis and avoid potential misdiagnosis as a deep tissue injury, for example. Documentation of a superficial thromboembolic process is important to confirm the etiology (McBride et al., 2020).

Chilblain lesions, or "pernio-like" lesions, appear as a localized inflammatory skin condition that involves swelling and discoloration in the extremities. Chilblain lesions are typically associated with exposure to cold temperatures or damp humid environments. Autoimmune diseases (e.g., lupus) and Raynaud's phenomenon are also associated with chilblain-like lesions. The presence of erythematous or violaceous discoloration of the toes in patients with COVID-19 has been informally labeled as "COVID toes" as illustrated in Plate 75. Unlike other COVID-19 cutaneous manifestations, chilblain-like lesions develop later in their course of the disease and in a small percent these lesions developed in patients who were asymptomatic carriers of COVID-19 (Rahimi & Tehranchinia, 2020). These chilblain-like lesions are typically located on acral area (i.e., toes, heels, and fingers), with the heels and toes most commonly affected (Rahimi & Tehranchinia, 2020). The hypothesized pathophysiologic mechanism in COVID-19 includes vasoconstriction, vasospasm leading to hypoxemia and inflammation, and hyperviscosity or endothelial damage (Singh et al., 2021). Pain and pruritis also accompanies chilblain-like lesions.

Livedoid lesions (i.e., livedo reticularis) have also been described with COVID-19, although uncommon. This is the presence of a reticular (net-like or lace-like) violaceous, hyperpigmented pattern on the skin that has an appearance of mottled discoloration (Rose, Saggar, Boyd, Patel, & McLellan, 2013). It is an indication of an underlying change in cutaneous blood flow and can be physiologic (such as a normal response to cold) or pathologic. Pathologic livedo reticularis can be caused by an impairment in cutaneous vasculature resulting in diminished blood flow and deoxygenated hemoglobin to the skin such as with vasospasm, reduced intravascular flow, endothelial damage, vessel obstruction, medications, and neurologic disorders (Rose et al., 2013; Singh et al., 2021). The primary pathology of the livedo reticularis is the inflammation in the arteriole. Anatomically these lesions have been reported in COVID-19 patients on the trunk, forearms, thighs, hands, and feet. The pathophysiologic process is theorized to be associated with hypercoagulability, endothelialitis (typical feature of COVID-19), and microthromboses in the subcutaneous and dermal layers. Table 32.1 provides a summary of COVID-19-related skin manifestations including type, morphology, description, related findings, and differential diagnosis considerations. Plate 75 presents a spectrum of COVID-19 dermatologic manifestations with severity of disease calculated by percentage of hospitalized patients with each condition.

SPIDER BITES

Spiders bite only in self-defense; most spiders are small and their fangs are too short to penetrate human skin. The toxin from the majority of spider bites causes pain, swelling, and inflammation. Typically, the swelling will be limited to the bite site and expand for a few centimeters; the presence of hive-like swelling distinguishes the bite from a bacterial cellulitis (Dinulos, 2021). Cool soaks and histamines are used to reduce itching and swelling.

Only 60 of the 20,000 species of spiders in the world are capable of inflicting a bite, and only 2 can cause significant reaction, the brown recluse and the black widow. The brown recluse spider is one of five species of spiders within the genus *Loxosceles*. This spider is about the size of a U.S. quarter, is yellow to brown in color, and has a characteristic dark fiddle-shaped marking on its back (Dinulos, 2021). The brown recluse spider usually is shy and nocturnal. It tends to avoid humans and seek shelter in abandoned or infrequently used buildings, attics, and basements. Bites generally occur

TABLE 32.1 COVID-19-Related Skin Manifestations[a]

Type	Morphology	Description	COVID-19-Related Findings	Differential Considerations
Inflammatory Rashes	Maculopapular	Morbilliform (resembles measles). Localized distribution Plates 6AB and 74A	Most common. Predominantly on trunk. May occur simultaneously with COVID-19 symptoms or 3 weeks later	Candidiasis
	Urticarial	Hives or angioedema, erythematous slightly raised papular rash accompanied by pruritis Plate 75		Adverse reaction to medications (many used to treat COVID-19)
	Vesicular	Clear fluid-filled blister lesions <1 cm Plates 6H and 75		Contact dermatitis, medications, bacterial or viral (e.g., HSV, HZV) infections
Vascular or thrombotic vasculopathy abnormalities	Chilblain or pernio-like	Localized swelling and discoloration typically on toes, heels, and fingers Plate 75	AKA COVID toes. Develops later in disease course Small percent reported in asymptomatic carriers	Autoimmune diseases, exposure to cold Atherosclerosis Embolism Medication reactions
	Petechiae (Plate 43) and purpura (Plate 42)	Petechia <2 mm Purpura >2 mm Often includes pain and pruritis Nonblanching	Petechia less common. Retiform purpuric areas have been reported on sacral and thigh areas may include necrosis (Plate 74C and D)	DTPI
	Livedoid (ischemic microangiopathy)	Reticular pattern (net-like or lace-like) of mottled appearing discolorations and can be a transient or persistent	Uncommon. Have been reported on the trunk, forearms, thighs, hands, and feet	DTPI

[a]Skin manifestations listed are not unique to COVID-19. A full medical work up, collaboration with a dermatologist and/or biopsy may be indicated for accurate differential diagnosis.

when a person disturbs a pile of wood or rocks, moves boxes that have been stored, or dresses in clothes that have been stored for a long period of time. The most common site for a *Loxosceles* spider bite is on the extremities, but they also can occur on the buttocks or genitalia.

The venom of the brown recluse spider is a mixture of enzymes that destroy cellular membranes, resulting in damage to the surrounding skin, fat, nerves, and blood vessels. Manifestations of a brown recluse spider bite can range from small lesions with erythema to full-thickness necrotic wounds (known as necrotic arachnidism). Fewer than 10% of patients develop severe skin necrosis or other systemic reaction (e.g., loxoscelism, which is characterized by fever, nausea, hemolysis, and thrombocytopenia) (Arnold, 2021; Zeglin, 2005). Severity of the reaction depends on the amount of venom injected, the site of the bite, and host susceptibility. However, it is the accumulation of activated neutrophils that is responsible for the cutaneous necrosis (Arnold, 2021). Accumulation of neutrophils occurs 24–72 h before skin necrosis and ulceration. The very young, the elderly, and individuals in poor physical condition are at highest risk for serious illness from a spider bite.

After a brown recluse spider bite, the person may experience a mild burning sensation or may experience no discomfort at all. Within 6–12 h, itching, pain, a central papule, and erythema may develop. Wounds that progress usually begin to do so within 48–72 h of the bite. As the tissue damage progresses, the characteristic "red, white, and blue" sign of a brown recluse bite develops; the sign consists of a ring of blanched skin (due to vasoconstriction) surrounded by erythema with gray-to-red-purple bullae at the site of the bite (Arnold, 2021; Zeglin, 2005) (see Plate 76). Severe necrosis is more likely when the bite is located in an area with significant adipose tissue, such as the thighs and buttocks. When the bite remains localized with a central blister, resolution occurs within 3 weeks. Severe bites that develop necrosis heal over a 2- to 3-month time span (Rhoads, 2007).

The standard treatment of spider bite lesions is RICE: (1) rest, (2) ice, (3) compresses, and (4) elevation. Oral anti-inflammatory medications and tetanus vaccine also may be given. The ice packs are important to reduce inflammation, slow lesion evolution, and enhance the effectiveness of the other treatments (Dinulos, 2021). Skin necrosis will typically be obvious within the first 24–48 h and antibiotics are warranted as infection prophylaxis. The site should be monitored for signs of deterioration and cellulitis (Rhoads, 2007).

Patients with severe and rapidly progressing lesions may be given dapsone (Avlosulfon) therapy, which is an inhibitor of neutrophil function and is effective even when given 48 h after the bite (Dinulos, 2021). Dapsone minimizes tissue necrosis by reducing leukocyte infiltration and perivasculitis (Dinulos, 2021; Zeglin, 2005). In moderate and severe lesions, early excision of necrotic areas is discouraged. Removal of eschar should be postponed until after the wound has stabilized and the inflammation has subsided 96–10 weeks (Dinulos, 2021). There is no antivenom available.

The black widow spider has a fat abdomen and a red hourglass marking on the underside of the abdomen. The bite itself may be painless or sharp pain with minimal subsequent reactions such as slight swelling at the site. The venom contains a neurotoxin that triggers increased concentration of catecholamines at the synapses resulting in migratory muscle cramps, malaise, and weakness. Muscle cramping may occur to involve the entire torso or any skeletal muscles. Symptoms persist for several hours and slowly subside over 2–3 days (Dinulos, 2021).

PYODERMA GANGRENOSUM

Pyoderma gangrenosum (PG) is a chronic neutrophilic, systemic autoinflammatory, ulcerating skin disease that most likely represents an aberrant immune response to an as-yet-unidentified antigen. It has been characterized by neutrophil dysfunction and overexpression of various leukocytes signaling cytokines such as IL-8, IL-16, and tumor necrosis factor (Ahronowitz, Harp, & Shinkai, 2012; Reguiaï & Grange, 2007). Histologically, the presence of numerous polymorphonuclear leukocytes creates a dense infiltrate of the dermis that can extend from the superficial dermis to the subcutaneous tissue.

These painful lesions often occur in patients with chronic underlying systemic diseases, such as inflammatory bowel disease, seropositive rheumatoid arthritis, chronic active hepatitis, ankylosing spondylitis, and monoclonal gammopathies (Ahronowitz et al., 2012) (Box 32.1). Almost 50% of cases occur in patients with no known associated systemic disease and are idiopathic (Snyder, 2008; Wollina, 2007). When PG accompanies a systemic disease, it does not necessarily parallel the underlying disease and instead may be triggered by trauma (Paparone, Paparone, & Paparone, 2009).

Pyoderma gangrenosum has several different manifestations, but generally, these extremely painful lesions begin with a painful nodule, pustule, or bulla that develops significant induration and erythema and proceeds to ulceration. Five subtypes of PG have been identified: classic (ulcerative), bullous, pustular, vegetative, and peristomal (Ahronowitz et al., 2012). The most common presentation is the classic ulcerative form. With this particular variation, ulcers usually occur on the lower extremities but may also occur on the abdomen, genitalia, trunk, head, and neck. It is commonly associated with inflammatory bowel disease (particularly Crohn's

---

BOX 32.1 Systemic Diseases Associated With Pyoderma Gangrenosum

- Ankylosing spondylitis
- Rheumatoid arthritis
- Sarcoidosis
- Chronic active hepatitis
- Inflammatory bowel disease (chronic ulcerative colitis and Crohn's disease)
- Monoclonal gammopathies
- Myeloma

disease), rheumatoid arthritis, and monoclonal gammopathy and may occur before, during, or after the disease (Aggarwal, 2012; Callen & Jackson, 2007).

Bullous PG is commonly associated with myeloproliferative disease, refractory anemias, and myelogenous leukemia (Callen & Jackson, 2007). These lesions begin as painful, rapidly enlarging vesicles and bullae with central necrosis that evolves into an erosion rather than a necrotic ulcer (Ruocco, Sangiuliano, Gravina, et al., 2009). The hands, arms, and face are more commonly affected than legs. This particular variation of PG is commonly misdiagnosed as cellulitis. Bullous PG in the patient with acute myeloid leukemia is suggestive of poor prognosis; thus it is important to rule out a hematologic malignancy in the patient who develops bullous PG (Ahronowitz et al., 2012). Treatment of the underlying malignancy results in improvement in the bullous PG.

Vegetative PG is characterized by a single superficial ulcer with a nonpurulent wound bed and the absence of undermining and periwound erythema (Ruocco et al., 2009). This is a nonaggressive form of PG, not associated with systemic disease, and responds well to topical therapy. The most common sites are the head and neck. Pustular PG develops as a painful pustular lesion with erythematous halo and is often associated with irritable bowel disease (IBD) and hepatobiliary disease (Ahronowitz et al., 2012). These lesions are most often found on the legs and upper trunk. Peristomal PG consists of lesions around a stoma commonly associated with IBD, monoclonal gammopathy, and connective tissue disease. At onset, the peristomal PG lesion is a painful, erythematous papule with violaceous borders that erodes into ulcers with undermined borders. These lesions are similar in appearance to classic PG.

Common characteristics of the ulcerative PG lesion include irregularly shaped wound edges that are elevated and violaceous (see Plate 77). Ulcers are exudative and extremely tender. The wound base is often filled with yellow slough and/or islands of necrosis; wound edges are undermined. A band of erythema may extend from the wound edge, which defines the direction in which the ulcer will extend. Healing may be present along one edge of the ulcer, whereas enlargement occurs along another edge. Ulcers heal slowly and leave an atrophic, irregular scar. A common and notable characteristic of PG is a phenomenon known as *pathergy*, which is the abnormal and exaggerated inflammatory response to noxious stimuli. Patients often report the lesion developing after minor trauma, such as a bump against a piece of furniture. Minor trauma preceding the development of the ulcer is an important piece of information to obtain during the patient interview (Paparone et al., 2009).

Pyoderma gangrenosum is difficult to diagnose; it is essentially a diagnosis by exclusion. As many as 10% of PG cases are misdiagnosed including vascular disease, vasculitis, malignancies, autoimmune disease, or infection (Box 32.2), thus delaying appropriate treatment (Ahronowitz et al., 2012). A history and physical examination, skin biopsy for histology and microbiology, and an investigation for an associated illness constitute a complete workup (Box 32.3). Diagnosis is largely based on clinical manifestations (rapidly enlarging,

---

BOX 32.2 Differential Diagnoses for Pyoderma Gangrenosum

- Vascular/neuropathic conditions
  - Venous insufficiency
  - Arterial insufficiency
  - Neuropathic disease
  - Antiphospholipid antibody syndrome
- Malignancy
  - Squamous cell carcinoma
  - Basal cell carcinoma
  - Cutaneous T-cell lymphoma
  - Metastatic carcinoma
- Systemic vasculitis
  - Polyarteritis nodosa
  - Behcet's disease
  - Cryoglobulinemic vasculitis
  - Rheumatoid vasculitis
  - ANCA-associated vasculitides
- Viral
  - Herpes zoster
  - Chronic herpes simplex virus
- Bacterial
  - Cutaneous tuberculosis
  - Impetigo
  - Buruli ulcer
  - Necrotizing fasciitis

BOX 32.3 Essential Data in Workup for Suspected Pyoderma Gangrenosum

1. Obtain history of onset of lesions
   - Rapidly enlarging, painful ulcer with violaceous, undermined edges and hemorrhagic/necrotic wound bed
2. Obtain skin biopsy from the erythematous margin of the wound for histology and microbiology
3. Obtain laboratory tests:
   - Routine tests to screen for hematologic, liver, or kidney disorder:
     - Complete blood count (CBC) with differential
     - Electrolytes
     - Urinalysis (UA)
     - Liver function
     - Erythrocyte sedimentation rate (ESR)
     - C-reactive protein (CRP)
   - Rule out systemic disorder
     - Antinuclear antibody
     - Coagulopathy panel
       - Antiphospholipid antibody test
       - Cryoglobulins
       - Rheumatoid factor
       - Antineutrophilic cytoplasmic antibodies (ANCA)
   - Rule out infectious etiology (if risk factors exist):
     - Rapid plasma reagin (RPR)
     - Hepatitis serologies
     - HIV

BOX 32.4 Proposed Diagnostic Criteria for Pyoderma Gangrenosum

Major Criteria (must satisfy both major criteria):
1. Rapid[*] progression of painful,[†] necrolytic, cutaneous ulcer[‡] with irregular, violaceous, undermined border
2. Exclusion of other causes of cutaneous ulceration

Minor Criteria (must also satisfy at least two minor criteria):
1. History suggestive of pathergy[§] or clinical finding of cribriform scarring
2. Systemic diseases associated with pyoderma gangrenosum[¶]
3. Histopathologic findings (sterile dermal neutrophilia ± mixed inflammation ± lymphocytic vasculitis)
4. Treatment response (rapid response to systemic glucocorticoid treatment)[**]

[*]Characteristic margin expansion of 1–2 cm/day, or 50% increase in ulcer size within 1 month.
[†]Pain usually out of proportion to size of ulceration.
[‡]Typically preceded by papule, pustule, or bulla.
[§]Ulcer development at sites of minor cutaneous injury.
[¶]Inflammatory bowel disease, polyarthritis, myelocytic leukemia, or preleukemia.
[**]Generally responds to dosage of 1–2 mg/kg/day, with 50% decrease in size within 1 month.
Adapted from Su, W. P., Davis, M. D., Weenig, R. H., et al. (2004). Pyoderma gangrenosum: Clinicopathologic correlation and proposed diagnostic criteria. *International Journal of Dermatology, 43*, 790–800.

painful ulcer with violaceous, undermined edges and hemorrhagic/necrotic wound bed), a thorough examination in which other ulcerative skin disorders (e.g., vasculitis, Behcet's disease, rheumatoid vasculitis, and infections) have been excluded, and pathologic features (Ratnagobal & Sinha, 2013; Tang, Vivas, Rey, et al., 2012). Proposed diagnostic criteria are listed in Box 32.4. While biopsy is often discouraged because it is of little discriminative value (Dinulos, 2021), it can be used to exclude malignancy and vasculitic, vasoocclusive, and infectious causes (Ratnagobal & Sinha, 2013). The biopsy must be full thickness and obtained from the erythematous margin of the wound for accurate histopathology. Laboratory tests such as antineutrophilic cytoplasmic antibodies (ANCA), rheumatoid factor, and antiphospholipid antibodies (anticardiolipin antibodies, lupus anticoagulant, and rapid plasma reagin) are important to exclude other diseases that could account for these lesions (Ratnagobal & Sinha, 2013). Inflammatory markers (erythrocyte sedimentation rate and C-reactive protein [CRP]) will also facilitate diagnosis. Because there is no definitive test to confirm the presence of PG, a diagnosis *consistent with* PG is appropriate, but only after a thorough workup is completed (Tang et al., 2012).

Treatment of PG consists of a combination of systemic therapy and local wound care. Table 32.2 summarizes topical medications that have been reported; the most commonly used and effective are corticosteroids, tacrolimus, and cyclosporine. Topical and intralesional corticosteroids may be effective for small early lesions (Dinulos, 2021).

Of the various treatments that have been used to manage PG, the most consistent, effective results have been obtained with systemic immunosuppression with corticosteroids and cyclosporine. Large, orally administered doses of prednisolone (60–120 mg) are given daily until the disease is under control as demonstrated by the reduction in pain and the presence of granulation tissue. Cyclosporine (oral 3–10 mg/kg/day and intravenous [IV] 4 mg/kg/day) appears to be particularly effective with PG in the presence of IBD (Ahronowitz et al., 2012). Although PG is not an infectious disease process, it can be complicated by infections. In fact, patients may receive treatment with antibiotics for cellulitis and may not improve because an initial biopsy was not obtained (Callen & Jackson, 2007; Wollina, 2007). Antineutrophillic therapies that interfere with neutrophil chemotaxis such as colchicine, sulfonamides, sulfones, and dapsone have demonstrated improvement in PG in small studies. Dapsone has been used alone or in combination with corticosteroids at doses of 50–200 mg/day; topical dapsone has also been effective in improving peristomal PG (Ahronowitz et al., 2012). Antitumor necrosis factor agents such as adalimumab, infliximab, and etanercept have also been successful in twice-weekly to twice-monthly administrations (Dinulos, 2021).

Topical wound management should address wound needs, which include exudate management, protection from trauma, a moist wound environment, and pain control. Slough and nonviable tissue present in PG ulcers gradually decrease and transition to a granular wound bed as immunosuppressive medications are implemented and wound exudate is contained. Typically, management of the wound is necessary before its cause is known. Because of the extreme pain that typifies PG, nonadhesive dressings are preferred. Debridement is achieved only through autolysis and regression of the disease process itself. Aggressive sharp debridement is contraindicated because it will lead to extension of the disease through the process of pathergy. In fact, local care should be delivered with great caution because of the tendency for pathergy to occur. Skin grafts also are to be avoided due to pathergy (Paparone et al., 2009). Antibacterial topical dressings are often warranted to manage the wound bioburden and potential secondary bacterial infections (Callen & Jackson, 2007).

VASCULITIS AND CONNECTIVE TISSUE DISORDERS

Vasculitis comprises a group of disorders that have in common the pathologic features of inflammation of the blood vessels, endothelial swelling, and necrosis. Damage to the blood vessels is attributed to the deposition of circulating immune complexes (Tang et al., 2012). Vessels of any size can be affected, so any organ or system may be involved, resulting in a wide array of symptoms and clinical presentations. Cutaneous vasculitic diseases are classified by the size and type of vessel involved and the type of inflammatory cell within the vessel walls (i.e., neutrophil, lymphocyte, or histiocyte) (Dinulos, 2021). Vasculitis ulcers usually are the sign of a

TABLE 32.2   Topical Medications for Pyoderma Gangrenosum

	Mechanism of Action	Dose	Comments

Corticosteroids	• Antiinflammatory and immunosuppressive action
	• Reduced neutrophil and macrophage activity
	• Reduced proliferation of T cells
	• Decreased cytokine production
	• Decreased histamine production
	• Decreased IgG production
		Topical:
		• Betamethasone 17 valerate lotion (0.1%)
		• Intralesional injection in combination with systemic corticosteroid:
		  ○ 100 mg triamcinolone acetonide
		  ○ Varying concentrations (up to 40 mg/mL)
		  ○ Varying dosing schedules (i.e., every 4–6 weeks)
			Healing occurred with topical in 5–8 weeks
			Transparent dressing applied over lotion corticosteroid
			Low level of evidence (case reports of very small number of patients)

Sodium cromoglycate	Inhibits mast cell degranulation, platelet activation, and neutrophil chemotaxis	1%–2% aqueous solution applied 3 × per day	Healing in 5–8 weeks Two case series
Topical 5-aminosalicylic acid (5-ASA)	Theorized to inhibit prostaglandin and leukotriene production by scavenging free radicals	10% 5-ASA cream applied daily	Healing in 5 weeks Limited evidence (case reports)
Topical nitrogen mustard	Immunosuppressive and antiinflammatory agent	Aqueous solution (20%) applied daily	Healing after 3 months Limited evidence (case report)
Topical cyclosporine	Reduced proliferation of T cells by inhibiting interleukin-2 release	35 mg cyclosporine in isotonic saline solution injected intralesionally twice in 1 week	Healing in 3 months
Tacrolimus	Immunosuppressive agent for primary organ transplantation	0.1%–0.3% (combined with carmellose sodium paste [Orabase])	May cover with thin hydrocolloid or ostomy pouch Reapply daily Healing has been reported in 5 weeks to 4 months More effective in PG lesions larger than 2 cm Highly absorbed through ulcerated tissue; apply to inflamed rim of lesion, not ulcer bed

complex process and may indicate a systemic disorder such as rheumatoid arthritis or lupus. However, vasculitis ulcers also can occur as a primary condition (Anderson, 2008; Armitage & Roberts, 2004). Most vasculitic syndromes are believed to have an immunologic etiology.

The size of the vessels involved (large, medium, or small) helps to characterize the skin manifestations. When a small vessel is affected, pinpoint areas of bleeding may develop, and small red or purple spots on the skin (petechiae) may appear, particularly on the legs. Inflammation of larger vessels causes the vessel to swell, producing a nodule that may be palpated. Blood flow will be impaired when the lumen of the blood vessel becomes narrowed or occluded from the edema; thus islands of ischemia or necrosis will develop on the skin, and the tips of digits may become cold or ischemic.

Leukocytoclastic vasculitis, Wegener granulomatosis, and rheumatoid factor are common. Other potential causes include systemic lupus erythematosus, polyarteritis nodosa, hypersensitivity vasculitis, Sjögren syndrome, cryoglobulinemia, scleroderma, and dermatomyositis (Hunter et al., 2002; Rubano & Kerstein, 1998). It is important to point out that leg

ulceration has been reported in up to 10% of patients with rheumatoid arthritis (RA) and that the underlying cause is most often vascular (arterial, venous, or mixed) and less commonly RA-specific vasculitis or PG (Seitz, Berens, Bröcker, et al., 2010).

The general signs and symptoms of vasculitis are fever, myalgias, arthralgias, and malaise. Patients sometimes describe a vague, flu-like illness. Peripheral neuropathy may be present. Other symptoms depend on the organ involved, which is determined by the specific disease. For example, cryoglobulinemic vasculitis likely will be associated with renal and skin problems; Wegener granulomatosis may lead to respiratory as well as renal involvement; and the vasculitis associated with Sjögren syndrome attacks the brain, lungs, and skin (Jennette & Falk, 1997).

Cutaneous features of vasculitis can vary depending on the disease, but certain characteristics are common. The lesions can range from erythematous, nonblanching macules and/or nodules to hemorrhagic vesicles and palpable purpura, to necrotic lesions and ulceration. Skin ulcers associated with vasculitis are frequently located on the lower extremities in

TABLE 32.3	**Characteristics of Skin Lesions With Vasculitis Disorders**	
Vasculitic Disorder	**Description**	**Ulcer Characteristics**
Rheumatoid arthritis	Not well understood Associated with high levels of rheumatoid factor (RF) Evidence of venous insufficiency Limited ankle movement contributes to poor calf muscle pump function and may place patient at risk for venous ulcer development	Begin as palpable purpura and ecchymosis May progress to ulceration Shallow, well demarcated, painful, slow to heal May require addition of compression therapy
Systemic lupus erythematosus (SLE)	Chronic immune disorder Characterized by periods of exacerbation and remission Affects multiple organs (skin, serosal surfaces, central nervous system, kidneys) and red blood cells Circulating immune complexes and autoantibodies cause tissue damage and organ dysfunction No single cause; influenced by environment, host immune responses, hormones Common symptoms include fatigue, weight loss, fever, malaise Butterfly rash (facial edema over cheeks, nose) is typical Potential manifestations include seizures, hemiparesis, pericarditis, pleuritis, renal failure, nausea, vomiting, abdominal pain, and arthralgias	Present as palpable purpura Progress to ulceration Occur on malleolar area Present as round lesions with erythematous borders Wound may have atrophy and loss of pigmentation
Polyarteritis nodosa (PAN)	Medium- and small-vessel vasculitis Necrotizing arteritis affecting small- and medium-sized arteries of most organs Involved organs commonly include kidney, liver, intestine, peripheral nerves, skin, muscle Characterized by fresh and healing lesions Clinical manifestations include anorexia, weight loss, fever, fatigue Organ-specific manifestations include abdominal pain, myalgia, arthralgia, paresthesia Subcutaneous painful nodules of lower extremities may develop	Skin involvement occurs in approximately 40% of patients Lesions have "punched out" appearance Painful Lesions may begin as purpura with urticaria before progressing to ulceration May have "starburst" pattern extending from ulcer Painful subcutaneous nodules present

the lateral malleolus or pretibial area, making them difficult to distinguish from venous ulcers (Seitz et al., 2010) (see Plate 78). Serum ANCA is a serologic marker for many forms of necrotizing vasculitis. Use of this test to diagnose and classify vasculitis has surpassed the value of biopsy in these patients (Dinulos, 2021).

The goal of treatment of vasculitis ulcers is control of the underlying disease process. The presence of these painful ulcers necessitates an evaluation for the underlying disease and identification of involved organs, which is then used to guide treatment. Bed rest, nonsteroidal antiinflammatory agents, antihistamines, corticosteroids, and biologic immunosuppressive agents often are necessary (Hunter et al., 2002). Plasmapheresis might be necessary in cases associated with circulating immune complexes. Topical therapy includes removal of necrotic tissue (often through autolysis), prompt identification and treatment of infection, maintenance of a moist wound base, absorption of excess exudate, packing of any dead space, insulation, and protection from further trauma.

The various vasculitis syndromes have many similarities but also have specific differences unique to some of the diseases. The unique features of RA, systemic lupus erythematosus, and polyarteritis nodosa are listed in Table 32.3.

Drug-Induced Vasculitis

One of the more common causes of vasculitis is a drug reaction rather than a disease process. Drug-induced vasculitis usually is confined to the skin and appears about 1 week after administration of the drug. The drug binds to serum proteins, causing an immune-complex vasculitis (Radic, Kaliterna, & Radic, 2012). The typical presentation is purpura and ulceration involving the lower extremities. Once systemic disease has been ruled out, treatment involves removal of the precipitating drug and symptomatic treatment. Antihistamines and NSAIDs are most often prescribed. Corticosteroids may be added for more severe symptoms. Wound care is based on wound needs, and ulcers resolve spontaneously once the drug is removed.

CALCIPHYLAXIS

Calciphylaxis is a condition that is characterized by calcification of small- and medium-sized dermal and subcutaneous blood vessels (Bajaj, Courbebaisse, Kroshinsky, Thadhani, & Nigwekar, 2018; Nigwekar, Thadhani, & Brandenburg, 2018). This rare, life-threatening condition results in intensely painful ischemic lesions and hyperesthesia; pain may precede the appearance of skin lesions. Calciphylaxis occurs most often in patients with end-stage renal disease (ESRD) but can also occur in patients with early stages of chronic kidney disease, acute kidney injury, and kidney transplant; occasionally it will occur in patients with normal kidney function (Nigwekar et al., 2018). Calciphylaxis is further classified as uremic (occurring in patients with ESRD) and nonuremic (in patients with normal renal function or early kidney disease) (Nigwekar et al., 2018). The condition is often underrecognized and has a high mortality. One-year mortality in patients without ESRD is 25%–45%, while patients with ESRD have a 1-year mortality rate of 45%–80% (McCarthy, El-Azhary, Patzelt, et al., 2016; Nigwekar et al., 2018).

Clinically, calciphylaxis is linked to hyperparathyroidism (secondary to ESRD) and hyperphosphatemia, which contribute to vascular, subcutaneous, and cutaneous calcification (Tang et al., 2012; Udomkarnjananun et al., 2019). As a chronic progressive syndrome of arteriolar media calcification, thrombotic ischemia, and necrotic ulcerative calciphylaxis develops when levels of calcium and phosphate in the blood are no longer solubilized, leading to deposits in the arteriolar wall. Risk factors for calciphylaxis include: obesity, female, hypercalcemia, hyperphosphatemia, hypoalbuminemia, hyperparathyroidism, vitamin K deficiency, elevated alkaline phosphatase, exposure to aluminum, hepatobiliary disease, and autoimmune disorders; and concomitant use of calcium-based phosphate binders, vitamin K antagonists, and heparin (Nigwekar et al., 2018).

Calciphylaxis lesions are characterized by induration, necrotic tissue, and a violaceous discoloration (see Plate 79). A significant feature of this condition is severe pain that is refractory to common analgesics. Initially, the lesions may appear to be serpiginous, indurated plaques with surrounding pallor or ecchymosis. The lesions progress to subcutaneous nodules and ulcerations that eventually become gangrenous. The distribution of lesions is usually bilateral and symmetric. A proximal distribution pattern (trunk, thighs, and upper arms) of either uremic or nonuremic calciphylaxis is associated with a 50%–70% mortality rate (Alavi, Mayer, Hafner, et al., 2012). In contrast, distal calciphylaxis is associated with a 10% mortality rate. A distinctive finding with calciphylaxis is intact peripheral pulses because blood flow distal to or deeper than the necrosis remains intact. This clinical assessment is critical in distinguishing the disease from other conditions such as warfarin-induced skin necrosis, ASVD, venous ulcers, pyoderma gangrenosum, necrotizing vasculitis, or Martorell's ulcer (Nigwekar et al., 2018). Elevated serum calcium or phosphate levels are nonspecific to the diagnosis of calciphylaxis.

When calciphylaxis has an atypical presentation, skin biopsy is critical for an accurate diagnosis despite the potential for worsening of the ulcers after biopsy (Nigwekar et al., 2018; Tang et al., 2012). Histologically, the smooth muscle cells of the vascular wall develop into osteoid-like cells (Wollina, 2013). These calcifications precipitate a narrowing of the lumen and hyperplasia. The combination of microvascular calcification of the media layer and hyperplasia within the intima of arterioles with a diameter of approximately 0.04–0.1 mm is considered a histologic marker for calciphylaxis. These findings assist in differentiating this disease from peripheral arterial occlusion.

Treatment of calciphylaxis is neither universally standardized nor necessarily effective and requires a multidisciplinary approach including experts in dermatology, nephrology, nutrition, pain management, and wound care (Malabu, Manickam, Kan, et al., 2012). Normalization of abnormal calcium and phosphorus levels is warranted. Therapy includes intensified hemodialysis with noncalcium/nonaluminum phosphate binders, sodium thiosulfate, cinacalcet, hyperbaric oxygen therapy, and parathyroidectomy (Malabu et al., 2012; Udomkarnjananun et al., 2019). Sodium thiosulfate (administered by either IV or intraperitoneal infusion) acts as a chelator of cations, converting the insoluble tissue deposits of cations (e.g., calcium) into more soluble cations. Antibiotics should be given to treat wound infection and prevent sepsis.

Topical wound management should address specific wound needs: fill dead space, provide a physiologic environment, and absorb exudate. Hyperbaric oxygen therapy has also been reported as beneficial (Ugandundrum et al., 2018). Aggressive debridement and skin grafting may be indicated to reduce the potential for wound infection; increased patient survival has been reported with aggressive early debridement (Malabu et al., 2012; Wollina, 2013). The severity of wound-related pain should be assessed regularly, and control measures for pain should be implemented routinely and during wound procedures.

MARTORELL HYPERTENSIVE ISCHEMIC LEG ULCER

Another type of ulcer with an ischemic subcutaneous arteriolosclerosis etiology is known as Martorell hypertensive ischemic leg ulcer (HYTILU). Because the manifestations of the Martorell HYTILU are quite similar to calciphylaxis and PG, they may be misdiagnosed as one of these conditions or as necrotizing leukocytoclastic vasculitis (Mansour & Alavi, 2019). An accurate diagnosis is, however, essential to avoid harmful and detrimental treatments. Table 32.4 presents common differential diagnoses for Martorell HYTILU.

Diagnosis of Martorell HYTILU is based on history and clinical presentation and then confirmed with biopsy. Patients with Martorell HYTILU have a long history of arterial hypertension. They may also have obesity and diabetes mellitus type II. Ulcers develop due to local skin infarctions caused by arteriosclerosis of the dermis and subcutaneous tissue. Ulcers are characterized by central necrosis and a progressive inflammatory violaceous border. Because Martorell HYTILU is a disease of the subcutaneous arterioles, necrosis may be superficial or deep into the subcutaneous tissue and tend to spread rather than extend into deeper tissue

TABLE 32.4 Common Differential Diagnoses for Hypertensive Ischemic Leg Ulcer

Cause	Common Location	Clinical Characteristics	Pain	Association	Tests
Venous	Middle malleolus Lateral malleolus/ lower gaiter area	Shallow, granulation tissue base Serpiginous margin Woody fibrosis Venous varicosities Pitting edema Hyperpigmentation	+	Varicose veins Previous surgery Deep vein thrombosis Obesity Multiple pregnancy	Venous Doppler to demonstrate incompetent valves; superficial perforator, or deep Occasionally venous disease is due to clots or occluded vessels
Arterial	Anterior shin or trauma/ infection location	Punched-out, fibrous base Deep ulcer	+++	Smoking Coronary artery disease	Arterial Doppler Computed tomography angiography Magnetic resonance angiography
Martorell	Lateral–dorsal of shin	Shallow, necrotic Rapidly enlarging Deep necrosis Palpable pulses	+++ +	Hypertension Diabetes	Often normal ankle-brachial index unless coexisting arterial disease Deep wedge biopsy to identify small-vessel changes and skin necrosis
Pyoderma gangrenosum	Any location	Rapidly enlarging Rolled (metal gray) border that evolves into a central ulcer	+++	Inflammatory bowel disease Rheumatoid arthritis Myeloproliferative disorders 50% idiopathic	Diagnosis of exclusion: clinical picture/associations with a skin biopsy to rule out other disorders (i.e., infections, vasculitis)
Vasculitis	Often distal with often symmetric lesions	Palpable purpuric lesions Fixed urticarial/blisters Necrosis, ulceration Usually bilateral	++	Hepatitis C/other infections Connective tissue disorders, drugs, malignancy 50% other organ involvement; common to involve joints, liver/kidney (e.g., Henoch–Schönlein purpura)	Biopsy for regular histology and immunofluorescence C-ANCA P-ANCA
Sickle cell	Medial malleolus	May have central necrosis and scarring with frequent coexisting venous disease or infections	+++ +	Sickle cell anemia Pulmonary hypertension	Sickle prep Hb electrophoresis
Malignant	Any location	Slow expanding Crusted for squamous cell carcinoma Rolled border and telangiectasia for basal cell carcinoma Pigmented lesion with asymmetry, irregular border, color variability (black, blue, red, white) for melanoma	+	Photodamage Previous osteomyelitis sinus Previous radiotherapy edge or a graft or other area of chronic inflammation	Diagnostic biopsy, >1 biopsy may be necessary to ascertain a diagnosis
Calciphylaxis	Any location	Livedo reticularis-like pattern peripherally that evolves into central necrosis bilateral symmetric	+++	Chronic renal failure and renal impairment or on dialysis Secondary hyperparathyroidism	Biopsy
Vasculopathy	Lower leg	Livedo reticularis of the vascular supply leading to local areas of atrophy and necrosis	++	Abnormal circulating proteins: anticoagulant, cryoglobulins, cold agglutinins	Biopsy Appropriate serum factors

From Alavi, A., Mayer, D., Hafner, J., et al. (2012). Martorell hypertensive ischemic leg ulcer: An underdiagnosed entity©. *Advances in Skin & Wound Care, 25*(12), 563–572.

(Mansour & Alavi, 2019). These necrotic skin ulcers only develop on the lateral–dorsal aspect of the leg or the Achilles tendon and may be unilateral or bilateral. As with PG and calciphylaxis, the Martorell HYTILU is extremely painful with either a spontaneous onset or triggered by minor trauma.

The differential diagnosis for Martorell HYTILU requires differentiation from arterial or venous disease, PG, and calciphylaxis. Peripheral arterial occlusive disease cooccurs in a majority of patients. Distinction between PG and Martorell HYTILU is critical because the treatment for one is harmful to the other. While both PG and Martorell HYTILU have necrotic tissue and a violaceous border, HYTILU will be dry eschar in appearance, while the PG ulcer is typically liquified necrotic tissue (Mansour & Alavi, 2019). All patients with Martorell HYTILU have hypertension and may have associated cardiovascular conditions. In contrast, the patient with PG may have inflammatory bowel disease, rheumatoid arthritis, neutrophilia, or an elevated serum CRP. In addition, a large, elliptical, deep tissue biopsy (extending to fascia) that crosses the area of necrotic tissue into normal skin is necessary to confirm subcutaneous arteriosclerosis. Martorell HYTILU is the favored diagnosis in the presence of cardiovascular risk factors, the lateral–dorsal aspect lower leg or the Achilles tendon ulcer location, and full-thickness biopsy demonstrating arteriosclerosis (Mansour & Alavi, 2019).

Treatment includes addressing underlying pathology (i.e., blood pressure control) and reducing factors that compromise peripheral perfusion (i.e., smoking cessation, blood glucose control, anticoagulants, vasodilators, and graduated compression therapy). Because of the inherent reduced perfusion with this type of ulcer, it is important to monitor and manage wound bioburden with topical antimicrobials and/or systemic antimicrobials. Surgical excision of necrotic tissue, sometimes requiring repeat debridement, followed by NPWT is advocated (Mansour & Alavi, 2019). Topical wound care before definitive treatment via grafting should include nontraumatic debridement via autolysis. Nonocclusive, nonadhesive dressings such as hydrogels, honey, alginates, hydrofibers, and foam are appropriate topical dressings to provide autolysis or maintain optimum wound environment when awaiting debridement or wound closure.

EPIDERMOLYSIS BULLOSA

Epidermolysis bullosa (EB) is a rare inherited disorder characterized by mechanical stress-induced blistering of the skin and mucous membranes (Fine, Bruckner-Tuderman, Eady, et al., 2014). Between 1986 and 2002, the Unites States estimated the incidence of the disease to be 19.57 per 1,000,000 individuals (Fine, 2016). EB is classified into four main types and numerous clinical subtypes: EB simplex (EBS), junctional EB (JEB), dystrophic EB (DEB), and Kindler EB (KEB) (Has et al., 2020). The types of EB are based on the level at which the skin layers separate and blister forms: EBS is at the intraepidermal layer, JEB is at the lamina lucida of the basement membrane, and DEB is at the sublamina densa below the basement membrane. KEB separates on multiple tissue planes

(Mariath, Santin, Schuler-Faccini, & Kiszewski, 2020). Epidermolysis bullosa can affect every epithelial structure in the body, including the eyelids, conjunctivae, corneas, bowels, skin, and gums.

EB manifestations range from discrete, almost undetectable cutaneous signs to severe cutaneous and extracutaneous lesions involving the dermis–epidermis adhesion. Distinctive characteristics of EB are listed in Box 32.5. Blisters can be superficial, as with EBS, or deeper leading to ulcerations as with JEB, DEB, and KEB (Mariath et al., 2020).

Extracutaneous manifestations—gastrointestinal, ophthalmologic (corneal abrasions and ulcerations), skeletal (osteoporosis due to decreased weight bearing), genitourinary (obstructive uropathy, immunoglobulin A nephropathy), and cardiac—are common. Chronic anemia may be present due to blood loss from open wounds and poor nutritional intake. The severity of these manifestations varies with the category of EB and the subtype within that category (Watkins, 2016). Gastrointestinal complications are a major

---

BOX 32.5   Characteristics of Epidermolysis Bullosa by Category

Epidermolysis Bullosa Simplex (EBS)
- Intraepidermal blisters
- Heals without scar formation
- Nails and teeth normal
- Occasional cutaneous blistering
- Autosomal-dominant trait

Junctional Epidermolysis Bullosa (JEB)
- Autosomal-recessive trait
- Blisters form at lamina lucida (between epidermis and basement membrane)
- Several subtypes with distinct clinical manifestations

Recessive Dystrophic Epidermolysis Bullosa (RDEB)
- Dystrophic scarring is distinctive feature that serves as clinical marker
- Separation at basement membrane zone deep to basement membrane
- Recessive inheritance
- Blister formation results from even minimal mechanical trauma
- Blisters may be hemorrhagic
- Blisters eventually rupture to form slow-to-heal superficial ulcers that continue to be exposed to minimal mechanical trauma
- Healing always involves scarring, so skin has atrophic and wrinkled appearance
- Elbows, knees, hands, feet are sites of repeated trauma
- Predisposes patient to squamous cell cancer

Dominant Dystrophic Epidermolysis Bullosa (DDEB)
- Formation of blisters below basement membrane
- Autosomal-dominant inheritance
- Trauma-induced blisters form at birth or shortly thereafter
- Blisters heal with scar formation but usually are less extensive than in recessive form
- Predisposes patient to squamous cell cancer

TABLE 32.5   Special Precautions to Minimize Cutaneous Trauma to Patients With Dystrophic Epidermolysis Bullosa During Select Clinical Procedures

Procedure	Suggestions
Blood pressure monitoring	Apply dressing under blood pressure cuff
Electrocardiogram monitoring	Use nonadhesive plastic film (e.g., Omiderm, which does not interfere with electrical conduction) as a barrier between patient's skin and adhesive of electrode pads
Urine collections (young children)	Wring out cloth diaper; do not apply urine bags containing adhesives
Blood drawing	To cleanse skin, allow alcohol or Betadine swab to remain in place for 5 min without rubbing; place tourniquet over padding to protect skin; or apply direct pressure on vein using thumb in parallel position to skin
Parenteral therapy	Cut piece of extrathin hydrocolloid dressing into horseshoe shape and put dressing with adhesive backing side in contact with skin. Start intravenous (IV) line between legs of horseshoe bandage and tape tubing onto dressing. Secure IV with roller gauze, or place snug-fitting piece of tube gauze (e.g., Bandnet) on extremity adjacent to IV and secure with tape to tube gauze
Preoperative preparations (operating room, table, surgical drapes, surgical scrubs)	Operating room table should be well padded. Sheepskin covered by table-sized burn pad (e.g., Exu-Dry, which has double layer of meshed material to minimize friction) is advised. If positioning with pillows is necessary for patient with joint contractures, place Exu-Dry pad between pillow and patient's skin Place sterile sheets of nonadherent mesh (e.g., Exu-Dry Mesh, N-Terface) under sterile drapes to protect exposed skin from friction. Fold mesh over edge of drape and secure with clamps. Adhesive drapes are contraindicated Apply antimicrobial solution to surgical site and allow to remain on skin for 5 min, then irrigate to rinse. Repeat this process three times
Mask-delivered anesthesia	Protect skin on face from possible shearing by using nonadherent foam, which adheres to any damp surface and is easily removed by rewetting; or apply copious amount of petrolatum to face before applying mask

From Caldwell-Brown, D., Gibbons, S., & Reid, M. (1992). Nursing aspects of epidermolysis bullosa: A comprehensive approach. In A. N. Lin & D. M. Carter (Eds.), *Epidermolysis bullosa: Basic and clinical aspects.* New York: Springer Verlag.

source of symptoms and morbidity for all EB patients. The most severe problems are associated with the oropharynx, esophagus, and proximal gut. The simple use of eating utensils and the passage of foods result in the formation of bullae that rupture, erode, and heal with scar formation. Strictures are inevitable, and nutritional problems develop. With recurrent mechanical trauma, skin lesions become chronic and result in contractures or strictures in the more severe cases of DEB and KEB.

Anemia is another major problem with EB and is multifactorial in origin. Poor nutrition resulting from painful oral blisters and esophageal strictures precipitates a deficiency in iron, trace metals, and protein, which contributes to anemia. Protein and blood are also lost through the chronic skin lesions typical of JEB and DEB.

The patient with EB is deprived of an epidermal barrier to bacterial invasion. *S. aureus* and other pathogens often colonize the chronic, nonhealing wound. Sepsis is a serious complication, especially in infants. Judicious use of topical antibiotics and antimicrobial dressings is warranted to decrease bacterial flora and minimize the risk of soft tissue infection (Shinkuma, 2015). Silver-impregnated dressings may be effective in reducing bioburden as well as cleansing the lesions with a noncytotoxic debriding hypochlorous solution.

The primary objective in the care of patients with EB is promoting healing and preventing trauma. Nursing considerations include wound care, nutrition, education, pain control, and social support. Wound-healing ability is often compromised in patients due to malnutrition, anemia, increased wound bioburden, and loss of protective functions of the skin (Watkins, 2016). Special precautions to minimize cutaneous trauma during select clinical procedures are listed in Table 32.5. Interventions such as the routine use of convoluted foam on pad rails, sheepskin, an air-fluidized support surface, and joint protectors are important. Nonadhesive or low-adherence foam dressings may be appropriate for protecting the patient's hands or feet. However, if these dressings are used, they should be left in place and allowed to fall off rather than being removed and reapplied on a regular basis.

There is no single approach to wound care for managing EB lesions; rather, interventions should strive to achieve key objectives: contain exudate, avoid trauma, prevent infection, and maintain a moist environment. Three layers of dressings are often recommended (DebRA, http://www.debra.org). The first layer is nonadherent such as contact layer dressings and hydrogels. The second layer stabilizes the first layer and provides padding and protection (e.g., impregnated cause, nonadherent roll gauze, foam dressings, hydrofiber dressings, and specialty absorptive dressings). The third layer is used to maintain the dressing in place and may provide some elasticity (e.g., gauze and retention gauze). Adhesives and compressive dressings can induce blisters and should be avoided (Shinkuma, 2015). Fenestrated, nonadherent dressings can be used so that wound moisture can pass through the fenestrations and be trapped by the cover dressing. Ointments can be applied over the fenestrated layer when trying to reduce wound bioburden. Creative dressing techniques often are necessary for difficult locations, such as the digits or face, particularly to prevent fusion of digits. To avoid sensitization, the use of topical antibiotics is not recommended in the absence of very strong evidence of an infection. When infection is suspected (i.e., presence of increased drainage, odor, or wound pain), antimicrobial dressings (e.g., silver or cadexomer iodine) are appropriate. Vesicles or bullae should be lanced and drained to prevent extension through defectively bound skin layers (Shinkuma, 2015). Temporary skin substitutes and bioengineered skin hold a great deal of promise for this dangerous disease.

Pruritus is a common problem with EB and is the source of new blister formation and breakdown of healing wounds (Watkins, 2016). Moisturizers (e.g., emollients) and oral anti-pruritics are often indicated. Atrophic scarring and contractures are common and result in fusion of digits (i.e., mitten deformity or pseudosyndactyly), which requires repeat surgical release of contractures. Additional complications include squamous cell cancer, which is almost inevitable, so constant monitoring with aggressive skin surveillance is essential (Shinkuma, 2015). Additional information about this disease is available from the Dystrophic Epidermolysis Bullosa Research Association of America (DebRA, http://www.debra.org).

EXTRAVASATION

The role of the wound care specialist in caring for the patient with an extravasation is to provide consultation in the management of the resulting wound. The initial necessary interventions immediately following extravasation of a chemotherapeutic agent are provided by the oncology staff as guided by best evidence (Gorski et al., 2021). Therefore, the wound care specialist is not expected to be familiar with each medication, irritant potential, or immediate post-extravasation intervention specific to each medication. However, the wound care specialist may be consulted for wound management once tissue damage is evident. This section will address risk factors, prevention, assessment, and treatment of extravasation injury.

Infiltration is the "…inadvertent administration of nonvesicant solution or medication into surrounding tissue" (Gorski et al., 2021; pS207). In most situations, leakage of IV fluids or medications into surrounding tissues is innocuous. The spectrum of cutaneous reactions depends on whether the solution that leaked is a nonvesicant, an irritant, or a vesicant. Nonvesicant extravasation creates swelling but no tissue damage. An irritant solution induces an inflammatory reaction but no persistent tissue damage. Nonpharmacologic interventions, such as elevation and applying either cold or warm cloths, are sufficient to reduce swelling and discomfort.

In contrast, extravasation is the "…inadvertent infiltration of vesicant solution or medication into surrounding tissue" (Gorski et al., 2021; pS207). A vesicant can be composed of

TABLE 32.6	**Common Vesicants**	
DNA-Binding Agents	**Non-DNA-Binding Agents**	**Nonantineoplastic Vesicants**
Anthracycline Agents	**Vinca Alkaloids**	Hyperosmotic solutions
Actinomycin D	Vincristine	Concentrated electrolyte solu-tions
Dactinomycin	Vinblastine	Agents altering intracellular pH (sodium bicarbonate)
Doxorubicin	Vindesine	
Daunorubicin	Vinorelbine	
Epirubicin	**Taxane**	Vasopressors
Idarubicin	**Agents**	Phenytoin
Mitoxantrone	Paclitaxel	Aminophylline
Antitumor	Docetaxel	Mannitol
Antibiotics		Chloramphenicol
Mitomycin C		Nafcillin
Bleomycin		Oxacillin
Doxorubicin		Vancomycin
Alkylating		
Agents		
Mechlorethamine		
Platinum analogs		

calcium, potassium, parenteral nutrition, acyclovir, and others. Vesicants may be nonantineoplastic agents (hyperosmolar solutions, vasopressor agents, and antibiotics), but most commonly are antineoplastic agents (Table 32.6). A vesicant generates a reaction in the surrounding tissues that ranges from swelling to blistering to an inflammatory reaction. Progressive tissue destruction with slough and tissue necrosis may be delayed for several days, weeks, and months as a result of diffusion of the drug into adjacent tissue (see Plate 80).

Risk factors for extravasation injury are listed in Box 32.6. The extent of tissue damage is determined by several factors: drug concentration, amount infiltrated, duration of tissue exposure, extravasation site, hyperosmolarity, nonphysiological pH, medication's ability to cause vasoconstriction and timeliness of postextravasation intervention (Gorski et al., 2021; Kreidieh, Moukadem, & Saghir, 2016). Vesicants cause tissue damage by either binding to DNA within cells or interfering with mitosis. When the vesicant binds with DNA and the cells die, the drug is released into surrounding tissue and binds to more DNA. This process repeats a chain of events such that the area of tissue damage continues to widen. The vesicant then interferes with mitosis, causes tissue damage, and results in cell death but to a lesser degree than expected with DNA-binding chemicals. It is important for the wound specialist to be aware of the potential for significant local reactions caused by nonantineoplastic agents because these medications are administered to many patients in a variety of health care settings.

Assessment

During administration of vesicants, the injection site must be monitored closely for sudden swelling, stinging, burning, palpable subcutaneous fluid, bleb formation, pain, and redness. Induration, or obvious ulcer formation, is not an immediate manifestation, and visual inspection cannot determine the potential for or extent of tissue impairment (Gorski et al., 2021). Lack of blood return may suggest extravasation but alone is not always an indicator. Because extravasation can occur without symptoms, periodic reassessment of the injection site after completion of the infusion is warranted. Manifestations of extravasation include localized erythema, inflammation, blanching, induration, vesicle formation, ulceration, and tissue sloughing (Kreidieh et al., 2016). Serious complications are also possible, requiring reconstructive surgery or amputation due to full-thickness skin loss, infection, compartment syndrome, and muscle/tendon necrosis (Kim, Park, Lee, & Cheon, 2020). Extravasation can be divided into four grades according to severity. Grade 2 is erythema with symptoms such as edema, pain, induration, and phlebitis. Grade 3 is ulceration or necrosis. Grade 4 is life-threatening consequences and urgent intervention indicated. Grade 5 is death (Kreidieh et al., 2016).

Extravasation must be distinguished from other local reactions, such as venous flare and recall. Venous flare is a self-limiting, localized hypersensitivity response that involves the development of an erythematous streak along the course of the vein with pruritus, patchy erythema, and/or urticaria. Venous flare is not uncommon and usually resolved within 1–2 h (Kreidieh et al., 2016).

Interventions

Early intervention after extravasation can lessen the severity of tissue injury. It is estimated that one-third of all extravasations will produce ulceration in the absence of therapy (Ener, Meglathery, & Styler, 2004). Treatment of extravasation of chemotherapy or biotherapy agents should be guided by best evidence. Standard interventions are as follows: (1) disconnect the IV tubing from the IV device; (2) leave the needle in place; (3) attach small syringe to the IV device and aspirate residual drug from the IV; (4) avoid pressure on the site; (5) apply cold or heat (depending on the extravasant) as indicated by published evidence and institutional policy; and (6) elevate the involved extremity for 24 h (Gorski et al., 2021). Local heat or cold applications are used to decrease the site reaction or absorption of the infiltrate. Cold packs are recommended for extravasation of most DNA-binding vesicants (except mechlorethamine) and hot packs are recommended for non-DNA-binding vesicants (Kim et al., 2020).

Antidotes for the extravasation of cytotoxic agents are used to neutralize the chemicals in the tissues. Professional organizations such as the Oncology Nursing Society and Infusion Nurses Society are important to access for the most recent guidelines as well as manufacturers. One drug specifically approved for extravasation is Totect (dexrazoxane), which is administered as an IV infusion into anthracycline extravasations within 6 h of extravasation (Gorski et al., 2021). Hyaluronidase, sodium thiosulfate, granulocyte–macrophage colony-stimulating factor, phentolamine, and terbutaline are indicated for specific drugs triggering the extravasation (Gorski et al., 2021; Kreidieh et al., 2016). Hyaluronidase is also an antidote for several antibiotics, total parenteral nutrition, calcium, potassium, and high-concentration dextrose. Additional interventions that have been used include making stab incisions in the involved tissue, flushing with normal saline, and placing drains (Kim et al., 2020; Kreidieh et al., 2016).

Topical Wound Care

During follow-up, the site should be monitored closely for 24 h, then at 1 week, 2 weeks, and as indicated for pain, redness, swelling, ulceration, and necrosis. Depending on the patient's overall health and immune status, more frequent monitoring of the site may be needed if necrosis and ulceration develop. A referral to a plastic surgeon may be warranted if a large volume of vesicant was extravasated or the area and depth of tissue damage were significant. However, routine surgical excision is not warranted because not all vesicant extravasations will cause tissue ulceration. Surgical debridement may be indicated for extensive tissue damage or overwhelming infection. CTP dressings or skin grafting may be necessary to achieve wound closure.

Topical care of extravasation wounds should be dictated by the characteristics of the wound. Key objectives for topical care include absorption of exudate, removal of nonviable tissue, prevention of infection, elimination of dead space, and pain management. As the extent of tissue damage is revealed, the characteristics of the wound will change, and the local wound care choices will require modification. The area should be protected from shear and trauma. Hydrogels or hyperosmolar gauze can be used to promote autolysis of slough and necrotic tissue.

Documentation and close follow-up with appropriate consultations are highly recommended. Photographic documentation of the extravasation may be mandated by institutional policy. It is important to record the date and time of the infusion, when extravasation was noted, the size and type of catheter, the drug and amount of drug administered, and the estimated amount of extravasated solution (Gorski et al., 2021).

IMMUNE REACTIONS

Toxic Epidermal Necrolysis

Toxic epidermal necrosis is a rare but severe exfoliating disorder characterized by epidermal sloughing at the dermal–epidermal junction. Up to 80% of TEN is caused by a reaction to medication (Poulsen, Nielsen, & Poulsen, 2013) (see Plate 81). Milder variants include erythema multiforme and Stevens–Johnson syndrome (SJS). The Severe Cutaneous Adverse Reaction classification system (Box 32.7) differentiates SJS from TEN based on total body surface area (TBSA) affected. SJS involves less than 10% of TBSA, whereas TEN involves greater than 30% of TBSA. From 10% to 30% of TBSA affected is described as *SJS/TEN overlap* (Dinulos, 2021; Jellinek-Cohen, 2021). Based on seven known adverse prognostic factors, the SCORe of Toxic Epidermal Necrosis (SCORTEN) severity of illness scale (Table 32.7) is used to stratify severity of illness and predict mortality of TEN. The average mortality of SJS is 1%–5%, whereas the estimated mortality of TEN ranges from

TABLE 32.7 SCORTEN Clinical Scoring System for Predicting Outcome in Toxic Epidermal Necrolysis

Clinical–Biologic Parameter	INDIVIDUAL SCORE	
	Yes	No
Age >40 years	1	0
Malignancy	1	0
Tachycardia (>120/min)	1	0
Initial surface of epidermal detachment >10%	1	0
Serum urea >10 mmol/L	1	0
Serum glucose >14mmo/L	1	0
Bicarbonate <20 mmol/L	1	0

SCORTEN (Sum of Individual Scores)	Predicted Mortality (%)
0–1	3.2
2	12.1
3	35.3
4	58.3
≥5	90

From Bastuji-Garin, S., Fouchard, N., Bertocchi, M., et al. (2000). SCORTEN: A severity-of-illness score for toxic epidermal necrolysis. *Journal of Investigative Dermatology, 115*, 149–153.

BOX 32.7 Severe Cutaneous Adverse Reaction (SCAR) Classification System

Erythema Multiforme (EM)
- Typically round targets with three different zones and well-defined borders
- Most prominent on distal portions of extremities (acral distribution)
- Less than 1% of total body surface area involved

Stevens–Johnson Syndrome (SJS)
- Widespread, irregularly shaped, erythematous or purpuric macules
- Blistering occurs on all or part of macule
- Confluence of lesions and epidermal detachment is limited, involving less than 10% of total body surface area

Overlap SJS and Toxic Epidermal Necrolysis (TEN)
- Same as SJS
- 10%–29% of body surface area involved

TEN "With Spots"
- Blisters become more confluent, resulting in detachment of epidermis and erosions on greater than 30% of total body surface area
- Mucosal surfaces usually involved

TEN "Without Spots"
- Widespread, large, erythematous areas with no discrete lesions (macules or blisters)
- Epidermal detachment involves greater than 10% of total body surface area

10% to 70% (Jellinek-Cohen, 2021). Death usually results from overwhelming sepsis and multisystem organ failure.

Both SJS and TEN are characterized by epidermal detachment. Mucosal tissue is also affected in greater than 90% of patients with TEN. The lesions affect the mouth, eyes, respiratory tract, and genitourinary tract and tend to be very painful. Mucosal tissue is much less common with SJS. Both SJS and TEN occur in adults and children.

Toxic epidermal necrosis is a T-cell-mediated immune reaction similar to graft-vs-host disease (GVHD) (Dinulos, 2021). The epidermal necrolysis that occurs appears to be an immune-mediated reaction against epithelial cells involving T cells, cytotoxic reactions, and delayed hypersensitivity (Jellinek-Cohen, 2021). The most common medications associated with SJS and TEN are antibiotics and anticonvulsants, but more than 100 drugs, including oxicam, NSAIDs, allopurinol, antiretroviral medications, and corticosteroids, also are associated with this condition. Of the antibiotics, sulfonamides are most strongly associated with SJS/TEN; aminopenicillins, quinolones, cephalosporins, tetracyclines, and imidazole antifungals have also been identified (Dinulos, 2021; Jellinek-Cohen, 2021). Cutaneous manifestations typically appear within 1–4 weeks after starting the medication; within hours, the skin becomes painful.

Shortly before clinical skin manifestations (1–3 days), the patient may experience a phase of fever and malaise resembling a viral illness. Generalized erythema and macules initially appear on the trunk and then spread to the neck, face, and upper arms. The palms and soles can be affected. An irregularly shaped erythematous, dark-red, or purpuric macular rash typically develops, and the macules gradually coalesce. Mucosal manifestations may include sloughing of stratified epithelium in the upper respiratory tract, mouth, vagina, anal canal, and eyes. These mucosal lesions in conjunction with the macular rash are strongly suspicious of TEN (Dinulos, 2021; Jellinek-Cohen, 2021). As epidermal involvement progresses, the macular lesions take on a translucent gray hue that can occur either rapidly (hours) or over several days. As the epidermis necroses, it begins to separate from the dermis, and the macular lesions evolve into flaccid blisters. Slight thumb pressure applied to intact skin next to blisters causes the skin to wrinkle and slide laterally, which indicates a positive Nikolsky sign (top layers of skin slip away from lower layers when slightly rubbed). Although not specific to TEN, a positive Nikolsky sign is a hallmark sign for TEN (Dinulos, 2021; Jellinek-Cohen, 2021). Large sheets of skin are sloughed, exposing fragile, bleeding dermis.

Punch biopsies from the border of intact epidermis surrounding bullous lesions are needed to make the TEN diagnoses. Necrosis of the epidermis is an essential component in making the definitive diagnosis (Dinulos, 2021). The differential diagnosis for TEN includes distinction from SSSS, which is distinguished by skin biopsy, and GVHD of the skin, which is distinguished by history.

Treatment of the patient with TEN requires prompt cessation of suspicious medications and supportive care (Dinulos, 2021). The standard of care for the patient with TEN is transfer to a burn center to best manage the complex and life-threatening complications, such as temperature regulation, electrolyte disturbances, significant nutrition needs, and propensity to wound or skin infections (Jellinek-Cohen, 2021). Delay in transfer of patients to a burn center has been associated with increased mortality. In general, systemic corticosteroids are not recommended, enteral rather than parenteral nutrition is recommended, IV administration of immunoglobulin-G may be beneficial but should be sucrose free, empiric prophylactic antibiotics are not recommended, and ophthalmologic consultation to manage ocular manifestations of TEN is recommended (Jellinek-Cohen, 2021).

The goal of wound care is preventing infection so that the epithelial cells can resurface the exposed dermis. Sloughed epidermis can be debrided, but a temporary antimicrobial dressing or skin substitute (biologic or biosynthetic) should be applied to exfoliated areas; these are discussed in detail in Chapter 22. Sulfa-based topical antibiotics are contraindicated because sulfonamides are strongly associated with TEN.

Graft-vs-Host Disease

After allogeneic bone marrow transplantation (bone marrow from another individual), the transferred immunocompetent cells have the potential to produce a severe reaction in the transplant patient. Clinically, acute GVHD can occur early after transplantation (<100 days), after 100 days (late acute GVHD) or develop later to manifest with chronic GVHD (cGVHD) (Ghimire et al., 2017). Risk factors for chronic GVHD following hematopoietic stem cell transplantation include acute GVHD, chronic myeloid leukemia, age (>40 years), use of mismatched or unrelated donors, use of peripheral blood stem cells instead of bone marrow stem cells, and sex mismatch between recipient and donor (Saidu et al., 2020).

GVHD affects the skin, gut, and liver. It is a clinical diagnosis that cannot be confirmed by laboratory findings (Antin & Deeg, 2005). In the skin, cutaneous manifestations include a maculopapular rash that usually begins on the palms and then spreads to the face, arms, shoulders, and ears (see Plate 82). These manifestations may be asymptomatic, pruritic, or painful. In severe cases, generalized erythema, bullae, and desquamation may be present. GVHD may have the appearance of SSSS, a drug reaction, or TEN. A skin biopsy is beneficial to differentiate between these three possibilities (Antin & Deeg, 2005).

Treatment of GVHD requires a combination of immunosuppressant and antiviral medications. To stimulate adequate neutrophil levels with these treatment regimens, granulocyte colony-stimulating factor is also given. Topical wound care requires attention to infection control, maintenance of a physiologic wound environment, and pain management. Adhesive occlusive dressings are seldom desirable. Topical wound management should be determined collaboratively with input and discussion from the marrow transplantation team.

FROSTBITE

Frostbite is a cold-related injury resulting from prolonged exposure to subfreezing temperatures. Frostbite occurs when skin temperature drops below −0.5°C (Fudge, 2016). Skin can freeze at 28°F (−2°C) when no wind is present (Mohr, Jenabzadeh, & Ahrenholz, 2009). Wind decreases the amount of time required for skin to freeze. For example, exposed skin freezes within 1 h when the temperature is 0°F (−18°C) and the wind is 10 mph (Fudge, 2016). However, the skin will freeze in only 30 min at the same temperature when the wind is 20 mph. Therefore, heat loss is accelerated by wind speed, a concept known as *wind chill temperature*. A wind chill temperature of −40°F will result in tissue freezing within minutes (Mohr et al., 2009). In general, frostbite is a condition of morbidity, not mortality. However, when frostbite is combined with hypothermia or wound-related sepsis, death is possible.

Risk factors for frostbite are listed in Box 32.8. The majority of frostbite patients are male (80%), and 20% have been reported to be homeless (Mohr et al., 2009). Not all cold exposure results in tissue freezing (i.e., frostbite). The spectrum of cold injury is given in Table 32.8.

Extent of tissue damage is influenced by several factors: (1) susceptibility of specific body tissues to cold; (2) rate of cooling; (3) lowest tissue temperature achieved; (4) duration of cold exposure; (5) duration of ischemia; and (6) rewarming condition (Mohr et al., 2009). Although skin freezes more quickly with lower temperatures, the speed of freezing does not affect the degree of irreversible damage; rather, the extent of damage is related to the length of time the tissue remained frozen. Ultimately, tissue damage occurs as a result of tissue freezing and tissue reperfusion (Fudge, 2016).

When freezing is slow (as occurs with frostbite), *extra*cellular ice crystals are formed; when freezing is quick (as occurs

BOX 32.8   Risk Factors for Frostbite

- Intoxication (alcohol or drugs decrease awareness of cold and impair judgment; alcohol inhibits shivering and causes cutaneous vasodilation)
- Psychiatric illness (e.g., individuals with schizophrenia may have impaired ability to assess tissue cooling or comprehend cold injury)
- Neuropathy
- People who are inexperienced with or new to cold climates
- Homelessness
- Individuals stranded in the cold
- Cold-weather rescuers, soldiers, people who work in the cold
- Winter and high-altitude athletes
- Use of nicotine or other vasoconstrictive drugs
- Inadequate or constrictive clothing
- Underlying conditions (e.g., malnutrition, infection, peripheral vascular disease, atherosclerosis, arthritis, diabetes, thyroid disease, and previous cold injury)

TABLE 32.8   Spectrum of Cold Injury

Frostnip	Mild cold injury Completely reversible Skin pallor, numbness Typical on face, hands No ice crystal formation, no tissue damage Warmed tissue becomes hyperemic; decreased sensation or tingling may persist for weeks
Chilblain (Pernio)	Results from repeated exposure to near-freezing temperatures No ice crystal formation Skin has violaceous color with plaques or nodules May experience pain and pruritus with cold exposure Usually located on face, anterior lower leg, hands, feet
Frostbite	Occurs when tissues freeze slowly and form extracellular ice crystals Injuries are circumferential and progress distal to proximal Potentially reversible
Flash freeze	Extremely rapid cooling and formation of intracellular ice crystals Mechanism is contact with cold metals (handles) or volatile liquids Rapid onset, almost never circumferential

with flash freeze injury), *intra*cellular and *extra*cellular crystals are formed, and cells lyse. Flash freeze injuries occur after contact with cold surfaces or volatile liquids. Cellular damage, vascular injury, and resulting thrombosis are key mechanisms in the pathophysiologic process of frostbite injury (Twomey, Peltier, & Zera, 2005).

Rapid rewarming is recommended because it results in less irreversible damage to the tissue. Blood flow is restored quickly, without vasospasm or clot formation. Within 20 min, venous stasis develops and progresses retrograde through the capillary bed to the arterioles. When arterial inflow to the capillary bed is unchanged, edema develops. Rapid rewarming results in less irreversible damage to the extremity, despite the inevitable vascular permeability and edema (Mohr et al., 2009). During the ensuing reperfusion, the damaged endothelial lining of the affected blood vessels releases inflammatory mediators (prostaglandins, thromboxanes, bradykinin, and histamine) that cause additional edema formation. Ischemic injury to the affected tissue is progressive as a result of (1) capillary compression from increasing edema; (2) stagnation of blood in the vessels; (3) vessel occlusion caused by shedding of damaged endothelium into the blood vessels; and (4) thrombus formation due to the thrombogenic nature of the exposed basement membrane in blood vessels.

Within 6–24 h of rewarming, blisters develop due to the accumulation of extravasated fluid under the detached epidermis. Little or no fluid in the blister implies poor blood flow. Clear blister fluid contains high levels of prostaglandin and thromboxane, which result in vasoconstriction, leukocyte adherence, and platelet aggregation, factors known to intensify dermal ischemia. Blister fluid may also contain blood, which indicates the superficial dermis is damaged and thus more serious tissues damage has occurred than with a clear fluid blister.

Classification of Skin Injury

Initially frozen skin has the same appearance: cold, white, and firm to touch. The digits, ears, nose, and exposed facial skin are the most commonly injured. To classify the severity of the frostbite, the tissue must first thaw, and even then, the extent of skin damage will not be apparent for 10 days or more (Mohr et al., 2009). Frostbite injuries can be classified by degree of injury as defined in Table 32.9. Superficial frostbite includes first- and second-degree frostbite injuries, which generally heal. Deep frostbite includes third- and fourth-degree injuries, which are associated with tissue loss and chronic disability. Hemorrhagic bullae located proximally on the limb and distal tissue that remains cold, ischemic, and insensate are indicators of poor prognosis (Mohr et al., 2009).

Management of Frostbite

Similar to burns, treatment of frostbite may occur in a variety of health care settings. The phases or levels of care required for frostbite depend on the severity of the injury. Initial care generally is given at the location at which the injury occurs and addresses life-threatening conditions. Wet clothing should be replaced with dry, soft clothing to minimize further heat loss. The affected area should not be rubbed with warm hands due to risk for further injury. Alcohol or sedatives should not be given because they may enhance heat loss. Rewarming of the affected area should be initiated as soon as possible *unless* there is a danger of refreezing. If refreezing is a risk, get to shelter before attempting to rewarm at the scene. Walking on frostbitten feet can cause tissue chipping or fracture. The affected body part should be wrapped in a blanket for protection during transport.

TABLE 32.9	**Classification System for Frostbite Injury**
Degree of Injury	**Classification**
First	Superficial injury
	Intact sensation
	Normal to hyperemic skin color
	No blister formation on rewarming
	Transient mild burning, stinging, throbbing
	Desquamation but no tissue loss
Second	Superficial injury
	Edema may be substantial
	Blisters filled with clear or milky fluid within 24 h of injury
Third	Deep injury that results in hemorrhagic blister
	Blood-filled blisters that progress to black eschar over weeks
	Blisters are located deeper in dermis and more proximal
	Skin color is violaceous, soft, or boggy
	Does not blanch to palpation
	Initially no pain, then progresses to shooting, throbbing, and burning pain
Fourth	Results in full-thickness, cyanotic skin appearance
	Full-thickness damage affects muscles, tendons, bone
	Edema forms proximal, not distal, to involved area and becomes line of demarcation between viable tissue and full-thickness infarction
	Distal parts undergo mummification over weeks

BOX 32.9 Standard Protocol for Frostbite Care

- Rapid rewarming with water at 104–108°F (40–42°C)
- Tetanus prophylaxis
- Narcotic analgesics
- Ibuprofen
- Antibiotics
- Topical aloe vera
- Limb elevation
- No ambulation until edema resolved
- No smoking
- Daily hydrotherapy

Data from Mohr, W. J., Jenabzadeh, K., & Ahrenholz, D. H. (2009). Cold injury. *Hand Clinics, 25*(4), 481–496.

much tissue as possible, achieving maximal return of function, optimizing nutrition for healing, and preventing sepsis. Box 32.9 gives the standard protocol for frostbite care. Thrombolytic therapy is also used within 24 h postwarming to correct the underlying pathology (thrombi formation) leading to delayed tissue necrosis. The goals of topical wound care are maintaining a moist wound environment, protecting the skin from further cold-related damage, and reducing bacterial bioburden (Varnado, 2008). Light compression may be used to manage edema. Splints are indicated to maintain proper immobilization of limbs, and range-of-motion exercises prevent long-term contractures. Neuropathic pain is common and challenging to alleviate.

Emergency department care first addresses life-threatening conditions, such as fluid resuscitation, to enhance blood flow and tissue perfusion. Rapid rewarming of the affected body part is attempted using water or wet packs at 40–42°C with a mild antibacterial soap. Warmer temperatures or dry heat should be avoided due to risk for thermal injury. Thawing usually takes 20–40 min and is complete when the distal tip of the affected area blanches with pressure. Associated dislocations are reduced as soon as thawing is complete. Fractures are managed conservatively until postthaw edema has resolved. The only indication for early surgical intervention is debridement of necrotic tissue and fasciotomy in the case of compartment syndrome. Hemorrhagic blisters are left intact to reduce risk of infection in the injured extremity (Mohr et al., 2009). Once thawed, the injury is kept in sterile nonadherent dressings, elevated, and splinted when possible. Clear fluid blisters usually are aspirated to remove the prostaglandins and thromboxane and thus prevent further dermal damage.

Weeks can pass before frostbitten tissue demarcates to reveal viable and nonviable tissue. Therefore, any decision about amputation should be delayed as long as possible. The goals of management for frostbite include salvaging as

MARJOLIN'S ULCER

Marjolin's ulcer (MU) is a rare but aggressive malignant transformation of scar or chronic wound that arises after a long-term chronic inflammatory or traumatic assaults. Conversion to a malignancy is a slow process, often more than 10 years after initial injury up to a mean of 21 years (Yu et al., 2013). The risk of malignancy increases with the length of time the presence of the scar or ulcer. Of chronic wounds, it is estimated that 1.7% will undergo malignant degeneration to develop SCC. Marjolin first described chronic ulcers arising from burn wounds (Iqbal, Sinha, & Jaffe, 2015). This malignant transformation has subsequently been observed in venous ulcers, pressure injuries, anal fistulae, sinus tracts secondary to osteomyelitis, and scar tissue. Among trauma patients, burn patients are at the highest risk for malignant transformation of chronic wounds. Marjolin's ulcers with SCC are more aggressive and have higher recurrence and metastatic rates compared with SCC that is not a Marjolin's ulcer (Iqbal et al., 2015). MUs have a malodorous exudate and can be mistaken for infection.

Any clinical cause for suspicion, such as raised borders, unusual wound base, chronic exposure to trauma/friction, unexplained pain, changes in scar shape or color, previous history, or family history of skin cancer, requires referral for biopsy. Ulcers or lesions that do not respond to optimal therapy also warrant a referral for biopsy (Yu et al., 2013).

TABLE 32.10 **Characteristics of Skin Lesions With Blood Dyscrasias**

Blood Dyscrasia	Pathology	Ulcer Characteristics	Treatment
Sickle cell anemia	Sickled blood cells are rigid May clump together, occluding microcirculation Damage to endothelium leads to thrombus formation Altered vasomotor response can lead to rise in capillary pressure and edema formation	Exact etiology of ulceration is unclear Located on lower leg near malleolus May be single or multiple Can range significantly in size Ulcers are well defined, vary in depth, have raised borders Tend to heal slowly High recurrence rate	Control of edema (compression therapy and/or bed rest) Systemic management of underlying disease process (address anemia either pharmacologically or by transfusion) Debridement Prevention of infection Protection from trauma Pain management Moist wound healing (e.g., with hydrocolloids)
Thalassemia	Microcytic anemia common in people of Mediterranean descent	Etiology related to decreased hemoglobin and increased iron loading, making patients more susceptible to trauma	Blood transfusions and iron chelation therapy Topical care based on wound needs and moist wound healing principles Emphasis on insulating wound to prevent hypothermia Protect wound from further trauma

Biopsy technique is critical to cancer detection. It is recommended that wounds be biopsied from multiple sites (i.e., at 12, 6, 3, and 9 o'clock positions) and from multiple depths (e.g., 2, 4, and 6 mm). The biopsy sites should be recorded because rebiopsy is indicated if the wound does not respond as expected to treatment (Snyder, 2006).

BLOOD DYSCRASIAS

Two types of blood dyscrasias may lead to chronic leg ulceration: sickle cell anemia and thalassemia. Their etiologies, ulcer characteristics, and treatments are summarized in Table 32.10.

CLINICAL CONSULT

A: A wound consult is received for a 36-year-old female breast cancer patient with a chemotherapy extravasation of Adriamycin that occurred 5 days earlier. Intravenous administration was immediately stopped when the patient reported stinging and pain in the IV site followed by an inability to obtain a blood return in the IV tubing. Initial care consisted of withdrawing residual chemotherapy, applying ice to the site, and site monitoring. A soft, boggy, necrotic tissue area began developing at the site during the first week. Currently extravasation site on right forearm is erythematous extending 5 cm from puncture site with central island of soft adherent gray-black necrosis measuring 4 cm × 3 cm. Lower arm slightly edematous. Recent WBC in normal limits. Patient reports she has good appetite and is meeting her protein intake needs.

D: Vesicant extravasation resulting from Adriamycin.

P: Implement moist wound therapy with hydrogel to wound bed to aid in autolysis. Monitor closely to reassess erythema and effectiveness of autolysis. Call clinic if erythema increases in intensity or dimension. Will consider adding antimicrobial if erythema persists. Revise topical dressing as wound conditions change following autolysis and consider CTPs as needed for closure.

I: (1) Apply skin protectant around wound bed. (2) Trim hydrogel sheet to size of wound and place over wound. Cover with a nonadherent dressing and secure with roll gauze or nonadherent wrap. (3) Patient instructed to keep arm at chest level to reduce edema and protect wound from pressure, trauma, and extremes in temperature.

E: Return to monitor autolysis in 4 days.

SUMMARY

- Although the wound specialist is not expected to be proficient in the overall care of patients with the unusual pathologies described in this chapter, the management of the resulting complex cutaneous wounds requires astute observation, close monitoring, and adherence to the principles of wound healing.

- As with other chronic wounds, the goals of treatment for these types of wounds range from healing to palliation to symptom management.

- Collaboration with the multidisciplinary team (medical staff, surgeons, nursing staff, physical therapy, and dietitians) is essential to identify these rare complications early during onset and implement interventions that are timely and appropriate to minimize tissue damage and maximize healing.

SELF-ASSESSMENT QUESTIONS

1. A condition in which the skin develops superficial blistering and a sandpaper feel and exfoliates after exposure to bacterial toxins is known as:
   a. toxic epidermis necrosis (TEN)
   b. epidermolysis bullosa
   c. staphylococcal scalded skin syndrome (SSSS)
   d. calciphylaxis

2. General signs and symptoms of vasculitis include which of the following?
   a. Sandpaper feel to skin
   b. Severe pruritus
   c. Fever and arthralgias
   d. Mental confusion and imbalance

3. The extent of irreversible tissue damage due to frostbite is primarily influenced by which of the following?
   a. Lowest tissue temperature achieved
   b. Rewarming process
   c. Body part that is involved
   d. Speed with which skin froze

REFERENCES

Aggarwal, S. (2012). Recognition and management of pyoderma gangrenosum. *Dermatology, 22*(5), 26–30.

Ahronowitz, I., Harp, J., & Shinkai, K. (2012). Etiology and management of pyoderma gangrenosum: A comprehensive review. *American Journal of Clinical Dermatology, 13*(3), 191–211.

Alavi, A., Mayer, D., Hafner, J., et al. (2012). Martorell hypertensive ischemic leg ulcer: An underdiagnosed entity. *Advances in Skin & Wound Care, 25*(12), 563–572.

Anaya, D. A., & Dellinger, E. P. (2007). Surgical infections and choice of antibiotics. In C. M. Townsend Jr., R. D. Beauchamp, B. M. Evers, et al. (Eds.), *Sabiston textbook of surgery* (18th ed., p. 2152). Philadelphia: Saunders.

Anderson, I. (2008). Mixed aetiology: Complexity and comorbidity in leg ulceration. *The British Journal of Nursing, 17*(15), S17–S23.

Antin, J. H., & Deeg, H. J. (2005). Clinical spectrum of acute graft-vs-host disease. In J. F. Ferrara, K. R. Cooke, & H. J. Deeg (Eds.), *Graft-vs-host disease* (3rd ed.). New York: Marcel Dekker.

Armitage, M., & Roberts, J. (2004). Caring for patients with leg ulcers and an underlying vasculitic condition. *British Journal of Community Nursing*, (Suppl), S16–S22.

Arnold, T. C. (2021). *Spider envenomation, brown recluse.* http://www.emedicine.com/DERM/topic598.htm. Accessed November 13, 2021.

Attinger, C. E., Janis, J. E., Steinberg, J., et al. (2006). Clinical approach to wounds: Debridement and wound bed preparation including the use of dressings and wound-healing adjuvants. *Plastic and Reconstructive Surgery, 117*(Suppl. 7), S72–S109.

Bajaj, R., Courbebaisse, M., Kroshinsky, D., Thadhani, R. I., & Nigwekar, S. U. (2018). Calciphylaxis in patients with normal renal function: A case series and systematic review. *Mayo Clinic Proceedings, 93*(9), 1202–1212.

Caldeira, M. B., Pestana, M., João, A. L., Fernandes, C., João, A., & Cunha, N. (2021). Retiform purpura and extensive skin necrosis as the single manifestation of SARS-CoV-2 infection. *European Academy of Dermatology and Venereology.* https://doi.org/10.1111/jdv.17562.

Callen, J. P., & Jackson, J. M. (2007). Pyoderma gangrenosum: An update. *Rheumatic Diseases Clinics of North America, 33,* 787–802.

Criado, P. R., Abdalla, B. M. Z., de Assis, I. C., de Graaff Mello, C. B., Caputo, G. C., & Vierira, I. C. (2020). Are the cutaneous manifestations during or due to SARS-CoV-2 infection/COVID-19 frequent or not? Revision of possible pathophysiologic mechanisms. *Inflammation Research, 69,* 745–756.

Dinulos, J. G. H. (Ed.). (2021). *Habif's clinical dermatology. A color guide to diagnosis and therapy* (7th ed.). St. Louis: Elsevier.

Ener, R. A., Meglathery, S. B., & Styler, M. (2004). Extravasation of systemic hemato-oncological therapies. *Annals of Oncology, 15,* 858–862.

Fine, J. D. (2016). Epidemiology of inherited epidermolysis bullosa based on incidence and prevalence estimates from the National Epidermolysis Bullosa Registry. *JAMA Dermatology, 152,* 1231–1238.

Fine, J. D., Bruckner-Tuderman, L., Eady, R. A., et al. (2014). Inherited epidermolysis bullosa: Updated recommendations on diagnosis and classification. *Journal of the American Academy of Dermatology, 70*(6), 1103–1126.

Freeman, E. E., McMahon, D. E., Lipoff, J. B., Rosenbach, M., Kovarik, C., Desai, S. R., et al. (2020). The spectrum of COVID-19-associated dermatologic manifestations: An international registry of 716 patients from 31 countries. *Journal of the American Academy of Dermatology, 83*(4), 1118–1129.

Fudge, J. (2016). Exercise in the cold: Preventing and managing hypothermia and frostbite injury. *Sports Health, 8*(2), 133–139.

Ghimire, S., Weber, D., Mavin, E., Wan, X. N., Dickinson, A. M., & Holler, E. (2017). Pathophysiology of GvHD and other HSCT-related major complications. *Frontiers in Immunology, 8,* 79. https://doi.org/10.3389/fimmu.2017.00079.

Gorski, L. A., Hadaway, L., Hagle, M. E., Broadhurst, D., Clare, S., Kleidon, R., et al. (2021). Infusion therapy standards of practice, 8th Edition. *Journal of Infusion Nursing, 44*(1S), S1–S204.

Habif, T. P., Campbell, J. L., Jr., Chapman, M. S., et al. (2005). *Skin disease: Diagnosis and treatment* (2nd ed.). St. Louis: Mosby.

Has, C., Bauer, J. Q., Bodemer, C., Bolling, M. C., Bruckner-Tuderman, L., Diem, A., et al. (2020). Consensus reclassification of inherited epidermolysis bullosa and other disorders with skin fragility. *The British Journal of Dermatology, 183*(4), 614–627.

Hunter, J. A. A., et al. (2002). *Clinical dermatology*. Oxford: Blackwell Science.

Iqbal, F. M., Sinha, Y., & Jaffe, W. (2015). Marjolin's ulcer: A rare entity with a call for early diagnosis. *BML Case Reports*. https://doi.org/10.1136/bcr-2014-208176.

Jellinek-Cohen, S. (2021). *Toxic epidermal necrolysis (TEN)*. Medscape. https://emedicine.medscape.com/article/229698-overview. Accessed November 6, 2021.

Jennette, J., & Falk, R. (1997). Small-vessel vasculitis. *The New England Journal of Medicine, 337*(21), 1512–1523.

Jeyakumari, D., Gopal, R., Eswaran, M., et al. (2009). Staphylococcal scalded skin syndrome in a newborn. *Journal of Global Infectious Diseases, 1*(1), 45–47.

Kim, J. T., Park, J. Y., Lee, H. J., & Cheon, Y. J. (2020). Guidelines for the management of extravasation. *Journal of Educational Evaluation for Health Professions, 17*(21). https://doi.org/10.3352/jeehp.2020.17.21.

King, R. W., Carone, H. L., & de Saint Victor, P. R. (2019). *Staphylococcal scalded skin syndrome*. http://emedicine.medscape.com/article/788199-overview. Accessed November 13, 2021.

Klejtman, T. (2020). Skin and COVID-19. *Journal de Médecine Vasculaire, 45*, 175–176.

Kreidieh, F. Y., Moukadem, H. A., & Saghir, N. S. E. (2016). Overview, prevention and management of chemotherapy extravasation. *World Journal of Clinical Oncology, 10*(7), 87–97.

Malabu, U. H., Manickam, V., Kan, G., et al. (2012). Calcific uremic arteriolopathy on multimodal combination therapy: Still unmet goal. *International Journal of Nephrology, 2012*, 390768.

Mansour, M., & Alavi, A. (2019). Martorell ulcer: Chronic wound management and rehabilitation. *Chronic Wound Care Management and Research, 6*, 83–88.

Mariath, L. M., Santin, J. T., Schuler-Faccini, L., & Kiszewski, A. E. (2020). Inherited epidermolysis bullosa: Update on the clinical and genetic aspects. *Anais Brasileiros de Dermatologia, 95*, 551–569.

Martin, D. A., Nanci, G. N., Marlowe, S. I., et al. (2008). Necrotizing fasciitis with no mortality or limb loss. *The American Surgeon, 74*(9), 809–812.

Mazzone, L., & Schiestl, C. (2013). Management of septic skin necroses. *European Journal of Pediatric Surgery, 23*(5), 349–358.

McBride, J. D., Narang, J., Simonds, R., Agrawal, S., Rodriquez, E. R., Tan, C. D., et al. (2020). Development of sacral/buttock retiform purpura as an ominous presenting sign of COVID-19 and clinical and histopathologic evolution during severe disease course. *Journal of Cutaneous Pathology, 48*, 1166–1172.

McCarthy, J. T., El-Azhary, R. A., Patzelt, M. T., et al. (2016). Survival, risk factors, and effect of treatment in 101 patients with calciphylaxis. *Mayo Clinic Proceedings, 91*(10), 1384–1394.

Mohr, W. J., Jenabzadeh, K., & Ahrenholz, D. H. (2009). Cold injury. *Hand Clinics, 25*(4), 481–496.

Nigwekar, S. U., Thadhani, R., & Brandenburg, V. M. (2018). Calciphylaxis. *The New England Journal of Medicine, 378*(18), 1704–1714.

Paparone, P. P., Paparone, P. W., & Paparone, P. (2009). Post-traumatic pyoderma gangrenosum. *Wounds, 21*(4), 89–94.

Park, J. R. C., Choi, J. R., Song, J. Y., et al. (2014). Necrotizing fasciitis of the thigh secondary to radiation colitis in a rectal cancer patient. *Journal of the Korean Society of Coloproctology, 28*(6), 325–329.

Poulsen, V. O. B., Nielsen, J., & Poulsen, T. D. (2013). Rapidly developing toxic epidermal necrolysis. *Case Reports in Emergency Medicine, 2013*, 985951.

Radic, M., Kaliterna, D. M., & Radic, J. (2012). Drug induced vasculitis: A clinical and pathological review. *The Netherlands Journal of Medicine, 70*(1), 12–17.

Rahimi, H., & Tehranchinia, Z. (2020). A comprehensive review of cutaneous manifestations associated with COVID-19. *BioMed Research International, 2020*. https://doi.org/10.1155/2020/1236520.

Ratnagobal, S., & Sinha, S. (2013). Pyoderma gangrenosum: Guideline for wound practitioners. *Journal of Wound Care, 22*(2), 68–73.

Reguiaï, A., & Grange, F. (2007). Therapy in pyoderma gangrenosum associated with inflammatory bowel disease. *American Journal of Clinical Dermatology, 8*(2), 67–77.

Rhoads, J. (2007). Epidemiology of the brown recluse spider bite. *Journal of the American Academy of Nurse Practitioners, 19*(2), 79–85.

Rose, A. E., Saggar, V., Boyd, K. P., Patel, R. R., & McLellan, B. (2013). Case presentation: Liveo retiularis. *Dermatology Online Journal, 19*(12), 1. Available at https://escholarship.org/uc/item/4rk7z79h. Accessed November 14, 2021.

Rubano, J., & Kerstein, M. (1998). Arterial insufficiency and vasculitides. *Journal of Wound, Ostomy, and Continence Nursing, 25*(3), 147.

Ruocco, E., Sangiuliano, S., Gravina, A. G., et al. (2009). Pyoderma gangrenosum: An updated review. *Journal of the European Academy of Dermatology and Venereology, 23*, 1008–1017.

Saidu, N. E. B., Bonini, C., Dickinson, A., Grce, M., Inngjerdingen, M., Koehl, U., et al. (2020). New approaches for the treatment of chronic graft-versus-host disease: Current status and future directions. *Frontiers in Immunology, 11*, 5758314. https://doi.org/10.3389/fimmu.2020.578314.

Seitz, C. S., Berens, N., Bröcker, E. B., et al. (2010). Leg ulceration in rheumatoid arthritis—An underreported multicausal complication with considerable morbidity: Analysis of thirty-six patients and review of the literature. *Dermatology, 220*, 268–273.

Shinkuma, S. (2015). Dystrophic epidermolysis bullosa: A review. *Clinical, Cosmetic and Investigational Dermatology, 8*, 275–284.

Singh, H., Kaur, H., Singh, K., & Sem, C. K. (2021). Cutaneous manifestations of COVID-19: A systematic review. *Advances in Wound Care, 10*(2), 50–80.

Snyder, R. (2006). Skin cancers and chronic wounds. In R. Norman (Ed.), *Handbook of geriatric dermatology*. New York: Cambridge University Press.

Snyder, R. J. (2008). "Immunopathic" ulcers. *Podiatry Management*, 185–188.

Tang, J. C., Vivas, A., Rey, A., et al. (2012). Atypical ulcers: Wound biopsy results from a university wound pathology service. *Ostomy/Wound Management, 58*(6), 20–29.

Twomey, J. A., Peltier, G. L., & Zera, R. T. (2005). An open-label study to evaluate the safety and efficacy of tissue plasminogen activator in treatment of severe frostbite. *The Journal of Trauma, 59*, 1350–1355.

Udomkarnjananun, S., Kongnatthasate, K., Praditpornsilpa, K., Eiam-Ong, S., Jaber, B. L., & Susantitaphong, P. (2019). Treatment of calciphylaxis in CKD: A systematic review and meta-analysis. *Kidney International Reports, 4*, 231–244. https://doi.org/10.1016/j.ekir.2018.10.002.

Varnado, M. (2008). Frostbite. *Journal of Wound, Ostomy, and Continence Nursing, 35*(3), 341–346.

Vyas, J. M. (2020). *Toxic shock syndrome.* http://www.nlm.nih.gov/medlineplus/ency/article/000653.htm. Accessed November 13, 2021.

Watkins, J. (2016). Diagnosis, treatment and management of epidermolysis bullosa. *The British Journal of Nursing, 25*(8), 428–431.

Wollina, U. (2007). Pyoderma gangrenosum—A review. *Orphanet Journal of Rare Diseases, 2,* 19.

Wollina, U. (2013). Update on cutaneous calciphylaxis. *Indian Dermatology, 58*(2):87–92

Yu, N., Long, X., Lujan-Hernandez, J. R., Hassan, K. Z., Bai, M., Wang, Y., et al. (2013). Marjolin's ulcer: A preventable malignancy arising from scars. *World Journal of Surgical Oncology, 11,* 313. http://www.wsjo.com/content/11/1/313.

Zeglin, D. (2005). Brown recluse spider bites. *The American Journal of Nursing, 105*(2), 64–68.

FURTHER READING

Alcoser, P. W., & Burchett, S. (1999). Bone marrow transplantation: Immune system suppression and reconstitution. *The American Journal of Nursing, 99*(6), 26–31.

Alexander, S. (2009). Malignant fungating wounds: Key symptoms and psychosocial issues. *Journal of Wound Care, 18*(8), 325–329.

Bazalinski, D., Przybek-Mita, J., Baranska, B., & Wiech, P. (2017). Marjolin's ulcer in chronic wounds—Review of available literature. *Contemporary Oncology, 21*(3), 197–202.

Chand, S., Rrapi, R., Lo, J. A., Song, S., Gabel, C. K., Desai, N., et al. (2021). Purpuric ulcers associated with COVID-19: A case series. *Journal of the American Academy of Dermatology Case Reports, 11,* 13–19.

Endorf, F. E., Cancio, L. C., & Gibran, N. S. (2008). Toxic epidermal necrolysis clinical guidelines. *Journal of Burn Care & Research, 29*(5), 706–712.

Ethridge, R. T., et al. (2007). Wound healing. In C. M. Townsend Jr., R. D. Beauchamp, B. M. Evers, et al. (Eds.), *Sabiston textbook of surgery* (18th ed.). Philadelphia: Saunders.

Ferrara, J. F., et al. (Eds.). (2005). *Graft-vs-host disease* (3rd ed.). New York: Marcel Dekker.

Hanley, J. (2011). Effective management of peristomal pyoderma gangrenosum. *The British Journal of Nursing, 20*(7), S12–S17.

Murphy, J. V., Banwell, P. E., Roberts, A. H., et al. (2000). Frostbite: Pathogenesis and treatment. *The Journal of Trauma, 48,* 171–178.

Pillay, E. (2008). Epidermolysis bullosa. Part 1: Causes, presentation and complications. *The British Journal of Nursing, 17*(5), 292–296.

Ringden, O. (2005). Introduction to graft-versus-host disease. *Biology of Blood and Marrow Transplantation, 11*(Suppl. 2), 17–20.

Schober-Flores, C. (2003). Epidermolysis bullosa: The challenges of wound care. *Dermatology Nursing, 15*(2), 135–138. 141–144.

Schulmeister, L. (2009). Vesicant chemotherapy extravasation antidotes and treatments. *Clinical Journal of Oncology Nursing, 13*(4), 395–398.

Smith, L. H. (2007). Toxic epidermal necrolysis. *Clinical Journal of Oncology Nursing, 11*(3), 333–336.

Smith, L. H. (2009). National patient safety goal #13: Patients' active involvement in their own care: Preventing chemotherapy extravasation. *Clinical Journal of Oncology Nursing, 13*(2), 233–234.

Snyder, R. J., Stillman, R. M., & Weiss, S. D. (2003). Epidermoid cancers that masquerade as venous ulcer disease. *Ostomy/Wound Management, 49*(4), 63–66.

Sullivan, K. M. (1999). Graft-versus-host disease. In E. D. Thomas, et al. (Eds.), *Hematopoietic cell transplantation* (2nd ed.). Malden, MA: Blackwell Science.

Thomas, E. D., et al. (1999). *Hematopoietic cell transplantation* (2nd ed.). Malden: Blackwell Science.

Trent, J. T., Kirsner, R. S., Romanelli, P., et al. (2004). Use of SCORTEN to accurately predict mortality in patients with toxic epidermal necrolysis in the United States. *Archives of Dermatology, 140,* 890–892.

Vujinovich, A. (2005). Clinical treatment options for peristomal pyoderma gangrenosum. *The British Journal of Nursing, 14*(16), S4–S8.

Wickham, R., Engelking, C., Sauerland, C., et al. (2006). Vesicant extravasation part II: Evidence-based management and continuing controversies. *Oncology Nursing Forum, 33*(6), 1143–1150.

Wickham, R., et al. (2007). Letters to the editor. Readers share comments and questions about extravasation management. *Oncology Nursing Forum, 34*(2), 275–280.

Wong, S. L., Schneider, A. M., Argenta, L. C., et al. (2010). Loxoscelism and negative pressure wound therapy (vacuum-assisted closure): An experimental study. *International Wound Journal, 7,* 488–492.

33

Traumatic Wounds: Bullets, Blasts, and Vehicle Crashes

Rex E. Atwood, Matthew J. Bradley, and Eric A. Elster

OBJECTIVES

1. Identify common mechanisms and patterns of war wounds.
2. Describe critical components of acute management of traumatic wounds.
3. List important considerations in the initial assessment of a traumatic wound.
4. Define compartment syndrome.

INTRODUCTION

Traumatic wounds result from any blunt or penetrating impact that results in tissue damage. Their etiology can vary widely: bullet or projectile wounds, blasts, industrial accidents, falls, and car crashes. Modern care for the trauma patient has its origins in military medicine. Practices developed to treat war injuries have been modified and refined to address civilian trauma. War injuries tend to be exaggerations of civilian injuries. For example, bullets fired from common military firearms such as the M16/M4 (5.56 mm/0.223) or AK-47 (7.62 mm/0.308) cause significantly more damage than common civilian pistols firing 0.22 and 0.45 caliber bullets, even though the mechanism is largely the same. For this reason, this chapter emphasizes treatment of war wounds. Although the severity of injury may be different, the principles guiding wound care remain the same. Box 33.1 lists the components of traumatic wound care.

ETIOLOGY OF WAR WOUNDS

Weapon-related injuries are of two basic types: those resulting from small arms fire and those resulting from explosive munitions. Small arms fire includes pistols, rifles, shotguns, and machine guns. Explosive munitions include mines, grenades, mortars, missiles, bombs, and improvised explosive devices (IEDs). The primary mechanism of injury among US troops has changed dramatically over the years. Gunshot wounds, which comprised nearly 30% of injuries in Vietnam, now only account for 25% (Champion et al., 2010). In comparison, blasts, which accounted for 60% in Vietnam, comprised the lion's share in Operation Enduring Freedom, accounting for nearly three-quarters of the injuries (Kelly et al., 2008). Regardless of the mechanism of injury, extremity wounds have comprised the majority of wounds among US and UK soldiers since World War I, followed by head and neck, thoracic, and abdominal injuries (Cubano et al., 2018). Blast injuries characteristically injure multiple organ systems, resulting in elevated Injury Severity Scores (ISS). The ISS was developed in 1974 as a way to quantify the injury burden in patients with multiple injury sites (Baker, O'Neill, Haddon, & Long, 1974). The formula breaks the body down into six areas and assigns a score of 1–6 to each of the sites. The scores from the three most injured sites are then squared and summed to provide the total ISS. Interestingly, the Case Fatality Rate (CFR), a measure of the overall lethality of a conflict, has fallen over subsequent conflicts despite increasingly more powerful firepower (Holcomb, Stansbury, Champion, Wade, & Bellamy, 2006). The mortality rate has fallen from its peak in World War II at 30% down to 25% in Vietnam. A recent review of casualties in Iraq and Afghanistan from 2001 to 2017 revealed a case fatality rate of 8.6% and 10.1%, respectively, in the latter half of the war (Howard et al., 2019.) Ongoing improvement in the care for wounded service members in the conflicts of the 21st century was largely supported by the Joint Trauma System, frequently creating and updating clinical practice guidelines relevant to traumatically injured patients. Multiple clinical practice guidelines are relevant for wound care, including amputation, compartment syndrome, and wound debridement and irrigation are available (Joint Trauma System Clinical Practice Guidelines, 2020).

Bullet Wounds

Small arms fire a projectile (aka, a bullet) at an object. When in motion, a projectile compresses the air in front of it and creates a shockwave. The shockwave contacts an object before the projectile. The overpressure of the initial shockwave, followed by the vacuum after it dissipates, can injure hollow viscera, such as the lungs, bowel, and eardrums. The shockwave also can knock a victim against surrounding objects, causing additional trauma. However, the shockwave is not known to cause direct injury to solid tissue.

BOX 33.1   Components of Traumatic Wound Care

- Stabilization of injured patient via Advanced Trauma Life Support (ATLS) protocol is first step in traumatic wound care.
- Wound treatment is same regardless of etiology, although etiology may help practitioner discover concurrent occult injuries.
- Blood vessels, nerves, and bones must be covered with soft tissue if exposed in a wound to prevent further injury.
- Surgical debridement, irrigation, and negative pressure therapy using vacuum-assisted closure repeated every 48–72 h until wound closure or coverage are the hallmarks of traumatic wound care.
- Negative pressure dressings facilitate healing, decrease patient stress, and reduce provider time commitments.
- Optimizing the wound base includes reducing bacterial load and improving blood supply.
- Wound closure may occur through a variety of techniques based on size and location. Techniques for soft tissue wounds include primary closure, delayed primary closure, secondary intention, muscle and fasciocutaneous flaps, skin grafting, and skin substitutes.
- Techniques to close open abdominal wounds (used alone or in combination) include primary fascial closure, delayed fascial closure, component separation, planned ventral hernia, and serial abdominal closure.
- Systemic disease, the inflammatory response, and poor nutrition adversely affect wound closure; normalization of physiology, provision of adequate nutrition, and treatment of local or systemic infection are integral parts of wound healing.
- Chronic wounds are treated by converting the wound to an acute wound and treating it accordingly.
- Amputation is necessary for limb injuries when limb salvage is impossible, treatment of life-threatening injuries precludes prompt treatment of severe limb injuries, and limb ischemia time exceeds 6 h.
- Tetanus vaccination should be standard practice for all patients with traumatic wounds.

Upon contact with tissue, a projectile creates two cavities: a permanent cavity and a temporary cavity. The temporary cavity is much larger than the permanent cavity. The temporary cavity is the effect of the transmitted energy on elastic tissue such as muscle, fat, and connective tissue. The temporary cavity expands and then rebounds, leaving only the permanent cavity. Nonelastic tissue, such as bone, will fracture secondary to the temporary cavity (Cubano et al., 2018).

Two additional aspects of bullets cause further damage. When traveling through tissue, bullets can fragment after several centimeters. This increases the diameter of the injured tissue beyond the diameter of the bullet. Bullets also yaw, or tumble, which greatly increases the damage by a round. While the principle determinant of a bullet's energy is its velocity, yaw and fragmentation more heavily influence the amount of damage inflicted (Cubano et al., 2018). Common misconceptions regarding bullets are that bullets yaw in flight (they spin around their long axis, like a football), that bullets with a full metal jacket do not fragment (the jacket often peels back to expose a softer core), and that exit wounds are larger than entrance wounds (either wound can be predominant).

Explosive Munitions (Ballistic, Blast, and Thermal)

Explosive munitions come in a large variety and inflict damage in multiple ways. The three types of damage inflicted by most explosive munitions are ballistic, blast, and thermal. Depending on a person's distance from an explosion, they can be exposed to any or all of these elements.

Ballistic injuries can be sustained far away from the blast and are caused by flying fragments, whether it is the shell casing of a grenade, the ball bearings in an antipersonnel bomb, or the random dirt and debris from the area near an explosion. Different weapons are designed to propel fragments of different masses and velocities. Most explosive munitions have been designed to disperse fragments evenly. However, some weapons are shaped to fire fragments in a particular direction.

Blast injuries are caused by the sonic shockwave produced by the explosion. The shockwave typically has a much smaller range than ballistic damage. As with bullets, the shockwave can inflict damage to hollow organs, which can present occultly without evidence of external trauma. The mechanism for this primary blast injury is due to the speed of the blast wave propagating through tissues of different density and compressibility. Fluid-containing organs, such as the bowel and lungs, are the most susceptible to this primary blast wave. Explosions produce a much larger shockwave than bullets. Therefore, injuries resulting from a body being thrown against an object are much more common.

Thermobaric devices are designed to cause much larger shockwaves. During the initial explosion, these devices disperse a volatile substance such as fuel vapor. The fuel vapor then ignites and produces a longer and more powerful secondary explosion. This technology is frequently used in "bunker-busting" devices (Buchanan, 2006). When explosives are detonated in a confined space (such as a building, bunker, or armored vehicle), the primary blast wave can reflect off hard surfaces and back toward the intended target, intensifying the effect of the blast.

Thermal injuries of varying thickness are the third type of injury inflicted by a blast. This damage is done in close proximity to the explosion. Thermal injuries can be either from direct exposure to the heat generated by the explosives or by interaction with the burning explosives that may be blown on or into the patient. Significant thermal injures compound the difficulty in caring for traumatically injured patients, given the metabolic response to burn injury and are a significant source of increased morbidity and mortality (Levi, Hemmila, & Wang, 2016). Burn wounds require specific treatment as discussed in Chapter 34.

Different types of explosive munitions have been developed for different uses. There are a wide variety of grenades. Fragmentary grenades are antipersonnel tools that inflict injuries primarily through ballistic damage. Concussion grenades are designed to inflict blast damage. An incendiary grenade disperses hot chemicals to cause thermal injuries.

Three types of antipersonnel land mines predominate. *Static* land mines are planted and activated when stepped on. These mines commonly result in traumatic amputations, usually (but not exclusively) to the lower extremities along with various degrees of fragmentation injury to the pelvis, abdomen, and perineum, creating the so-called *dismounted IED injury pattern* that has characterized the conflicts in Iraq and Afghanistan (Cannon et al., 2016; Singleton, Gibb, Hunt, Bull, & Clasper, 2013). Further injury is caused by the contaminants that are driven up between fascial planes. This results in treatment regimens that center on serial operative debridement; a practice that brings substantial discomfort to both patient and family, and significantly increases overall morbidity and hospital length of stay. *Bounding* land mines bounce 1–2 m after being stepped upon. They then spray fragments, which enable them to injure multiple targets simultaneously. *Horizontal spray* land mines propel fragments in one direction and typically are remotely or tripwire activated.

Several types of antiarmor devices exist. A shaped charge is designed to direct an explosion at a target. Two types of fragments can injure people in an armored vehicle: fragments from the charge and spall, which is debris knocked off the armor plating. Rocket-propelled grenades (RPGs) and tube-launched, optically tracked, wire-guided (TOW) missiles are two types of shaped charges. An explosively formed projectile (EFP) is a specialized shaped charge that has been used by insurgents in Iraq. Kinetic energy rounds are aerodynamically shaped pieces of metal, usually depleted uranium or tungsten. Two common types of kinetic energy rounds are armor-piercing, fin-stabilized, discarding sabots (APFSDS) and high-explosive, antitank (HEAT) shells. Antitank mines are similar to land mines except the former are more powerful and are designed to disable vehicles. In Iraq and Afghanistan, the most common antitank mine is the IED or roadside bomb. These blasts transfer large amounts of energy through the floor to the occupants, resulting in characteristic injuries to the lower extremities, spine, and head (Ramasamy et al., 2011). Coalition forces have mitigated these effects through several vehicular improvements, such as adding V-shaped hulls, reinforcing floorboards, and adding passenger restraints.

Any of these explosive mechanisms have the ability to propel fragments deep into the patient. While most bullets are made of lead (Pb), they may be a wide variety of different metal types present within a patient with significant fragmentation injuries. In most cases, fragments are removed if they are easily accessible at the time of debridement or other operations but are otherwise not disturbed out of concern for worsening the injury. However, recent evidence has shown an association with high blood levels of lead in patients with significant retained fragment burden (Apte, Bradford, Dente, & Smith, 2019). This has led certain centers to obtain a baseline CT scan to determine the volume of metal fragments and to refer these patients for frequent hematologic and lead labs (Nickel, Steelman, Sabath, & Potter, 2018).

Vehicle Crashes

Vehicle crashes are yet another type of injury. Although some soft tissue injury may be due to penetrating trauma, much of the damage sustained is due to blunt trauma. Closed head injuries, fractures, cardiac contusions, pneumothoraces, spinal cord injuries, and spleen and liver injuries typically result from blunt trauma. Most of these blunt injuries are deceleration injuries. Organs in hollow cavities (brain, heart, and abdominal viscera) are injured by contacting soft tissue or shearing off of relatively fixed ligaments and vessels. Traumatic brain injury and traumatic aortic rupture are two frequently fatal deceleration injuries. Crush injuries may result when a patient is trapped in a vehicle after a crash. The lower extremities and pelvis are particularly vulnerable in these situations.

ACUTE MANAGEMENT OF TRAUMATIC WOUNDS

Advanced Trauma Life Support

The acute management of traumatic wounds is a component of the Advanced Trauma Life Support (ATLS) guidelines. Treatment of any wounded patient should follow these guidelines. Failure to recognize and correct life-threatening problems early post injury will make wound care meaningless. ATLS guidelines emphasize an organized and methodical approach to trauma. A brief overview of the guidelines is given here, but a more comprehensive review can be found in most general surgery texts. Anyone caring for acutely traumatized patients should take the Advanced Trauma Life Support (ATLS) course offered by the American College of Surgeons.

Any trauma can be managed using the ABCDE method: airway, breathing, circulation, disability, and exposure. The airway and breathing components of the ATLS guidelines emphasize that a person who is not able to breathe cannot oxygenate his or her tissues. This situation quickly leads to tissue ischemia, organ failure, and death. Priority should be given toward securing the patient's airway. If the patient is unconscious, has an altered consciousness, or has injuries that compromise the airway, a temporary airway (e.g., nasopharyngeal tube, oropharyngeal tube, cricothyroidotomy) should be established until a definitive airway (e.g., endotracheal tube or tracheostomy tube) can be placed. Next, any injuries that prevent adequate oxygenation or ventilation should be addressed immediately. This includes simple or tension pneumothorax or hemothorax. All are addressed with a tube thoracostomy (chest tube).

Once a person is able to oxygenate and ventilate, attention should be given to circulation. Organs and tissue that are not perfused will become ischemic. Beyond the obvious risk of death, ischemia has profound negative effects on wound healing. Ischemia results in larger wounds, longer healing times, and higher incidences of wound failure and infection. Some of the problems that can compromise circulation include cardiac tamponade, shock, and bleeding. Cardiac tamponade can be treated emergently by pericardiocentesis. In trauma, shock (the inability to maintain end organ perfusion) is predominantly secondary to hemorrhage, but a patient also may present with neurogenic shock, septic shock, cardiogenic shock, or adrenal insufficiency.

Control of Bleeding

Hemorrhage remains the number-one cause of preventable death on the battlefield, accounting for over 90% of such injuries (Eastridge, Mabry, Seguin, et al., 2012). Hemorrhagic shock is treated by first resuscitating the patient with crystalloid solutions (e.g., 0.9% NaCl or lactated Ringer's solution) and then blood products. Trauma patients are notoriously challenging to treat because their injuries make them susceptible to multiple coagulopathies (Hess et al., 2008). A new generation of diagnostic adjuncts, collectively known as thromboelastrometry (TEM), are helpful in guiding resuscitation in coagulopathic patients (Holcomb et al., 2012; Wikkelsø, Wetterslev, Møller, & Afshari, 2016). Using this technology, a provider can determine exactly what component is deficient and can replete it accordingly. Second, the source of bleeding is identified and controlled. A significant portion of trauma-related bleeding is internal. Fatal internal bleeding can occur in the thorax, abdomen (to include the retroperitoneum), pelvis, and long bones (e.g., femur). Identifying the bleeding source requires knowledge of the mechanism of injury and the use of various imaging modalities or surgical exploration. If a patient is hemodynamically unstable, surgical correction of the bleeding is necessary. Once bleeding control has been established, the patient can be assessed for neurologic disability and treated accordingly. The patient's clothing should be removed to ensure that no injury has been overlooked. The management of trauma is team oriented and multidisciplinary, and several steps of the ATLS guidelines may progress simultaneously depending on the resources of the hospital (Henry et al., 2018). To control hemorrhage, direct pressure should be the initial therapy. Direct pressure is noninvasive, requires no supplies other than a hand, and prevents further damage to the injured vessel and other tissue. Packing the wound can increase the amount of pressure that is applied to the bleeding area in conjunction with direct pressure. When a wound is not responsive to direct pressure or packing, use of a tourniquet should be considered.

Use of Tourniquets

When a wound is too large or the bleeding is too brisk, control of bleeding can be attempted with a tourniquet. A tourniquet circumferentially applies pressure proximal to damaged, bleeding tissue. The pressure is transferred to the underlying vessels, causing occlusion of the arteries and veins. Tourniquets are more effective than direct pressure in stopping hemorrhage. These can be purchased or constructed out of something as simple as a belt or a bed sheet. Tourniquet use comes at a price, however. When applied, hypoperfusion and subsequent ischemia occur to all tissue distal to the point of compression. Prolonged tourniquet use (as short as 90 min) can result in ischemia, compartment syndrome,

and nerve damage. Use for more than 6 h can result in limb loss (Beekley et al., 2008; Kam, Kavanagh, & Yoong, 2001).

However, in a combat theater, multiple factors may lead to delayed casualty evacuation. Environmental (e.g., sandstorms), geographic (e.g., mountain ranges), and tactical (e.g., ongoing combat) factors can delay evacuation for hours, if not days. Among combat fatalities, 30%–40% result from hemorrhage (Perkins, Cap, Weiss, Reid, & Bolan, 2008). In patients who are not killed immediately, hemorrhage is the most preventable cause of death. Advanced Trauma Life Support protocol should be followed as strictly as field capabilities allow. Placement of a tourniquet can temporarily halt bleeding, allowing perfusion of crucial organs and survival until an adequate surgical facility can be reached. Recent research derived from US experiences in Iraq and Afghanistan, suggests tourniquets are safe and limb loss is low when tourniquets are applied judiciously (Beekley et al., 2008; Kragh et al., 2009). US Tactical Combat Casualty Care guidelines encourage the use of tourniquets in their teaching, which is standard of care for all medical personnel deploying to combat theatres (Joint Trauma System Tactical Combat Casualty Care, 2020). A recent study showed that tourniquet use was one of the interventions responsible for a 44% reduction in mortality over the conflicts in Iraq and Afghanistan from 2001 to 2017 (Howard et al., 2019).

With the recent increase in civilian mass casualty events and deaths due to active shooter situations or improvised explosive devices, the relative prohibition on civilian use of tourniquets has come into question. The American College of Surgeons, in conjunction with the Hartford Consensus, formalized recommendations for bystander training and intervention for bleeding patients in a course known as Stop the Bleed (Pons & Jacobs, 2017). The objective of the course is to teach the general public how to identify and treat life-threatening bleeding. As previously described in this chapter, bleeding is best stopped by direct pressure over the wound, followed by packing the wound and continued pressure. If the bleeding fails to respond to these measures, a dedicated or improvised tourniquet may be used to stop extremity bleeding. Thus, the Stop the Bleed course brings lessons learned on the battlefield to the general population to reduce preventable deaths from uncontrolled hemorrhage.

Upon the patient's arrival to an operating room, tourniquets should be removed, and the patient's wounds explored for sites of bleeding. Blind clamping of vessels can lead to ischemia of healthy tissue and therefore should be avoided. Damaged vessels can be addressed with ligation or graft repair, depending on the structure and degree of collateral flow. If external bleeding occurs where a tourniquet cannot be applied (e.g., the groin, neck, or axilla) or if a tourniquet inadequately stops hemorrhage, a hemostatic dressing can be applied. Table 33.1 lists examples and descriptions of hemostatic agents and dressings (Kozen, Kircher, Henao, Godinez, & Johnson, 2008; Neuffer et al., 2004; Perkins et al., 2008; Pusateri et al., 2003; Rhee et al., 2008). Evidence from the CRASH-2 trial suggests that tranexamic acid (TXA) significantly reduces death due to hemorrhage (in patients

TABLE 33.1	Examples of Hemostatic Agents and Dressings		
Component	**Brand Name**	**Manufacturer**	**Formulation**
Zeolite/kaolin	QuikClot	Z-Medica	Powders and beads
			Zeolite is a mineral
Gelatins	Gelfoam	Pfizer	Absorbable foam dressing
	FloSeal	Baxter Health Care	Absorptive granules
	Surgifoam	Johnson and Johnson	Foam
Collagen	Avitene	CR Bard	Sponge
Microporous polysaccharides	TraumaDEX	Bleed-X	Plant-based powder
	BioHemostat	Hemodyne	Absorptive granules in a dressing
	Surgicel	Johnson and Johnson	Powder or gauze dressing
	Blood stop	LifeScience PLUS	Wrapped strips
Chitosan derived from shrimp shells	Celox	Medtrade	Granular powder or gauze dressing
	HemCon	HemCon Medical Technologies	Patch or bandage
	ChitoFlex	Tricol	Impregnated packing
	ChitoGauze	Tricol	Impregnated gauze
Fibrin sealant	Tisseel VH	Baxter Health Care	Tissue adhesive
	Evicel	Johnson and Johnson	Liquid
Polyethylene glycol	CoSeal	Baxter	Tissue adhesive
Cyanoacrylate	Dermabond	Ethicon	Tissue adhesive

with severe hemorrhagic injuries) and improves 28-day all-cause mortality if administered within 3 h of injury; administration of the antifibrinolytic outside of this window is associated with decreased survival (Roberts et al., 2013).

Immunization

Once a patient has been stabilized, tetanus prophylaxis should be administered. Tetanus, a disease characterized by intense muscle contractions and autonomic dysfunction, is caused by a toxin produced by the anaerobic bacteria *Clostridium tetani*. These contractions can be fatal if they affect the diaphragm (Birch & Bleck, 2020). Wounds necessitating tetanus prophylaxis include wounds older than 6 h, those with significant contamination or associated necrotic or ischemic tissue, puncture wounds, stab and gunshot wounds, and wounds resulting from burns or frostbite (Birch & Bleck, 2020). Patients who were immunized within the past 5 years or who have received a tetanus booster during this period may be exempt. Due to the significant contamination of war wounds and the difficulties in verifying medical records in a combat environment, many trauma surgeons recommend immunizing all wounded patients.

Irrigation and Assessment

Once a patient's life- and limb-threatening injuries have been addressed, it is appropriate to start wound care. Regardless of the etiology, traumatic wounds almost always occur in a non-sterile environment. Therefore, by definition, traumatic wounds are contaminated by debris and foreign objects from the surrounding environment. Many weapons are designed to embed foreign objects in their targets. Explosive munitions displace large volumes of dirt and debris upon detonation. To treat a traumatic wound, one must first assess the nature

and extent of wounding, including size; depth; and nerve, bone, or blood vessel exposure. Irrigation of the wound with sterile saline or water facilitates proper assessment and removes gross debris and contaminants and chemicals that could lead to further tissue injury (EPUAP, NPIAP, PPPIA, 2019). Mechanisms of irrigation for wound care are discussed later in this chapter and further in Chapter 21, In general, gentle lavage with sterile saline should be adequate at the initial assessment. Care should be taken to prevent injury to the operative team, as fragments may cut or stab providers during the injury. Special care should be taken in wounds contaminated with glass, as small fragments are radiolucent and difficult to see intraoperatively.

Coverage and Repair of Vital Structures

There are three types of nerve injury. *Neuropraxia,* the most minor nerve injury, is a conduction block of the nerve. These injuries are common in blunt trauma and compartment syndrome. Function lost secondary to neuropraxia usually returns in 3 months. *Axonotmesis* is an intermediate injury to the nerve that results from damage to the axon. The surrounding endoneurium and perineurium remain intact. The damaged axon will undergo Wallerian degeneration (degeneration of the axon distal to the injury) but then slowly grow back (about 1 cm/month). Most function will return after this type of injury. Both neuropraxia and axonotmesis will heal without specific intervention. The most severe type of nerve injury is *neurotmesis,* or complete transaction of the nerve. If the injury is secondary to penetrating trauma, it usually can be repaired. Neurotmesis secondary to gunshot wounds has a less favorable outcome. The gunshot wound results in thermal and shockwave injuries in addition to the penetrating injury, making functional recovery after surgical repair less likely. Optimally, a nerve should be repaired with a tension-free anastomosis. If this cannot be done because of a substantial defect in the nerve, grafting can be attempted. Autologous nerve grafting, usually using a patient's sural nerve as the donor, is the most common technique. Autologous vein grafts also can be used to guide regenerating nerves over defects. The timing of nerve repair depends on the degree of contamination and the need for subsequent operations to the same wound. Regardless of the degree of injury, an exposed nerve should be covered with soft tissue (Parnes, Carey, & Marmor, 2017). The exposed nerve is at higher risk for infection and iatrogenic injury during subsequent surgery. A nerve that is allowed to heal without soft tissue coverage becomes highly susceptible to even minor blunt trauma.

Traumatic wounds may contain open fractures that need to be reduced and stabilized. Open fractures are at risk for infection, bleeding, increased soft tissue damage, delayed union, and nonunion. Bone infections (osteomyelitis) are difficult to treat because of the density of the bone and the paucity of adjacent blood vessels supplying the cortical bone. After the wound is irrigated and debrided, open fractures are stabilized, either temporarily or definitively. Depending on the fractured bone, fixation can be achieved by a variety of methods, most commonly screw and/or plate fixation for periarticular fractures and intramedullary nails or external fixators for diaphyseal fractures. After fixation, open fractures require soft tissue coverage with either local tissue or transferred flaps. This typically is performed at a subsequent, definitive operation. Because coverage often cannot be performed at the initial operation due to contamination, infection, or physiologic reasons, a sterile dressing is placed over the bone until a later time when surgery can be performed under more favorable conditions (Dawson, Naga, & Atassi, 2017).

A wound should be explored for exposed traumatized blood vessels. Similar to nerves, exposed vessels are at risk for infection and iatrogenic injury during subsequent operations. Furthermore, any compromise to the blood supply compromises all the tissue it supplies. Medium and large arteries that supply an area of soft tissue without adequate collateral flow require repair around the time of injury. Examples include the superficial femoral, common femoral, and brachial arteries. Due to the presence of collateral veins, most major veins can be ligated following injury. If needed, repair can be performed using a variety of techniques, depending on the vessel and degree of injury. Most exposed vessels in open wounds will occur in the extremities. Repair of these vessels is by autologous or prosthetic graft. In the acute setting, a patient may be too unstable to tolerate a long operation. If this is the case and the patient has a large defect to a vessel supplying a limb, a temporary vascular shunt can be placed to maintain blood flow to the limb until definitive vascular repair can be achieved. Once a patient is able to tolerate a longer operation, the injured vessel should be repaired with an autologous vein graft, typically the saphenous vein, or an artificial conduit such as polytetrafluoroethylene. In most cases, an autologous vein graft is preferred over an artificial graft

because of superior patency rates and lower rates of infection. Next, consideration should be given to coverage of the exposed vessel. In addition to the risks of infection and iatrogenic injury, vessel walls will desiccate, erode, and possibly disrupt if wounds are allowed to heal without coverage. Coverage of a blood vessel can be provided by myocutaneous flap or fasciocutaneous flap as discussed in Chapter 35. When the wound is too large for flap coverage or is too contaminated for a viable flap, an extra anatomic bypass of the injured vessel should be performed, directing a graft to route the blood vessel around the wound in an uninjured tissue plane. When an injured vessel is being repaired, the graft should be similarly routed through uninjured, well-perfused tissue planes (Shackford & Sise, 2017).

Debridement

Once a wound has been irrigated copiously and assessed, all nonviable tissue should be debrided to prevent its negative effects on the wound bed (see Chapter 20). For the patient with a traumatic wound, the continued presence of nonviable tissue poses significant threats systemically by releasing toxic oxygen radicals, chemokines, cytokines, electrolytes, myoglobin, and other muscle breakdown products. These molecules lead to deleterious inflammatory responses that are exacerbated by resuscitation, leading to systemic inflammatory responses such as systemic inflammatory response syndrome (SIRS) and multiorgan dysfunction syndrome (MODS) (Table 33.2) (Bone et al., 1992). The SIRS response can become a maladaptive and hypermetabolic physiologic state that leads to prolonged healing times, poor wound healing, and various other complications. Multiorgan dysfunction syndrome is the end result of an exaggerated or prolonged SIRS response, which is characterized by multisystem organ failure and high morbidity and mortality rates. Further injury caused by necrotic tissue includes kidney damage secondary to myoglobin released by necrotic muscle. Lysis of cells releases a large volume of electrolytes and metabolic products. Of particular concern is hyperkalemia, which can lead to fatal cardiac dysrhythmias.

Although some surgeons advocate the use of bedside wound exploration for smaller wounds, most traumatic wounds should be irrigated and debrided in the operating room to minimize patient discomfort and allow for adequate exploration. If the patient requires an operation for a traumatic injury, irrigation and debridement of the wound can take place during the operation once the patient is stable and all life-threatening injuries have been addressed. A standardized method of debridement, with standard intervals of 48–72 h between trips to the operating room improved rates of closure when compared with a nonstandardized approach in a recent study (Lisboa et al., 2019).

Fasciotomy

Fasciotomies are performed for compartment syndrome or prophylactically for patients at risk for compartment syndrome. Compartment syndrome occurs after a crush injury or vascular injury with subsequent reperfusion in a closed

TABLE 33.2	Criteria for Definition of the qSOFA Score, Sepsis, Septic Shock, and MODS		
(Quick) Sequential Organ Failure Assessment (SOFA/qSOFA)	Sepsis	Septic Shock	Multiple Organ Dysfunction Syndrome (MODS)
qSOFA	An increase in the SOFA score by 2 with infection	Sepsis requiring vasopressor support to maintain MAP >65 or a lactate >2	Failure of two or more organs so homeostasis cannot be sustained without support
Respiratory rate>22/min			
Systolic blood pressure <100 mmHg			
Altered mental status			
The full SOFA score takes the following into account: PaO₂/FiO₂, Bilirubin, platelet count, mean arterial pressure (MAP), Glasgow Coma Score (GCS), creatinine/urine output			

Singer et al. (2016).

fascial space. The leg, forearm, and hand are the most commonly affected, although any muscular compartment bound by fascia can become affected. Tissue edema following injury places increased pressure directly on capillaries, resulting in decreased perfusion and ischemia. Additionally, external pressure on veins reduces capillary flow and further diminishes perfusion (Clayton, Hayes, & Barnes, 1977). If ischemia continues, permanent nerve damage, renal failure, and loss of limb can ensue. Unlike open wounds, compartment syndrome has a more occult presentation. Symptoms include pain, paresthesias (e.g., tingling or pricking), paresis (muscle weakness or partial paralysis), poikilothermia (inability to regulate temperature), and pallor of the affected extremity. The most common exam finding is pain out of proportion to physical exam findings, and pain on passive stretching of affected compartment muscles. An absence of pulses may be noted in an affected limb but typically is a late finding. Compartment pressure can be measured using a needle attached to an Intracompartmental Pressure Monitor System or a modified arterial line kit that is inserted through the fascia. Normal compartment pressures range from 0 to 15 mmHg, whereas an elevated pressure mandating treatment is either a compartment pressure greater than 30 mmHg or compartment pressure 35 mmHg less than arterial diastolic pressure (Witmer, Marshall, & Browner, 2017). Treatment involves surgical decompression of compartments by incising the muscular fascia of all of the compartments in the injured area. Failing to decompress all compartments, or delaying the fasciotomy, can lead to significant myonecrosis and possible need for amputation. Fasciotomy rates increased throughout the conflicts in Iraq and Afghanistan, likely due to increased use of tourniquets (Kragh et al., 2016), the significant morbidity associated with missed compartment syndrome or inadequate fasciotomy, lower extremity fasciotomy training is now standardized in the ASSET course organized by the American College of Surgeons Committee on Trauma (Fildes et al., 2010). In trauma, fasciotomies are performed prophylactically in patients at risk for compartment syndrome (e.g., those with severe crush injuries

or with prolonged ischemia). Once the fasciotomy is performed, subacute management of the open wound begins, with subsequent attention to debridement of necrotic muscle and fascia, and eventual closure with a combination of delayed primary closure, negative pressure wound therapy, and occasional skin grafts.

SUBACUTE MANAGEMENT OF TRAUMATIC WOUNDS

Usually, the degree of contamination, the severity of the wound, and the local and systemic inflammatory response to the critically ill state of the wounded patient do not allow for wound closure after initial evaluation, irrigation, and debridement because care must be focused on lifesaving procedures, ensuring adequate airway and ventilation, stopping blood loss, and preventing further organ injury. Therefore, wound bed preparation and wound closure are planned during the subacute phase of traumatic wound management.

Serial Irrigation and Debridement

Although a wound bed may appear to be free of necrotic tissue after initial debridement, repeat evaluation during subacute management may reveal additional necrosis. Patients with traumatic wounds tend to have physiologic, immunologic, and nutritional derangements that predispose them to infection. On a local level, wounds are predisposed to colonization. Therefore, traumatic wounds typically require serial irrigation, evaluation, and debridement. Traditionally, open traumatic wounds are evaluated on a daily or twice-daily basis.

Debridement should be performed using an atraumatic surgical technique (Attinger et al., 2006). Examples include sharp dissection and bipolar cautery, which allow for minimal destruction of underlying, healthy tissue. Descriptions and examples of healthy and unhealthy tissue is described in Chapter 10. Healthy tissue is well vascularized and bleeds. Other hallmarks of viable tissue depend on the tissue type. Healthy fascia appears white and glistens. Fat is bright yellow. Viable muscle can be recognized by the 4 Cs: red *Color*,

Contraction upon stimulation with forceps or electrocautery, strong *Consistency*, and *Capacity* to bleed (Volgas, 2007). Most bleeding resulting from surgical debridement can be stopped with direct pressure. If direct pressure is inadequate, suture ligation or pinpoint electrocautery can be used. Extra attention must be paid to patients who are severely coagulopathic or on active antiplatelet medications or anticoagulation. Topical hemostatic agents, described in Table 33.1, can serve as an adjunct to the above hemostatic methods, especially in tissue where further manipulation will lead to more bleeding (muscle, friable granulation tissue, and solid organs).

Reevaluation of a traumatic wound with repeat irrigation and debridement should occur at least twice per week even if no grossly necrotic or nonviable tissue is noted in the wound bed (Attinger et al., 2006). As wound healing progresses, the extent of debridement needed decreases. Once a bed of granulation tissue is present throughout the wound, debridement may no longer be needed. At this point, gentle wound irrigation and the use of negative pressure dressings can maintain the bacterial load at sufficiently low levels.

Many traumatic wounds have exposed bone. Although radiographs and magnetic resonance imaging are the standard techniques for diagnosing osteomyelitis, the presence of exposed bone in a wound or the ability to probe to bone should be considered clinical evidence of infection (Fritz & McDonald, 2008). Infected or nonviable bone is friable and should be debrided. Curettes, Cobb elevators, and rongeurs are sharp surgical instruments typically used for bone debridement. Once bone has been adequately debrided, it should be covered with soft tissue (Attinger et al., 2006). Occasionally, adjacent tissue can be sutured over the defect. Otherwise, a rotational or free myocutaneous flap is needed. In cases where anatomic or physiologic restrictions contraindicate a flap procedure or ongoing infection is suspected, bone will granulate. Secondary intention is suboptimal because granulation is slow and takes several weeks. Early flap reconstruction is associated with shorter hospital stays for patients with traumatic wounds and is feasible in even complicated polytraumatic injury (Celiköz et al., 2005; Stanec et al., 1993).

Should a traumatic wound become infected, the infection can travel very quickly along fascial planes, a condition known as *necrotizing fasciitis*. Tendon necrosis or infection can be difficult to manage. Overzealous debridement of a tendon can lead to loss of muscle function. Care should be taken to preserve as much healthy tissue as possible. If the paratenon surrounding the tendon requires debridement, the tendon must be kept moist to prevent desiccation and necrosis. Because infection can quickly spread along tendons, small incisions should be made in the healthy tendon or muscle proximal and distal to the infected or necrotic tissue. Small tendons may require sacrifice if they become infected. Larger tendons should be preserved as much as possible. Reconstruction of certain large tendons (e.g., Achilles tendon) is possible using pedicle or free flaps (Attinger et al., 2006).

Following debridement, irrigation (see Chapter 19) should be performed to remove bacteria and loose debris. Tangential

hydrosurgery is a technique that combines pulsed lavage irrigation and debridement. A pulsed lavage device (e.g., Versajet ™ Smith and Nephew) debrides tissue by shooting a stream of water across a small gap. The stream is very high pressure, up to 15,000 psi. The high-pressure stream creates a vacuum that pulverizes surrounding necrotic tissue, removes it from the wound bed, and preserves adjacent healthy tissue (Granick, Tenenhaus, Knox, & Ulm, 2007; Klein et al., 2005). Due to the high pressure generated by the device, the procedure is associated with a significant amount of discomfort and anxiety to the patient. Subsequently, adequate anesthesia in the form of conscious sedation, spinal, or general anesthesia is recommended. Recent literature has argued against the use of high-pressure irrigation (pulsed lavage) systems due to its high rate of tissue damage and bacterial rebound. Because of this, low-pressure systems, like the bulb syringe, have returned to favor (Fry, 2017; Tintle, Keeling, Shawen, Forsberg, & Potter, 2010).

Dressings

After the wound is irrigated and debrided, it should be covered with a sterile dressing. Different types of dressings perform different functions (Stojadinovic, Carlson, Schultz, Davis, & Elster, 2008). In acute traumatic wounds, wet to dry dressings are no longer the standard of care. In wounds that are heavily colonized, dressings moistened with diluted sodium hypochlorite (i.e., Dakin's solution) instead of water or saline may still be utilized. Sodium hypochlorite is a bleach that is bactericidal but has cytotoxic effects on healthy cells (Wilson, Mills, Prather, & Dimitrijevich, 2005). Depending on the degree of colonization, either half-strength or quarter-strength Dakin's solution can be used until the level of contamination decreases.

Negative pressure wound therapy (NPWT) between 75- and 150-mmHg is the most commonly used dressing for traumatic wounds following debridement of necrotic tissue and all eschar. Negative pressure wound therapy is described in detail in Chapter 24. It removes effluent from the wound which subsequently reduces wound edema and fosters faster healing. Additionally, negative pressure wound therapy dressings are occlusive, thus preventing contamination of the wound by additional bacteria or debris. Evidence demonstrates this therapy will also stimulate granulation tissue by promoting capillary growth. Intermittent instead of continuous negative pressure has been shown to further increase the rate of granulation tissue formation (Lindstedt, Malmsjö, Gesslein, & Ingemansson, 2008; Malmsjö, Gustafsson, Lindstedt, Gesslein, & Ingemansson, 2012; Ubbink, Westerbos, Nelson, & Vermeulen, 2008).

Different variants of wound filler dressings can be used for NPWT as described in Chapter 24. A silver-impregnated sponge is warranted for infected wounds or wounds with a heavy bacterial load. Silver ions are bacteriocidal and have potency against multidrug-resistant bacteria, such as methicillin-resistant *Staphylococcus aureus,* vancomycin-resistant *Enterococcus,* and *Pseudomonas aeruginosa* (Tredget, Shankowsky, Groeneveld, & Burrell, 1998; Yin,

Langford, & Burrell, 1999). A nonadherent sponge is instrumental in the care of wounds that contain structures such as tendons, nerves, or viscera, to prevent adherence to vulnerable structures and to provide moisture. An alternative to the nonadherent sponge is to apply a nonadherent contact layer over the top of the vulnerable structure such as bone, tendon, nerves, and blood vessels to protect the tissues from the foam. This technique is may be preferred over the top of skin grafts to take advantage of increased capillary growth while preventing graft removal. Two randomized control trials demonstrated decreased graft loss (Llanos et al., 2006) and improved cosmetic outcome (Moisidis, Heath, Boorer, Ho, & Deva, 2004) when NPWT was placed over grafts.

For small, shallow wounds not amenable to NPWT, numerous alternative dressings may be used (see Chapters 19, 21, and 22). Dressings that reduce bacterial load and provide gentle debridement are generally preferred for traumatic wounds.

Local Antibiotics

An additional adjunct that has been used for treatment of traumatic wounds with open fractures has been direct application of antibiotics in the form of powders, cement, or beads. Osteomyelitis is hard to treat due to the difficulty in achieving therapeutic levels of antibiotics in bone. Treatment generally requires 6 or more weeks of intravenous antibiotics. As an adjunct to systemic antibiotics, several German orthopedic surgeons placed antibiotics in bone cement used for hip arthroplasty (Buchholz & Engelbrecht, 1970). A reduction in postoperative arthroplasty infections was noted, leading to more widespread use of antibiotic impregnated bone cement. Antibiotic-impregnated beads subsequently were developed for temporary placement at sites of bone debrided for osteomyelitis. The beads are created by mixing bone cement powder, typically polymerized polymethylmethacrylate (PMMA), with powdered antibiotics before adding liquid methylmethacrylate to make the adhesive cement. Before hardening, the beads can be threaded on a permanent suture to facilitate removal. In settings where reoperation to remove the beads would be undesirable, some surgeons utilize the powdered antibiotics directly on the wound bed. This is often done when placing hardware in wounds, in conjunction with healthy soft tissue coverage. Only a few antibiotics are available in powdered form, limiting the choice to aminoglycosides, vancomycin, and β-lactams (Hake et al., 2015; Wininger & Fass, 1996).

In traumatic wounds with open fractures, antibiotic beads have been used to decrease the bacterial load of the wound. In a study of 1085 patients with compound limb fractures requiring debridement and stabilization, 845 received gentamicin-impregnated antibiotic beads plus systemic antibiotics versus 240 treated with systemic antibiotics alone. The rate of infection decreased from 12% to 3.7% in the group that received the beads (Ostermann, Seligson, & Henry, 1995). Due to the high incidence of multidrug-resistant Acinetobacter infections in US service members with traumatic wounds sustained in Iraq and Afghanistan, antibiotic beads have become a frequently used method for treating and preventing osteomyelitis (Weintrob et al., 2018). Hake et al. (2015) provide a relevant review of antibiotic impregnated beads in orthopedic trauma as well as detailed instructions on how to mix, form, and use the beads.

Wound Closure

The timing of wound closure is an important clinical decision. The goal of closure is to protect the underlying tissue, restore the innate immunologic barrier of skin, and provide a cosmetically acceptable outcome. Although most healthy wounds will granulate and close by secondary intention, surgical closure reduces the duration of closure, produces a cosmetically superior appearance, decreases the need for wound care resources, and decreases the time burden on the patient. Improper timing of closure leads to dehiscence and failure. Dehiscence results when a closed wound reopens. Failure includes dehiscence, but also may include failure of a wound to accept a graft (e.g., skin graft). Currently, no laboratory tests or imaging modalities can predict the optimal time for wound closure. Providers are forced to rely on clinical factors, including wound appearance and patient physiology, as well as their own clinical experience. A recent study by the senior author of this chapter established a clinical decision support tool, using cytokines from the effluent of the NPWT device on traumatic wounds in addition to other clinical and laboratory values, to help determine optimal time to closure of traumatic wounds (Lisboa et al., 2019).

Current criteria used to determine timing of wound closure include the patient's general condition, injury location, adequacy of perfusion, and gross appearance of the wound bed. Factors related to the patient's general condition include nutritional and nonspecific systemic inflammatory parameters. Relevance of injury location and visual assessment of the wound, such as the appearance of granulation tissue, are subjectively determined by the surgeon. However, considerable interobserver variability exists in wound assessment.

Once a wound has a base of healthy granulation tissue without evidence of infection, the wound can be closed. Several techniques are used to close traumatic wounds. As previously stated, secondary intention is one method. Secondary intention involves the growth of skin over the top of a granulated wound from the wound edge. No surgical intervention is necessary for secondary intention; however, the long duration (several months), resources needed (wound dressings), and cosmetic outcome do not favor its use, especially for large traumatic wounds.

For wounds with healthy skin edges, primary or delayed primary closure can be attempted. See Table 33.3 for characteristics influencing the choice between primary, delayed primary closure, and closure by secondary intention. The term *delayed* refers to the time lapse between initial wound care and the time of closure. Delayed primary closure involves approximating the edges of a wound and fixating them together.

Multiple methods for approximating skin exist, including skin adhesives, sutures, and staples. In general, adhesives in

TABLE 33.3 Patient and Wound Characteristics Influencing Method of Closure

Patient Factors	Primary Closure	Delayed Primary Closure	Closure by Secondary Intention
Nutritional status	Good	Stable, or improving	Poor
Septic burden/wound contamination	None	Low	High
Wound location	Clean surgical incision	Sensitive areas (joints, face, hands)	Intertriginous areas
Need for further debridement	None	None	Concern for further necrosis or infection
Tension on wound edges	Low	Low	High
Amount of undermining	Low	Low	High
Delicate structures in wound bed	Yes	Yes	No

gel or strip form are reserved for clean wounds. Sutures and staples are often interchangeable in practice. Sutures have the benefit of being able to be tightened by hand to select the correct amount of wound tension and can be placed in various methods and layers to decrease tension on high-risk areas of the wound. Skin staples are advantageous due to their ease of deployment and ability to close large wounds quickly. Regardless of the mechanism used, skin closures should be under low tension. High-tension closures result in failure and dehiscence.

In general, wounds that have been approximated with sutures or staples are covered with a dry, sterile dressing which is typically not removed unless visibly soiled for the first 72 h postoperatively. Patients may then leave the wounds open to air, or with a simple gauze dressing for comfort. No lotions, emollients, or creams should be applied to the wound, and the patients are instructed not to submerge the wound under water for at least two weeks. Wounds in intertriginous areas or those being closed in clean contaminated fields (e.g., bowel resection without frank spillage) may benefit from negative pressure wound therapy placed over an appropriate barrier dressing over the incision, (incisional NPWT) as this has been shown to decrease wound dehiscence and infection in certain settings (Curran et al., 2019; Kwon et al., 2018).

Occasionally, larger wounds cannot be surgically closed due to unacceptably high tension, so a skin graft must be considered. As previously discussed, the provider must first analyze a wound for exposed bone, nerve, or blood vessel. If one of these structures appears in the wound base, a muscle, myocutaneous, or fasciocutaneous flap should be used for cover. Coverage protects nerves and vessels from subsequent trauma and bone from skin erosion. As described in Chapter 35, many types of tissue flaps exist, including pedicle flaps, rotational flaps, and free flaps. Choice of flap type and procedure usually requires an experienced plastic surgeon. Flaps, especially free flaps, require frequent monitoring in the first 48 h to ensure adequate perfusion. Most flaps also contain a segment of skin. If the flap does not, a skin graft may be performed once the flap is viable and secure. Skin grafts are

described in Chapter 35. Several artificial skin substitutes have been developed (see Chapter 22). Although none of these substitutes can replace an autograft, they can promote graft acceptance. These products, in combination with NPWT, have proven useful in wounds with exposed tendon, allowing for granulation over tendon and eventual skin grafting (Helgeson, Potter, Evans, & Shawen, 2007).

Open Abdomen

Visceral swelling results secondary to trauma and is caused by massive cytokine release, increased vascular permeability, and loss of fluid to the interstitial space, most notably following resuscitation. Although the swelling typically resolves in 1 to 2 weeks, the bowel becomes so large that the abdominal wall cannot be reapproximated. Closure of the abdominal wall also can be difficult if a trauma results directly in a large soft tissue defect, or a "loss of domain."

Regardless of the cause, closure of the abdomen is necessary to contain and protect the viscera, prevent desiccation of the bowel, and prevent peritonitis. Multiple techniques have been developed to close the abdomen. The simplest method is primary fascial closure. To close an abdomen by primary fascial closure, a component separation is often performed to lessen tension of the reapproximated fascia. Component separations involve separating individual muscular layers of the abdominal wall from eachother to allow for improved ability to close midline defects. Generally, component separations grouped into anterior or posterior separations, depending on the muscular layer used. Anterior component separation dissects skin off the anterior rectus sheath and incises the external oblique fascia, allowing for increased mobilization of the fascia and closure (Ramirez, Ruas, & Dellon, 1990). Posterior component separation dissects the transverse abdominis from the underlying transversalis fascia and peritoneum, lateral to the semilunar line (Novitsky, Elliott, Orenstein, & Rosen, 2012). To reduce the amount of dissection needed and resultant large soft tissue flaps, laparoscopic versions of these procedure have been developed (Jensen,

Henriksen, & Jorgensen, 2014; Milburn et al., 2007). Major complications of the procedure include wound infection and recurrent hernia.

One technique is the planned ventral hernia. In this technique, an absorbable mesh is used to close the fascial defect. Once the mesh granulates, a split-thickness skin graft is placed over the wound. Over time, the mesh is absorbed and a ventral hernia results. The ventral hernia is then surgically repaired 6 to 12 months after the trauma, usually requiring a component separation (Fabian et al., 1994; Jernigan et al., 2003; Weinberg et al., 2008). Due to the high rate of enterocutaneous fistula formation (approximately 8% of patients) and the need for future major abdominal surgeries, this technique is less popular than delayed fascial closure.

Delayed fascial closure involves placement of an NPWT dressing such as a visceral layer dressing (e.g., ABThera™ 3M/KCI, Minneapolis MN) over the open abdomen until bowel swelling reduces enough to allow closure by component separation and/or a mesh. Decreased adhesions between the abdominal wall and bowel have been noted. A negative pressure dressing is created by placing a plastic sheet or towel over the viscera and under the abdominal wall. The dressing is placed over the towel and is covered by an occlusive dressing. The dressing is connected to continuous negative pressure at 75 mmHg. Every 2 to 3 days, the patient returns to the operating room and the dressing is changed under sterile conditions until abdominal closure is technically viable (Argenta et al., 2006; Bee et al., 2008; Morykwas, Argenta, Shelton-Brown, & McGuirt, 1997; Schecter, Ivatury, Rotondo, & Hirshberg, 2006). While the patient remains with an open abdomen, the viscera begin to lateralize in the abdominal wall, making repeat exploration and fascial closure difficult. For this reason, temporary abdominal closures are usually kept on for as short of a time period as possible, with a 3–4 days being an optimal goal for closure. Many methods of closure exist, including primary fascial closure, formal hernia repair with mesh, or various forms of planned ventral hernias such as skin only closures or closures incorporating absorbable mesh over viscera. While this process may appear time intensive, the incidence of complications with this method is reduced: fistula (5%), bowel obstruction (2%), and abscess formation (4%) (Barker et al., 2007).

Another technique used to close the open abdomen is serial abdominal closure (Kafie et al., 2003). Serial abdominal closure requires placement of a temporary mesh or in the open abdomen. As bowel edema lessens, the mesh loosens. During serial operations, the central portion of the loose mesh is cut, and the edges are sewn together. Eventually, the residual mesh is removed, and the abdomen is closed (Barker et al., 2007; Vertrees et al., 2008). Similar results can be achieved with commercially available hook and loop devices which are sewn to fascial edges and sequentially tightened.

A variety of rotational and free muscle flaps have been used to cover large abdominal wounds. Muscle flaps typically are used when an ostomy, drain site, or multiple prior procedures have distorted or destroyed the normal anatomic planes. The rectus abdominis and tensor fascia lata are the two most commonly used muscles for flaps (Mathes, Steinwald, Foster, Hoffman, & Anthony, 2000).

Combination techniques have been attempted. For soldiers with large abdominal wounds resulting from blast injuries in Iraq and Afghanistan, a combined technique called *early-delayed fascial closure* has been described. The method combines delayed fascial closure, serial abdominal closure, and use of temporary and permanent meshes (Vertrees et al., 2008).

Choice of closure technique is largely based on anatomic factors, complication rates, and surgeon's experience and preference. Technique choice should emphasize protecting the bowel, closing the abdominal wall in a timely manner to allow rehabilitation, and preventing complications such as enterocutaneous fistulas and recurrent hernias.

Amputation

Extremely severe blast and crush injuries may result in mangled extremities with unsalvageable wounds. In these situations, amputation may be the only viable option. The decision to amputate can be extremely difficult due to the resulting cosmetic, functional, and psychological defects. Reasons to amputate include prolonged limb ischemia, irreparable peripheral nerve injury with no hope of meaningful limb rehabilitation, and presence of concurrent life-threatening injuries. Usually, the need to amputate is fairly straightforward. However, in a subset of trauma patients, the duration of limb ischemia or degree of nerve injury may cause a surgeon to attempt limb salvage when amputation is warranted. However, limb salvage is not without risks. In the LEAP trial comparing limb salvage to amputations, a significantly increased incidence of complications was noted in the limb salvage group (37.7% vs 24.8%) (Harris et al., 2009).

In order to predict which patients would benefit from limb salvage, a series of different limb injury scoring systems have been developed (Table 33.4). One system is the Mangled Extremity Severity Score (MESS). The MESS ranks the degree of soft tissue/skeletal injury, limb ischemia, shock, and age; a score of 7 correlates with a need to amputate (Johansen et al., 1990). Other scoring systems include the Limb Salvage Index (LSI); Predictive Salvage Index (PSI); Hannover Fracture Scale-97 (HFS-97); and Nerve Injury, Ischemia, Soft Tissue Injury, Skeletal Injury, Shock, and Age of Patient Score (NISSSA). Two large studies evaluated the utility of these scoring systems. In a large prospective study, Bosse et al. (2001) found that none of these scores could accurately predict limb salvage potential. A retrospective study by Ly et al. (2008) found that no available scoring system was predictive of functional recovery of patients undergoing limb salvage.

Approximately 80% of combat-related amputations are performed within the zone of injury and therefore typically require delayed closure and result in frequent wound-healing

TABLE 33.4	**Lower Extremity Injury Classifications**		
Limb Injury Scoring System	**Acronym**	**Components**	**Citation**
Mangled extremity severity score	MESS	Skeletal and soft tissue injury, limb ischemia, systemic hypotension, patient age	Johansen, Daines, Howey, Helfet, and Hansen (1990)
Limb salvage index	LSI	Injury to artery, deep vein, bone, skin, muscle, warm ischemia time	Russell, Sailors, Whittle, Fisher, and Burns (1991)
Predictive salvage index	PSI	Arterial injury, bone injury, muscle injury, time to surgery	Howe et al. (1987)
Hannover fracture scale	HFS-98	Bone loss, skin injury, muscle injury, contamination, periosteal injury, local circulation, systemic circulation, nerve injury	Krettek, Seekamp, Köntopp, and Tscherne (2001)
Nerve injury, ischemia, soft tissue injury, skeletal injury, shock, and age of patient score	NISSSA	Nerve injury, soft tissue injury, skeletal injury, shock, patient age	McNamara, Heckman, and Corley (1994)

problems. Often, we have seen an increasing number of individuals returning after 1 or more years of living with a limb that went through multiple salvage procedures but just was not functioning at the level desired by the individuals, so they present for an elective amputation. Due to increasing progress in prosthesis design and limb reconstruction (including areas such as hand transplantation, and osteointegration) and faster patient evacuation times, limb salvage will continue to be a complex decision. Patients should be made aware, however, that they can have meaningful recoveries following amputation.

Heterotopic Ossification

Heterotopic ossification is the formation of lamellar bone in nonosseous tissue. Multiple events have been associated with its formation, including traumatic amputation, spinal cord trauma, severe head injuries, total hip arthroplasty, thermal or electrical burns, acetabular or elbow fractures, familial disorders, and neoplasm. Heterotopic ossification is a source of discomfort and disability in patients when it occurs around joints and can frequently require reoperative intervention for these symptoms (Tintle et al., 2014). Heterotopic ossification is a particular problem for amputees, as it can increase limb pain, causes breakdown of overlying skin, and interferes with prosthesis fitting and use (Potter, Burns, Lacap, Granville, & Gajewski, 2006). An excellent review of the pathophysiology, proposed prophylaxis, and current directions in research and treatment for this condition is presented by Hoyt, Pavey, Potter, and Forsberg (2018)

Heterotopic ossification in the extremities remains a common complication in the setting of high-energy wartime extremity trauma. Recent literature suggests that the incidence may be higher than previously reported, particularly in blast-injured amputees and in those in whom the definitive

amputation was performed within the zone of injury. A 63% incidence has been noted in the residual limbs of US soldiers injured in Iraq and Afghanistan (Potter, Burns, Lacap, Granville, & Gajewski, 2007).

An area of concern regarding heterotopic ossification and high-energy long bone fractures is the method of definitive fixation. Heterotopic ossification is a known complication of both external fixation and internal fixation. Because heterotopic ossification formation may result following muscle injury that occurs during surgical fixation, it is possible that in the patient with multiple injuries, internal fixation carries an increased risk of developing heterotopic ossification compared with definitive external fixation, especially when definitive internal fixation is delayed.

Prophylaxis against ectopic bone formation is well established in patients undergoing arthroplasty and operative treatment of acetabular fractures. Local radiation therapy and nonsteroidal antiinflammatory drugs (NSAIDs) have been found to reduce the incidence of heterotopic ossification. After a severe trauma, many patients are too unstable to undergo radiation therapy and have contraindications against NSAID use, including renal failure and increased bleeding risks. In a combat zone, providing radiation is logistically difficult (Potter et al., 2006, 2007).

Surgical excision is a mainstay of treatment. However, in amputees, excision may require limb revision. In most patients with heterotopic ossification, ectopic bone is removed once it has matured and become symptomatic. Orthopedic surgeons in the US military have found that early excision results in faster recovery times and quicker prosthesis rehabilitation (Forsberg et al., 2008; Potter et al., 2006, 2007). Ongoing research in the field is focusing on novel medications to inhibit ectopic bone growth and the potential for phage mediated therapies (Pavey et al., 2016).

CLINICAL CONSULT

A: Consulted for a 25-year-old male 2 days s/p exploratory laparotomy for splenectomy after a stab wound with a dirty knife who presents with pain at his surgical wounds with foul smelling discharge. Patient is febrile to 39, with a significant leukocytosis to 20,000 and evidence of hyponatremia and hyperglycemia. Physical exam reveals a midline laparotomy wound draining cloudy tan appearing fluid. Surrounding skin is tender to palpation with dusky, purple-red erythema. There is extensive crepitus on exam.

D: Potential for necrotizing fasciitis given concerning findings of crepitus, diffuse dusky skin changes and brown, thin discharge from recent surgical intervention.

P: Emergent surgical consult for operative debridement. Transfer the patient to an intensive care unit, obtain blood cultures, start broad-spectrum IV antibiotics and initiate crystalloid resuscitation.

I: General surgery was contacted, and the patient was emergently taken to the operating room for wound exploration revealing full-thickness necrosis of skin and underlying soft tissues. Muscular fascia of abdominal wall was involved with tracking of infection along fascial planes with diffuse edema and foul-smelling fluid in wound, however, with intact underlying musculature and abdominal closure. Resulting wound spans from inframammary fold to pubis and laterally to the anterior axillary line bilaterally with exposed muscle throughout. Tissue and fluid culture was sent for examination. The wound was dressed with dry gauze soaked with dilute Daikin's solution with plans for frequent changes given extensive edema and possible need for further operative intervention.

E: The patient recovered well in the intensive care unit postoperatively. Frequent wound checks revealed areas concerning for further involvement at the wound edges and the patient was serially debrided at 3-day intervals for the next week until there was no evidence of further necrosis or infection, after which he was transitioned to negative pressure wound therapy. After a week of negative pressure wound therapy there was extensive granulation tissue in the base of the wound with healthy surrounding skin flaps. Subsequently, the skin flaps were sutured to the underlying granulating tissue over surgical drains, and the resulting defect was skin grafted.

SUMMARY

- In acute trauma, stabilization of the patient according to ATLS principles takes priority over initial wound care.
- Stop life-threatening bleeding by using direct pressure, wound packing, or a tourniquet.
- The most critical aspects of acute traumatic wound care are debridement of devitalized tissues, thorough irrigation, and identifying additional injuries that require subspecialty care (open fractures, neurovascular injury).
- Compartment syndrome is a clinical emergency that should be suspected in patients with ischemic or crush injuries. Pain out of proportion to the injury and pain with passive stretch should raise concern for the diagnosis.
- Postacute management of traumatic wounds focuses on maintaining a clean wound environment until healthy tissue is present in the wound bed. Wound closure methods depend on the size and location of the wound. Closure methods can range from the simple, such as delayed primary closure to the complex, including free flaps and use of prosthetics.

SELF-ASSESSMENT QUESTIONS

1. Which of the following organs are most at risk from blast over pressure?
   a. Liver
   b. Soft Tissue
   c. Hollow Viscus Organs
   d. Bone
2. What is the initial priority in management of the patient with traumatic wounds?
   a. Advanced Trauma Life Support
   b. Assessment of the wounds
   c. Wound irrigation and debridement
   d. All of the above
3. Which of the following have been shown to positively impact the healing of traumatic wounds?
   a. High-pressure pulse irrigation

   b. Negative Pressure Wound Therapy
   c. A standardized method of wound debridement every 48–72 h
   d. b and c
   e. All of the above
4. What step is critical to the success of wound care over exposed critical structures (nerves, blood vessels, or tendons)?
   a. Frequent irrigation with Dakin's solution
   b. Negative Pressure Wound Therapy
   c. Coverage with well-vascularized tissue
   d. Allowing the critical structures to be exposed in the wound be for frequent inspection

REFERENCES

Apte, A., Bradford, K., Dente, C., & Smith, R. N. (2019). Lead toxicity from retained bullet fragments: A systematic review and meta-analysis. *Journal of Trauma and Acute Care Surgery, 87*(3), 707–716.

Argenta, L. C., Morykwas, M. J., Marks, M. W., DeFranzo, A. J., Molnar, J. A., & David, L. R. (2006). Vacuum-assisted closure: State of clinic art. *Plastic and Reconstructive Surgery, 117*(7 Suppl), 127S–142S.

Attinger, C. E., Janis, J. E., Steinberg, J., Schwartz, J., Al-Attar, A., & Couch, K. (2006). Clinical approach to wounds: Debridement and wound bed preparation including the use of dressings and wound-healing adjuvants. *Plastic and Reconstructive Surgery, 117*(7 Suppl), 72S–109S.

Baker, S. P., O'Neill, B., Haddon, W., Jr., & Long, W. B. (1974). The injury severity score: A method for describing patients with multiple injuries and evaluating emergency care. *The Journal of Trauma, 14*(3), 187–196.

Barker, D. E., Green, J. M., Maxwell, R. A., Smith, P. W., Mejia, V. A., Dart, B. W., et al. (2007). Experience with vacuum-pack temporary abdominal wound closure in 258 trauma and general and vascular surgical patients. *Journal of the American College of Surgeons, 204*(5), 784–793.

Bee, T. K., Croce, M. A., Magnotti, L. J., Zarzaur, B. L., Maish, G. O., 3rd, Minard, G., et al. (2008). Temporary abdominal closure techniques: A prospective randomized trial comparing polyglactin 910 mesh and vacuum-assisted closure. *The Journal of Trauma, 65*(2), 337–344.

Beekley, A. C., Sebesta, J. A., Blackbourne, L. H., Herbert, G. S., Kauvar, D. S., Baer, D. G., et al. (2008). Prehospital tourniquet use in operation Iraqi freedom: Effect on hemorrhage control and outcomes. *The Journal of Trauma, 64*(2 Suppl), S28–S37.

Birch, T. B., & Bleck, T. P. (2020). Teatnus (*Clostridium tetani*). In J. E. Bennett, et al. (Eds.), *Mandell, Douglas, and Bennett's principles and practice of infectious diseases*. Philadelphia: Elsevier.

Bone, R. C., Balk, R. A., Cerra, F. B., Dellinger, R. P., Fein, A. M., Knaus, W. A., et al. (1992). Definitions for sepsis and organ failure and guidelines for the use of innovative therapies in sepsis. The ACCP/SCCM Consensus Conference Committee. American College of Chest Physicians/Society of Critical Care Medicine. *Chest, 101*(6), 1644–1655.

Bosse, M. J., MacKenzie, E. J., Kellam, J. F., Burgess, A. R., Webb, L. X., Swiontkowski, M. F., et al. (2001). A prospective evaluation of the clinical utility of the lower-extremity injury-severity scores. *The Journal of Bone and Joint Surgery, 83*(1), 3–14.

Buchanan, B. (2006). *Gunpowder, explosives and the state*. Aldershot: Ashgate.

Buchholz, H. W., & Engelbrecht, H. (1970). Uber die Depotwirkung einiger Antibiotica bei Vermischung mit dem Kunstharz Palacos (Depot effects of various antibiotics mixed with Palacos resins). *Chirurg, 41*(11), 511–515.

Cannon, J. W., Hofmann, L. J., Glasgow, S. C., Potter, B. K., Rodriguez, C. J., Cancio, L. C., et al. (2016). Dismounted complex blast injuries: A comprehensive review of the modern combat experience. *Journal of the American College of Surgeons, 223*(4), 652–664.e8.

Celiköz, B., Sengezer, M., Işik, S., Türegün, M., Deveci, M., Duman, H., et al. (2005). Subacute reconstruction of lower leg and foot defects due to high velocity-high energy injuries caused by gunshots, missiles, and land mines. *Microsurgery, 25*(1), 3–15. https://doi.org/10.1002/micr.20049.

Champion, H. R., Holcomb, J. B., Lawnick, M. M., Kelliher, T., Spott, M. A., Galarneau, M. R., et al. (2010). Improved characterization of combat injury. *The Journal of Trauma, 68*(5), 1139–1150.

Clayton, J. M., Hayes, A. C., & Barnes, R. W. (1977). Tissue pressure and perfusion in the compartment syndrome. *The Journal of Surgical Research, 22*(4), 333–339.

Cubano, M. A., et al. (Eds.). (2018). *Emergency war surgery* (5th ed.). Fort Sam Houston: The Borden Institute.

Curran, T., Alvarez, D., Pastrana Del Valle, J., Cataldo, T. E., Poylin, V., & Nagle, D. (2019). Prophylactic closed-incision negative-pressure wound therapy is associated with decreased surgical site infection in high-risk colorectal surgery laparotomy wounds. *Colorectal Disease, 21*(1), 110–118. https://doi.org/10.1111/codi.14350.

Dawson, J. R., Naga, A. E., & Atassi, O. (2017). Lower extremity. In E. E. Moore, et al. (Eds.), *Trauma*. New York: McGraw-Hill.

Eastridge, B. J., Mabry, R. L., Seguin, P., et al. (2012). Death on the battlefield (2001–2011): Implications for the future of combat casualty care. *Journal of Trauma and Acute Care Surgery, 73*(6 Suppl. 5), S431–S437.

European Pressure Ulcer Advisory Panel, National Pressure Injury Advisory Panel, and Pan Pacific Pressure Injury Alliance. (2019). *Prevention and treatment of pressure ulcers/injuries*. EPUAP/NPIAP/PPPIA.

Fabian, T. C., Croce, M. A., Pritchard, F. E., Minard, G., Hickerson, W. L., Howell, R. L., et al. (1994). Planned ventral hernia. Staged management for acute abdominal wall defects. *Annals of Surgery, 219*(6), 643–653.

Fildes, J., et al. (Eds.). (2010). *ASSET: Advanced Surgical Skills for Exposure in Trauma*. Chicago: American College of Surgeons.

Forsberg, J. A., Elster, E. A., Andersen, R. C., Nylen, E., Brown, T. S., Rose, M. W., et al. (2008). Correlation of procalcitonin and cytokine expression with dehiscence of wartime extremity wounds. *The Journal of Bone and Joint Surgery. American Volume, 90*(3), 580–588. https://doi.org/10.2106/JBJS.G.00265.

Fritz, J. M., & McDonald, J. R. (2008). Osteomyelitis: Approach to diagnosis and treatment. *The Physician and Sportsmedicine, 36*(1), nihpa116823.

Fry, D. E. (2017). Pressure irrigation of surgical incisions and traumatic wounds. *Surgical Infections, 18*(4), 424–430.

Granick, M. S., Tenenhaus, M., Knox, K. R., & Ulm, J. P. (2007). Comparison of wound irrigation and tangential hydrodissection in bacterial clearance of contaminated wounds: Results of a randomized, controlled clinical study. *Ostomy/Wound Management, 53*(4), 64–72.

Hake, M. E., Young, H., Hak, D. J., Stahel, P. F., Hammerberg, E. M., & Mauffrey, C. (2015). Local antibiotic therapy strategies in orthopaedic trauma: Practical tips and tricks and review of the literature. *Injury, 46*(8), 1447–1456.

Harris, A. M., Althausen, P. L., Kellam, J., Bosse, M. J., Castillo, R., & Lower Extremity Assessment Project (LEAP) Study Group. (2009). Complications following limb-threatening lower extremity trauma. *Journal of Orthopaedic Trauma, 23*(1), 1–6.

Helgeson, M. D., Potter, B. K., Evans, K. N., & Shawen, S. B. (2007). Bioartificial dermal substitute: A preliminary report on its use for the management of complex combat-related soft tissue wounds. *Journal of Orthopaedic Trauma, 21*(6), 394–399.

Henry, S., et al. (2018). *ATLS advanced trauma life support* (10th ed.). Chicago: American College of Surgeons.

Hess, J. R., Brohi, K., Dutton, R. P., Hauser, C. J., Holcomb, J. B., Kluger, Y., et al. (2008). The coagulopathy of trauma: A review of mechanisms. *The Journal of Trauma, 65*(4), 748–754.

Holcomb, J. B., Minei, K. M., Scerbo, M. L., Radwan, Z. A., Wade, C. E., Kozar, R. A., et al. (2012). Admission rapid thrombelastography can replace conventional coagulation tests in the emergency department: Experience with 1974 consecutive trauma patients. *Annals of Surgery, 256*(3), 476–486.

Holcomb, J. B., Stansbury, L. G., Champion, H. R., Wade, C., & Bellamy, R. F. (2006). Understanding combat casualty care statistics. *The Journal of Trauma, 60*(2), 397–401. https://doi.org/10.1097/01.ta.0000203581.75241.f1.

Howard, J. T., Kotwal, R. S., Stern, C. A., Janak, J. C., Mazuchowski, E. L., Butler, F. K., et al. (2019). Use of combat casualty care data to assess the US military trauma system during the Afghanistan and Iraq conflicts, 2001–2017. *JAMA Surgery, 154*(7), 600–608.

Howe, H. R., Jr., Poole, G. V., Jr., Hansen, K. J., Clark, T., Plonk, G. W., Koman, L. A., et al. (1987). Salvage of lower extremities following combined orthopedic and vascular trauma. A predictive salvage index. *The American Surgeon, 53*(4), 205–208.

Hoyt, B. W., Pavey, G. J., Potter, B. K., & Forsberg, J. A. (2018). Heterotopic ossification and lessons learned from fifteen years at war: A review of therapy, novel research, and future directions for military and civilian orthopaedic trauma. *Bone, 109*, 3–11. https://doi.org/10.1016/j.bone.2018.02.009.

Jensen, K. K., Henriksen, N. A., & Jorgensen, L. N. (2014). Endoscopic component separation for ventral hernia causes fewer wound complications compared to open components separation: A systematic review and meta-analysis. *Surgical Endoscopy, 28*(11), 3046–3052.

Jernigan, T. W., Fabian, T. C., Croce, M. A., Moore, N., Pritchard, F. E., Minard, G., et al. (2003). Staged management of giant abdominal wall defects: Acute and long-term results. *Annals of Surgery, 238*(3), 349–357.

Johansen, K., Daines, M., Howey, T., Helfet, D., & Hansen, S. T., Jr. (1990). Objective criteria accurately predict amputation following lower extremity trauma. *The Journal of Trauma, 30*(5), 568–573.

Joint Trauma System Clinical Practice Guidelines. (2020). https://jts.amedd.army.mil/index.cfm/PI_CPGs/cpgs. Accessed 14 August 2020.

Joint Trauma System Tactical Combat Casualty Care Collection. (2020). https://www.deployedmedicine.com/market/11. Accessed 28 February 2020.

Kafie, F. E., Tessier, D. J., Williams, R. A., Podnos, Y. D., Cinat, M., Lekawa, M., et al. (2003). Serial abdominal closure technique (the "SAC" procedure): A novel method for delayed closure of the abdominal wall. *The American Surgeon, 69*(2), 102–105.

Kam, P. C., Kavanagh, R., & Yoong, F. F. (2001). The arterial tourniquet: Pathophysiological consequences and anaesthetic implications. *Anaesthesia, 56*(6), 534–545.

Kelly, J. F., Ritenour, A. E., McLaughlin, D. F., Bagg, K. A., Apodaca, A. N., Mallak, C. T., et al. (2008). Injury severity and causes of death from Operation Iraqi Freedom and Operation Enduring Freedom: 2003–2004 versus 2006. *The Journal of Trauma, 64*(2 Suppl), S21–S27.

Klein, M. B., Hunter, S., Heimbach, D. M., Engrav, L. H., Honari, S., Gallery, E., et al. (2005). The Versajet water dissector: A new tool for tangential excision. *The Journal of Burn Care & Rehabilitation, 26*(6), 483–487.

Kozen, B. G., Kircher, S. J., Henao, J., Godinez, F. S., & Johnson, A. S. (2008). An alternative hemostatic dressing: Comparison of CELOX, HemCon, and QuikClot. *Academic Emergency Medicine, 15*(1), 74–81.x.

Kragh, J. F., Jr., Dubick, M. A., Aden, J. K., 3rd, McKeague, A. L., Rasmussen, T. E., Baer, D. G., et al. (2016). U.S. Military Experience from 2001 to 2010 with extremity fasciotomy in war surgery. *Military Medicine, 181*(5), 463–468.

Kragh, J. F., Jr., Walters, T. J., Baer, D. G., Fox, C. J., Wade, C. E., Salinas, J., et al. (2009). Survival with emergency tourniquet use to stop bleeding in major limb trauma. *Annals of Surgery, 249*(1), 1–7. https://doi.org/10.1097/SLA.0b013e31818842ba.

Krettek, C., Seekamp, A., Köntopp, H., & Tscherne, H. (2001). Hannover Fracture Scale '98—Re-evaluation and new perspectives of an established extremity salvage score. *Injury, 32*(4), 317–328. https://doi.org/10.1016/s0020-1383(00)00201-1.

Kwon, J., Staley, C., McCullough, M., Goss, S., Arosemena, M., Abai, B., et al. (2018). A randomized clinical trial evaluating negative pressure therapy to decrease vascular groin incision complications. *Journal of Vascular Surgery, 68*(6), 1744–1752. https://doi.org/10.1016/j.jvs.2018.05.224.

Levi, B., Hemmila, M. R., & Wang, W. C. (2016). Burns. In M. W. Mulholland (Ed.), *Greenfields surgery: Scientific principles and practice*. Philadelphia: Lippincott, Williams & Wilkins.

Lindstedt, S., Malmsjö, M., Gesslein, B., & Ingemansson, R. (2008). Evaluation of continuous and intermittent myocardial topical negative pressure. *Journal of Cardiovascular Medicine (Hagerstown, Md.), 9*(8), 813–819.

Lisboa, F. A., Dente, C. J., Schobel, S. A., Khatri, V., Potter, B. K., Kirk, A. D., et al. (2019). Utilizing precision medicine to estimate timing for surgical closure of traumatic extremity wounds. *Annals of Surgery, 270*(3), 535–543.

Llanos, S., Danilla, S., Barraza, C., Armijo, E., Piñeros, J. L., Quintas, M., et al. (2006). Effectiveness of negative pressure closure in the integration of split thickness skin grafts: A randomized, double-masked, controlled trial. *Annals of Surgery, 244*(5), 700–705.

Ly, T. V., Travison, T. G., Castillo, R. C., Bosse, M. J., MacKenzie, E. J., & LEAP Study Group. (2008). Ability of lower-extremity injury severity scores to predict functional outcome after limb salvage. *The Journal of Bone and Joint Surgery, 90*(8), 1738–1743.

Malmsjö, M., Gustafsson, L., Lindstedt, S., Gesslein, B., & Ingemansson, R. (2012). The effects of variable, intermittent, and continuous negative pressure wound therapy, using foam or gauze, on wound contraction, granulation tissue formation, and ingrowth into the wound filler. *Eplasty, 12*, e5.

Mathes, S. J., Steinwald, P. M., Foster, R. D., Hoffman, W. Y., & Anthony, J. P. (2000). Complex abdominal wall reconstruction: a comparison of flap and mesh closure. *Annals of Surgery, 232*(4), 586–596.

McNamara, M. G., Heckman, J. D., & Corley, F. G. (1994). Severe open fractures of the lower extremity: A retrospective evaluation of the mangled extremity severity score (MESS). *Journal of Orthopaedic Trauma, 8*(2), 81–87. https://doi.org/10.1097/00005131-199404000-00001.

Milburn, M. L., Shah, P. K., Friedman, E. B., Roth, J. S., Bochicchio, G. V., Gorbaty, B., et al. (2007). Laparoscopically assisted components separation technique for ventral incisional hernia repair. *Hernia, 11*(2), 157–161.

Moisidis, E., Heath, T., Boorer, C., Ho, K., & Deva, A. K. (2004). A prospective, blinded, randomized, controlled clinical trial of topical negative pressure use in skin grafting. *Plastic and Reconstructive Surgery, 114*(4), 917–922.

Morykwas, M. J., Argenta, L. C., Shelton-Brown, E. I., & McGuirt, W. (1997). Vacuum-assisted closure: A new method for wound control and treatment: animal studies and basic foundation. *Annals of Plastic Surgery, 38*(6), 553–562.

Neuffer, M. C., McDivitt, J., Rose, D., King, K., Cloonan, C. C., & Vayer, J. S. (2004). Hemostatic dressings for the first responder: A review. *Military Medicine, 169*(9), 716–720.

Nickel, W. N., Steelman, T. J., Sabath, Z. R., & Potter, B. K. (2018). Extra-articular retained missiles; is surveillance of lead levels needed? *Military Medicine, 183*(3–4), e107–e113.

Novitsky, Y. W., Elliott, H. L., Orenstein, S. B., & Rosen, M. J. (2012). Transversus abdominis muscle release: A novel approach to posterior component separation during complex abdominal wall reconstruction. *American Journal of Surgery, 204*(5), 709–716. https://doi.org/10.1016/j.amjsurg.2012.02.008.

Ostermann, P. A., Seligson, D., & Henry, S. L. (1995). Local antibiotic therapy for severe open fractures. A review of 1085 consecutive cases. *The Journal of Bone and Joint Surgery, 77*(1), 93–97.

Parnes, N., Carey, P. A., & Marmor, M. (2017). Upper extremity. In E. E. Moore, et al. (Eds.), *Trauma*. New York: McGraw-Hill.

Pavey, G. J., Qureshi, A. T., Tomasino, A. M., Honnold, C. L., Bishop, D. K., Agarwal, S., et al. (2016). Targeted stimulation of retinoic acid receptor-γ mitigates the formation of heterotopic ossification in an established blast-related traumatic injury model. *Bone, 90*, 159–167. https://doi.org/10.1016/j.bone.2016.06.014.

Perkins, J. G., Cap, A. P., Weiss, B. M., Reid, T. J., & Bolan, C. D. (2008). Massive transfusion and nonsurgical hemostatic agents. *Critical Care Medicine, 36*(7 Suppl), S325–S339. https://doi.org/10.1097/CCM.0b013e31817e2ec5.

Pons, P. T., & Jacobs, L. (2017). *Save a life: What everyone should know to stop bleeding after and injury*. Chicago: American College of Surgeons.

Potter, B. K., Burns, T. C., Lacap, A. P., Granville, R. R., & Gajewski, D. (2006). Heterotopic ossification in the residual limbs of traumatic and combat-related amputees. *The Journal of the American Academy of Orthopaedic Surgeons, 14*(10), S191–S197.

Potter, B. K., Burns, T. C., Lacap, A. P., Granville, R. R., & Gajewski, D. A. (2007). Heterotopic ossification following traumatic and combat-related amputations. Prevalence, risk factors, and preliminary results of excision. *The Journal of Bone and Joint Surgery. American Volume, 89*(3), 476–486.

Pusateri, A. E., Modrow, H. E., Harris, R. A., Holcomb, J. B., Hess, J. R., Mosebar, R. H., et al. (2003). Advanced hemostatic dressing development program: Animal model selection criteria and results of a study of nine hemostatic dressings in a model of severe large venous hemorrhage and hepatic injury in Swine. *The Journal of Trauma, 55*(3), 518–526.

Ramasamy, A., Hill, A. M., Phillip, R., Gibb, I., Bull, A. M., & Clasper, J. C. (2011). The modern "deck-slap" injury—Calcaneal blast fractures from vehicle explosions. *The Journal of Trauma, 71*(6), 1694–1698.

Ramirez, O. M., Ruas, E., & Dellon, A. L. (1990). "Components separation" method for closure of abdominal-wall defects: An anatomic and clinical study. *Plastic and Reconstructive Surgery, 86*(3), 519–526.

Rhee, P., Brown, C., Martin, M., Salim, A., Plurad, D., Green, D., et al. (2008). QuikClot use in trauma for hemorrhage control: Case series of 103 documented uses. *The Journal of Trauma, 64*(4), 1093–1099.

Roberts, I., Shakur, H., Coats, T., Hunt, B., Balogun, E., Barnetson, L., et al. (2013). The CRASH-2 trial: A randomised controlled trial and economic evaluation of the effects of tranexamic acid on death, vascular occlusive events and transfusion requirement in bleeding trauma patients. *Health Technology Assessment (Winchester), 17*(10), 1–79.

Russell, W. L., Sailors, D. M., Whittle, T. B., Fisher, D. F., Jr., & Burns, R. P. (1991). Limb salvage versus traumatic amputation. A decision based on a seven-part predictive index. *Annals of Surgery, 213*(5), 473–481. https://doi.org/10.1097/00000658-199105000-00013.

Schecter, W. P., Ivatury, R. R., Rotondo, M. F., & Hirshberg, A. (2006). Open abdomen after trauma and abdominal sepsis: A strategy for management. *Journal of the American College of Surgeons, 203*(3), 390–396.

Shackford, S. R., & Sise, M. J. (2017). Peripheral vascular injury. In E. E. Moore, et al. (Eds.), *Trauma*. New York: McGraw-Hill.

Singleton, J. A., Gibb, I. E., Hunt, N. C., Bull, A. M., & Clasper, J. C. (2013). Identifying future "unexpected" survivors: A retrospective cohort study of fatal injury patterns in victims of improvised explosive devices. *BMJ Open, 3*(8), e003130.

Singer, M., et al. (2016). The third international consensus definitions for sepsis and septic shock (sepsis-3). *JAMA, 315*(8), 801–810. https://doi.org/10.1001/jama.2016.0287.

Stanec, Z., Skrbić, S., Dzepina, I., Hulina, D., Ivrlac, R., Unusić, J., et al. (1993). High-energy war wounds: Flap reconstruction. *Annals of Plastic Surgery, 31*(2), 97–102.

Stojadinovic, A., Carlson, J. W., Schultz, G. S., Davis, T. A., & Elster, E. A. (2008). Topical advances in wound care. *Gynecologic Oncology, 111*(2 Suppl), S70–S80.

Tintle, S. M., Keeling, J. J., Shawen, S. B., Forsberg, J. A., & Potter, B. K. (2010). Traumatic and trauma-related amputations: part I: General principles and lower-extremity amputations. *The Journal of Bone and Joint Surgery, 92*(17), 2852–2868.

Tintle, S. M., Shawen, S. B., Forsberg, J. A., Gajewski, D. A., Keeling, J. J., Andersen, R. C., et al. (2014). Reoperation after combat-related major lower extremity amputations. *Journal of Orthopaedic Trauma, 28*(4), 232–237. https://doi.org/10.1097/BOT.0b013e3182a53130.

Tredget, E. E., Shankowsky, H. A., Groeneveld, A., & Burrell, R. (1998). A matched-pair, randomized study evaluating the efficacy and safety of Acticoat silver-coated dressing for the treatment of burn wounds. *The Journal of Burn Care & Rehabilitation, 19*(6), 531–537.

Ubbink, D. T., Westerbos, S. J., Nelson, E. A., & Vermeulen, H. (2008). A systematic review of topical negative pressure therapy for acute and chronic wounds. *The British Journal of Surgery, 95*(6), 685–692.

Vertrees, A., Greer, L., Pickett, C., Nelson, J., Wakefield, M., Stojadinovic, A., et al. (2008). Modern management of complex open abdominal wounds of war: A 5-year experience. *Journal of the American College of Surgeons, 207*(6), 801–809.

Volgas, D. A. (2007). Care of the soft tissue envelope. In J. P. Stannard, et al. (Eds.), *Surgical treatment of orthopaedic trauma*. New York, NY: Thieme Medical Publishers.

Weinberg, J. A., George, R. L., Griffin, R. L., Stewart, A. H., Reiff, D. A., Kerby, J. D., et al. (2008). Closing the open abdomen: improved success with Wittmann Patch staged abdominal closure. *The Journal of Trauma, 65*(2), 345–348.

Weintrob, A. C., Murray, C. K., Xu, J., Krauss, M., Bradley, W., Warkentien, T. E., et al. (2018). Early infections complicating the care of combat casualties from Iraq and Afghanistan. *Surgical Infections, 19*(3), 286–297.

Wikkelsø, A., Wetterslev, J., Møller, A. M., & Afshari, A. (2016). Thromboelastography (TEG) or thromboelastometry (ROTEM) to monitor haemostatic treatment versus usual care in adults or children with bleeding. *Cochrane Database of Systematic Reviews, 2016*(8), CD007871. https://doi.org/10.1002/14651858. CD007871.pub3. Accessed 4/10/2020.

Wilson, J. R., Mills, J. G., Prather, I. D., & Dimitrijevich, S. D. (2005). A toxicity index of skin and wound cleansers used on in vitro fibroblasts and keratinocytes. *Advances in Skin & Wound Care, 18*(7), 373–378.

Wininger, D. A., & Fass, R. J. (1996). Antibiotic-impregnated cement and beads for orthopedic infections. *Antimicrobial Agents and Chemotherapy, 40*(12), 2675–2679.

Witmer, D. K., Marshall, S. T., & Browner, B. D. (2017). Emergency care of musculoskeletal injuries. In C. M. Townsend, et al. (Eds.), *Sabiston textbook of surgery*. Philadelphia: Elsevier.

Yin, H. Q., Langford, R., & Burrell, R. E. (1999). Comparative evaluation of the antimicrobial activity of ACTICOAT antimicrobial barrier dressing. *The Journal of Burn Care & Rehabilitation, 20*(3), 195–200.

34

Burns

Marc Robert Matthews

OBJECTIVES

1. Discuss mechanisms of burn injury, epidemiology, and pathophysiology of burn injury.
2. Describe the three phases of burn care and key management objectives for each phase including early emergency room care, initial intravenous resuscitation.
3. Discuss potential complications associated with burns such as compartment syndrome, inhalation injury, and hypertrophic scarring.
4. List the American Burn Association burn injury transfer criteria.
5. Identify assessment parameters for burn injury including depth, zone, and size.
6. Discuss appropriate topical management for burn wounds and donor site care including antimicrobials, eschar excision, debridement, wound dressings (i.e., CTPs).
7. Identify the role of outpatient care, physical/occupational therapy, and rehabilitation.

EPIDEMIOLOGY

A burn injury is primarily the result of heat (thermal) but is also caused by radiation, radioactivity, electricity, friction or contact with chemicals (World Health Organization, 2018). As the fourth most common type of civilian trauma worldwide, burns are a global public health problem. The incidence of burn injuries exceeds the combined incidence of HIV/AIDS and tuberculosis, approaching the incidence of malignant neoplasms (GBD 2019 Disease and Injuries Collaborators, 2020). Burns account for as many as 180,000 deaths annually with almost 90% occurring in low- or middle-income countries and almost two-thirds of those burn injuries occurring in the African and South-East Asia WHO regions.

In the United States, there is one home fire every 93 s (Hall & Everts, 2022). Burns do not always require referral to a burn center or unit. On average, 90% seek emergency treatment within the first few hours after a burn injury and are then discharged (American Burn Association, 2018). A key reason for this is that most burns are small (less than 10% of total body surface area) (Greenhalgh, 2019; American Burn Association, n.d.). In 2016 approximately 486,000 burn injuries were treated in an emergency department, doctor's office, or outpatient clinic. Of these, an estimated 40,000 required hospitalization due to burn injury, 60% (30,000) of whom were admitted to one of the 128 burn centers (American Burn Association, n.d.). These burn centers average over 200 annual admissions of thermally injured patients. The patient survival rate for burn injuries is 96.8% (American Burn Association, n.d.).

More recently, over the 3-year period of 2016 through 2018, civilian burn injuries were estimated at 10,390 (Miller, 2021). Similarly, 11,100 civilian burn injuries were reported in 2021 (Hall & Everts, 2022).

Burn injuries resulting in death occur every 2 h and 41 min (American Burn Association, n.d.). In 2016 alone, estimated burn fatalities from residential fires were 2745, vehicular crash-related fires resulted in 310 deaths, and there were 220 deaths from other sources (America Burn Association, n.d.). The estimated fire related deaths from residential fires between 2016 and 2018 averaged 2370 (Miller, 2021). Additional epidemiological factors describing burn injuries are listed in Box 34.1.

Over the past 50 years burn injury as a disease entity has been a major success story in the United States (Litt, 2018). There have been major environmental and manufacturing improvements, with more safety regulations, stricter building codes, and wider use of sprinkler systems in the United States. Burn treatment has improved due to advances in surgical critical care, early burn excision with improved grafting techniques, intravenous fluid resuscitation, infection control, metabolic, nutrition, and ventilatory support (Jeschke & Herndon, 2017). The current Burn Team is comprised of a burn surgeon, critical care intensivist, indispensable nursing personnel, pharmacist, physical/occupational, respiratory and speech therapists, nutritionist, psychologist, child life specialist, anesthesiologist, physiatrist, social service worker, and case manager.

Burn injury is still a major trauma concern, since the United States population has been increasing in terms of absolute numbers, even though there is a decrease in the percent of burn injuries overall (American Burn Association, n.d.; Grand View Research, 2023). While burn survival has increased over the past half century (Branski, Herndon, & Barrow, 2012), burn mortality has remained stable for the past few years. One study found that mortality is based on the three factors: age >60 years, burn size >40% and inhalation injury. Mortality increased as the risk factors increased from a low of 0.3% with zero factors to a high of 90% with the presence of all three factors (Ryan et al., 1998).

MECHANISMS OF INJURY

Burn injuries may occur secondary to a variety of sources but thermal injuries (the presence of too much heat) such as scalding water or burning materials (e.g., wood or other substances in a house fire) are the most common. Thermal injuries also occur when tissue is in direct cutaneous contact with a medium that carries heat away such as snow, ice or cold water. The hypothermic (frostbite) injury itself causes less damage. The thawing of the frozen tissue or limb results in more significant harm including vessel thrombosis, tissue ischemia, and necrosis (Tintinalli, 2016). Frostbite is discussed in more detail in Chapter 32.

Electrical

Electrical injury, often called the great masquerader, may result from any multitude of sources but accounts for approximately 3% of all burn injuries (Waldmann, Narayanan, Combes, & Marijon, 2017). This type of injury is caused by the strength of the electrical current, electroporation, thermal injury production or from a fall after being thrown at the scene. The electrical current, as the most important determinant of tissue damage, enters the body as a small contact wound but exits in a much larger wound pattern; both should

be identified, explored, and adequately treated. Higher voltage electricity produces a larger burn injury. Burn injuries are also proportional to the duration of contact, the tissue resistance between the entry and exit sites and the cross-sectional area of contact.

Electrical injuries may damage the skin but also penetrate and affect the underlying tissues of less resistance such as muscle, nerve and vessels which lead to cardiac asystole or even a traumatic amputation (Tintinalli, 2016). Skin, fat and bones have a higher resistance to electricity, thus the heat released destroys the adjacent lower-resistance tissue (Kidd et al., 2007; Skoog, 1970). Blood vessels and nerves are great conductors of electrical current because of their lower resistance but can still sustain severe damage (Spies & Trohman, 2006). If the skin becomes wet, electrical conduction drops a thousand-fold (Spies & Trohman, 2006; Skoog, 1970). After an electrical injury, the skin may appear only slightly damaged, but the affected muscles and nerves may develop muscle destruction, nervous paresthesias and paralysis, respectively (Bryan, Andrews, Hurley, & Taber, 2009; Spies & Trohman, 2006). Electroporation is the cellular disruption by membrane damage, producing pores that release cellular content and destroy the cells (Bryan et al., 2009; Spies & Trohman, 2006). This can also occur in intimal layers of blood vessels, producing external hemorrhage and vessel thrombosis. Over time, the injured muscle may necrose from the initial injury and not from inadequate debridement.

As the injured extremity swells from tissue destruction and intravenous fluid (IVF) resuscitation, it may become pulseless distal to the circumferential electrical burn injury prompting the need for a fasciotomy to release that muscular compartment pressure to allow distal blood flow. If not recognized in time, the patient's distal digits and the affected extremity will become ischemic (Davis & Graham, 1981; Hettiaratchy & Papini, 2004). After 6 h, there is a high likelihood for the need for an amputation. If the electrical injury crosses the chest, cardiac asystole may result from ventricular fibrillation (Kroll, Fish, Lakkireddy, Luceri, & Panescu, 2012; Spies & Trohman, 2006). Neurologic signals may disrupt the respiratory system leading to apnea. If the electrical injury enters or exits at the cranial level, the brain and cervical spine must be evaluated with a CT scan, frequent neurologic checks, a mini-mental status examine, and a baseline eye assessment for possible subsequent traumatic cataract formation.

Chemical

Chemical injuries occur as a result of contact with an acid, base, or organic substance, such as hydrocarbons, each potentially leading to cutaneous damage. Most injuries occur in younger-aged males in the workplace or at home (Friedstat, Brown, & Levi, 2017). There are six types of chemical burns: (1) reduction by binding to free electrons of proteins, for example, hydrochloric acid; (2) oxidation by oxidizing proteins, for example, sodium hypochlorite acid (bleach); (3) corrosion by denaturing proteins on contact, for example, phenols, white phosphorous; (4) protoplasmic poisoning by binding calcium, magnesium or other organic ions, for example, hydrofluoric acid; (5) vesicants which produce ischemia and necrosis, for example, mustard gas or Lewisite and (6) desiccation by dehydrating tissue and releasing exothermic energy, for example, sulfuric or muriatic acid (Herndon & Tompkins, 2004). The degree of chemical burn injury and depth of penetration is dependent on duration of contact, volume of the chemical in contact with the skin, chemical concentration, and whether the chemical was washed off completely. As the skin is typically either denatured or liquefied, the depth and rate of chemical absorption into the tissues becomes erratic. Systemic absorption can also occur. The clinician must monitor for indications of adverse effects to internal organs: cardiac irregularities, renal impairment and anuria, electrolyte disturbances, and mental status changes (Herndon & Tompkins, 2004; Mayer & Werman, 2019). Classically, acid injuries (pH < 2) destroy by protein coagulation and protein denaturation. Whether ingested or topical, alkali injuries (pH > 11.5) penetrate deeper, more extensively, and cause more damage by liquefaction necrosis (Tintinalli, 2016). The result is a soapy texture to the skin secondary to cutaneous saponification. Prior to irrigation, for acid and alkaline burns, water irrigations regulated by the litmus paper test, are required as soon as possible until the cutaneous pH is close to normal (pH 5.5) and rechecked in the emergency department. If a transfer occurs, and the pH is still aberrant, further irrigations are required. Hydrocarbons such as petrol and organic solutions damage cellular membranes and the exposed skin should be irrigated as well. Antidotes to the chemical, such as bacitracin to remove tar or water to remove most chemicals, should not be used if an exothermic reaction is expected but certainly should be considered if an exothermic reaction is *not* expected. White phosphorous granules ignite on exposure to air, so gloves, gown, and eyewear are essential attire during removal from the cutaneous wound. Forceps should be utilized to place the granules in a water bath to prevent further ignition once extracted. It is recommended to wait 48–72 h to allow the chemical burn to declare its fullest extent of injury prior to debridement.

UNDERLYING PRINCIPLES OF ACUTE BURN CARE

Most wound care and emergency department providers are proficient in the treatment of burn injuries and other skin disorders. It is a fundamental tenet that all burn wounds must be debrided to remove dead tissue clinging to the burn wound: superficial burn eschar, un-sloughed burned tissue, and blistered skin (ABLS, 2018). This traumatized tissue is invaded by prokaryotic organisms and requires prompt removal because it is adjacent to open cutaneous wounds and therefore susceptible to infection. If this tissue is not removed, the burn wound may become infected and develop surrounding cellulitis of the unburned skin. Subsequently, fever and chills may ensue with the onset of bacteremia and sepsis. The initial debridement by the practitioner exposes the full extent of the injury and protects against infection. All blisters should remain in place as a

"biologic dressing" until the patient is promptly transferred to a burn center where the blisters will be subsequently debrided. However, if the patient is not to be transferred, then the blisters must be immediately debrided and covered with an appropriate dressing with close follow-up. The wound is covered with a topical antimicrobial dressing and frequently monitored if the patient is admitted. Systemic antibiotics are not needed in the acute burn setting because all wounds are colonized but not infected. If the burn wound is several days old and develops cellulitis accompanied with a fever, systemic antibiotics may be required. Every patient should receive a tetanus vaccination or booster (within 5 years) to prevent burn wound associated with *Clostridium tetani* infection.

Initial burn care in any emergency department must be swift and purposefully utilize Advanced Trauma Life Support (ATLS) protocols (ATLS COT; Rosenkranz and Sheridan, 2002). As with all trauma patients, a primary survey is initiated, the airway is assessed and stabilized, followed by the patient's breathing and cardiovascular systems (Hettiaratchy & Papini, 2004). Intravenous access is essential and can be placed through burned skin if unburned tissue is not available. If necessary, a central venous catheter may be placed but the thermally injured patient may have such a low intravascular volume, venous cannulation may not be immediately attainable. An intraosseous infusing line may be placed in an unbroken bone of a child or an adult allowing for immediate volume instillation until adequate intravenous cannulation can be obtained. Once other life-threatening, traumatic injuries are found and addressed, the secondary survey is initiated during which the skin should be assessed for depth and size of the burn injury (Matthews et al., 2019)

Compartment Syndrome, Escharotomy, and Fasciotomy

All rings, jewelry, piercings and tight-fitting clothing must be removed to prevent a tourniquet effect secondary to the ensuing edema. The practitioner must be alert to the presence of the circumferentially burned extremities, torso or neck (Bezuhly & Fish, 2012). With inflammation and resuscitation, increased edema will occur resulting in a compartment syndrome. As blood flow becomes limited distally and ischemia develops, this can cause nervous and muscle damage (Brown, Greenhalgh, Kagan, & Warden, 1994). Escharotomy, an incision made through the length of the burn eschar into the normal subcutaneous tissue, or possible fasciotomy, a deeper incision through the fascial levels covering the muscles of the extremity, must be performed to release the elevated tissue pressures. These incisions are required to establish normal blood flow to the distal forearms, hands, fingers, legs, feet, or toes. Subsequent to these decompressive procedures, the patient is assessed for a return of a palpable pulse, capillary refill, or Doppler signals in the major arterial blood vessels. Additional escharotomies may be required for the release of compartment syndrome in the chest when associated with decreased oxygen saturations, decreased lung tidal volumes, increased peak airway pressures, or a decrease in urine output. Abdominal compartment syndrome, manifested by hypotension with increased tachycardia, a tense abdomen on physical examination, and elevated bladder pressures, will also require release with a laparotomy incision with the patient is under general anesthesia. If there is a fixed acidosis, as noted by an elevated lactic acidosis, decreased bicarbonate levels, a depressed pH level below 7.20 or an elevated base deficit, during the assessment for abdominal compartment syndrome, the clinician must be concerned for ischemic bowel until proven otherwise. While decompressive escharotomies and fasciotomies have been well-described in the literature, missed or delayed presentation remains an issue in the clinical care of the burn patients (Orgill & Piccolo, 2009).

Inhalation Injury

The thermally injured patient may require an endotracheal tube for an inhalation injury (Esnault et al., 2014; Onishi, Osuka, Kuroki, & Ueyama, 2017). Once the burning process has been stopped with either removal of the patient from the environment or the irrigation of the wound on-scene, the airway must be evaluated. Inhalation injury must be suspected in all patients with a history of being exposed to smoke in an enclosed environment (Grabowska, Skowronek, Nowicka, & Sybirska, 2012). Patients with singed facial hair (beard, mustaches, eyebrows or eyelashes, burns to the face, eyes, or neck) must be evaluated for loss of airway (Pruitt & Wolf, 2009). In addition, complaints of stridor, dyspnea, tachypnea, or carbonaceous sputum production are indicative of an airway injury. Progression of hoarseness or gasping for air mandates immediate intubation with an endotracheal tube or potentially a cricothyrotomy with placement of a tube beyond the vocal cords for a definitive airway. Patients with COPD or asthma may only have a finite amount of time before the airway is lost. The majority of airway injuries to pulmonary parenchyma occur when patients inhale incomplete products of combustion during a fire, such as carbon monoxide, cyanide, arsenicals, phosgenes, and other products. Steam can damage the mucosa of the airway above the vocal cords and possibly down to the upper trachea leading to edema requiring intubation. In large, total body surface area (TBSA) burns with a concomitant infusion of resuscitation fluid, the airway can become edematous and should be secured prior to progressive airway loss. After securing the airway, carbon monoxide and cyanide levels should be obtained. Carbon monoxide binds to hemoglobin 240 times that of oxygen and displaces it from hemoglobin (Ernst & Zibrak, 1998). Therefore, the pulse oximeter which only registers whatever is bound to hemoglobin, becomes inaccurate. The patient should be kept on 100% FiO_2 from 45 min to 4 h to decrease the half-life potential of carbon monoxide poisoning (Mayer & Werman, 2019). Hydroxycyanocobalamin can be administered intravenously to counteract the effects of cyanide toxicity in the patient if cyanide poisoning is suspected (Alharbi et al., 2012; Kaita, Tarui, Shoji, Miyauchi, &

Yamaguchi, 2018). All patients with a suspected inhalation injury leading to intubation should have a bronchoscopy performed postintubation to identify and assess the extent of airway injury.

Guidelines for Referral

Since most burn injuries can be handled as an outpatient, a limited number of burn patients require referral and transfer to a burn center. Referral criteria, as established by the American Burn Association (ABA), are listed in Box 34.2. Based on a combination of burn mechanism, burn depth, extent and anatomic location, the overall severity of the burn injuries may can be categorized as minor, moderate or major (Jeschke et al., 2020; Rice & Orgill, 2021) (Table 34.1). These categories provide general guidance on preferred disposition. Communication with a regional burn center is often helpful to discern appropriate care and transfer if warranted. If patients do not fit the advocated criteria for transfer, most of the smaller burns can be treated with topical agents and over the counter nonsteroidal pain medications or occasionally a small number of narcotics. Larger burns, that is, greater than 20% TBSA, require admission for intravenous resuscitation, possible endotracheal intubation (if there is a suspicion of inhalation injury), adequate sedation, and opioid pain medications (Onishi et al., 2017). Clinicians in all settings must also be vigilant to identify the signs of nonaccidental pediatric burns during physical examination and be prepared to treat the nonaccidental pediatric burn patients (Box 34.3).

Other Skin Disorders

Burn centers possess resources for the necessary surgical intervention and treatment for numerous other nonburn-related skin disorders. Such conditions include necrotizing fasciitis,

---

BOX 34.2 American Burn Association Referral Criteria[a]

(1) Full-thickness thermal burns
(2) Partial thickness thermal burns that are equal to or greater than 10% total body surface area
(3) Any deep partial or full thickness thermal burns that involves the hands, face, feet, genitalia, perineum or over any joints
(4) Patients with thermal burns and other comorbidities
(5) Patients with thermal burns and concomitant traumatic injuries
(6) Thermal burns with poorly controlled pain
(7) Suspected inhalational injuries
(8) All pediatric burns
(9) All chemical burns
(10) All high voltage ($\geq$1000 V) electrical injuries and lightening injuries

[a]For more information, see the detailed Guidelines for Burn Patient Referral. (Advice on Transfer and Consultation). https://ameriburn.org/burnreferral.

TABLE 34.1 Overall Severity of Burn Injury[a]

Minor Burns	Moderate Burns	Major Burns
Adults: <10% TBSA	Adults: 10%–20% TBSA, mixed partial/full thickness	Adult: >20% TBSA
Young children and elderly: <5% TBSA	Young children or elderly 5% to 10% TBSA; 2–5% if full thickness burn	>10% TBSA in young children and elderly
<2% TBSA full-thickness burns not involving cosmetic or functional risk or impairment of face, ears, eyes, feet, hands, perineum	High voltage injury; possible inhalation injury; circumferential burn; other health problems	>10% TBSA full thickness burn All burns of face, eyes, ears, hands, or perineum, especially if functional or cosmetic impairment exists All high-voltage burns Known inhalation injury Associated injuries

TBSA, total body surface area.
[a]Minor burns are often managed in outpatient setting while major burns require hospitalization.
Adapted from Collins, SW: Burns (2019). https://www.infectiousdiseaseadvisor.com/home/decision-support-in-medicine/hospital-infection-control/burns/

BOX 34.3 Nonaccidental Burn Criteria

- Multiple hematomas, broken bones and scars in various stages of healing
- Concurrent injuries or evidence of neglect (e.g., malnutrition)
- History of prior hospitalization for "accidental" trauma
- Unexplained delay between time of injury and first attempt to obtain medical attention
- Burns appear older than the alleged time of the accident
- Account of accident not compatible with age and ability of patient
- Adults in charge allege that there are no witnesses to the "accident" and that the child was merely discovered to have been burned
- Relatives other than parents bring injured child to the hospital
- Burn is attributed to the action of a sibling or other child
- Injured child is excessively withdrawn, submissive, or overly polite or does not cry during painful procedures
- Scalds on hands or feet, often symmetric, appear to be full thickness in depth, suggesting extremities were forcibly immersed and held in hot liquid
- Isolated burns of buttocks that could hardly be produced by accidental means in children

necrotizing soft tissue infections, Stevens-Johnson syndrome, toxic epidermal necrolysis, calciphylaxis, extensive pressure injuries, cutaneous infection (cellulitis), large abscess, distal extremity vasopressor-induced ischemia, scalded skin syndrome, and purpura fulminans. Cutaneous diseases such as pemphigoid diseases coupled with a variety of other epidermal skin sloughing diseases, such as psoriasis, do not usually meet admission criteria because they do not require surgical intervention or large fluid resuscitations. Although these entities only require medical management with local or regional wound care, consultation with a regional burn center is advised. Chapter 32 provides a description of many of these conditions.

Burn Pathophysiology

Initial burn injury does not lead to immediate shock. When burns are greater than 20% TBA in the adult patient, there is a massive release of inflammatory mediators that can lead to systemic inflammatory response syndrome (SIRS) and increased vasodilatation (Nielson, Duethman, Howard, Moncure, & Wood, 2017). After 4–6 h, burn shock can develop due to third spacing of intravascular fluids into the soft tissues throughout the entire body even in areas not affected by the burn. Such third-spacing does not include red blood cells unlike that seen with traumatic injuries. Third spacing must be replaced with intravenous fluid due to intravascular fluid leakage which contributes to subsequent tissues and organ hypoperfusion. After a major burn injury, mast cells undergo a massive release of histamine in the systemic tissue vascular tree causing vascular fluid leakage (Santos et al., 2000), while eicosanoids and serotonin release cause vascular leakage in the pulmonary vascular tree (Zhang, Irtun, Zheng, & Wolfe, 2000). Other products may negatively affect the coagulation system leading to a hypercoagulable state. Patients with such thermal injury have not only increased inflammation and hypermetabolism but also have subsequent problems with glycolysis, lipolysis, proteolysis, and insulin utilization (Herndon & Tompkins, 2004). In this hypermetabolic and catabolic state, the patient subsequently becomes tachycardic and hypotensive despite an initial increase in systemic vascular resistance. Myocardial depressant effect is produced from the release of these systemic inflammatory mediators leading to a reduced cardiac output. With adequate resuscitation, the patient should have a return to improved hemodynamic levels within 24–48 h. The hypermetabolic response to the burn injury may continue, albeit to a lesser degree, for up to a year. The patient with a large burn can no longer thermoregulate and losses temperature quickly to the environment leading to hypothermia. The large surface area burned patient is also at risk for renal failure and sepsis, but classically, after the first 24 h, will become hypermetabolic, develop malnutrition from catabolism, loss of muscle mass, and eventual graft loss, if the patient does not receive adequate calories enterically. Most burn centers start feeding the patient on admission unless there are contraindications present.

Extent of Burn Injury
Depth of Burn Injury

Three levels of thermal burn injury depth are classically described. Approximately 70% of physical examinations are accurate when describing burn depth by the experienced, clinical practitioner, but recent developments in technology can increase the accuracy of depth (Bezuhly & Fish, 2012). This includes the use of laser doppler which can assist in measuring the depth of the thermally injured tissue (Shin and Yi, 2016; Hop et al., 2013). However, burn injuries can also evolve into deeper burn eschar if not adequately treated or become infected.

Superficial burn (formally first degree). The first layer of thermal injury is called a superficial burn, formerly denoted as first degree, which includes penetrating thermal energy down into the epidermis. The skin is unbroken, warm, and red as a result of vasodilatation and blanches easily when depressed. Equivalent to a mild to moderate sunburn or kitchen scald with unbroken skin, and painful to touch, it heals in 4–7 days if no further thermal energy is transmitted to the skin surface. In subsequent days, the skin will eventually desquamate and may even start peeling the most superficial stratum corneum and granulosum layers, but it never blisters. There is no scaring as a result this depth of injury. A superficial burn area is not counted when calculating total burn surface area.

Partial thickness (formerly second degree). The next level of injury can be divided into two categories called superficial partial thickness and deep partial-thickness burns.

- Superficial Partial Thickness: A superficial partial thickness burn extends through the epidermis into the upper half of the papillary dermis producing blisters or sloughing at the epidermal/dermal interface. When this tissue is debrided in the emergency department, it is pink and shiny secondary to the serum oozing through damaged but viable dermal tissue. It blanches to digital depression, and hair follicles are present. It is rarely a source of bleeding but if the burn wound is large enough, it can result in significant fluid loss. Because the nerve endings are directly involved and damaged but not destroyed, the wound surface is very painful. Healing occurs during the next 21 days with topical medications and dressing changes but does not necessitate eschar excision and skin grafting. Only slight surface discoloration might be evident in the long-term. The wound reepithelializes from the retained epidermal elements in the hair follicular shaft, sweat glands, and rete ridges of the skin in the reticular dermis.
- Deep Partial Thickness: A deep partial-thickness burn may appear whitish, tan with a reddish/pinkish hue just below the injured surface. This injury extends down to the deep dermis and reticular dermis. It may be dry or slightly moist, but this is based on the depth of damage into the dermis. There is either no or very slow capillary refill with digital depression. The skin is painful, but hair follicles may still be present. Inadequate or delayed resuscitation, subsequent skin infection, or continued chemical penetration into the dermis may go on to develop a deeper injury resulting in a full-thickness burn. Healing occurs in 21 to 28 days and more evident scarring may be the result of this thermal injury.

Full thickness (formerly third degree). Full-thickness burns, formerly considered 3rd degree, involve all layers of the epidermis and dermis and extend into the subcutaneous tissue. The full-thickness burn is insensate because the nerve endings are severely damaged or destroyed, and the wounds are not painful. There is no blood flow and the eschar will not blanch with digital depression. In addition, the burn eschar is dry and leathery to the touch and may appear white, tan, brown, black, purple or possibly cherry-red but dry (Alharbi et al., 2012). Because of tissue destruction and coagulated capillaries in the full-thickness burn, it is dry and there is no serous ooze through the eschar. Third degree thermal burns require excision and grafting as the burned tissue cannot regenerate itself. There is no reticular dermis, which contains the organelles such as sweat glands and hair follicles, which provide the necessary epidermal cells for skin regeneration. This damaged skin may become a reservoir for prokaryotic organisms that can lead to overwhelming infection, sepsis and death. If the patient does survive without excision and grafting, severe contractures will develop, causing limitations in extremity/torso function and scar disfigurement.

Fourth-degree burns are more challenging to accurately describe as the burn depth is not fully identified until the patient is in the operating room. Although there is a clinical classification called the Index of Deep Burn Injury (IDBI) (Zhu, Donelan, & Sheridan, 1997), and laboratory models (Zelt, Daniel, Ballard, Brissette, & Heroux, 1988), a classification of two distinct levels is simpler and based on the fascial anatomy.

TYPE A fourth-degree burns are full-thickness burn injuries that extend beyond the epidermis and dermis into the adipose tissue but remain above the level of the fascia. Such burns occur in isolated segmental regions of the extremity or torso in direct contact with a thermal source for a prolonged time period. Examples are a patient with diabetic foot neuropathy in contact with hot asphalt and a burn which extends to the plantar fascia; road rash friction injuries which involve adipose tissue and extend to the fascia.

TYPE B fourth-degree burns are full-thickness burns which destroy all epidermal and dermal layers above as well as muscles, nerves, blood vessels and bone below the fascia. This can be secondary to (1) mechanical injury such as road rash, (2) direct cutaneous contact such as an intensely hot surface, for example, molten metals, or (3) a blast that tears soft tissue away, for example, a traumatic amputation, concomitant with thermal energy destruction from the explosion. While thermally injured internal organs are rare, they can occur with further extension into the abdomen, chest, neck, or extremities from such intense heat seen with industrial incidents or combat. An example includes the eyes which are the only exposed portion of the brain. The use of the term fifth-degree burn is considered a thermal injury including the bone.

Burn Zones

An additional burn model exists in describing zones of the burn injury initially described by Jackson (1953) (see Plate 84). The center of the area injured is considered the zone of coagulation, an irreversibly damaged region that will never return to function despite resuscitation efforts. Immediately adjacent is the zone of stasis with decreased perfusion. The zone of stasis has the potential to return to be functional if the tissue is adequately resuscitated and if not, will undergo necrosis because of vascular thrombosis. Resuscitation delivers the necessary nutrients required for survival including oxygen, glucose and other products coupled with the removal of waste products. Immediately around the zone of stasis is the zone of hyperemia that represents a minimally injured and vasodilated region that will most likely survive and is akin to that of a superficial burn. It is engorged and erythematous in appearance and facilitates the delivery of blood and nutrients to the zone of stasis.

Burn Size

Burn size can be measured using the classic description in the Lund Browder chart (Fig. 34.1). This chart has percent total body surface area (%TBSA) assigned by age and injured body regions and is applied to the Parkland or other resuscitation formulas. In an average adult, a Rule of Nines quick calculation shows upper extremity 9%; lower extremity 18%; front torso

and back, each 18%; the head and neck 9%; the perineum and genitalia 1% TBSA. If the burn is scattered, small or covers the surfaces atypically, the hand model using the outstretched palm and extended fingers can be utilized and equates to one percent in the average adult. Children do not fit into the rule of nines as the body proportions are different as children mature into adulthood. The infant's head is 18%, while the lower extremities are shorter and only account for 13% to 14% body surface area. The Lund-Browder chart categorizes children developmentally from the time of birth to adulthood, providing a more accurate burn assessment for intravenous fluid administration. For individuals with morbidly obesity, %TBSA also changes and is different between males and females with BMI greater than 40 mg/kg^2.

Intravenous Fluid Resuscitation

Adult patients burned ≥20% of their TBSA will require a large volume intravenous fluid resuscitation (Monafo, 1996; Pham, Cancio, & Gibran, 2008). This increase in intravenous fluid resuscitation also applies to children (<8 years old) and the elderly (≥65 years old) burned >15% TBSA because of their thinner skin. Many burn resuscitation formulas have been described but the most well known and most utilized globally is the Parkland burn resuscitation formula (Alvarado, Chung, Cancio, & Wolf, 2009). This formula is calculated as follows: 4 cc crystalloid x patient's body weight (kgs) × percent TBSA,

Burn Area Chart

Area	Birth - 1 yr	1 – 4 yrs	5 – 9 yrs	10 – 14 yrs	15	Adult	Second Degree	Third Degree	Total
Head	19	17	13	10	9	7			
Neck	2	2	2	2	2	2			
Anterior Trunk	13	13	13	13	13	13			
Posterior Trunk	13	13	13	13	13	13			
Right Buttock	2.5	2.5	2.5	2.5	2.5	2.5			
Left Buttock	2.5	2.5	2.5	2.5	2.5	2.5			
Genitalia	1	1	1	1	1	1			
Right Upper Arm	4	4	4	4	4	4			
Left Upper Arm	4	4	4	4	4	4			
Right Lower Arm	3	3	3	3	3	3			
Left Lower Arm	3	3	3	3	3	3			
Right Hand	2.5	2.5	2.5	2.5	2.5	2.5			
Left Hand	2.5	2.5	2.5	2.5	2.5	2.5			
Right Thigh	5.5	6.5	8.5	8.5	8.5	9.5			
Left Thigh	5.5	6.5	8.5	8.5	8.5	9.5			
Right Leg	5	5	5.5	6	6.5	7			
Left Leg	5	5	5.5	6	6.5	7			
Right Foot	3.5	3.5	3.5	3.5	3.5	3.5			
Left Foot	3.5	3.5	3.5	3.5	3.5	3.5			
Total Body Surface Area (*complete all percentages and totals in yellow and gray boxes)									

Table header spans: **Description of Injury (Maximum Percentage Allowed by Patient Age)**

Fig. 34.1 Lund and Browder Chart. Adapted from Sabeston, D. C., Jr., (Ed.). (1977). *Textbook of surgery: The biographical basis of modern surgical practice*, (11th ed.). Philadelphia: Saunders.

which equals a specific intravenous volume to be administered over a defined time period. This total volume of crystalloid is divided in half, of which the first half is given intravenously during the first 8 h and the second half delivered during the next 16 h. (The ABA has recently suggested that initial formula should be adjusted to 2–3 cc's to avoid complications of volume overload, however, this is not universally accepted because of the concern for complications arising from under-resuscitation leading to organ failure; ABLS, 2018.) The fluid of choice is Lactated Ringer's solution that most closely reapproximates serum electrolytes with a sodium of 132 mEq/L, potassium of at 4 mEq/L, magnesium at 2 mEq/L and acetate at 110 mEq/L. Some burn centers add albumin drips at various times during the initial 48 h of resuscitation, which increases intravascular oncotic pressure. Large volume intravenous normal saline administration can lead to a hyperchloremic metabolic acidosis and should be avoided if possible. Urine output should be monitored hourly with a guideline for minimum output being 0.5 cc's/kg/h in the adult and 1 cc/kg/h in children. A bladder catheter is critical to monitor urine output, especially in males with a circumferentially burned penis. Resuscitation is vital to prevent the development of burn shock which is denoted by tachycardia, hypotension, and anuria. Although somewhat controversial, heart rate, blood pressure and urine output have remained the steadfast triumvirate for monitoring adequate intravascular volume resuscitation (Dries & Waxman, 1991). Electrolytes such as magnesium, calcium, phosphorous, and glucose must also be monitored during this critical time of resuscitation.

Navigator

Despite the plethora of burn resuscitation formulas, the most recent and most advanced option was developed by the United State Army Institute of Surgical Research (USAISR) called the Burn Navigator (Cancio, 2014). This computer-guided system is a decisional support making tool used by a burn center to assist in the hourly adjustment in intravenous resuscitation (Salinas et al., 2011). Previous fluids given by pre-hospital providers and other patient parameters are entered into this computer algorithm. Fluids are adjusted based on these clinical parameters to arrive at a more balanced and more even resuscitation by analyzing not only what is clinically happening at that moment but also based on what has happened in the immediate past. This real-time electronic process seems to work better than the standard modified Brooke or Parkland burn resuscitation formulas and assists with preventing over- or under-resuscitating the burned patient.

Topical Dressings
Superficial Burns

In the emergency department, topical antimicrobial dressings are applied to the burn wound based on the depth of injury (Greenhalgh, 2009; Norman et al., 2017) in both the adult and pediatric patient (Cartotto, 2017). For superficial burns that only penetrate the epidermis without skin sloughing or blistering, any number of topical, fragrance-free, nonoily, or

desiccating agents may be used to rehydrate the skin. The key is to remove the patient from the thermal source, usually sun exposure, for several days until the redness resolves.

Partial- and Full-Thickness Burns

Deeper injuries into the dermis and beyond require an antimicrobial agent to protect from prokaryotic organism invasion and are used for more than just cutaneous hydration. Silver Sulfadiazine (AgSD) is a topical antimicrobial agent that contains silver and a well-known antiprokaryotic agent as it binds to the DNA of prokaryotic organisms. Application is soothing to the burn wound and can be effective for up to 24 h, but AgSD is not a chemical debrider and has only limited tissue penetration. In addition, the mechanical action for the removal of the AgSD by wiping the cream off the wound provides the removal of the dead but sloughing tissue. A possible transient decrease in the patient's white blood cell count (WBC) is the main complication of AgSD, which does not deter from its benefit for the burn. AgSD will penetrate and destroy cartilage; therefore, it should not be used on the ears and nose. AgSD can also develop a topical build-up referred to as a "psuedoeschar." Pseudoeschar presence may confuse the practitioner who falsely believes that the wound is deeper than it actually is. Subsequent removal requires painful debridements with metal-edged debriders. In cases where the pseudoeschar is too thick, operative management while under heavy sedation or general anesthesia may be required for its removal utilizing a curette.

Mafenide acetate, Sulfamylon (Mylan Institution, Inc., Rockford, IL) cream, is another effective topical antimicrobial agent. This cream applied twice a day will penetrate the burn eschar and act as a chemical debrider. With larger burns, widespread application can cause a metabolic acidosis by inhibiting carbonic anhydrase, and protracted administration can favor *Candida albicans* overgrowth in the tissue. It is also painful when applied topically to the burn wound. Mafenide acetate is sparingly applied to cartilaginous structures such as the nose and ears secondary due to decreased perfusion in these areas.

Xeroform (Bismuth Tribromophenate, DeRoyal Industries, Inc., Powell, TN) and Bacitracin (Dynarex Corporation, Orangeburg, NJ) cream are additional soothing topical agents that can be utilized together on superficial partial-thickness burns for their antimicrobial effects. Xeroform has bismuth, which is a well-known antimicrobial agent and bacitracin, made from *Bacillus subtilis*, has gram-positive cocci-cidal effects. Without the bismuth tribromophenate component (stains the dressing yellow), Xeroform is essentially a petrolatum gauze dressing.

Silver nitrate (0.5% solution) is nontoxic and does not injure regenerating epithelium. It cannot penetrate the burn eschar and may lead to hyponatremia and hypochloremia. Silver nitrate is light sensitive and turns the wound black. While an older agent, it is very effective and can be used as a second-line agent on infected burn wounds.

A relatively recent addition to the roster of topical antimicrobials includes Plurogel (Medline Industries,

Northfield, IL). This is a nontoxic amorphous hydrogel that is soothing on the wound, decreases inflammation (Curry, Wright, Lee, Kang, & Frim, 2004; Hunter, Luo, Zhang, Kozar, & Moore, 2010), and improves capillary blood flow to the wound bed (Birchenough, Rodeheaver, Morgan, Peirce, & Katz, 2008). Plurogel is unique in that it is a cross-linked micelle salve in an aqueous phase at low temperatures but becomes a gel at warmer temperatures, which helps keep the wound bed moist. Additionally, plurogel blocks adhesion to certain proteins to prevent microbial adhesions, disrupts the development of biofilm, and facilitates necrotic tissue/burn eschar skin slough removal (Tharmalingam, Ghebeh, Wuerz, & Butler, 2008; Yang, Larose, Della Porta, Schultz, & Gibson, 2017).

Finally, Santyl, a collagenase (Smith & Nephew, Inc., Fort Worth, TX), is used to debride burn eschar and fibrinous exudate and promote granulation tissue formation. It has also been used in deep second-degree burns to prevent a compartment syndrome development. The enzymatic activity is strongest when the wound has a pH between 6 and 8. There is minimal systemic risk except for hypersensitivity, which is extremely rare. A local slightly transient cutaneous erythema might be noted in the surrounding healthy tissue. Santyl can be deactivated by povidone iodine.

Absorptive dressings such as a foam, alginate or hydrofiber, impregnated with silver, benzethonium chloride, or ethylenediaminetetraacetic acid are indicated to prevent wound colonization and infection. These dressings absorb, contour to the wound bed and kill organisms trapped in the dressing. Sterile roll gauze is often applied to secure the dressing and replaced as needed. See Chapters 19 and 21 for further description of topical dressings and antimicrobial products (Metcalf, Parsons, & Bowler, 2017).

INTERMEDIATE PHASE OF BURN CARE

Debridement

After the initial 48 h of resuscitation and stabilization, if the burn eschar matures to include a full thickness injury of dead cutaneous tissue colonized by prokaryotic organisms, excision is necessary (Engrav, Heimbach, Reus, Harnar, & Marvin, 1983; Gray et al., 1982). The burn eschar places a tremendous metabolic stress on the human body and early excision reduces the systemic effects caused by the inflammatory mediators released by the burn eschar. The aim is to prevent possible overwhelming infection/sepsis and multisystem organ failure. Tangential excision using the standard Goulian (small guarded blades) and Watson (large guarded blades) knives is required to excise the burn-injured tissue. For thinner superficial or deep partial-thickness burn eschar, the hydrosurgical debridement may be utilized as a fine water-pressure knife that lifts and debrides the dead tissue. The wound is then covered with either an antimicrobial dressing or porcine xenograft for immediate wound coverage and pain control. Porcine xenograft is utilized for superficial debrided

wounds where a topical graft may not be needed; the expectation is that the body will heal underneath the xenograft and eventually reject the xenograft. Porcine xenograft is typically covered with Xeroform and bacitracin dressings to simplify the dressing care and changed daily.

Excisional Hemostasis

Deep and extensive excised surface areas can bleed briskly. The surgeon must be in constant communication with the anesthesiologist or certified nurse anesthetist to make sure that the patient is hemodynamically stable, that blood products are available, and that such products are being administered to keep up with blood loss. If the wound is full thickness or deeper and has been tangentially excised, hemostasis is achieved intraoperatively to initiate clot formation using one of the following techniques: (1) electrocautery; (2) epinephrine-soaked gauze (1 L of normal saline with 20 cc's of 1:1000 concentration of epinephrine) plus or minus the addition of recombinant thrombin; (3) Combat Gauze, (Z-medica, Wallingford, CT); (4) extremity tourniquets; (5) Tissel, a fibrin spray (Johnson and Johnson, New Brunswick, NJ). Additional pressure to the bleeding wound bed is achieved by the application of elastic wrap bandages. In areas or missions with limited resources or available blood banks, a mixture of one liter of injectable, normal saline with 2 cc of 1:1000 epinephrine solution can be injected with a small needle on a 60 cc syringe subcutaneously to tumesce the tissue below the eschar that requires excision. This will minimize the acute blood loss and can also be used subcutaneously for split-thickness skin graft harvest. The patient's wounds can then be wrapped in the epinephrine-soaked gauze/nonadherent pad and secured with an elastic wrap for additional pressure, prior to autografting.

Burn Wound Excision

At the first excisional operation, a decision must be made to either provide temporary wound coverage with human cadaveric allografts or a permanent autograft by split thickness or full-thickness skin grafting. These options contain an epidermis and thin upper portion of dermis together. When the burn eschar excision is taken down to the fat layer, it is not advisable to immediately close the wound with an autograft, because the wound bed is unlikely to accept the graft. This is particularly significant because the burn patient will have limited sites from which to harvest an autograft. Such decisions regarding type of wound coverage are predicated on the nature of the wound bed: (1) clean of infection with noncellulitic surrounding skin; (2) evidence of a granulating tissue bed which is usually not present on first excision; (3) not a deep wound that needs to fill-in prior to closure, so as not to leave a disfiguring closure; and (4) does not necessitate subsequent reexcision for continued eschar or for infection. Sequential, tangential debridements for deep or large burns are typically required to assure that the wound has had complete removal of all burned and necrotic tissue and that the wound will accept an autograft. While waiting for a vascular autograft acceptable wound surface, human cadaveric allografts can serve as a temporary cover and are relatively inexpensive compared with the use and then possible loss of the patient's own skin. The allograft is applied for 3 to 7 days. If a reddish to pinkish hue is transmitted through the allograft with firm adherence, the provider is relatively assured that an autograft will be accepted by the wound bed. If the ensuing days does not reveal improved granulation tissue under the cadaveric allograft, then the older allograft should be removed, and new allograft applied to await the development of granulation.

The sequence for burn eschar and dead tissue excision is based on burn location. The upper extremities are excised first before the lower extremities. This is followed by the anterior torso before the posterior torso which is excised last. Hands and feet (distal structures) are excised before the proximal extremities under tourniquet control, if possible, to decrease hemorrhage. Once the decision to excise the back is made and to prevent hemodynamic instability during the posterior torso excision, the patient may be placed on their side while under general anesthesia. This obviates the need for prone positioning, as it may not be tolerated from a hemodynamic standpoint in the hypermetabolic patient. The face, neck, and head deserve special attention and are observed daily to assess the optimal time for definitive excision. Facial excisions are usually held off until there is a declared need for excision. In the meantime, the face can be treated with Xeroform and Bacitracin for more superficial burns or AGSD or topical antimicrobial products (e.g., Medi-honey; Derma Sciences, Princeton, NJ) for deep burn injuries.

Burned hands and feet often require a multidisciplinary approach to the care and functionality of these specialized anatomic structures: the burn team, physical and occupational therapists, hand surgeons, podiatrists, plastic surgeons, and physiatrists (Sterling et al., 2009). With hand and finger burn eschar excisions, elevation to reduce edema coupled with splinting is recommended postoperatively and followed closely by the occupational therapist (OT). Daily adjustments and range of motion passive stretching exercises are required to prevent contractures. Active/passive range of motion exercises and splinting are important for the early mobilization of the hand to achieve normal function. Axillary splinting places the upper extremity at 90 degrees of abduction to the torso to help prevent axillary contractures. The elbow is splinted in extension while the hand is placed at 70 to 90 degrees at the metacarpophalangeal joints with the wrist and interphalangeal joints splinted at 30 degrees.

Autografting

Once excised, open wounds beds should be covered with the patient's own skin as quickly as possible. Use of the patient's own skin at the earliest possible time will result in better functional and cosmetic outcomes. Typically, a thin intermediate skin graft with a depth between 0.01 and 0.014 inches, with 0.012 being the gold standard, is harvested using a dermatome (Zimmer, Biomet, Warsaw, IN or Padgett, Integra Life Sciences, Plainsboro, Township, NJ) from an unburned and least visible portion of the patient's body. Hand and foot wounds are usually covered with unmeshed skin grafts to allow for less

skin contracture; these areas may benefit from full thickness skin grafting or thicker split thickness skin grafts. Full-thickness skin grafts are primarily reserved for eyelid reconstruction to prevent ectropions or eyelid contractures. Because mesh patterns are readily noticeable, meshed autografts are usually not utilized in exposed areas such as the hands, face or any cosmetically sensitive area. While meshed grafts may allow for more area coverage, one complication is that the larger the mesh size, the more wound contracture will occur. Therefore, sheet grafts have the least amount of contracture and even more so for full thickness grafts. A 1 to 1 meshed graft will have the least amount of contracture compared with a 9 to 1 meshed graft that will contract the most. When the burn wound requires large eschar excisions, the meshing pattern is 3:1 or as large as 9:1. This typically is harvested from either of the bilateral thighs and buttock regions. Nonetheless, if the burn is a large TBSA, harvest sites may include any other areas available that are unburned such as the back, legs, and even the scalp. Harvesting of thinner autografts helps in a quicker healing process with faster vascular ingrowth. Thinner autografts can lead to more scar contracture as can the size of graft meshing. While either 1:1 to 1:2 meshing is standard., meshing also allows for the egress of serum from the wound bed throughout the autograft to prevent a contained seroma or hematoma trapped below an autograft, leading to subsequent graft loss. Once the patient's own skin is ready to be applied to the tissue bed, these autografts are typically stapled in place. A more dilute, topical fibrin spray (e.g., Artiss; Baxter Healthcare Corp., Deerfield, IL) may be applied to the wound bed to allow an additional securing of the graft to the wound bed beyond the traditional use of staples and/or suture. In addition to staples and fibrin spray, a topical skin adhesive and/or wound closure adhesive strips (e.g., Steri-Strips; 3M, St. Paul, MN) can be applied on skin graft edges.

Adjuvant Modalities for Autografting: CEA, ReCell

CEA (cultured epithelial autografts), (Epicell, Boston, MA) placement or ReCell, (Avita, Australia), which is a skin spray of keratinocytes and melanocytes, assist with wound closure over the autograft interstices, or in areas where autografting is not available because of no donor areas. Both are grown from the patient's own skin commercially.

CEA should be considered when enough skin is not readily available with the harvest of autografts from unburned skin. At the bedside or in the operating room under sterile conditions, the skin is harvested and subsequently cloned and grown into sheets of skin (approximately 3 weeks) in the manufacturing laboratory. Unfortunately, success is not high because the CEA are fragile, predisposed to infection, and can be easily dislodged and removed with dressing changes or inadvertent pressure or shearing.

For *ReCell,* harvested skin is placed in a trypsin bath and allowed to soak which loosens skin attachments which is then minced and reprocessed through the trypsin solution. The final product is immediately sprayed over a previously placed meshed autograft or harvest site wound bed. Even the autograft harvest sites have been reported to heal faster with ReCell "spray on skin" and the donor harvest sites can be used again more rapidly (Holmes et al., 2018, 2019).

The reason for graft loss is most commonly the result of an inadequately excised wound bed as there can be no neovascularization into the skin graft. For similar reasons, hematomas or seromas that separate the skin graft from the wound bed prevent ingrowth of the neovascular tissue to support graft survival. Shear injuries to the skin graft also sever the attachments and neovascularity between the wound bed and the autograft. Finally, infections will destroy the skin graft before it is incorporated into the body with its defenses in the immune system. Proper dressing application with appropriate bolsters applies pressure to the graft annealing it to the wound bed to help minimize shear while improving contact.

The autograft is initially without a blood supply for several days and is hindered from fighting an infection. Once an autograft is placed on the wound bed, a topical antimicrobial solution on a gauze dressing is needed over the fresh autograft. Before an antimicrobial dressing is applied, a nonadherent contact layer is placed over the autograft to prevent its removal or dislodgement with dressing changes. An antimicrobial soaked gauze is then applied over the nonadherent contact dressing. Classically, sulfamylon solution has been routinely used for antimicrobial coverage as it is effective in killing prokaryotic organisms. Unfortunately, sulfamylon solution is painful to the patient, has to be made in the pharmacy with each application which takes time and planning before each dressing placement, and is very expensive (Foster, Richey, Champagne, & Matthews, 2019).

Gaining popularity is the antimicrobial wound cleanser, hypochlorous acid. Unique features of this product are that it is not painful when applied to a graft on top of a wound bed, kills all prokaryotic organisms within 15 s of sustained contact with gauze application and is very inexpensive (Hiebert & Robson, 2016). Hypochlorous acid reduces wound bed microbial counts to less than 10^{-2} with consistent use and does not damage the eukaryotic organism tissue.

DABS, a debridement antibiotic solution, utilizes three antibiotics. The three antibiotics can vary but are classically gentamicin (Pfizer, Sanford, NC), neomycin (LGM Pharma, Boca Raton, FL), and bacitracin. This antimicrobial solution is effective against gram-negative rods and gram-positive cocci. Polymyxin B Sulfate (Xellia Pharmaceuticals, Copenhagen, Denmark) is another antimicrobial solution that is effective against some microbes and is not painful on contact. Sodium hypochlorite solution (0.5%) (Dakin's solution, (Century Pharmaceuticals, Indianapolis, IN) has been used on autografts; it is extremely effective against prokaryotic organisms, but it is toxic to eukaryotic cells (Cardile et al., 2014). Dakin's solution is useful during initial dressing changes for necrotizing fasciitis or soft tissue infections on a freshly debrided, infected wound bed. After 24 h, it is beneficial to switch to an antimicrobial solution that is not as harmful to eukaryotic macrophages, neutrophils, and keratinocytes while the wound bed granulates.

Donor Site Dressings

The dressing selected to cover a donor site (sites used to harvest autografts) requires covering with a dressing that will absorb exudate, promote wound healing, cause minimal pain with removal, and provide a superior cosmetic effect. While traditionally xeroform, petroleum gauze, and nonadherent gauze pad coated with bacitracin have been used to cover the donor site, many other options exist. Absorptive dressings containing alginates and a soft tack silicone adhesive are desirable in that they facilitate transfer of fluid with minimal adherence to the wound bed or ingrowth of granulation tissue and can be changed every other day depending on the amount of exudate

Epidermal and Dermal Replacement Tissue

Various tissues and cellular-based tissues (CTPs) are also available as cutaneous (epidermal and dermal) replacement substitutes with minimal morbidity. These are discussed in more detail in Chapter 22.

Integra

Integra (Integra LifeSciences, Princeton, NJ) placement reduces scarring and contracture formation especially to the hands and face. Integra is a well-known dermal substitute and is made from bovine collagen and shark chondroitin sulfate forming a cytoskeleton with a silicone film backing that makes it a bilaminate covering. As the body granulates into the dermal matrix, this skin substitute forms granulation tissue in the deeply debrided wounds, which may have exposed tendons, fascial planes/muscles or bones. Once completely granulated after 2 to 3 weeks, the silicone backing is removed for subsequent autograft placement. The major drawback with Integra is the propensity to develop an infection before it granulates. For this reason, Integra must be treated with an antimicrobial solution such as hypochlorous acid, sulfamylon, or DABS. A silver-coated antimicrobial barrier dressing (e.g., Acticoat; Smith & Nephew, Fort Worth, TX) has also been applied around the Integra graft edges to prevent antimicrobial invasion from the periphery. If an infection is detected, prompt removal of the silicone backing or the entire piece of Integra is necessary.

PriMatrix

Another dermal substitute is PriMatrix (TEI BioSciences, Inc., Boston, MA) which is an acellular dermal tissue matrix derived from fetal bovine dermis (Parcells). While similar to Integra it only contains the bovine scaffolding that can be placed on a wound to become incorporated with the ingrowth of granulation tissue. Concerns for infection also exist with PriMatrix, and PriMatrix AG (the same product with impregnated silver). Nonetheless, the use of an antimicrobial topical dressing is still useful and keeps the environment moist.

ACell

ACell, Matristem (ACell Inc., Columbia, MD), is ground-up porcine urinary bladder that can be placed as a powder or as a matrix scaffolding over a deep wound bed for granulation development and site-specific tissue remodeling to prevent scarring. However, while this product does not contain growth factors, it does contain epithelial basement membranes and collagen. Nonetheless, providers have found good clinical success in multiple surgical fields with tissue regeneration.

AmnioFill and EpiBurn

AmnioFill and EpiBurn (MiMedx Group, Inc., Marietta, GA) are dehydrated human amnion/chorion products with evidence of rapid generation of granulation tissue necessary for autografting in a variety of wounds. These dehydrated amnion/chorion products contain more than 300 growth factors, chemokines and cytokines, promote fibroblast and endothelial cell proliferation, growth factor stimulation in native tissues and neovascularization (Koob, Lim, Massee, Zabek, & Denoziere, 2014). Once applied to the wound bed, a hydrocolloid dressing is used to cover these products followed by the application of a negative pressure wound therapy device (NPWT). Within a week to ten days, the NPWT device is removed in the OR and reapplication of these products may be necessary versus autografting over a well-vascularized dermal wound bed. Such use may not only salvage limbs with exposed tendon and bone but may also heal chronic wounds (Koob et al., 2013) and decrease the need for free tissue flap transfers with concomitant risk of failure and increased morbidity.

Deep burn injuries that result in exposed bone or tendons after debridement may be covered with free tissue transfers as described in the plastic surgical literature. This has been especially true for open and exposed tibial bones in the distal half to two-thirds of the leg. Free tissue flap transfers must rely on tissues, for example, the latissimus muscle with its overlaying skin and subcutaneous tissues, which will provide a good vascular source with an arterial and venous anastomosis. The presence of arteriosclerosis in the arteries proximal to the planned anastomotic site in the leg's arterial tree can be dealt with by interventional radiology with angioplasty or stenting to improve blood flow to the free tissue flap. Physical examination and ultrasound are coupled with CT angiography to delineate any arteriosclerotic lesions that may require intervention.

Biodegradable Temporizing Matrix (BTM)

BTM (PolyNovo North America, Carlsbad, CA) is a new wound dressing that is bioabsorbable and designed to facilitate dermal growth under polyurethane foam. This polyurethane dressing is applied over a hemostatic, freshly excised wound bed and covered with an NPWT for over several weeks. Once the wound bed is healed, the BTM sealing membrane is removed revealing a freshly granulated, smooth, well-vascularized dermis that can support an autograft. The BTM dressing has been utilized in small and large TBSA burns, once the burn eschar has been excised.

Negative Pressure Wound Therapy (NPWT)

NPWT can be used to secure epidermal and dermal tissue coverings or to prepare a wound bed for tissue covering. NPWT

has been demonstrated to actively promote granulation tissue after deep burn wound excisions by creating macrostrain and microstrain in the wound tissue bed (Saxena et al., 2004). Macrostrain is advantageous to the burn wound in that it draws the wound edges together, removes infectious material such as prokaryotic organisms and pro-inflammatory substances, reduces edema, and promotes wound bed perfusion. Microstrain results in microdeformation and cell stretch which stimulates cellular activity and granulation tissue formation (McNulty, Schmidt, Feeley, Villanueva, & Kieswetter, 2009).

The NPWT sponge is typically placed over the nonadherent contact layer covering the autograft and left in place for five days. Prior to autograft placement, a silver foam sponge can be used with the NPWT to reduce bacterial load in the wound bed. Additionally, NPWT with automated instillation of fluid can be advantageous to lift devitalized tissue, facilitate granulation tissue formation in a deep wound bed and stimulate vascularity prior to graft placement temporarily. The type of foam used with this automatic instillation of fluid is a hydrophilic, large reticulated open-cell foam and the irrigant can be normal saline, hypochlorous acid or an antimicrobial solution (Matthews, Hechtman, Quan, Foster, & Fernandez, 2018). Further discussion of NPWT can be found in Chapter 24.

Hyperbaric Oxygen Therapy (HBO)

Increasing oxygen delivery can help cellular and tissue viability in thermally injured patients with burns that are still perfusing. It is theorized that HBO will maintain the cell's ability to manufacture adenosine-triphosphate (ATP) to help maintain the cells ability to fight injury and maintain cellular viability (Yamaguchi et al., 1990). ATP manufactured by the cell is only capable by the delivery of oxygen through the microvasculature. In addition, high-dose oxygen delivery to the tissue decreases edema in the damaged tissue secondary to vasoconstriction (Boykin, Eriksson, & Pittman, 1980). It has also been shown to decrease proinflammatory cytokines and the inflammatory response (Chen, Yu, Cheng, Yu, & Lo, 2007). Literature indicates that burn surgery operative requirements decreased (8–3.7) with HBO therapy (Cianci et al., 1988). In another study, the mean healing time decreased from 43.8 days to 19.7 days (Hart et al., 1974).

HBO therapy should be strongly considered for failing autografts or surgical flaps. Inhalation injury carbon monoxide poisoning can be dealt with effectively with HBO treatment (Buckley, Juurlink, Isbister, Bennett, & Lavonas, 2011). However, the logistics of placing a large TBSA burn patient inside the chamber while maintaining frequent bedside interventions and access to cardiopulmonary resuscitation without disruption of the HBO treatment can be logistically daunting and not recommended.

REHABILITATION AND RECONSTRUCTION PHASE OF BURN CARE

As more burn patients are surviving with even larger burns, functional return to the preburn state, or as close as possible, is the goal in the third phase of burn care. This entails appropriate psychological and social function beyond just physical wound healing. Occupational and physical therapists play a key role in this return to function with repeated clinical follow-up appointments and adjustments in the rehabilitation plan where indicated (Young, Dewey, & King, 2019). The therapist's role includes but are not limited to strengthening, balance, ambulation, returning the patient to activities of daily living, splinting, scar message, and range of motion exercises. The goal is to return the patient to school, college or work at as high a functioning level as possible from the initial burn admission through predischarge and subsequent clinic follow-up.

Stocking compression of the hands, feet, extremities, neck, face and torso, coupled with scar message, are necessary to ameliorate the effects of hypertrophic scaring. Silicone sheeting and tight garments and topical moisturizers can help prevent hypertrophic scarring formation and maintain skin hydration (Steinstraesser et al., 2011). However, all too frequently, patients develop hypertrophic scarring after burn injuries that require further surgical excision, reconstructive flaps, or local tissue rearrangements. Hypertrophic scarring especially across joints may require surgical techniques such as Z-plasty or regrafting with full-thickness skin grafts. Z-plasty rearranges the local tissues to disrupt tension across scar bands that may form and thereby allow joint mobility in the hands, feet, neck, shoulders/axillae, and extremities to reach their full and natural range of motion. Z-plasty can be utilized in a sequential, temporal fashion or in a preplanned series of operations. Such reconstructive efforts should be done in concert with the physical and occupational therapists who monitor the patient's progress and physical hinderances pre- and postoperatively. In addition, local injection of steroids may be performed to help decrease the local inflammatory response coupled with cutaneous message in scar tissue. One to two mL of Kenalog (Bristol-Myers-Squibb, Lawrence Township, NJ) (40 mg/mL) placed in 10 mL of 0.25% Marcaine (Pfizer, Sanford, NC) is injected into the scar coupled with injected site massage.

Pruritus

Pruritus in the postburn period is a common complaint for both adult and pediatric patients and can last for years. One study found that pruritis was prevalent for 87% of large burn area adult patients at 3 months and decreased to only 67% at 24 months (Van Loey et al., 2008). Another study found that burn size, areas grafted, and donor were correlated to pruritis intensity. While more common in the pediatric population, pruritis is typically treated with cutaneous massage and oral antihistamines such as diphenhydramine or atarax as well as topical hydrating lotions. Doxepin cream has also been applied with success. If not treated adequately, patients with continued and severe itching can scratch these symptomatic areas leading to cutaneous excoriations and new wounds over older healed wounds. Unfortunately, pruritis will persist in long-term burn survivors and can affect many aspects of their sleep and quality of life. Some relief of clinical symptoms has been achieved with CO_2 laser therapy.

Pain Control

Pain control in the acute setting is critical as superficial partial and deep partial-thickness burn injuries are characterized by exposed nerve endings in the wound bed. Depending on the size and depth of these burns, patients may require heavy intravenous drips of narcotics including fentanyl and dilaudid coupled with antianxiety medications such as benzodiazepines, ketamine, propofol, or dexamedetomidine while hospitalized in the ICU. Chronic pain may develop with closed or reconstructed wounds, and a pain specialist or physical medicine and rehabilitation specialist assistance may be necessary to wean intermediate and long acting narcotics such as MS Contin, methadone and sedative medications to prevent addiction. Nonsteroidal antiinflammatory medications may be appropriate as well as neurontin to alleviate the neuropathic pain associated with these healing injuries.

Laser Scar Therapy

Laser scar therapy can be used in burn patients with hypertrophic scarring. Pulsed dye lasers using a 585-nm wavelength and CO_2 lasers have shown good results in early scar management. Shorter pulsed durations can also treat the scar effectively. Lasers create collagen bundle realignment, and decreased fibroblast formation. Treatments generally require 3–8 sessions which can be performed in a clinic or as an outpatient, operating room procedure. The laser-treated areas are initially covered with a topical steroid cream for 48 h or can be injected with Kenalog but then transitioned to nonprescription Aquaphor (Beiersdorf AG, Hamburg, Germany). Immediate side effects are localized pain, erythema, and later, pigmentation changes. Pain at the treated site may require a brief hospitalization.

Heterotopic Ossification

Unfortunately, patients may develop heterotopic ossification or the pathologic bone formation in the soft tissues including muscles and joint capsules (Chen, Yang, Chuaung, Huang, & Yang, 2009). This occurs as a result of the initial burn injury and can limit range of motion by contractures or cause chronic pain especially with nerve tissue involvement. These areas may require excision for better range of motion when coupled with operative reconstructive efforts by the plastic, orthopedic or burn providers.

School and Societal Reintegration

Reintegration into the community (school or work) can be startling and difficult for the burn survivor, especially for children (American Academy of Pediatrics Child Life Council and Committee on Hospital Care & Wilson, 2006). This may require the help of child-life specialists and psychologists for the recovering burn patient who may also be suffering from posttraumatic stress disorder from the initial burn event or from the trauma of the hospitalization. Loss of personal identity or loss of significant others from the initial burn incident should be address with the psychologist to deal with such bereavement issues and loss of the prior self-image. Programs dealing with school reintegration can also be beneficial especially for the young burn survivor who may fall victim to bullying.

CLINICAL CONSULT

A: MM is a 18-month-old female who was burned 20 min ago when she pulled a pot of boiling water off the stove. She has deep partial- and full-thickness burns to her face, upper body, bilateral upper extremities, left hand, and left leg. The left arm and left hand are burned circumferentially; there is no stocking/glove distribution. MM is directly admitted to the pediatric burn intensive care unit (PICU). She weighs 18 kg on admission, has no past medical history, and is up to date on immunizations. Initial assessment and stabilization have been completed. Endotracheal intubation (secondary to facial burns and large fluid resuscitation), fluid resuscitation (Lactated Ringer's Solution) and maintenance fluids (D5 containing fluid) are initiated. Tetanus vaccination administered, indwelling urinary catheter, naso-jejunal feeding tube and oxygen saturation monitor placed, vital signs (VS) every hour and admission labs completed. Parents are at the bedside; no additional family members were injured.

D: 35% total body surface area (TBSA) accidental scald burn injury; 20% partial thickness to face, chest, back; and 15% full thickness to left arm, left hand, left leg.

P: Burn wound assessment and dressing application at bedside per pediatric burn surgical team under moderate to heavy sedation. Initiate supportive care for patient and family.

I: (1) Partial-thickness and full-thickness burns debrided and initially PleuroGel topical dressings applied; bacitracin ointment to face after debriding and loose cutaneous eschar. (2) Position with head of bed elevated to 30 degrees on pressure redistribution support surface and burned extremities elevated. (3) Circulation stks every hour to areas of full-thickness circumferential burns to left arm, hand, and leg for possible escharotomy placement. (4) After feeding tube placed, enteral feeds immediately initiated per protocol. (5) Pain and anxiety management per continuous narcotics and benzodiazepine infusions with boluses during procedures. (6) Stress ulcer prophylaxis and nutritional supplementation began. (7) Consults: physical therapy (PT), occupational therapy (OT), pediatric dietician, pediatric clinical pharmacologist, social work, child life, pediatric intensive care, ophthalmology. (8) Plan for operating room (OR) for burn eschar debridement and possible escharotomies and possible skin grafting or skin-substitute for full-thickness wounds in 2–3 days.

E: Daily wound assessment per burn team. Strict I and O's. Follow-up labs: comprehensive metabolic panel (CMP), Mg, Phos, complete blood count (CBC) with differential, ABG every morning, every morning and T and C for operative intervention. Plan of care and ICU/operative consents reviewed with parents.

SUMMARY

Regardless of clinical setting or severity of burn, health-care practitioner's must be able to:

- identify the difference between the superficial, superficial partial-thickness, deep partial-thickness, and full-thickness burns and the appropriate therapy based on those injuries,
- calculate the burn size and need for further fluid resuscitation,
- immediately treat burn injuries and identify the possibility of further end-organ deterioration,

- understand that various topical burn care products and understand the benefits and potential risks,
- surgically intervene based on the burn patient's initial presentation (escharotomy or fasciotomy) or subsequent burn injury progression that requires definitive operations (tangential excision and grafting) and
- understand the three phases of burn care and recovery and the appropriate care to optimize therapeutic and psychosocial outcomes.

SELF-ASSESSMENT QUESTIONS

1. Thermal injuries may occur from:
   a. snow
   b. ice
   c. scalding water
   d. All of the above

2. Which of the following statements describing electrical injuries is TRUE?
   a. Wet skin slows the conduction of electrical current.
   b. The extent of visible skin damage is a direct correlation with the extent of internal damage.
   c. Fat and bones are severely damaged by electrical current.
   d. Vessel thrombosis, muscle destruction, paresthesia and paralysis may develop.

3. How is burn size most commonly measured?
   a. With a measuring guide, length, width, and depth in centimeters (cm)
   b. By calculating total body surface area (%TBSA)
   c. With use of a camera and integrated digital 3D wound measurement
   d. None of the above

4. Phases of burn care and recovery include:
   a. Emergent, Rehabilitation, Recovery
   b. Acute, Emergent, Rehabilitation and Reconstruction
   c. Resuscitation, Wound Management, Psychosocial Support
   d. Resuscitation, Debridement, Wound Management

REFERENCES

Alharbi, Z., Piatkowski, A., Dembinski, R., Reckort, S., Grieb, G., Kauczok, J., et al. (2012). Treatment of burns in the first 24 hours: Simple and practical guide by answering 10 questions in a step-by-step form. *World Journal of Surgery, 7*(1), 1–10.

Alvarado, R., Chung, K. K., Cancio, L. C., & Wolf, S. E. (2009). Burn resuscitation. *Burns, 35*(1), 4–14.

American Academy of Pediatrics Child Life Council and Committee on Hospital Care, & Wilson, J. M. (2006). Child life services. *Pediatrics, 188*(4), 1757–1763. https://doi.org/10.1542/peds.2006-1941

American Burn Association–ABLS Advisory Committee. (2018). *Advance burn life support course. Provider manual. 2018 update.* American Burn Association. Accessed 4/14/20201 from: http://ameriburn.org/wp-content/uploads/2019/08/2018-abls-providermanual.pdf.

American Burn Association. (n.d.). *Burn Incidence Fact Sheet. Burn incidence and treatment in the United States: 2016.* Retrieved 01/15/2023 from: https://ameriburn.org/who-we-are/media/burn-incidence-fact-sheet/.

Bezuhly, M., & Fish, J. S. (2012). Acute burn care. *Plastic and Reconstructive Surgery, 130*(2), 349e–358e.

Birchenough, S. A., Rodeheaver, G. T., Morgan, R. F., Peirce, S. M., & Katz, A. J. (2008). Topical poloxamer 1888 improves blood flow following thermal injury in rat mesenteric microvasculature. *Annals of Plastic Surgery, 60*(5), 584–588.

Boykin, J. V., Eriksson, E., & Pittman, R. N. (1980). In vivo microcirculation of a scald burn and the progression of postburn dermal ischemia. *Plastic and Reconstructive Surgery, 66*(2), 191–198.

Branski, L. K., Herndon, D. N., & Barrow, R. (2012). A brief history of acute burn care management. In D. N. Herndon (Ed.), *Total burn care* (4th ed., pp. 1–7). Elsevier.

Brown, R. L., Greenhalgh, D. G., Kagan, R. J., & Warden, G. (1994). The adequacy of limb escharotomies-fasciotomies after referral to a major burn center. *Journal of Trauma, 37*(6), 916–920.

Bryan, B. C., Andrews, C. J., Hurley, R. A., & Taber, K. H. (2009). Electrical injury, Part I: Mechanisms. *The Journal of Neuropsychiatry and Clinical Neurosciences, 21*(3), iv–244.

Buckley, N. A., Juurlink, D. N., Isbister, G., Bennett, M. H., & Lavonas, E. J. (2011). Hyperbaric oxygen for carbon monoxide poisoning. *Cochrane Database Systematic Reviews, 2011*(4), CD002041.

Cancio, L. C. (2014). Initial assessment and fluid resuscitation of burn patients. *Surgical Clinics North America, 94*(4), 741–754.

Cardile, A. P., Sanchez, C. J., Jr., Hardy, S. K., Romano, D. R., Hurtgen, B. J., Wenke, J. C., et al. (2014). Dakin solution alters macrophage viability and function. *Journal of Surgical Research, 192*(2), 692–699.

Cartotto, R. (2017). Topical antimicrobial agents for pediatric burns. *Burns & Trauma, 5*(1).

Chen, H. C., Yang, J. Y., Chuaung, S. S., Huang, C. Y., & Yang, S. Y. (2009). Heterotopic ossification in burns: Our experience and literature reviews. *Burns, 35*(6), 857–862.

Chen, S. J., Yu, C. T., Cheng, Y. L., Yu, S. Y., & Lo, H. C. (2007). Effects of hyperbaric oxygen therapy on circulating interleukin-8, nitric oxide, and insulin-like growth factors in patients with type 2 diabetes mellitus. *Clinical Biochemistry, 40*(1–2), 30–36.

Cianci, P. E., Lueders, H., Lee, H., Shapiro, R., Sexton, J., Williams, C., et al. (1988). Adjunctive hyperbaric oxygen reduces the need for surgery in 40–80% burns. *The Journal of Hyperbaric Medicine, 3,* 97.

Curry, D. J., Wright, D. A., Lee, R. C., Kang, U. J., & Frim, D. M. (2004). Poloxamer 188 volumetrically decreases neuronal loss in the rat in a time-dependent manner. *Neurosurgery, 55*(4), 943–949.

Davis, T. S., & Graham, W. I. (1981). Escharotomies. *Journal of Trauma, 21*(1), 83–84.

Dries, D. J., & Waxman, K. (1991). Adequate resuscitation of burn patients may not be measured by urine output and vital signs. *Critical Care Medicine, 19*(3), 327–329.

Engrav, L. H., Heimbach, D. M., Reus, J. L., Harnar, T. J., & Marvin, J. A. (1983). Early excision and grafting vs. nonoperative treatment of burns of indeterminant depth: a randomized prospective study. *Journal of Trauma and Acute Care Surgery, 23*(11), 1001–1004.

Ernst, A., & Zibrak, J. D. (1998). Carbon monoxide poisoning. *New England Journal of Medicine, 339*(22), 1603–1608.

Esnault, P., Prunet, B., Cotte, J., Marsaa, H., Prat, N., Lacroix, G., et al. (2014). Tracheal intubation difficulties in the setting of face and neck burns: Myth or reality? *The American Journal of Emergency Medicine, 32*(10), 1174–1178.

Foster, K. N., Richey, K. J., Champagne, J. S., & Matthews, M. R. (2019). Randomized comparison of hypochlorous acid with 5% sulfamylon solution as topical therapy following skin grafting. *Eplasty, 19,* e16. PMID: 31217832; PMCID: PMC6554702.

Friedstat, J., Brown, D. A., & Levi, B. (2017). Chemical, electrical, and radiation injuries. *Clinics in Plastic Surgery, 44*(3), 657.

GBD 2019 Disease and Injuries Collaborators. (2020). Global burden of 369 disease and injuries in 204 countries and territories, 1990–2019: A systematic analysis for the Global Burden of Disease Study 2019. *Lancet, 396*(10258), 1204.

Grabowska, T., Skowronek, R., Nowicka, J., & Sybirska, H. (2012). Prevalence of hydrogen cyanide and carboxyhaemoglobin in victims of smoke inhalation during enclosed-space fires: A combined toxicological risk. *Clinical Toxicology, 50*(8), 759–763.

Grand View Research. (2023). *U.S. burn care centers market size, share, & trends analysis report by facility type (in-hospital, standalone), by treatment type, by burn severity, by service type, and segment forecasts, 2022–2030.* Report ID: GVR-4-68039-950-2. Retrieved 01/14/2023 from: https://www.grandviewresearch.com/industry-analysis/us-burn-care-centers-market-report.

Gray, D. T., Pine, R. W., Harnar, T. J., Marvin, J. A., Engrav, L. H., & Heimbach, D. M. (1982). Early surgical excision versus conventional therapy in patients with 20 to 40 percent burns: a comparative study. *The American Journal of Surgery, 144*(1), 76–80.

Greenhalgh, D. G. (2009). Topical antimicrobial agents for burn wounds. *Clinics in Plastic Surgery, 36*(4), 597–606.

Greenhalgh, D. G. (2019). Management of burns. *The New England Journal of Medicine, 380,* 2349–2359. https://doi.org/10.1056/NEJMra1807442.

Hall, S., & Evarts, B. (September 2022). News & Research. Fire loss in the United States. In *National Fire Protection Association (NFPA).* https://www.nfpa.org/News-and-Research/Data-research-and-tools/US-Fire-Problem/Fire-loss-in-the-United-States#.

Hart, G. B., O'Reilly, R. R., Broussard, N. D., Cave, R. H., Goodman, D. B., & Yanda, R. L. (1974). Treatment of burns with hyperbaric oxygen. *Surgery, Gynecology and Obstetrics, 139*(5), 693–696.

Herndon, D. N., & Tompkins, R. G. (2004). Support of the metabolic response to burn injury. *The Lancet, 363*(9424), 1895–1902.

Hettiaratchy, S., & Papini, R. (2004). Initial management of a major burn: II—Assessment and resuscitation. *The British Medical Journal, 329*(7457), 101–103.

Hiebert, J. M., & Robson, M. C. (2016). The immediate and delayed post-debridement effects on tissue bacterial wound counts of hypochlorous acid versus saline irrigation in chronic wounds. *Eplasty, 16*.

Holmes, J. H., Molnar, J. A., Carter, J. E., Hwang, J., Cairns, B. A., King, B. T., et al. (2018). A comparative study of the ReCell® device and autologous split-thickness meshed skin graft in the treatment of acute burn injuries. *Journal of Burn Care & Research, 39*(5), 694–702.

Holmes, J. H., Molnar, J. A., Shupp, J. W., Hickerson, W. L., King, B. T., Foster, K. N., et al. (2019). Demonstration of the safety and effectiveness of the ReCell® System combined with split-thickness meshed autografts for the reduction of donor skin to treat mixed-depth burn injuries. *Burns, 45*(4), 772–782.

Hop, M. J., Hiddingh, J., Stekelenburg, C. M., Kuipers, H. C., Middelkoop, E., Nieuwenhuis, M. K., et al. (2013). Cost-effectiveness of laser Doppler imaging in burn care in the Netherlands. *BioMed Central Surgery, 13*(1), 2.

Hunter, R. L., Luo, A. Z., Zhang, R., Kozar, R. A., & Moore, F. A. (2010). Poloxamer 188 inhibition of ischemia/reperfusion injury: Evidence for a novel anti-adhesive mechanism. *Annals of Clinical & Laboratory Science, 40*(2), 115–125.

Jackson, D. M. (1953). The diagnosis of the depth of burning. *The British Journal of Surgery, 3*, 988–996.

Jeschke, M. G., & Herndon, D. N. (2017). Burns. In C. M. Townsend Jr., R. D. Beauchamp, B. M. Evers, & K. L. Mattox (Eds.), *Sabiston textbook of surgery* (20th ed.). Philadelphia: Elsevier.

Jeschke, M. G., van Baar, M. E., Choudhry, M. A., Chung, K. K., Gibran, N. S., & Logsetty, S. (2020). Burn injury. *Nature Reviews Disease Primers, 6*(1), 11. https://doi.org/10.1038/s41572-020-0145-5.

Kaita, Y., Tarui, T., Shoji, T., Miyauchi, H., & Yamaguchi, Y. (2018). Cyanide poisoning is a possible cause of cardiac arrest among fire victims, and empiric antidote treatment may improve outcomes. *The American Journal of Emergency Medicine, 36*(5), 851–853.

Kidd, M., Hultman, C. S., van Aalst, J., Calvert, C. T., Holms, C., Peck, M., et al. (2007). The contemporary management of electrical injuries: Resuscitation, reconstruction, rehabilitation. *Annals of Plastic Surgery, 58*, 273–278.

Koob, T. J., Lim, J. J., Massee, M., Zabek, N., & Denoziere, G. (2014). Properties of dehydrated human amnion/chorion composite grafts: Implications for wound repair and soft tissue regeneration. *Journal of Biomedical Materials Research Part B: Applied Biomaterials, 102*(6), 1353–1362.

Koob, T. J., Rennert, R., Zabek, N., Massee, M., Lim, J. J., Temenoff, J. S., et al. (2013). Biological properties of dehydrated human amnion/chorion composite graft: Implications for chronic wound healing. *International Wound Journal, 10*(5), 493–500.

Kroll, M. W., Fish, R. M., Lakkireddy, D., Luceri, R. M., & Panescu, D. (2012). Essentials of low-power electrocution: Established and speculated mechanisms. In *2012 Annual International Conference of the IEEE Engineering in Medicine and Biology Society* (pp. 5734–5740). IEEE.

Litt, J. S. (2018). Evaluation and management of the burn patient: A case study and review. *Missouri Medicine, 115*(5), 443.

Matthews, M. R., Hechtman, A., Quan, A. N., Foster, K. N., & Fernandez, L. G. (2018). The use of vac veraflo cleanse choice in the burn population. *Cureus, 10*(11).

Matthews, M. R., Van Sant, L. M., Bollenbach, S. E., Swanson, S. D., Hollingworth, A. K., & Foster, K. N. (2019). Why trauma must trump burn injuries: The spectre of missed injuries. *Burns Open, 3*(3), 112–115.

Mayer, C. L., & Werman, H. A. (2019). Management of burn injuries. *Trauma Reports, 20*(1). Accessed 9/21/2020 from: https://www.reliasmedia.com/articles/143698-management-of-burn-injuries.

McNulty, A. K., Schmidt, M., Feeley, T., Villanueva, P., & Kieswetter, K. (2009). Effects of negative pressure wound therapy on cellular energetics in fibroblasts grown in a provisional wound (fibrin) matrix. *Wound Repair and Regeneration, 17*(2), 192–199.

Metcalf, D. G., Parsons, D., & Bowler, P. G. (2017). Clinical safety and effectiveness evaluation of a new antimicrobial wound dressing designed to manage exudate, infection and biofilm. *International Wound Journal, 14*(1), 203–213.

Miller, D. (2021). 2016–2018 Residential Fire Loss Estimates. U.S. National estimates of fires, deaths, injuries, and property losses from unintentional fires. In *U.S. Consumer Product Safety Commission*. Retrieved 01/16/2023 from: https://www.cpsc.gov/content/2016-to-2018-Residential-Fire-Loss-Estimates-Final.

Moiser, M. J., Bernal, N., & Farakas, I. (2017). *National burn repository 2017 update: Report of data from 2008–2017* (13th ed.). American Burn Association.

Monafo, W. W. (1996). Initial management of burns. *New England Journal of Medicine, 335*(21), 1581–1586.

Nielson, C. B., Duethman, N. C., Howard, J. M., Moncure, M., & Wood, J. G. (2017). Burns: pathophysiology of systemic complications and current management. *Journal of Burn Care & Research, 38*(1), e469–e481.

Norman, G., Christie, J., Liu, Z., Westby, M. J., Jefferies, J. M., Hudson, T., et al. (2017). Antiseptics for burns. *Cochrane Database of Systematic Reviews, 7*.

Onishi, S., Osuka, A., Kuroki, Y., & Ueyama, M. (2017). Indications of early intubation for patients with inhalation injury. *Acute Medicine & Surgery, 4*(3), 278–285.

Orgill, D. P., & Piccolo, N. (2009). Escharotomy and decompressive therapies in burns. *Journal of Burn Care & Research, 30*(5), 759–768.

Pham, T. N., Cancio, L. C., & Gibran, N. S. (2008). American burn association practice guidelines burn shock resuscitation. *Journal of Burn Care & Research, 29*(1), 257–266.

Pruitt, B. A., & Wolf, S. E. (2009). An historical perspective on advances in burn care over the past 100 years. *Clinics in Plastic Surgery, 36*(4), 527–545.

Rice, P. L., Jr., & Orgill, D. P. (2021). *Assessment and classification of burn injury*. UpToDate. https://www.uptodate.com/contents/assessment-and-classification-of-burn-injury?topicRef=350&source=see_link.

Rosenkranz, K. M., & Sheridan, R. (2002). Management of the burned trauma patient: Balancing conflicting priorities. *Burns, 28*(7), 665–669.

Ryan, C. M., Schoenfeld, D. A., Thorpe, W. P., Sheridan, R. L., Cassem, E. H., & Tompkins, R. G. (1998). Objective estimates of the probability of death from burn injuries. *New England Journal of Medicine, 338*(6), 362–366.

Salinas, J., Chung, K. K., Mann, E. A., Cancio, L. C., Kramer, G. C., Serio-Melvin, M. L., et al. (2011). Computerized decision support system improves fluid resuscitation following severe burns: An original study. *Critical Care Medicine, 39*(9), 2031–2038.

Santos, F. X., Arroyo, C., García, I., Blasco, R., Obispo, J. M., Hamann, C., et al. (2000). Role of mast cells in the pathogenesis of postburn inflammatory response: Reactive oxygen species as mast cell stimulators. *Burns, 26*(2), 145–147.

Saxena, V., Hwang, C. W., Huang, S., Eichbaum, Q., Ingber, D., & Orgill, D. P. (2004). Vacuum-assisted closure: microdeformations of wounds and cell proliferation. *Plastic and Reconstructive Surgery, 114*(5), 1086–1096.

Shin, J. Y., & Yi, H. S. (2016). Diagnostic accuracy of laser Doppler imaging in burn depth assessment: Systematic review and meta-analysis. *Burns, 42*(7), 1369–1376.

Skoog, T. (1970). Electrical injuries. *Journal of Trauma and Acute Care Surgery, 10*(10), 816–830.

Spies, C., & Trohman, R. G. (2006). Narrative review: Electrocution and life-threatening electrical injuries. *Annals of Internal Medicine, 145*(7), 531–537.

Steinstraesser, L., Flak, E., Witte, B., Ring, A., Tilkorn, D., Hauser, J., et al. (2011). Pressure garment therapy alone and in combination with silicone for the prevention of hypertrophic scarring: Randomized controlled trial with intraindividual comparison. *Plastic and Reconstructive Surgery, 128*(4), 306e–313e.

Sterling, J., Gibran, N. S., & Klein, M. B. (2009). Acute management of hand burns. *Hand Clinics, 25*(4), 453.

Tharmalingam, T., Ghebeh, H., Wuerz, T., & Butler, M. (2008). Pluronic enhances the robustness and reduces the cell attachment of mammalian cells. *Molecular Biotechnology, 39*(2), 167–177.

Tintinalli, J. (2016). *Tintinallis emergency medicine: A comprehensive study guide.* McGraw-Hill Education.

Van Loey, N. E. E., Bremer, M., Faber, A. W., Middelkoop, E., Nieuwenhuis, M. K., & Research Group. (2008). Itching following burns: Epidemiology and predictors. *British Journal of Dermatology, 158*(1), 95–100.

Waldmann, V., Narayanan, K., Combes, N., & Marijon, E. (2017). Electrical injury. *BMJ, 357,* j1418.

World Health Organization. (2018). Burns. In *World Health Organization.* Retrieved 01/15/2023 from: https://www.who.int/news-room/fact-sheets/detail/burns.

Yamaguchi, K. T., Hoffman, C., Stewart, R. J., Cianci, P. A., Vierra, M., & Naito, M. (1990). Effect of oxygen on bum wound tissue levels of ATP and collagen [abst]. *Undersea Biomedical Research, 17,* 65.

Yang, Q., Larose, C., Della Porta, A. C., Schultz, G. S., & Gibson, D. J. (2017). A surfactant-based wound dressing can reduce bacterial biofilms in a porcine skin explant model. *International Wound Journal, 14*(2), 408–413.

Young, A. W., Dewey, W. S., & King, B. T. (2019). Rehabilitation of burn injuries: An update. *Physical Medicine and Rehabilitation Clinics of North America, 30*(1), 111–132.

Zelt, R. G., Daniel, R. K., Ballard, P. A., Brissette, Y., & Heroux, P. (1988). High-voltage electrical injury: Chronic wound evolution. *Plastic and Reconstructive Surgery, 82*(6), 1027–1039.

Zhang, X. J., Irtun, O., Zheng, Y., & Wolfe, R. R. (2000). Methysergide reduces nonnutritive blood flow in normal and scalded skin. *American Journal of Physiology-Endocrinology and Metabolism, 278*(3), E452–E461.

Zhu, X., Donelan, M., & Sheridan, R. (1997). The index of deep burn injury: An analysis of 66 extremity sites in 15 children. *Burns, 23*(1), 11–14.

FURTHER READING

American College of Surgeons—Committee on Trauma. (2014). *Resources for optimal care of the injured patient* (6th ed.). American College of Surgeons. Accessed 4/14/20201 from: https://www.facs.org/-/media/files/quality-programs/trauma/vrc-resources/resources-for-optimal-care.ashx.

Carrougher, G. J., Martinez, E. M., McMullen, K. S., Fauerbach, J. A., Holavanahalli, R. K., Herndon, D. N., et al. (2013). Pruritus in adult burn survivors: Postburn prevalence and risk factors associated with increased intensity. *Journal of Burn Care and Research, 34*(1), 94–101.

Fernandez, L. G., Matthews, M. R., Alvarez, P. S., Norwood, S., & Villarreal, D. H. (2019). Closed incision negative pressure therapy: Review of the literature. *Cureus, 11*(7).

Frim, D. M., Wright, D. A., Curry, D. J., Cromie, W., Lee, R., & Kang, U. J. (2004). The surfactant poloxamer-188 protects against glutamate toxicity in the rat brain. *Neuroreport, 15*(1), 171–174.

MacLennan, L., & Moiemen, N. (2015). Management of cyanide toxicity in patients with burns. *Burns, 41*(1), 18–24.

Matthews, M. R., Quan, A. N., Shah, A. R., Tugulan, C. I., Nashed, B. A., Goldberg, R. F., et al. (2018). Hypochlorous acid for septic abdominal processes using a unique negative pressure wound therapy system: A pilot study. *Surgical Science, 9*(11), 412.

Mustoe, T. A., & Gurjala, A. (2011). The role of the epidermis and the mechanism of action of occlusive dressings in scarring. *Wound Repair and Regeneration, 19,* s16–s21.

Song, J., Hornsby, P., Stanley, M., Abdel Fattah, K. R., & Wolf, S. E. (2014). Porcine urinary bladder extracellular matrix activates skeletal myogenesis in mouse muscle cryoinjury. *Journal of Tissue Engineering and Regenerative Medicine, 3*(3).

35

Reconstructive Surgery for Wounds

Richard Simman

OBJECTIVES

1. State key factors to be considered in surgical decision-making.
2. Differentiate between flaps and grafts and their indications.

3. Describe interventions and tactics to optimize surgical outcomes.
4. Describe preoperative and postoperative interventions for patients undergoing surgical grafts or flaps.

Surgical intervention for chronic wounds is seldom the first choice. In general, much local care of the wound has preceded any decision for surgery. However, some chronic wounds deteriorate and require operative management, and some wounds reach a point in the healing trajectory where surgery is indicated to aid wound closure. This chapter addresses the wounds that may benefit from operative treatment, decisions about surgical closure, and care of the patient and the wound before and after surgery.

HISTORY OF SURGERY FOR WOUNDS

Traumatic wounds have existed since the beginning of man. The Edwin Smith Papyrus, which was written more than 5000 years ago, is the oldest known surgical treatise. It contains 142 different references to the management of sores and wounds. Surgical management of wounds is nearly as old. Hippocrates said, "He who wishes to be a surgeon should go to war." His words highlight the relationship between surgical advances and war-related injury. Modern reconstructive surgery had its beginnings with traumatic injury, at a time when the nose was cut off as a form of punishment or destroyed by syphilis. In Italy during the 16th century, noses were reconstructed in two stages using the skin of the inner upper aspect of the arm. This flap is known as the Tagliacozzi flap and even today is the emblem for the American Association of Plastic Surgeons. Modern plastic surgery came into its own during World War II when the sulfa antibiotic allowed many wounded soldiers to survive their injuries, and consequently they required reconstructive surgery. Today, surgery remains an important aspect of wound care and advances in surgical options continue to be made.

SURGICAL DECISION MAKING

Assessment of the Patient

A comprehensive patient assessment is required to determine the risk-to-benefit ratio and the type of surgical procedure indicated. The patient's condition and comorbidities form the primary aspect of the risk portion of the risk-to-benefit ratio. Although it is always ideal to have a closed wound, the patient must be able to tolerate anesthesia, surgery, blood loss, and postoperative restrictions and accept the risks involved. An estimation of anesthetic risk, such as the American Society of Anesthesiologists classification, provides an objective measure of relative risk for surgery. The patient must also be able to tolerate the pain and accept immobility after surgery, and the facility must be willing to keep the patient as long as the surgeon deems necessary for safe healing. Finally, the consequences of leaving a wound open must also be identified and considered as a potential benefit to operative intervention.

Assessment of the Wound

A successful wound closure requires deep understanding of wound anatomy and physiology as well as the healing phases of the wound. The basic principles of wound closure, diabetes control, wound perfusion, normal nutrition status, infection control, mechanical stress avoidance, and local wound care are all important elements in achieving healing of acute and chronic wounds. A number of wound closure techniques are available to the reconstructive surgeon. This armamentarium includes a variety of techniques, from simple primary wound closure (delayed primary closure, Plate 85 A and B) to more sophisticated and costly free flap reconstructive techniques. Logic dictates that the closure choice should start with the simple approach, if applicable, while the surgeon bears in mind that in certain circumstances, more sophisticated techniques are needed for a better outcome. Traumatic contaminated wounds should be debrided and irrigated, their foreign bodies removed, and hemostasis obtained in preparation for closure. Other wounds, such as iatrogenic, which may result after cancer resection, are presumed clean and may be closed without further preparatory wait. To reduce the rate of dehiscence, scaring, skin necrosis, and infection, tension should be avoided at all costs when closing a wound (European Pressure Ulcer Advisory Panel, National Pressure Injury Advisory Panel, Pan Pacific Pressure Injury Alliance [EPUAP, NPIAP, PPPIA], 2019; Simman, 2009). Further understanding of the causative factors and the missing tissues is important to optimize the outcome.

Causative Factors

Acute traumatic wounds may be missing fragments of skin, but with removal of these devitalized tissues and mobilization of surrounding skin, the laceration may be closed primarily. In the chronic wound, it is important to identify and ameliorate factors contributing to the chronic nature of the wound. The underlying etiology of the wound must be corrected or minimized (e.g., pressure) and cofactors treated (e.g., infection, ischemia, malnutrition) before healing can ensue. For example, the wound complicated by an ischemic process will require improvement of blood flow in order to heal. Likewise, an ischial pressure injury will not heal if the patient continues to sit on the wound. Surgical reconstruction of wounds in which the causative factor has not been addressed is not likely to succeed (EPUAP, NPIAP, PPPIA, 2019).

Missing/Needed Tissue

When planning surgical reconstruction of a wound, a full understanding of exactly what tissues are missing is needed in order to reconstruct the area for restoration of both form and function. Replacing like by like is a basic principle in reconstructive surgery. If a wound lacks only skin, replacing the skin (skin graft) may be a reasonable option, provided other patient conditions are well managed. However, simply putting skin on a wound without controlling infection, ischemia, or pressure is a doomed enterprise. Frequently, tissue padding (e.g., subcutaneous tissue and muscle) is needed to protect a bony prominence from recurrent breakdown, therefore a flap containing these elements would be necessary.

SELECTION OF WOUND CLOSURE METHOD

Several approaches are available to achieve wound closure ranging from least complex to most complex, often referred to as the reconstructive ladder (Fig. 35.1). This ladder serves as a guide for plastic and reconstructive surgery. Secondary intention wound healing (see Plate 86 A and B) is defined and described in Chapter 8. The surgical approach selected is made with consideration of complexity (i.e., prioritize the simplest method that accomplishes the patient's goals), and donor site morbidity. For example, if a person lost a thumb, transplantation of the

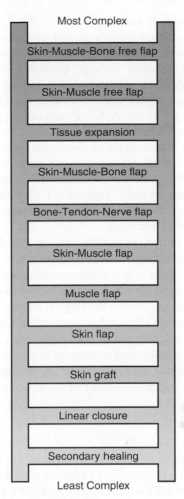

Fig. 35.1 Reconstructive ladder.

great toe to replace the thumb would be considered; however, the thumb would not be used to replace a great toe.

When considering donor site morbidity for pressure injury surgery, it is important to keep in mind that tissues usually can be moved or donated only once. Therefore, the choice of which tissue to use is important. Surgeons try to select donor areas that will not interfere with future potential flap donor sites, especially in patients with paralysis because this patient population often requires more than one operation during their lifetime. Large wounds of the entire perineum or pelvis in patients with paralysis may require hip disarticulation which includes removal of the femur and filleting of the remaining lower extremity tissues to form an adequately sized flap of muscle and skin that will sufficiently close the wound. This situation is a dramatic example of donor site morbidity.

Skin Grafts

During skin graft procedure, the skin is detached from a native donor site and transplanted to a different area of the body to cover a defect that resulted from a burn, surgery, or other injuries. The skin graft can be a split-thickness or full-thickness skin graft. When the defect is too large to close primarily, split-thickness skin grafts (STSGs) are available to cover the wound. The STSG will contain epidermis and variable amounts of dermis (Plate 87 A–F). A full-thickness skin graft will contain epithelium and a full thickness of dermis and contracts less than an STSG. In addition, a FTSG is not as readily available in large quantities. Therefore, the FTSG is reserved for relatively small wounds, such as on the face, hands, and feet, to provide better functional and cosmetic results (Plate 88 A–C). Preauricular, postauricular, supraclavicular, inguinal, antecubital skin, thigh, buttocks, and trunk are all examples of donor sites (Simman, 2009). Grafts in general are placed over the prepared wound bed and secured with a bolster dressing for 5–7 days to ensure contact with the recipient bed; NPWT may also be used to secure the graft. The donor site heals spontaneously in 12–14 days by epithelialization.

Skin grafts provide superficial coverage but do not replace deeper tissue layers, such as subcutaneous tissue and muscle; thus, they are unable to provide the padding needed to protect bony prominences from recurrent breakdown. Therefore, skin grafts are rarely used in the surgical management of pressure injuries, except to close donor sites (that cannot be closed primarily) from flaps containing multiple layers of tissue. Skin grafts are commonly used to manage burn wounds and are described in greater detail in Chapter 34. Skin grafts have also been used in the management of venous ulcers (Marston et al., 2017).

Skin Flaps

Skin flaps refer to the process whereby tissue is transferred from its bed to an adjacent area while retaining its native vascular attachment. This technique is used to fill a defect, pad a prominent bone, or protect underlying vital structures. Flaps differ from skin grafts in that they carry their own blood supply with them. Tissue flaps are either local (native nutrient vessels are moved with the flap) or distant (free) in which nutrient vessels are reestablished via microsurgery once the flap is transferred. Arterial–venous vessels remain in their native bed in a pedicle flap or are anastomosed by microvascular technique in free flap. Flaps are categorized by the anatomic structures, method used to move the flap, or method used to perfuse the flap (Box 35.1).

BOX 35.1 Categories of Surgical Tissue Flaps

Local Flaps
Classified by anatomic structures and tissue included in flaps:
- Skin flap
- Fasciocutaneous
- Perforator free flaps
- Myocutaneous or musculocutaneous flap

Classified by method used to move flap:
- Advancement flap
- Rotation flap
- Transposition flap

Classified by methods of retaining perfusion:
- Random flap
- Axial flap

Distant (Free) Flaps
- Fasciocutaneous
- Myocutaneous
- Osteocutaneous

Anatomic Structures

Types of flaps based on anatomic structure include skin, muscle, musculocutaneous, fascial, fasciocutaneous, and osteocutaneous. Myocutaneous (also called musculocutaneous) flaps involve rotation of all soft tissue layers (skin, subcutaneous tissue, fascia, muscle). As shown in Fig. 35.2, these flaps provide optimal coverage for bony prominences and therefore are frequently used in the surgical reconstruction of chest wall defects, cancer excision defects, complex leg wounds, pressure injuries, and other full-thickness wounds. Myocutaneous flaps carry along with them the native arterial and venous blood supplies to the muscle and the overlying skin. Because these flaps must survive on their original blood flow, their reach is limited by their nutrient vessel(s). When the flaps are pulled or stretched beyond their limits, the blood vessels also are stretched and are not able to perfuse the flaps. Therefore, tension-free closure and postoperative monitoring of arterial inflow and venous outflow is crucial for flap survival.

The area of potential reach for each muscle flap is known. For example, the biceps femoris muscle (one of the lateral

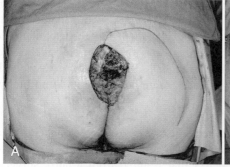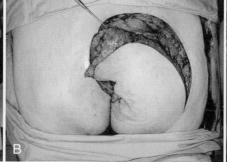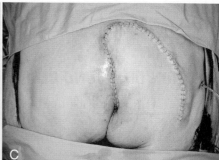

Fig. 35.2 Sacral ulcers can be closed with a gluteus maximus myocutaneous flap. (A) Gluteus muscle is identified using landmarks guided by the ischial tuberosity and the posterior iliac spine. (B) Segment of the muscle is rotated into the wound and is fed by the superior gluteal artery. (C) Muscle is divided and moved into the wound. The wound is closed primarily with a long incision to avoid tension. (From Song, D. H. (2013). Lower extremity, trunk, and burns. In P. C. Neligan (Eds.), *Plastic surgery* (3rd ed., Vol. 4). Philadelphia: Elsevier.)

hamstring muscles) is supplied with blood via arteries from the profunda femoris. The flap has an arc of rotation that can cover defects of the ischium and groin.

Local flaps are most commonly used for pressure injuries (EPUAP, NPIAP, PPPIA, 2019; Hansen, Young, Lang, et al., 2013). Local flaps used maybe fasciocutaneous or myocutaneous preserving their native blood supply. They are moved into the defect to obliterate the dead space and to replace the lost tissue.

Method Used to Move the Flap

Methods used to move local skin flaps include rotation, transposition, interpolation, and advancement (V-Y or rectangular). A rotation flap is a semicircular flap of skin and subcutaneous tissue that is rotated about a pivot point into the defect. A transposition flap, such as a rhomboid flap, is elevated and transposed into an adjacent defect. The donor site is closed primarily, or skin grafted. An advancement flap is raised and advanced into the defect in a straight line. The degree of advancement depends on the amount of stretching of the skin. A rectangular flap and a V-Y advancement flap are examples of these types of flaps.

Distant/rotational flaps with direct transfer are performed by the flap being raised based on a pedicle, which brings blood supply, and being placed to cover the defect. An interpolation flap is an example in which the base of the flap is located away from the wound bed resulting in a bridge of tissue flap base providing perfusion to the wound bed. Once vascularity is established between the wound and the flap, this pedicle is removed in a second surgical procedure (Ramsey, 2021). Local vessels from the defect bed grow into the flap, which no longer depends on its pedicle, by inserting the flap into

the defect. Here at least two-stage reconstruction is required. Groin flap for the reconstruction of hand defects and the forehead for the reconstruction of nasal defects are examples of this kind of flap (Simman, 2009).

A *free flap* contains a mass of composite tissue, with its vascular pedicle, that is transferred surgically from its native body location to a distant defect recipient site where vessel continuity is restored by microvascular anastomosis. This free flap is indicated when a large defect is seen with or without bone, vessel, or nerve exposure in an area where local pedicle flaps are compromised, unavailable, or too small to cover a large defect. They are most commonly used in trauma or cancer defect with or without radiation insult (see Plate 89 A and B).

Methods of Retaining Perfusion

The perfusion of the flap is important in the design of the flap. All flaps of tissue carry with them a blood supply (unlike a skin graft). *Random flaps* depend on the dermal and subdermal vessels for their blood supply. Because these vessels are small, the blood supply to these flaps is tenuous. *Axial flaps* are designed to include an artery, which increases vascularity and the chances for flap survival. These vessels nourish the flap until new collateral capillary systems are established between the flap and the wound bed. Common axial muscle flaps include the pectoralis flap to reconstruct the neck after radical neck surgery and the tensor fascia lata flap (Fig. 35.3) used to close ischial pressure injuries. When tissue is not available locally, it can sometimes be brought in using a free flap. This type of operation is more technically challenging because it requires microvascular surgical techniques. In this approach, the donor tissue, along with its blood supply, is

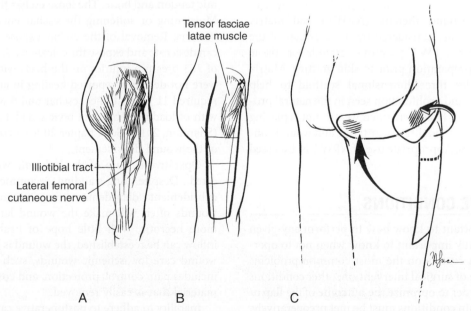

Fig. 35.3 Ischial and trochanteric ulcers can be closed using a tensor fasciae latae flap. (A) Muscle is found on the lateral thigh and fed by the femoral circumflex artery, which enters at the superior anterior iliac spine. (B) Advantage of the flap is the long muscle and skin cover. (C) Arc of rotation can provide coverage for both ischial and trochanteric ulcers. (From Cohen, S. (1990). Pressure sores. In J. McCarthy (Ed.), *Plastic surgery*. Philadelphia: Saunders.)

completely removed from the donor site and transferred to the recipient site. The artery and vein that supply the flap are attached by microvascular techniques to vessels near the wound. These types of flaps can be used to repair wounds of the head and neck, breast, or lower third of the leg. For example, recalcitrant venous ulcers with severe lipodermatosclerosis may benefit from free flap transfer by allowing wide excision of diseased tissue and replacing it with healthy tissue with its own microvasculature and uninjured venous valves (Marston et al., 2017).

Tissue Expansion

In tissue expansion, the skin responds to mechanical stress when it is applied by proliferating. During pregnancy, the lower abdominal skin responds rapidly to expansion. By expanding local skin surrounding the defect, wound coverage is provided with tissue that carries similar color and texture without compromising the donor area. The tissue expander is placed adjacent to the future defect when a congenital birth mark, burn scar, or hair baring scalp is excised. When the target volume is reached, the device is removed, and the skin is advanced into the defect for coverage. The device is placed under the muscle and skin when a breast is reconstructed after mastectomy. Sterile fluid is injected into the expander at routine intervals until the pouch is fully expanded. When the target volume is reached, the expander is removed and replaced with a permanent saline or silicone implant. For example, a scalp wound with alopecia may be treated with tissue expanders placed alongside the bare area to expand the hair-bearing scalp. Once fully expanded the bare area is excised and the expanded hair-bearing tissue is moved to cover the defect (Simman, 2009).

Negative Pressure Wound Therapy and Matrix Replacement

Negative pressure wound therapy (NPWT) and matrix replacement products are considered by some as part of the reconstructive ladder. NPWT promotes granulation tissue during wound bed preparation prior to skin grafting. Matrix replacement provides three-dimensional scaffold to help native cell migration and proliferation seen in the natural process of wound healing. However, since we are not replacing like by like, using these modalities, scar tissue and wound contractures may develop. Appropriate use of NPWT is discussed in Chapter 24.

NONOPERATIVE CONDITIONS

Although it is important to know how to perform any given operation, it is equally important to know when not to operate. This discussion centers on the most common problems that rule out the use of surgical intervention; other conditions also may exist. In order to optimize the outcome of the flap or graft coverage, certain conditions must be met preoperatively.

A pressure injury in a malnourished patient should not be repaired until the underlying malnutrition is controlled and the patient is anabolic again (EPUAP, NPIAP, PPPIA, 2019). If malnutrition is a volitional decision, then surgery

should not be an option. If the pressure injury did not heal due to malnutrition, then the surgical wound will not heal for the same reason.

Recalcitrant venous insufficiency ulcers require a bed of well-oxygenated granulation tissue to nourish a skin graft especially in patients with mixed vascular disease. If the edema cannot be controlled or the patient is unable to wear an external compression device, a skin graft will not survive. Chapters 15 and 16 provide a comprehensive review of assessment and management of venous insufficiency ulcers including details related to compression devices and option.

Calciphylaxis is due to ischemia in the skin and subcutaneous tissue from vascular acute calcification and occlusion. It is most commonly seen in patients with renal failure, hypercalcemia, and hyperphosphatemia. It may be seen in patients with hyperparathyroidism. Lesions usually develop on the legs and trunk and begin as areas of mottled skin that progress into painful, firm areas of necrosis. Surgery, if considered, usually consists of debridement of the lesion to prevent sepsis. However, until the underlying problems are controlled, the wounds often worsen or reappear (Magro, Simman, & Jackson, 2011; Maroz, Mohandes, Field, Kabakov, & Simman, 2015; Nigwekar, Thadhani, & Brandenburg, 2018). More information related to calciphylaxis is described in Chapter 32.

Stable eschar on the heel frequently presents as a nonoperative condition. Stable eschar is dry, hard, and firmly attached to the underlying skin; indications of an infection (induration, erythema, pain) are absent. Stable eschar on the heels should be offloaded, left intact and not debrided (EPUAP, NPIAP, PPPIA, 2019). Slowly, the eschar will release at the edges as the underlying tissue heals while the eschar forms a barrier to protect underlying relatively ischemic tendon and bone. The loose eschar then can be trimmed. Moistening or softening the eschar encourages invasion of bacteria. Removal of the eschar exposes the fat pad, which can desiccate and expose the calcaneus. A retrospective review of 263 pressure injuries on the heels with stable eschar that were not debrided reported healing in all but one patient. It required 11 weeks to heel eschar and 6 weeks to heal blisters with offloading. This data review had 41% lost to follow-up (Shannon, 2013). See Chapter 20 for a comprehensive review of the wound debridement.

Operative closure of the ischemic wound is contraindicated. Despite long-standing recommendations for serial debridement, debridements on ischemic lower extremity wounds often will make the wound larger, and eventually more necrotic, with little hope of healing. Unless arterial inflow can be reestablished, the wound is best left alone. Local wound care for ischemic wounds, such as arterial wounds, includes pain control, protection, and coverage with dressing material that is easily removed.

Inability to adhere to postoperative care requirements can be a significant deterrent to healing of a surgical wound. If the patient cannot remain off the flap, consume adequate calories, and control fecal and/or urinary contamination of the incision, the skin graft or flap likely will fail. It is important to keep in mind that only a given number of flap options can be used in a lifetime. Once a muscle is used, it cannot be used again. Therefore, the decision to operate should be made only after the patient is adequately educated regarding the interventions necessary postoperatively to reduce complications and prevent recurrence. Complications following surgical repair of pressure injuries have been reported as high as 35% and includes sepsis, wound dehiscence, and mortality (Kwok et al., 2018). Independent risk factors for postop complications were obesity, elderly, and diabetes. A review of 227 flaps to close ischial pressure injuries reported 88 recurrences (39%). Recurrence was highest in patients who were younger than 45 years, had low albumin, and had elevated hemoglobin A1C (Keys, Daniali, Warner, et al., 2010). Not surprisingly, two studies in 2017 identified surgery on an ischial pressure injury as a significant risk factor for recurrence (Bamba et al., 2017; Chiu et al., 2017).

Pyoderma gangrenosum is a rare condition that causes painful wounds on the lower extremities. Its cause is unknown and thought to be immune related. It is associated with other immunologic disorders, including rheumatoid arthritis and inflammatory bowel disease. It evolves from a small wound and is often confused by patients as a spider bite. These wounds often have a characteristic purple discoloration. A skin biopsy is typically performed showing a dense infiltration of neutrophils. Corticosteroids and other immunologic therapies are used for treatment. These ulcers are not treated surgically, as this tends to enlarge and exacerbate the ulcers (Dinulos, 2021). More information related to pyoderma gangrenosum is described in Chapter 32.

URGENT OPERATIVE CONDITIONS

Traumatic Wounds

Patients with traumatic wounds must undergo a thorough assessment to be certain they do not have major vessel, nerve, tendon injury, or bone fracture; therefore, the examination must be completed before the administration of local anesthetics. The wound is closed primarily, when possible, without creating donor site morbidity; for example, pulling the lower eyelid down and exposing the eye because the lid cannot close creating ectropion. Facial wounds require precision closure with small sutures to avoid excess scar formation. The timing of suture removal is dependent on the anatomic location and method of closure. For example, sutures on the face are generally removed sooner than sutures on the lower leg or buttocks. Details about linear closure and care of the surgical incision are described in Chapter 31.

When patients are severely injured, their wound issues may become the second priority to airway, breathing, and circulation. Clean wounds should be dressed with normal saline gauze and, if possible, closed within 12–24 h. After that time, they are considered contaminated. Operative closure should be a delayed primary closure, or the wound should be allowed to heal secondarily, with scar revision at a later date. Chapter 33 further discusses the care of the trauma patient with complex wounds.

Abscess

An abscess is a local collection of pus and sometimes infected hematoma. Abscesses are incised and drained. The remaining cavity may require packing to prevent healing from occurring at the surface before healing occurs in the deeper tissues. Culture is obtained and the patients are treated with antibiotics.

Wet Gangrene

Wet gangrene is infected soft tissue necrosis that develops from a sudden interruption in blood supply, as occurs with burns, freezing, hematoma, injury that becomes infected, or from primary infection of tissues from certain bacteria. Wet gangrene from any organism can quickly spread into surrounding tissues as a result of the bacteria and destroy muscle and other tissues. The patient has pain and fever. Malodor is often the most obvious sign. The tissue becomes discolored, blistered, and boggy and may have crepitus if the wound is infected with gas-forming organisms such as *Clostridium perfringens* (formerly known as *Clostridium welchii*). Frequently no line of demarcation exists between normal and infected tissue. Anaerobic infections can develop into gas gangrene within 1–2 days, and if the patient develops bacteremia, the mortality rate increases. If the gangrene is recognized and treated early and aggressively, mortality rates range from 25% to 35% (Bonne & Kadri, 2017). Surgery for wet gangrene includes radical removal of infected tissues or amputation. Hyperbaric oxygen therapy (HBOT) may also be used. Spreading gangrene is a surgical emergency. The wounds from these operations can be large and deep, with extensive areas of tissue loss.

In contrast, *dry* gangrene develops slowly from progressive loss of arterial supply, commonly in the extremities. A coagulative necrosis develops, and the tissue becomes black, dry, scaly, and greasy. A clear line of demarcation exists between viable and gangrenous tissue. The body will slowly slough the gangrenous tissue at the line of demarcation. Surgery may not be needed unless the area becomes infected. Although the gangrene is not painful at this stage, it likely was painful earlier in the process because of ischemia, and adjacent compromised tissue may exhibit ischemic pain. Dry gangrene should be covered with dry dressings and the tissue not moistened to prevent conversion to wet gangrene. An area of dry gangrene should never be soaked.

Necrotizing Fasciitis

Necrotizing fasciitis is a rapidly spreading, inflammatory infection of the deep fascia, with secondary necrosis of the subcutaneous tissues. The causative bacteria may be aerobic or anaerobic. Frequently, the cause is two synergistic bacteria that thrive in the hypoxic tissues. Because of the common presence of gas-forming organisms, subcutaneous air is classically described in necrotizing fasciitis and readily seen on radiograph. Pain out of proportion to the physical findings is a hallmark sign. The infection spreads rapidly along the fascial plane. These infections can be difficult to recognize in their early stages, but they rapidly progress to septic shock and organ failure. Emergency aggressive surgical debridement is required to remove all the necrotic tissue. Empiric broad-spectrum intravenous antibiotics are used until culture findings are known; however, the shock does not improve until the involved tissue is debrided (Dinulos, 2021). HBOT is an important adjunct to treatment where available. Two systematic reviews (Hua, Bosc, Sbidian, et al., 2018; Wang, Schwaitzberg, Berliner, et al., 2003) reported that HBOT may be helpful for some wounds, but there is insufficient evidence to ascertain the appropriate time to initiate therapy and to establish criteria that determine whether patients will benefit.

PREOPERATIVE MANAGEMENT OF PLANNED SURGERIES

Reducing Comorbid Factors and Improving Outcomes

When the health care team has the luxury of time, improving the patient's underlying condition will improve surgical wound healing (EPUAP, NPIAP, PPPIA, 2019; Keys et al., 2010). Many comorbid conditions can delay healing of both chronic and acute wounds. Some of the most common conditions that require correction or mitigation in this patient population (perfusion, oxygenation, bioburden, corticosteroids, diabetes, malnutrition, nicotine) are discussed in detail within chapters throughout this text. Permanent or temporary fecal and urinary diversions are sometimes needed to obtain a healed wound. Use of a bowel program or catheterization can divert urine and fecal material without the need for additional surgery (EPUAP, NPIAP, PPPIA, 2019; Gray, 2010).

Spasms and Contractures

Patients with paraplegia, quadriplegia, or other neurologic diseases have spasms that can lead to friction damage or traction on the incision, which can cause dehiscence. Spasms and fixed contractures also may limit postoperative positioning and leave patients at risk for the development of new pressure injuries. Management of muscle spasm and contractures should begin preoperatively and continue until the wound is completely healed (EPUAP, NPIAP, PPPIA, 2019).

Social Support

Closure of pressure injuries with flaps is technically possible in many cases. However, maintaining a closed wound is difficult unless the patient has a social network that can encourage adherence to postoperative restrictions and promote a lifetime of self-care (EPUAP, NPIAP, PPPIA, 2019; Keys et al., 2010; Tadiparthi, Hartley, Alzweri, Mecci, & Siddiqui, 2016). The individual's wheelchair, wheelchair cushion, and other mechanical devices are assessed before surgery.

Wound Bed Preparation

Successful closure of any wound requires a clean, well-vascularized wound bed. Excisional debridement helps prepare the wound bed that is likely to heal either by secondary intention or by attachment of surgically transferred

tissues. A recurring criticism of sharp and surgical debridement is that it is nonselective where viable and nonviable tissues are removed. Although this statement is true from a broad-brush perspective, most surgical debridements are done until the wound bed is clean and bleeding. Even though some layers of viable tissue may be sacrificed, there is a greater likelihood of removing all nonviable tissue, senescent cells, and avascular biofilm protective to bacteria. Failure to remove these factors often leads to failure of the surgical effort. Newer debridement instruments can debride in thin layers less than 1 mm thick. Techniques for wound debridement are discussed in Chapter 20.

NPWT is especially useful for accelerating the process of wound bed preparation for flaps and grafts, treating dehisced wounds, and preparing wounds for skin grafts or delayed linear closure (Chowdhry & Wilhelmi, 2019; Marston, Tang, Kirsner, & Ennis, 2016). NPWT may be used as a bridge between wound preparation and surgery, which allows time for the health care team to optimize the patient's condition for success of the reconstruction. It should be noted, however, that wounds healed with just NPWT and allowed to close via contracture may create unstable scarring over time, seen as scar tissue ulceration and pain with any stretching of the scar.

OPERATIVE MANAGEMENT OF PRESSURE INJURIES

International pressure injury guidelines recommend surgical consultation for operative repair in individuals with Stage 3 or 4 pressure injuries that are not closing with conservative treatment and for individuals who desire more rapid closure of the wound (EPUAP, NPIAP, PPPIA, 2019). Pressure injury excision and closure are commonly completed with patients under general anesthesia, even in those with paralysis, to reduce spastic and reflexic muscle movement and to control their vasomotor instability. Blood loss is anticipated, and patients should have blood typed and cross-matched for intraoperative administration.

Sacral Pressure Injuries

The sacrum is the most common location for pressure injuries. Large skin defects in the sacral area are not uncommon and can be associated with even larger areas of undermining. Fortunately, these injuries rarely are deep. Ostectomy of the sacral prominence is necessary if bone is infected. Coverage is most commonly obtained with a large gluteal myocutaneous flap (see Fig. 35.2) or fasciocutaneous rotational or gluteal fasciocutaneous V-Y advancement flaps (Fig. 35.4A and B).

Greater Trochanteric Pressure Injuries

Pressure injuries on the greater trochanter are seen in patients, many of whom have severe contractures and can only lie on their sides. The tensor fascia lata myocutaneous flap (see Fig. 35.2A–C) is the workhorse of wound covering in this region. It is most commonly designed as a transposition flap with a large resultant dog-ear. V-Y advancement

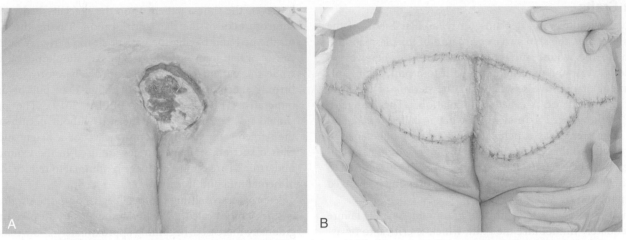

Fig. 35.4 (A) Stage 3 sacral pressure injury. (B) Bilateral gluteal V-Y advancement flaps used to close pressure injury.

(described in the next section) and rotation of the tensor fasciae latae flap often give an excellent functional and better aesthetic result. Other flaps include the rectus femoris myocutaneous flap and random bipedicle or unipedicle fasciocutaneous flaps.

Ischial Pressure Injuries

Ischial pressure injuries occur from prolonged erect sitting without changes in position and are most common in patients with lower limb paralysis. Usually, a small skin wound with a large cavity beneath the surface is present. The ischial tuberosity is the pressure point and is always involved. Ischial ostectomy is avoided if the bone is not infected because this procedure distributes the body weight onto the perineum, and the resulting ulcers are very difficult to manage.

Many options for flaps to cover ischial ulcers exist, including the tensor fasciae latae (Fig. 35.3A–C) and the posterior thigh fasciocutaneous flap. Another flap that can be used for patients with recurrent ulcerations in extremely large defects because thorough dissection yields 10–12 cm of advancement, is called a *V-Y flap* because the flap is raised with V-shaped incisions and then closed as a Y. This flap is well vascularized by segmental perforators from the hamstrings originating from the deep femoral artery. However, because the origins and insertions of the muscles are severed, this flap cannot be used in an ambulatory patient. Additional myocutaneous flaps for ischial ulcer closure include the rectus abdominis flap and the gracilis flap.

The gluteus maximus muscle flap offers a large amount of well-vascularized tissue with which to fill the defect. Even in the patient with a spinal cord injury, significant muscle mass still exists. Skin closure of the donor site can be obtained by linear closure in some cases or by a separate, inferiorly based fasciocutaneous rotation flap. It can be designed as a split muscle flap preserving donor site function in the ambulatory patient. Medially based posterior thigh advancement fasciocutaneous flaps can also be used to cover the defect over the ischium. Ischial ulcers in paralyzed patients are difficult

wounds. The recurrence of ulcers in this population can be high. The acute surgical wound can be delayed in healing, and the psychosocial components in the patient can lead to recurrence. However, the odds of having a recurrent pressure injury are reduced with a healthy lifestyle, being employed, and having a positive social network (Saunders & Krause, 2010).

Multiple Pressure Injuries

Extensive ulcerations of the sacrum, trochanters, and ischium are not uncommon, particularly in paralyzed patients. Removal of the femur combined with amputation of the leg allows the use of the skin and muscle from the thigh, called a *total thigh flap,* and has sometimes been necessary to provide enough tissue to close these extensive multiple wounds. Before surgery, urologic evaluation is completed because of the frequency of urinary infection. Urinary diversion may be required. Fecal diversion (temporary colostomy) also may be necessary. Common complications after surgery include hemorrhage and infection. Prolonged immobilization on special pressure redistribution beds is needed postoperatively, or these flaps will fail.

POSTOPERATIVE MANAGEMENT

Immobilization of the wound site while a skin graft is taking is crucial for adherence, inosculation, and neovascularization. Sliding or direct pressure can cause separation of a graft from its new vascular bed. This separation can be complicated by seroma, hematoma, fibrin, or purulent secondary effects. There are many methods of immobilization: splinting, restricted motion, bolster dressing, NPWT dressing and pinning, or external fixation. A sterilized wound bed and antibiotics may be needed to prevent skin graft loss from infection. Drain placement is important to prevent fluid collection under the flap. Appropriate dressing choice and team communication in flap and graft monitoring is key in successful outcome.

Skin Grafts

Survival of skin grafts depends on revascularization of the grafts. Initially, the skin survives because of the plasma imbibition on the wound surface. Within 48–72 h, new vessels should traverse the graft and change it to a pink color. This alignment of microvessels between the dermis of the graft and the wound bed is called "inosculation." The change in color of the grafted skin signifies what is called a *take* and often is expressed as a percentage of take or adherence to the wound bed that occurs through the ingrowth of new capillaries and fibrin bands. For example, an STSG is reported to have a 90% take after 72 h when the first dressing is changed (Simman, 2009).

The factors associated with skin graft failure are (1) failure to adequately immobilize the graft, which is critical to revascularization, (2) inadequate wound bed preparation (debridement and adequate blood flow), (3) infection, and (4) hematoma or seroma. One of the most common clinical problems after lower extremity skin grafting is failure to prevent edema in the wound bed. The patient must keep the skin graft site elevated for at least 72 h. All too often, the patient tries to get to the bathroom quickly or to sit briefly on the edge of the bed, and the grafted site becomes engorged with blood despite stented dressings and wraps. Clear instructions are imperative.

NPWT is sometimes used over skin grafts to promote adherence. Although the actual mechanism of action is not completely understood, it is likely that NPWT immobilizes the graft and reduces edema in the wound bed (Chowdhry & Wilhelmi, 2019; Evangelista, Kim, Evans, & Wirth, 2013; Marston et al., 2016; Simman, Forte, Sliverbug, & Moriera-Gonzalez, 2004). The graft may be meshed for NPWT to be more effective, especially in large surface area grafts. The NPWT foam should not be placed directly on the graft, so nonadherent wound contact dressings are usually placed directly on the graft site. Continuous negative pressure must be applied for 5–7 days. Appropriate use of NPWT is discussed in Chapter 24.

Once the graft has taken, the site is dry and prone to pruritus, dermatitis, or folliculitis. These conditions occur because sweat and oil glands are located in the deep dermis and are not transferred with partial-thickness skin grafts. Patients must be taught to develop lifelong strategies to protect and moisturize the skin.

Flaps

After flap surgery, the patient is placed on a specialty bed that provides pressure redistribution and eliminates shear (e.g., low air-loss bed or air-fluidized bed) (EPUAP, NPIAP, PPPIA, 2019; Fleck & Simman, 2010; Qaseem, Humphrey, Forciea, Starkey, Denberg, & Clinical Guidelines Committee of the American College of Physicians, 2015). A minimum requirement is 10–14 days on a specialty bed;

however, the time a patient is on the specialty bed varies by surgeon, take of the flap and location. Taking the patient off the bed and having the patient sit too early are common causes of flap injury or failure. The flap should not be pulled while the patient is being positioned. Therefore, the use of turning sheets to lift the patient rather than pull or drag is imperative (EPUAP, NPIAP, PPPIA, 2019). The patient should not be moved from the bed without permission of the surgeon, for example, onto a cart for a diagnostic test. Closed suction drainage devices are used in the wound and undermined areas until drainage is minimal to reduce the risk of hematoma and infection.

A progressive sitting protocol begins once the surgical site is sufficiently healed. Mobility and exposure to pressure are gradually increased, beginning approximately 2–5 weeks after the procedure, with careful monitoring of skin and suture lines (Ahluwalia, Martin, & Mahoney, 2010; EPUAP, NPIAP, PPPIA, 2019; Keys et al., 2010). Evaluation for an appropriate pressure redistribution chair cushion for the seating surface (chair or wheelchair) should be provided before surgery to reduce the risk of ischemia (see Chapter 11). Inadequate pressure redistribution might have been the cause of the ulceration to begin with and will recur if the seat cushion is not revised or replaced. Consider using pressure mapping to assist in selection and chair cushion evaluation. The patient should be reeducated on methods for reducing skin pressure and for monitoring skin daily for early signs of breakdown. Methods used by paraplegics to transfer from bed to chair (e.g., slide boards) should be discouraged until the flap is fully healed due to the shearing from the lateral movement (EPUAP, NPIAP, PPPIA, 2019).

Complications include flap necrosis due to spasm or stretch of the feeding blood vessels to the flap. The tissue appears pale and is cool or cold. Assessment of the vascular status of a flap can be improved by having two nurses examine the flap together at shift change to establish a baseline appearance. Seldom is surgery performed to close the dehisced area; most often, the open area is allowed to heal secondarily using moist wound healing principles and advanced wound care technology such as NPWT.

The most common complication is recurrence of the ulcer. Early recurrences are due to mobilizing the patient too much and too early, which frequently is done in an effort to reduce hospital length of stay. Late recurrences are often due to failure to change the previous lifestyle behaviors that caused the first ulcer. Support, equipment, and educational needs must be addressed and in place before patient discharge to facilitate adaptation (see Chapter 5) and prevent reoccurrence. Flaps are not as resilient as native tissue, and periods of time sitting on the flaps must be limited in duration for the patient's lifetime. Remember that only a few flap sites are available for reconstruction of any given area; once they are all used, the prognosis is grim.

CLINICAL CONSULT

A: Patient seen in wound clinic with plastic surgeon. 34-year-old male with paraplegia asking for surgical closure of a nonhealing sacral pressure injury of 3 months' duration. Wound 5 × 6 × 2 cm, wound base primarily nonviable adherent yellow slough, with moderate exudate and mild periwound erythema. Patient is currently afebrile with no other local signs of infection. Followed by home care. Patient is sitting slumped in his chair on a foam cushion but demonstrates ability to raise himself off the chair effectively.

D: Unstageable sacral pressure injury related to limited mobility.

P: Optimize local wound care, nutrition, and offloading prior to evaluation for surgical closure.

I: (1) Sharp debridement followed by alginate dressing covered with foam to promote autolysis and manage exudate.

(2) Instructions provided to home care to change daily initially then every other day as exudate decreases. (3) Sent for nutrition evaluation and recommendations. (4) Patient declined low air-loss bed due to difficulties with transferring. He states he can and will stay off his back; on foam viscoelastic mattress at home. (5) An appointment with physical therapy (PT) was made for a seating evaluation. (6) Surgeon explained flap surgery process in detail including need to commit postoperatively to bed rest on an advanced therapy support surface for several weeks followed by short seating trials on a specialized seating surface with slow incremental increases.

E: Return to clinic in 1 week for sharp debridement if needed, discuss dietary and PT evaluations, and evaluate effectiveness of local wound care. Consider trial of specialty mattress prior to considering surgical wound closure.

SUMMARY

- Many surgical wound closure techniques are available. However, surgical closure of wounds is not a panacea and is not appropriate for all wounds or all patients.
- The success of a surgical wound closure is contingent upon management of several issues, such as the causative factors

of the wound, the type of tissue missing and needed, the patient's general physiologic condition, the type of wound closure technique selected, preoperative nutritional status, postoperative care, and lifestyle behaviors.

SELF-ASSESSMENT QUESTIONS

1. A wheelchair-bound patient is most likely to develop which type of pressure injury?
   a. Sacral pressure injury
   b. Ischial pressure injury
   c. Trochanteric pressure injury
   d. Gluteal pressure injury
2. A bedridden patient presents to the clinic with large sacral pressure injury mostly covered with black eschar needing debridement. At the edge of the ulcer and through a small opening, the gluteal muscle fascia is visible. Which of the following statements is TRUE about this ulcer?
   a. The ulcer should be staged as Stage 3.

   b. The ulcer should be staged as Stage 4.
   c. The ulcer is unstageable until it's debrided and the necrotic tissue is removed.
   d. The ulcer is a deep tissue injury.
3. The most reliable choice of coverage of Stage 4 sacral pressure injury is:
   a. Split-thickness skin graft.
   b. Full-thickness skin graft.
   c. Fasciocutaneous flap.
   d. Myocutaneous flap.

REFERENCES

Ahluwalia, R., Martin, D., & Mahoney, J. L. (2010). The operative treatment of pressure wounds: A 10-year experience in flap selection. *International Wound Journal, 7*(2), 103–106.

Bamba, R., Madden, J. J., Hoffman, A. N., Kim, J. S., Thayer, W. P., Nanney, L. B., et al. (2017). Flap reconstruction for pressure ulcers: An outcomes analysis. Plastic and Reconstructive Surgery. *Global Open, 5*(1), e1187. https://doi.org/10.1097/GOX.0000000000001187.

Bonne, S. L., & Kadri, S. S. (2017). Evaluation and management of necrotizing soft tissue infections. *Infectious Disease Clinics of North America, 31*(3), 497–511. https://doi.org/10.1016/j.idc.2017.05.011.

Chiu, Y. J., Liao, W. C., Wang, T. H., et al. (2017). A retrospective study: Multivariate logistic regression analysis of the outcomes after pressure sores reconstruction with fasciocutaneous, myocutaneous, and perforator flaps. *Journal of Plastic Reconstructive & Aesthetic Surgery, 70*(8), 1038–1043.

Chowdhry, S., & Wilhelmi, B. (2019). Comparing negative pressure wound therapy with instillation and conventional dressings for sternal wound reconstructions. *Plastic and Reconstructive Surgery. Global Open, 7*, e2087.

Dinulos, J. G. H. (Ed.). (2021). *Habif's clinical dermatology. A color guide to diagnosis and therapy* (7th ed.). St. Louis: Elsevier.

European Pressure Ulcer Advisory Panel, National Pressure Injury Advisory Panel, Pan Pacific Pressure Injury Alliance (EPUAP, NPIAP, PPPIA). (2019). In E. Haesler (Ed.), *Prevention and treatment of pressure ulcers/injuries.* Osborne Park: Cambridge Media.

Evangelista, M. S., Kim, E. K., Evans, G. R., & Wirth, G. A. (2013). Management of skin grafts using negative pressure therapy: The effect of varied pressure on skin graft incorporation. *Wounds,* *25*(4), 89–93.

Fleck, C., & Simman, R. (2010). Use of alternatives to air-fluidized support surfaces in the care of complex wounds, post-flap and post-graft patients. *The Journal of the American College of Certified Wound Specialists,* *2*(1), 4–8.

Gray, M. (2010). Optimal management of incontinence-associated dermatitis in the elderly. *American Journal of Clinical Dermatology,* *11*(3), 201–210. https://doi.org/10.2165/11311010-000000000-00000.

Hansen, S. L., Young, D. M., Lang, P., et al. (2013). Flap classification and applications. In P. Neligan (Ed.), *Plastic surgery* (3rd ed.). St. Louis: Elsevier.

Hua, C., Bosc, R., Sbidian, E., et al. (2018). Interventions for necrotizing soft tissue infections in adults. *Cochrane Database of Systematic Reviews,* *5*(5), CD011680. https://doi.org/10.1002/14651858.CD011680.

Keys, K. A., Daniali, L. N., Warner, K. J., et al. (2010). Multivariate predictors of failure after flap coverage of pressure ulcers. *Plastic and Reconstructive Surgery,* *125*, 1725–1734.

Kwok, A. C., Simpson, A. M., Willcockson, J., Donato, D. P., Goodwin, I. A., & Agarwal, J. P. (2018). Complications and their associations following the surgical repair of pressure ulcers. *American Journal of Surgery,* *216*, 1177–1181.

Magro, C., Simman, R., & Jackson, S. (2011). Calciphylaxis: A review. *The Journal of the American College of Clinical Wound Specialists,* *2*(4), 66–72.

Maroz, N., Mohandes, S., Field, H., Kabakov, Z., & Simman, R. (2015). Calciphylaxis in patients with preserved kidney function. *The Journal of the American College of Clinical Wound Specialists,* *6*(1–2), 24–28. https://doi.org/10.1016/j.jccw.2015.08.002. 26442208. PMC4566866.

Marston, W. W., Ennis, W. J., Lantis, II, J. C., Kirsner, R. S., Galiano, R. D., Vanscheidt, W., et al. (2017). Baseline factors affecting closure of venous leg ulcers. *Journal Vascular Surgery: Venous and Lymphatic Disorders,* *5*(6), 829.e1–835.e1.

Marston, W., Tang, J., Kirsner, R. S., & Ennis, W. (2016). Wound Healing Society 2015 update on guidelines for venous ulcers. *Wound Repair and Regeneration,* *24*(1), 136–144. https://doi.org/10.1111/wrr.12394. 26663616.

Nigwekar, S. U., Thadhani, R., & Brandenburg, V. M. (2018). Calciphylaxis. *New England Journal of Medicine,* *378*(18), 1704–1714. https://doi.org/10.1056/nejmra1505292.

Qaseem, A., Humphrey, L. L., Forciea, M. A., Starkey, M., Denberg, T. D., & Clinical Guidelines Committee of the American College of Physicians. (2015). Treatment of pressure ulcers: A clinical practice guideline from the American College of Physicians. *Annals of Internal Medicine,* *162*(5), 370–379. https://doi.org/10.7326/M14-1568.

Ramsey, M. L. (2021). Pedicle/interpolation flaps. *Medscape. Drugs & Diseases. Clinical Procedures.* Available at: https://emedicine.medscape.com/article/1128874-overview. Accessed 12/08/2021.

Saunders, L. L., & Krause, J. S. (2010). Personality and behavioral predictors of pressure ulcer history. *Topics in Spinal Cord Injury Rehabilitation,* *16*(2), 61–71. https://doi.org/10.1310/sci1602-61.

Shannon, M. M. (2013). A retrospective descriptive study of nursing home residents with heel eschar or blisters. *Ostomy/Wound Management,* *59*(1), 20–27.

Simman, R. (2009). Wound closure and the reconstructive ladder in plastic surgery. *The Journal of the American College of Certified Wound Specialists,* *1*(1), 6–11.

Simman, R., Forte, R., Sliverbug, B., & Moriera-Gonzalez, A. (2004). A comparative histological study of skin graft take with tie-over bolster dressing versus negative pressure wound therapy in a pig model: A preliminary study in a pig. *Wounds,* *16*(2), 76–80.

Tadiparthi, S., Hartley, A., Alzweri, L., Mecci, M., & Siddiqui, H. (2016). Improving outcomes following reconstruction of pressure sores in spinal injury patients: A multidisciplinary approach. *Journal of Plastic, Reconstructive & Aesthetic Surgery,* *69*(7), 994–1002. https://doi.org/10.1016/j.bjps.2016.02.016. Epub 2016 Mar 10 27117674.

Wang, C., Schwaitzberg, S., Berliner, E., et al. (2003). Hyperbaric oxygen for treating wounds: A systematic review of the literature. *Archives of Surgery,* *138*(3), 272–280.

FURTHER READING

Bolton, L. L., Girolami, S., Corbett, L., & van Rijswijk, L. (2014). The Association for the Advancement of Wound Care (AAWC) venous and pressure ulcer guidelines. *Ostomy/Wound Management,* *60*(11), 24–66.

Brenner, M., Hilliard, C., Peel, G., et al. (2015). Management of pediatric skin-graft donor sites: A randomized controlled trial of three wound care products. *Journal of Burn Care & Research,* *36*(1), 159–166.

Erba, P., Ogawa, R., Vyas, R., & Orgill, D. P. (2010). The reconstructive matrix: A new paradigm in reconstructive plastic surgery. *Plastic and Reconstructive Surgery,* *126*, 492–498.

Finnegan, M., Gazzerro, L., Finnegan, J. O., et al. (2008). Comparing the effectiveness of a specialized alternating air pressure mattress replacement system and an air-fluidized integrated bed in the management of post-operative flap patients: A randomized control pilot study. *Journal of Tissue Viability,* *17*(1), 2–9.

Franz, M. G., Robson, M. C., Steed, D. L., et al. (2008). Guidelines to aid healing of acute wounds by decreasing impediments of healing. *Wound Repair and Regeneration,* *16*, 723–748.

Knobloch, K., & Vogt, P. (2011). The reconstructive ladder in light of evidence-based medicine. *Plastic and Reconstructive Surgery,* *127*, 1017–1018.

Mari, W., Younes, S., Naqvi, J., Issa, A. A., Oroszi, T. L., Cool, D. R., et al. (2019). Use of a natural porcine extracellular matrix with negative pressure wound therapy hastens the healing rate in stage 4 pressure ulcers. *Wounds,* *31*(5), 117–122. Epub 2019 Mar 15 30990777.

Mills, M. K., Faraklas, I., Davis, C., et al. (2010). Outcomes from treatment of necrotizing soft-tissue infections: Results from the National Surgical Quality Improvement Program database. *American Journal of Surgery,* *200*(6), 790–794.

Schryvers, O. I., Stranc, M. F., & Nance, P. W. (2000). Surgical treatment of pressure ulcers: 20-year experience. *Archives of Physical Medicine and Rehabilitation,* *81*(12), 1556–1562.

Simman, R., Mari, W., Younes, S., & Wilson, M. (2018). Use of hyaluronic acid-based biological bilaminar matrix in wound bed preparation: A case series. *Eplasty,* *18*, e10. 29527248. PMC5828938.

36

Skin Care Needs of the Patient With Obesity

Joshua R. Dilley, Lucian G. Vlad, and Joseph A. Molnar

OBJECTIVES

1. Define obesity.
2. Describe necessary accommodations in the physical environment for the patient with obesity.
3. Identify risk factors for three common skin complications in the obese patient population.
4. Discuss two common pulmonary complications in the obese patient population.

Over 70% of Americans are overweight, more than one-third of all Americans are obese, and roughly 7% are morbidly obese (Flegal et al., 2012; National Institute of Diabetes and Digestive and Kidney Diseases, 2017; Strum & Hattori, 2013). Obesity prevalence in the United States from 2013 to 2016 was estimated to be 36.5% for men and 40.8% for women (Hales et al., 2018). Worldwide the prevalence of obesity doubled in 73 countries and increased in nearly all the remaining countries between 1980 and 2015 (Abarca-Gómez et al., 2017; NCD Risk Factor Collaboration, 2016). Morbid obesity (body mass index [BMI] >40), once a rare occurrence in America, has essentially quadrupled since the 1980s (Gallagher, 2014). The proportion of the population with a BMI >50 has increased 10-fold since 1986 (Strum & Hattori, 2013). Research also shows that the heaviest Americans have become even heavier in the past decade (Beydoun & Wang, 2009). Studies suggest a substantial increase in obesity among all age, ethnic, racial, and socioeconomic groups (Lanz et al., 1998). In the early 1960s, only one-fourth of Americans were overweight; today, more than two-thirds of US adults are overweight, as are 31% of US children (Flegal et al., 2012; Ogden et al., 2012). By 2030, projections estimate 1 in 2 US adults will be obese, and 1 in 4 adults will have severe obesity (Ward et al., 2019).

Worldwide, the number of individuals who are overweight or obese, which totals over 2 billion (30% of the world's population), now exceeds the number of those suffering from starvation (Barrios & Jones, 2007; Tremmel et al., 2017; World Health Organization, 2015). Over the past 40 years, the world has transitioned from where underweight prevalence was twice as high as obesity to a world where more people are obese than underweight (NCD Risk Factor Collaboration, 2016).

Obesity has an economic, physical, and emotional impact on our patients. Americans spend close to $150 billion on obesity-related health problems, and over $70 billion is spent annually in attempts to control or lose weight (Kim & Basu, 2016; Marketdata Enterprises, Inc., 2020). The medical costs of obesity-related illnesses in the United States have been estimated at $315 billion annually (in 2010 dollars) (Biener et al., 2017). For example, obesity is associated with a more than 13-fold increase in the cost of antidiabetic medications (Apovian, 2013). The cost of absenteeism to employers has been estimated to exceed $8.6 billion annually (Andreyeva et al., 2014). Despite efforts at weight loss, Americans continue to gain weight, with obesity reaching epidemic proportions. Obesity has been implicated as a contributor to two-thirds of the globally leading causes of death from noncommunicable diseases by increasing the risk of diseases such as diabetes, kidney disease, and heart disease (Censin et al., 2019). Obesity is a factor in 5 of the 10 leading causes of death and is considered the second most common cause of preventable death in the United States only behind smoking (West Virginia Department of Health and Human Resources, 2014). In addition to the physiologic costs, obesity is associated with emotional conditions such as depression, altered self-esteem, eating disorders, substance abuse, and social isolation (Rotenberg et al., 2017; Sarwer & Polonsky, 2016). Furthermore, obesity is associated with stigma in education, healthcare, and employment (O'Brien et al., 2013). Obesity has been noted to negatively impact recruitment for the armed forces because an increasing proportion of the population does not meet the fitness standards (Cawley & Maclean, 2012). Major comorbidities associated with obesity include type 2 diabetes, cardiovascular disease, hypertension, sleep apnea or obesity hypoventilation syndrome, increased risk of cancers, and lipid disorders, including metabolic syndrome. Other associated conditions include other specific dietary insufficiencies, immobility, and depression. These comorbidities affect the patient who is morbidly obese disproportionately and at a younger age. Diagnosis in the patient with obesity is difficult, and procedures are technically more complicated, which ultimately places the patient at a disadvantage (Al-Mulhim et al., 2014; Nightingale et al., 2015). In addition, many hospitals, clinics, and home care settings are not prepared to meet the needs of this patient group because of inadequate equipment and insufficient personnel to accommodate the needs of the larger patient, factors known to contribute to the patient's risk of mechanical skin damage due to pressure, shear, or adhesives. However, advances in information, intervention, equipment, and education have helped reduce some of these risks (Gallagher, 2014).

DEFINING OBESITY

Obesity is defined as a BMI of 30 or greater; morbid obesity is defined as BMI greater than 40 (Box 36.1). *Bariatrics* is a term derived from the Greek word *baros* and refers to the practice of health care relating to the treatment of obesity and associated conditions. The Obesity Medicine Association defines obesity as chronic, relapsing, multifactorial, neurobehavioral disease, wherein an increase in body fat promotes adipose tissue dysfunction and abnormal fat mass physical forces, resulting in adverse metabolic, biomechanical, and psychosocial health consequences (Obesity Medicine Association, 2017). Others describe obesity simply as the excessive accumulation of body fat, which manifests as slow, steady, progressive increase in body weight. However, recent discoveries suggest that obesity is more than simply overeating or lack of control. In the broadest sense, obesity is at least in part a form of malnutrition as over nutrition is also malnutrition. Genetics, gender, physiology, biochemistry, neuroscience, and cultural, environmental, and psychosocial factors influence weight and its regulation (Lee et al., 2019; Ludwig & Pollack, 2009). As far back as 1994, the National Institutes of Health regarded obesity simply as a diagnostic category that represents a complex and multifactorial disease. However, obesity is most recently viewed as a chronic, multifactorial disease. In 2013, the American Medical Association voted to consider obesity as a treatable disease (Kyle et al., 2016).

Misunderstandings about the etiologies of obesity are common among health care providers. For example, obesity has long been perceived as a problem of self-discipline. Such misunderstandings can fuel prejudice and discrimination. Patients with obesity experience discrimination in schools, the workplace, and health care settings (O'Brien et al., 2013). As early as 1997, health care clinicians were often noted as biased against the larger patient (Thone, 1997).

Some practitioners view obesity as a symptom stemming from underlying issues. There is an increased understanding of Adverse Childhood Experiences (ACEs) in the pathophysiology of obesity (Felitti & Anda, 2010). In a 2010 study, it was suggested that obesity was not the problem but rather a compensatory solution for the underlying unaddressed adverse experiences (Felitti & Anda, 2010). The ACE study run by CDC from 1995 to 1997 enrolled 17,000 participants from Kaiser Permanente health plan and looked at seven categories of ACEs: psychological, physical, sexual abuse, violence against mother, living in household with substance abusers, mentally ill or suicidal members, or imprisoned (Felitti et al., 1998). This study has found strong correlation between ACEs and chronic conditions including obesity. An ACE score was described and a score of 4 or more was considered to be critical. Other studies have also noticed association between exposure to sexual and physical abuse during childhood and increased risk of severe obesity (Richardson et al., 2014).

Prejudice and discrimination pose barriers to care, regardless of practice setting or professional discipline. The overwhelming misunderstanding of obesity likely interferes with preplanning efforts, access to services, and resource allocation. This misunderstanding is not universal, but is pervasive enough to pose obstacles, and clinicians interested in making changes will need to recognize these barriers (Camden et al., 2008; Gallagher, 2011; Phelan et al., 2015).

ALTERED SKIN FUNCTION

In the obese person, a greater percentage of centralized and cutaneous adiposity is responsible for a number of changes in skin physiology and comorbidities that directly affect the skin. For example, the obese individual must perspire more when overheated in order to cool the body adequately due to the thick subcutaneous adipose layer (Lottenberg & Jensen, 2018). The barrier function of the skin is altered to have increased transepidermal water loss than in skin with less adiposity. Dry skin is characteristic of obesity as a consequence of a fundamentally altered epidermal lipid profile due to changes in the amount and composition of ceramides (Mori et al., 2017). Levels of androgens, insulin, growth hormone, and insulin-like growth factors frequently are elevated, triggering sebaceous gland activity, altered skin pH, and an increased prevalence of inflammatory or noninflammatory papules, pustules, nodules, or cystonodules over the head, face, neck, back, or arms (Hirt et al., 2019; Pokorny, 2008).

UNIQUE NEEDS

Common problems associated with the patient with obesity that interfere, at least potentially, with skin integrity include pressure injuries, intertrigo, incontinence-associated

BOX 36.1	**Body Mass Index Categories**
Underweight	<18.5
Normal weight	18.5–24.9
Overweight	25–29.9
Obesity	≥30
Morbid obesity	≥40

Source: National Heart, Lung, and Blood Institute, Bethesda, MD.

dermatitis (IAD), and foot dysfunction. Risk factors, manifestations, and prevention and management are described in Chapters 5, 7, 14, and 15; however, unique aspects occur in this patient population.

Pressure Management

Pressure injuries are considered areas of localized injury to the skin and/or underlying tissue because of pressure, or pressure in combination with shear (National Pressure Injury Advisory Panel, European Pressure Ulcer Advisory Panel, and Pan Pacific Pressure Injury Alliance [NPIAP/EPUAP/PPPIA], 2019). Pressure injuries typically occur over a bony prominence and develop because of the inability to adequately offload the pressure; this is particularly true among very heavy patients who may have limited mobility (Walden et al., 2013). To compound this problem, friction and pressure can exist in locations unique to the obese person (Gallagher, 2011; Pokorny, 2008). Atypical or unusual pressure injuries can result from tubes or catheters, an ill-fitting chair or wheelchair, or pressure within skin folds or over a point of contact not typically observed among patients who are not obese (Beitz, 2014).

Tubes and catheters can burrow into skin folds and ulcerate the skin surface. Pressure from side rails and armrests not designed to accommodate an obese individual can cause pressure injuries on the patient's hips. Patients often develop pressure injury over the buttocks rather than over the sacrum, an area that frequently is the point of maximum contact with the surface, because of the patient's atypical body configuration. Shearing/pressure damage can develop lateral to the gluteal cleft over the fleshy part of the buttocks due to insufficient repositioning or transfer onto a stretcher or the operating room table. Interventions to prevent these types of mechanical injuries are listed in Table 36.1.

Bariatric beds with a pressure redistribution mattress will reduce the risk of pressure injuries, promote patient independence, improve clinical outcomes, decrease staff workload, and help control unnecessary costs (Gallagher, 2012). As described in Chapter 12, bariatric support surfaces are available in foam, air, gel, and water. They offer features with or without microclimate and moisture control that include low friction covers. These devices are useful for reducing friction and shear and dissipating moisture. In addition to benefiting the patient, bariatric beds provide specific features that affect the staff and facility, as listed in Table 36.2 (Gallagher, 2011; Kramer, 2004). The support surface with lateral rotation therapy, often used for select pulmonary situations, has been used to help with repositioning a very large patient whose need for frequent turning may otherwise pose a realistic challenge (Camden, 2008). Additional precautions during lateral rotation to prevent friction and shear are well advised. The patient should be fitted to the appropriately sized surface with correct pressure settings, and frequent assessments for skin changes must be implemented (Gallagher, 2012; NPIAP/EPUAP/PPPIA, 2019).

TABLE 36.1   Management of Skin Damage in the Patient With Obesity

Type of Skin Damage	Causative Factor	Prevention Intervention
Pressure	Tubes and catheters burrow into skin folds	Reposition tubes and catheters every 2 h
	Pressure between skin folds or under large breasts	Place tubes so that patient does not rest on them
		Use tube and catheter holders
		Reposition large abdominal panniculus every 2 h to prevent pressure injury beneath panniculus
		Physically reposition pannus off suprapubic area every 2 h
		Use side-lying position with pannus lifted away from underlying skin surface, allowing air flow to regions
		Reposition breasts every 2 h
	Pressure injury on hips or lateral thighs from side rails and armrests	Use properly sized bariatric equipment
	Pressure injury occurs in slightly lateral fleshy areas of the buttocks rather than midline (directly over the sacrum) because it is difficult to prevent excess skin on buttocks from being folded and compressed when repositioning the patient	Bariatric support surface Proper repositioning Trapeze Establish, communicate, and implement safest transfer and positioning method to prevent shear that can be used during handoffs
Moisture-associated skin damage (e.g., intertrigo)	Excess perspiration to cool the body more efficiently when overheated Redundant skin creating skin folds Severe pruritus, burning, local pain between skin folds	Use cotton clothing (particularly undergarments) Maintain weight Avoid tight clothing Avoid corticosteroids and antibiotics

TABLE 36.2	Benefits of Bariatric Bed Features for Patient, Care Staff, and Facility		
Feature	Patient Benefit	Staff Benefit	Cost Benefit/Risk Reduction
600–1000-lbs capacity	Safely supports weight Eliminates fear of bed breaking	Reduces risk of injury during care	Reduces risk of patient injury (and possible litigation) if bed breaks Reduces risk of worker's compensation injury
Integrated scale	Safety Retained dignity More accurate than portable, under-mattress scales	Less time consuming than using a loading dock More accurate	Reduces risk of inappropriate treatment due to inaccurate weights
Expandable	Enhances patient participation by providing sufficient room in bed for proper repositioning	Bed width is a safe surface distance to prevent back injuries from overreaching Reduces risk of nosocomial pressure injury development from railings, skin fold pressure	Reduces risk of worker's compensation injury Reduces risk for litigation and citations from regulating agencies for nosocomial pressure injuries
Trendelenburg/ reverse Trendelenburg	Decreases friction on back when bring patient to top of bed	Helps with gravity-assisted movement of patient for fewer lifting injuries	Reduces risk of worker's compensation injury
Cardio-Chair	Increases mobility Decreases cardiac and pulmonary decomposition Facilitates faster recovery	Facilitates patient mobility Decreases staff lifting Simplifies transfers	Reduces risk of worker's compensation injury Reduces length of stay by decreasing effects of immobility
Trapeze	Increases mobility Facilitates patient independence Decreases friction on skin Facilitates deep breathing and pulmonary hygiene	Decreases staff lifting Facilitates mobility Reduces risk for nosocomial pressure injury development	Reduces risk of worker's compensation injury Reduces length of stay by decreasing effects of immobility or staff injury Reduces risk for litigation and citations from regulating agencies for nosocomial pressure injuries
Therapeutic mattress with microclimate control	Redistributes pressure appropriately to reduce risk of mechanical trauma (pressure, shear, friction) Facilitates moisture evaporation to reduce moisture entrapment in skin folds and sweating	Eases transfers and turning of patients Saves additional linen changes due to adequate control of perspiration Reduces risk for nosocomial pressure injury development	Reduces risk of worker's compensation injury Reduces risk for litigation and citations from regulating agencies for effects of immobility Reduces length of stay by decreasing nosocomial pressure injuries

Data from Kramer, K. (2004). WOC nurses as advocates for patients who are morbidly obese: A case study promoting use of bariatric beds. *Journal of Wound, Ostomy, and Continence Nursing, 31*(6), 379–384; Gallagher, S. M. (2012). Special patient populations. In W. Charney (Ed.), *Epidemic of medical errors and hospital-acquired infections.* Boca Raton: CRC Press; Gallagher, S. M. (2014). The intersection of ostomy and wound management, obesity, and associated science. *Ostomy/Wound Management, 60*(1), 6–7.

Skin Fold Management

Moisture-associated skin damage (MASD), pressure, and intertrigo can develop between skin folds of the patient with obesity. Common sites include the inner thighs, axilla, underside of breasts, and panniculus. Pressure from the weight of the pannus over the suprapubic area or breasts against the chest wall and upper abdomen are sufficient to cause skin breakdown (see Plate 90).

Because the patient with obesity experiences increased perspiration and sebum production and a change in skin pH, the barrier function of the skin is compromised (Hirt et al., 2019). In addition, coexisting medical conditions in the patient with

obesity such as diabetes mellitus, immunosuppression and infection will further increase the risk of MASD and intertrigo. Intertrigo (inflammation within skin folds) can become an intertriginous infection with bacterial, viral, or fungal organisms alone or in combination (Nobles & Miller, 2018). The main factor leading to the development of intertrigo is the mechanical friction between the skin folds (Metin et al., 2018). Unsurprisingly, the prevalence of intertrigo appears to increase with the degree of obesity (García-Hidalgo et al., 1999). Clinical manifestations of intertrigo in this patient population include scaling, erythema, and small pustules. Left untreated, the lesions can progress to fissures, macerations and erosions. Intertrigo usually has an insidious onset and can give symptoms of itching, burning, or prickling (Metin et al., 2018). Patients may scratch the skin surface to relieve the sensation of itching, further compromising skin integrity and leading to a secondary bacterial invasion. When an individual is hospitalized, moisture from urine, perspiration, or wound drainage exacerbates this chronic but otherwise mild condition (Beitz, 2014).

Knowing the patient with obesity is at risk for MASD and intertrigo, preventive interventions should be implemented upon admission and discussed in the outpatient wound clinic. In addition to the interventions presented in Box 9.4, management strategies unique to the patient with obesity are presented in Table 36.1.

Intertrigo, by itself, does not indicate a secondary infection (fungal, dermatophytes, and bacterial). If the area fails to improve or worsens within a reasonable time frame with conservative measures such as keeping the area dry, clean, and cool and minimizing friction, a superimposed infection should be considered (Nobles & Miller, 2018). Satellite lesions may suggest candida involvement, while clinical signs of cellulitis (increased redness, pain, and drainage) could suggest bacterial infection. A KOH skin scraping, or fungal culture can identify candida (Metin et al., 2018). Bacterial culture can identify pathological bacteria in the area. Prompt treatment of secondary infection is important to avoid worsening of the condition. Topical antimicrobial dressings, such as silver-impregnated textile products, may be appropriate at this point. Biopsy should be considered to rule out other pathologies if the condition fails despite appropriate treatment.

Incontinence-Associated Dermatitis

Increased BMI has a direct association with urinary incontinence and is a risk factor for urinary incontinence independent of age (Osborn et al., 2013). Subak et al. (2009) demonstrated a dose–response effect of weight on urinary incontinence as each 5 unit increase in BMI increased the risk of incontinence by 20%–70%. Increased weight raises the intraabdominal pressure, which stresses the pelvic floor leading to incontinence (Fuselier et al., 2018). Sleep apnea, another condition associated with obesity, can lead to decreases in oxygen tension and relative central nervous system hypoxia, both of which cause increased excitability of autonomic neurons and thus trigger urgency. Continuous positive pressure ventilation has been reported to improve symptoms associated with urinary incontinence, such as urgency and enuresis (Steers & Suratt, 1997).

Many otherwise continent persons develop short-term acute incontinence when they are physically dependent or acutely ill in a health care setting. This condition may occur because of medication, confusion, infection, delays in locating a caregiver to place the patient on the bedpan, or because the patient cannot access a commode in time to prevent an incontinent episode. It is critical that health care providers attempt to identify an underlying etiology of the incontinence (medications, infection, constipation, debility, etc.) and treat the underlying cause if possible. Additional barriers to maintaining continence include inadequate staffing, negative attitudes by the staff (American Nurses Association, 2013; Dingwall & Mclafferty, 2006; Ostaszkiewicz et al., 2008), and reluctance on the part of the patient to ask for assistance. The health care team should collaborate with the patient and family to address and minimize any barriers. Maintaining clean, dry skin is the objective, and if the patient needs assistance in this effort, caregivers must be available to help.

After each incontinent episode, the entire affected area should be cleansed with a gentle incontinence cleanser, dried, and appropriate skin protector or moisture barrier applied (Woo et al., 2017). Skin irritation can occur as early as 1 h after exposure to urinary or fecal irritants and is dependent upon their concentration, so it is important to clean the skin promptly (Larner et al., 2015). A recent review found that perineal skin cleansers may be more effective at preventing IAD compared with soap and water, however, this was based on limited, low-quality evidence (Beeckman et al., 2016; Lachance & Argaez, 2019). The pH of skin is approximately 5–5.5 so avoiding alkaline products (cleansers or soaps) is important as they can alter the skin surface pH and promote bacterial growth (Woo et al., 2017). Table 9.4 and Box 9.4 list strategies and products used for the prevention and management of IAD. Patients report that drying the buttocks and the perineal area and between folds with an institutionally approved blow dryer on the cool setting is more comfortable than towel drying. This technique may be less traumatic to the outermost layer of skin (Blackett et al., 2011). If IAD develops despite preventive efforts, the skin care protocol must be reassessed and updated to include a moisture barrier ointment or fecal containment with either an external fecal pouch (in conjunction with a skin barrier paste or barrier strip), or an internal fecal device, all of which are described in Chapter 9.

Foot and Lower Leg Pathology

Individuals with obesity are prone to place excess stress on their joints and feet due to their increased weight. In these individuals, the most common dermatological finding is plantar hyperkeratosis due to excess pressure on the heel during walking (García-Hidalgo et al., 1999). Studies have demonstrated patients are at increased risk of foot pain with increasing BMI (Dufour et al., 2017). The reason for this is potentially twofold—both mechanical and metabolic. Individuals with obesity have flatter feet, less range of motion and cause larger forces under the feet when walking which places excess stress on the foot structures (Dufour et al., 2017). The excess adipose tissue increases proinflammatory cytokines and may lead to development of foot symptoms (Tanamas et al., 2012). Foot pain could signal other serious medical conditions, such as arthritis, nerve and circulatory disorders, and diabetes. Among the obese population, foot discomfort or dysfunction requires prompt attention. Foot pain can delay a patient with obesity from seeking care due to ambulation and transportation difficulties. Accommodations in the physical environment that promote patient safety and comfort may overcome some of these obstacles (Checklist 36.1). As described in Chapters 14 and

15, when the joints of the feet are involved, medication, physical therapy, exercise, orthotics, braces, specially designed shoes, and surgery are among the tools that can be used to restore feet to as near-normal function as possible.

Obesity is a major risk factor for the development of lower extremity venous disease (LEVD) through several mechanisms (Meulendijks et al., 2020). Increased abdominal pressure from adipose tissue is transmitted to the femoral veins leading to external venous obstruction and reflux. Cytokines released from adipose tissue contribute to increased endothelial permeability and microcirculation dysfunction. Finally, obesity can lead to decreased mobility which reduces activation of the calf muscle and consequently reduces venous flow (Meulendijks et al., 2020). Obesity is associated with impaired wound healing, altered collagen formation and higher risk of infection (Hirt et al., 2019; Pence & Woods, 2014). Patients with LEVD are encouraged to stay mobile, exercise, and get plenty of physical activity as physical activity appears to improve wound healing by reducing systemic inflammation (Pence & Woods, 2014).

Lymphedema is a chronic, incurable disorder that is caused either by the abnormal development of the lymphatic system (primary lymphedema) or injury to the lymphatic system (secondary lymphedema). The lymphatic system transport lymph fluid, which is composed of white blood cells, bacteria, cell debris, protein, and water. Around 5 million Americans suffer from lymphedema (Rockson & Rivera, 2008). The most common symptom of lymphedema is swelling in the distal extremities. Individuals with a BMI >50 are at risk for obesity-induced lymphedema and those with a BMI >60 likely have the disease (Greene et al., 2012). The link between obesity and lymphedema appears to be reciprocal where obesity impairs lymphatic transport, and this impaired transport/function promotes adiposity deposition (Mehrara & Greene, 2014). The uncontrolled swelling can lead to ulceration and make the extremity more prone to develop a chronic wound from minor trauma. The mainstays of treatment are weight loss and manual lymph therapy performed by a trained therapist and compression.

Lower extremity arterial disease (LEAD) is considered common among the obese individual mostly due to the associated comorbidities, predominantly diabetes, coronary artery disease and kidney disease. Recently, obesity has been identified as a strong, independent risk factor for LEAD. Individuals with obesity are 1.5× more likely to develop LEAD with critical limb ischemia than normal weight individuals (Hicks et al., 2018). Further, the obese person with LEAD is at increased risk of functional decline (McDermott et al., 2006). There is growing evidence of an "obesity paradox" where these individuals have more favorable cardiovascular mortality outcomes compared with normal weight individuals, but evidence is conflicting (Ludhwani & Wu, 2019). Weight loss may improve functional outcomes in individuals with obesity with LEAD, but further studies are needed (Polonsky et al., 2019). See Chapter 4 for additional reading on LEAD.

Regardless of the foot or leg pathology, self-assessment and professional assessment and treatment can be challenging.

CHECKLIST 36.1   Accommodations in Physical Environment for the Patient With Obesity

✓ Larger, wider blood pressure cuff
✓ Long needles
✓ Larger tracheostomy ties
✓ Longer abdominal binders
✓ Large gowns/drapes
✓ Elbow-length gloves for incontinence cleanup
✓ Bed frame wide enough for effective repositioning
✓ Pressure redistribution support surface
✓ Overhead trapeze to facilitate repositioning when appropriate
✓ Bariatric ceiling or floor-based lift for safely moving the patient (e.g., ceiling lifts)
✓ Bedside commode (appropriate size)
✓ Wide wheelchair with specialized cushion
✓ Walker with proper support
✓ Size-friendly art and magazines
✓ Larger clinic examination tables anchored to floor with adequate step
✓ Sturdy, armless chair for clinic waiting rooms
✓ Air displacement lateral transfer devices
✓ Mechanical lifts with provisions for limb band, pannus sling, turning band, lithotomy band, repositioning sling

---

Obesity and/or decreased flexibility can prevent a patient from seeing his or her feet. Self-inspection can be difficult, with these limitations often requiring family or outside help (Game, 2013). Physical inspection can be a real-life challenge because positioning larger, heavier individuals poses threats to caregiver safety (Walden et al., 2013). Arnold (2014) describes trends in the emerging science of safe patient handling and mobility that serve the wound care provider either in the clinic or at the bedside. Specially designed slings, bands, and devices to position heavier patients safely are available and serve as an adjunct to dignified, comprehensive care (Gallagher, 2011). Specialized training to how to transport and maneuver the patient with obesity can improve patient and safety (Gable et al., 2014).

THE SURGICAL EXPERIENCE

The surgical experience predisposes the patient to skin injury due to intraoperative mechanical factors (shear, friction, and pressure) and postoperative factors (immobility, pain, sedation, fear of falling, and inadequate staffing). In addition, the patient with obesity is at increased risk for impaired healing of the surgical incision and complications from the anesthesia and from the surgical procedure itself (e.g., cardiovascular, and respiratory complications) that can further jeopardize wound healing (Martindale & Deveney, 2013; Pierpont et al., 2014).

Addressing Mechanical Threats to Skin Integrity

Although the patient may be awake and alert shortly after surgery, extra personnel and supportive equipment are required to transfer the patient, particularly to prevent shearing injury or placing undue stress on the incision. Early activity is encouraged to decrease the chances of immobility-related complications (Gallagher, 2011). Using bariatric equipment that will convert into a chair will facilitate achieving early mobilization. Deconditioning can occur rapidly in the patient with obesity when mobilization after surgery is delayed, thus increasing the risk for skin- and wound-related complications (Padwal et al., 2012). A physical therapy consultation within 24 h of admission may be valuable to (1) evaluate for and demonstrate immobility-related equipment and (2) provide passive and active exercises to slow deconditioning (Gallagher, 2011; Morris et al., 2008). The larger patient typically has several comorbid conditions, so postoperative recovery can be complicated and require close monitoring. However, it is important to assess and reassess the skin frequently (at least every 8 h) so that potential complications can be prevented or identified, and interventions applied early (Gallagher, 2012). Preplanning for the patient with obesity by having proper bariatric equipment and appropriate staffing available is essential to providing competent, safe postoperative care.

After surgery, elevating the head of the bed to 30 degrees (semi-Fowler's position) can improve ventilatory effort and tidal volumes in the patient with obesity by reducing the adipose tissue pressing against the diaphragm (Johnson & Meyenburg, 2009). The challenge in terms of skin care is that the 30-degree elevation at the head of the bed can increase the risk of sacral pressure injuries without adequate position changes (Sideranko et al., 1992). Introducing pressure redistribution early in the admission may reduce some of this risk, along with patient and clinical education designed to improve awareness about the risk. An appropriate bariatric support surface, such as an air or foam mattress, and trapeze should be in place to reduce shear on the sacrum and adequately redistribute pressure (Johnson & Meyenburg, 2009). The patient should be encouraged to offload and shift his or her weight at regular intervals, including reducing the head of the bed when possible, to prevent prolonged pressure to the sacrum. Similarly, the lower back should be monitored frequently for signs of friction or shear.

Incisions and Sutured Wounds

Obesity is associated with a higher incidence of wound complications, such as surgical site infection and wound dehiscence (Glance et al., 2010; Martindale & Deveney, 2013; Pierpont et al., 2014). A possible contributing factor is hypoperfusion of adipose tissue due to the higher ratio of tissue mass to capillaries in adipose tissue. The resulting decreased oxygen tension in adipose tissue can be inadequate to meet the oxygen needs of the healing surgical incision although evidence is conflicting (Anaya & Dellinger, 2006; Lempesis et al., 2020). Additional factors that contribute to the increased rate of surgical site infections in the patient with obesity include perioperative hyperglycemia (obesity is associated with insulin resistance and hyperglycemia), prolonged operative time (operative time is an independent

predictor of surgical site infection), obesity-related decreased immune function, increased operative blood loss and suboptimal doses of prophylactic antibiotics to achieve therapeutic tissue concentrations (Anaya & Dellinger, 2006; Hourigan, 2011; Thelwall et al., 2015). In addition to optimizing tissue oxygen tension, as discussed in Chapters 28 and 34, tight perioperative glucose control, larger doses of prophylactic antibiotics to maximize serum and tissue concentrations intraoperatively, layered suture closure and performance of minimally invasive surgeries whenever feasible may reduce incidence of infections (Anaya & Dellinger, 2006; Lang et al., 2017).

Incised and sutured wounds are expected to create a watertight seal within 48 h; however, wound healing can be delayed in some patients due to malnutrition if the patient has a diet that lacks essential vitamins and nutrients. When the incision is within a skin fold, wound healing can be delayed due to moisture entrapment and bioburden in the skin fold (Lang et al., 2017). A well-placed and well-constructed stoma will be critical to prevent postoperative peristomal and stoma complications that can be aggravated by irregularities in abdominal topography (Colwell, 2014).

To reduce the occurrence of abdominal wound separation, a surgical binder can be used to support the surgical incision. The binder should rest no higher than 4 cm below the xiphoid process and should allow 2.5 cm of space between the skin and binder to avoid constricting the chest wall and hampering ventilation. Abdominal binders have been shown to decrease postoperative pain and psychological stress, improve respiratory function, prevent abdominal wall dehiscence, and improve mobility (Saeed et al., 2019). Regular and routine skin assessments of the area under the binder are important to monitor for signs of early pressure-related breakdown.

Hypoventilation Syndrome and Sleep Apnea

Patients with morbid obesity tend to have pulmonary problems; two in particular: obesity hypoventilation syndrome and sleep apnea. Obesity hypoventilation syndrome is an acute respiratory condition in which the weight of adipose tissue on the rib cage and abdomen prevents the chest wall from expanding fully by causing impaired diaphragm motion (Masa et al., 2019). Because patients are unable to breathe in and out fully, there is an increased work of breathing and ventilatory insufficiency can occur (Gallagher, 2012; Masa et al., 2019).

Sleep apnea usually occurs when the patient is asleep in the supine position. The weight of the excess fatty tissue in the neck causes the throat to narrow, severely restricting or even cutting off breathing for seconds or even minutes at a time. Obesity is the strongest risk factor for development of sleep apnea. Symptoms of sleep apnea include snoring, headaches, daytime sleepiness, sleep disruption, pulmonary hypertension and arrythmias (Lang et al., 2017). Breathing can be made easier by keeping the patient in the semi-Fowler's position, which takes some of the pressure off the diaphragm. Mobilizing the patient as early as possible also will help. At home, many patients manage the problems of nighttime sleep apnea by using a continuous positive airway pressure machine (Lang et al., 2017). However, in the health care setting, some patients use bilevel positive airway pressure for a short time after extubation.

Tracheostomy Care

Tracheostomy dependence is increased in the patient with obesity due to disordered breathing and obesity hypoventilation syndrome. Increased cervical and submental adipose tissue decreases visualization and access to the airway which increases the challenge of performing a tracheostomy (Gross et al., 2002). A large incision may be needed to locate the trachea. This larger wound can lead to complications such as bleeding, infection, or damage to the surrounding tissue. Postoperative tracheostomy care, therefore, must include steps to protect the peristomal skin, manage the tracheostomy, and contain wound drainage. Locally, a nonadhesive absorptive wound dressing is appropriate. Compounding the potential skin-related problems associated with a tracheostomy in the patient with obesity is the inadequacy of standard-sized tracheostomy tubes for use in patients with larger necks. In addition, narrow cloth tracheostomy ties can burrow deep within the folds of the neck, further damaging the skin. Wider tracheostomy tie material should be used to accommodate the patient with obesity. When additional pressure relief is needed under the tracheostomy tie, padding such as a gauze or foam dressing can be applied between the skin and the tie.

NUTRITIONAL CONSIDERATIONS

It is important to recognize that excess weight does not reflect adequate or normal nutritional status. Frequently, nutritional evaluation of the patient with obesity can be incorrectly deferred due to assuming excess weight excludes nutrition inadequacy. Malnutrition can be divided into two subcategories: undernutrition and overnutrition (Tanumihardjo et al., 2007). Classically, malnourishment is thought as undernutrition and lack of appropriate intake. However, overnutrition, including obesity, is a form of malnutrition. Obesity arises from people having excess calories to meet their energy requirements but lacking dietary quality to promote optimal health. Micronutrient deficiencies and protein deficiencies are increasingly common among the obese population due to a refined western diet (Kaidar-Person et al., 2008). The refined diet is higher in fat, carbohydrates, and caloric value but overall nutrient poor. The combination of obesity and malnutrition, in the form of micronutrient deficiency, has been termed the "obesity paradox" and is associated with poverty and food insecurity (Tanumihardjo et al., 2007). Food insecure households have the highest BMI and prevalence of obesity (Olson, 1999).

Research suggests that 7%–12% of the obese population in general is malnourished (Moize et al., 2003). A study of critically ill patients found as much as 60% of patients with obesity suffered from malnutrition in the intensive care unit (Robinson et al., 2015). Macronutrients and micronutrients have long been recognized as essential in skin integrity and wound healing among all individuals, but especially in those at risk, such as patients with obesity, whose nutritional status may be compromised because of repeated dieting and weight cycling, simple misunderstanding of proper nutrition, or weight loss surgery (Bal et al., 2012). Weight loss surgery is a metabolic surgery designed to produce malnutrition. Energy deficit occurs due to decreased food intake, food intolerance, and nutrient malabsorption. The goal in weight loss surgery or any weight loss program is to achieve monitored weight loss without adverse complications (Valentino et al., 2011). Bariatric surgery places patients at risk for iron, calcium, vitamin B12, vitamin D, vitamin A, vitamin E, vitamin K, thiamine, and folate deficiencies. These nutrients play an important role in wound healing. Chapter 29 discusses the role and dietary sources of these nutrients; Table 29.7 lists their specific relevance to the wound repair process. Most importantly, surgery can place the patient at risk for protein malnutrition which causes a host of problems including delayed wound healing. In order to combat malnutrition after bariatric surgery, a high-protein diet and micronutrient supplementation is recommended.

QUALITY IMPROVEMENT

In managing the skin care needs of the patient with obesity, a comprehensive, interdisciplinary patient care approach is necessary to provide safe patient care in a timely and effective manner. This approach should include (1) a bariatric task force; (2) a criteria-based protocol, which includes preplanning equipment; (3) competencies/skill set; and (4) outcome measurement efforts (Gallagher, 2012).

The Bariatric Task Force should consist of multiple disciplines who develop the plan on best practices to care for the patient with obesity. The task force should be instrumental in creating a criteria-based protocol. A patient's weight, BMI, body width and clinical condition can serve as criteria to help arrange special equipment or ensure the expertise of certain clinical staff are involved in a patient's care. Once the criteria have been established, it is important that all staff are trained to ensure competency in caring for the patient with obesity. Training could include how to safely reposition a patient or urinary catheter placement. Training should be individualized on the needs on the staff. Finally, the bariatric program's outcomes should be measured. Potential outcomes include patient/staff satisfaction, safety, and adverse events.

CLINICAL CONSULT

A: Patient is 55-year-old female with past medical history of obesity (BMI 35) admitted to the hospital for pancreatitis; wound care is consulted regarding management of an abdominal pressure injury. The patient works full time as a teacher, is quite active, and has no pressure injuries anywhere but her abdomen. The patient has been applying bacitracin and gauze every day after her shower. She has been doing her best to lose weight in hopes to reduce the pressure from her pannus. She has lost 30 lbs in the past 2 weeks by drastically cutting calories. The patient consented to a wound assessment despite her obvious discomfort. She is currently on an appropriately sized foam pressure redistribution mattress. Skin inspection under pannus revealed 10 × 4 cm of erythema and both dry and moist desquamation, satellite lesions noted, patient complains of intense itch/burn sensation.

D: Pannus intertrigo dermatitis (ITD) secondary to moisture and friction on opposing skin surfaces. Satellite lesions are indicative of secondary candidiasis. Possible malnutrition given significant recent weight loss despite obesity.

P: Optimize nutrition with a focus on high protein intake up to 2 g/kg/day, minimize moisture and friction at apposing skin folds, treat candidiasis, and teach the patient how to manage skin folds to prevent future recurrences.

I: (1) Consult nutrition services. (2) Discontinue bacitracin to help restore normal flora. (3) Twice daily, gently rinse with cleaner and dry completely, apply antifungal moisture barrier to clean dry skin followed by soft moisture wicking soft textile or cloth to keep opposing skin free from friction and moisture.

E: Plan to return in 3 days to evaluate effectiveness of interventions and discuss realistic management strategies for the home and work environment, which will most likely include daily pH balanced cleansing, moisture-wicking soft textile or cloth, and dietician-guided weight loss.

SUMMARY

- Obesity is increasing in prevalence in the United States and the world.
- Caring for the obese population requires special equipment to protect them from developing wounds including appropriately sized wheelchairs, beds with offloading capabilities and lifts to help transfer.
- Excess weight places patients with obesity at higher risk of moisture-associated dermatitis and incontinence-associated dermatitis. Care of these conditions focuses on keeping the skin dry and clean.
- Individuals with obesity are at higher risk for surgical complications and appropriate planning could help reduce chance of complications.
- Do not forget to assess the nutritional status of these individuals as overnutrition is associated with malnutrition and micronutrient deficiencies.

SELF-ASSESSMENT QUESTIONS

1. Individuals with obesity are more prone to pressure injury formation because:
   a. Limited mobility
   b. Excess, friction, and pressure
   c. Ill-fitting beds and chairs
   d. All of the above
2. Obesity places a patient at risk for which of the following surgical complications?
   a. Increased mortality
   b. Increased skin and soft tissue infection
   c. Weight loss
   d. Gastrointestinal upset
3. What intervention can help reduce the risk of abdominal wound dehiscence in the obese patient population?
   a. Abdominal binder
   b. Incentive spirometer
   c. Delayed mobility after surgery
   d. Fowler's position (head of bed at 30 degrees)

REFERENCES

Abarca-Gómez, L., Abdeen, Z. A., Hamid, Z. A., Abu-Rmeileh, N. M., Acosta-Cazares, B., Acuin, C., et al. (2017). Worldwide trends in body-mass index, underweight, overweight, and obesity from 1975 to 2016: A pooled analysis of 2416 population-based measurement studies in 128·9 million children, adolescents, and adults. *The Lancet*, 390(10113), 2627–2642.

Al-Mulhim, A. S., Al-Hussaini, H. A., Al-Jalal, B. A., Al-Moagal, R. O., & Al-Najjar, S. A. (2014). Obesity disease and surgery. *International Journal of Chronic Diseases*, 2014, 652341.

American Nurses Association. (2013). *ANA principles for nurse staffing* (2nd ed.). Silver Spring: ANA.

Anaya, D. A., & Dellinger, E. P. (2006). The obese surgical patient: A susceptible host for infection. *Surgical Infections*, 7, 473–480.

Andreyeva, T., Luedicke, J., & Wang, Y. C. (2014). State-level estimates of obesity-attributable costs of absenteeism. *Journal of Occupational and Environmental Medicine/American College of Occupational and Environmental Medicine, 56*(11), 1120.

Apovian, C. M. (2013). The clinical and economic consequences of obesity. *The American Journal of Managed Care, 19*(Suppl. 10), S219–S228.

Arnold, M. (2014). Maximizing mobility, preserving skin integrity and preventing complications during the care of the obese patient. One hospital's solutions for patient and caregiver safety. A pictorial narrative of care tasks. *Ostomy/Wound Management, 60*(1), 24–29.

Bal, B. S., Finelli, F. C., Shope, T. R., et al. (2012). Nutritional deficiencies after bariatric surgery. *Nature Reviews. Endocrinology, 8*(9), 544–556.

Barrios, L., & Jones, D. B. (2007). Healthcare economics of weight loss surgery. *Bariatric Times, 4*(8). 1, 16–17, 20–21.

Beeckman, D., Van Damme, N., Schoonhoven, L., Van Lancker, A., Kottner, J., Beele, H., et al. (2016). Interventions for preventing and treating incontinence-associated dermatitis in adults. *Cochrane Database of Systematic Reviews, 11.*

Beitz, J. (2014). Providing quality skin and wound care for the bariatric patient: An overview of clinical challenges. *Ostomy/Wound Management, 60*(1), 12–21.

Beydoun, M. A., & Wang, Y. (2009). Gender-ethnic disparity in BMI and waist circumference distribution shifts in U.S. adults. *Obesity, 17*(1), 169–176.

Biener, A., Cawley, J., & Meyerhoefer, C. (2017). The high and rising costs of obesity to the US health care system. *Journal of General Internal Medicine, 32*(Suppl. 1), 6–8. https://doi.org/10.1007/s11606-016-3968-8. 28271429. PMCID: PMC5359159.

Blackett, A., Gallagher, S., Dugan, S., et al. (2011). Caring for persons with bariatric health care issues. *Journal of Wound, Ostomy, and Continence Nursing, 38*(2), 133–138.

Camden, S. G. (2008). Pressure ulcers, CMS, and patients of size. *Bariatric Times, 5*(12), 1, 8–13.

Camden, S. G., Brannan, S., & Davis, P. (2008). Best practices for sensitive care and the obese patient: Task report. *Bariatric Nursing and Surgical Patient Care, 3*(3), 189–196.

Cawley, J., & Maclean, J. C. (2012). Unfit for service: The implications of rising obesity for US military recruitment. *Health Economics, 21*(11), 1348–1366.

Censin, J. C., Peters, S. A., Bovijn, J., Ferreira, T., Pulit, S. L., Mägi, R., et al. (2019). Causal relationships between obesity and the leading causes of death in women and men. *PLoS Genetics, 15*(10), e1008405.

Colwell, J. (2014). The role of obesity in the patient undergoing colorectal surgery and fecal diversion: A review of the literature. *Ostomy/Wound Management, 60*(1), 24–28.

Dingwall, L., & Mclafferty, E. (2006). Do nurses promote urinary continence in hospitalized older people? An exploratory study. *Journal of Clinical Nursing, 15*(10), 1276–1286.

Dufour, A. B., Losina, E., Menz, H. B., LaValley, M. P., & Hannan, M. T. (2017). Obesity, foot pain and foot disorders in older men and women. *Obesity Research & Clinical Practice, 11*(4), 445–453.

Felitti, V. J., & Anda, R. F. (2010). The relationship of adverse childhood experiences to adult health, well-being, social function, and healthcare. In R. Lanius, E. Vermetten, & C. Pain (Eds.), *The impact of early life trauma on health and disease: The hidden epidemic* (pp. 77–87). New York: Cambridge University Press.

Felitti, V. J., Anda, R. F., Nordenberg, D., Williamson, D. F., Spitz, A. M., Edwards, V., et al. (1998). Relationship of childhood abuse and household dysfunction to many of the leading causes of death in adults: The Adverse Childhood Experiences (ACE) Study. *American Journal of Preventive Medicine, 14*(4), 245–258.

Flegal, K. M., Carroll, M. D., Kit, B. K., et al. (2012). Prevalence of obesity and trends in the distribution of body mass index among U.S. adults, 1999–2010. *Journal of the American Medical Association, 307*(5), 491–497.

Fuselier, A., Hanberry, J., Lovin, J. M., & Gomelsky, A. (2018). Obesity and stress urinary incontinence: Impact on pathophysiology and treatment. *Current Urology Reports, 19*(1), 10.

Gable, B. D., Gardner, A. K., Celik, D. H., Bhalla, M. C., & Ahmed, R. A. (2014). Improving bariatric patient transport and care with simulation. *Western Journal of Emergency Medicine, 15*(2), 199.

Gallagher, S. M. (2011). Exploring the relationship between obesity, patient safety, and caregiver injury. *American Journal of Safe Patient Handling & Movement, 1*(2), 8–12.

Gallagher, S. M. (2012). Special patient populations. In W. Charney (Ed.), *Epidemic of medical errors and hospital-acquired infections* (pp. 225–238). Boca Raton: CRC Press.

Gallagher, S. M. (2014). The intersection of ostomy and wound management, obesity, and associated science. *Ostomy/Wound Management, 60*(1), 6–7.

Game, F. (2013). Obesity and the diabetic foot. *Diabesity in Practice, 2*, 112–117.

García-Hidalgo, L., Orozco-Topete, R., Gonzalez-Barranco, J., Villa, A. R., Dalman, J. J., & Ortiz-Pedroza, G. (1999). Dermatoses in 156 obese adults. *Obesity Research, 7*(3), 299–302.

Glance, L. G., Wissler, R., Mukamel, D. B., et al. (2010). Perioperative outcomes among patients with the modified metabolic syndrome who are undergoing noncardiac surgery. *Anesthesiology, 113*(4), 859–872.

Greene, A. K., Grant, F. D., & Slavin, S. A. (2012). Lower-extremity lymphedema and elevated body-mass index. *The New England Journal of Medicine, 366*(22), 2136–2137.

Gross, N. D., Cohen, J. I., Andersen, P. E., & Wax, M. K. (2002). Defatting tracheotomy in morbidly obese patients. *The Laryngoscope, 112*(11), 1940–1944.

Hales, C. M., Fryar, C. D., Carroll, M. D., Freedman, D. S., & Ogden, C. L. (2018). Trends in obesity and severe obesity prevalence in US youth and adults by sex and age, 2007–2008 to 2015–2016. *Journal of the American Medical Association, 319*(16), 1723–1725.

Hicks, C. W., Yang, C., Ndumele, C. E., Folsom, A. R., Heiss, G., Black, J. H., III, et al. (2018). Associations of obesity with incident hospitalization related to peripheral artery disease and critical limb ischemia in the ARIC study. *Journal of the American Heart Association, 7*(16), e008644.

Hirt, P. A., Castillo, D. E., Yosipovitch, G., & Keri, J. E. (2019). Skin changes in the obese patient. *Journal of the American Academy of Dermatology, 81*(5), 1037–1057.

Hourigan, J. S. (2011). Impact of obesity on surgical site infection in colon and rectal surgery. *Clinics in Colon and Rectal Surgery, 24*(4), 283.

Johnson, K. L., & Meyenburg, T. (2009). Physiological rationale and current evidence for therapeutic positioning of critically ill patients. *AACN Advanced Critical Care, 20*(3), 228–240.

Kaidar-Person, O., Person, B., Szomstein, S., & Rosenthal, R. J. (2008). Nutritional deficiencies in morbidly obese patients: A new form of malnutrition? *Obesity Surgery, 18*(7), 870–876.

Kim, D. D., & Basu, A. (2016). Estimating the medical care costs of obesity in the United States: Systematic review, meta-analysis, and empirical analysis. *Value in Health, 19*(5), 602–613.

Kramer, K. (2004). WOC nurses as advocates for patients who are morbidly obese: A case study promoting use of bariatric beds. *Journal of Wound, Ostomy, and Continence Nursing, 31*(6), 379–384.

Kyle, T. K., Dhurandhar, E. J., & Allison, D. B. (2016). Regarding obesity as a disease: Evolving policies and their implications. *Endocrinology and Metabolism Clinics, 45*(3), 511–520.

Lachance, C. C., & Argaez, C. (2019). *Perineal skin cleansers for adults with urine incontinence in long-term care or hospital settings: A review of the clinical effectiveness and guidelines.*

Lang, L. H., Parekh, K., Tsui, B. Y. K., & Maze, M. (2017). Perioperative management of the obese surgical patient. *British Medical Bulletin*, 1–21.

Lanz, P., House, J. S., Lepkowski, J. M., et al. (1998). Socioeconomic factors, health behaviors, and mortality. *Journal of the American Medical Association, 279*(2), 1703–1708.

Larner, J., Matar, H., Goldman, V. S., & Chilcott, R. P. (2015). Development of a cumulative irritation model for incontinence-associated dermatitis. *Archives of Dermatological Research, 307* (1), 39–48. https://doi.org/10.1007/s00403-014-1526-y.

Lee, A., Cardel, M., & Donahoo, W. T. (2019). Social and environmental factors influencing obesity. In *Endotext (Internet)*. MDText.com, Inc.

Lempesis, I. G., van Meijel, R. L., Manolopoulos, K. N., & Goossens, G. H. (2020). Oxygenation of adipose tissue: A human perspective. *Acta Physiologica, 228*(1), e13298.

Lottenberg, A. M. P., & Jensen, N. S. O. (2018). Hyperhidrosis and obesity. In *Hyperhidrosis* (pp. 19–25). Cham: Springer.

Ludhwani, D., & Wu, J. (2019). Obesity paradox in peripheral arterial disease: Results of a propensity match analysis from the national inpatient sample. *Cureus, 11*(5).

Ludwig, D. S., & Pollack, H. A. (2009). Obesity and the economy. *Journal of the American Medical Association, 301*(5), 533–535.

Marketdata Enterprises, Inc. (2020). *$71 Billion weight loss market pivots amid Covid-19*. Marketdata Enterprises. https://www.marketdataenterprises.com/71-billion-weight-loss-market-pivots-amid-covid-19/.

Martindale, R. G., & Deveney, C. W. (2013). Preoperative risk reduction: Strategies to optimize outcomes. *The Surgical Clinics of North America, 93*(5), 1041–1055.

Masa, J. F., Pépin, J. L., Borel, J. C., Mokhlesi, B., Murphy, P. B., & Sánchez-Quiroga, M.Á. (2019). Obesity hypoventilation syndrome. *European Respiratory Review, 28*(151).

McDermott, M. M., Criqui, M. H., Ferrucci, L., Guralnik, J. M., Tian, L., Liu, K., et al. (2006). Obesity, weight change, and functional decline in peripheral arterial disease. *Journal of Vascular Surgery, 43*(6), 1198–1204.

Mehrara, B. J., & Greene, A. K. (2014). Lymphedema and obesity: Is there a link? *Plastic and Reconstructive Surgery, 134*(1), 154e.

Metin, A., Dilek, N., & Bilgili, S. G. (2018). Recurrent candidal intertrigo: Challenges and solutions. *Clinical, Cosmetic and Investigational Dermatology, 11*, 175.

Meulendijks, A. M., Franssen, W. M. A., Schoonhoven, L., & Neumann, H. A. M. (2020). A scoping review on chronic venous disease and the development of a venous leg ulcer: The role of obesity and mobility. *Journal of Tissue Viability, 29*(3), 190–196.

Moize, V., Geliebter, A., Gluck, M. E., et al. (2003). Obese patients have inadequate protein intake related to protein status up to 1 year following Roux-en-Y gastric bypass. *Obesity Surgery, 13*, 23–28.

Mori, S., Shiraishi, A., Epplen, K., Butcher, D., Murase, D., Yasuda, Y., et al. (2017). Characterization of skin function associated with obesity and specific correlation to local/systemic parameters in American women. *Lipids in Health and Disease, 16*(1), 214.

Morris, P. E., Goad, A., Thompson, C., Taylor, K., Harry, B., Passmore, L., et al. (2008). Early intensive care unit mobility therapy in the treatment of acute respiratory failure. *Critical Care Medicine, 36*(8), 2238–2243.

National Institute of Diabetes and Digestive and Kidney Diseases. (2017). *Overweight & obesity statistics*. Retrieved 10/1/2020 from: https://www.niddk.nih.gov/health-information/health-statistics/overweight-obesity.

National Pressure Injury Advisory Panel, European Pressure Ulcer Advisory Panel, and Pan Pacific Pressure Injury Alliance (NPIAP/EPUAP/PPPIA). (2019). In E. Haesler (Ed.), *Prevention and treatment of pressure ulcers/injuries: Clinical practice guideline. The international guideline.*

NCD Risk Factor Collaboration. (2016). Trends in adult body-mass index in 200 countries from 1975 to 2014: A pooled analysis of 1698 population-based measurement studies with 19·2 million participants. *The Lancet, 387*(10026), 1377–1396.

Nightingale, C. E., Margarson, M. P., Shearer, E., Redman, J. W., Lucas, D. N., & Skues, M. (2015). Peri-operative management of the obese surgical patient. Association of Anesthetists of Great Britain and Ireland Society for Obesity and Bariatric Anaesthesia. *Anaesthesia, 70*(7), 859–876.

Nobles, T., & Miller, R. A. (2018). Intertrigo. In *StatPearls (Internet)*. StatPearls Publishing.

Obesity Medicine Association. (2017). *Definition of obesity*. https://obesitymedicine.org/definition-of-obesity/.

O'Brien, K. S., Latner, J. D., Ebneter, D., & Hunter, J. A. (2013). Obesity discrimination: The role of physical appearance, personal ideology, and anti-fat prejudice. *International Journal of Obesity, 37*(3), 455–460.

Ogden, C. L., Carroll, M. D., Kit, B. K., et al. (2012). Prevalence of obesity and trends in body mass index among U.S. children and adolescents, 1999–2010. *Journal of the American Medical Association, 307*(5), 483–490.

Olson, C. M. (1999). Nutrition and health outcomes associated with food insecurity and hunger. *The Journal of Nutrition, 129*(2), 521S–524S.

Osborn, D. J., Strain, M., Gomelsky, A., et al. (2013). Obesity and female stress urinary incontinence. *Urology, 82*(4), 759–763.

Ostaszkiewicz, J., O'Connell, B., & Millar, L. (2008). Incontinence: Managed or mismanaged in hospital settings? *International Journal of Nursing Practice, 14*(6), 495–502.

Padwal, R. S., Wang, X., Sharma, A. M., & Dyer, D. (2012). The impact of severe obesity on post-acute rehabilitation efficiency, length of stay, and hospital costs. *Journal of Obesity, 2012.*

Pence, B. D., & Woods, J. A. (2014). Exercise, obesity, and cutaneous wound healing: Evidence from rodent and human studies. *Advances in Wound Care, 3*(1), 71–79.

Phelan, S. M., Burgess, D. J., Yeazel, M. W., Hellerstedt, W. L., Griffin, J. M., & van Ryn, M. (2015). Impact of weight bias and stigma on quality of care and outcomes for patients with obesity. *Obesity Reviews, 16*(4), 319–326.

Pierpont, Y. N., Dinh, T. P., Salas, R. E., Johnson, E. L., Wright, T. G., Robson, M. C., et al. (2014). Obesity and surgical wound healing: A current review. *ISRN Obesity, 2014.*

Pokorny, M. E. (2008). Lead in: Skin physiology and disease in the obese patient. *Bariatric Nursing and Surgical Patient Care, 3*(2), 125–128.

Polonsky, T. S., Tian, L., Zhang, D., Bazzano, L. A., Criqui, M. H., Ferrucci, L., et al. (2019). Associations of weight change with changes in calf muscle characteristics and functional decline in peripheral artery disease. *Journal of the American Heart Association, 8*(13), e010890.

Richardson, A. S., Dietz, W. H., & Gordon-Larsen, P. (2014). The association between childhood sexual and physical abuse with incident adult severe obesity across 13 years of the National Longitudinal Study of Adolescent Health. *Pediatric Obesity, 9*(5), 351–361.

Robinson, M. K., Mogensen, K. M., Casey, J. D., McKane, C. K., Moromizato, T., Rawn, J. D., et al. (2015). The relationship among obesity, nutritional status, and mortality in the critically ill. *Critical Care Medicine, 43*(1), 87–100.

Rockson, S. G., & Rivera, K. K. (2008). Estimating the population burden of lymphedema. *Annals of the New York Academy of Sciences, 1131*(1), 147–154.

Rotenberg, K. J., Bharathi, C., Davies, H., & Finch, T. (2017). Obesity and the social withdrawal syndrome. *Eating Behaviors, 26,* 167–170.

Saeed, S., Rage, K. A., Memon, A. S., Kazi, S., Samo, K. A., Shahid, S., et al. (2019). Use of abdominal binders after a major abdominal surgery: A randomized controlled trial. *Cereus, 11*(10).

Sarwer, D. B., & Polonsky, H. M. (2016). The psychosocial burden of obesity. *Endocrinology and Metabolism Clinics, 45*(3), 677–688.

Sideranko, S., Quinn, A., Burns, K., & Froman, R. D. (1992). Effects of position and mattress overlay on sacral and heel pressures in a clinical population. *Research in Nursing & Health, 15*(4), 245–251.

Steers, W. D., & Suratt, P. M. (1997). Sleep apnea as a cause of daytime and nocturnal enuresis. *The Lancet, 349*(9069), 1604.

Strum, R., & Hattori, A. (2013). Morbid obesity rates continue to rise rapidly in the US. *International Journal of Obesity (London), 37*(6), 889–891.

Subak, L. L., Richter, H. E., & Hunskaar, S. (2009). Obesity and urinary incontinence: Epidemiology and clinical research update. *The Journal of Urology, 182*(6S), S2–S7.

Tanamas, S. K., Wluka, A. E., Berry, P., Menz, H. B., Strauss, B. J., Davies-Tuck, M., et al. (2012). Relationship between obesity and foot pain and its association with fat mass, fat distribution, and muscle mass. *Arthritis Care & Research, 64*(2), 262–268.

Tanumihardjo, S. A., Anderson, C., Kaufer-Horwitz, M., Bode, L., Emenaker, N. J., Haqq, A. M., et al. (2007). Poverty, obesity, and malnutrition: An international perspective recognizing the paradox. *Journal of the American Dietetic Association, 107*(11), 1966–1972.

Thelwall, S., Harrington, P., Sheridan, E., & Lamagni, T. (2015). Impact of obesity on the risk of wound infection following surgery: Results from a nationwide prospective multicentre cohort study in England. *Clinical Microbiology and Infection, 21*(11). 1008.e1–8.

Thone, R. R. (1997). *Fat: A fate worse than death.* New York: Harrington Park Press.

Tremmel, M., Gerdtham, U. G., Nilsson, P. M., & Saha, S. (2017). Economic burden of obesity: A systematic literature review. *International Journal of Environmental Research and Public Health, 14*(4), 435.

Valentino, D., Sriram, K., & Shankar, P. (2011). Update on micronutrients in bariatric surgery. *Current Opinion in Clinical Nutrition and Metabolic Care, 14*(6), 635–641.

Walden, C. M., Bankard, S. B., Cayer, B., Floyd, W. B., Garrison, H. G., Hickey, T., et al. (2013). Mobilization of the obese patient and prevention of injury. *Annals of Surgery, 258*(4), 646–651.

Ward, Z. J., Bleich, S. N., Cradock, A. L., Barrett, J. L., Giles, C. M., Flax, C., et al. (2019). Projected US state-level prevalence of adult obesity and severe obesity. *The New England Journal of Medicine, 381*(25), 2440–2450.

West Virginia Department of Health and Human Resources. (2014). *Obesity and mortality.* Retrieved 8/8/2020 from: http://www.wvdhhr.org/bph/oehp/obesity/mortality.htm.

Woo, K. Y., Beeckman, D., & Chakravarthy, D. (2017). Management of moisture-associated skin damage: A scoping review. *Advances in Skin & Wound Care, 30*(11), 494.

World Health Organization. (2015). *Obesity and overweight.* Retrieved 15/8/2020 https://www.who.int/en/news-room/fact-sheets/detail/obesity-and-overweight.

37

Unique Skin Care Needs of the Neonatal and Pediatric Patient

Ann Marie Nie, Ruth A. Bryant, and Denise P. Nix

OBJECTIVES

1. Define the terms *neonate, premature, preterm, late preterm infant, toddler, school age, adolescent, and young adult.*
2. Identify assessment tools designed for neonatal and pediatric patients.
3. Discuss special considerations for premature and neonatal skin care, including bathing and use of cleansers, antiseptics, and emollients.
4. List risk factors for skin breakdown for pediatric patients.
5. Describe common pediatric skin conditions and age-related, developmentally sensitive interventions.
6. Identify two key patient factors the influence safety of wound care products in the pediatric patient population.

The physiology of wound repair, principles of wound care, and common skin conditions are the same for pediatric and adult patients. However, there are significant differences in morphologic and functional skin characteristics as well as developmental phases that influence assessment and intervention strategies. This chapter focuses on *unique* considerations for neonatal and pediatric skin care and should not be read in isolation of related chapters throughout the text that detail critical information applicable to both adults and children.

NEONATAL TERMINOLOGY

Many terms are used to describe stages of infant development (Table 37.1). *Infancy* refers to the first year of life. During the first 28 days of life, an infant is referred to as a *neonate*. If born before 37 weeks of gestational age, the neonate is *premature* or *preterm* (Alderman & Breuner, 2019; CDC, 2021; WHO, 2018b).

NEONATAL SKIN CHARACTERISTICS

Stratum Corneum

Developmental and structural differences in neonatal skin are significant compared with adult skin. Chapter 7 describes the unique characteristic of fetal skin (Box 37.1) and compares morphologic and functional differences between the premature newborn, the neonate, and adults (see Tables 7.1 and 7.2). Differences according to weeks gestation are discussed in this section.

At 23–24 weeks gestation, only 1–2 layers of the *stratum corneum* is present in the neonate compared with the 16–20 layers in the full-term neonate (Boyar, 2020b). The connections between cells are weak and the protective skin covering present at birth known as the *vernix caseosa* (described later) is very thin to nonexistent in neonates born less than 28 weeks or neonates weighing less than 1000 g (Boyar, 2020b; Eichenfiled, Frieden, & Esterly, 2015; Kusari et al., 2019). The *skin pH* is neutral to mildly acidic which increases their risk for bacterial colonization. The skin's decreased *fatty acids and antioxidants* increases their risk for skin irritation. *Transepidermal water loss* (TEWL) in a neonate born at 25 weeks can be 10–15× that of a full-term infant (Hardman, Sisi, Banbury, & Byne, 1998; Kusari et al., 2019). Infants less than 28 weeks gestation are more suited to the "aquatic environment" in utero than to atmospheric conditions. Neonate TEWL normalizes with skin maturation according to gestational weeks (Kusari et al., 2019). For example

- 8 weeks when born at 23 weeks,
- 3 weeks when born at 28 weeks,
- 2 weeks when born less than 30 weeks,
- 1 week when born at 30–33 weeks, and
- 4 h or less when born 34–41 weeks.

Maturation and barrier function of neonatal skin continues to evolve throughout the first year of life. When the skin barrier is not fully developed, the protective functions of the stratum corneum are compromised. The premature infant has significantly reduced protection against toxins, and infectious agents such as bacteria, fungi, and viruses (Fluhr et al., 2010; Kalia, Nonato, Lund, & Guy, 1998).

Dermal Layer

Compared with the full-term infant, the *dermal layer* is not fully developed and thinner for the premature infant skin. *Collagen* fibers are shorter and fewer, the *reticular layer* is absent and there are fewer *sebaceous glands*. The *fibrils* that connect the epidermis and dermis have wider spacing between the connecting points further decreasing skin layer

TABLE 37.1 Definition of Terms

Premature or preterm infant	Infant born before 37 weeks' gestation
• Extremely preterm	• <28 weeks gestation
• Very preterm	• 28–32 weeks gestation
• Late preterm infant	• 34–37 weeks' gestation
• Full-Term Infant	• 37–42 weeks gestation
Neonate	Birth to 28 days of life
Infant	Birth to 12 months
Toddler	1–3 years of age
Preschool	3–5 years of age
Middle childhood	6–11 years
Teenager	12–18 years
Adolescence	11–21 years

From World Health Organization (WHO) (2018a). *Preterm Birth* Retrieved 6/10/2022 from: https://www.who.int/news-room/fact-sheets/detail/preterm-birth; Centers for Disease Control and Prevention (CDC) (2021). *Child development*. Retrieved 6/10/2022 from: https://www.cdc.gov/ncbddd/childdevelopment/positiveparenting/toddlers.html; Alderman, E.M., & Breuner, C.C. (2019). AAP Committee on Adolescence. Unique needs of the adolescent. *Pediatrics*, 144(6), e20193150. Retrieved 6/10/2022 from: https://publications.aap.org/pediatrics/article/144/6/e20193150/37985/Unique-Needs-of-the-Adolescent?autologincheck=redirected; Child Development.

BOX 37.1 Neonatal Skin Condition Scale

Dryness
1. Normal, no sign of dry skin
2. Dry skin, visible scaling
3. Very dry skin, cracking/fissures

Erythema
1. No evidence of erythema
2. Visible erythema, ≤50% body surface
3. Visible erythema, ≥50% body surface

Breakdown
1. None
2. Small, localized areas
3. Extensive

From the Association of Women's Health, Obstetric and Neonatal Nurses, 2018.

cohesion (Reed, Johnson, & Nie, 2021). The premature neonate is at risk for medical adhesive-related skin injury (MARSI) when removing adhesive products from the skin (AWHONN, 2018) because the bond between the epidermal layer and the adhesives may be stronger than the bond between the epidermis and the dermal layer. MARSI prevention is discussed later in the chapter, a comprehensive review is provided in Chapter 9.

Absorption

The barrier function of the epidermis in the premature infant is under-developed which increases the risk of *transdermal absorption* of chemicals and medications commonly used in the older neonate, due to their greater ratio of surface area to volume and immature barrier function compared with the full-term infant, percutaneous absorption of topically applied

agents (soaps, lotions, antiseptics, alcohol, etc.) place the premature infant at greater risk for skin complications and systemic toxicities (Kusari et al., 2019; Sardesai, Kornacka, Walas, & Ramanathan, 2011). Risk may also increase due to the premature infant's alterations in metabolism, excretion, distribution, and protein binding of chemical agents and drugs (AWHONN, 2018; Darmstadt & Dinulos, 2000). Infant care must include specific skin care practices that protect the developing stratum corneum and protect the infant from toxic substances. Table 37.2 describes products and chemicals that should be avoided in this population.

TABLE 37.2 Examples of Transcutaneous Absorption of Topical Products in Neonates, Infants, and Children[a]

Compound	Toxicity
Alcohols under occlusion	Hemorrhagic skin necrosis
Aniline (dye used in laundry)	Methemoglobinemia
Benzocaine and prilocaine (topical anesthetics)	Methemoglobinemia, seizures
Boric acid (baby powder)	Vomiting, diarrhea, erythroderma, seizures, severe dermatitis, death
Chlorhexidine gluconate (CHG)	Hemorrhagic necrosis of the dermis of newborns <28 weeks gestation
Hexachlorophene (topical antiseptic)	Vacuolar encephalopathy
Methylene blue (dye)	Methemoglobinemia
Neomycin	Ototoxicity, deafness (premature infants)
Pentachlorophenol (laundry disinfectant)	Tachycardia, sweating, hepatomegaly, metabolic acidosis
Povidone-iodine (topical antiseptic)	Hypothyroidism, goiter, skin necrosis
Salicylic acid	Metabolic acidosis
Silver-sulfadiazine	hyperbilirubinemia and/or kernicterus Not recommended for infants <2 months
Topical corticosteroids (overuse)	Cushing's syndrome, systemic toxicity, dermal atrophy
Urea (exfoliating, emollient ingredient)	Uremia

[a]Not an all inclusive list.
From Fernandes, J.D., Machado, M.C.R., & de Oliveira, Z.N.P. (2011). Children and newborn skin care and prevention. *Anais brasileiros de dermatologia*, 86(1), 102–110; Sardesai, S., Kornacka, M., Walas, W., & Ramanathan, R. (2010). Iatrogenic skin injury in the neonatal intensive care unit. *The Journal of Maternal-Fetal and Neonatal Medicine, 24*(2), 197–203. https://doi.org/10.3109/14767051003728245; Association of Women's Health, Obstetric and Neonatal Nurses (AWHONN) and National Association of Neonatal Nurses. (2018). *Neonatal skin care evidence-based clinical practice guideline* (4th ed.). Washington, DC: AWHONN.

BATHING AND MOISTURIZING

Infants are born with a protective covering called vernix caseosa. This substance consists of fatty secretions from the sebaceous glands and dead epidermal cells. The purpose of this covering is skin protection of the developing fetus while in utero. Vernix is 81% water, 9% protein containing lipids and 10% other (Smith & Shell, 2017). Of the proteins, 39% have components of immunity and 29% have direct antimicrobial properties. The vernix acts as an antibacterial barrier to protect the infant during childbirth. It also protects against loss of fluids and electrolytes. Recognizing the significance of the vernix, the World Health Organization (World Health Organization, 2018a) announced a standard for delaying the first bath for 24 h. AWHONN (2018) recommends delayed bathing for uncompromised *full-term infants* for at least 6 h of age and after two consecutive axillary temperatures of at least 98.2°F.

For *late preterm* infants, the first bath should be delayed until thermal and cardiorespiratory stability is insured at least until 6 h of age but ideally 24 h. Vernix should be left in place. Gently remove blood, meconium etc. but do not vigorously scrub to remove vernix (AWHONN, 2018). *Preterm infants* should be bathed infrequently (e.g., every 4 days) using warm water only (Kusari et al., 2019) during the first week of life (AWHONN, 2018). Use soft materials (e.g., cotton). In the presence of skin breakdown, consider warm sterile water (AWHONN, 2018).

Less frequent bathing and strict attention to heat loss and avoidance of cold minimizes behavioral and physiologic instability in infants. Infants immersed in water at the correct temperature (between 100 and 104°F) are calmer, quieter, and experience less heat loss than infants receiving a sponge bath. The infant bath should be in a draft-free, warm room (between 79° and 81°F). Warm towels should be used for drying. Procedures for bathing and drying should be as brief as possible to facilitate thermoregulation (AWHONN, 2018; Loring et al., 2012). When skin cleansers are indicated, a mild liquid baby cleanser used sparingly with a neutral pH (5.5–7.0) is recommended. Preservatives demonstrated to be safe for newborns are needed to prevent bacterial growth with the product container (AWHONN, 2018; Blume-Peytavi et al., 2009).

Bathing introduces changes to the stratum corneum that can dry the skin. Moisturizing creams or ointments may be indicated for dry, flaking, or fissured skin. Encourage caregivers to apply emollients at least once daily at the first sign of dryness, fissures, cracking, or cradle cap (AWHONN, 2018). Emollients promote and restore skin barrier function. Ointments are often preferred formulations particularly to prevent diaper dermatitis because of the ability to penetrate the subcutaneous cells. While occlusive products such as petrolatum have been used on the preterm baby to prevent evaporation (Boyar, 2020b), topical ointment petrolatum has also been reported to increase the risk of candidemia and coagulase-negative *Staphylococcus* infection in the preterm infant (Kusari et al., 2019). Dimethicone is another common occlusive but thinner than petrolatum and with better water vapor permeability. Many oils are known for their irritant potential and pro-inflammatory action, thus not recommended for newborns. Oils to be avoided are those with high oleic acid content: olive, mustard, corn, soybean, and vegetable oils (AWHONN, 2018; Boyar, 2020a). Safe oils are sunflower and safflower oil due to their high linoleic acid content (Boyar, 2020a). Products should be fragrance free with only a few ingredients.

Topical Antiseptics and Antimicrobial Agents

Topical applications of antiseptics and antimicrobial agents have been known to create irritant contact dermatitis, sensitization, and systemic toxicity in the infant population. Neonates born 32 weeks gestation or earlier are at greatest risk of skin complications related to disinfectants. Examples of topical products (including some antimicrobials) at risk for transcutaneous absorption and toxicity in neonates, infants, and children are included in Table 37.2. Hemorrhagic necrosis of the dermis from the absorption of isopropyl alcohol and chlorhexidine gluconate (CHG) under occlusion has been reported (Sardesai et al., 2011) and has been mistaken as bruising or pressure. Povidone iodine has been associated with skin injury and carries the risk of systemic toxicity involving thyroid function (Fernandes, Machado, & de Oliveira, 2011). CHG contains alcohol and is NOT recommended in newborns <28 weeks gestation. Betadine is used in this age group and wiped off completely after the insertion of lines and catheters (Children's Hospitals' Solutions for Patient Safety (SPS), 2021a, 2021b; Vanzi et al., 2018).

Organic, Natural, and Herbal Products

"Natural" products are often considered harmless; however, because of the poor regulations that exist in monitoring these products, adverse reactions do occur. There is little incentive for pharmaceutical companies to investigate or standardize these preparations because it is unlikely patents would be applicable. Herbs that are known for causing contact dermatitis include aloe, arnica, bromelain, calendula, chamomile, goldenseal, tea tree oil, and yarrow. However, more serious events such as Stevens-Johnson syndrome have occurred when combination preparations were used. Therefore, experts recommend avoiding their use with infants and children because of the uncertainty of adverse reactions that could occur (Boyar, 2020a). Natural fragrances such as essential oils may also be allergens and irritants and are not necessarily safer than synthetic fragrances. Interestingly, a product can be labeled "fragrance free" if the scented ingredient is added for a purpose other than fragrance. Likewise, products labeled "unscented" may contain a fragrance if it is added to mask the odor of a product (AWHONN, 2018).

SKIN INSPECTION AND RISK ASSESSMENT

Preventing skin complications always starts with understanding the potential etiologies and conditions that place an individual at risk. Both AWHONN (2018) and EPUAP, NPUIP,

PPPIA (2019) guidelines recommend considering the use of a reliable and valid pediatric risk assessment tool *as one component of* a structured skin injury risk assessment. Researchers from Japan (Fujii, Sugama, Okuwa, Sanada, & Mizokami, 2010) evaluated risk factors for 81 infants in NICU incubators at gestational ages from 24 to 41 weeks, and from seven hospitals. Using multivariate analysis, the risk of pressure injuries in the neonate was increased four times by two factors: skin texture, as defined by the *Dubowitz neonatal maturation assessment* ($P = 0.012$), and endotracheal intubation ($P = 0.042$) (OR = 4.0; 95% CI 1·04–15·42, $P = 0.042$). Age-appropriate pressure injury risk and skin assessments should be performed and documented on admission, daily and with a change in condition that may alter pressure, friction, shear, and/or moisture. Table 37.3 summarizes several neonatal and pediatric skin condition and risk assessment scales/tools that have undergone reliability and validity studies for their use in neonatal and pediatric populations.

A head-to-toe skin inspection should be conducted at least daily; more frequently as needed with change in condition (AWHONN, 2018; EPUAP, NPUIP, PPPIA, 2019). Children's Hospitals' Solutions for Patient Safety (SPS, 2021a, 2021b) advocate every shift change for high-risk patients, every 4 h in children with compromised perfusion, and after surgery cases lasting 4 h or more.

Inspection around and under medical devices should occur routinely and more often (e.g., more than twice daily in the presence of edema) at least twice daily according to International Pressure Injury Guidelines (EPUAP, NPIAP, PPPIA, 2019). AWHONN (2018) recommends device-related skin inspection at least every 12 h, more frequently, as needed with change in condition. As detailed in Chapter 10, skin inspection must include adequate lighting and palpation, especially in the presence of darkly pigmented skin or hair on the occipital region. Skin folds need to be gently separated, and medical devices may require careful repositioning for an adequate assessment.

PEDIATRIC CONDITIONS THAT AFFECT THE SKIN

Throughout this text, a variety of types of skin damage have been presented and appropriate prevention and management tactics applicable to both adults and children discussed. In the care of the neonate and/or the pediatric patient population, additional interventions and precautions are often warranted. In the following sections additional considerations regarding pressure injury, diaper dermatitis, gastrostomy, fecal and urinary diversion, medical adhesive–related skin damage, burns, and extravasation will be presented.

Pressure Injuries

Components for creating and maintaining a quality pressure injury prevention program (PIPP), including medical device–related pressure injury prevention, are described in Chapter 11 and should be thoroughly reviewed for pressure injury prevention in any patient population. Information related to risk assessment, support surface selection, and repositioning for the small yet rapidly growing neonate and pediatric patients are included in this section.

As with adults, significant variability of methodologies exists for pressure injury prevalence and incidence data collection among the pediatric population. However, pressure injuries present a clinically significant problem. Pediatric pressure injury incidence ranges from 0.47% to 35%. Like adults, the highest incidence occurs in critical care. Delmore, Deppisch, D'Nurs, Luna-Anderson, and Nie (2019) reported a pressure injury prevalence ranging from 1.4% to 27% in pediatrics.

Prevention bundles and active surveillance have been shown to be effective in reducing pressure injuries in the pediatric population. For example, Frank et al. (2017) reported the results of 33 children's hospitals over a 2-year period after implementation of the Children's Hospitals Solutions for Patient Safety (SPS) pediatric pressure injury prevention bundle (Table 37.4) along with a pressure injury risk assessment tool. Results showed a statistically significant 50% reduction of stage 3 and stage 4 pressure injuries (P < 0.001 and $P = 0.02$), respectively (Children's Hospitals' Solutions for Patient Safety (SPS), 2021a, 2021b).

Although the etiology and classification for pressure injuries are the same for adults and children (see Chapter 11), there are some special considerations for the pediatric population that are described in the chapter.

Occipital Pressure Injuries

Children under the age of 6 have a greater surface area to the head than older children and adults. With this increase in surface are, the occiput will absorb more of body weight while supine (Manning, Gatuvreau, & Curley, 2015). Children in a supine position need to have their occiput offloaded (e.g., hourly manual lifts, fluidized head pillow). When repositioning a pediatric patient, the head should be moved in the direction of the turn. Progressive mobility techniques, including slow incremental turning as discussed in Chapter 11, should be used whenever possible for pressure injury prevention in children and adults (Alderden, Rondinelli, Pepper, Cummins, & Whitney, 2017).

Pressure Redistribution, Holding, Positioning

Chapter 11 provides a detailed overview of pressure redistribution surfaces. Support surface considerations in PI prevention include chair cushions, overlays for standard beds and cribs, and elbow and heel protectors. Positioning devices can be purchased to offload pressure for the child with impaired mobility. In teaching parents and caregivers about pressure injury prevention, it is pertinent to emphasize that pressure redistribution is one of the many benefits to holding the infant (Razmus & Bergquist-Beringer, 2017; Schindler et al., 2011; Turnage-Carrier, McLane, & Gregurich, 2008). Evidence for an ideal turn angle in the neonates, infant, and toddlers is lacking. With their smaller body width, a 30-degree turn could position them onto the trochanter. Palpating the coccyx can

TABLE 37.3 Pediatric and Neonatal Skin Condition and Risk Scales/Tools

Risk Assessment Tool	Outcome Measure	Age	Brief Description	Reference
Braden Q	Risk of pressure injury in pediatric patient	21 days to 8 years	Adapted from Braden pressure scale, all 6 Braden subscales plus 7th Tissue Perfusion and Oxygenation. Scores range from 28 (lowest risk) to 7 (highest risk). Score <16 at risk for skin breakdown. Subscale scores 1 (least favorable) to 4 (most favorable) Other: no cost, no modifications allowed, translations available Research populations: pediatric acute care Demonstrated reliability and validity for pediatric ICU patients 3 weeks to 8 years on bed rest at least 24 h. With score of 16, sensitivity is 88%; specificity is 58%	Curley, Quigley, and Lin (2003); Curley, Razmus, Roberts, and Wypij (2003) Available at http://www.marthaaqcurley.com/braden-q.html (accessed August 25, 2020)
Braden QD	Risk of pressure Injury (device related and decreased mobility related)	Preterm to 21 years of age in ICU, non-ICU and on bedrest at least 4 h	Revised Braden Q scale to include risk from medical device (D). Estimates risk for both MDRPI and Mobility related PIs. Comprised of 3 overall categories and 7 subscales: intensity and duration of pressure (2 subscales: mobility and sensory perception), skin and tissue tolerance (3 subscales: friction/shear, nutrition, tissue perfusion and oxygenation), and medical devices (2 subscales: number of devices and repositionability/skin protection). Subscale scores range from 0 to 3. Overall scores range from 0 (lowest) to 20 (highest risk). Scores of 13 or higher indicate risk for skin breakdown. Reliability and validity established in preterm to 21 years on bedrest for at least 2 h, ICU and non-ICU and had a medical device in place. With cutoff of 13, sensitivity is 86% and specificity is 59%	Curley et al. (2018) Chamblee et al. (2018)
Braden Q + P	Comprehensive pediatric PI risk assessment and interventions		Adapted from the Braden Q for use in pediatric patients in the OR setting Quality improvement project; no reliability or validity testing	Galvin and Curley (2012)
Glamorgan	Predict immobility-related and device related pressure injuries in pediatric patient	Birth to 18 years	Developed using expert opinion of relevant factors from a literature review and statistical analysis of collected inpatient data. The higher the score, the greater the risk: 0 not at risk 10+ at risk, 15+ high risk, 20+ very high risk Interrater reliability and reliability tests indicate this tool provides little additional discrimination information about PI risk in a general pediatric patient population. Scale publically available, permission to reprint requested	Willock, Baharestani, and Anthony (2008); Kottner, Kenzler, and Wilborn (2012)

Continued

TABLE 37.3 Pediatric and Neonatal Skin Condition and Risk Scales/Tools—cont'd

Risk Assessment Tool	Outcome Measure	Age	Brief Description	Reference
AWHONN/NANN Neonatal Skin Condition Score Association of Women's Health, Obstetric and Neonatal Nurses and National Association of Neonatal Nurses (NANN)	Skin condition	Birth to 28 days	Observation of dryness, erythema, and breakdown on a 1–9 scale; higher the skin score = greater potential for systemic infection, breakdown, and longer hospitalization Sample size 2820 infants from 51 NICU and well-baby nurseries in 27 states in the United States More applicable to infants >1000 g Pressure ulcer risk not measured directly; breakdown not specific to pressure ulcer	Lund and Osborne (2004) (see Box 37.1)
NS Neonatal Skin Risk Assessment Scale	NICU PU Risk	26–40 weeks' gestation	Specific for neonatal population at risk for skin breakdown, based on the Braden Scale for Predicting Pressure Sore Risk and includes gestational age category. Developed in 1997; subscale descriptor revision at later date 6 subscales; lower scores = higher risk, higher scores = lower risk. Piloted on 32 neonates Sensitivity 83% Specificity at 81% Reliable for general physical condition, activity and nutrition	Huffines and Logsdon (1997)
Starkid Skin Scale	Skin Condition	Hospitalized children	Adapted from the Braden Q: 6 subscales rated on scale 1 to 4 with lower scores representing higher risk: mobility/activity, sensory perception, moisture, friction/shear, nutrition and tissue perfusion/oxygenation Request permission to reprint Sensitivity low at 17.5%, high specificity of 98.5% Internal reliability 0.71, interrater reliability is 0.85	Suddaby, Barnett, and Facteau (2006)

TABLE 37.4 Prevention Bundle Elements and Care Descriptions

Prevention Bundle Element-Maintenance	Care Descriptions
Standard Elements	
Skin and Risk Assessment	• Within 24 h of admission (consensus best practice is within 8 h) and at least every 24 h but consensus best practice—recommend every 8 h (every 4 h in perfusion compromised patients), Operating Room (OR) at end of cases lasting 4 h or more and/or on arrival PACU/ICU's, and with change in condition
Medical Device Rotation/Reposition, Padding	• Assess skin in contact with medical devices a minimum of each shift or more frequently with other care; rotate pulse-ox probe at least every 8 h; remove C-collars at least twice daily (unless medically contraindicated); change collar padding when soiled. Assess proper fit of respiratory device minimum every 6 h, preferred every 4 h; follow manufacturers instructions
Patient Positioning	• Reposition or turn all immobile and limited mobility patients at least every 2 h; synchronize care with routine NICU care (e.g., standardized turning schedule, clock at bedside) • Maintain HOB less than or equal to 30 degrees (unless medically contraindicated) Note: Patients in chairs or upright in bed greater than 2 h must be repositioned to redistribute pressure (consider appropriate surface and consider time limit) Note: "Do Not Turn" instructions should require a provider order and be reevaluated every 24 h
Appropriate Bed Surface	• Evaluate need for specialty bed based on Skin Risk Assessment • Use gel pads, fluidized positioners, and/or pressure redistribution device to cushion bony prominences
Moisture Management	• Apply moisture barrier and/or wicking product to keep skin dry • Keep skin clean dry and hydrated

Adapted from Children's Hospitals' Solutions for Patient Safety (SPS) Prevention Bundles: Pressure Injuries (2021). Retrieved 1/2/2023 from: https://www.solutionsforpatientsafety.org/wp-content/uploads/SPS-Prevention-Bundles_FEB-2021.pdf.

help ensure that the bone is not being used as a pivot point and the patient is adequately offloaded (Nie, 2020).

When selecting a pressure redistribution support surface for children, critical selection criteria are size and weight. A child below the manufacturer's minimum weight requirement of >70 pounds may sink in between cushions of a low-air-loss surface, lodge between alternating air cells, or slide through the oversized side rails, creating the potential for entrapment and other safety concerns (EPUAP, NPIAP, PPPIA, 2019; McLane, Krouskip, McCord, & Fraley, 2002). There are no studies to support a low air loss surface for an immobile child. The child does not have enough weight for envelopment and will lay on the surface as if on a regular mattress. However, a variety of media have been trialed and used for pressure redistribution with pediatric patients, including fluid, gel, and foam as described in Chapter 12 (García-Molina et al., 2012; McInnes, Jammali-Blasi, Cullum, & Leung, 2018; McLane et al., 2002; Turnage-Carrier et al., 2008).

Medical Devices Related Pressure Injury

Prevention measures related to medical devices are discussed in Chapter 11. As with adults, a team approach is critical to medical device-related skin damage recognizing a deference in expertise within the interdisciplinary team (see Table 11.5). PI incidence is highest in the pediatric critical care areas, up to 43.1% (Delmore et al., 2019).

In the NICU, respiratory devices, such as masks, nasal cannula, percutaneous tracheostomy, and endotracheal tubes, are the most common causes of MDRPIs. Infants do not have length to their neck and thus have skin folds present that will press against devices, such as a tracheostomy, and cause pressure (Boesch et al., 2012; Jaryszak, Shah, Amling, & Pena, 2011). To prevent pressure injuries in the NICU population, it is important to recognize that premature infants are put in environments with high humidity to assist in skin maturity; thus moisture, a known pressure injury risk factor, must be considered. Consequently, any prophylactic dressing used under a respiratory device for pressure redistribution must also allow for moisture evaporation and proper application of the device.

As with adults, other medical devices (e.g., video EEG leads, cervical collars, ID bands, pulse oximetry, IVs, nasogastric tubes, and g-j tubes) require frequent surveillance and the judicious use of prophylactic dressings (EPUAP, NPIAP, PPPIA, 2019). Skin inspection around and under medical devices should be conducted at least twice daily; more often as need such as in the presence of edema (AWHONN, 2018).

Iatrogenic Anetoderma of Prematurity

Another skin condition that is device related is iatrogenic anetoderma of prematurity (Maffeis et al., 2014). Although relatively uncommon, congenital and acquired forms of iatrogenic anetoderma have been reported in extremely premature infants. The congenital form has been reported in babies at 24–25 weeks of gestation and is hypothesized to be the result of a congenital defect in the production of elastic fibers in the dermis. Acquired iatrogenic anetoderma has been reported in premature infants between 24 and 32 weeks' gestation with a prolonged stay in the neonatal intensive care unit and the use of monitoring devices such as leads, electrodes and transcutaneous oxygen.

Anetoderma is a benign dermatosis characterized by the focal loss of mid-dermal elastic tissue. Manifestations include isolated or patches of well-defined areas of macular depressions or pouchlike herniations of the skin (Maffeis et al., 2014). This condition most often becomes clinically apparent months or years after medical devices have been discontinued. Eruptions have been described as atrophic, round-flat, skin colored or violaceous, brown or gray depressions localized on the ventral surface of the chest, abdomen, upper arms, and proximal thighs. Despite being benign, significant aesthetic damage can develop over time and require surgical repair. Familiarity with the condition is important for accurate diagnosis as well as to heighten awareness to adopt strategies to reduce stress to immature skin by the cautious use of these devices.

Diaper Dermatitis

Diaper dermatitis, also known as *perineal dermatitis, diaper rash,* and *irritant diaper dermatitis*, broadly refers to skin inflammation that occurs in the diaper area (Cohen, 2017) that is caused by the presence of urine and feces. Diaper dermatitis may also develop secondary to chafing triggered by diaper materials, or an allergy to the diaper materials or skin cleansing diaper wipes (Merrill, 2015). Additional skin eruptions can develop in the diaper area with or without the skin inflammation and should be excluded as a potential cause. See Table 9.3 for a list of differential diagnoses (Cohen, 2017; Merrill, 2015). For the purposes of this chapter, the term *diaper dermatitis* will be used to describe this condition in the pediatric population where continence is not developmentally or medically anticipated or expected.

In the United States, diaper dermatitis occurs in as many as 35% of the general population (Merrill, 2015) and typically lasts approximately 2–4 days (Carr et al., 2019). Internationally, estimates of diaper dermatitis range from 16% to 65% (Carr et al., 2019). Although one of the most common skin conditions in an infant, diaper dermatitis is rarely a serious condition from a medical perspective yet causes considerable discomfort for the infant and the caregivers. Among hospitalized pediatric patients, the prevalence of diaper dermatitis has been reported between 16% and 42% (McLane, Bookout, McCord, McCain, & Jefferson, 2004; Noonan, Quigley, & Curley, 2006). Diaper dermatitis in children (see Plate 15) generally affects the skin in greatest contact with the diaper, including the buttocks, perianal, intertriginous, female genitals and male genitals (Carr et al., 2019; Shin, 2014). As with the adults, candidiasis may also develop in the presence of diaper dermatitis particularly during a course of antibiotic therapy.

Common risk factors for diaper dermatitis include frequent stooling, antibiotic use, malabsorption, opiate withdrawal, chemotherapy, and weak or under-developed anal sphincter tone. Conditions that increase the risk of diaper

dermatitis in the pediatric population include spina bifida, Hirschsprung's disease, anorectal malformation, imperforate anus, opiate withdrawal, malabsorption syndromes, inflammatory bowel disease, short bowel disease, neonatal abstinence syndrome, and necrotizing enterocolitis (NEC) (Boyar, 2020a, 2020b).

The key to preventing diaper dermatitis is appropriate skin cleansing, skin protection, and containment. With the availability of superabsorbent modern disposable diapers, urine is wicked away from the skin reducing the risk of saturating the skin. In addition, dermatitis due to allergic reactions has diminished since the introduction of hypoallergenic products including laundry detergents and perineal cleaning wipes (Cohen, 2017). Table 9.4 provides examples and descriptions of products available to prevent and manage IAD. Although commonly used for adults and children, many of these products are not appropriate for infants and premature neonates.

Cleansing must be gentle with water and a soft cloth or non scented diaper wipe at every diaper change and limited to the removal of the soiled layer of the skin protectant only. Vigorously rubbing to the skin protectant moisture barrier product is not necessary and should be avoided. Appropriate methods to cleanse the diaper area must include only those products that have been tested on neonates such as soft cloths, water, disposable diaper wipes, and gentle cleansers designed for use in the pediatric/neonate population in the perineal area (AWHONN, 2018). Diaper wipes have been found to be superior to washcloths on both healthy and damaged skin with regards to skin gentleness and minimal disruption to the stratum corneum. Similarly, the use of soaps also results in skin barrier disruption and should be avoided (Shin, 2014). As discussed previously, temperature control during cleansing and bathing is critical with the neonate, and perineal cleansing is no exception.

A moisture barrier skin protectant should be applied at every diaper change universally with or without diaper dermatitis. In neonates, preference should be given to formulations with fewer additives and chemicals that are potentially absorbed through the skin (AWHONN, 2018).

Skin protectants are formulated as creams, pastes, lotions, or films and packaged into wipes, wands, packets, sprays, and tubes. To function as a skin protectant, it must contain a known barrier as an active ingredient (e.g., petrolatum, zinc oxide, dimethicone) alone or in combination (Beeckman et al., 2015). The active ingredients in FDA-approved topical moisture barrier skin protectants must be present in certain concentrations to be designated as an over-the-counter moisture barrier skin protectant, including those marketed for pediatric use. Active ingredients frequently found in products labeled for pediatric use and their FDA-specified concentrations include zinc oxide (1%–25%), petrolatum (30%–100%), and dimethicone (1%–30%). Other ingredients must be listed in order of their amount unless they are 1% or less. In that case, they can be listed in any order (US Food and Drug Administration, 2022).

Moisture barrier skin protectant *pastes* are a mixture of absorbent material (e.g., carboxymethylcellulose) which facilitate adherence to moist denuded skin, and ointments. As stated previously, it is appropriate to remove only the soiled layer of the barrier during cleansing. All barriers should be removed once per day for assessment of the skin.

Moisture barrier skin protectant *films* are liquids that contain a polymer (e.g., acrylate based) dissolved in a solvent. Upon application, films form a transparent protective coating on the skin. They are not labeled as having an active ingredient (Beeckman et al., 2015). The FDA has approved alcohol-free barrier films as treatment of diaper dermatitis in neonates older than 28 days old can be applied every 24 h (AWHONN, 2018). Barrier films are generally not an effective barrier to gastrointestinal enzymes typical of the infant or child with short bowel syndrome. In these situations, a thick zinc oxide paste should be utilized for prevention and management.

Treatment of diaper dermatitis complicated by a yeast or bacterial infection is discussed in Chapter 8. Commercially prepared diaper dermatitis ointments that contain an antifungal agent can safely be used in the treatment of candidiasis. Combination products that treat the candidiasis and the dermatitis that accompanies the infection are also effective. Antifungal powders should be kept away from the child's airway. If the skin is weepy, the antifungal powder can be covered with a skin-protectant sealant. Conventional baby powders with talcum and corn starch are not recommended for neonates because of the potential of inhaled powder particles and respiratory irritation (AWHONN, 2018; Kuller, 2016).

Topical corticosteroids in the diaper area should be avoided, except in unique circumstances, and then only under the direction of a provider and for a short time. Overuse of topical corticosteroids has been linked to Cushing syndrome, systemic toxicity, and dermal atrophy in infants (AWHONN, 2018; Heimall, Storey, Stellar, & Finn Davis, 2012). If diaper dermatitis does not improve with appropriate evidence-based care, allergic contact dermatitis should be considered due to enhanced sensitizations to allergens in the moist environment and increasing frequency of diaper dye dermatitis. Dye-free diapers should be implemented when diaper dye dermatitis is suspected. Occasionally, topical corticosteroids may be used for a short time interval (AWHONN, 2018; Wiley, Smith, & Jacob, 2009).

When diaper dermatitis is present, diaper changes every 1–3 h during the day and at least once at night are recommended (AWWOHN, 2018). A breastfed infant will have increased stooling frequency than the bottle-fed infant due to the ease of metabolism of the breast milk. Tight-fitting diapers hold irritants against the skin and should be avoided. Advances in the design and manufacturing process of both reusable and disposable diapers provide consumers with more options for effective products that contain urine and stool thus reducing the risk of diaper dermatitis. These products also eliminate the negative environmental impact of disposable diapers.

Disposable diapers may vary in quality but in general are designed to keep the baby's skin dry. Optimal absorption of urine and feces is achieved by the use of specialized polymer materials arranged in different layers contained between a "back sheet" and a "top sheet" (Counts, Weisbrod, & Yin, 2017). The back sheet is constructed from waterproof polyethylene film and microporous barrier allowing for water vapor to be released while the outside of the diaper remains dry. A small amount of barrier ointment (containing petrolatum, stearyl alcohol, and aloe) is included in the diaper top sheet and has been demonstrated to reduce skin wetness, reduce erythema, and maintain skin health (Counts et al., 2017). Diaper products with a plastic outer layer can cause overhydration of the skin and increase the risk of diaper dermatitis, thus are not recommended. An ointment or paste should be applied directly to the skin, never to the diaper itself. Similarly, it is important to follow the manufacturer's directions regarding the thickness of the application so that the ointment or paste does not block or limit fluid uptake of the diaper material causing overhydration of the stratum corneum, leakage, and increased risk of diaper dermatitis (Counts et al., 2017).

Experts encourage and support breastfeeding when possible, through infancy because stool and urine of breastfed infants have a lower pH than formula-fed infants. The stool of breastfed infants also contains lower levels of enzymes, resulting in less perineal irritation (AWHONN, 2018).

Medical Adhesive–Related Skin Injury

Medical adhesive–related skin injury (MARSI) occurs in all ages and patient care settings. However, the risk of MARSI in neonates is significant due to the diminished cohesion between the epidermal and dermal layers characteristic of skin development at this age. MARSI is reported as the primary cause of skin breakdown in neonatal intensive care units (AWHONN, 2018). Silicone tape and paper tape have been demonstrated to cause minimal skin damage when used with healthy children ages 9–47 months (Grove, Zerweck, Ekholm, Smith, & Koski, 2014). Unfortunately, they are not appropriate in all situations. Securement of tubes and catheters considered critical, such as endotracheal tubes, chest, or extracorporeal membrane oxygenation (ECMO) catheters, need a tape that causes minimal skin stripping but are strong enough to keep the tubes in place without dislodgement (McNichol, Lund, & Osborne, 2013). Chapter 9 provides a comprehensive review of prevention and management of MARSI. Box 9.3 lists strategies for the prevention of MARSI.

Application of a nonalcohol-based protective barrier film may be applied to the skin before tape application to protect the epidermis from stripping with tape removal. Use of alcohol-free protective barrier films is common in all pediatric settings and situations. While oil-based adhesive removers should not be used with neonates due to skin reaction, silicone-based adhesive removers are safe and gentle. Water can also be used to ease adhesive removal, but petrolatum and mineral oil is discouraged because these products will prevent retaping to the same area of skin. One randomized controlled trial with 50 low birth weight neonates in NICU demonstrated both skin-to-skin care and expressed breast milk administration were effective nonpharmacologic strategies for pain control during adhesive tape removal (Nanavati, Balan, & Kabra, 2013).

Gastrostomy Tubes

Enteral nutrition in the pediatric patient population is indicated for a variety of clinical conditions once aggressive oral interventions have been ruled out. Pediatric enteral nutrition (EN) is warranted for insufficient oral intake, such as children over 1 year of age achieving less than 60%–80% of individual requirements for 5 days or more; in children less than 1 year the time frame is 3 days. Additionally, EN is indicated for failure to thrive, wasting and stunting. (Boullata et al., 2017). Enteral nutrition in pediatric patients can be provided via nasal and oral routes for short-term use (4–6 weeks). Long-term access can be achieved through the percutaneous endoscopic or laparoscopic placement of a balloon or nonballoon tube or button (Boullata et al., 2017; Thompson, 2019). Most often a low-profile button with a balloon or bumper will be selected to minimize the risk of dislodgement during childcare or self-exploration.

Care of the tube and the tube site in the pediatric patient and the adult patient are quite similar in terms of strategies to prevent and manage peritubular leakage, peristomal complications, and tube stabilization (see Chapter 40). Children may develop peritubular leakage due to a number of factors including balloon failure, delayed gastric emptying, dysmotility, increased volume of feedings, constipation, weight loss, and enlarged stoma (McSweeney et al., 2021; Thompson, 2019). Additional complications include infection/candidiasis, MASD, hypergranulation tissue, buried bumper syndrome, and tube dislodgement (Thompson, 2019).

Infants and children are generally fed by nasogastric tubes before gastrostomy placement. After surgery, children may return to their presurgical feeding rates within a few days. Others, however, may take 2–3 weeks before they tolerate the same rate without leaking. These are often children with a history of difficulty tolerating feedings, such as those with complex cardiac anomalies, gastroesophageal reflux, or short bowel syndrome. It is critically important to lengthen the time over which the feedings are given in order to allow the tract to heal and prevent peritubular skin breakdown. A child receiving feedings over 45 min may need to have feedings given over 1.5 h. Some children need a period of continuous feedings. The onset of an acute illness such as a respiratory infection and cough or intestinal infection and diarrhea may require adjustments in standard tube-feeding regimens until the illness resolves.

When the child is able to meet their nutritional needs orally, the gastrostomy tube can be removed and will heal without surgical intervention. When the tube is removed, the stoma tract is treated with silver nitrate; prior to this, however, the site is prepared by applying lidocaine jelly 2% to the stoma tract. A pressure dressing can then be applied and a foam adherent dressing. This can be left in place for several days to promote healing. The stoma site is monitored for healing and silver nitrate reapplied if needed. Surgical closure may be necessary in some cases when healing does not occur within 1–2 months (Thompson, 2019).

Urinary and Fecal Diversions

The most common conditions in the neonate and infant that typically require the creation of an ostomy include congenital malformations and medical conditions such as Hirschsprung's disease, imperforate anus and urogenital malformations, and NEC. In school age child and teenager, the most common reason for a fecal diversion is Crohn's disease, familial adenomatous polyposis (FAP), ulcerative colitis, trauma, intraabdominal abscess and tumors. Urinary diversion can also be performed to preserve renal function for children with poorly functioning urinary system or malignancy of the bladder (Baker, Phearman, & McIltrot, 2022).

Pouching is always recommended for containment of stool and urine. In the infant with a mitrofanoff, allowing the urine to flow in the diaper is normally recommended. This is an easier task for parents. Referral to a certified ostomy nurse (www.wocn.org) for preop stoma marking, ostomy education, and ongoing assessment and management recommendations will facilitate patient and family satisfaction, cost-effective utilization of ostomy supplies, and follow-up for ongoing needs and changes as the child grows.

The benefits of stoma site marking before surgery for children is to identify body contours that might complicate or jeopardize successful pouch adherence. Preoperative stoma site selection, although recommended in pediatric practice, can be limited by the nature of the surgery. Stoma surgery in the newborns is typically emergent due to a congenital condition therefore presurgical site selection is seldom feasible. Planned surgical procedures in which an ostomy is anticipated, however, should allow time for preoperative stoma site selection and consultation. Depending on the surgical procedure, type of stoma planned and the surgeon's preference, the certified ostomy specialist should be consulted to select and mark an appropriate site for the ostomy (WOCN Society, AUA and ASCRS, 2021). Many additional factors impact pouch effectiveness, wear time, and peristomal skin breakdown in infants and children and must be considered when managing a pediatric patient with an ostomy, including:

1. Nature of the surgical procedure: Infants born with Hirschsprung's disease, anorectal malformation and imperforate anus usually undergo surgery shortly following birth. A diverting ileostomy is often temporarily required when an infant develops NEC. Older children with myelomeningocele usually undergo an ACE (Antegrade Continence Enema) procedure related to the neurogenic bowel for bowel continence. An ileostomy may be required to manage Inflammatory Bowel Disease (IBD) in the older child.

2. Stoma placement: An ostomy may be created through an incision due to limited abdominal space or a desire to minimize scarring. Infants with NEC can have multiple stomas brought through the incision. In some conditions, the functioning stoma (i.e., proximal bowel) will be positioned away from the nonfunctioning stoma (i.e., mucous fistula or distal bowel) to prevent migration of fecal contents into the distal bowel.

3. Abdominal surface geography and characteristics. Limited surface area for a stoma placement, lack of muscular development, proximity to additional monitoring devices, and changes in abdominal contours when crying are all factors to consider with stoma placement. Children with many genetic abnormalities also have difficulty with oral feeding. Due to this concern, these children may require a gastrostomy or a gastrostomy/jejunostomy tube. The site is typically in the left upper abdominal quadrant which can pose a significant concern for pouching in a pediatric patient who has an existing ostomy or may require a colostomy.

Pouching

To protect peristomal skin, promote a reliable wear time, and prevent leakage, the following considerations are essential (Baker et al., 2022):

- Select an appropriate pouching system with features that will accommodate the unique parameters of the child's abdomen.
- Use a consistent technique for preparation (both the pouch and skin), application, and removal of the pouching system.
- Empty pouch regularly when one-third to one-half full of flatus, liquid, or stool.
- Encourage regular and routine appointments with the WOC nurse for reevaluation as the child grows (larger pouch sizes are often required to adequately contain output and prevent leakage). This can be every 3–6 months until 3 or 4 years of age.
- A soft cloth should be used to clean peristomal skin with tap water, rather than wipes and other products with emollients which can impair pouch adhesion.
- Use alcohol-free skin barrier paste or a barrier ring around the stoma or pouch opening. A syringe may be used for a more precise application of the barrier paste.
- Apply barrier paste or barrier strips into abdominal folds or crevices to create a flat pouching surface.
- Change the pouch at routine intervals to avoid leakage, such as every 24–72 h for infants and twice a week for older pediatric patients. Examine the integrity of the pouch barrier upon removal can help determine whether a pouch wear time (schedule change) needs to be adjusted.

Box 37.2 contains pouching tips for infant/pediatric ostomies. Box 37.3 contains organizations and websites that provide free and noncommercial educational tools and procedures for health care providers, patients, and families. The importance of routine follow-up with a board-certified ostomy nurse who can anticipate the child's ostomy-related needs as they grow and thereby avoid complications or treat them promptly, cannot be understated.

If pouching is unsatisfactory, absorptive products and moisture barrier skin protectants (see Table 9.4) can be used as described earlier in this chapter. However, this should be a temporary and last resort intervention as the stool is no longer contained without a pouching system and can be disruptive to social development.

BOX 37.2 Pouching Tips for Infant/Pediatric Stomas

- Avoid use of pastes that contain alcohol, which can irritate skin. A syringe can be filled with skin barrier paste to ease the application of a thin bead of paste to the wafer or skin.
- Barrier strips and rings have gentle adhesives and can be cut or molded to specific shape.
- Apply pouch to clean, dry skin absent of wrinkles and creases.
- Change pouch on routine basis (do not wait for it to leak).
- Teach caregivers to assess skin barrier for signs of erosion upon removal.
- Inform parents that another pouch size may be necessary as child grows.
- Cotton balls can be put in pouch to wick effluent off wafer, extending wear time.
- Position pouch so that tail of pouch empties toward infant's side to facilitate emptying into diaper when in a supine position.
- Urinary pouch with antireflux will increase wear time when used to contain liquid output from ileostomy.
- Do not rinse pouch, they are odor proof and waterproof.

BOX 37.3 Ostomy Online Resources

- Wound, Ostomy and Continence Nurses Society™ http://www.wocn.org/ accessed 1/1/2023
- United Ostomy Association of America (UOAA) www.uoaa.org accessed 1/1/2023

Refeeding Ostomy Output

Infants with short gut syndrome and high fecal output can lead to feeding and nutritional imbalances such as dehydration, electrolyte imbalances, poor growth, and exposure to the long-term effects of parenteral nutrition as described in Chapter 29. Children and infants with a patent distal intestinal limb (i.e., mucous fistula) may be able to have their stool collected from the ostomy pouch and administered (refed) through their distal stoma. A pouch is applied over this distal stoma and a catheter inserted through an opening in the pouch (Baker et al., 2022; Richardson, Banerjee, & Rabe, 2006). The catheter can be secured either in a window in the ostomy pouch or sandwiched between two ostomy barrier rings. See chapter 39 for additional options for securing catheters though ostomy pouches. For safety, initial placement of the catheter under radiograph may be required. A pump is used to control refeeding administration. Strict labeling of all tubes and lines as well as accurate intake and output measurement should be implemented. A WOC nurse should be part of the team to help secure the tubing and prevent stomal and peristomal skin complications and leakage (Baker et al., 2022).

Burn/Thermal Injury

Chapter 34 provides a detailed discussion related to burn care. Children through age four years are more likely to sustained scald injuries, while the older children are more likely to have flame injuries (Moiser, Bernal, & Farakas, 2017). Toddlers are at high risk for sustaining burns to their chest, arms, face, hands, and abdomen as they begin to walk and explore their environment, grabbing onto tables, tablecloths, and radiators to pull themselves up to standing. Hot liquids pulled down from tables result in burns to the head, face, and chest. Burns to the hands are common, especially in cold climates and homes with radiator heat. Hot water tanks set above 120 degrees put children at risk during bathing (Shields et al., 2013). Approximately 10% of child abuse cases involve burning, and up to 20% of pediatric burn admissions involve abuse or neglect. Criteria for nonaccidental burn injuries that are suspicious for abuse or neglect are listed in Chapter 34, Box 34.2. Keeping dressings in place when children are burned is particularly challenging because of their location and because children are so active. Unaffected thumbs should be kept out of the dressing whenever possible. Flexible tube net dressing or socks over the hand can also be used to keep the dressings in place.

Intravenous Extravasation Injury

Extravasation injury is the inadvertent leaking or infusing of vesicant or nonvesicant solution into the surrounding tissue instead of into the vascular pathway (AWHONN, 2018). Neonates, especially premature infants, are at very high risk for serious skin damage from extravasation due to immature skin structures, lack of subcutaneous tissue, and the small size of their blood vessels.

Careful and frequent assessment of the intravenous (IV) insertion site (at least every hour) is vital for prevention of infiltration and extravasation (AWHONN, 2018; Children's Hospitals Solution for Patient Safety, 2019a, 2019b). Infusion pumps alone are not reliable for detecting an infiltrate; in fact, severe consequences have been reported to progress unnoticed for up to 72 h. Injuries range from cosmetic to functional and from ischemia to compartment syndrome requiring surgery, prolonged hospitalization, and significant morbidity (Amjad, Murphy, Nylander-Housholder, & Ranft, 2011).

Checklist 37.1 contains a list of extravasation prevention strategies. Risk is minimized with the use of vascular access devices made of plastic instead of steel in places that are easier to immobilize. If an arm board is used, prevent obstruction of venous return by placing tape loosely over the bony prominence and do not completely encircle the extremity with adhesive tape (AWHONN, 2018). Correct fluid concentrations and diluents before IV medicines should be administered. Securing the IV site with a transparent adhesive dressing is preferred so that the site can be frequently monitored (Beall, Hall, Mulholland, & Gephart, 2013). Avoid placing a vascular device in areas of flexion, surrounding tendons, nerves or arteries or near the face or forehead (AWHONN, 2018).

In children, negative blood return in the tubing does not confirm infiltration because small catheters can prevent withdraw of blood even when patent. Likewise, blood return into the tubing does not rule out extravasation (AWHONN, 2018). Signs and symptoms of extravasation include swelling, pain, blanching, or coolness, inability to flush, leakage, erythema, blistering, or skin sloughing. Several infiltration grading

---

CHECKLIST 37.1 Extravasation Prevention Strategies

✓ Use small enough plastic/silicone catheter to avoid restriction of blood flow.
✓ Avoid repeated use of a vein.
✓ Avoid placing an IV in an area difficult to immobilize.
✓ Use transparent tape to secure.
✓ Cover the site with a sterile semipermeable transparent dressing that will permit ongoing visualization of the insertion site.
✓ Upper extremities less likely to infiltrate or leak compared with peripheral IV in lower extremities or scalp veins.
✓ Place tape loosely over bony prominences to avoid restricting blood flow to the extremity. Do not encircle around the arm.
✓ Limit IV glucose to 12.5%.
✓ Dilute medications as much as possible before administration of other solutions to prevent extravasation.

---

scales have been developed including the Milliam Scale, developed by the Infusion Nurses Society. In classifying severity, these grading scales refer to joints involved rather than inches of infiltration of involved skin, thus reflecting the degree of severity relative to the size of the patient. Another infiltration grading scale is the Thigpen Grading Scale, which incorporates treatment options (Amjad et al., 2011; AWHONN, 2018; Thigpen, 2007).

Once symptoms are noted, swift action may minimize adverse outcomes and the degree of skin damage: (1) disconnect the tubing from the IV device; (2) leave the needle in place; (3) attach a 1- to 3-mL syringe to the IV device and aspirate residual drug from the IV; (4) avoid pressure on the site; (5) elevate the involved extremity as soon as possible.

If applicable, appropriately trained clinicians may administer a recommended antidote for that particular medication (e.g., hyaluronidase), subcutaneously, not through the IV catheter, to neutralize chemicals as soon as possible. Aseptic puncture techniques have been used by qualified providers to remove fluid and toxic agents from under the skin (Gopalakrishnan, Goel, & Banerjee, 2017). These techniques have been reported to dramatically decrease swelling and complications; however, risk for infection and further tissue damage must be considered. Unlike adults, topical application of heat or cold is not recommended for neonates due to risk of thermal injury in already immature, compromised, and perhaps hypoperfused skin (AWHONN, 2018).

Ongoing local wound care will depend on the characteristics of the wound and maintaining a physiologic environment. Often, extravasation wounds require time before the full extent of the tissue damage is apparent. Thus, as the wound characteristics change, adjustments in the topical wound management will be required. As with adults, it is not unusual to use a variety of dressings to manage the pediatric extravasation wound site (Lehr, Lulic-Botica, Lindblad, Kazzi, & Aranda, 2004; Sawatzky-Dickson & Bodnaryk, 2006).

SUPPORT FOR HEALING

Chapters 18 to 20 provide details for wound bed preparation and principles of wound management, including infection, debridement, and topical management, to create a physiologic wound environment. Maximizing nutrition and reducing or eliminating other cofactors such as pain, nutrition, perfusion, and oxygenation are described throughout this textbook. Additional pediatric-specific considerations are provided in this section.

Nutritional Support

Nutritional assessment and monitoring, as well as diet, supplements, and feeding strategies, are vital components of any skin integrity care plan. Neonates and children, however, are generally at higher risk for nutritional deficiencies than adults due to the greater demands generated during the phase of life that the body grows most rapidly, while at the same time having smaller appetites and less ability for food and supplement intake. Premature infants have even greater nutritional requirements than term infants due to their diminished nutrient stores at birth (Ditzenberger, 2010). Additionally, children with actual or potential skin breakdown tend to have coexisting conditions and illnesses that increase nutritional needs while further compromising the ability to meet nutritional needs. A pediatrician, dietitian, or other qualified health professional should perform an age-appropriate nutritional assessment, which may include strategies discussed in Chapter 27, such as anthropometric (with head circumference) measurements; growth charts; nutritional screening tools; and consideration of hydration, fluid shifts, and needs associated with any existing comorbidities and skin conditions (Mehta et al., 2009; Ranade & Collins, 2011; Skillman & Wischmeyer, 2008).

Anxiety and Discomfort

Any condition that affects the skin of a child will most likely involve procedures and interventions that create anxiety and/or discomfort. Examples range from changing dressings, pouches, and tube/device stabilizers to debridement, intubation, or surgery. Skin assessment alone, especially in the presence of skin breakdown, can also be painful and frightening to a child. Regardless of the type of procedure, age and developmentally appropriate assessment of pain and discomfort must be accomplished. Features of development, such as how a child of a particular age thinks, fears, and learning styles (Table 37.5), are critical to developing an effective care plan to facilitate coping with procedures and associated pain. Tools for assessing pain in neonatal and infants are presented in Chapter 28 and Table 28.1.

Pain management in preemies, neonates, and infants include *nonpharmacologic* interventions beginning with preprocedure preparation, caregiver/parent presence and participation during the procedure. The use of cognitive-based interventions and distraction (Table 37.6) during tend after the procedure are commonly used to facility child coping and mastery, both physically and emotionally (Baharestani,

2007; Hockenberry et al., 2011). As previously described, skin-to-skin (e.g., kangaroo) care and expressed breast milk administration have demonstrated pain reduction during adhesive tape removal (Nanavati et al., 2013). *Sucrose 24%* given orally directly on the tongue by syringe, if the infant is intubated, according to post conceptual age, or by pacifier dipped in the sucrose solution and repeated as needed for pain for minor procedures such as heel stick, venipuncture, venous catheterization, nasogastric insertion, bladder catheterizations, intramuscular or subcutaneous injections, eye examinations, dressing changes, and tape removal. Sucrose combined with additional analgesic agents may be moderately painful procedures, such as lumbar puncture, circumcision, chest tube insertion, percutaneous central venous catheter insertion, or intraosseous access (Stevens, Yamada, Ohlsson, Haliburton, & Shorkey, 2016).

Topical local anesthetics are effective for local pain control over the skin for some procedures used either as adjuncts or alternatives to oral, intravenous, and intranasal medications. Common examples include *Eutectic Mixture of Local Anesthetics* (EMLA; Astra-Zeneca, Wilmington, DE) and *Liposomal lidocaine products* (e.g. LMX-4; EBSA Laboratories Inc, Jupiter, Florida). Critical to the success of these products is to allow time up to 30 minutes to take effect (Chumpitazi et al., 2022).

According to the manufacturer's instructions (https://www.accessdata.fda.gov/drugsatfda_docs/label/2000/19941s11lbl.pdf), EMLA is not recommended for neonates with a gestational age less than 37 weeks nor with infants under the age of twelve months who are receiving treatment with methemoglobin-inducing agents. Controlled studies of EMLA cream in children under the age of 7 years have shown less overall benefit than in older children or adults. These results illustrate the importance of emotional and psychological support of younger children undergoing medical procedures. Maximum dose recommendations to avoid toxicity is based on age, body weight, application area and time exposed to intact skin on a child with normal renal and hepatic function.

Liposomal lidocaine products are lidocaine formulated in liposomes sold over the counter (OTC) for minor skin irritations in adults and children over 2 years of age. As always, it is important to read manufacturer's instructions as age limits vary by brand and % Lidocaine. Initially thought to be safer than EMLA (Eidelman, Weiss, Lau, & Carr, 2005; Taddio, Soin, Schuh, Koren, & Scolnik, 2005), a 2012 study (Oni, Brown, & Kenkel, 2012) compared five common topical lidocaine prescriptions and OTC products. Results showed the highest serum lidocaine and monoethylglycinexylidide (MEGX) levels with the OTC products and significant discrepancies with lidocaine absorption and metabolizes for even a single OTC product. Results showed significant differences between the 4% lidocaine preparations ($P = 0.0439$); the 2.5% preparation had a greater absorption than the 4% lidocaine preparation and the 6% lidocaine preparation ($P = 0.0016$). There were three adverse reactions with the OTC preparations, one of which resulted in postinflammatory hyperpigmentation. Authors concluded that although topical anesthetics are considered safe, some individuals have

TABLE 37.5   Features of Development That Are Pertinent to Helping Children Cope With Procedures

	Birth to 2 Years	2–7 Years	7–12 Years	Adolescence
How the child thinks and solves problems	Sensory motor experience develops schema (well-defined and repeated sequences of actions and perceptions) Memory is obvious by 3–4 months Begins using symbols for thought reasoning between 18 and 24 months	Thinking is dominated by perceptions rather than logic Verbal communication important for learning Exploratory manipulations helps child learn Child watches, listens, asks questions (Why? How?) Classifies similar things Perceptions limited to single salient feature, so difficult for child to differentiate unessential from essential properties of an experience Difficulty distinguishing pain from cooling or heat sensation Uses memory to reconstruct past events Uses imagination to cope Egocentric point of view	Learns from interacting with peers and own experiences Able to understand viewpoints of others Able to see relative nature of things (e.g., this hurts a little; that hurts a lot) Uses deductive logic with respect to tangible (concrete) experiences (if this, then that) Able to view things in context (e.g., "the shot hurt, but it will make me better") Evaluates painful intensive actions in terms of logical function rather than punishment Understands unseen body mechanics/functions Makes use of sensory and procedural information	Uses reason and logical thinking Interested in theoretically possible problems and questions Able to engage in self-reflection Learns from verbally presented ideas and arguments
Major fears and worries	Separation from parents Anything unfamiliar, especially when not with a parent	Separation from parents Harm to body Punishment for wrongdoing	Body injury Loss of body functions Loss of control	Uncertain about self as person Concerned if body, thoughts, feelings are "normal"
Understanding cause and effect	By about 3 months, may associate an action with a result In second year: magical thinking; believes that what is wished for happens	Everything happens by intention Misbehavior is followed by punishment Interprets unrelated events to be related	Before about 9 years, views illness as a consequence of transgressions of rules At about 9 years, begins to understand that illness may have multiple causes	Uses formal rules of logic and evidence to assess cause and effect

From Pridham, K.F., Adelson, F., Hansen, M.F. (1987). Helping children deal with procedures in a clinic setting: A developmental approach. *Journal of Pediatric Nursing, 2*(1), 13–22. PMID: 3643261.

unpredictably high absorption levels demonstrating that concentration, formulation, and the individual patient all have significant effects on serum levels. The authors recommend using OTC topical anesthetics under the supervision of a health care professional to avoid adverse effects.

Pediatric Dressing Selection

Factors that guide dressing selection in the adult will also guide dressing selection in the pediatric patient population.

Fewer studies comparing the effectiveness and safety of dressings with children when compared with adults exist. Primarily, dressings should be selected based on the characteristics of the wound (size, depth, location, exudate, and periwound skin) and treatment goals. Dressings commonly used for pediatric patients with a variety of wounds include transparent, hydrocolloids, foams, silicones, medical grade honey, hydrogels and hydrofibers (King, Stellar, Blevins, & Shaw, 2014; Steen et al., 2020). Unless specified, children have

TABLE 37.6	**Distraction Techniques for the Neonate and Child**
Age	**Distraction Techniques**
Infant 0 to 12 months	• Parental presence (touch, soft voice, singing) • Swaddling • Pacifier • Feeding (breast or bottle) • Massage • Books with lights/sounds • Music • Rattles
Toddler 1 to 3 years	• Same as infants • Music: singing, musical instruments • Pinwheels • Storytelling • Peek-a-boo • Toys and books that light up or play music • Blowing bubbles • Sensory toys (such as Play-Doh, balls with interesting textures, glitter wands, rain sticks)
Preschool age 3 to 5 years	• Pinwheels, feathers • Storytelling, books: Pop-up, I-spy or find-it books • Noise makers • Music, singing, musical instruments and toys • Comfort items (stuffed animals, blankies) • Electronic tablet applications or games • Sensory toys (see above) • Blowing bubbles • Familiar movies/TV shows
School age 6 to 12 years	• Electronic tablet applications or games • Storytelling, Books: pop-up, I Spy • Guided imagery, relaxation • Breathing techniques • Participation in procedure • Familiar movies/TV shows • Brain teasers or puzzles • Fidget items • Virtual reality
Adolescent	• Electronic tablet applications or games • Familiar movies/TV shows • Web surfing/social media/online videos • Talking/texting with friends or family • Guided imagery, relaxation • Trivia games or brain teasers • Fidget items

From Boles, J. (2018). The powerful practice of distraction. *Pediatric Nursing, 44*(5), 247–249, 253; Hockenberry, M.J., McCarthy, K., Taylor, O., et al. (2011). Managing painful procedures in children with cancer. *Journal of Pediatric Hematology/Oncology, 33*(2), 119–127.

the same indications and reimbursement parameters as described for adults in Chapter 21. Unique considerations may be required to secure dressings to prevent the inadvertent loosening or removal of the dressing due to the child's exploration of their body.

Neonatal Dressing Selection

Single and multiple case studies with *term and preterm* infants have noted safe treatment of a variety of wounds (e.g., chemical burns, thermal burns, and pressure injuries) using medical grade honey and silver-impregnated dressings (August, Ireland, & Benton, 2015; AWHONN, 2018; Oquendo et al., 2015; Tenenhaus, Greenberg, & Potenza, 2014).

Silver-impregnated dressings were originally avoided in the neonatal population due to concerns of silver absorption to toxic levels; however, publications including multiple and single case studies have demonstrated safe uses of ionic silver in neonates (August et al., 2015; AWHONN, 2018; Oquendo et al., 2015; Rustogi, Mill, Fraser, & Kimble, 2005; Tenenhaus et al., 2014).

Successful use of medical grade honey in preterm infants have been presented in case studies involving preterm infants for a stage 3 pressure injury, dehisced and infected surgical wounds, and extravasation (Boyar, Handa, Clemens, & Shimborske, 2014; Esser, 2017; Mohr, Reyna, & Amaya, 2014). A multicenter, retrospective chart review of 115 neonatal and pediatric patients of which 34 were preterm and 38 were between 0 and 6 months of age, medical grade honey was a safe and effective treatment option for wounds requiring debridement (Amaya, 2015). AWHONN (2018) recommends considering the use of medical grade honey especially with wounds requiring debridement.

Hydrogels have been shown to be effective in neonatal and pediatric case studies describing the management of toxic epidermal necrolysis, wound dehiscence, extravasation injuries, pressure ulcers, fungating lesions, and burns (Caniano, Ruth, & Teich, 2005; Cisler-Cahill, 2006; McCord & Levy, 2006).

Negative Pressure Wound Therapy (NPWT)

There is a lack of robust literature dedicated to NPWT use in infants and children. In fact, safety and efficacy has not yet been approved by the FDA for use with children less than 8-year-old. However, in a literature review through 2017, 115 articles were generated that focused in NPWT in the pediatric patient population ranging in ages from less than one year old to 18 years of age (Santosa et al., 2019). In these 115 studies, the most common age group was 0–1 years of age ($n = 47$), 23 studies reported use in children aged 2–11 years old, and 11 studies reporting use in the older child ages 12–17 years. While these were case studies or small case series, the leading indication was for major abdominal surgery (e.g., gastroschisis) and cardiothoracic surgical problems. In an analysis of 3184 administrative health care claims, however, NPWT was more common for musculoskeletal indications in the older child and very few were placed in the child under 2 years old. From this analysis, researchers concluded that NPWT use in infants and children appear to have low rates of serious complications.

NPWT continues to be used off-label in both infants and children for a variety of acute and chronic wounds (Baharestani, 2007; Bütter, Emran, Al-Jazaeri, & Ouimet, 2006; McCord et al., 2007; Mooney, Argenta, Marks, Morykwas, & DeFranzo, 2000; Rentea, Somers, Cassidy, Enters, & Arca, 2013).

Due to lack of FDA approval, guidelines for the use of NPWT in neonates, infants, and children cannot be found in manufacturer's instructions. However, Baharestani et al. (2009) proposed age and wound-specific recommendations for pressure settings and choice of foam dressing in the pediatric population (Table 37.7). Several of the authors, correlated negative pressure settings to −25 mmHg above the mean arterial blood pressure of the patient in the neonate, infant, and toddler population and adjusted as needed based on comorbidities, perfusion status, wound location, and pain tolerance. Providers should consider that neonates and infants are at risk for fluid loss and dehydration during treatment with NPWT (King et al., 2014). Despite the limitations of existing research on the use of NPWT in

TABLE 37.7 **Recommended Negative Pressure Settings for Children**	
Newborn (birth to 1 month)	50–75 mmHg
Infants (>1 month to 2 years)	50–75 mmHg
Children (>2–12 years)	75–125 mmHg
Adolescents (>12 years)	75–125 mmHg

Adapted from Baharestani, M.M. (2007). Use of negative pressure wound therapy in the treatment of neonatal and pediatric wounds: A retrospective examination of clinical outcomes. *Ostomy Wound Manage, 53*(6):75–83.

the pediatric population, NPWT is widely used for many indications across different ages. Following a population based analysis of the pediatric literature, researchers observed a low incidence of serious complications (Santosa et al., 2019). The study concluded NPWT use in infants and children is safe and can be effectively utilized by both surgical and nonsurgical disciplines. See Chapter 24 for more discussion of NPWT.

CLINICAL CONSULT

A: Consulted for 4-year-old boy in the emergency department after falling off his tricycle. Immunizations current. No known allergies. Patient was crying and agitated until his parents were brought into the treatment room, encouraged to stay and assist in age-appropriate distraction techniques. Tightly secured dry gauze was soaked off with warm saline (to avoid painful removal). Bilateral knees with large 5 × 5 cm irregularly shaped abrasions. Initial cleanse with hypochlorous solution. No foreign body (dirt/gravel) noted in the wounds. Moderate dried exudate. Periwound skin without erythema. No local signs of infection. No other signs of injury.

D: Road abrasions.
P: Cleanse with normal saline or shower per patient and parent preference. Dress wound with gentle silicone foam dressing to promote moist wound healing while minimizing periwound exudate and pain. Change every 5 days, or sooner for strike through exudate.
I: (1) Parent teaching with demonstration using adequate technique for removal and application of dressings. (2) Parents verbalize signs and symptoms of infection.
E: Follow-up planned with the patient's pediatrician in 7–10 days or sooner if wound shows signs of infection or deterioration.

SUMMARY

- Infants and children suffer many skin-related problems.
- Caring for neonatal skin and wounds requires knowledge of skin properties to prevent absorption of toxic chemicals.
- Research into all areas of pediatric wound care and prevention is needed.

- Ongoing education of staff and parents related to wound healing is essential.
- Nurses experienced in wound care can improve the lives of sick children with their knowledge of skin health, skin maintenance, wound healing, and expertise using advanced wound care products.

SELF-ASSESSMENT QUESTIONS

1. Infant refers to a child:
   a. Birth to 12 months
   b. Less than 28 weeks gestation
   c. 34–37 weeks gestation
   d. Birth to 6 months.
2. True or False. A neonate is birth to 3 months.

3. What is a key factor to consider that will influence determination of product safety when used with an infant?
   a. Skin pigmentation
   b. Maturity of the skin
   c. Duration of product application
   d. Preference of the parents

4. Which of the following pressure injury risk assessment scales are valid or reliable in the pediatric patient population?
   a. Munro Scale
   b. Braden and Norton
   c. Glamorgan and Braden Q
   d. NSARS and Hunters Hill Marie Curie Centre

5. According to AWHONN, how often should skin inspection under a medical device occur?
   a. Daily
   b. At change of shift
   c. At least every 12 h (e.g., edema, deterioration in health)
   d. Every 1–4 h

REFERENCES

Alderden, J., Rondinelli, J., Pepper, G., Cummins, M., & Whitney, J. A. (2017). Risk factors for pressure injuries amount critically ill patients: A systematic review. *International Journal of Nursing Studies, 71*, 97–114. https://doi.org/10.1016/j.ijnurstu.2017.03.012.

Alderman, E. M., & Breuner, C. C. (2019). AAP Committee on adolescence. Unique needs of the adolescent. *Pediatrics, 144*(6), e20193150. Retrieved 6/10/2022 from: https://publications.aap.org/pediatrics/article/144/6/e20193150/37985/Unique-Needsof-the-Adolescent?autologincheck.redirected.

Amaya, R. (2015). Safety and efficacy of active *Leptospermum* honey in neonatal and paediatric wound debridement. *Journal of Wound Care, 24*, 95–103.

Amjad, I., Murphy, T., Nylander-Housholder, L., & Ranft, A. (2011). A new approach to management of intravenous infiltration in pediatric patients: Pathophysiology, classification, and treatment. *Journal of Infusion Nursing, 34*(4), 242–249. https://doi.org/10.1097/NAN.0b013e31821da1b3.

Association of Women's Health, Obstetric and Neonatal Nurses (AWHONN) and National Association of Neonatal Nurses. (2018). *Neonatal skin care evidence-based clinical practice guideline* (4th ed.). Washington, DC: AWHONN.

August, D. L., Ireland, S., & Benton, J. (2015). Silver-based dressing in an extremely low-birth-weight infant: A case study. *Journal of Wound, Ostomy, and Continence Nursing, 42*, 290–293.

Baharestani, M. M. (2007). Use of negative pressure wound therapy in the treatment of neonatal and pediatric wounds: A retrospective examination of clinical outcomes. *Ostomy/Wound Management, 53*(6), 75–83. https://pubmed.ncbi.nlm.nih.gov/17586874/.

Baharestani, M., Amjad, I., Bookout, K., Fleck, T., Gabriel, A., Kaufman, D., et al. (2009). V.A.C. therapy in the management of paediatric wounds: Clinical review and experience. *International Wound Journal, 6*(Suppl. 1), 1–26. https://doi.org/10.1111/j.1742-481X.2009.00607.x.

Baker, C., Phearman, L. A., & McIltrot, K. (2022). In J. Carmel, J. Colwell, & M. Goldberg (Eds), *Wound Ostomy and Continence Nurses Society Core Curriculum: Ostomy Management* 2nd ed. (pp. 252–264). Philadelphia, PA: Wolters Kluwer.

Beall, V., Hall, B., Mulholland, J. T., & Gephart, S. M. (2013). Neonatal extravasation: An overview and algorithm for evidence-based treatment. *Neonatal and Infant Nursing Review, 13*(4), 189–195. https://doi.org/10.1053/j.nainr.2013.09.001.

Beeckman, D., et al. (2015). Proceedings of the Global IAD Expert Panel. Incontinence associated dermatitis: Moving prevention forward. *Wounds International, 2015*. Available to download from www.woundsinternational.com; Retrieved 6/112022 from: https://www.academia.edu/20000855/Beeckman_D_et_al_2015_Incontinence_Associated_Dermatitis_Addressing_evidence_gaps_for_best_practice.

Blume-Peytavi, U., Cork, M. J., Faegemann, J., Szczapa, J., Vanaclocha, F., & Gelmetti, C. (2009). Bathing and cleansing in newborns from day 1 to first year of life. *Recommendations From a European Round Table Meeting, 23*(7), 751–759. https://doi.org/10.1111/j.1468-3083.2009.03140.x.

Boesch, P. R., Myers, C., Garrett, T., Nie, A. M., Thomas, N., Chima, A., et al. (2012). Prevention of tracheostomy-related pressure ulcers in children. *Pediatrics, 129*(3), e792–e797. https://doi.org/10.1542/peds.2011-0649.

Boullata, J. I., Carrera, A. L., Harvey, L., Escuro, A. A., Hudson, L., Mays, A., et al. (2017). ASPEN safe practice for enteral nutrition therapy. *Journal of Parenteral and Enteral Nutrition, 41*(1), 15–103.

Boyar, V. (2020a). Diaper dermatitis: What products are appropriate? *Wound Management & Prevention, 66*(2), 12–15.

Boyar, V. (2020b). New year, old problem: Diaper dermatitis. *Wound Management and Prevention, 66*(1), 8–10.

Boyar, V., Handa, D., Clemens, K., & Shimborske, D. (2014). Clinical experience with Leptospermum honey use for treatment of hard to heal neonatal wounds: Case series. *Journal of Perinatology, 34*, 161–163. https://doi.org/10.1038/jp.2013.158.

Bütter, A., Emran, M., Al-Jazaeri, A., & Ouimet, A. (2006). Vacuum-assisted closure for wound management in the pediatric population. *Journal of Pediatric Surgery, 41*(5), 940–942. https://doi.org/10.1016/j.jpedsurg.2006.01.061.

Caniano, D. A., Ruth, B., & Teich, S. (2005). Wound management with vacuum-assisted closure: Experience in 51 pediatric patients. *Journal of Pediatric Surgery, 40*, 128–132. https://doi.org/10.1016/j.jpedsurg.2004.09.016.

Carr, A. N., DeWitt, R., Cork, M. J., Eichenfield, L. F., Fölster-Holst, R., Hohl, D., et al. (2019). Diaper dermatitis prevalence and severity: Global perspective on the impact of caregiver behavior. *Pediatric Dermatology, 37*, 130–136.

Centers for Disease Control and Prevention (CDC). (2021). *Child Development*. Retrieved 6/10/2022 from: https://www.cdc.gov/ncbddd/childdevelopment/positiveparenting/toddlers.html.

Chamblee, T. B., Paske T. A., Caillouette, C. N., Stellar, J. J., Quigley, S. M., & Curley, M. A. Q. (2018). How to predict pediatric pressure injury risk with the Braden QD Scale. *American Journal of Nursing 118*(11), 34–43.

Children's Hospitals' Solutions for Patient Safety (SPS). (2021a). Peripheral IV infiltration and extravasation (PIVIE). In *SPS prevention bundles*. Retrieved 1/1/2023 from: https://www.solutionsforpatientsafety.org/wp-content/uploads/SPS-Prevention-Bundles.pdf.

Children's Hospitals' Solutions for Patient Safety (SPS). (2021b). *Pressure injuries in SPS prevention bundles*. Retrieved 1/1/2023 from: https://www.solutionsforpatientsafety.org/wp-content/uploads/SPS-Prevention-Bundles.pdf.

Chumpitazi, C. E., Chang, C., Atanelov, Z., Dietrich, A. M., Lam, S. H., Rose, E., et al. (2022). Managing acute pain in children presenting to the emergency department without opioids. *Journal of the American College of Emergency Physicians open*, *3*(2), e12664. https://doi.org/10.1002/emp2.12664.

Cisler-Cahill, L. (2006). A protocol for the use of amorphous hydrogel to support wound healing in neonatal patients: An adjunct to nursing skin care. *Neonatal Network*, *25*(4), 267–273. https://doi.org/10.1891/0730-0832.25.4.267.

Cohen, B. (2017). Differential diagnosis of diaper dermatitis. *Clinical Pediatrics*, *56*(5S), 16S–22S.

Counts, J., Weisbrod, A., & Yin, S. (2017). Common diaper ingredient questions: Modern disposable diaper materials are safe and extensively tested. *Clinical Pediatrics*, *56*(SS), 23S–27S.

Curley, M. A. Q., Hasbani, N. R., Quigley, S. M., Stellar, J. J., Pasek, T. A., Shelley, S. S., et al. (2018). Predicting pressure injury risk in pediatric patients: The Braden QD scale. *The Journal of Pediatrics*, *192*, 189–192e2. https://doi.org/10.1016/j.jpeds.2017.09.045.

Curley, M. A., Quigley, S. M., & Lin, M. (2003). Pressure ulcers in pediatric intensive care: Incidence and associated factors. *Pediatric Critical Care Medicine*, *4*(3), 284–290. https://doi.org/10.1097/01.PCC.0000075559.55920.36.

Curley, M. A., Razmus, I. S., Roberts, K. E., & Wypij, D. (2003). Predicting pressure ulcer risk in pediatric patients: The Braden Q scale. *Nursing Research*, *52*(1), 22–33. https://doi.org/10.1097/00006199-200301000-00004.

Darmstadt, G. L., & Dinulos, J. G. (2000). Neonatal skin care. *Pediatric Clinics of North America*, *47*(4), 757–782. https://doi.org/10.1016/s0031-3955(05)70239-x.

Delmore, B., Deppisch, M., D'Nurs, C. S., Luna-Anderson, C., & Nie, A. M. (2019). Pressure injuries in the pediatric population: A national pressure injury advisory panel white paper. *Advances in Skin & Wound Care*, *32*(9), 394–408. https://doi.org/10.1097/01.ASW.0000577124.58253.66.

Ditzenberger, G. R. (2010). Nutritional management. In M. Walden (Ed.), *Core curriculum for neonatal intensive care nursing* (4th ed., pp. 182–207). St. Louis: Elsevier.

Eichenfiled, L. F., Frieden, I. H., & Esterly, N. B. (2015). *Neonatal dermatology* (3rd ed.). Philadelphia: Saunders Elsevier.

Eidelman, A., Weiss, J. M., Lau, J., & Carr, D. B. (2005). Topical anesthetics for dermal instrumentation: A systematic review of randomized, controlled trials. *Annals of Emergency Medicine*, *46*(4), 343–351. https://doi.org/10.1016/j.annemergmed.2005.01.028.

Esser, M. (2017). Leptospermum honey for wound care in an extremely premature infant. *Advances in Neonatal Care*, *17*, 27–32. https://doiorg/101097/ANC0000000000000331.

European Pressure Ulcer Advisory Panel, National Pressure Injury Advisory Panel, and Pan Pacific Pressure Injury Alliance. (2019). In E. Haesler (Ed.), *Prevention and treatment of pressure ulcers/injuries: Clinical practice guideline* The International Guideline 2019.

Fernandes, J. D., Machado, M. C. R., & de Oliveira, Z. N. P. (2011). Children and newborn skin care and prevention. *Anais Brasileiros de Dermatologia*, *86*(1), 102–110. https://doi.org/10.1590/s0365-05962011000100014.

Fluhr, J. W., Darlenski, R., Taieb, A., Hachem, J. P., Baudouin, C., Msika, P., et al. (2010). Functional skin adaptation in infancy—Almost complete but not fully competent. *Experimental Dermatology*, *19*, 483–492. https://doi.org/10.1111/j.1600-0625.2009.01023x.

Frank, G., Walsh, K. E., Wooton, S., Bost, J., Dong, W., Keller, L., et al. (2017). Impact of a pressure injury prevention bundle in the solutions for patient safety network. *Pediatric Quality & Safety*, *2*(2), e013. https://doi.org/10.1097/pq9.0000000000000013.

Fujii, K., Sugama, J., Okuwa, M., Sanada, H., & Mizokami, Y. (2010). Incidence and risk factors of pressure ulcers in seven neonatal intensive care units in Japan: A multisite prospective cohort study. *International Wound Journal*, *7*(5), 323–328. https://doi.org/10.1111/j.1742-481X.2010.00688.x.

Galvin, P. A., & Curley, M. A. Q. (2012). The Braden Q+P: A pediatric perioperative pressure ulcer risk assessment and intervention tool. *AORN Journal*, *96*(3), 261–270. https://doi.org/10.1016/j.aorn.2012.05.010.

García-Molina, P., Balaquer-López, E., Torra I Bou, J. T., Alvarez-Ordiales, A., Quesada-Romos, C., & Verdu-Soriano, J. (2012). A prospective longitudinal study to assess use of continuous and reactive low-pressure mattresses to reduce pressure ulcer incidence in a pediatric intensive care unit. *Ostomy/Wound Management*, *58*(7), 32–39. http://hdl.handle.net/10045/36196.

Gopalakrishnan, P. N., Goel, N., & Banerjee, S. (2017). Saline irrigation for management of skin extravasation injury in neonates (review). *Cochrane Database of Systematic Reviews*, *7*, CD008404. https://doi.org/10.1002/14651858.CD008404.pub3.

Grove, G. L., Zerweck, C. R., Ekholm, B. P., Smith, E. S., & Koski, N. I. (2014). Randomized comparison of a silicone tape and a paper tape for gentleness in healthy children. *Journal of Wound, Ostomy, and Continence Nursing*, *41*(1), 40–48. https://doi.org/10.1097/WON.000436669. 79024.b0.

Hardman, M. J., Sisi, P., Banbury, D. N., & Byne, C. (1998). Patterned acquisition of skin barrier function during development. *Development*, *125*(8), 1541–1552. PMID: 9502735.

Heimall, L. M., Storey, B., Stellar, J. J., & Finn Davis, K. (2012). Beginning at the bottom: Evidence-based care of diaper dermatitis. *MCN: American Journal of Maternal Child Nursing*, *37*(1), 10–16. https://doi.org/10.1097/NMC.0b013e31823850ea.

Hockenberry, M. J., McCarthy, K., Taylor, O., Scarberry, M., Franklin, Q., Louis, C. U., et al. (2011). Managing painful procedures in children with cancer. *Journal of Pediatric Hematology/Oncology*, *33*(2), 119–127. https://doi.org/10.1097/MPH.0b013e3181f46a65.

Huffines, B., & Logsdon, M. C. (1997). The neonatal skin risk assessment scale for predicting skin breakdown in neonates. *Issues in Comprehensive Pediatric Nursing*, *20*(2), 103–114. https://doi.org/10.3109/01460869709026881.

Jaryszak, E. M., Shah, R. K., Amling, J., & Pena, M. T. (2011). Pediatric tracheotomy wound complications: Incidence and significance. *Archives of Otolaryngology—Head & Neck Surgery*, *137*(4), 363–366. https://doi.org/10.1001/archoto.2011.33.

Kalia, Y. N., Nonato, L. B., Lund, C. H., & Guy, R. H. (1998). Development of skin barrier function in premature infants. *The Journal of Investigative Dermatology*, *111*(2), 320–326. https://doi.org/10.1046/j.1523-1747.1998.00289.x.

King, A., Stellar, J. J., Blevins, A., & Shaw, K. N. (2014). Dressings and products in pediatric wound care. *Advances in Wound Care*, *3*(4), 324–334. https://doi.org/10.1089/wound.2013.0477.

Kottner, J., Kenzler, M., & Wilborn, D. (2012). Interrater agreement, reliability and validity of the Glamorgan Paediatric Pressure Ulcer Risk Assessment Scale. *Journal of Clinical Nursing*, *23*, 1165–1169. https://doi.org/10.1111/jocn.12025.

Kuller, J. M. (2016). Infant skin care products: What are the issues? *Advances in Neonatal Care*, *16*(Suppl. 5S), S3–S12. https://doi.org/10.1097/ANC.0000000000000341.

Kusari, A., Han, A. M., Virgen, C. A., Matiz, C., Rasmussen, M., Friedlander, S. F., et al. (2019). Evidence-based skin care in preterm infants. *Pediatric Dermatology*, *36*, 16–23. https://doi.org/10.1111/pde.13725.

Lehr, V. T., Lulic-Botica, M., Lindblad, W. J., Kazzi, N. J., & Aranda, J. V. (2004). Management of infiltration injury in neonates using duoderm hydroactive gel. *American Journal of Perinatology*, *21*(7), 409–414. https://doi.org/10.1055/s-2004-835309.

Loring, C., Gregory, K., Gargan, B., LeBlanc, V., Lundgren, D., Reilly, J., et al. (2012). Tub bathing improves thermoregulation of the late preterm infant. *Journal of Obstetric, Gynecologic, and Neonatal Nursing*, *41*(2), 171–179. https://doi.org/10.1111/j.1552-6909.2011.01332.x.

Lund, C. H., & Osborne, J. W. (2004). Validity and reliability of the neonatal skin condition score. *Journal of Obstetric, Gynecologic, and Neonatal Nursing*, *33*(3), 320–327. https://doi.org/10.1177/0884217504265174.

Maffeis, L., Pugni, L., Pietrasanta, C., Ronchi, A., Fumagalli, M, Gelmetti, C., et al. (2014). Iatrogenic anetoderma of prematurity: A case report and review of the literature. *Case Reports in Dermatological Medicine*, *2014*, Article ID 781493. https://doi.org/10.1155/2014/781493.

Manning, M. J., Gatuvreau, K., & Curley, M. A. Q. (2015). Factors associated with occipital pressure ulcers in hospitalized infants and children. *American Journal of Critical Care*, *24*(4), 342–348. https://doi.org/10.4037/ajcc2015349.

McCord, S., & Levy, M. L. (2006). Practical guide to pediatric wound care. *Seminars in Plastic Surgery*, *20*(3), 192–199. https://doi.org/10.1055/s-2006-949119.

McCord, S., Naik-Mathuria, B. J., Murphy, K. M., Murphy, K. M., Mclane, K. M., Gay, A. N., et al. (2007). Negative pressure wound therapy is effective to manage a variety of wounds in infants and children. *Wound Repair and Regeneration*, *15*(3), 296–301. https://doi.org/10.1111/j.1524-475X. 200700229. x.

McInnes, E., Jammali-Blasi, A., Cullum, N., & Leung, V. (2018). Support surfaces for treating pressure injury. *Cochrane Database of Systematic Reviews*. https://doi.org/10.1002/14651858. CD009490.pub2.

McLane, K., Bookout, K., McCord, S., McCain, J., & Jefferson, L. S. (2004). The 2003 national pediatric pressure ulcer and skin breakdown prevalence survey: A multisite study. *Journal of Wound, Ostomy, and Continence Nursing*, *31*(4), 168–178. https://doi.org/10.1097/00152192-200407000-00004.

McLane, K., Krouskip, T., McCord, S., & Fraley, K. J. (2002). Comparison of interface pressures in the pediatric population among various support surfaces. *Journal of Wound, Ostomy, and Continence Nursing*, *29*, 243–251. https://doi.org/10.1067/mjw.2002.127208.

McNichol, L., Lund, C., & Osborne, C. (2013). Medical adhesives and patient safety: State of the science: consensus statements for the assessment, prevention, and treatment of adhesive-related skin injuries. *Journal of Wound, Ostomy, and Continence Nursing*, *40*(4), 365–380. https://doi.org/10.1097/NOR.0b013e3182a39caf.

McSweeney, M. E., Mitchell, P. D., Smithers, C. J., Doherty, A., Perkins, J., & Rosen, R. (2021). A retrospective review of primary percutaneous endoscopic gastrostomy and laparoscopic gastrostomy tube placement. *Journal of Pediatric Gastroenterology and Nutrition*, *73*(5), 586–591.

Mehta, N. M., Compher, C., & A.S.P.E.N. Board of Directors. (2009). A.S.P.E.N. clinical guidelines: Nutrition support of the critically ill child. *JPEN Journal of Parenteral and Enteral Nutrition*, *33*(3), 260–276. https://doi.org/10.1177/0148607109333114.

Merrill, L. (2015). Prevention, treatment and parent education for diaper dermatitis. *Nursing for Women's Health*, *19*(4), 326–336.

Mohr, L. D., Reyna, R., & Amaya, R. (2014). Neonatal case studies using active Leptospermum honey. *Journal of Wound, Ostomy, and Continence Nursing*, *41*, 213–218. https://doi.org/10.1097/WON0000000000000028.

Moiser, M. J., Bernal, N., & Farakas, I. (2017). *National Burn Repository 2017 update: Report of data from 2008–2017* (13th ed.). American Burn Association.

Mooney, J. F., Argenta, L. C., Marks, M. W., Morykwas, A. J., & DeFranzo, A. J. (2000). Treatment of soft tissue defects in pediatric patients using the V.A.C. system. *Clinical Orthopaedics and Related Research*, *376*, 26–31. https://doi.org/10.1097/00003086-200007000-00005.

Nanavati, R. N., Balan, R., & Kabra, N. S. (2013). Effect of kangaroo mother care vs expressed breast milk administration on pain associated with removal of adhesive tape in very low birth weight neonates: A randomized controlled trial. *Indian Pediatrics*, *50*, 1011–1015.

Nie, A. M. (2020). Pressure injury prevention and treatment in critically ill children. *Critical Care Nursing Clinics of North America*, *32*(4), 521–531. https://doi.org/10.1016/j.cnc.2020.08.003.

Noonan, C., Quigley, S., & Curley, M. A. Q. (2006). Skin integrity in hospitalized infants and children: A prevalence survey. *Journal of Pediatric Nursing*, *21*(6), 445–453. https://doi.org/10.1016/jpedn.2006.07.002.

Oni, G., Brown, S., & Kenkel, J. (2012). Comparison of five commonly-available, lidocaine-containing topical anesthetics and their effect on serum levels of lidocaine and its metabolite monoethylglycinexylidide (MEGX). *Aesthetic Surgery Journal*, *32*(4), 495–503. https://doi.org/10.1177/1090820X12442672

Oquendo, M., Agrawal, V., Reyna, R., Patel, H., Emran, M. A., & Almond, P. S. (2015). Silver-impregnated hydrofiber dressing followed by delayed surgical closure for management of infants born with giant omphaloceles. *Journal of Pediatric Surgery*, *50*, 1668–1672. https://doi.org/10.1016/j jpedsurg 2015 06 011.

Ranade, D., & Collins, N. (2011). Nutrition 411: Children with wounds: The importance of nutrition. *Ostomy Wound*, *57*(10), 14–24. https://www.o-wm.com/article/nutrition-411-children-wounds-importance-nutrition.

Razmus, I., & Bergquist-Beringer, S. (2017). Pressure ulcer risk and prevention practices in pediatric patients: A secondary analysis of date from the national database of nursing quality indicators. *Ostomy Wound Management*, *63*(2), 28–32. PMID: 28267681.

Reed, R. C., Johnson, D. E., & Nie, A. M. (2021). Preterm infant skin structure is qualitatively and quantitatively different from that of term newborns. *Pediatric and Developmental Pathology: The Official Journal of the Society for Pediatric Pathology and the Paediatric Pathology Society*, *24*(2), 96–102. https://doi.org/10.1177/1093526620976831.

Rentea, R. M., Somers, K. K., Cassidy, L., Enters, J., & Arca, M. J. (2013). Negative pressure wound therapy in infants and children: A single-institution experience. *The Journal of Surgical Research*, *184*(1), 658–864. https://doi.org/10.1016/j.jss.2013.05.056.

Richardson, L., Banerjee, S., & Rabe, H. (2006). What is the evidence on the practice of mucous fistula refeeding in neonates with short bowel syndrome? *Journal of Pediatric Gastroenterology and Nutrition, 43*(2), 267–270.

Rustogi, R., Mill, J., Fraser, J. F., & Kimble, R. M. (2005). The use of acticoat in neonatal burns. *Burns, 31*, 878–882. https://doi.org/10.1016/jburns2005 04 030.

Santosa, K. B., Keller, M., Olsen, M. A., Keane, A. M., Sears, E. D., & Snyder-Warwick, A. K. (2019). Negative-pressure wound therapy in infants and children: A population-based study. *The Journal of Surgical Research, 235*, 560–568. https://doi.org/10.1016/j.jss.2018.10.043.

Sardesai, S., Kornacka, M., Walas, W., & Ramanathan, R. (2011). Iatrogenic skin injury in the neonatal intensive care unit. *The Journal of Maternal-Fetal and Neonatal Medicine, 24*(2), 197–203. https://doi.org/10.3109/14767051003728245.

Sawatzky-Dickson, D., & Bodnaryk, K. (2006). Neonatal intravenous extravasation injuries: Evaluation of a wound care protocol. *Neonatal Network, 25*(1), 13–19. https://doi.org/10.1891/0730-0832.25.1.13.

Schindler, C., Mikhailov, T. A., Kuhn, E. M., Christopher, J., Conway, P., Riddling, D., et al. (2011). Protecting fragile skin: Nursing interventions to decrease development of pressure ulcers in pediatric intensive care. *American Journal of Critical Care, 20*(1), 26–34. https://doi.org/10.4037/ajcc2011754.

Shields, W. C., McDonald, E., Frattaroli, S., Perry, E. C., Zhu, J., & Gielen, A. C. (2013). Still too hot: Examination of water temperature and water heater characteristics 24 years after manufacturers adopt voluntary temperature setting. *Journal of Burn Care & Research, 34*(2), 281–287. https://doi.org/10.1097/BCR.0b013e31827e645f.

Shin, H. T. (2014). Diagnosis and management of diaper dermatitis. *Pediatric Clinics of North America, 61*(2), 367–382. https://doi.org/10.1016/j.pcl.2013.11.009.

Skillman, H. E., & Wischmeyer, P. E. (2008). Nutrition therapy in critically ill infants and children. *JPEN Journal of Parenteral and Enteral Nutrition, 32*(5), 520–534. https://doi.org/10.1177/0148607108322398.

Smith, E., & Shell, T. (2017). *Delayed Bathing, International Childbirth Education Association (ICEA) position paper.* Retrieved 8/29/2020 from: https://icea.org/wp-content/uploads/2018/02/ICEA-Position-Paper-Delayed-Bathing.pdf.

Steen, E. H., Want, X., Boochoon, K. C., Ewing, D. E., Strang, H. E., Kaul, A., et al. (2020). Wound healing and wound care in neonates: Current therapies and novel options. *Advances in Skin & Wound Care, 33*(6), 294–300. https://doi.org/10.1097/01.ASW.0000661804.09496.8c.

Stevens, B., Yamada, J., Ohlsson, A., Haliburton, S., & Shorkey, A. (2016). Sucrose for analgesia in newborn infants undergoing painful procedures. *Cochrane Database of Systematic Reviews, 7*(7), CD001069. https://doi.org/10.1002/14651858.CD001069.pub5.

Suddaby, E. C., Barnett, S. C., & Facteau, L. (2006). Skin breakdown in acute care pediatrics. *Dermatology Nursing, 18*(2), 155–161. PMID: 16708678.

Taddio, A., Soin, H. K., Schuh, S., Koren, G., & Scolnik, D. (2005). Liposomal lidocaine to improve procedural success rates and reduce procedural pain among children: A randomized controlled trial. *CMAJ : Canadian Medical Association journal = journal de l'Association medicale canadienne, 172*(13), 1691–1695. https://doi.org/10.1503/cmaj.045316.

Tenenhaus, M., Greenberg, M., & Potenza, B. (2014). Dehydrated human amnion/chorion membrane for the treatment of severe skin and tissue loss in an preterm infant: A case report. *Journal of Wound Care, 23*, 492–495.

Thigpen, J. L. (2007). Peripheral intravenous extravasation: Nursing procedure for initial treatment. *Neonatal Network, 26*(6), 379–384. https://doi.org/10.1891/0730-0832.26.6.379.

Thompson, N. M. (2019). Nursing care and management of gastrostomy and gastrojejunostomy tubes in the pediatric population. *Journal of Pediatric Surgical Nursing, 8*(4), 97–111.

Turnage-Carrier, C., McLane, K. M., & Gregurich, M. A. (2008). Interface pressure comparison of healthy premature infants with various neonatal bed surfaces. *Advances in Neonatal Care, 8*(3), 176–184. https://doi.org/10.1097/01.ANC.0000324342.32464.83.

U.S. Food and Drug Administration. (2022). Part 347—Skin protectant drug products for over-the-counter human use. Active ingredients. *Code of Federal Regulations. Title 21.* Retrieved January 3, 2023 from: https://www.accessdata.fda.gov/scripts/cdrh/cfdocs/cfcfr/cfrsearch.cfm?fr=347.10.

Vanzi, V., & Pitaro, R. (2018). Skin injuries and chlorhexidine gluconate-based antisepsis in early premature infants: A case report and review of the literature. *The Journal of Perinatal & Neonatal Nursing, 32*(4), 341–350. https://doi.org/10.1097/JPN.0000000000000334.

Wiley, J., Smith, W. J., & Jacob, S. E. (2009). The role of allergic contact dermatitis in diaper dermatitis. *Pediatric Dermatology, 26*(3), 369–370. https://doi.org/10.1111/j.1525-1470.2009.00934.x.

Willock, J., Baharestani, M. M., & Anthony, D. (2008). The development of the glamorgan paediatric pressure ulcer risk assessment scale. *Journal of Wound Care, 18*(1), 17–21. https://doi.org/10.12968/jcyn.2007.1.5.27446.

World Health Organization (WHO). (2018a). *Preterm Birth.* Retrieved 6/10/2022 from: https://www.who.int/news-room/fact-sheets/detail/preterm-birth.

World Health Organization. (2018b). *WHO recommendations: intrapartum care for a positive childbirth experience.* Geneva: WHO. Retrieved 10/9/2020 from: https://apps.who.int/iris/bitstream/handle/10665/260178/9789241550215-eng.pdf;jsessionid=7E800B590A164DC7FC879E73B480D6FC?sequence=1.

Wound, Ostomy and Continence Nurses Society (WOCN). (2016). *Guideline for management of pressure ulcers (WOCN® clinical practice guideline series no. 2).* Mt. Laurel: WOCN®.

Wound, Ostomy and Continence Nurses Society (WOCN), American Urological Association (AUA), and American Society of Colorectal Surgions (ASCRS) Position Statement on Preoperative Stoma Site Marking for Patients Undergoing Ostomy Surgery. (2021). *Journal of Wound, Ostomy, and Continence Nursing, 48*(6), 533–536.

FURTHER READING

Bissinger, R. L., & Annibale, D. J. (2010). Thermoregulation in very low-birth-weight infants during the golden hour. *Advances in Neonatal Care, 10*(5), 230–238. https://doi.org/10.1091097/ANC.0b013e31811f0ae63.

Dedmond, B. T., Kortesis, B., Punger, K., Simpson, J., Argenta, J., Kulp, B., et al. (2007). The use of negative-pressure wound therapy (NPWT) in the temporary treatment of soft-tissue injuries associated with high-energy open tibial shaft fractures. *Journal of Orthopaedic Trauma, 21*(1), 11–17. https://doi.org/10.1097/BOT.0b013e31802cbc54.

Dolack, M., Huffines, B., Stikes, R., Hayes, P., & Logsdon, M. C. (2013). Updated neonatal skin risk assessment scale (NSRAS). *Kentucky Nurse, 61*(4), 6. PMID: 24260847.

Hickey, K. J., Anderson, C. J., & Vogel, L. C. (2000). Pressure ulcers in pediatric spinal cord injury. *Topics in Spinal Cord Injection Rehabilitation, 6*(Suppl), 85–90. https://doi.org/10.1310/1C86-7L96-1JAR-7Y3N.

Horn, P. L., Ruth, B., & Kean, J. R. (2007). Use of wound V.A.C. therapy in pediatric patients with infected spinal wounds: A retrospective review. *Orthopedic Nursing, 26*(5), 317–324. https://doi.org/10.1097/01.NOR.0000295960.94450.69.

Kelechi, T. J., Arndt, J. V., & Dove, A. (2013). Review of pressure ulcer risk assessment scales. *Journal of Wound, Ostomy, and Continence Nursing, 40*(3), 232–236. https://doi.org/10.1097/WON.0b013e31828f2049.

Murray, J. S., Noonan, C., Quigley, S., et al. (2013). Medical device-related hospital-acquired pressure ulcers in children: An integrative review. *Journal of Pediatric Nursing, 28*(6), 585–595.

Neri, I., Ravaioli, G. M., Faldella, G., Capretti, M. G., Arcuri, S., & Patrizi, A. (2017). Chlorehexidine-induced chemical burns in very low birth weight infants. The Journal of Pediatrics, 191, 262–265.e2. https://doi.org/10.1016/jpeds.2017.08.002.

Noonan, C., Quigley, S., & Curley, M. A. Q. (2011). Using the Braden Q scale to predict pressure ulcer risk in pediatric patients. *Journal of Pediatric Nursing, 26*(6), 566–575. https://doi.org/10.1016/j.pedn.2010.07.006.

Odio, M., & Thaman, L. (2014). Diapering, diaper technology, and diaper area skin health. *Pediatric Dermatology, 31S*(S1), 9–14. https://doi.org/10.1111/pde.12501.

Sandberg, F., Viktorsdóttir, M. B., Salö, M., Stenström, P., & Arnbjörnsson, E. (2018). Comparison of major complications in children after laparoscopy-assisted gastrostomy and percutaneous endoscopic gastrostomy placement: A meta-analysis. *Pediatric Surgery International, 34,* 1321–1327.

Vender, R. B. (2003). Adverse reactions to herbal therapy in dermatology. *Skin Therapy Letter, 8*(3), 5–8. PMID: 12858233.

Wesner, E., Vassantachart, J. M., & Jacob, S. E. (2019). Art of prevention: the importance of proper diapering practices. *International Journal of Women's Dermatology, 5,* 233–234.

38

Managing Wounds in Palliative Care and End of life

Ruth A. Bryant and Victoria Nalls

Palliative care is a medical competency associated with serious illness and with patient-centered goals such as relief from distressing symptoms, easing of pain, and enhanced quality of life. When healing the wound is not an appropriate or realistic goal, the goal is palliation or maintenance. Many factors influence whether the goal is wound healing or palliation. This chapter describes the patient situations in which palliative wound care would be appropriate, the types of wounds that may be associated with palliation, and the principles of palliative wound care. Among the many challenges facing patients in palliative or hospice care are the issues surrounding skin and wound care. Because untreated wounds can lead to physical discomfort and impair quality of life, it is appropriate that they receive attention.

DEFINITION OF TERMS

Palliative care refers to a holistic approach that includes physical, functional, psychological, practical, and spiritual concerns of patients with serious illness and their caregivers through expert management of pain and other symptoms along with supporting caregiver needs (National Consensus Project, 2018). Palliative care is not synonymous with the abandonment of hope or treatment options. No specific therapies are excluded if they can improve the patient's quality of life and align with the patient's goals of care (National Consensus Project, 2018; Tippett, Sherman, Woo, Swezey, & Posthauer, 2012/2018). In fact, palliative care is ideally a general approach to patient care that should be routinely integrated into primary care and should occur concurrently with other treatments. Palliative care is not limited to end-of-life

situations. Although it is indicated for patients with a life-threatening condition, it is also relevant for those with a debilitating illness that encompasses a broad range of diagnoses, including people who are living with a persistent or recurring illness that adversely affects their daily functioning or will predictably reduce life expectancy (National Consensus Project, 2018). Palliative care focuses on the palliative journey from diagnosis onward rather than focusing on the last days of life (Westwood, 2014). Therefore, palliative care services are indicated across the trajectory of a patient's illness and are not restricted to the end-of-life phase (National Consensus Project, 2018). Specialists in palliative care, those who have received formal education in palliative care and are credentialed in the field, may be consulted to provide specialty-level palliative care when the complexity of the situation warrants (National Consensus Project, 2018).

Hospice care is a specific type of palliative care and focuses on alleviation of distressing symptoms and maximizing quality of life; however, Medicare and Medicaid regulations state that patients must have a defined, time-limited prognosis of 6 months or less to live and forego curative therapies to be eligible for hospice (National Consensus Project, 2018).

When the patient enters the terminal stage of an illness or condition, curative treatments are no longer effective, and/or the patient no longer desires to continue them, hospice becomes the care of choice. Hospice provides comprehensive biomedical, psychosocial, and spiritual support as patients face the end of life (AAHPM, 2008; National Consensus Project, 2018). The key difference between palliative care and hospice is that palliative care is appropriate, regardless of the stage of the disease or the need for other therapies and can be rendered along with life-prolonging treatment as the main focus of care (Westwood, 2014).

PALLIATIVE WOUND CARE

The International Palliative Wound Care Initiative (Ferris, Khateib, Fromantin, et al., 2007) defines palliative wound care as "the evolving body of knowledge and skills that take a holistic approach to relieving suffering and improving quality of life for patients and families living with chronic wounds, whether the wound is healable or not." In a concept analysis, Emmons and Lachman (2010) described palliative wound care as a holistic and integrated approach to care that addresses symptom management and psychosocial well-being, is multidisciplinary, is driven by patient/family goals, and is integrated into everyday wound care principles and practice. An important aspect of palliative wound care is the management of symptoms such as odor, exudate, bleeding, pain, and infection and maintenance of skin integrity. Prevention of wound deterioration is desirable but is not always realistic, as with a fungating wound (Cornish, 2019; Tilley, Lipson, & Ramos, 2016). Palliative care is elected care rather than care that is forced on the patient; the focus is on physical, psychosocial, and spiritual issues during end of life (National Consensus Statement, 2018).

Indications

Palliative wound care as a goal of wound management is often related to terminal illness or end of life when healing interventions are inconsistent with the patient's goals. However, palliative wound care may also be indicated when the underlying etiology or existing cofactors cannot be overcome as a result of advanced illness and poor physical state. Although malignancies and metastases are commonly associated with palliative wound care, the patient's condition and situation will also dictate the need for palliative wound care. Palliation as a goal for wound management may be indicated in the following situations:

1. *The patient is terminally ill.* Most often this is a patient who has cancer, but it could just as well be a patient who has end-stage renal disease or end-stage congestive heart failure. The wound could be an open surgical wound, pressure injury, neuropathic foot ulcer, venous ulcer, burn, malignant fungating wound, radiation dermatitis, etc.

2. *Overwhelming comorbidities are present.* As an example, a patient may have significant hypotension after a massive cardiac arrest and require high doses of a vasopressor medication to achieve an adequate blood pressure. The resulting vasoconstriction may be sufficient enough to cause a gradual transition in the fingertips or toes to cyanosis and then necrosis. Clearly the comorbidities dictate that the priority is sustaining adequate blood pressure.

3. *Patient choice.* This is the situation where a patient does not have overwhelming comorbidities, or a terminal illness yet simply chooses palliation as a goal. Possible reasons may include a preference to continue a certain lifestyle that jeopardizes wound healing, a realization that the

modifications needed for treatment are not feasible or consistent with other priorities, a financial burden, or a decision based on the patient's age.

Types of Wounds Common to Palliative Care

The etiology of wounds in the patient receiving palliative care can be nonmalignancy or malignancy related. The nonmalignant wound common in palliative care is the wound that develops from mechanical trauma (e.g., unrelieved pressure, shear, friction, skin stripping), moisture-associated skin damage (MASD) (urinary incontinence, fecal incontinence, etc.), or infection (e.g., candidiasis or herpes). These nonmalignant wounds are prevented and managed with the same interventions, resources, and tools described throughout this textbook. Malignancy-related wounds may be a primary tumor, metastasis, or malignant transformation. Malignancy-related wounds have common wound characteristics that warrant unique kinds of care.

NONMALIGNANCY-RELATED WOUNDS

Any type of wound can be observed in a patient receiving palliative or hospice care. Some of the most common include nonpressure related ulcers, skin tears, and chemical or radiation dermatitis; pressure injuries are the most common wound in palliative care (Dale & Emmons, 2014; Ferris, Price & Harding, 2019; Tippett et al., 2012/2018). Ferris and colleagues (2019) report that the sacrum is the most common site of pressure injuries in palliative care patients.

The frequency of pressure injuries in the patient receiving palliative or hospice care is varied, with a prevalence reported as high as 47% (Hendrichova, Castelli, Mastroianni, et al., 2010; Moore, Johanssen, & van Etten, 2013; Tippett, 2005). Galvin (2002) found 26.1% of patients admitted to a palliative care program over a 2-year timeframe had a pressure injury, and 12% of all patients admitted to the palliative care setting developed a pressure injury during their stay. Within hospice programs, the literature reports an incidence of pressure injuries ranging from 10% to 17.5%; prevalence is reported at 27% (Reifsnyder & Magee, 2005; Tippett, 2005). In a small study of a single hospice program, a total of 35% of patients had some type of skin issue, 50% of them being pressure injuries (Tippett, 2005).

Pressure Injury Prevention

While skin deterioration or "failure" may occur at the end of life, the development of a pressure injury should not be expected or assumed to be unavoidable. Pressure injury prevention and skin care are critically important components of palliative care (Beldon, 2011; Sibbald, Krasner, & Lutz, 2010; Vickery et al., 2020; Westwood, 2014). As many as 10% of patients develop a new pressure injury within the first 3 months of admission to a hospice program (Reifsnyder & Magee, 2005). Of interest, however, in a survey of inpatient palliative care units, only 61% had a written policy for pressure injury prevention, 17.6% indicated their policy was under development, and 19.6% reported they did not have a policy. A pressure injury prevention program has been presented in detail in Chapter 11. In the palliative care setting, risk assessment and prevention have a few unique considerations.

Risk Assessment

International guidelines recommend pressure injury risk assessment for palliative care patients on a regular basis using a structured, consistent approach (EPUAP, NPIAP, & PPPIA, 2019). Rather than assessing pressure injury risk solely by completing a risk assessment tool, it is also recommended to use a validated risk assessment tool, a comprehensive skin assessment, *and* clinical judgment with regard to key risk factors. The Marie Curie Centre's Hunters Hill Risk Assessment tool (recommended by the EPUAP, NPIAP, and PPPIA guideline), Palliative Performance Scale (PPS), the F.R.A.I.L. Healing Probability Assessment Tool and the Hospice Pressure Ulcer Risk Assessment Scale (HoRT) were designed and tested specifically for the individual at or near the end of life (Baik et al., 2018; Chaplin, 2000; Chrisman, 2010; EPUAP, NPIAP, & PPPIA, 2019; Henoch & Gustaffson, 2003; Woo, Krasner, Kennedy, et al., 2015). In contrast, many experts suggest that *every* palliative care patient should be considered at "high risk" for pressure injury development (Richards et al., 2007; Walding, 2005). Risk assessment should be obtained within 6 to 12 hours of admission and reassessed on a daily basis because of the speed with which the palliative patient's condition can change (Chaplin & McGill, 1999).

Factors that contribute to pressure injury formation in palliative care patients include fragile skin condition, older age, decreasing food and fluid intake, altered sensation, poor general physical condition, decreased mobility, pain, compromised immunity, poor oxygenation, and lean body type (Naylor, 2005; Woo et al., 2015). Of interest, Artico et al. (2018) found that being obese or severely thin and having a low PPS were some of the predictors of pressure ulcers in home palliative care. It has also been shown that palliative patients with advanced age, advanced wound age, and low PPS are more likely to suffer from unhealed wounds (Lai, Yip, & Sham, 2019). One-fourth of all palliative home care patients experienced the inability to lie flat because of shortness of breath, which increased the patient's risk for pressure injury. Thus repositioning may exacerbate shortness of breath and require a modification in the standard of care to utilize a higher level of support surface so that repositioning can be less frequent.

Prevention

Pressure injury prevention interventions are vital for the palliative care patient population, particularly because the development and resulting treatment often are painful (Navaid, Melvin, Berube, & Dotson, 2010). At the same time, the pressure injury prevention plan of care must be reflective of and consistent with the patient's clinical picture and end-of-life goals. Reducing or eliminating some risk factors may not

be achievable or in accordance with the comfort-focused goals of palliative care (Navaid et al., 2010; Vickery et al., 2020). For example, maintaining the head of the bed lower than 30 degrees or turning the patient every 2 hours may not be realistic or consistent with the patient's wishes. In these instances, complete patient and family education becomes more critical than ever so that the patient and family are fully informed before they make decisions that may increase the risk for pressure injury. At the same time, it is the responsibility of the wound care provider to recommend the support surface that would best redistribute coccyx pressure while accommodating the patient's need for an elevated head of bed. The challenge is to accommodate the patient's unique needs by using creative and potentially less common pressure injury prevention interventions. The international pressure ulcer treatment guidelines (EPUAP, NPIAP, & PPPIA, 2019) instruct the care provider to consider changing the support surface to improve pressure redistribution and comfort.

Prevention measures that are most universally appropriate in palliative care include (1) adequate and appropriate offloading with a support surface; (2) adequate pain control so that optimal positioning is possible; and (3) incontinence management (containment and skin protection). However, good pain management is critical to being able to provide these basic prevention interventions (Dale & Emmons, 2014). The international guidelines stipulate the patient should be premedicated 20–30 min before a scheduled position change when he or she experiences significant pain with movement (EPUAP, NPIAP, & PPPIA, 2019).

Although there is no validated algorithm to determine whether a pressure injury is preventable or unavoidable, the Centers for Medicare and Medicaid (CMS), along with the National Pressure Injury Advisory Panel (NPIAP) and the Wound, Ostomy, and Continence Nurses Society (WOCN Society), has provided definitions and consensus statements in support of the concept of an unavoidable pressure injuries at end of life (Ayello et al., 2019). The CMS State Operations Manual for Long Term Care Facilities also acknowledges the Kennedy Terminal Ulcer as a potential outcome at end of life and an unavoidable pressure injury. Lastly, the Trombley Brennan Terminal Tissue Injury is also being described in palliative care literature (Trombley, Brennan, Thomas, & Kline, 2012; Brennan, Thomas, & Kline, 2019; Ayello et al., 2019). Despite this support, the debate continues whether pressure injuries in palliative and hospice patients can be prevented. Regardless of the outcome of this debate, it is incumbent on the wound specialist to provide care that is compliant with national guidelines for the prevention of pressure injuries and to diligently avoid withholding preventive interventions based on the designation of palliative or end-of-life care. Furthermore, documentation should record the implementation of assessments and interventions reflective of the guidelines, as well as when interventions were withheld and why. A nosocomial pressure injury then can be considered inevitable when it develops even though the care provided met the standard of care for pressure injury prevention.

Pressure Injury Care

Pressure injury care in the palliative care patient should closely follow the international guidelines on pressure injury treatment and deviate from that standard only as needed and indicated by the international guidelines (EPUAP, NPIAP, & PPPIA, 2019). Overall, the palliative care guidelines encourage comfort, prompt symptom management, consistency between care provided and the patient's goals, and change guided by the values and goals of the patient and family. Specific and unique issues relative to exudate control, pain control, odor control, debridement, assessment and monitoring of healing, and dressing selection are discussed later in this chapter.

MALIGNANCY-RELATED WOUNDS

Malignancy-related wounds can be a primary cutaneous tumor, a metastasis, or a malignant transformation of an existing ulcer. The common primary cutaneous tumors that can present as a wound are untreated basal cell cancer (see Plate 92), squamous cell cancer (see Plate 93a), and malignant melanoma (Gerlach, 2005). A primary tumor also can invade through the skin layers and erode through the skin to form a malignant wound (Hampton, 2008). Although any tumor left untreated can cause a malignant wound, the most common cancers are breast and soft tissue sarcoma (Tilley et al., 2016). A tumor can metastasize to the skin when it has invaded blood or lymph vessels; consequently, circulating malignant cells become trapped in the tiny skin capillaries. Seeding of malignant cells can occur during surgery to the abdominal wall, for example. Cancer of the ovary, cecum, and rectum can infiltrate the anterior wall of the abdomen (Grocott, 2007).

Malignant Cutaneous Wounds

Collectively, any wound that is a primary or metastatic skin lesion is referred to as a *malignant cutaneous wound,* also commonly known as a *fungating malignant wound* (see Plate 93b). These malignant cutaneous wounds usually are chronic, ulcerating, open, and draining (Recka, Montagnini, & Vitale, 2012).

A malignant cutaneous wound begins as a small, firm nodule under the surface of the skin that may be flesh colored, pink, red, violet, or brown (Tandler & Stephen-Haynes, 2017). As the malignant cells proliferate, they interfere with the capillaries and lymph vessels. Although the tumor develops its own microcirculation, it is disorganized and has impaired blood-clotting abilities (Tilley et al., 2016). These lesions can develop into necrotic "cauliflowerlike" eruptions on the skin that progress to become exudative and hemorrhagic. Anaerobic organisms (usually *Bacteroides*) flourish on the necrotic tissue and produce volatile fatty acids as metabolic end-products that are responsible for the characteristic pungent and penetrating odor; this odor is a source of great embarrassment and distress to the patient, family, and caregivers (Draper, 2005; Tandler & Stephen-Haynes, 2017). One in ten patients with a metastatic disease has cutaneous metastases (Recka et al., 2012). The patient with a malignant cutaneous wound may have no symptoms or may experience pruritus, pain, stinging, exudate, odor, and thickening and hardening of the skin (Alexander, 2010; Tandler & Stephen-Haynes, 2017; Tilley et al., 2016).

Patients with malignant cutaneous wounds have a poor outcome. Treatment options for patients with fungating malignant wounds are aimed at the underlying pathology and include radiotherapy, chemotherapy, hormone therapy, surgery, cryotherapy, or laser therapy. External beam radiation therapy may be used to control local metastases, which in turn may help control malignant cutaneous wound symptoms.

Malignant cutaneous wounds are often misinterpreted initially as an ulcer with an etiology of pressure, arterial insufficiency, or pyoderma. When the wound fails to progress despite appropriate topical therapy, cancer should be suspected, and biopsies obtained from at least four different locations in the base of the wound. These kinds of wounds will appear abnormal (e.g., thickened, rolled wound edges) and should be thoroughly assessed (Gerlach, 2005).

Marjolin Ulcer

Malignant transformation of an existing ulcer occurs in approximately 2% of all chronic wounds (e.g., pressure ulcer, sinus tract, irradiated skin, burn wound, venous ulcer). The site of chronic irritation and inflammation is a common location for this malignant transformation, otherwise called a *Marjolin ulcer,* which tends to be an aggressive tumor. Treatment is based on the size and extent of the wound and the condition of the patient (Khan, Schafer, & Wood, 2020).

OBJECTIVES IN THE CARE OF THE MALIGNANT CUTANEOUS WOUND

Wound management decisions are a balance of meeting the patient's priorities and achieving the identified aims arising from the comprehensive assessment (Tilley et al., 2016; Woo et al., 2015). Goals of care and treatment priorities are negotiated with each patient based on the stage of the underlying disease process and the potential for available therapeutic options to be beneficial and meet personal preferences (Woo, 2017). Above all, quality of life is the guiding principle when planning patient care (British Columbia Cancer Agency, 2015).

In most situations, the quality of care given to the patient with a malignant fungating wound is the most important factor in determining their quality of life (Tilley et al., 2016). The priorities of topical care address the common symptoms of a malignant wound: odor, exudate, pain, bleeding, and pruritus. Interventions include control of bioburden, debridement, exudate-absorbent dressings, wound cleansing, and protection of the surrounding skin, as summarized in Table 38.1 and described in the following sections.

TABLE 38.1   Interventions for Palliative Wound Care

Pain Management	Odor Management	Exudate Control
• Nontraumatic Dressing Changes – Contact layer – Gauzes, nonadherent or coated – Foam – Protective barrier films – Nontraumatic tapes	• Wound Cleansing – Ionic cleansers – Sodium-impregnated gauze – Antimicrobials	• Exudate Absorption or Containment – Foam, alginates, hydrofiber dressings, absorptive powders – Wound drainage pouch
• Periwound Skin Management – Nontraumatic tapes – Skin sealants (alcohol free) – Barrier ointment or cream – Hydrocolloid wafer	• Deodorizers – Charcoal dressings – Chloromycetin solution – Metronidazole gel	• Indicators for Dressing Changes – When pooling on intact skin occurs – When strikethrough occurs
	• Debridement – Hydrogel and enzymes for dry, hard, necrotic tissue – Absorptive dressings, copolymer dressings, polysaccharide beads or starch for exudative, slough filled wounds	• Control of Bleeding – Hemostatic dressings – Nonadherent gauze – Alginates – Sliver nitrate – Monsel's solution
	• Reduction of Bacterial Burden – Irrigation with ionic cleansers – Antimicrobial dressings and creams – Absorptive dressings – Sodium-impregnated gauze – Oral antimicrobials	

Control Pain and Pruritus

Causes of pain in the malignant wound may be multiple and include emotional factors, neuropathic pain (due to nerve damage from the tumor), and procedural pain, as occurs with dressing removal (Tilley et al., 2016) (see Chapter 28) for detailed information related to pain assessment and management). When pain is related to underlying disease, practitioners, including interventional radiologists, anesthesiology pain specialists, radiation oncologists, surgical oncologists, and pharmacists, should be part of the team helping to manage complex pain issues (Krouse, 2008). In addition to systemic analgesia and rapid-onset, short-acting analgesics administered before beginning dressing changes, topical anesthetics can be used to control pain (Brinker, Protus, & Kimbrel, 2018). Topical lidocaine or benzocaine or ice packs applied before or after wound care may be beneficial (Woo, 2017; Woo et al., 2015). Topical eutectic mixture of local anesthetic cream (EMLA 5%) (containing lidocaine with prilocaine) has been used to reduce pain intensity (Brinker et al., 2018). EMLA should be applied in a thick layer and covered with plastic film, for 30–45 min before dressing change to allow time for anesthetic effects to develop (Chrisman, 2010). Diligence is required in the use of EMLA cream because it has a pH of 9.4 and can penetrate damaged skin. Daily application of a topical opioid-infused amorphous hydrogel (10 mg morphine sulfate in 8 g of hydrogel) has been used anecdotally to manage painful pressure ulcers

and malignant wounds (Ashfield, 2005; Back & Finlay, 1995), as well as in randomized controlled studies (Zeppetella, Paul, & Ribeiro, 2003; Zeppetella & Ribeiro, 2005), with significantly improved pain control compared with pretreatment medications. Similar results have been reported with use of either crushed oxycodone or meperidine topically in two patients with sickle cell ulcers (Ballas, 2002). Nociceptive pain should also be managed with nonsteroidal antiinflammatory medications (Woo et al., 2015). Nonpharmacologic measures for pain management include heat or cold, energy therapies (i.e., Reiki, healing touch), relaxation and deep breathing, mindfulness meditation, hypnosis, and the use of "time-outs" (Woo et al., 2015).

Although a malignant or fungating wound is characteristically painful, a key source of pain is the trauma associated with dressing changes. Consequently, controlling or minimizing pain requires attention to the reduction or elimination of mechanical trauma and preventing medical adhesive–related skin injury (MARSI). Two primary interventions are (1) minimization of trauma associated with dressing changes by using nonadhesive dressings and (2) infrequent dressing changes. The malignant or fungating wound site has an increased tendency to bleed when disturbed, which may aggravate the presence of pain. Infrequent dressing changes reduce the potential for bleeding. When bleeding is a concern, appropriate dressings that do not adhere to the wound surface will reduce the potential for a bleeding episode and must be selected.

The malignant wound often triggers pruritus at the wound site as the skin tissues stretch in response to the growing tumor. Diphenhydramine or hydroxyzine may be warranted to manage the pruritus and moisturizers applied to keep the periwound skin supple (Brinker et al., 2018).

Atraumatic Dressing Changes

Nonadhesive but absorbent dressings are recommended to achieve atraumatic dressing removal. Dressing selection options include a contact-layer dressing, nonadherent gauze, impregnated gauze (e.g., hydrogel- or petrolatum-impregnated gauze), and semipermeable foam dressings. To eliminate unnecessary dressing changes, dressings that have a long wearing time should be selected and preferably changed no more often than every 3 days (Brinker et al., 2018). However, once-daily dressing changes may be necessary for the highly exudative wound. Protective barrier films, particularly those without alcohol, can be applied to the surrounding skin to further decrease trauma to periwound skin. Atraumatic tapes and mesh netting can be used to secure dressings, thereby avoiding trauma to the surrounding skin on removal.

Control or Prevent Bleeding

Erosion of capillaries can lead to significant spontaneous bleeding. Atraumatic dressing removal is critical to avoid precipitating a bleeding episode. If bleeding occurs even with the use of atraumatic dressing removal techniques, direct pressure, and an ice pack can be applied initially. If these are ineffective, many different types of dressings and products are available that assist in the control of bleeding (see Table 38.1). Monsel's solution (ferric subsulfate) has been shown to be an effective adjunct to compression for hemostasis (Alvarez, Kalinski, Nusbaum, et al., 2007). A comprehensive wound assessment should direct the choice of which dressing is most appropriate. Absorbable hemostatic dressings and silver nitrate cautery sticks can be used to specifically control small bleeding points. Alginates have been demonstrated to exhibit hemostatic effects and have been useful for heavily exudative wounds. Nonadherent gauze is an option that will absorb exudate without adhering to the wound bed. Significant bleeding events may require oral antifibrinolytics, radiotherapy, and embolization. Although vasoconstrictive effects can result in ischemia and consequently necrosis, gauze saturated with topical adrenaline 1:1000 may be applied for emergent situations; however, the patient should be monitored for systemic absorption of the medications (Grocott, 1999; Seaman, 2006). These more aggressive options are appropriate if they will improve the quality of life in patients with a malignant wound (Seaman, 2006).

Manage Periwound Skin

The nature of wounds occurring in palliative care predisposes toward maceration and denudement, and care should focus on preventing epidermal stripping, maceration, contact dermatitis, infection, and moisture-associated skin damage (Beers, 2019; Stephen-Haynes, 2008; Woo et al., 2015). Routine skin assessments should be obtained to monitor for signs and symptoms of bacterial infection (induration, localized erythema, heat, pain) and fungal infection (erythematous, papular rash). Interventions to protect the fragile periwound skin include nonadhesive dressings, alcohol-free protective barrier films, and bracketing the wound bed with skin barrier strips to serve as a barrier to exudate and an anchor for adhesives. Additional measures to protect periwound skin are described in Chapter 9.

Control Odor

Malodor is recognized as having a physical and psychological impact by reducing appetite, affecting well-being, causing social isolation, and distorting body image (Fletcher, 2008; Tilley et al., 2016; West, 2007). Odor can be caused by necrotic tissue, bacterial burden, infection, or saturated dressings. Objective assessment for the presence of odor is difficult, so subjective reporting by the patient should guide interventions; odor is often reported as the most distressing symptom to patients and caregivers (Cornish, 2019; Tilley et al., 2016).

Interventions appropriate for the management of odor include wound cleansing, topical deodorizers, room deodorizers, topical and oral antimicrobials, debridement, carbon dressings, and manuka honey (Chrisman, 2010; Tilley et al., 2016). Many of these interventions can be used simultaneously to aggressively attack the problem of odor. Topical metronidazole gel (0.75%–0.80%) is associated with control of anaerobic bacteria and protozoal infections. It is applied directly to the wound once daily for 5 to 7 days or more as needed. Metronidazole tablets may also be crushed and placed on the wound bed (Chrisman, 2010; Winardi & Irwan, 2019). In a systematic review of the literature examining topical agents to reduce odor in malignant wounds, da Costa Santos, de Mattos Pimenta, and Nobre (2010) found that topical metronidazole, sodium-impregnated gauze, charcoal or activated charcoal dressings, and curcumin ointment yielded a grade B (moderate level) recommendation. Grades C and D recommendations, the lowest level of evidence that are mostly based on case studies and expert opinion, included the use of topical arsenic trioxide, essential oils, green tea extract, hydropolymer dressings, antiseptic solutions, hydrogels, and debridement enzymes. Despite the volume of literature on managing odor, there is still a lack of high-quality rigorous studies to provide high-level recommendations.

Wound Cleansing

Gentle removal of exudate and debris from the wound base can aid in odor management (EPUAP, NPIAP, & PPPIA, 2019). Wound cleansing with gentle irrigations and atraumatic technique rather than swabbing the surface is recommended. Normal saline, ionic irrigants, and commercial wound cleansers with surfactants can be used (Tilley et al., 2016). A daily shower with the water aimed slightly above the wound may be an effective method for cleansing the wound.

Deodorizers

Deodorizers can be used topically as well as within the room to control odor. Strategies such as aromatherapy oils, expensive aftershave lotions, room deodorizers, and scented candles tend to mask the odor of the malignant wound and overall yield unsatisfactory results (Tilley et al., 2016; Woo, 2017). Use of a "sugar paste" has been reported in the literature as an effective deodorizing preparation by reducing bioburden and necrotic tissue. However, the commercially available manuka honey is preferred because its processing is standardized so that the product is sterilized, thus eliminating the risk of botulism, and it is safe from toxins that are present in certain nectars (Wilson, 2005).

Although not appropriate when the objective is wound healing, Chloromycetin solution has been reported to be an effective wound deodorant. Gauze is moistened with the Chloromycetin solution and applied to the wound surface; it is generally changed twice daily so that the dressing will remain moist. Skin protection should be implemented to keep the solution from contacting the surrounding skin because Chloromycetin will cause an irritant reaction to intact skin. A gauze dressing saturated with a wound cleanser solution containing a low-toxicity antiseptic agent may effectively control odor (Sibbald et al, 2021).

Antimicrobials

Antimicrobial creams and sodium-impregnated gauze both may assist in reducing bacterial numbers, thereby reducing odor. Dressings with an antimicrobial component that assist in controlling the wound bioburden include those that contain silver, iodine, or honey (Cornish, 2019; Tilley et al., 2016). Exudate can increase and become viscous and malodorous when a wound becomes infected (Stephen-Haynes, 2008). Infections are treated systemically, locally, or both.

Oral (systemic) metronidazole can be given to reduce the anaerobic bacterial load in the wound. Although this treatment has been reported to be successful, notable adverse effects are metallic taste in mouth, furred tongue, nausea and vomiting, and intolerance to alcohol, in addition to development of resistance to the bacteria (Tandler & Stephen-Haynes, 2017).

In contrast, topical metronidazole decreases bacterial load at the wound site but without the nausea and vomiting that sometimes accompanies oral metronidazole (Tandler & Stephen-Haynes, 2017). Metronidazole has been applied directly to the wound or on petrolatum gauze and can be used in combination with calcium alginate, hydrofiber, or foam dressings (Alvarez et al., 2007). A systematic review by Winardi and Irwan (2019) found metronidazole evaluated in 4 studies with level of evidence 2B, and formulations found to be effective were topical metronidazole 0.8%, metronidazole gel 0.75%, and metronidazole topical power.

Metronidazole gel (0.75%) is commercially available and can be applied to the wound bed and then covered with a saline-soaked gauze or hydrogel. Topical metronidazole is changed daily, and odor should be eradicated or greatly diminished between 3 and 7 days (Chrisman, 2010; Winardi & Irwan, 2019). Contact layers are often used in combination with antimicrobials (e.g., metronidazole gel or crushed tablets), which significantly reduce the bacteria that cause the odor and drainage.

Debridement

Necrotic tissue can be extremely pungent and malodorous, so removing nonviable tissue is beneficial to controlling odor. Sharp debridement is not usually recommended for fungating wounds due to tissue friability (Strohal et al., 2013); however, it may be appropriate for trimming loose-hanging necrotic tissue by a trained clinician (Woo, 2017). Surgical debridement of these wounds should be avoided because of the risk of bleeding (Woo, 2017). However, when extensive necrotic tissue is present or the size of the fungating wound affects quality of life, surgical debridement (i.e., debulking) may be warranted if it is compatible with the patient's palliative goals of care (Seaman, 2006). As discussed in Chapter 20, mechanical debridement is not recommended because of the tendency for wounds to bleed and because of the pain that is triggered by wet-to-dry dressings.

Conservative debridement (e.g., with autolysis or enzymes) is preferred. Hydrogel dressings are a gentle method of debridement because they soften the necrotic tissue (see Plates 62–64) and facilitate its separation from the wound bed (Tandler & Stephen-Haynes, 2017) (see Chapters 20 and 21 for further discussion of debridement and contraindications). These dressings have the additional benefit of providing a soothing effect and providing pain control. Realistically, the malignant cutaneous wound is quite exudative, however, so a hydrogel dressing (a dressing designed to donate, not absorb, moisture) often is inappropriate. Absorptive dressings (polysaccharide beads, sodium-impregnated gauze, starch copolymer beads, alginates, hydrofibers) are most appropriate and can be combined with superabsorbent dressings to increase the absorptive capacity of the dressing and extend the time between dressing changes.

Charcoal Dressings

Charcoal dressings can reduce odor by filtering out the chemicals that cause the odor and by absorbing bacteria (Tandler & Stephen-Haynes, 2017); these dressings do not address contributing factors such as odor-causing bacteria. Odor with each dressing change will continue. Therefore, carbon dressings are typically used as an adjunctive method of odor reduction along with treatments such as topical antimicrobials that address the cause of bacterial overload.

As an outer covering, charcoal-impregnated dressings can be used either as a primary dressing (when the wound is not exudative) or as a secondary dressing (over a primary absorptive dressing) to suppress odor. These dressings are changed when they become moist (moisture inactivates the charcoal) and when the charcoal is saturated so that it is no longer effective. Charcoal dressings are effective only when they are "sealed" around all four edges so that odor is forced to pass through the charcoal filter. Because some wounds are so irregularly shaped and the topography is so varied, securing the charcoal dressing may be too difficult to attain. Charcoal dressings may require changes ranging from daily to every 2 or 3 days depending on the extent of the odor. Charcoal dressings combined with an antimicrobial are available and serve the dual purpose of reducing bioburden and odor.

Collect and Contain Exudate

High levels of exudate from the malignant cutaneous wound are the result of abnormal capillary permeability within the wound (due to disorganized tumor vasculature), secretion of vascular permeability factor by tumor cells, and autolysis of necrotic tissue by bacterial proteases (Tandler & Stephen-Haynes, 2017). The surrounding tissue of a malignant or fungating wound often is edematous such that even a small ulcer or nodule can produce prolific amounts of exudate. In addition to topical antimicrobials, interventions that aid in exudate control include (1) absorptive atraumatic dressings and (2) containment devices.

Moderately or highly exudative wounds require dressings that are capable of absorbing high volumes of exudate. Moderate to large amounts of exudate can be contained with semipermeable foam dressings and alginates. Very heavily exudative wounds may require a superabsorbent pad in conjunction with an alginate dressing, a hydrofiber dressing, or maltodextrin powder (see Wound Dressing Formulary in Table 21.4). If further protection of the wound bed is necessary to control pain, a contact-layer dressing can be used to line the wound. Two-layer permeable vented dressings also may be used. With these dressings, the perforated nonadherent layer protects the wound surface and permits passage of exudate to an absorbent and permeable layer (Letizia, Uebelhor, & Paddack, 2010; Chrisman, 2010).

Dressing change frequency is primarily a function of the volume of exudate produced, the volume of necrotic tissue present, and the patient's hydration status and activity level. As with other wounds, dressings for malignant or fungating wounds should be changed when exudate is pooling over intact skin or when "strikethrough" occurs. Ideally, dressings should not require changing more often than once per day.

Wound drainage pouches are available from most ostomy manufacturers. These pouches are indicated when the volume of exudate produced exceeds the capabilities of the dressings. Pouching should be considered when dressings must be changed more often than two to three times daily, when the skin begins to show early signs of damage, when the patient's ability to ambulate is hampered, or when odor is uncontrolled. These products have various desirable features, such as an attached skin barrier, flexible adhesive surface, and an access window over the wound site. Many wound pouches also have an attached tubular drain spout that facilitates connecting the pouch to a drainage container so that the fluid does not pool over the wound site or over fill the pouch, a common source of leakage. Chapter 39 describes various techniques for pouching the draining wound.

Negative pressure wound therapy (NPWT) devices have been reported in palliative wound care to contain exudate, control odor, and decrease the number of painful dressing changes (Beers, 2019; Letizia et al., 2010). However, reimbursement for these devices when used in the palliative care wound is seldom approved and therefore not affordable. Manufacturer's recommendations for use of NPWT in *malignant* wounds should be carefully reviewed before use in palliative wounds. More information regarding the use of NPWT is found in Chapter 24.

EVALUATION

Reviewing wound management decisions regularly is essential because the condition of any wound is dynamic, especially in palliative care (Dale & Emmons, 2014). Toward this end, care is targeted to the areas of most concern to the patient and family while maximizing the effects of the intervention (Beers, 2019). It is useful to begin the assessment by asking the patient what aspects of the wound or wound care interventions are of greatest concern. It may be surprising to learn that dressing changes as often as two to three times daily do not upset the patient as much as the odor from the wound or the constant drainage.

CLINICAL CONSULT

A: Wound consult ordered to the home of an 88-year-old female who is in hospice and accepting of dying but has a large metastatic fungating cutaneous wound over the right breast. The family—a daughter, son-in-law, and granddaughter—are caring for the patient in her home. The wound measures 10 × 6 cm, cauliflower appearance of mixed gray/yellow and white exudative tissue. The surrounding skin has MARSI with skin stripping. Currently dressings are being changed twice daily to control odor and exudate and the family is using gauze and ABD pads with microporous tape. The patient and family acknowledge the dressing changes are extremely painful.
D: Patient with a fungating malignant wound at end of life.
P: Goals for this patient and family are to contain odor and exudate and reduce pain at the site.
I: (1) Apply topical mixture of lidocaine 2.5% and prilocaine 2.5% to wound, cover with nonadherent pad solution 30 min prior to dressing change. (2) Rinse off wound with NS or hypochlorous solution and dab very lightly to dry. (3) Apply no-sting skin sealant to entire periwound skin. (4) Sprinkle crushed metronidazole over wound surface to reduce anaerobic bacteria load and control odor. (5) Apply nonadherent silicone-based wound liner. (6) Cover with alginate or hydrofiber dressings to contain exudate. (7) Place super absorbent wound dressing over alginate/hydrofiber. (8) Secure with tubular stockinette applied around chest if patient is able to raise both arms; may need to use "Montgomery straps" to secure dressings if stockinette not feasible.
E: Consider adding charcoal cover dressing over super absorbent wound dressing if odor continues to permeate. Change dressings once per day if exudate saturating cover dressing; goal is to change dressing every other day. The hospice team notified of the change in plan of care and will reconsult if new plan fails to improve comfort for patient and family.

SUMMARY

- The American Academy of Hospice and Palliative Medicine (AAHPM, 2008) position statement maintains that all seriously ill patients who have symptoms that are difficult to treat or who face challenging decisions about goals of care should have access to palliative care consultation and/or hospice. Efforts to enhance quality of life should be offered alongside curative and or restorative medical care, with palliative care a fundamental component of excellent medical care and not an alternative after other approaches have been pursued.

- Palliative wound care is a holistic approach to care that shifts the primary outcome from wound closure to symptom management, aimed at maximizing the quality of life for an individual with advanced or terminal illness.

- The potential skin complications associated with palliative wounds are amenable to the application of wound-healing principles. As with other chronic wounds, the goals for these types of wounds range from healing to palliation and symptom management.

- Practitioners must advocate for changes in policy, regulations, and reimbursement guidelines that may limit palliative wound care practice (Tippett et al., 2012/2018).

SELF-ASSESSMENT QUESTIONS

1. Palliative wound care has goals focused on
   a. Wound healing
   b. Aggressive debridement
   c. Symptom management like odor or exudate
   d. All of the above
2. An existing ulcer that develops a malignancy would be called which of the following?
   a. Marjolin's ulcer
   b. Pressure injury
   c. Fungating tumor
   d. Metastasis
3. Odor control options for a malignant cutaneous wound include:

   a. TNF (tumor necrosis factor) applied topically every day
   b. Prednisone applied topically every day
   c. Metronidazole powder applied topically with every dressing change
   d. Topical bacitracin applied to the wound twice a day
4. Ideally, wound dressings for palliative wounds are changed
   a. Twice a day
   b. As ordered by the provider
   c. Once a week
   d. Tailored to the unique wound conditions and patient status

REFERENCES

Alexander, S. (2010). An intense and unforgettable experience: The lived experience of malignant wounds from the perspectives of patients, caregivers and nurses. *International Wound Journal*, *7*(6), 456–465.

Alvarez, O., Kalinski, C., Nusbaum, J., et al. (2007). Incorporating wound healing strategies to improve palliation (symptom management) in patients with chronic wounds. *Journal of Palliative Medicine*, *10*(5), 1161–1189.

American Academy of Hospice and Palliative Medicine (AAHPM). (2008). *Position statement on access to palliative care and hospice.* Glenview: AAHPM. Retrieved from http://aahpm.org/positions/access. Accessed 8/7/2021.

Artico, M., Dante, A., D'Angelo, D., Lamarca, L., Mastroianni, C., Petitti, T., et al. (2018). Prevalence, incidence and associated factors of pressure ulcers in home palliative care patients: A retrospective chart review. *Palliative Medicine*, *32*(1), 299–307.

Ashfield, T. (2005). The use of topical opioids to relieve pressure ulcer pain. *Nursing Standard*, *19*(45), 90–92.

Ayello, E. A., Levine, J. M., Langemo, D., Kennedy-Evans, K. L., Brennan, M. R., & Sibbald, G. R. (2019). Reexamining the literature on terminal ulcers, SCALE, skin failure, and unavoidable pressure injuries. *Advances in Skin & Wound Care*, *32*(3), 109–121. https://doi.org/10.1097/01.ASW.0000553112.55505.5f.

Back, I., & Finlay, I. (1995). Analgesic effects of topical opioids on painful skin ulcers. *Journal of Pain and Symptom Management*, *10*(7), 493.

Baik, D., et al. (2018). Using the palliative performance scale to estimate survival for patients at the end of life: A systematic review of the literature. *Journal of Palliative Medicine*, *21*(11), 1651–1661.

Ballas, S. (2002). Treatment of painful sickle cell leg ulcers with topical opioids. *Blood*, *99*, 1096.

Beers, E. H. (2019). Palliative wound care: Less is more. *Surgical Clinics of North America*, *99*(5), 899–919.

Beldon, P. (2011). Managing skin changes at life's end. *Wound Essentials*, *6*, 76–79.

Brennan, M. R., Thomas, L., & Kline, M. (2019). Prelude to death or practice failure? Trombley-Brennan terminal tissue injury update. *American Journal of Hospice & Palliative Medicine*, *36*(11), 1016–1019.

Brinker, J., Protus, B. M., & Kimbrel, J. M. (2018). *Wound care at end of life* (2nd ed.). Optum Hospice Pharmacy Services.

British Columbia Cancer Agency. (2015). *Symptom management guidelines: Care of malignant wounds.* Retrieved from http://www.bccancer.bc.ca/nursing-site/documents/10.%20malignant%20wounds.pdf. Accessed 8/13/2021.

Chaplin, J. (2000). Pressure sore risk assessment in palliative care. *Journal of Tissue Viability*, *10*(1), 27–31.

Chaplin, J., & McGill, M. (1999). Pressure sore prevention. *Palliative Care Today*, *8*(3), 38–39.

Chrisman, C. (2010). Care of chronic wounds in palliative care and end-of life patients. *International Wound Journal, 7*(4), 214–235.

Cornish, L. (2019). Holistic management of malignant wounds in palliative patients. *British Journal of Community Nursing, 24* (Suppl. 9), S19–S23. Retrieved from https://pubmed.nvbi.nlm.nig.gov/31479334/. Accessed 6/12/2021.

da Costa Santos, C., de Mattos Pimenta, C., & Nobre, M. (2010). A systematic review of topical treatments to control the odor of malignant fungating wounds. *Journal of Pain and Symptom Management, 39*(6), 1065–1076.

Dale, B., & Emmons, K. (2014). Palliative wound care: Principles of care. *Home Healthcare Nurse, 32*(1), 47–53.

Draper, C. (2005). The management of malodour and exudates in fungating wounds. *The British Journal of Nursing, 14*(11), S4–S12.

Emmons, K., & Lachman, V. (2010). Palliative wound care: A concept analysis. *Journal of Wound, Ostomy, and Continence Nursing, 37*(6), 639–644.

European Pressure Ulcer Advisory Panel (EPUAP), National Pressure Injury Advisory Panel (NPIAP), & Pan Pacific Pressure Injury Alliance. (2019). Prevention and treatment of pressure ulcers/injuries: Clinical practice guideline. In E. Haesler (Ed.), *The International Guideline.* EPUAP/NPIAP/PPPIA.

Ferris, A., Khateib, A., Fromantin, I., et al. (2007). Palliative wound care: Managing chronic wounds across life's continuum: A consensus statement from the International Palliative Wound Care Initiative. *Journal of Palliative Medicine, 10*(1), 37–39.

Ferris, A., Price, A., & Harding, K. (2019). Pressure ulcers in patients receiving palliative care: A systematic review. *Palliative Medicine, 33*(7), 770–782. https://doi.org/10.1177/0269216319846023.

Fletcher, J. (2008). Malodorous wounds, assessment and management. *Wound Essentials, 3,* 14–17.

Galvin, J. (2002). An audit of pressure ulcer incidence in a palliative care setting. *International Journal of Palliative Nursing, 8*(5), 214–221.

Gerlach, M. (2005). Wound care issues in the patient with cancer. *The Nursing Clinics of North America, 40*(2), 295–323.

Grocott, P. (1999). The management of fungating malignant wounds. *Journal of Wound Care, 8*(5), 232–234.

Grocott, P. (2007). Care of patients with fungating malignant wounds. *Nursing Standard, 21*(24), 57–58, 60.

Hampton, S. (2008). Malodorous fungating wounds: How dressings alleviate symptoms. *British Journal of Community Nursing, 13*(6), S31–S32. S34, S36 passim.

Hendrichova, I., Castelli, M., Mastroianni, C., et al. (2010). Pressure ulcers in cancer palliative Care patients. *Palliative Medicine, 24,* 669–673.

Henoch, I., & Gustaffson, M. (2003). Pressure ulcers in palliative care: Development of a hospice pressure ulcer risk assessment scale. *International Journal of Palliative Nursing, 9*(11), 474–484.

Khan, K., Schafer, C., & Wood, J. (2020). Marjolin ulcer: A comprehensive review. *Advances in Skin & Wound Care, 33*(12), 629–634.

Krouse, R. (2008). Palliative care for cancer patients: An interdisciplinary approach. *Cancer Chemotherapy Review, 3*(4), 152–160.

Lai, T., Yip, O., & Sham, M. (2019). Clinical parameters of wound healing in patients with advanced illness. *Annals of Palliative Medicine, 8*(Suppl. 1), S5–S14.

Letizia, M., Uebelhor, J., & Paddack, E. (2010). Providing palliative care to seriously ill patients with nonhealing wounds. *Journal of Wound Ostomy & Continence Nursing, 37*(3), 277–282.

Moore, Z., Johanssen, E., & van Etten, M. (2013). A review of PU prevalence and incidence across Scandinavia, Iceland, and Ireland (Part 1). *Journal of Wound Care, 22,* 361364–362368.

National Consensus Project. (2018). *Clinical practice guideline for quality palliative care* (4th ed.). Richmond: National Coalition for Hospice and Palliative care.

Navaid, M., Melvin, T., Berube, J., & Dotson, S. (2010). Principles of wound care in hospice and palliative medicine. *American Journal of Hospice & Palliative Medicine, 27*(5), 337–341.

Naylor, W. (2005). A guide to wound management in palliative care. *International Journal of Palliative Nursing, 11*(11), 572–579.

Recka, K., Montagnini, M., & Vitale, C. (2012). Management of bleeding associated with malignant wounds. *Journal of Palliative Medicine, 15*(8), 952–954.

Reifsnyder, J., & Magee, H. (2005). Development of pressure ulcers in patients receiving home hospice care. *Wounds, 17*(4), 74–79.

Richards, A., Lelechi, T., Hennessy, W., et al. (2007). Risk factors and wound management for palliative care patients. *Journal of Hospice and Palliative Nursing, 9*(4), 179–181.

Seaman, S. (2006). Management of malignant fungating wounds in advanced cancer. *Seminars in Oncology Nursing, 22*(3), 185–193.

Sibbald, R. G., Elliott, J. A., Persaud-Jaimangal, R., Goodman, L., Armstrong, D. G., Harley, C., et al. (2021). Wound bed preparation 2021. *Advances in Skin & Wound Care, 34*(4), 183–195. https://doi.org/10.1097/01.ASW.0000733724.87630.d6. PMID: 33739948. PMCID: PMC7982138.

Sibbald, R., Krasner, D., & Lutz, J. (2010). SCALE: Skin Changes at Life's End: Final Consensus Statement. *Advances in Skin & Wound Care, 23*(5), 225–236.

Stephen-Haynes, J. (2008). An overview of caring for those with palliative wounds. *British Journal of Community Nursing, 13*(12), S2–S4.

Strohal, R., Dissemond, J., Jordan O'Brien, J., Piaggesi, A., Rimdeika, R., Young, T., et al. (2013). An updated overview and clarification of the principle role of debridement. *Journal of Wound Care, 22*(Suppl), S1–S52.

Tandler, S., & Stephen-Haynes, J. (2017). Fungating wounds: Management and treatment options. *British Journal of Nursing (Mark Allen Publishing), 26*(12 Suppl), S6–S14.

Tilley, C., Lipson, J., & Ramos, M. (2016). Palliative wound care for malignant fungating wounds: Holistic considerations at end-of-life. *The Nursing Clinics of North America, 51*(3), 513–531. https://doi.org/10.1016/j.cnur.2016.05.006. Retrieved from https://pubmed.ncbi.mln.nih.gov/27497023/. Accessed 6/19/2021.

Tippett, A. (2005). Wounds at the end of life. *Wounds, 17*(4), 91–98.

Tippett, A., Sherman, R., Woo, K., Swezey, L., & Posthauer, E. (2012/2018). Perspectives on palliative wound care: Interprofessional strategies for the management of palliative wounds. *Wound Source.* White papers from https://www.woundsource.com/whitepaper/perspectives-palliative-wound-care-interprofessional-strategies-management-palliative. Accessed 8/7/2021.

Trombley, K., Brennan, M. R., Thomas, L., & Kline, M. (2012). Prelude to death or practice failure? Trombley-Brennan terminal tissue injuries. *American Journal of Hospice & Palliative Medicine, 29*(7), 541–545.

Vickery, J., Compton, L., Allard, J., Beeson, T., Howard, J., & Pittman, J. (2020). Pressure injury prevention and wound management for the patient who is actively dying: Evidence-based recommendations to guide care. *Journal Wound, Ostomy, Continence Nursing, 47*(6), 569–575. https://doi.org/10.1097/WON.0000000000000702.

Walding, M. (2005). Pressure area care and the management of fungating wounds. In C. Faull, Y. Carter, & L. Daniels (Eds.), *Handbook of palliative care* (2nd ed.). Oxford: Blackwell.

West, D. (2007). A palliative approach to the of malodour from malignant fungating tumours. *International Journal of Palliative Nursing, 13*(3), 137–142.

Westwood, R. (2014). The principles behind end of life care and the implications for patients' skin. *Journal of Clinical Nursing, 28*(3), 58–64.

Wilson, V. (2005). Assessment and management of fungating wounds: A review. *British Journal of Community Nursing, 10*(3), S28–S34.

Winardi, A., & Irwan, A. (2019). Topical treatment for controlling malignant wound odour. *Journal of the European Wound Management Association, 20*, 7–13.

Woo, K. (2017). Hopes for palliative wounds. *International Journal of Palliative Nursing, 23*(6), 264–268.

Woo, K., Krasner, D., Kennedy, B., et al. (2015). Palliative wound care management strategies for palliative patients and their circles of care. *Advances in Skin & Wound Care, 28*(3), 130–140.

Zeppetella, G., Paul, J., & Ribeiro, M. (2003). Analgesic efficacy of morphine applied topically to painful ulcers. *Journal of Pain and Symptom Management, 25*, 555–558.

Zeppetella, G., & Ribeiro, M. (2005). Morphine in intrasite gel applied topically to painful ulcers. *Journal of Pain and Symptom Management, 29*, 118–119.

Draining Wounds and Fistulas

Ruth A. Bryant and Kathleen Borchert

OBJECTIVES

1. Identify medical conditions associated with fistula formation.
2. Distinguish between a draining wound and a fistula.
3. Distinguish between an enteric fistula and an enteroatmospheric fistula.
4. List three complications that contribute to mortality from fistulas.
5. Identify proper terminology of a fistula according to involved structures.
6. Describe three ways to classify fistulas.
7. List the risk factors for postoperative fistula development and radiation-induced fistulas.
8. Identify the six objectives of medical management for the patient with a fistula.
9. List factors known to correlate with spontaneous closure and known to impede spontaneous closure of fistula tracts.
10. Describe surgical procedures commonly used to close or bypass fistula tracts.
11. List eight nursing management goals for the patient with a fistula.
12. Describe four essential assessments that guide the management of the patient with a fistula.
13. Explain the role of four different types of skin barriers and their indications for use.
14. Identify features to be considered when selecting a fistula pouching system.
15. Briefly describe the "isolation" technique (formerly known as the bridging technique) and indications for use.
16. Identify options for odor control in a wound managed with dressings and managed with pouching.
17. Describe the role of negative pressure wound therapy (NPWT) and closed wound suction in the management of enteroatmospheric fistulae.

The presence of a draining wound or fistula can be a frustrating and disheartening experience for the patient and family because it typically represents a major complication. It can also present a significant financial burden; the typical cost of fistula care is more than $500,000 per patient (Gribovskaja-Rupp & Melton, 2016). Fistula management can also be a difficult experience for caregivers. However, management can be quite rewarding when effluent is successfully contained, odor is controlled, the patient is comfortable, and realistic resolution is attained. Management for this patient population requires astute assessment skills, knowledge of pathophysiology, competent technical skills, diligent follow-up, persistence, and knowledge of management alternatives.

Fistula management is more than skin protection and containment. In this chapter, the pathophysiology of fistula formation, the medical and surgical aspects of managing a patient with a fistula, and the nursing management (i.e., skin protection, odor control, and containment techniques) of the patient with a fistula will be presented. The techniques discussed in this chapter are also applicable to other types of wounds and drain sites that are not adequately contained by dressings.

EPIDEMIOLOGY AND ETIOLOGY

Gastrointestinal (GI) fistulas are serious complications associated with high morbidity, high mortality (5.5%–33%), extended hospital stays, and increased costs (Dudrick & Panait, 2011; Gribovskaja-Rupp & Melton, 2016; Kassis & Makary, 2008). Mortality rates increase to as high as 40% when the fistula occurs in middle of an open abdominal wound; the enteroatmospheric fistula (Marinis, Gkiokas, Argyra, et al., 2013). Malnutrition, sepsis, and electrolyte imbalance are the predominate causes of death. Fistulas develop in a wide array of complex patient conditions and often are concentrated in large medical centers. Frequency data (i.e., incidence and prevalence) therefore tend to be skewed and difficult to interpret. Factors affecting the prognosis of the patient with a fistula, however, are well known, with evidence derived from retrospective studies and increasingly rigorous case series.

Causative factors and conditions for fistula formation include unintended operative injury to the intestine; disruption of an anastomotic leak; technical difficulties with anastomosis; abscess at the site of the anastomosis; and coexisting disease such as inflammatory bowel disease, cancer, or diverticulitis (Dudrick & Panait, 2011). The following are risk factors that increase the likelihood of fistula formation when these medical conditions are present: severe malnutrition, sepsis, hypotension, vasopressor therapy, and steroid therapy. Enterocutaneous fistulas are either spontaneous (15%–25%) or iatrogenic (75%–85%) (Cowan & Cassaro, 2021; Gribovskaja-Rupp & Melton, 2016). Approximately 50% of the iatrogenic enterocutaneous fistulas that occur postoperatively represent a leak in the anastomosis (Nussbaum & Fischer, 2007). Ischemia, tension, poor surgical technique, extensive lysis of adhesives, inadequate bowel prep such as with emergency surgery or trauma surgery, and preexisting conditions such as morbid obesity, systemic hypotension, local sepsis, and prior radiation therapy contribute to the risk of anastomotic complications (Kassis & Makary, 2008; Pfeifer, Tomasch, & Uranues, 2011). To reduce the risk of this complication, Maykel and Fischer (2003) advocate specific prevention strategies when faced with emergency surgery: provide adequate intravenous fluids, ensure adequate circulatory support, keep the patient warm, and provide appropriately timed broad-spectrum antibiotics. In addition, when surgery is planned, they consider adequate nutritional preparation to be the most important step in preventing an anastomotic breakdown. Patients at highest risk for an anastomotic breakdown are the severely malnourished patients as manifested by a hydrated serum albumin level less than 3 g/dL and weight loss of 10%–15% over a 4- to 6-month period (Kassis & Makary, 2008).

Approximately 25% of fistulas are acquired, that is, they develop spontaneously and are associated with an intrinsic intestinal disease (cancer, radiation, diverticulitis, inflammatory bowel disease, and appendicitis) or external trauma (Cowan & Cassaro, 2021). Spontaneous fistulas are generally resistant to spontaneous closure. Patients who have been treated for a pelvic malignancy are particularly vulnerable to fistula formation because of radiation damage to the rectum, anal canal, and gynecologic organs (Tran & Thorson, 2020; Tuma, McKeown, & Al-Wahab, 2021). Irradiation triggers occlusive vasculitis, fibrosis, and impaired collagen synthesis, a process termed *radiation-induced endarteritis*. Because the endarteritis persists, complications may develop immediately after radiation (within 6 months) or years later (as much as 30 years), although the majority will develop within 1–5 years (Pfeifer et al., 2011). Additional risk factors for irradiation-induced fistulas include coexisting processes such as atherosclerosis, hypertension, diabetes mellitus, advanced age, cigarette smoking, pelvic inflammatory disease, and previous pelvic surgery. Pelvic radiation doses exceeding 50 Gray (Gyr) increase the incidence of bowel injury (Hollington, Mawdsley, Lim, et al., 2004; Viswanathan et al., 2014).

The three most common and highly significant complications associated with fistulas are sepsis, malnutrition, and fluid and electrolyte imbalance (Berry & Fischer, 1996; Fischer, 1983). The loss of hypertonic protein-rich fistula effluent contributes to fluid and electrolyte depletion and malnutrition because of the loss of sodium bicarbonate and

amino acids (Nussbaum & Fischer, 2007). Sepsis occurs as a result of abscess formation and compromised immune response due to poor nutritional status (Makhdoom, Komar, & Still, 2000). Uncontrolled sepsis and coexisting malnutrition are primarily responsible for the mortality in patients with enterocutaneous fistulas (Hollington et al., 2004; Nussbaum & Fischer, 2007; Yanar & Yanar, 2011).

TERMINOLOGY

Definitions

Fistula is a Latin word meaning "pipe" or "flute." A fistula is an abnormal passage between two or more epithelialized surfaces so that a communication tract develops from one hollow organ to another hollow organ or to the external environment allowing the loss of nutrients, fluids, and/or secretions (Dudrick & Panait, 2011) (Figs. 39.1 and 39.2). An enterocutaneous fistula communicates specifically between the lumen of the GI tract and the skin. A fistula that develops in the base

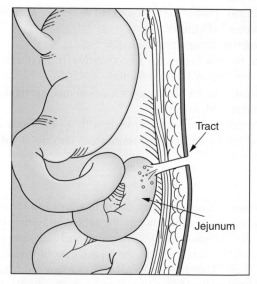

Fig. 39.1 Simple enterocutaneous fistula.

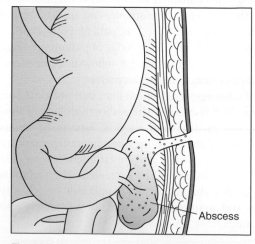

Fig. 39.2 Complex fistula with associated abscess.

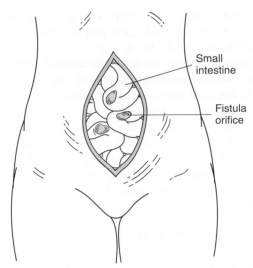

Fig. 39.3 Enteroatmospheric fistula with multiple openings in large abdominal wall defect.

of an open abdominal wound bed is referred to as an *enteroatmospheric fistula* (EAF) (Fig. 39.3) (Marinis et al., 2013).

It is important to distinguish between a fistula and a drain site or draining wound. Not all wounds that drain are fistulas. The term *draining wound* may refer to a surgical site that is draining, a tube site that is draining, or a puncture site (e.g., paracentesis, needle-guided intervention). Drain tubes may be placed either surgically or by interventional radiology to drain a pocket of fluid (e.g., abscess or seroma). For example, a drain tube, such as a Penrose, sump catheter, or Jackson Pratt, may be placed in a surgical incision or through a stab wound to facilitate drainage of pooled fluid. A draining wound, surgically placed drain site, or wound dehiscence should not be misinterpreted as a fistula.

Classification

Several methods are used to classify fistulas. These classification schemes are useful in predicting the morbidity rate, mortality rate, and potential for spontaneous closure (Wong, Buie, & Annamaneni, 2004).

From an anatomic perspective, the fistula may be *simple, complex,* or an *EAF* (Box 39.1). The simple fistula has a short, direct tract; no abscess; and no other organ involved. The complex fistula is associated with an abscess and has multiple organ involvement, and the EAF which opens into the base of

BOX 39.1 Classification of Fistulas by Complexity

Simple
- Short, direct tract
- No associated abscess
- No other organ involvement

Complex
- Associated with abscess
- Multiple organ involvement
- Opens into base of disrupted wound

an open abdominal wound and requires specific and unique management techniques.

A fistula may be classified according to *organ of origin.*: type 1 (abdominal, esophageal, and gastroduodenal), type II (small bowel), type III (large bowel), and type IV (enteroatmospheric, regardless of origin) (Schein & Decker, 1991). A fistula may be differentiated based on whether it is *internal or external*. The internal fistula exists between internal structures, whereas the external fistula communicates between an internal organ and the skin, vagina, or rectum. This classification system is more specific in that the site of origin and site of termination are identified. Examples of such terminology are listed in Table 39.1.

A fistula may also be classified according to *volume of output* (Table 39.2). A high-output fistula is most commonly

TABLE 39.1 Fistula Terminology

From	To	Name	Internal/External
Pancreas	Colon	Pancreatico-colonic	Internal
Jejunum	Rectum	Jejunorectal	External
Intestine	Skin	Enterocutaneous	External
Intestine	Colon	Enterocolonic	Internal
Intestine	Bladder	Enterovesical	Internal
Intestine	Vagina	Enterovaginal	External
Intestine	Wound bed or surface	Enteroatmospheric	External
Colon	Skin	Colocutaneous	External
Colon	Colon	Colocolonic	Internal
Colon	Bladder	Colovesical	Internal
Rectum	Vagina	Rectovaginal	External
Bladder	Skin	Vesicocutaneous	External
Bladder	Vagina	Vesicovaginal	External

Modified from Irrgang, S., & Bryant, R. (1984). Management of the enterocutaneous fistula. *Journal of Enterostomal Therapy*, 11, 211–228.

TABLE 39.2 Fistula Classification

	Designation	Characteristics
Location	Internal	Tract contained within body
	External	Tract exits through skin or wound bed
Involved structures	Colon	Colon
	Entero-	Small bowel
	Vesico-	Bladder
	Vaginal	Vagina
	Cutaneous	Skin
	Recto-	Rectum
Volume	High output	>500 mL per 24 h
	Moderate output	200–500 mL per 24 h
	Low output	<200 mL per 24 h

Modified from Boarini, J., Bryant, R. A., & Irrgang, S. J. (1986). Fistula management. *Seminars in Oncology Nursing, 2*(4), 287–292.

defined as producing more than 500 mL per 24 h, a moderate-output fistula is associated with output of 200–500 mL per 24 h, and a low-output fistula produces less than 200 mL per 24 h (Maykel & Fischer, 2003; Nussbaum & Fischer, 2007). The frequencies of sepsis, malnutrition, and fluid and electrolyte imbalance are directly related to fistula output. Fistula output is a direct reflection of the fistula's site of origin. Distal large-bowel fistulas typically have low output (<200 mL per 24 h), whereas most proximal small-bowel fistulas are considered high output because they may produce from 1000 to as much as 3000 mL per 24 h, at least initially. Consequently, the high-output fistula is associated with severe malnutrition, significant fluid and electrolyte disturbance, higher morbidity and mortality rates, and lower spontaneous closure rate (Kassis & Makary, 2008; Wong et al., 2004).

MANIFESTATIONS

Fever and abdominal pain are the initial indicators of a possible fistula (Nussbaum & Fischer, 2007). The passage of GI secretions or urine through an unintentional opening onto the skin heralds the development of a cutaneous fistula. Manifestations of a fistula exiting through the vagina (i.e., rectovaginal or vesicovaginal) include passage of gas, feces, purulent material, or urine through the vagina and discharge that is extremely malodorous (Tuma, Crespi, Wolff, et al., 2020). Irradiation-induced rectovaginal fistulas often are preceded by diarrhea, passage of mucus and blood rectally, a sensation of rectal pressure, and a constant urge to defecate (Das & Snyder, 2016; Tran & Thorson, 2020; Tuma et al., 2021). An initial manifestation of a fistula between the intestinal tract and the urinary bladder (e.g., colovesical fistula) is the passage of gas or stool-stained urine through the urethra.

MEDICAL MANAGEMENT

The desired endpoint of the medical management of a fistula is spontaneous closure. Approximately 19%–40% of all fistulas will close spontaneously with conservative medical management, but only when sepsis is controlled and nutrition support is adequate and appropriate (Kassis & Makary, 2008). Of the fistulas that do heal spontaneously, 80%–90% do so within 5 weeks, provided the patient is adequately nourished (Kassis & Makary, 2008; Maykel & Fischer, 2003). Factors known to correlate with spontaneous fistula closure include absence of sepsis, adequate nutritional support, low output, and classification as a postoperative fistula (Campos, Andrade, Campos, et al., 1999; Nussbaum & Fischer, 2007). Small enteric fistulas (<1 cm) and long fistula tracts (>2 cm) are conditions that favor spontaneous closure. Factors associated with failure of spontaneous closure include intestinal discontinuity, adjacent abscess, stricture or inflamed bowel, radiation therapy, foreign bodies, or distal obstruction (Evenson & Fischer, 2006). Approximately 90% of simple fistulas close spontaneously, whereas the EAF will always require some type of surgical intervention to achieve closure (Marinis et al., 2013; Shecter, 2011; Whelan Jr &

Ivatury, 2011; Wong et al., 2004). The reason for this is that there is no fistula tract, and lack of well-vascularized overlying tissue (Di Saverio et al., 2015).

Achievement of the medical management goals requires patience, astute assessment skills, and the cooperation of many health care specialists. Appropriate management is based on the four key themes: optimize nutrition, delineate fistulous tract anatomy, skin care, and manage underlying disease (Tuma et al., 2020). Medical management can be divided into nonsurgical treatment and surgical treatment. A comprehensive and effective interdisciplinary and multidisciplinary team approach is vital to achieve closure and reduce mortality and morbidity.

Nonsurgical Treatment

The nonsurgical treatment of fistulas requires a comprehensive plan of care with attention to six specific objectives. These objectives are easily recalled by using the acronym "SNAP" which describes the essential elements of an ECF care protocol (Kaushal & Carlson, 2004; Samad, Anele, Akhtar, & Doughan, 2015). "S" indicates skin and sepsis; "N" represents nutrition; "A" indicates anatomy is defined, and "P" indicates a procedure is proposed for managing the fistula conservatively and potentially surgically.

Objective 1: Fluid and Electrolyte Replacement

From 5 to 9 L of fluid rich in sodium, potassium, chloride, and bicarbonate is secreted into the GI tract daily. The loss of fluid and electrolytes that accompanies the presentation of a high-output fistula may result in hypovolemia and circulatory failure. Such blood volume imbalances must be corrected before initiating nutritional support or definition of the fistula tract. Adequate tissue perfusion and urine output must be maintained. Potential electrolyte imbalances should be anticipated and can be inferred from an understanding of the usual electrolyte composition of GI secretions. Electrolyte replacement can also be guided by measuring the electrolyte composition of the fistula output and serum (Shecter, 2011).

Objective 2: Control of Infection

Sepsis is the major cause of death in patients with enteric fistulas. The bacteria proliferate rapidly in the poorly vascularized tissue typically surrounding a fistula tract (Kassis & Makary, 2008). Pooling of bowel contents as a result of the dehiscence of a suture line precipitate localized and then diffuse abdominal pain, ileus, fever, and, ultimately, septic shock. The presence of systemic or local sepsis must be evaluated, typically with computed tomographic scanning or ultrasound. Effective drainage can be accomplished by use of percutaneous radiographic techniques or surgery. The specific approach depends on abscess location, patient status, and available resources. Surgical laparotomy for control of sepsis should be limited to proximal diversion and drainage of the abscess. Definitive repair of the fistula is undertaken later only after inflammation has receded and nutrition is restored. Abscess contents should be cultured (aerobic and anaerobic) and Gram stained to identify the causative organisms and sensitivities. Organisms are most commonly of bowel origin: coliform, *Bacteroides*, and enterococci. Staphylococci also may be present. Antibiotics are only appropriate in the presence of an infection and in conjunction with adequate drainage of the abscess (Wong et al., 2004).

Objective 3: Control of Fistula Output and Skin Protection

Drainage of intestinal contents onto the skin will result in epidermal erosion and pain within only a few hours. Aggressive skin protection is essential and should be initiated at once. This is discussed specifically in the "Nursing Management" section.

Intestinal output must be minimized. Conventional methods for achieving this goal are giving the patient nothing by mouth (NPO) and administering proton pump inhibitors (H_2 antagonists or PPIs) and medications to slow intestinal transit. NPO status decreases luminal contents, GI stimulation, and pancreaticobiliary secretion. Administering PPIs reduces stress ulcerations and decreases gastric, biliary, and pancreatic secretions. The dose is titrated to achieve a fistula output less than 1 L per day and effluent pH greater than 6 (Bleier & Hedrick, 2010). Despite reducing GI secretions, H_2 receptors have not been shown to speed closure of the enterocutaneous fistula (Maykel & Fischer, 2003). In addition, sucralfate can be used for its gastric neutralizing and constipating affect (Evenson & Fischer, 2006). None of the acid reduction therapies have been shown to increase rate of fistula closure. Medications that slow intestinal transit are the priority in reducing fistula output (Table 39.3). Of these, loperamide is the most effective and should be taken 30 min before meals when the patient is eating (Bleier & Hedrick, 2010).

Octreotide is a synthetic analog of somatostatin, which is a naturally occurring hormone present throughout the body. More than two-thirds of somatostatin is derived from the GI tract, especially the distal portion of the stomach, duodenum, jejunum, and pancreas. In the presence of fat, protein, and carbohydrates with a meal, somatostatin secretion significantly increases. Somatostatin release is inhibited by the release of acetylcholine from cholinergic neurons

(Nussbaum & Fischer, 2007). It has extensive, well-known biologic effects that include inhibition of gastric, biliary, pancreatic, and salivary secretions and reduced GI motility, gastric emptying, and gallbladder emptying. When used in combination with *total parenteral nutrition* (TPN), a synergistic effect on reduced GI secretions can be expected. The short half-life of 1–2 min requires that somatostatin be administered through continuous intravenous infusion (250 mcg/h). The analog octreotide has a half-life of almost 2 h, so it can be administered three times daily subcutaneously (300 mcg/day). Results from available prospective controlled studies and randomized controlled studies of octreotide have been mixed. The most encouraging results of octreotide are seen with postoperative, high-output, small-bowel fistulas in which fluid-, electrolyte-, and protein-store depletion is prevented. Fistula output reductions of 40%–90% after 48 h and reduced time to closure (50 days to 5–10 days) have been reported (Fagniez & Yahchouchy, 1999; Hesse, Ysebaert, & de Hemptinne, 2001; Shecter, 2011). These medications are less effective with fistulas associated with intrinsic bowel diseases, such as ulcerative colitis or Crohn's disease (Hild, Dobroschke, Henneking, et al., 1986; Shecter, 2011). Somatostatin or octreotide do not improve mortality, but they can significantly decrease fistula output, allow for faster spontaneous fistula closure and therefore result in a shorter hospital stay (Gribovskaja-Rupp & Melton, 2016). Octreotide should be used with caution due to reports of villous atrophy, interruption of intestinal adaptation, acute cholecystitis, and inhibition of growth hormone thereby potentially inhibiting immune function (Maykel & Fischer, 2003; Shecter, 2011). Considering the risk/benefits of this medication a reasonable course of action is to trial somatostatin analogue medication for 3 days if current fistula output >1 L/day and if this 72-h trial is successful then utilize this treatment for a longer period of time (Gribovskaja-Rupp & Melton, 2016). Use somatostatin or somatostatin analog when patient has high-output (>500 mL/d) ECF as a method to reduce effluent drainage and enhance spontaneous closure (Kumpf et al., 2017).

Objective 4: Nutritional Support

Malnutrition is a significant complication experienced by most patients with a fistula. Several factors contribute to the fistula patient's poor nutritional status. Often the patient is malnourished before the fistula develops. Additional factors contributing to negative nitrogen balance include reduced protein intake, inefficient nutrient use, excessive losses of protein-rich fluids (especially from pancreatic and proximal jejunal fistulas), and muscle protein breakdown (hypercatabolism) that occurs with sepsis. Daily small-bowel secretions contain as much as 75 g of protein (12 g of nitrogen); desquamated cells; and pancreatic, biliary tract, small-bowel, and gastric secretions, all of which are normally reabsorbed by the bowel (Yanar & Yanar, 2011).

Clinical Guidelines for Nutrition Support of Adult Patients with Enterocutaneous Fistula (Kumpf et al., 2017) state malnutrition should be diagnosed by physical exam, nutrition

TABLE 39.3 Antimotility Medications for High-Output Fistulas	
Medication	**Dose**
Loperamide	Up to 4 mg four times daily
Diphenoxylate	2.5–5 mg up to four times daily
Tincture of opium	0.3–1.0 mL up to four times daily
Codeine	15–100 mg up to four times daily
Paregoric	5–10 mL two to four times daily
Proton pump inhibitors	Dosage varies by agent
Octreotide	50–500 micrograms (mg) subcutaneously up to three times daily

Bleier, J. I., & Hedrick, T. (2010). Metabolic support of the enterocutaneous fistula patient. *Clinics in Colon and Rectal Surgery, 23*(3), 142–148.

history, including unintentional weight loss, and estimation of energy/nutrient intake. Nutritional assessment should be conducted upon diagnosis of the ECF. If malnutrition does not present at baseline, periodic reassessments are critical as malnutrition is likely due to nutrient malabsorption, fluid and electrolyte losses, and sepsis. Serum protein concentrations prior to and during nutrition therapy are helpful since they are prognostic outcome indicators although not sensitive nutrition markers (Kumpf et al., 2017).

Adequate nutritional support is achieved when the patient is maintained in a state of positive nitrogen balance and receives adequate vitamin and trace mineral replacement. The number of calories and amount of protein required will depend on the patient's preexisting status, sepsis, and fistula output (Kumpf et al., 2017). It is important to initiate nutritional support without delay because lean body mass is lost at a rate of 300–900 g per 24 h depending on the degree of stress (Maykel & Fischer, 2003). Trace elements (e.g., copper, zinc, and magnesium), multivitamins, and vitamins (B, C, and K) must be supplemented (Maykel & Fischer, 2003; Wong et al., 2004). González-Pinto and González (2001) recommend twice the recommended daily allowance (RDA) for vitamins and trace minerals and up to 10 times the RDA for vitamin C. Nutritional recommendations for calories, protein, vitamins, and elements are provided in Table 39.4.

The route of nutritional support is contingent upon the patient's ability to ingest sufficient quantities, the location of the fistula tract, the absorptive capacity of the bowel mucosa, and the patient's tolerance. Patients with high output (e.g., >500 mL/day) may require TPN to meet fluid, electrolyte and nutrient requirements to support spontaneous or surgical closure of the ECF (Kumpf et al., 2017). TPN is often initiated on the second or third day of fistula management and is often associated with a decreased fistula output (by as much as 30%–50%), as well as modification of the composition of GI and pancreatic sections (Yanar & Yanar, 2011). Unfortunately, there are serious complications associated with TPN, such as bacterial translocation, access site infections, and metabolic disorders. The oral route of nutritional support is appropriate for colonic fistulas, whereas the preferred route for distal ileal fistulas is enteral nutrition accompanied by simultaneous "bowel rest." This may not be feasible in the presence of feeding intolerance, inability to access the GI tract, or high fistula output, all of which may require TPN to improve spontaneous closure rates (Shecter, 2011). In general, TPN is indicated for patients with duodenal, pancreatic, or jejunoileal fistulas (Yanar & Yanar, 2011). Based on expert consensus, TPN at home may be considered if the patient is medically stable and the fistula output is manageable (Kumpf et al., 2017).

Enteral nutrition (EN) is the preferred route of nutritional support in recognition that even small amounts will maintain the normal structural, immunologic, and hormonal integrity of the GI tract and prevent translocation of bacteria. However, enteral nutrition requires approximately 4 feet of small intestine between the ligament of Treitz and the fistula orifice (Dudrick, Maharaj, & McKelvey, 1999; Knechtges & Zimmermann, 2015; Maykel & Fischer, 2003). Many types of enteral solutions are available, and a dietitian should be consulted to recommend the most appropriate solution and administration procedure so that GI intolerance (e.g., diarrhea, and abdominal distention) can be avoided.

When the GI tract is functional and the patient is cooperative, enteral nutrition may also be achieved when the fistula is located in the most proximal bowel by placing the feeding tube distal to the fistula orifice (Kumpf et al., 2017; Yanar & Yanar, 2011). *Fistuloclysis* is defined as the infusion of enteral nutrition formula via the distal stoma of an enterocutaneous fistula with OR without reinfusion of the output from the proximal fistula opening. This technique be implemented when the infusion ECF site is not expected to close spontaneously and should NOT be implemented until AFTER confirmation of integrity and patency of the small intestine beyond the most distal fistula opening (Kumpf et al., 2017). The central idea for implementing this technique is to feed both the gut mucosa and the patient, to minimize the need for parenteral nutrition. Tolerance is two-fold; whether there is an increase in ECF output and ability for this method to maintain patient hydration and provide adequate nutrition.

There is a lack of evidence that multicomponent immune-enhancing formulas improve ECF outcomes of ECF. Nutrition guidelines (Kumpf et al., 2017) recommend the use of a polymeric formula initially with a change to a semi-elemental (oligomeric) diet if tolerance occurs. Oral glutamine in addition to TPN may improve mortality and fistula closure rates.

Objective 5: Definition of Fistula Tract

After the patient is stabilized (fluid and electrolytes balanced and infection controlled), the fistula must be examined to ascertain (1) the origin of the fistula tract; (2) the condition of adjacent bowel; (3) the presence of additional abscess pockets; and (4) the presence of distal obstruction or bowel discontinuity. Water-soluble contrast agents (e.g.,

TABLE 39.4   Nutrition Needs of Patient With ECF

	Calorie Requirement (kcal/kg/day)	Protein (g/kg/day)	Vitamin C	Other Vitamins	Elements Requirement (Zinc, Copper, Selenium) (g/kg/day)
Low-output fistula	20–30	1–1.5	5–10 times normal	At least normal	At least normal
High-output fistula	25–35	1.5–2.5	10 times normal	2 times normal	2 times trace elements

Adapted from Gribovskaja-Rupp, I., & Melton, G. B. (2016). Enterocutaneous fistula: Proven strategies and updates. *Clinics in colon and rectal surgery, 29*(2), 130–137. https://doi.org/10.1055/s-0036-1580732.

Renografin, Hypaque, and Gastrografin) are preferred to visualize the fistula tract and are administered through the fistula orifice using a soft-tip catheter. A computed tomographic scan is indicated only when the patient is not responding to conservative treatment. If other organs are involved, additional tests (e.g., cystoscopy or intravenous pyelogram) should be pursued (Wong et al., 2004).

Objective 6: Conservative Management

As already described, most enterocutaneous fistulas will heal spontaneously with patience, time, and conservative management (positive nitrogen balance with nutritional support, sepsis-free state). The challenge is trying to shorten the time to spontaneous healing and increasing the number of fistulas that heal spontaneously.

Fistula closure is sometimes successful with the insertion of clotting substances into the fistula tract. The concept of using fibrin for anastomosis of tissue was first used for hemostasis in 1909 (Migaly & Rolandelli, 2007). Fibrin sealants (also referred to as *fibrin glue*) are composed of a concentrated allotment of fibrinogen/factor XIII/fibronectin and thrombin that congeals to form an insoluble fibrin clot when mixed with calcium chloride, a process that essentially replicates the last step of the coagulation cascade (Kassis & Makary, 2008; Tuma et al., 2021). The mechanism of action consists of fibrin glue providing a "matrix" for the influx of various cells and collagen formation (Buchanan, Bartram, Phillips, et al., 2003).

Fibrin sealant products can be created from the patient's own plasma (autologous) or from human plasma that has been collected and pooled from many donors (heterologous) after screening and viral testing. The fibrin glue is applied endoscopically at the origin of the fistula to seal the fistula (Migaly & Rolandelli, 2007). Gribovskaja-Rupp and Melton (2016) identify the "ideal" fistula to treat with fibrin sealant as long, narrow, low output, devoid of distal obstruction and IBD. Despite variable success rates, their overall opinion was that fibrin sealant therapy should be used for selective cases. In contrast, the current role of fibrin glue in rectovaginal fistula repair is limited due to inconsistent and marginal results of success (Das & Snyder, 2016).

Endoscopic clip technology is available for acute fistulas, but currently this technology has little application in the cure of chronic ECF. Another technique for closing the fistula is the fistula plug which was first reported in 2008; this procedure involves debridement of the fistula tract and then suture fixation of the plug within the fistula tract (Das & Snyder, 2016). Lyon, Hoddle, Hucks, and Changkuon (2013) used the fibrin plug to treat 6 different patients with an enteroatmospheric fistula and reported closure in all patients, with recurrence in two patients at 9 and 12 months. Often several repeat plug procedures are required resulting in a lower first time procedure success rate compared with the overall success rate. However, because the plug is easy to insert, well tolerated by the patient and associated with little risk, utilization even if successful for only a short time, spare tissue for future surgical procedures (Das & Snyder, 2016).

Surgical Treatment

Immediate surgery is imperative when (1) a septic focus has been identified; (2) uncontrolled hemorrhage has developed; (3) bowel necrosis has developed; or (4) an evisceration is present. However, closure of the fistula or excision of the fistula tract should *not* be attempted under these circumstances.

Surgical intervention to close the fistula will be required when impediments to spontaneous closure have been identified. Factors known to prevent spontaneous closure are listed in Box 39.2 (Nussbaum & Fischer, 2007). If any of these factors are present and closure of the fistula is the ultimate goal for the patient, surgical intervention will eventually be necessary. Surgical procedures may also be indicated for palliation.

The exact timing for surgical intervention is variable, depending on the patient's status. In general, operative interventions to close the fistula tract should be delayed until the patient is in a positive nitrogen balance and control of infection is established. Corrective surgery for a simple or complex fistula that continues to produce effluent is commonly undertaken within 4 to 6 weeks when the patient is nutritionally and metabolically stable and, in a sepsis-free environment (Redden, Ramsay, Humphries, et al., 2013). However, it is important that definitive surgery such as this be delayed until the abdominal wall is soft and supple; tissues should return to a normal soft, pliable state, particularly in the presence of irradiated tissue (Shecter, 2011; Wong et al., 2004).

Enteroatmospheric fistulas invariably require definitive surgery; however, the timing of surgery is not well defined. Nutritional status, metabolic status, and immunocompetence should be normalized, and the obliterative peritonitis and inflammation associated with chronic peritoneal contamination resolved (Marinis et al., 2013; Shecter, 2011; Wong et al., 2004). Judicious timing of surgery for enteroatmospheric fistulas is warranted. The most often reported timing ranges from 3 to 6 months.

The surgical interventions available for management of enterocutaneous fistulas will either divert the GI tract (without resection of the fistula) or provide definitive resection of the fistula tract (Nussbaum & Fischer, 2007). Factors such as location, size, and cause of the fistula; the patient's overall status; and the presence of irradiated tissue will influence the approach selected. However, Maykel and Fischer (2003) warn that the best results occur with resection of the fistula and end-to-end anastomosis and those other surgical procedures represent a compromise.

BOX 39.2 FRIEND: Factors That Prevent Spontaneous Fistula Closure

F = Foreign body in fistula tract or suture line
R = Radiation (previous irradiation) to the site
I = Infection (abscess) or inferior distal suture line/anastomosis
E = Epithelium-lined tract contiguous with skin or wound bed
N = Neoplasm, tumor or disease (Crohn's) in site
D = Distal obstruction

Adapted from Cowan, K. B., Cassaro, S. (2022). Enterocutaneous fistula. In StatPearls [Internet]. Treasure Island: StatPearls Publishing; Available from: https://www.ncbi.nlm.nih.gov/books/NBK459129/. [Updated 2022 Aug 8].

Diversion techniques divert the fecal stream away from the fistula site; removal of the fistula is not accomplished. Resection of the fistula is not always appropriate or possible in the presence of extensive or recurrent malignancy or when tissue perfusion is inadequate in the vicinity of the fistula (secondary to numerous surgical resections, scar formation, uncontrolled diabetes, or prior irradiation).

Diversion can be achieved by creating a stoma proximal to the fistula or by anastomosing (end to end or side to side) the two segments of bowel on both sides of the fistula (e.g., ileotransverse anastomosis when the fistula communicates with the right colon). This latter procedure may be referred to as an *intestinal bypass* in which the segment of bowel containing the fistula is completely isolated and separated from the fecal stream.

When closure of the fistula is the goal, resection will be necessary. The advantage of this technique is that the diseased tissue is removed. An end-to-end anastomosis of the intestine with resection of the fistula tract is performed. To protect the anastomosis, diversion of the fecal stream through a temporary stoma may be indicated. If the distal part of the rectum is not suitable for anastomosis or the anal sphincters are not competent, a permanent stoma with a Hartmann's pouch may be the safest procedure.

Enteric fistulas communicating with the urinary tract will always require diversion of the fecal stream proximal to the fistula site to prevent urinary tract infections and pyelonephritis.

NURSING MANAGEMENT

The occurrence of a fistula lengthens recovery time, whether closure is spontaneous or occurs with surgical repair. This section focuses on the technical management of the patient with a fistula. The principles and techniques presented are applicable to all types of draining wounds and drain sites. Principles are presented so that management can be tailored to achieve effective solutions. However, the care plan must also include detailed attention to patient and family needs, involvement, education, and emotional support.

Technically, the patient with a fistula is one of the most challenging patients encountered by wound and ostomy care providers. Critical thinking skills are necessary to synthesize assessment data, product knowledge (advantages, disadvantages, effectiveness, and guidelines for use), patient needs, and physiology into realistic goals. Principles of wound care and principles of ostomy management are applied to the management of these clinical problems. There is also an art involved in the techniques presented in this chapter.

Following a comprehensive review of the literature, the Nurses Specialized in Wound, Ostomy and Continence Canada (NSWOCC) (formerly the CAET) developed a best practice document as a resource for nurses managing the patient with an ECF and EAF in the adult population in all care settings. Recommendations are presented in Table 39.5. These recommendations are intended as guidance for the entire

---

TABLE 39.5 Nurses Specialized in Wound, Ostomy and Continence Canada (NSWOCC) Best Practice Recommendations for Nursing Management of Fistulas

1. Collaborate with Leadership	1.1. Ensure the provision of policies, procedures, and related interdisciplinary education in order to standardize assessment and management approaches
	1.2. Ensure the provision of programs that facilitate care for the patient across the continuum of care
2. Perform a Comprehensive Nursing Assessment	
3. Determine Goals of Care in Collaboration with the Integrated Team	
4. Prevent Malnutrition and Optimize Nutritional Status	4.1. Consult a registered dietitian
	4.2. Correct fluid and electrolyte imbalances
	4.3. Provide nutritional support using one or more strategies
	4.4. Provide ongoing monitoring and reevaluation
5. Recognize the Importance and Impact of Potential Adjunctive Pharmaceutical Therapies	
6. Support and Enhance the Emotional Well-being and Quality of Life of the Patient	
7. Provide Educational Support to the Patient	
8. Select an ECF/EAF Management Method that Effectively Contains Output	8.1. Dressings
	8.2. Pouching systems (ostomy and wound managers)
	8.3. Troughing
	8.4. Saddlebagging
	8.5. Bridging
	8.6. Pouching for fistuloclysis
	8.7. Negative-pressure wound therapy (NPWT)

Nurses Specialized in Wound, Ostomy and Continence Canada (NSWOCC). (2018), Nursing Best Practice Recommendations: Enterocutaneous Fistula and Enteroatmospheric Fistula. Retrieved 8/27/2021 from: http://nswoc.ca/ecf-best-practices/.

BOX 39.3 **Eight Nursing Goals for Fistula Management**

1. Containment of effluent
2. Protection of perifistula skin or healing of surrounding open wound
3. Odor control
4. Patient comfort
5. Accurate measurement of effluent
6. Patient mobility
7. Ease of care
8. Cost containment

BOX 39.4 **Fistula Assessment and Documentation Guide**

1. Source (e.g., small bowel, bladder, esophagus)
2. Characteristics of effluent
   a. Volume
   b. Odor? (If yes, describe)
   c. Consistency (e.g., liquid, semiformed, formed, gas)
   d. Composition
      I. Color (e.g., clear, yellow, green, brown)
      II. Active enzymes
      III. Extremes in pH
3. Topography and size
   a. Number of sites
   b. Location(s)
   c. Length and width of each (include patterns)
   d. Openings (e.g., below skin level, at skin level, above skin level)
   e. Proximity to bony prominences, scars, abdominal creases, incision, drain(s), stoma
   f. Muscle tone surrounding opening (e.g., firm, soft, flaccid)
   g. Contours at the fistula opening (e.g., flat, shallow depth (<1/16 inch), moderate depth (1/16 to 1/4 inch), or deep (>1/4 inch))
4. Perifistular skin integrity at each location (e.g., intact, macerated, erythematous, denuded or eroded, ulcerated, infected)

interdisciplinary team, but especially for nurses, in the care of the adult population in all care settings (Brooke, El-Ghaname, Napier, & Sommerey, 2019).

Goals

Effective nursing management of the enterocutaneous fistula strives to achieve eight goals, as listed in Box 39.3. The primary goal of fistula management is containment of effluent. By doing that, the remaining goals are often also achieved. Interventions to achieve the goals begin as soon as the patient is noted to have a fistula; they are not contingent upon medical diagnosis.

When containment of fistula effluent is obtained by pouching, the following four (4) guidelines are important to attain success (Rolstad & Wong, 2004):

1. Assess the pouching system and seal frequently; expect changes.
2. Build flexibility into the care plan.
3. Innovate, using the easiest, most practical approach first.
4. Recognize that care of the patient is frequently provided by inexperienced caregivers.

Assessment

Distinct behavior, manifestations, and characteristics of the fistula are significant when selecting a management method. These are discussed in this section and outlined in Box 39.4. Because fistulas change in shape and contour over time, repeat assessment and monitoring are necessary. Modifications to the initial containment system are invariably necessary (Scardillo & Folkedahl, 1998; Wiltshire, 1996; Zwanziger, 1999).

Source

Initially, little information may be available regarding the origin of the fistula or the involved organs (if diagnostic studies have not yet been conducted). However, it may be possible to identify the probable origin of the fistula based on the assessment of fistula output (volume, odor, consistency, and composition) (Table 39.6). This information provides insight into the patient's risk for altered skin integrity and provides decision points for selection of the management approach. For example, a fistula producing semiformed, odorous effluent likely is communicating with the left transverse or descending

colon. Effluent from the transverse or descending colon will be less damaging to the skin than the output from the ileum. Therefore, in this situation, the primary goals of nursing management will be containment of effluent and odor control.

Characteristics of Effluent

Characteristics of effluent that must be considered in fistula management include volume, odor, consistency, and composition. In general, the fistula with output volumes greater than 100 mL over 24 h requires containment using a pouch or suction.

Odor is another factor when selecting a management method. The patient with a malodorous output of only 10 to 20 mL per 24 h may still require a pouching system to contain odor. However, there are dressings that can be used for odor control of low volume high odor output fistula management. Odor may originate from numerous sources, including exudate, necrotic or infected tissue, soiled dressings, dressing materials, and chemicals used during treatment.

Consistency of effluent is particularly important when pouching because it affects the type of drainage spout needed and subsequently the type of pouch selected. It also influences the need for additional skin barriers. Liquid effluent is much more corrosive than thick effluent and results in premature erosion of the skin barrier.

The color of effluent acts as an indicator of fistula source (see Table 39.6). In the presence of effluent with active enzymes or extremes in pH, the perifistular skin will require aggressive protection. However, all perifistular skin should be monitored and protected from moisture, even when effluent composition does not include active enzymes. Until

TABLE 39.6   Characteristics of Gastrointestinal Secretions

Source	Secretions	pH	24-h Volume (cc)	Color	ELECTROLYTE CONCENTRATION			
					Na (mg)	K (mEq)	Cl (mg)	HCO₃ (mg)
Saliva	Ptyalin, maltase	6–7	1000–1200	Clear	20–80	16–23	24–44	20–60
Gastric juice	Pepsin, rennin (chymosin) lipase, hydrochloric acid	1–3.5	2000–3000	Clear/ green	20–100	4–12	52–124	0
Pancreatic juice	Amylase, trypsin, chymotrypsin, lipase, sodium bicarbonate	8–8.3	700–1200	Clear/ milky	120–150	2–7	54–95	70–110
Bile	Bile salts, phospholipids	7.8	500–700	Golden brown to greenish yellow	120–200	3–12	80–120	30–50
Duodenum, jejunum, ileum	Peptidase, trypsin, lipase, maltase, sucrase, lactase	7.8–8	2000–3000	Gold to dark gold	80–130	11 to 21	48 to 116	20 to 30
Colon		7.5–8.9	50–200	Brown	4	9	2	—

Cl, Chloride; *HCO₃,* bicarbonate; *Na,* sodium; *K,* potassium.

radiographic studies are performed, the enzymatic and pH composition of the effluent can be inferred from the volume and consistency of the drainage.

Fistula Opening

The size of the fistula opening is determined by measuring the length and width in centimeters or inches. A pattern is always useful because the fistula orifice may be irregularly shaped. The pattern should be kept in the patient's room with supplies. The fistula opening may occur within a wound bed (EAF) or directly on the skin surface (ECF).

Abdominal Topography

Assessment is performed with the patient in a supine and semi-Fowler's position. The cutaneous fistula locations are identified and documented. The area is assessed for the presence of irregular skin surfaces that are created by scars or creases. This assessment indicates how flexible the adhesive in contact with the skin must be and whether filling agents, such as skin barrier paste or strips, are needed to level irregular surfaces (see Plates 94 and 95). In addition, the number of cutaneous fistula openings, the location of each, and the proximity to a bony prominence or other obstacles (e.g., retention sutures or stoma) are assessed and documented. These characteristics will help to determine the size and shape of the adhesive surface needed to secure the sites but not impinge on the prominence or protrusion. If two cutaneous sites are too far apart to be pouched in one system, two pouches may be necessary.

Muscle tone in the area and skin contours should be assessed. Decreased abdominal muscle tone can be expected in the patient who lacks exercise or is overweight, in the elderly, and in the infant. Aging affects subcutaneous tissue support. Muscle tone may be characterized as firm, soft, or flaccid.

It is important to assess the level at which the fistula opening exits onto the skin. Contours of the skin surrounding the fistula opening may be classified as flat, shallow ($<^1/_{16}$ inch), moderate depth ($^1/_{16}$ to $^1/_4$), or deep ($>^1/_4$ inch) (Rolstad & Boarini, 1996). The EAF requires assessment of both the fistula opening and the surrounding wound bed.

Protection of Perifistula Skin or Healing of Surrounding Wound Bed

Perifistular skin condition should be assessed and documented at each dressing or pouch change. Constant exposure of the epidermis to moisture, active enzymes, extremes in pH of fluids, and mechanical trauma frequently lead to breaks in skin integrity. Denudation of perifistular skin is a common complication in fistula management. Skin constantly bathed in fluid causes maceration, whereas effluent with enzymatic drainage or extremes in pH levels creates erythema and denuded or eroded perifistular skin. The perifistular skin may also develop an infection because of moisture entrapment against the skin and antibiotic-precipitated changes in the normal skin flora. Candidiasis is a common secondary complication as depicted in Plate 16. Chapter 9 provides additional information to facilitate delineation of fungal infection from irritant, chemical, or contact dermatitis.

Although visual inspection of the skin is best, data can also be obtained from the nursing staff and patient to aid assessment. For example, when frequent dressing changes (every 4 h) are reported, skin will deteriorate quickly as a result of moisture, chemical, and mechanical injury. Patient reports of burning or stinging sensations around the fistula or wound commonly indicate denudation of the epidermis.

The ideal management of the EAF is isolation of the effluent from the surrounding wound bed. However, this is not always possible. Various methods of effluent containment are described later in this chapter.

Planning and Implementation

Four key questions should be asked when planning the technical management of a fistula:

1. Is the output volume more than 100 mL in 24 h?
2. Is odor a problem?
3. Is the fistula (ECF) opening or fistula + surrounding wound less than 3 inches? (if unable to isolate EAF)
4. Is an access cap/window needed?

Fig. 39.4 shows an algorithm that incorporates these four questions to guide decision making for managing a fistula. Note, if the volume is >100 cc then according to this algorithm the question about odor is not relevant as the algorithm directs the clinician to use a pouching system, which will contain odor.

Fistula output can be contained with pouches, dressings, suction, or all three. When planning the specific fistula management approach, the four key questions and the goals that have been identified by the health care team and patient must be considered. In most situations, the priority goals are containment of effluent, odor control, and perifistular skin protection. Initially some goals may be compromised, such as

ease of care, patient mobility, and cost containment because of the acuteness of the situation. This section presents nursing interventions that facilitate attainment of each goal for the nursing management of fistulas.

Skin Protection

The potential for skin breakdown (either perifistular in the cutaneous fistula or periwound in the EAF) is always present when a fistula exists. Preventive strategies should be implemented early and be accompanied by frequent monitoring. Strategies include atraumatic adhesive removal and protection of the skin from exposure to effluent. Dressings alone do not offer skin protection, so concurrent use of a skin barrier is necessary. Skin barriers are available in various forms (Table 39.7). Table 39.7 summarizes the characteristics and indications of each type of skin barrier.

If pouching is selected as the management approach, pectin-based skin barriers usually are integrated into the pouching system during manufacturing. Additional pectin-based skin barriers may be required to caulk edges, fill creases, and/or add convexity. Skin protectants may also be used to

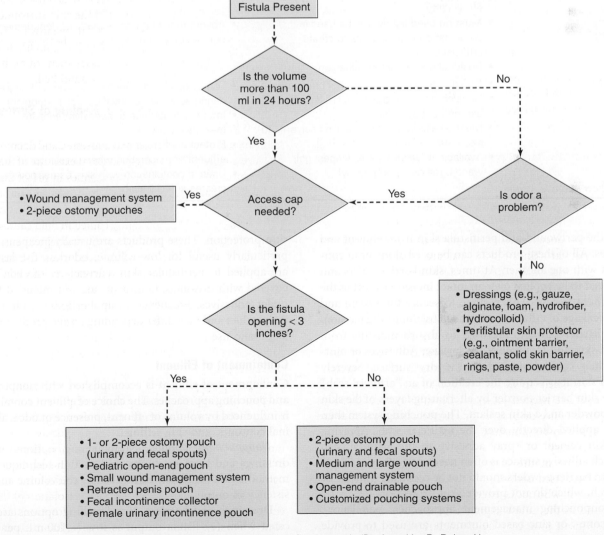

Fig. 39.4 Algorithm for selecting a fistula pouch. (Designed by B. Rolstad.)

TABLE 39.7	Guide to Use of Skin Barriers in Fistula Management	
Type of Skin Barrier	**Characteristics**	**Indications**
Solid wafers (4 inch × 4 inch or 8 inch × 8 inch) Plate 90	• Pectin-based wafers with adhesive surface • Available as wafers or rings • Have moist tack • Have varied flexibility • May be cut into wedges, rings, or strips • Have varied durability to effluent • Changed only when they loosen from perifistular edges or once every 7 days	• Provide skin protection, referred to as laying down a protective platform • Level irregular skin surfaces • Protect perifistular skin from effluent when dressings are used or skin is exposed • Gauze dressings are applied over the skin barrier wafer and taped to wafer rather to skin
Skin barrier rings Plate 70	• Available in hydrocolloid and karaya formulations • Have moist tack • Have varied flexibility • Have varied durability to effluent • Recommended for fistula management	• Level irregular skin surfaces • Protect perifistular skin from effluent when dressings are used or skin is exposed
Paste (tube or strip) Plate 95	• Commercial preparations may contain alcohol, which can create burning sensation if skin is denuded • Extremely tacky; should be applied as thin bead and smoothed into place with damp gloved finger or tongue blade • Contains solvents; allow to dry briefly so that solvents can escape before other products are applied	• Level irregular skin surfaces • Protect exposed skin from effluent (i.e., with pouching) • Extend duration of solid-wafer barrier when pouching
Powder Plate 70	• Must be used lightly; can be used in combination with sealants to create artificial scab • Residual powder alters adhesion	• Absorb moisture from superficial denudement before applying ointments or adhesives
Skin protectant Plate 52	• Liquid, nonalcohol, and alcohol preparations • Nonalcohol skin protectants are indicated for use on denuded skin • Must be allowed to dry to permit solvents to dissipate • Available in various forms (wipes, gel, wands, roll-ons, pump spray)	• Can be used under adhesives to protect fragile skin during adhesive removal (i.e., skin stripping) • Improve adherence of adhesives to skin (particularly oily skin) • Protect perifistular and periwound skin from effluent or maceration when dressings are used • Used in combination with skin barrier powders; creates artificial scab

protect the periwound and perifistula skin from effluent and adhesives. All of these products can be used alone or in conjunction with one another. At times, skin barrier wafers and pastes need to be applied over an intact incision as part of the management system. This is done to secure the system and prevent leakage of effluent from the fistula onto the incision.

Skin barrier powders are used to absorb moisture from denuded skin and to create a dry surface. Adhesives or ointments then can be applied to the dry surface. Severely denuded skin may require the creation of an "artificial scab" with the skin barrier powder by alternating layers of the skin barrier powder and a skin sealant. The pouching system then may be applied directly over the artificial scab. Applying either skin cement or spray adhesive to the artificial scab and pouch adhesive surface is often needed to enhance adherence. Skin barrier powders should not be confused with talc or cornstarch, which do not provide skin protection.

In nonpouching management approaches, petroleum-, dimethicone-, or zinc-based ointments are used to provide skin protection. These products are usually inexpensive and particularly useful for low-volume, odorless fistulas. They are applied to perifistular skin, particularly the edges, and covered with dressings. Ointments are not intended for use under adhesives. Frequency of application is indicated on the product and may differ depending on the product formulation and use.

Containment of Effluent

Containment of effluent is accomplished with nonpouching and pouching approaches. The choice of effluent containment is influenced by volume of effluent, presence of odor, abdominal contours, and care setting.

Nonpouching options. Nonpouching options include dressings and barriers, drains, and suction techniques. The method chosen is greatly influenced by the volume and consistency of output.

Dressings and barriers. Nonpouching options are indicated when (1) fistula output is low (<100 mL per 24 h);

(2) odor is not present; and (3) skin contours or location of the fistula makes pouching impossible. Containment of effluent can be achieved with dressings intended for absorption, which include gauze (sponges or strip packing), alginates, foam, and combinations of dressings. Packing should be done only with dressing materials that can be retrieved from the wound. For example, a strip packing material may be gently packed into a low-volume drain site. A 2-inch tail of dressing material is left outside the wound and is used to retrieve the packing at dressing changes. Entrapment of effluent against the skin may cause maceration and breakdown; therefore, skin barriers may be needed in conjunction with the dressings to protect the skin (see Table 39.7).

If, despite best efforts, the skin becomes compromised or output volume exceeds 100 mL in 24 h, dressings become less effective and more time intensive to manage. The application of additional dressings will not increase the absorbency of the dressing or lengthen the time between dressing changes. As a rule, a pouching system should be used when dressings must be changed more often than every 4 h.

Vaginal fistula management options. Vaginal fistulas (Fig. 39.5) occasionally develop secondary to pelvic irradiation or obstetric trauma; as a result the patient is incontinent of feces or urine through the vagina. The uncontrolled passage of feces or urine vaginally results in severe perivaginal skin denudation and discomfort. Aggressive nursing care is essential to prevent these complications.

Skin protection can be achieved with barrier ointments, pastes, and pads. Frequent dressing changes are necessary to prevent entrapment of caustic drainage contents against the skin. These options for vaginal fistulas are less than optimal because they are labor intensive, do not promote patient mobility, do not adequately contain the fecal contents, and fail to control odor. A female urinary incontinence pouch may be useful in these situations and may be connected to straight drainage. However, the difficult location and moist surface surrounding the vaginal orifice make application of an adhesive pouching system challenging.

One option that does not require adhesives is to create a vaginal drain device modified from the procedure initially described by Adrien (1983). A vaginal/menstrual cup can be inserted a short distance into the vagina to contain low-output fistula drainage. To allow continuous drainage of a higher fistula output, a cruciate incision can be made through a reusable vaginal cup, through which a catheter is threaded. Because the vaginal cup occludes the vagina, the drainage is either collected and contained by the cup or directed down the catheter.

The discomfort to the patient created by such manipulation of the labia and vagina can be minimized by lubricating the device with lidocaine jelly (Xylocaine). Tubing is attached to the device to channel the fistula contents into a straight drainage collection bag. The drainage tubing should be secured to the patient's inner thigh.

A vaginal drain device will remain in place effectively while the patient is reclining. As the patient becomes more ambulatory, the device may have a tendency to become dislodged; however, because the procedure is so easy, the patient can reinsert the vaginal cup as needed. Gentle irrigation of the tubing may be indicated if the tubing becomes occluded by fistula material. A vaginal drain device may be a temporary or permanent management technique depending on the patient's status.

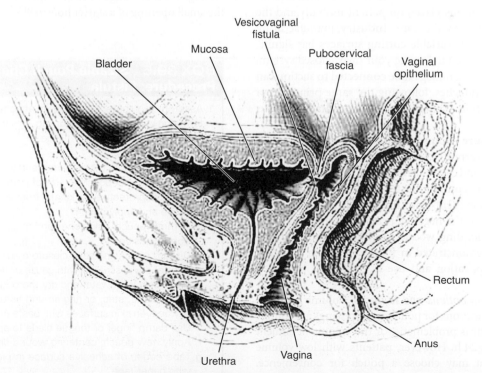

Fig. 39.5 Vaginal fistula between vagina and bladder.

Closed suction systems. Closed suction systems continue to be a viable, reliable, and cost-effective method for managing high-output fistulas, especially with EAF (Davis, Dere, & Hadley, 2000; Jones, Harbit, & Anderson, 2003; Kordasiewicz, 2004). Catheters attached to low intermittent suction may be used when routine pouching is ineffective or overwhelmed by the volume of output (Beitz & Caldwell, 1998; Lange, Thebo, Tiede, et al., 1989). However, suction does not provide complete containment of effluent; dressings and skin protection still are necessary. Effluent must be liquid for suction to be effective; thick or particulate drainage will occlude the catheter. The wound is cleansed, and a layer of saline-moistened gauze or nonadherent contact layer is placed in the wound bed. The catheter is laid in the wound and directed toward the bottom of the setup. Another layer of moist gauze may be applied over the catheter, and a large transparent dressing may be applied as a secondary dressing (Hollis & Reyna, 1985; Jeter, Tintte, & Chariker, 1990). Skin barrier paste, strips, or rings are sometimes necessary to fill in irregular skin surfaces and to seal around the catheter as it exits from the transparent dressing. Suction tubing is then attached to the suction catheter and set at a low level of continuous suction. A Hemovac can provide the suction for short periods to increase the patient's mobility. This dressing usually is changed every 1 to 2 days.

A catheter that is inserted into the fistula tract will act as a foreign body and may interfere with healing and even increase fistula output (Welch, 1997). On the other hand, a catheter coiled in a defect above the orifice or in the open wound surrounding the fistula opening will not inhibit closure. Because firm tubes can injure fragile tissue, only soft, flexible suction catheters should be used with fistulas (Welch, 1997). Suction catheters should be considered a short-term intervention because of the limitations placed on patient mobility and the time-intensive nature of the care. Industry manufacturing pouching systems with variable cutting surfaces has significantly impacted the need to "create your own" closed system, as mentioned above. A drainage tube connected to suction can be used with these pouches, following the same principles of wound bed protection with gauze and/or contact layer, as discussed.

Negative pressure wound therapy. Negative pressure wound therapy is warranted for use with an EAF to facilitate healing of the wound bed surrounding the fistula orifice. NPWT, however, is contraindicated over the fistula orifice itself or to contain effluent from the fistula. Isolation of the fistulized bowel from the negative pressure system is critical and only the surrounding wound bed has contact with the NPWT foam, as demonstrated in Plate 70 Further information about the application and use of NPWT is presented in Chapter 24.

Pouching system options and features. Volume and odor are the primary indications for pouching. Dressings are contraindicated when odor is problematic, or the volume of effluent exceeds 100 mL in 24 h. However, patients with low volume nonodorous output may choose a pouch for convenience. The pouch may be changed once per week and is less expensive than dressings.

Numerous techniques for managing fistulas have been reported in the literature (Boarini, Bryant, & Irrgang, 1986; Davis et al., 2000; Di Saverio et al., 2015; Irrgang & Bryant, 1984; Jones et al., 2003; Kordasiewicz, 2004; O'Brien, Landis-Erdman, & Erwin-Toth, 1998; Rolstad & Wong, 2004; Skingley, 1998; Smith, 1982, 1986). Ostomy pouches (fecal or urinary; adult or pediatric) can be used, as well as pouches specifically designed for managing complex wounds. Pouching preserves patient dignity by containing embarrassing odor and drainage. Pouching is an effective strategy for pain control because it requires less manipulation of the wound and protects the surrounding skin from painful denudement caused by caustic effluent. An effective pouching system also offers a sense of control to the caregivers because effluent is contained and emptied at specific intervals. Finally, a successful pouching system allows for accurate output measurement. Pouch changes are scheduled at convenient times before leakage occurs. Intervening to prevent the embarrassment of odor and leaking dressings can protect a patient's dignity. A routine pouch change procedure and fistula pouching tips are listed in Boxes 39.5 and 39.6, respectively.

Historically, frequent modifications of skin barriers, adhesives, and/or pouches were required to effectively manage the complicated fistula. Few alternatives were available to manage the fistula with a large cutaneous opening, irregular contours of the skin, and other unique situations. Materials used for pouches included garbage bags, colostomy irrigation sleeves, and sandwich bags. Today, manufactured wound management systems are designed for the difficult-to-manage site. Solid-wafer skin barriers with durable formulations that provide longer wear time are integrated into most pouching systems. Cutting surfaces of the skin barriers are available to manage a broad range of fistula opening sizes, ranging from the small opening of a starter hole to 9½ × 6 inches. However,

---

BOX 39.5 Sizable Pouch Change Procedure: Fistula

1. Assemble equipment: pouch with attached skin barrier, pattern, skin barrier strip, paste or ring, scissors, paper tape, closure clip, water, gauze, or tissue.
2. Prepare pouch.
   a. Trace pattern onto skin barrier surface of pouch.
   b. Cut skin barrier pouch to size of pattern.
   c. Remove protective backing(s) from pouch.
3. Remove and apply pouch.
   a. Remove pouch, using one hand to gently push skin away from adhesive.
   b. Discard pouch and save closure clip.
   c. Control any discharge with gauze or tissue.
   d. Clean skin with water and dry thoroughly.
   e. Apply paste, strip, or ring around fistula or stoma. Fill in any uneven skin surfaces with paste or skin barrier strips. Use damp finger or tongue blade to apply paste.
   f. Apply new pouch, centering wound site in opening.
   g. Tape edges of adhesive surface in picture frame effect with paper tape.
   h. Close bottom of pouch with clip.

BOX 39.6 Fistula Pouching Tips

1. Schedule the procedure, if possible, to allow education and participation from nursing staff and other caregivers.
2. Set up all equipment before starting procedure. Fistula function is unpredictable and may otherwise occur when adhesives are not completely set up.
3. Cut opening in pouch adhesive approximately $1/8$ inch larger than fistula cutaneous opening.
4. Protect exposed periwound skin with skin barrier paste (see Plate 95).
5. Apertures much larger than actual fistula opening may be necessary with severe, deep depressions that create irregular skin surfaces.
6. Follow universal precautions with clean technique during procedures. Sterile products are an unnecessary expense and are not shown to control infection.
7. To remove adhesives from skin, gently roll off adherent material with dry gauze. Solvents may be used, but must be cleansed thoroughly from skin before adhesive application. Do not scrub or abrade skin. It may be necessary to leave small amounts of residual paste or cement on skin but should not hinder pouch adhesion.
8. Cleanse skin with tap water or commercially available skin cleanser and gauze. Cleansers will emulsify fecal material and are primarily indicated when fistula drainage is adherent to surrounding skin. Cleansers should be nongreasy and rinsed thoroughly; use on denuded skin is discouraged. Dry thoroughly.
9. Minimize pooling of corrosive effluent over skin barrier by angling tail of pouch off to reclining patient's side, or attach drainage tubing to enable continuous drainage.
10. Empty pouch when one-third to half full. Encourage patient to monitor.

BOX 39.7 Features of Fistula Pouches

Adhesive Surface
- Integrated skin barrier
- Size and shape of cutting surface
- Sizable versus presized adhesive surface
- Presence or absence of starter hole
- Degree of flexibility of skin barrier wafer

Pouch Capacity
- Volume (3- to 4-hour capacity preferred)

Pouch Outlet
- Fecal outlet (clamp closure)
- Spout for liquids (urinary outlet)
- Wide drain for viscous material
- Wide tubular outlet can be converted to open-end drain

Wound Access
- Two-piece pouch
- Access window on wound management system
- Wide tubular outlet can be converted to open-end drain

Pouch Film
- Odorproof or odor-resistant pouch film
- Transparent versus opaque film

---

it remains essential to fill irregular skin surfaces so that a flat, stable surface is attained for the pouching system.

Selecting a pouching system that supports the perifistular tissue and stabilizes soft skin may be necessary. In general, if the skin is soft or flaccid, a firm skin barrier adhesive and possibly a belt may be indicated. In contrast, firm skin surrounding the fistula site is best managed with a flexible, soft adhesive surface. Examples of soft, pliable materials include skin barrier paste, wafers, strips, and rings. Methods for achieving firm support include firm rings, convexity in ostomy pouching systems, and belts.

Knowledge of available features of products is essential to make appropriate choices. Features include adhesive skin barrier surface, pouch capacity, pouch material (film and outlet), and wound access (Box 39.7).

Adhesive skin barrier surface. When the cutaneous opening is less than 3 inches, a one- or two-piece ostomy pouch may be used. For fistulas larger than 3 inches, commercially available wound management systems or modifications of larger pouches are warranted. In either case, the adhesive skin barrier surface must be large enough to accommodate the fistula opening and generally allow for 1–2 inches of adhesive contact around the fistula. The adhesive surface should be applied in such a fashion as to avoid obstacles in the perifistular skin area, such as a bony prominence or drain site. If this

is not possible, a pouch with a smaller adhesive surface may be needed.

Conversely, a large amount of adhesive contact (over 4–5 inches) with the surrounding skin is generally not necessary and may be detrimental. Movement-induced skin changes under the adhesive surface will precipitate leakage and disruption of the pouch seal. Also, having a large amount of adhesive contact subjects the patient to being at higher risk for medical adhesive-related skin injury (MARSI).

Pouching systems may have a starter hole for cutting the opening into irregular shapes or may be presized (e.g., for round, regular shapes). Although starter holes are convenient for cutting, they restrict the positioning of the opening in the adhesive because the opening includes the starter hole. In some situations, the opening may have to be covered with a skin barrier so that other locations on the adhesive may be cut to fit the size of the fistula.

Pouch capacity. The capacity of the pouch is predetermined by the size of the adhesive surface; typically pouches with larger adhesive surfaces have larger pouch capacities. Generally, a pouch with the capacity to contain at least 3–4 h worth of effluent is recommended so that the risk of leakage is minimized. A smaller-capacity pouch may be used if the caregiver or patient is willing to empty the pouch more frequently or if the pouch can be connected to straight drainage. Small-volume, closed-end pouches may also be indicated for the patient with minimal malodorous output. Ideally, this pouch would be changed and discarded once or twice per week, although it could be changed as frequently as daily if needed.

Pouch outlet. Effluent consistency and volume dictate the best type of outlet spout for pouch management. Pouches are designed with either a urinary (or liquid) outlet/spigot or a fecal outlet. The urinary outlet is indicated for liquid effluent. It is convenient because it may be connected to straight drainage. When a urinary pouch is used for fistula care, the antireflux mechanism may obstruct flow; therefore, the antireflux mechanism may be pulled apart prior to application. Some wound pouches and "high output" fecal pouches have a larger drainage spigot. This allows for more particulate or thicker output to pass through the outlet. Fecal outlets (or open-end drains) are appropriate for thick, mushy effluent. The closure mechanism on this pouch is either integrated into the tail of the pouch or the pouch is closed with a clamp.

The two-piece ostomy system, fecal incontinence collectors, and wound management systems offer the benefit of having a urinary outlet that can be attached to a bedside bag. As the effluent thickens, the outlet can be trimmed off and secured with a clamp, transforming the pouch from a urinary to a fecal pouch without having to remove the pouch from the skin.

Two-piece high-output pouching systems are available that combine the desirable features of an ostomy system (e.g., presized adhesive surface with or without convexity) with outlets that can accommodate the varying consistency of effluent typical of a fistula.

Adaptations can be made to pouches to accommodate fistula consistency. For example, when formed output becomes liquid, urinary pouch–adapter latex drainage tubing can be attached to a fecal pouch. If the output begins to thicken or form particulate matter, wider respiratory tubing can be attached to the tail of an open-end drain (Box 39.8).

Wound access. At times, access to the fistula site may be desirable so that tubes can be advanced, the fistula can be assessed easily, or skin barrier pastes can be reinforced. Access

to the site without disruption of the pouch adhesive can be achieved with a two-piece pouch or with a pouch that has an attached "access window." When such access features are not available or have an inadequate adhesive surface size, wide open-end drains can be used. Cuffing the pouch film back can facilitate limited access to the fistula site.

Pouch film. Urinary drainage equipment and some fecal pouches may be more odor resistant than odorproof. More frequent pouch changes may be necessary to prevent the odor from permeating the pouch film, or more aggressive odor management techniques (e.g., oral or pouch deodorizers) may be required. It is critical to keep the pouch tail or exterior spigot clean from effluent. Verify the odor is not due to effluent on the tail closure before exploring an alternative pouching system for odor control. Pouching systems marketed as wound management systems are transparent to allow for visual inspection. Ostomy pouches adapted for fistula care provide choices in film color (transparent, opaque, beige tone).

Pouching system adaptations

Adhesives. Additional adhesive is available as cement, medical adhesive spray forms, and sheet forms. Cements and sprays are applied according to the manufacturer's instructions; most require time to become tacky. They are used to enhance the tack of an existing adhesive and to extend the adhesive surface on a pouch. Adhesives may also be warranted to improve the tack when several applications of skin barrier powder are required in the presence of severe denudation. Occasionally, liquid adhesive is used in combination with skin barrier powders to protect exposed skin from caustic effluent. This procedure is similar to the artificial scab discussed previously.

Because fistulas vary in size and shape and abdominal contours can be dramatic, large and unusually shaped pouch apertures may be necessary. One option is to create a pouch (Box 39.9). The advantage to this technique is that it offers immediate skin protection and containment of affluent using readily available supplies. Although this is a temporary

---

BOX 39.8 Addition of Continuous Drainage Tube to Fecal Outlet Pouch

Equipment
- Fecal pouch or open-end drain.
- Connector to fit tubing and bedside system.
- Five inches of wide-lumen tubing or respiratory tubing.
- Rubber band.
- Bedside drainage system.

Procedure
1. Cut desired size for fistula in skin barrier adhesive of fecal pouch or open-end drain.
2. Insert wide-lumen tubing or respiratory tubing into drain spout.
3. Working at adhesive surface, reach inside pouch and pull drain spout and tubing through opening cut in skin barrier adhesive.
4. Wrap rubber band securely around tubing to secure.
5. From bottom of pouch, pull tubing through so that outlet spout is in its normal location. Tail of pouch now is cuffed around tubing inside pouch.
6. Attach to bedside drainage system.

Note: If wide respiratory tubing is used, a condom catheter can be used to connect the pouch to bedside drainage.

BOX 39.9 Procedure for Making Temporary Fistula Pouch

Equipment
- Plastic bag.
- Skin barrier wafer.
- Double-faced adhesive sheet or double-faced tape.

Procedure
1. Remove protective paper from one side of adhesive sheet and apply to area of pouch where adhesive and barrier are intended to be (in absence of adhesive sheets, substitute with overlapping strips of double-sided tape).
2. Remove other side of adhesive sheet or tape.
3. Attach skin barrier wafer (top side toward exposed adhesive on pouch).
4. Cut barrier of pouch to desired size.
5. Remove skin barrier wafer protective paper backing.
6. Continue in usual fashion.

intervention, it allows the care provider time to design a management system and to obtain commercially available products with the desirable features identified in the plan of care.

Another method that can be used to acquire a large adhesive surface is to attach two open-end drainable pouches, a technique called *saddlebagging* (Fig. 39.6). Pouch features that facilitate saddlebagging include no attached solid-wafer skin barrier, and no floating collar. A large solid-wafer skin barrier is then attached to the new combined adhesive surface, and the pouch is prepared in the usual fashion. Box 39.10 describes the saddlebagging technique.

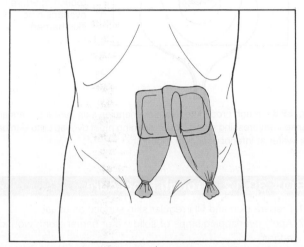

Fig. 39.6 Saddlebagging technique in which two open-ended drainable pouches is connected along the adhesive surface to create a large adhesive surface.

BOX 39.10 Saddlebagging Technique

Equipment
- Two open-end drains (without floating collar or attached skin barrier or starter hole).
- Solid-wafer skin barrier (8 × 8 inches).
- Skin barrier paste.

Procedure
1. Align pouches as final product is intended to appear on abdomen.
2. Peel protective backing away from adhesive along common edges of pouches approximately 1/2 to 1 inch.
3. Attach two pouches along this 1/2- to 1-inch margin only.
4. Trace pattern of wound onto new adhesive surface (combined pouch adhesive surfaces).
5. Cut out pouch opening; do not cut into "seam" created by combining pouches.
6. Trace pattern onto solid-wafer skin barrier and cut out.
7. Remove protective paper backing from pouch adhesive surface and attach to solid-wafer skin barrier.
8. Prepare skin as indicated by wound contours and continue pouching procedure.

Note: Both pouches will fill with drainage and will require emptying.

Isolation technique. The isolation technique, previously known as "bridging," is a procedure that can be used to isolate the EAF from the wound bed. This technique may be achieved in a variety of ways. Solid-wafer skin barriers or convex barrier rings can be applied in layers to isolate the fistula opening, or section of wound with fistulas (Fig. 39.7). A routine pouch or more complicated pouching system can then be applied over this section of the wound and allow independent wound care to the area of the wound without a fistula. Box 39.11 describes the steps involved in this technique. A second isolation procedure is using NPWT to the surrounding wound and isolating the fistula and applying a pouch for output containment (see Plate 70). Commercial products for fistula isolation in an open wound are now available (Wirth et al., 2018) (see Plate 69).

Catheter ports. When a catheter or tube is in place at a fistula site, leakage onto perifistular skin may occur. A pouching system with an attached catheter port may be used to collect the drainage. A catheter port is a nipple-shaped device that attaches to the external wall of a pouch. The catheter is

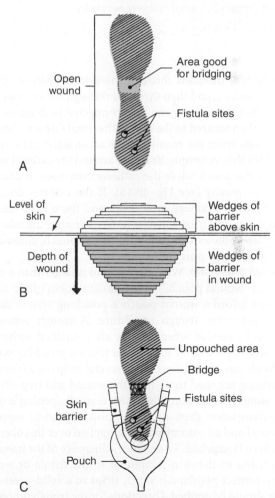

Fig. 39.7 Isolation technique. (A) Area of wound where fistula sites are located and identified can be separated from remainder of wound. (B) Cross-sectional view of tapered skin barrier wedges used to fill wound defect and to extend slightly above level of skin. (C) Demonstration of how a pouch is applied over a bridge and fistula, leaving the area of the wound that is not draining available for more appropriate wound care.

BOX 39.11 Isolation Technique

1. Assess wound and determine most appropriate location for "bridge." Be sure all sites from which drainage is produced are included on the side of wound to be pouched. For simplification of bridging procedure, areas that are narrower or shallower should be selected.
2. Apply layered wedges of solid-wafer skin barrier and paste to create bridge. Wedges must be custom cut to fit dimensions of wound at that level; usually the bottom wedge is narrowest because the deepest part of the wound typically is the narrowest area. Each successive wedge is a little wider until the skin barrier wafer wedges reach skin level.
3. Continue to layer solid-wafer barrier wedges above skin level, using progressively smaller and narrower wedges (to create pressure dressing effect).
4. Apply solid-wafer skin barrier to cover newly created bridge and extend onto intact skin. Paste may be needed to smooth "seams."
5. Continue with routine or complex pouching procedure as indicated.

Note: Skin barrier paste, adhesive spray, or cement can be used between wedges but is not routinely necessary.

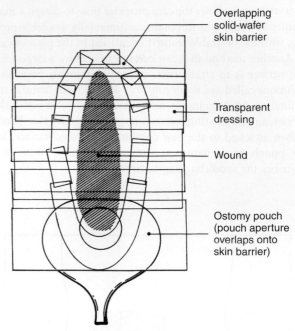

Fig. 39.8 Trough procedure. Note overlapping skin barrier wafers and transparent dressing strips. Pouch opening must overlap onto skin barrier wafer at inferior aspect of wound.

disconnected, threaded through the pouch opening on the adhesive surface, and then threaded through the catheter port itself so that the catheter can be reconnected to drainage. The pouch is then secured to the skin in the usual fashion. Detailed instructions from the manufacturer accompany the catheter port. With this technique, drainage around the catheter is collected in the pouch while the catheter continues to drain by suction or gravity (see Fig. 40.16). If the catheter does not require gravity drainage or suction, and there is no need to record the output from the tube or from around the tube separately, the catheter can be left inside the pouch, eliminating the need to add a port to the pouch.

Trough procedure. When the wound is larger than a manufactured "wound pouch," or the patient doesn't have access or cannot afford a wound pouch a pouching system can be created using the trough procedure. A trough procedure may also be needed when fistulas are contained within the depressions of a wound such that a routine pouching system fails. With this procedure, one or several strips of a transparent dressing are used to occlude the wound and trap effluent in the wound depression (Fig. 39.8). A small opening is made in the transparent dressing at the most dependent aspect of the wound and an ostomy pouch is applied over this opening. No pattern is required. To enhance adherence of the transparent dressing to the skin peripheral to the fistula or wound (and to protect perifistular skin), strips of a solid-wafer skin barrier should be applied. Directions for the trough procedure are given in Box 39.12.

Odor control. In general, odor control measures are indicated any time the patient and/or family perceive an odor to be objectionable, even if the odor seems almost imperceptible.

BOX 39.12 Trough Procedure

1. Prepare skin and fill irregular skin surface as usual.
2. Apply overlapping strips of solid-wafer barrier along wound edges.
3. Apply skin barrier paste to smooth "seams" (between barrier edges and along skin edges). *Note:* Inferior aspect of wound should be bordered with a solid piece of barrier instead of overlapping strips to prevent leakage.
4. Cut strips of transparent dressing wide enough to cover wound and skin barrier strips. Calculate length of strips so that strips overlap intact skin with 1- to 2-inch margins.
5. Reserve one strip of transparent dressing to be applied to the most inferior aspect of wound.
6. Attach a drainable pouch (can be urinary or fecal) to this one strip of transparent dressing.
7. Cut hole in pouch or transparent dressing adhesive surface so that it is lower than inferior wound margins (should clear wound edges to provide adequate drainage).
8. Beginning at top of wound, apply transparent dressing in overlapping strips.
9. Attach final strip of transparent dressing (with attached pouch) so that bottom of pouch opening is secured onto skin barrier wafer.

The method of odor control depends on whether dressings or pouches are being used. Gauze dressings do not control odor; therefore charcoal-impregnated dressings may be needed over the gauze dressings. However, charcoal becomes inactivated with moisture, so these dressings should not come into contact with wound drainage. Charcoal dressings are most cost effective with low-output fistulas, for which the dressings remain intact for 24–48 h. These dressings are effective only when all edges of the dressing are secured with tape. Intact pouches provide odor control. However, when the pouch is emptied, odor may be noticeable. Therefore, odor management must be a component of the care plan.

Odor is best controlled by use of a pouch to contain the effluent. A pouch may be the preferred management technique simply to contain the odor, regardless of the volume of output. Although most pouches have an odorproof film, the film's ability to contain odor varies. For example, many urinary pouches and urinary drainable systems are not odorproof and may become saturated with odor quickly.

To control odor, (1) dispose of soiled linens and dressings from the room promptly; (2) use care in emptying pouches to prevent splashing effluent on the patient or on linens; (3) cleanse the tail of drainable fecal pouches after emptying; and (4) use deodorants appropriately.

Deodorants can be taken internally (orally) or used externally (in the pouch or as a room spray). Internal deodorants are available in tablet form but are generally discouraged in the presence of a pathologic condition such as a fistula. External deodorants are available in liquids, powders, and tablets and are placed in the pouch after each emptying. Room deodorants are particularly useful when emptying the pouch, changing the pouch, or changing dressings. The room deodorant selected should eliminate rather than mask odor. At home a patient may also elect to light a fragrant candle or use a plug-in or infuser to mask odor. With the many types of deodorants now available, patients, families, and caregivers should not have to tolerate the odor that often accompanies a fistula.

Patient Comfort

Areas to address to promote patient comfort include prevention and early treatment of perifistular skin irritation, pain control, and education to decrease anxiety. Leaking pouches, wet dressings on the skin and odor in the patient's room all negatively affect morale. Medicating the patient before dressing or pouch changes may be indicated. Factors contributing to skin irritation include damp dressings, presence of caustic effluent in contact with the skin, and frequent tape application and removal. When selecting and evaluating a management technique, interventions appropriate to prevent unnecessary patient discomfort should be considered. It may be something as simple as the patient not knowing the schedule of when someone is going to come and change her pouch that is anxiety producing. In this situation, developing a time for the visit twice weekly would be identified as a comfort measure.

Accurate Measurement of Effluent

Accurate measurement of effluent from a fistula or drain site is critical to the success of fluid and electrolyte resuscitation and nutritional support. As the patient becomes stabilized, accurate measurement of the effluent is less important. Pouching offers the most objective method for monitoring output, and suction is accurate only if the effluent does not leak around the catheters or pouch. Dressings can provide an estimate of volume if the dressings are weighed; however,

this method is time consuming, messy, and inconsistent from caregiver to caregiver.

Patient Mobility

Consideration for optimizing the patient's activity should be of paramount importance when a fistula management method is being selected. Restrictions on physical activity predispose the patient to physical complications such as pneumonia, pressure injuries, and thrombophlebitis, as well as to psychosocial complications such as depression and withdrawal. Because limitations on a patient's physical activity are sometimes necessary when suction or dressings are used to contain effluent, these interventions should be used only on a temporary basis. Pouches are less likely to restrict mobility. When a tube with suction is used with the fistula, temporary suction can be maintained with the portable devices such as a Hemovac, or the suction tubing can be clamped off for a short period such as during ambulation. The drawback, however, to clamping off the suction tubing is that effluent production by the fistula is unpredictable and can occur suddenly, causing the pouching system adhesive to fail.

Ease of Use

Complex patient situations may necessitate unique pouching systems that may be expensive and labor intensive. These unique adaptations often set up hurdles to the successful participation of care providers. These complicated systems increase the chance of error in application and the time required of the caregiver. Therefore, management may be complex initially and require the expertise of a certified ostomy care nurse (COCN) or wound, ostomy, continence nurse (CWOCN). As care progresses, the method of pouching should be simplified as much as possible to a more user-friendly system so that care can be delegated. Several conveniences are available and should be considered as long as effectiveness is not compromised (Box 39.13).

Cost Containment

Accountable, appropriate fistula management requires selection of treatment options that are cost effective. For example, a fistula pouch with a wound access window is more costly than a sizable ostomy pouch, which probably would yield

---

BOX 39.13 User-Friendly Considerations in Fistula Care

1. Use presized pouch rather than sizable pouch whenever possible.
2. Avoid suction when pouching is effective.
3. Fill skin defects with strip paste rather than tube paste in patients with manual dexterity problems.
4. Use pouching systems with convexity rather than creating convexity with layers of skin barriers.
5. Use one-piece rather than two-piece pouches.
6. Select equipment that is easy to access in the community. Mail order of products is a convenience as long as orders are placed before patient's supplies are depleted.

the same wear time. However, if use of a pouch with an access window prolongs wear time by providing access for wound care and paste application, it may be the most cost-effective option, even if the pouch is changed every other day. Cost containment implies attention not only to products and materials but also to labor and time.

Evaluation

Accomplishment of Goals

The nurse should take time to reflect on the eight nursing management goals and evaluate how well they have been accomplished. Can steps in the procedure be omitted? Is the skin intact? Is odor controlled? As the fistula stabilizes, the technical approach should be reevaluated and simplified as much as possible. One management system is seldom effective from the onset of the fistula until closure. For example, one fistula may be managed over its course with a pouch, dressings, suction, or all three. While the patient is in the hospital, suction may be a workable option; however, mobility is compromised, and plans for home care are complicated. Therefore, developing a pouching system that does not require suction would be an important simplification. Similarly, using products that are difficult to obtain is a

complicating step and may be expensive. Planning to use an effective system that is easy and readily available is essential to facilitate the delivery of care.

Making Changes

It is important to expect changes in fistula care and to modify interventions as needed. Seldom will the first pouch applied to a complex fistula be effective. Generally, modifications are necessary in the pouch pattern, size of adhesive surface, and use of skin barrier pastes or wafer strips. Changes are best made one at a time so that the effect of each modification can be accurately assessed. The addition of a belt may be warranted to add security to the pouch system, particularly on obese patients or when the perifistular skin is mobile (i.e., flaccid abdomen).

The nurse must provide close monitoring for the duration of the fistula, regardless of the health care setting. An inquisitive, analytic approach will facilitate identifying steps to improve the duration of the pouching system. For example, if the pouch leaks, is the leak between the skin and the barrier or between the barrier and the pouch? Is the pouch being emptied when it is one-third to one-half full to prevent overfilling?

CLINICAL CONSULT

A: A 36-year-old female patient is seen in consult for recommendations to address three enterocutaneous fistulas on her abdomen from metastatic cervical cancer. The patient is terminal and wants to go home for her last days. However, despite multiple trials of pouching the draining abdominal fistulas, all attempts have failed and leaked caustic stool on her skin. The patient's oral intake is very limited and her volume of effluent is approximately 150 cc per 24 h

D: Metastatic cervical cancer resulting in small-bowel fistula.

P: The goal for care is to contain the fistula output and protect her skin. After meeting the patient, a simple plan was developed that

the patient and caregivers could demonstrate apply a thin skin barrier wafer to encircle fistulas. She then will layer superabsorbent nonadherent dressings over the site to wick effluent away from her skin and secure them in place with mesh panties. A full incontinence brief can be used over the mesh panties to add security for drainage containment.

I: The patient is given the dressings and instructions for care. She is instructed she can shower off the dressings at any time.

E: The patient will be given phone contact for any added support or changes in plan of care.

SUMMARY

- Successful management of a patient with a fistula requires close monitoring and a plan of care that addresses the technical, educational, and emotional needs of the patient.
- Care often crosses many health care settings with varying levels of expertise in the unique containment and skin protection vital to the patient's well-being.

- In these situations, special arrangements must be made for appropriate follow-up of these complex patients.

SELF-ASSESSMENT QUESTIONS

1. Which of the following terms is the best to describe the fistula that empties into the base of a wound?
   a. Colovesical fistula
   b. Enteroatmospheric fistula
   c. Simple fistula
   d. Type 1 fistula

2. Which of the following factors are known to contribute to bowel fistula formation?
   a. Hypotension, tension on the suture line, distal bowel obstruction
   b. Diabetes mellitus, anemia, hematoma formation at site of anastomosis

c. Compromised blood flow to area of anastomosis, distal bowel obstruction, presence of foreign body close to suture line

d. Hypoalbuminemia, electrolyte imbalance, tension at the suture line

3. Define the involved structures for the following fistulas:
   a. Enterocutaneous. (small bowel to skin)
   b. Colocutaneous
   c. Vesicovaginal
   d. Rectovaginal
   e. Colovesical

4. Which of the following is the major cause of death in the patient with a fistula?
   a. Malnutrition
   b. Sepsis
   c. Fluid and electrolyte imbalance
   d. Hypotension

5. Which of the following fistulas in an adult would be appropriately managed with a pouching system?
   a. Output during the past 4 h required four dressing changes and skin is inflamed.
   b. Output during past 24 h was 50 mL and nonodoros.
   c. Output is noncorrosive and skin is intact.
   d. Output is nonodorous, contained with dressings, and skin is intact.

6. Skin barrier ring or paste used when pouching a fistula achieves which of the following objectives?
   a. Absorb moisture from denuded skin.
   b. Increase tack of pouch adhesive.
   c. Level irregular skin surfaces.
   d. Protect the skin from adhesives.

REFERENCES

Adrien, L. (1983). Vaginal fistulas: Adaptation of management method for patients with radiation damage. *Journal of Enterostomal Therapy, 10*(6), 229–230.

Beitz, J. M., & Caldwell, D. (1998). Abdominal wound with enterocutaneous fistula: A case study. *Journal of Wound, Ostomy, and Continence Nursing, 25*(2), 102–106.

Berry, S. M., & Fischer, J. E. (1996). Classification and pathophysiology of enterocutaneous fistulas. *The Surgical Clinics of North America, 76*(5), 1009–1018.

Bleier, J. I., & Hedrick, T. (2010). Metabolic support of the enterocutaneous fistula patient. *Clinics in Colon and Rectal Surgery, 23*(3), 142–148.

Boarini, J., Bryant, R. A., & Irrgang, S. J. (1986). Fistula management. *Seminars in Oncology Nursing, 2*(4), 287–292.

Brooke, J., El-Ghaname, A., Napier, K., & Sommerey, L. (2019). Executive summary: Nurses Specialized in Wound, Ostomy and Continence Canada (NSWOCC) nursing best practice recommendations: Enterocutaneous fistula and enteroatmospheric fistula. *Journal of Wound, Ostomy, and Continence Nursing, 46*(4), 306–308.

Buchanan, G. N., Bartram, C. I., Phillips, R. K., et al. (2003). Efficacy of fibrin sealant in the management of complex anal fistula: A prospective trial. *Diseases of the Colon and Rectum, 46*(9), 1167–1174.

Campos, A. C., Andrade, D. F., Campos, G. M., et al. (1999). A multivariate model to determine prognostic factors in gastrointestinal fistulas. *Journal of the American College of Surgeons, 188*(5), 483–490.

Cowan, K. B., & Cassaro, S. (2022). Enterocutaneous fistula. In StatPearls [Internet]. Treasure Island: StatPearls Publishing; Available from: https://www.ncbi.nlm.nih.gov/books/NBK459129/. [Updated 2022 Aug 8].

Das, B., & Snyder, M. (2016). Rectovaginal fistulae. *Clinics in Colon and Rectal Surgery, 28*, 50–56.

Davis, M., Dere, K., & Hadley, G. (2000). Options for managing an open wound with draining enterocutaneous fistula. *Journal of Wound, Ostomy, and Continence Nursing, 27*(2), 118–123.

Di Saverio, S., Tarasconi, A., Inaba, K., Navsaria, P., Coccolini, F., Navarro, D. C., et al. (2015). Open abdomen and concomitant enteroatmospheric fistula: Attempt to rationalize the approach to surgical nightmare and proposal of a clinical algorithm. *Journal of the American College of Surgeons, 220*(3), e23–e33.

Dudrick, S. J., Maharaj, A. R., & McKelvey, A. A. (1999). Artificial nutritional support in patients with gastrointestinal fistulas. *World Journal of Surgery, 23*(6), 570–576.

Dudrick, S. J., & Panait, L. (2011). Metabolic consequences of patients with gastrointestinal fistulas. *European Journal of Trauma and Emergency Surgery, 37*(3), 215–225.

Evenson, A. R., & Fischer, J. E. (2006). Current management of enterocutaneous fistula. *Journal of Gastrointestinal Surgery, 10*(3), 455–464.

Fagniez, P. L., & Yahchouchy, E. (1999). Use of somatostatin in the treatment of digestive fistulas. Pharmacoeconomic issues. *Digestion, 60*(Suppl. 3), 65–70.

Fischer, J. E. (1983). The pathophysiology of enterocutaneous fistulas. *World Journal of Surgery, 7*, 446–450.

González-Pinto, I., & González, E. M. (2001). Optimizing the treatment of upper gastrointestinal fistula. *Gut, 49*(Suppl. 4), 22–31.

Gribovskaja-Rupp, I., & Melton, G. B. (2016). Enterocutaneous fistula: Proven strategies and updates. *Clinics in Colon and Rectal Surgery, 29*, 130–137.

Hesse, U., Ysebaert, D., & de Hemptinne, B. (2001). Role of somatostatin-14 and its analogues in the management of gastrointestinal fistulae: Clinical data. *Gut, 49*(Suppl. 4), 11–21.

Hild, P., Dobroschke, J., Henneking, K., et al. (1986). Treatment of enterocutaneous fistulas and somatostatin. *Lancet, 2*(8507), 626.

Hollington, P., Mawdsley, J., Lim, W., et al. (2004). An 11-year experience of enterocutaneous fistulas. *The British Journal of Surgery, 91*(12), 1646–1651.

Hollis, H. W., & Reyna, T. M. (1985). A practical approach to wound care in patients with complex enterocutaneous fistulas. *Surgery, Gynecology & Obstetrics, 161*(2), 179–180.

Irrgang, S., & Bryant, R. (1984). Management of the enterocutaneous fistula. *Journal of Enterostomal Therapy, 11*, 211–228.

Jeter, K. F., Tintte, T., & Chariker, M. (1990). Managing draining wounds and fistulae: New and established methods. In D. Krasner (Ed.), *Chronic wound care: A clinical source book for healthcare professionals* (pp. 240–246). King of Prussia: Health Management.

Jones, E. G., Harbit, M., & Anderson, R. (2003). Management of an ileostomy and mucous fistula located in a dehisced wound in a patient with morbid obesity. *Journal of Wound, Ostomy, and Continence Nursing, 30*(6), 351–356.

Kassis, E. S., & Makary, M. A. (2008). Enterocutaneous fistula. In J. S. Cameron (Ed.), *Current surgical therapy* (9th ed.). St. Louis: Mosby.

Kaushal, M., & Carlson, G. I. (2004). Management of enterocutaneous fistulas. *Clinics in Colon and Rectal Surgery, 17*(2), 79–88.

Knechtges, P., & Zimmermann, E. M. (2015). Intra-abdominal abscesses and fistulae. In T. Yamada, D. H. Alpers, L. Laine, et al. (Eds.), *Vol. II. Textbook of gastroenterology* (6th ed.). Philadelphia: Lippincott Williams & Wilkins.

Kordasiewicz, L. M. (2004). Abdominal wound with fistula and large amount of drainage status after incarcerated hernia repair. *Journal of Wound, Ostomy, and Continence Nursing, 31*(3), 150–152.

Kumpf, V. J., deAguilar-Nascimiento, J. E., Diaz-Pizarro Graf, J. I., McKeever, L., Steiger, E., Winkler, M. F., et al. (2017). American Society for Parenteral and Enteral Nutrition ASPEN-FELANPE Clinical Guideline: Nutrition support of adult patients with enterocutaneous fistula. *Journal of Parenteral and Enteral Nutrition, 41*(1), 104–112.

Lange, M. P., Thebo, L. M., Tiede, S. M., et al. (1989). Management of multiple enterocutaneous fistulas. *Heart & Lung, 18*(4), 386–390.

Lyon, J. W., Hoddle, J. P., Hucks, D., & Changkuon, D. I. (2013). First experience with the use of collagen fistula plug to treat enterocutaneous fistulas. *Journal of Vascular Interventional Radiology, 24*(10), 1559–1565.

Makhdoom, Z. A., Komar, M. J., & Still, C. D. (2000). Nutrition and enterocutaneous fistulas. *Journal of Clinical Gastroenterology, 31*(3), 195–204.

Marinis, A., Gkiokas, G., Argyra, E., et al. (2013). "Enteroatmospheric fistulae"—Gastrointestinal openings in the open abdomen: A review and recent proposal of a surgical technique. *Scandinavian Journal of Surgery, 102*(2), 61–68.

Maykel, J. A., & Fischer, J. E. (2003). Current management of intestinal fistulas. In J. L. Cameron (Ed.), *Advances in surgery*. St. Louis: Mosby.

Migaly, J., & Rolandelli, R. H. (2007). Suturing stapling and tissue adhesives. In C. J. Yeo, D. T. Dempsey, A. S. Klein, et al. (Eds.), *Shackelford's surgery of the alimentary tract* (6th ed.). St Louis: Saunders.

Nussbaum, M. S., & Fischer, D. R. (2007). Gastric, duodenal and small intestinal fistulas. In C. J. Yeo, D. T. Dempsey, A. S. Klein, et al. (Eds.), *Shackelford's surgery of the alimentary tract* (6th ed.). St Louis: Saunders.

O'Brien, B., Landis-Erdman, J., & Erwin-Toth, P. (1998). Nursing management of multiple enterocutaneous fistulae located in the center of a large open abdominal wound: A case study. *Ostomy/Wound Management, 44*(1), 20–24.

Pfeifer, J., Tomasch, G., & Uranues, S. (2011). The surgical anatomy and etiology of gastrointestinal fistulas. *European Journal of Trauma and Emergency Surgery, 37*, 209–213.

Redden, M. H., Ramsay, P., Humphries, T., et al. (2013). The etiology of enterocutaneous fistula predicts outcome. *The Ochsner Journal, 13*, 507–511.

Rolstad, B., & Boarini, J. (1996). Principles and techniques in the use of convexity. *Ostomy/Wound Management, 42*(1), 24–26, 28–32.

Rolstad, B., & Wong, W. D. (2004). Nursing management of cutaneous intestinal fistulas. In P. A. Cataldo, & J. M. MacKeigan (Eds.), *Intestinal stomas: Principles, techniques and management* (6th ed.). New York: Marcel Dekker.

Samad, S., Anele, C., Akhtar, M., & Doughan, S. (2015). Implementing a proforma for multidisciplinary management of enterocutaneous fistula: A case study. *Ostomy/Wound Management, 61*(6), 46–52.

Scardillo, J., & Folkedahl, B. (1998). Management of a complex high-output fistula. *Journal of Wound, Ostomy, and Continence Nursing, 25*(4), 217–220.

Schein, M., & Decker, G. A. (1991). Postoperative external alimentary tract fistulas. *American Journal of Surgery, 161*(4), 435–438.

Shecter, W. P. (2011). Management of enterocutaneous fistulas. *The Surgical Clinics of North America, 91*(3), 481–491.

Skingley, S. (1998). The management of a faecal fistula. *Nursing Times, 94*(16). 64–66, 68.

Smith, D. B. (1982). Fistulas of the head and neck. *Journal of Enterostomal Therapy, 9*(5), 20–24.

Smith, D. B. (1986). Multiple stomas, fistulas and draining wounds. In D. B. Smith, & D. R. Johnson (Eds.), *Ostomy care and the cancer patient: Surgical and clinical considerations*. New York: Grune & Stratton.

Tran, N. A., & Thorson, A. G. (2020). The management of rectovaginal fistula. In J. L. Cameron, & A. M. Cameron (Eds.), *Current surgical therapy* (13 ed.). St. Louis: Elsevier.

Tuma, F., Crespi, Z., Wolff, C. J., et al. (2020). Enterocutaneous fistula: A simplified clinical approach. *Cureus, 12*(4), e7789. https://doi.org/10.7759/cureus.7789.

Tuma, F., McKeown, D. G., & Al-Wahab, Z. (2021). Rectovaginal fistula. In *StatPearls [Internet]*. Treasure Island: StatPearls Publishing. Retrieved 9/3/2021 from: https://www.ncbi.nlm.nih.gov/books/NBK535350/.

Viswanathan, A. N., Lee, L. J., Eswara, J. R., Horowitz, N. S., Konstantinopoulos, P. A., Mirabeau-Beale, K. L., et al. (2014). Complications of pelvic radiation in patients treated for gynecologic malignancies. *Cancer, 120*, 3870–3883.

Welch, J. P. (1997). Duodenal, gastric, and biliary fistulas. In M. J. Zinner, et al. (Eds.), *Vol. 1. Maingot's abdominal operations* (10th ed.). Stamford: Appleton & Lange.

Whelan, J. F., Jr., & Ivatury, R. R. (2011). Enterocutaneous fistulas: an overview. *European Journal of Trauma and Emergency Surgery, 37*, 251–258.

Wiltshire, B. L. (1996). Challenging enterocutaneous fistula: A case presentation. *Journal of Wound, Ostomy, and Continence Nursing, 23*(6), 297–301.

Wirth, U., Renz, B. W., Andrade, D., Schiergens, T. S., Arbogast, H., Andrassy, J., et al. (2018). Successful treatment of enteroatmospheric fistulas in combination with negative pressure wound therapy: Experience on 3 cases and literature review. *International Wound Journal, 15*(5), 722–730. https://doi.org/10.1111/iwj.12916.

Wong, W. D., Buie, W. D., & Annamaneni, R. K. (2004). Management of intestinal fistulas. In P. A. Cataldo, & J. M. MacKeigan (Eds.), *Intestinal stomas: principles, techniques, and management* (2nd ed.). New York: Marcel Dekker.

Yanar, F., & Yanar, H. (2011). Nutritional support in patients with gastrointestinal fistula. *European Journal of Trauma and Emergency Surgery, 37*, 227–231.

Zwanziger, P. J. (1999). Pouching a draining duodenal cutaneous fistula: A case study. *Journal of Wound, Ostomy, and Continence Nursing, 26*(1), 25–29.

FURTHER READING

Nurses Specialized in Wound, Ostomy and Continence Canada (NSWOCC). (2018). *Nursing best practice recommendations:* *enterocutaneous fistula and enteroatmospheric fistula*. Retrieved 8/27/2021 from: http://nswoc.ca/ecf-best-practices/.

Polk, T. M., & Schwab, C. W. (2012). Metabolic and nutritional support of the enterocutaneous fistula patient: A three-phase approach. *World Journal of Surgery, 36*(3), 524–533.

Percutaneous Tube Management

Ruth A. Bryant

OBJECTIVES

1. Identify two primary reasons for using percutaneous tubes.
2. Distinguish among the placement approaches for gastrostomy and jejunostomy, including indications and overview of technique.
3. Explain the rationale for tube stabilization.
4. Describe at least two options for stabilizing gastrostomy or jejunostomy tubes. A nephrostomy tube is a percutaneous GU tube that is placed in the kidney to divert the urine above an obstruction in the ureter.
5. Identify a prevention and management approach for: peritubular leakage, tube migration, candidiasis, and tube occlusion.
6. Identify percutaneous tubes that can be irrigated and those that cannot be irrigated.
7. Describe routine site care for the patient with a percutaneous tube.

Percutaneous tubes are placed for a variety of purposes, including feeding, decompression, and drainage. They can be placed in the gastrointestinal tract, genitourinary tract, and in spaces such as the pleural space and abdomen, on a temporary or long-term basis. For example, a nephrostomy tube may be placed percutaneously into the kidney pelvis temporarily to divert the urine above an obstructed or dilated ureter. Percutaneous tubes can be placed by a range of providers: gastroenterologists, urologists, surgeon, interventional radiologists (IRs), and interventional pulmonologists (IPs) (Alsunaid, Holden, Kohli, Diaz, & O'Meara, 2021; Yarmus, Gilbert, Lechtzin, et al., 2013).

The most familiar and common percutaneous tubes are gastrointestinal (GI) tubes, or GI tubes. Although described in the 13th century, planned surgical gastrostomy as a procedure was first proposed in 1837 and performed 12 years later in 1849, with the first reported survival of the procedure performed by S. Jones in 1876 (Jones, 2004). This chapter will describe the various GI tubes and the management of the percutaneous tube. Principles that guide the stabilization and management of percutaneous GI tubes can be applied to any percutaneous tube.

Malfunction of these tubes can result in skin erosion, denudement, inflammation, leakage, and pain such that referral to the wound care specialist becomes necessary. This chapter reviews common percutaneous tubes; their purpose; and procedures for placement, nursing management, and potential complications.

Effective nursing management of the patient with a percutaneous tube requires an understanding of the anatomy and physiology of the affected body system, the pathology involved, the rationale for tube placement, the method of tube insertion, and the anticipated length of time that the tube will be necessary. Nursing management of the patient with a percutaneous tube should always include routine care designed to maintain tube function and prevent peritubular complications, patient/caregiver education, and routine surveillance for tube dysfunction or complications. Comprehensive care is best provided with a collaborative team approach.

GASTROSTOMY AND JEJUNOSTOMY DEVICES

A *gastrostomy* is an opening into the stomach, and a *jejunostomy* is an opening into the jejunum. Such procedures may be used to provide decompression or enteral support for a patient unable to ingest or absorb adequate nutrients (Lord, 2018; Rahnemai-Azar, Rahnemaiazar, Naghshizakdian, Kurtz, & Farkas, 2014). Enteral nutrition is considered superior to parenteral nutrition for many reasons, including lower rates of infectious and metabolic complications, decreased hospital length of stay, reduced cost, and preservation of gut integrity (histologic structure and physical viability) (Blumenstein, Shastri, & Stein, 2014; Vudayagiri, Hoilat, & Gemma, 2021). Short-term enteral support through nasal placed tubes with distal tips positioned in the stomach or small intestine may be used for a few days up to 4 weeks (D'Cruz & Cascella, 2022; Lord, 2018; Wei, Ho, & Hegde, 2021). Placement of the nasal feeding tube beyond the stomach is warranted for gastric or duodenal conditions such as gastric outlet obstruction, proximal fistula or obstruction.

BOX 40.1 **Risk Factors for Aspiration**

- Altered mental status
- Swallowing dysfunction
- History of aspiration
- Severe gastroesophageal reflux
- Gastric outlet obstruction
- Gastroparesis

From Gorman, R. C., Nance, M. L., & Morris, J. B. (1995). Enteral feeding techniques. In M. H. Torosian (Ed.), *Nutrition for the hospitalized patient: Basic science and principles of practice.* New York: Marcel Dekker.

When a high risk of aspiration exists, small bowel placed feeding tube is preferred (Lord, 2018). Box 40.1 lists the risk factors for aspiration.

PLACEMENT APPROACHES

For more than a century, gastrostomy placement required surgical intervention involving anesthesia and the traditional preoperative preparation for abdominal surgery. Historically, a suture was placed around the base of the tube at skin level and then through the skin to immobilize the gastrostomy tube. Gastrostomy tubes usually were connected to suction for 12–24 hours to reduce tension on the suture line. Feedings were delayed until bowel sounds, tube patency, and proper placement of the tube were confirmed.

Today, a gastrostomy or jejunostomy is created by one of three approaches: surgical, endoscopic, or interventional radiologic. Open laparotomy is rarely performed due to the success of the much less invasive endoscopic and laparoscopic techniques (D'Cruz & Cascella, 2022). Fig. 40.1 presents an algorithm for determining the most appropriate means of enteral access.

Surgical Approaches

A surgically placed gastrostomy or jejunostomy tube can be accomplished through an open surgical procedure or a laparoscopic procedure. Surgical placement is relatively expensive, requires anesthesia and the use of sterile dressings, and exposes the patient to many potential complications. Generally, the surgical approach is reserved for the patient in whom abdominal surgery is already being performed (DeLegge, 2018). Surgical placement is also performed when endoscopic placement has failed. Although these procedures are less common today, they may still be placed in unique situations and therefore it is important to have an understanding of their purpose.

Open Surgical Procedure

The most common open surgical procedures for gastrostomy tube placement are the Stamm, the Witzel, and the Janeway. The Stamm and the Witzel are the simplest procedures and are considered temporary; the Janeway is more of a long-term or permanent procedure.

Stamm Gastrostomy. Stamm gastrostomy is the standard open gastrostomy, the gold standard for transabdominal gastric access (Shapiro & Montgomery, 2019). Creation of a Stamm gastrostomy begins by making a small incision in the left upper quadrant of the abdomen. Another small incision is made over and through the body of the stomach, through which a catheter (Foley, mushroom, Malecot, or gastrostomy replacement tube) is inserted (Fig. 40.2). Several purse-string sutures are used to invaginate the stomach around the tube. The stomach is then fixed to the abdominal wall at the catheter site, and traditionally a nonabsorbable suture is used to secure the catheter to the skin. Although the Stamm gastrostomy is the simplest surgical technique to perform and remove, it is frequently difficult to manage

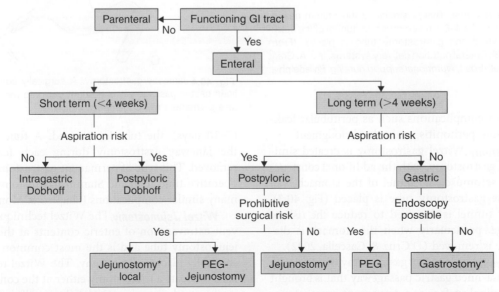

Fig. 40.1 Enteral access algorithm for selecting the most appropriate technique for an individual patient. (From Gorman, R. C., & Morris, J. B. (1997). Minimally invasive access to the gastrointestinal tract. In J. L. Rombeau & R. H. Rolandelli (Eds.), *Clinical nutrition: Enteral and tube feeding* (3rd ed.). Philadelphia: Saunders.)

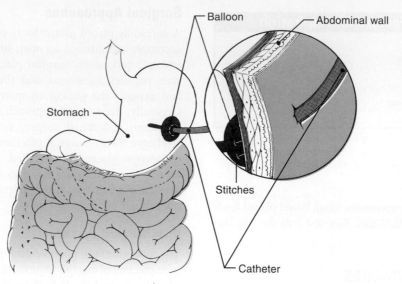

Fig. 40.2 Stamm gastrostomy tube technique, oblique view. An incision is placed through the abdominal wall into the stomach, through which a catheter is passed.

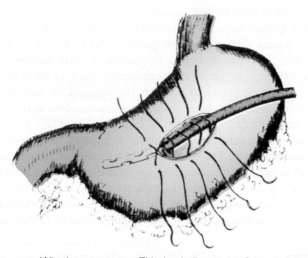

Fig. 40.3 Witzel gastrostomy. This is similar to the Stamm gastrostomy with the addition of a 4–6-cm seromuscular tunnel of the stomach wall, through which the gastrostomy tube is placed. (From Patterson, R. S. (1988). Enteral nutrition delivery systems. In J. A. Grant & C. Kennedy-Caldwell (Eds.), *Nutritional support nursing*. Philadelphia: Grune & Stratton.)

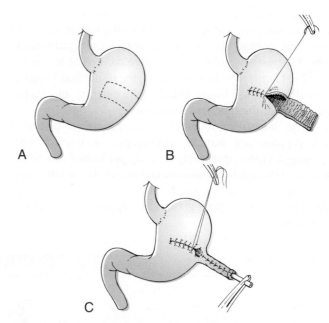

Fig. 40.4 Janeway gastrostomy. A surgically constructed, mucosa-lined gastric passageway is brought out onto the abdominal surface as a permanent mucocutaneous stoma.

and is plagued with complications such as peritubular leakage, wound infection, peritonitis, and tube dislodgment.

Witzel Gastrostomy. Witzel gastrostomy is created similarly to the Stamm gastrostomy, with the additional construction of a 4–6-cm seromuscular tunnel of the stomach wall through which the gastrostomy tube is placed (Fig. 40.3). The seromuscular tunnel is designed to reduce the risk of peritubular leakage, particularly when the stomach is distended or the tube is removed (D'Cruz & Cascella, 2022).

Janeway Gastrostomy. Janeway gastrostomy is a surgically constructed, mucosa-lined gastric passageway that is brought out onto the abdominal surface as a permanent mucocutaneous stoma. Fig. 40.4 illustrates how the Janeway gastrostomy is constructed. Postoperatively, an inflated balloon-tip catheter is placed in the tract. Once the tract has matured

(7–10 days), the tube is removed. A tube is inserted into the Janeway gastrostomy during each feeding and then removed. This type of permanent gastrostomy requires more operative time than the Stamm gastrostomy and results in many similar complications (Shapiro & Montgomery, 2019).

Witzel Jejunostomy. The Witzel technique is used to prevent extravasation of enteric contents at the exit site of the jejunostomy tube and is the most common technique for a surgically placed jejunostomy. The Witzel technique can be used to create a jejunostomy either at the conclusion of a surgical procedure or as an isolated procedure. The usual site is the left upper quadrant. A loop of jejunum 15–20 cm from the ligament of Treitz is brought up to the wound, and a circular purse-string suture is placed in the antimesenteric border. An

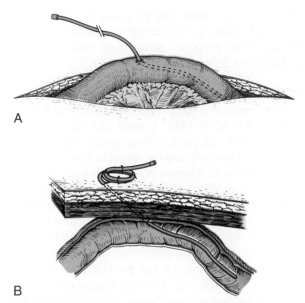

Fig. 40.5 Technique for placement of a needle catheter jejunostomy. (A) The catheter is inserted into the lumen of the jejunum for a distance of 40–50 cm and secured into place with a purse-string suture. (B) The jejunum is secured to the anterior abdominal wall. The feeding catheter is removed postoperatively when the patient can tolerate oral feedings. (From Bland, K. I., et al. (1995). *Atlas of surgical oncology*. Philadelphia: Saunders.)

incision through the center of the purse-string suture is made, and a 14-French (14-Fr) feeding catheter is inserted into the jejunal lumen and advanced. A serosal tunnel is constructed at the exit site in the jejunal wall, extending approximately 5–6 cm proximally. The catheter is brought to the skin through a separate incision and secured, typically with sutures. The loop of intestine is then anchored to the anterior abdominal wall (DeLegge, 2018).

Needle Catheter Jejunostomy. The needle catheter jejunostomy is often used in conjunction with a laparotomy and major gastrointestinal resection when prolonged enteral support is anticipated. At approximately 30–40 cm distal to the ligament of Treitz, a 14- to 16-gauge needle is used to create a submucosal tunnel in the jejunal wall. A feeding catheter is advanced through the needle 30–40 cm distally, and the needle is withdrawn. A purse-string suture is made around the tube to close the jejunal opening around the catheter. The loop of bowel is anchored to the anterior abdominal wall, and the catheter is secured to the skin (Fig. 40.5) (D'Cruz & Cascella, 2022; DeLegge, 2018).

Laparoscopic Surgical Approach

The laparoscopic approach for insertion of the gastrostomy or jejunostomy has been possible since the introduction of high-resolution video cameras and has the advantages of minimal invasion and few surgical side effects (Saberi et al., 2021; Siow, Mahendran, Wong, Milaksh, & Nyunt, 2017). This approach also provides the opportunity to selectively determine the site of the tube within the stomach (e.g., lesser-curvature gastrostomy rather than the more commonly selected greater-curvature), which may be important in the patient who is

at high risk for reflux or aspiration. In addition, biopsy specimens can be obtained if necessary or malignancy staging can be conducted (Siow et al., 2017). This technique requires a smaller incision than the open surgical approach, but local or general anesthesia is still needed.

Laparoscopic Gastrostomy. The indication for laparoscopic gastrostomy for feeding is the inability to perform percutaneous endoscopic gastrostomy (PEG), such as with a morbidly obese patient. A small supraumbilical incision is made through which the camera port is placed, and a 5-mm port is placed in the epigastrium. An atraumatic instrument is used to grasp the stomach, and the site for the proposed gastrostomy is identified. An 18-gauge angiocatheter is passed through the anterior abdomen, at the site chosen for the gastrostomy, and into the stomach. The needle is removed, and a soft J-wire is passed into the stomach. Dilators (12 and 14 Fr) are placed over this J-wire. A 16-Fr peel-away catheter is placed over the dilator, and a 16-Fr catheter is inserted through the sheath. The catheter is positioned against the stomach wall by inflating the balloon or securing the internal bumper. This particular type of gastrostomy is less commonly used than the Stamm due to technical requirements and pneumoperitoneum (Shapiro & Montgomery, 2019).

Laparoscopic Jejunostomy. Specific indications for laparoscopic jejunostomy include concomitant laparoscopy for other problems and difficult laparoscopic gastrostomy. It is a minimally invasive procedure with desirable advantages of reduced postoperative pain and shortened recuperative time; general anesthesia is required.

The laparoscope is inserted through a small incision above the umbilicus. The proximal small bowel is identified and traced 25 cm distal to the ligament of Treitz, and the antimesenteric border is withdrawn into the umbilical wound. At this location in the small bowel, a Witzel tunnel is created or concentric purse-string sutures are placed, and a 12-Fr catheter is inserted into the bowel. The bowel is secured to the fascia around the tube and returned to the abdominal cavity, and the fascia and skin are closed. The catheter is tunneled subcutaneously to exit the skin at the site previously selected on the abdomen.

In another technique, T-fasteners (or tacks) are inserted through the skin into the bowel lumen to anchor and retract the bowel against the abdominal wall (Siow et al., 2017). Once the bowel is anchored, a percutaneous jejunostomy tube can be placed directly through the abdominal wall (Fig. 40.6).

Endoscopic Approach

The endoscopic approach to gastrostomy tube placement, known as *percutaneous endoscopic gastrostomy*, was first described in 1980 and is today the procedure of choice (Hitawala & Mousa, 2022; Wei et al., 2021). This can be placed under local anesthesia and conscious sedation in the endoscopy suite, in the operating room, or at the bedside in a critical care unit if necessary (Rothrock & Alexander, 2012).

Contraindications to PEG include inability to perform upper endoscopy, inability to illuminate the abdominal wall, ascites, esophageal obstruction, hepatomegaly, hemodynamic instability, sepsis, previous gastric resection, gastric

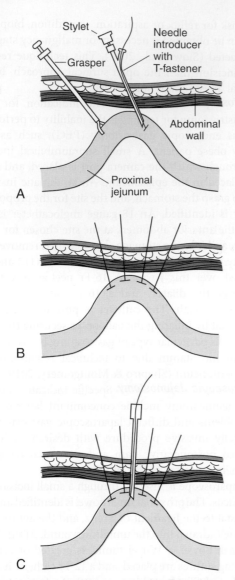

Fig. 40.6 Laparoscopic jejunostomy with T-fasteners, which are inserted through the skin into the bowel lumen to anchor and retract the bowel against the abdominal wall before a percutaneous jejunostomy tube is inserted directly through the abdominal wall.

outlet obstruction and severe gastroparesis, peritoneal carcinomatosis, and uncorrectable coagulopathy (Vudayagiri et al., 2021). Morbid obesity may present an obstacle to PEG placement, due to the difficulty in transillumination through the thickness of the overlying adipose tissue without the use of an 8-in-long spinal needle and 240-cm-long guidewire commonly used in endoscopic retrograde cholangiopancreatography procedures to overcome the problem of transillumination (Senadhi et al., 2012).

Various techniques can be used to insert a gastrostomy tube endoscopically. Three techniques are most commonly used: peroral pull technique, peroral push technique and the direct (Russell) technique. All techniques involve a complete esophagogastroduodenoscopy, insufflation of air into the stomach, and transillumination of the stomach. After application of a topical pharyngeal anesthetic and sedation, an endoscope is passed into the stomach. Air is insufflated into the stomach, which distends the stomach against the anterior abdominal wall. The proposed gastrostomy site is then transilluminated. The endoscopy assistant indents the abdomen at the proposed gastrostomy site, which should be at least 2 cm below the costal margin.

Per-oral Pull (Ponsky) Technique

This "pull" method is most widely used and was introduced by Gauderer et al. in 1980. A small incision is made over the illuminated site, and a large-gauge angiocatheter is inserted percutaneously into the stomach. The needle is withdrawn, and 60 in of a suture is passed through the catheter into the stomach. With a biopsy snare, the endoscopist grasps the suture and pulls so that the endoscope is removed with the suture attached (Fig. 40.7). The gastrostomy tube is attached to the suture. By pulling on the suture at the abdominal gastrostomy site, the endoscopist draws the tube through the esophagus into the stomach and positions it snugly against the anterior stomach wall. To verify proper position of the PEG, an endoscope is passed again. Once placement is confirmed, the endoscope is removed, and the PEG secured at the skin level (DeLegge, 2018; Shapiro & Montgomery, 2019).

Per-oral Push (Sachs-Vine) Technique

With this technique, a long, flexible guidewire is inserted through the angiocatheter into the stomach. With a biopsy snare and endoscope, the wire is snared and pulled up through the esophagus and out the patient's mouth (Fig. 40.8). The PEG tube is pushed over the guidewire and advanced through the esophagus to the stomach and positioned against the anterior stomach wall. As with the "pull" technique, PEG placement is checked with the endoscope, which is then removed, and the PEG secured.

Direct Introducer (Russell) Technique

In this modification of the above techniques, a guidewire is placed transabdominally into the stomach and a dilating catheter and sheath is passed over the guidewire. The endoscopist confirms the position of the dilator, the dilator is removed, and a well-lubricated catheter is advanced through the peel-away sheath. The endoscopist verifies adequate placement of the catheter against the anterior stomach wall, and the endoscope is removed (Blumenstein et al., 2014; Hitawala & Mousa, 2022).

Percutaneous Endoscopic Jejunostomy

Techniques to achieve postpyloric enteral access via an endoscopic approach include the PEG-J and the direct percutaneous endoscopic jejunostomy (DPEJ). The PEG-J is the insertion of a jejunal extension tube through a previously established PEG that is advanced to the jejunum (Hitawala & Mousa, 2022). Under endoscopic visualization, a biopsy forceps is used to grasp the weighted tip and attached heavy suture tie on the feeding tube and guide the tube into the duodenum (Fig. 40.9). The endoscope is then withdrawn. An excess amount of tubing is left within the stomach to allow peristalsis to pull the weighted tip past the ligament of Treitz.

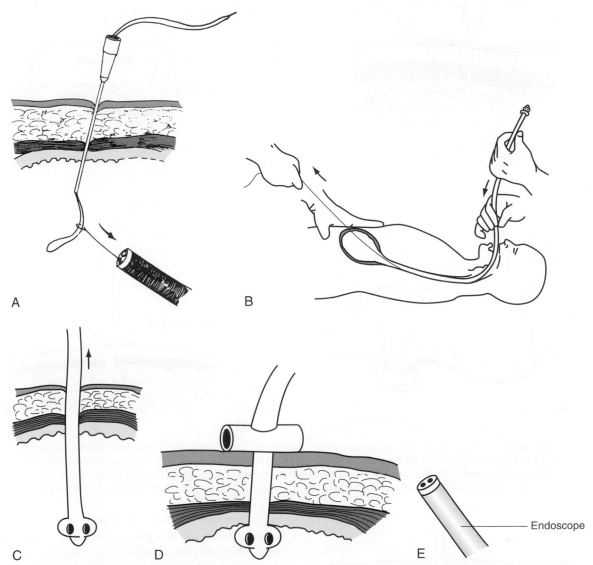

Fig. 40.7 Ponsky (pull) percutaneous endoscopic gastrostomy (PEG) technique. (A) After local anesthesia is instilled, a 10-mm transverse incision is made, through which a tapered cannula needle is introduced under direct endoscopic vision. A looped heavy suture is directed through the catheter into the stomach, secured with a polypectomy snare, and withdrawn from the patient's mouth. (B) The well-lubricated PEG catheter is now secured to the suture, and steady traction is directed down the posterior pharynx into the esophagus. (C) The endoscope is reintroduced (see E), and under direct vision the catheter is pulled across the gastroesophageal junction and then approximated to the anterior gastric wall. It is imperative that the inner cross-bar gently approximates the mucosa without excess tension to avoid ischemic necrosis. The stomach is decompressed by aspiration, and the gastroscope is withdrawn. (D) The outer cross-bar is gently approximated to the skin level and secured with two 0–0 Prolene sutures. (From Gorman, R. C., & Morris, J. B. (1997). Minimally invasive access to the gastrointestinal tract. In J. L. Rombeau & R. H. Rolandelli (Eds.), *Clinical nutrition: Enteral and tube feeding* (3rd ed.). Philadelphia: Saunders.)

Directed PEJ. Using a modification of the Ponsky pull procedure, the feeding tube can be inserted directly into the jejunum under endoscopic visualization. In this approach, the endoscope is advanced past the pylorus approximately 20 cm distal to the ligament of Treitz, and the abdominal wall is transilluminated. Using a small-gauge needle, the jejunum is cannulated through the abdominal wall, a heavy thread is inserted, a biopsy forceps is used to grasp the thread, and the thread is withdrawn through the mouth. The thread is tied to a feeding tube (typically mushroom tipped), which is pulled into position under endoscopic observation. The directed PEJ seems to alleviate the problems associated with transpyloric placement (tube migration, clogging, and aspiration) (Strong et al., 2017; Zhu, Shi, Hao, & Tao, 2012)

Interventional Radiologic Approach
Percutaneous Gastrostomy via Radiologic Intervention
Recent advances have led to the development of a radiographic approach to percutaneous gastrostomy tube placement. Percutaneous tubes placed by the interventional

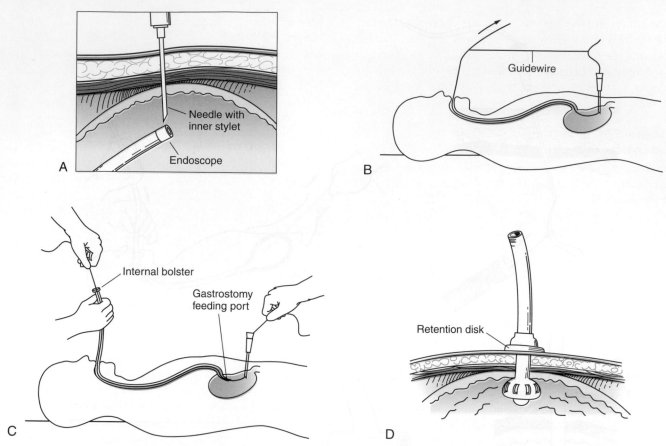

Fig. 40.8 Sachs-Vine technique for percutaneous endoscopic gastrostomy (PEG) insertion. (A) Needle is inserted through abdomen into the stomach under visualization by endoscopist. (B) Endoscope is withdrawn, pulling guidewire up through the esophagus, out the patient's mouth. (C) PEG tube is pushed over the guidewire and advanced through the esophagus to the stomach. (D) PEG is positioned against the anterior stomach wall.

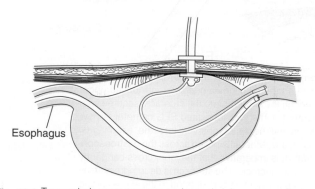

Fig. 40.9 Transpyloric percutaneous endoscopic jejunostomy. Endoscopist guides the weighted tip of the feeding tube into the duodenum.

radiologist are an alternative when surgical or endoscopic procedures are not feasible. In many hospitals, it is the preferred method of tube placement. The interventional radiology nurse takes the lead in preparing the patient for the procedure, providing patient education, and monitoring the patient's recovery.

In the radiographic approach, the stomach is dilated with air, and a needle is percutaneously inserted into the stomach. A J-wire is threaded into the stomach under fluoroscopic guidance, and the needle is withdrawn. A 1-cm-long incision is made into the skin at the exit site of the wire. When

entry into the stomach has been determined, the tract is slowly dilated and the permanent catheter inserted. These catheters usually have a balloon that is inflated and positioned snugly against the gastric wall. Stabilization at the skin surface is achieved using a suture or a tube stabilization device.

- T-tacks are small anchors that are deployed into the stomach during the beginning phase of gastrostomy or gastrostomy–jejunostomy tube placement.
- T-tacks pull and hold the stomach firmly against the abdominal wall. This helps the radiologists so that they do not have to work through "dead" space when placing the tube into the stomach.
- T-tacks *must* be cut within 7–10 days of placement to prevent reverse crater ulcerations in the stomach mucosal lining.
- Metal "T"s simply pass through the patient's GI tract.

Percutaneous Jejunostomy via Radiologic Intervention

This technique first requires radiologic access to the stomach as is done for percutaneous gastrostomy placement via radiology. A guidewire is passed through the duodenum and into the jejunum. A balloon occluder catheter is inserted over the guidewire and placed in the jejunum. The balloon is inflated with air and water-soluble contrast so that the position can be checked by fluoroscopy. Still under fluoroscopic surveillance, an 18-gauge needle is inserted into the jejunum, and the balloon is punctured. A guidewire is passed into the tract, and the tract is dilated to approximately 10 Fr size so that a feeding catheter can be inserted. The balloon occluder catheter is removed, and the feeding catheter is secured to the skin.

Conversion of Gastrostomy to Gastrostomy–Jejunostomy Tube

Repeat aspirations may necessitate conversion of an existing gastrostomy tube to a gastrostomy–jejunostomy tube. This can be done using endoscopy or radiology with a combined gastrostomy–jejunostomy tube, or by inserting a smaller-diameter feeding tube through the gastrostomy tube. When a combined gastrostomy–jejunostomy tube is used, the gastrostomy tube is removed, and an angiocatheter and guidewire are inserted and advanced through the pylorus. The guidewire is further advanced distal to the ligament of Treitz, and the angiocatheter is removed. A gastrostomy–jejunostomy tube is inserted over the guidewire and advanced into the jejunum, and the guidewire is removed. The gastrostomy internal bumper or balloon is secured snugly against the stomach mucosa. An external securing device (bumper, flange, or commercial device) is used to secure the tube against the skin. Three ports will be apparent: gastric (proximal) port, duodenal or jejunal (distal) port, and balloon port (Fig. 40.10).

When a combined gastrostomy–jejunostomy tube is not available, a jejunal tube can be placed, and the external end of the jejunal tube can be threaded into a gastrostomy tube. The gastrostomy tube is advanced over the jejunal tube, and the internal gastrostomy bumper is positioned against the anterior stomach wall. External stabilization of the tube to the skin is necessary.

Summary of Placement Techniques

The type of patient who typically requires these tubes is a major reason for the high morbidity rate. Patients commonly have multiple medical problems and are malnourished. For these reasons, the surgical approach to tube placement has quickly been replaced by the endoscopic or radiographic approach. Endoscopic techniques for enteral tube placement have a lower complication rate, are more cost effective than surgical methods, and can be performed on an outpatient basis. Performance of these techniques requires the ability to insert an endoscope. Laparoscopic and radiologic techniques are used less frequently but are options when endoscopy is not anatomically feasible or when surgery is too risky.

A key consideration for the type of tube placed is whether prepyloric or postpyloric delivery of enteral feedings is preferred (Lord, 2018; Shapiro & Montgomery, 2019). PEG tube placement into the stomach preserves the integrity of the cardiac sphincter, decreasing the risk of gastroesophageal reflux and pulmonary aspiration. However, in the presence of significant gastroesophageal reflux, impaired gastric emptying, or resection of the esophagus, stomach, pancreas or duodenum, postpyloric placement (i.e., in the proximal duodenum or jejunum) is often preferred (D'Cruz & Cascella, 2022; DeLegge, 2018).

FEEDING TUBE FEATURES

Material Composition

Historically, gastrostomy and jejunostomy tubes were made from rubber, polyvinyl chloride, and latex, which are very stiff and uncomfortable. Because the softer and more pliable polyurethane and silicone tubes are associated with less soft tissue reaction and longer wear time, they are preferred. However, polyurethane tubes are more resilient and less likely to deteriorate. In addition, aspiration of intestinal or gastric contents from silicone tubes is difficult because the walls of the tube collapse.

Tube Diameter

The outer diameter (OD) of the lumen is referred to in French units. A 1-Fr tube is 0.33 mm across. However, the internal diameter (ID) can vary for any OD French size depending on the material used. For example, silicone tubes have thicker walls than polyurethane tubes, so their internal diameter will be smaller even though they are labeled with the same French size.

The risk of the tube becoming clogged decreases as ID increases (Lord, 2018). However, for the patient's comfort,

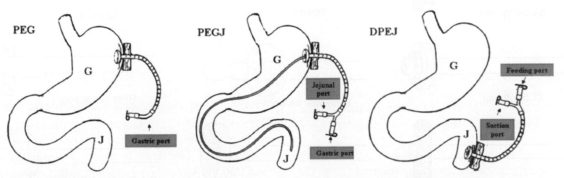

Fig. 40.10 Various types of feeding tubes. Percutaneous gastrostomy tube (PEG, *left*); PEG with jejunal extension (PEG-JET, *middle*); direct percutaneous endoscopic jejunostomy (DPEJ, *right*). (From Zhu, Y., Shi, L., Tang, H., et al. (2012). Current considerations of direct percutaneous endoscopic jejunostomy. *Canadian Journal of Gastroenterology, 26*(2), 92–96.)

the smallest ID nasogastric tube possible that allows unimpeded flow of formula should be used. When enteral formulas containing fiber or viscous formulas will be administered, an 8-Fr or larger tube is recommended. Gastrostomy tubes most often are 12 Fr, jejunostomy tubes should be 6 Fr, and needle catheter jejunostomy tubes should be smaller than 8 Fr.

Tip Configurations

Several tip configurations are illustrated in Fig. 40.11. Foley catheters are not designed for use as gastrostomy tubes and should not be used because the balloon of the Foley catheter is subject to decay from gastric acid, necessitating periodic and regular replacement. In addition, Foley catheters do not have an external bumper and will migrate if an external tube stabilization device is not applied. Migration can cause gastric outlet obstruction by blocking the pylorus. Specifically designed gastrostomy tubes, many silicone based, commonly known as a *G-tube* or *replacement gastrostomy tube,* are essential to use.

Another tip configuration (and one used to a great extent on the PEG) is the disk. This tip cannot be removed by simple extraction through the skin; it must be cut off. The tip is passed through the GI tract or retrieved endoscopically. The PEG tip may also have a cross-bar or bulb tip, which cannot be extracted through the skin.

Tubes may have a type of mushroom catheter known as a *Pezzer tip.* These rubber tubes have stiff, round, pointed tips. The Pezzer tip has only minimal tiny holes and becomes easily plugged. This type of tip cannot be removed easily. The Malecot tube, also considered a mushroom catheter, has a bulbous tip with much larger openings. This type of tube can be removed more easily and is less likely to become obstructed than the Pezzer tip.

Ports

Tubes with multiple ports are available. Some gastrostomy tubes have three ports: balloon, feeding, and medication. A triple-lumen tube may be used when patients require both proximal decompression and enteral feeding. This tube has four outlets or ports: a gastric lumen for gastric suction, a proximal duodenal lumen for duodenal suction, a distal duodenal lumen for feeding, and a gastric balloon. To maintain proper tube placement, the gastric balloon is inflated with sterile water or air (depending on the manufacturer's specific recommendation), and a retaining disk or tube stabilization device is applied at skin level. These tubes may be confusing to the staff because the tubes are placed in the anticipated location for a gastrostomy tube but deliver feedings to the jejunum. Ports should be clearly labeled, and a diagram of the tube should be available in the patient's care plan to provide clarity.

LOW-PROFILE GASTROSTOMY TUBE (BUTTON)

A skin-level gastric conduit that is flush with the abdominal surface is known as a *gastrostomy button* or a "button" G-tube (Gauderer & Stellato, 1986). The button was first developed for use in children who require long-term gastrostomy feedings. It is a short silicone tube with a flip-top opening, a one-way antireflux valve (to prevent leakage of stomach contents around the tube), and a radiopaque dome that fits snugly against the stomach wall (Fig. 40.12). Some devices have special tubing that opens the reflux valve to permit decompression of the stomach.

To administer feedings, an adapter is passed through the one-way valve and connected to a feeding catheter. When

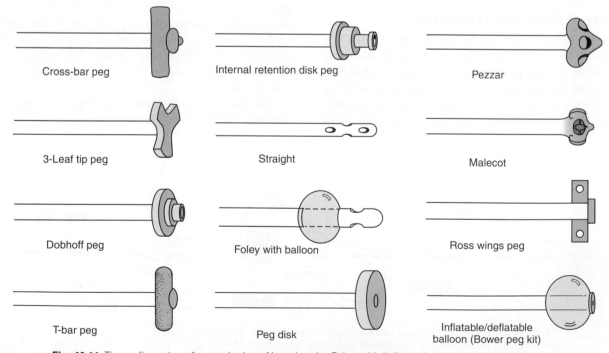

Fig. 40.11 Tip configuration of enteral tubes. Note that the Foley with balloon tip is included to provide comparison in tip designs; it is not an appropriate tube for enteral feedings.

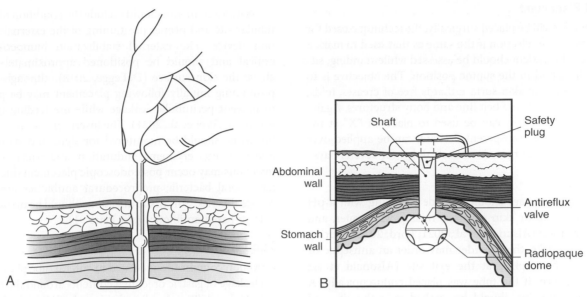

Fig. 40.12 Gastrostomy button. (A) Correct gastrostomy button size is determined by using a device to measure the width of the abdominal wall. (B) Gastrostomy feeding button in place.

the feeding is completed, the tube is flushed with water, the adapter is removed, and the flip-top opening is closed.

A button can be inserted in a clinic setting in an established gastrostomy tract and does not require patient anesthesia. Otherwise, placement is a minimally invasive surgical procedure using a percutaneous endoscopic (blind) approach or via laparoscopic technique (Saberi et al., 2021). The device is available in different shaft lengths and diameters. Correct shaft length is critical to ensure proper positioning of the dome of the button against the anterior stomach wall and prevent gastric reflux around the button. The appropriate shaft length is determined by inserting a special measuring device into the tract. An obturator is inserted into the button to straighten the dome of the button, making insertion of the button into the tract possible. The button should be lubricated to facilitate insertion. Once the button is in place, the obturator is removed and the flip-top opening closed. The device may have to be resized if the patient's weight changes.

Key advantages of the low profile button include being less visible, lighter, less impact on mobility or activity and no external tubing that requires taping for securement or could become dislodged (Lord, 2018). The internal stabilizing bumper may be a balloon- or mushroom-shapeddome. Disadvantages of the button include the potential for dysfunction of the antireflux valve with subsequent leakage and the need for replacement every 3–4 months.

NURSING MANAGEMENT: ENTERAL TUBES

Optimal management of patients requiring an enteral feeding tube long-term begins in the preplacement phase. Assessment of each patient should include the reason for each tube alternative, the risks and benefits associated with various treatment options, and the commitment of the patient or caregiver to long-term management. Preplacement information and instructions are critical to adequately prepare the patient and family for what will be expected.

Nursing staff play a vital role in preparing the patient for enteral tube placement and teaching self-care following placement (Berman et al., 2017). Much of the success of enteral feeding tubes depends on proper care. Topics that must be addressed include preplacement site selection, site care, tube patency, tube stabilization, and management of complications. It is advisable to develop a competency checklist for the nursing staff who care for a significant number of patients with feeding tubes.

Preplacement Site Selection

Tube exit sites should be considered preoperatively to reduce the potential for complications and to facilitate self-care. Site selection is commonly based on vague guidelines such as "3–5 cm below the costal margin" and "avoidance of the costal margin." However, in the patient who has a protuberant hernia or is malnourished or confined to a wheelchair, this location may present a substantial problem such that it affects the integrity of the skin. Preplacement site selection is even more important in the infant and particularly when an ostomy is present.

Endoscopic Placement

When the tube is placed by the endoscopic approach, the location of the tube depends on transillumination. Therefore, the specific site for the tube cannot be determined before the procedure. Nonetheless, by marking important abdominal landmarks (e.g., skin crease, fold, or scar; costal margin; belt line; prosthetic equipment; hernia), the endoscopist can attempt to place the tube in a site that will avoid these landmarks. An indelible marker should be sufficient for these markings.

Surgical Placement

When the tube will be placed surgically, the technique used for preplacement site selection is the same as that used to mark a stoma site. The patient should be assessed while standing, sitting, bending, and in the supine position. The objective is to find 1 in of smooth skin surface that is free of creases, folds, and scars and avoids the belt line and bony structures. Again, a surgical marking pen can be used to place an "X" at the desired location. A transparent dressing can be applied over the marking when surgery is not scheduled for several days.

Site Care

Initially, daily site care should include cleansing with a pH neutral mild soap or skin cleanser, rinsing with water, and drying (Box 40.2) (Alsunaid et al., 2021; Lord, 2018). During the first 1–2 weeks, the provider may order an antiseptic or antibiotic to be applied at the exit site (Alsunaid et al., 2021) particularly if the tube was placed endoscopically. A sterile gauze dressing should be applied over the site and changed daily to protect the site from external contamination and infection during this period while the gastrocutaneous tract is forming. A split gauze may be applied under the external retention device only if it does not cause extra tension to the site (Lord, 2018). Long term, a dressing is not necessary over the tube site, although some individuals may prefer the padding of a dressing under the external securement device. Once the tract is healed, tap water can be used to cleanse the exit site using a cotton-tipped applicator. Hydrogen peroxide may be used to remove dried drainage and then rinsed with tap water. When drainage is present, a moisture barrier may be used after cleansing around the tube to prevent moisture-associated skin damage (MASD) as long as the cause of the drainage is addressed and corrected (e.g., bacterial or fungal infection, hypergranulation tissue, and excessive gastric acid production). Nonadhesive absorptive dressings can be applied over the external fixation portion of the percutaneous tube if drainage is present. However, best practice regarding placement of dressings under the external bumper of the PEG tube is unclear. Dressings should not be applied under the external fixation disk or bumper that will trap moisture or exert excess tension on the internal bumper against the gastric mucosal surface (Box 40.2).

BOX 40.2 Site Care for Drainage Tubes

- Change dressing every day.
- Remove dressing from site.
- Use a clean washcloth to cleanse the area around the tube with gentle soap or pH neutral skin cleanser and water.
- Use a dry washcloth to pat dry skin around tube.
- If necessary, reposition tube so that it does not kink or twist sharply.
- Secure fresh, split wound care dressing around tube site and over the retention disk using tape.
- Covering the tube site is not necessary while showering. These steps can be done in the shower or after the shower.

Note: Never submerge the tube site under water. No tub baths or swimming is permitted.

Daily assessments should include the condition of the peritubular site and proper positioning of the external stabilization device. The external stabilization bumper/device is critical and should be positioned approximately 1–2 cm above the skin surface (DeLegge, 2018), although a tighter positioning initially following placement may be preferable to prevent peritubular leakage while the feeding tube tract is healing (Wei et al., 2021). The insertion site and surrounding tissue should be monitored for signs and symptoms of infection (e.g., erythema, induration, and pain). Superficial infections may occur postendoscopic placement due to transfer of oral bacteria; preprocedural antibiotics are used to reduce this risk. Soft tissue infections should be managed with culture-based antibiotics (see Plate 91).

Tube Stabilization

Common complications related to enteral tube placement are (1) leakage of gastric or jejunal contents around the tube onto the skin and (2) tube dislodgment, both of which are frequently attributed to inadequate tube stabilization. Therefore, postplacement nursing management must include measures to stabilize the tube.

Adequate tube stabilization requires proper internal positioning and proper external (skin-level) positioning. To achieve proper internal positioning, a tube that has a balloon, bumper, mushroom, or disk tip is used. These devices are positioned lightly against the anterior wall of the stomach (Fig. 40.13). When a balloon tip is used, it must be inflated with an adequate volume of sterile water or air (in accordance with the manufacturer's guidelines) (Lord, 2018). Although saline may be readily available, it should not be used for balloon inflation because saline can crystallize and cause the balloon to rupture. Because water and air will diffuse through the walls of the balloon, adequacy of inflation should be checked weekly and whenever peritubular leakage is noted. Tubes with balloon tips are never used as jejunal tubes because an inflated balloon within the jejunum is sufficient to cause a bowel obstruction in the jejunum.

Adequate skin-level stabilization of the tube is necessary to prevent (1) lateral movement in the tube at skin level and (2) tube migration (in-and-out movements). Lateral movement of the tube contributes to leakage of gastric or intestinal contents onto the skin by eroding the tissue along the tract. Inflammation of the site can also develop from the presence of this chronic irritant. A stabilized tube should allow minimal lateral movement.

To maintain proper tube positioning in the stomach or small bowel, migration of the tube in and out of the tract must be prevented. Nonstabilized tubes are subject to migration as a result of gastric and intestinal motility and abdominal wall motion. The tube can migrate and obstruct the gastric outlet (causing gastric distention, nausea, and vomiting) and compromise tube function.

Historically, sutures were used to stabilize tubes. However, sutures can cause tearing of the skin, with subsequent inflammation and significant pain at the suture site. In addition, sutures prevent tube migration, but they do not eliminate

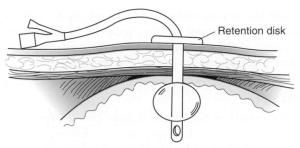

Fig. 40.13 Proper stabilization of gastrostomy tube. Tube is secured between the anterior wall of the stomach and abdomen by a properly inflated internal balloon and externally with a tube stabilization device. Side-to-side mobility of the tube and tube migration are thus prevented.

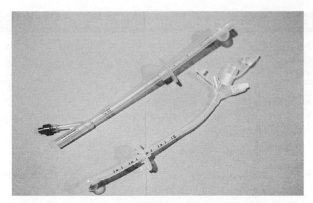

Fig. 40.15 Sample replacement gastrostomy tubes.

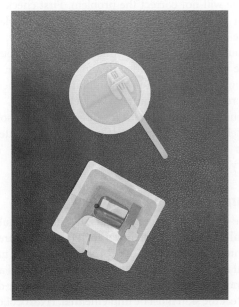

Fig. 40.14 Commercial external tube stabilization devices.

lateral tube movement. When sutures are used, an external tube stabilization device should be applied to provide more secure stabilization and comfort to the patient.

Commercial external tube stabilization devices are readily available and should be used to secure percutaneous tubes (Fig. 40.14). The commercial tube stabilization device is changed as needed; frequency is determined by the need to assess the tube site or provide site care. When frequent site care is required (as with newly placed tubes), a stabilization system that allows easy visualization of the site without removal of adhesives is desirable. The Hollister vertical drain/tube attachment device effectively holds tubes. The dressing is designed so that the tube comes straight out of the tract and is secured by the strap. Because the tube does not lie against the skin, there is no concern for development of a pressure ulcer/injury along the tract. For smaller abdomens, the tape ring can be removed. The vertical drain/tube attachment device can be left in place for 5–7 days.

Many tubes are being created specifically as gastrostomy tubes complete with stabilization features inherent in the design, thereby eliminating the need for commercial external stabilization devices. For example, the button has an internal dome, limited shaft length, and a flip-top cap to ensure stabilization of the tube. PEG tubes are designed with an internal bolster and an external bolster. The internal bolster can be a bumper, disk, or balloon that, when properly positioned, lies against the anterior stomach wall. Exteriorly, on the abdominal surface, the bolster is a bumper or disk that can be adjusted to lie rest loosely against the abdominal wall. This stabilization is critical to prevent dislodgment of the tube, excess mobility, obstruction, and peritubular leakage. A few Silastic catheter feeding tubes (with a balloon to secure the tube against the anterior stomach wall) have an adjustable external flange (Fig. 40.15). Once the Silastic catheter is in position and the balloon is inflated, the flange is slid down against the skin, stabilizing the catheter without the use of adhesives.

Regardless of the type of stabilization device or bolster used, adequate stabilization is critical to the success of the tubes. The devices secure the tube against the abdominal wall and against the anterior stomach wall. The tension between the internal and external securing devices should allow slight leeway from the skin to prevent erosion of the skin (i.e., device-related pressure ulcer) or gastric mucosa (known as buried bumper syndrome (BBS)) (Lord, 2018; Alsunaid et al., 2021). This leeway should be monitored daily because changes in abdominal girth, as occurs with ascites, can develop, which exposes the patient to excess pressure under the external stabilization device. Modifications should be made as necessary.

Tube Patency

To maintain patency, all enteral feeding tubes require routine flushing (see Box 40.3). In adults, the tube should be flushed with 30 mL of water (3–5 mL in pediatrics) every 4 hours during continuous feeding, before and after intermittent feedings, and after measuring residual volume (Lord, 2018). It is also imperative that each medication be instilled separately and flushed with 15 mL of water before, in between, and after each medication (Lord, 2018). When the safety of tap water is questioned, distilled or sterile water should be used. Medications should be in liquid form or crushed and dissolved in tap water; enteric-coated, time-released, or sustained-release medications are not appropriate (Tong, 2010).

Occlusion of a feeding tube can result from administration of powdered or crushed medications in the feeding tube, viscous formulas, and poor or inadequate flushing techniques, partially digested proteins, yeast, and aspiration of gastric or intestinal contents into the tube. Instillation of 50 mL tepid water from a 60-mL syringe should be used initially to dislodge an occlusion allowing the water to dwell. This process can also assist in distinguishing a kinked tube from a clogged tube in that kinked tubes allow slow passage of water, whereas clogged tubes do not allow any passage of water. When irrigation with water fails, activated pancreatic enzymes can be used as a declogging solution following the same technique. The declogging solutions consist of a crushed tablet of on-enteric-coated sodium bicarbonate (650 mg) or baking soda (1/4 teaspoon) dissolved in 10 mL of warm water. Added to this is an opened capsule of pancrelipase (12,000 U) or a crushed pancrelipase tablet (10,440 U). These are allowed to dissolve and then instilled into the tube in a manner described above.

Commercially available declogging products include enzymes and mechanical products. Clog Zapper, a powder containing a combination of enzymes (e.g., papain, cellulose, and α-amylase), is reconstituted with water, instilled into the clogged tube, and allowed to dwell for 30–60 minutes. Two methods for the mechanical dislodgement of a clog include a machine-operated declogger with a flexible wire encased in a sheath (e.g., Bionix Enteral Feeding Tube Declogger) and a corrugated plastic rod (e.g., Bard PEG cleaning brush). Limited evidence is available in the use of these declogging strategies. The use of cranberry juice, chymotrypsin, carbonated drinks, and meat tenderizers is discouraged because they tend to precipitate in the feeding solution and cause adverse effects in patients with severe hepatic, renal, or coagulation abnormalities (Tong, 2010).

COMPLICATIONS

Complications associated with percutaneous enteral tubes include local complications such as peristomal leakage, MASD, hyperplasia, peritubular site infection, and BBS. The wound specialist may see a patient with an enteral feeding tube for the first time when a skin complication develops. In addition to addressing the skin problem, investigation and correction of the underlying problem precipitating the skin irritation is essential.

Leakage

Small amounts of peritubular leakage can be expected with newly placed tubes. Excessive leakage, however, warrants investigation (Alsunaid et al., 2021). Factors often associated with peritubular leakage include: delayed healing of the tract, gastric hypersecretion, BBS, excessive torsion on the feeding tube, and instability of the tube. Steps must be taken to correct any possible cause of the leakage. Replacing the tube with a larger size will not correct the problem. First check the adequacy of tube stabilization, appropriate balloon placement, adequate inflation of the balloon, and tube patency. The balloon should be deflated and reinflated with the amount of air or sterile water recommended by the manufacturer. Antacid medications (e.g., proton pump inhibitors) to reduce gastric acid secretion are warranted (Wei et al., 2021). Leakage may occur as a result of bolus feedings and may resolve with slower delivery or continuous delivery. When all attempts to halt the leakage fail, replacement of the tube may be necessary.

Moisture-Associated Skin Damage

Moisture-associated skin damage surrounding a tube most commonly results from chemical irritation (exposure to gastric or intestinal contents), the chronic presence of moisture, or fungal infection. If all attempts to halt leakage fail and tube replacement is not an option, methods to contain the drainage and protect the skin must be implemented. Hydrocolloids and absorbent dressings are often not appropriate because they will trap drainage and moisture against the skin, exacerbating MASD; foam dressings are an alternative.

To contain excessive drainage around a tube site, an ostomy pouch and catheter port can be applied. By attaching a catheter port to the pouch, the tube can exit the wall of the pouch through the port, which allows for feeding, suction, or gravity drainage to continue. The ostomy pouch then contains peritubular drainage (Fig. 40.16). Such a pouching system is cost effective and allows collection, identification, and measurement of the drainage, as well as skin protection. Instructions for containing peritubular leakage are outlined in Box 40.4. The frequency of pouch changes is determined by the duration of the pouch seal, but on average, the pouch is changed every 4–7 days. If a urinary pouch is selected, it may be necessary to "pop" the antireflux mechanism within the pouch, particularly when drainage is thick or contains particulate matter.

Fungal infections (e.g., candidiasis) can result when moisture is trapped at the insertion site. Corrective measures include protecting the skin from moisture with skin sealants or ointments or containing the moisture with appropriate dressings. Antifungal medications (e.g., powders) may be necessary when extensive candidiasis is present.

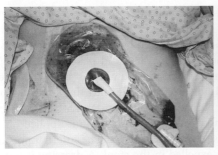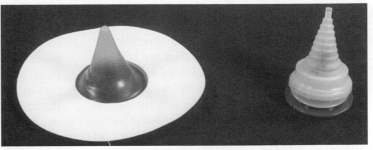

Fig. 40.16 Catheter access port attached to drainable ostomy pouch (*left*). Two examples of a catheter access port (*right*). (Courtesy NuHope and Hollister.)

BOX 40.4   Pouching Procedure for Leakage Around Tube

1. Assemble pouch and catheter access device.
   a. Cut opening in barrier and pouch to accommodate tube site.
   b. Make small slit in anterior surface of pouch.
   c. Attach access device to anterior surface of the pouch.
   d. Tear paper backing on pouch or wafer but leave in place.
2. Prepare skin.
   a. Cleanse and dry skin.
   b. Treat any denuded skin (skin barrier powder to denuded area; skin sealant if needed).

   c. Apply skin barrier ring immediately around insertion site, if needed.
3. Disconnect and plug tube.
4. Feed catheter through opening in pouch. Use water-soluble lubricant to pass tube, and use hemostat to pull tube through the pouch or barrier opening, anterior wall of the pouch, and access device.
5. Reconnect tube.
6. Ensure skin is dry. Remove paper backing from wafer and secure pouch to skin.
7. Secure tube to stabilization device with tape.

Allergic contact dermatitis can occur when a patient's skin is sensitive to anchoring devices, tapes, soaps, or other commercial products. Medical adhesive-related skin injury in the form of mechanical trauma or folliculitis can also develop as a result of traumatic removal of adhesives used to anchor the tube. These issues are discussed further in Chapter 5.

Peristomal Hyperplasia

An overgrowth of granulation tissue at the tube exit site can develop and is commonly referred to as *hyperplasia*. This overgrowth of granulation tissue occurs in response to chronic irritation of the tissue lining the tract. The source of the chronic irritation can be the type of tube material used (latex is more irritating than Silastic material), tube mobility (particularly in-and-out movements of the tube), and the chronic presence of excessive moisture (Lord, 2018; Wei et al., 2021). Hyperplasia may or may not be uncomfortable. However, when hyperplasia is allowed to persist, seepage from the overgrowth will develop and compromise the integrity of the external stabilization and skin integrity. Treatment should address the underlying causative factor (e.g., tube stability and peritubular leakage). If chronic moisture is present, medications to reduce gastric reflux may be warranted. Adequacy of tube stabilization should be reevaluated. Once the cause is corrected, the hyperplasia should resolve. Debridement and cautery with silver nitrate sticks are often warranted and the continued ongoing management with the application

of topical corticosteroid. Because it can be painful for the patient, cautery with silver nitrate sticks should be done infrequently and only by an experienced care provider.

PERITUBULAR SITE INFECTION

The peritubular site should be assessed daily for erythema, drainage, and pain at the site. However, the cause for the erythema may or may not be infection. Faint peritubular site erythema is to be expected following new placement of a percutaneous enteral tube. Peritubular erythema may also accompany peritubular leakage and chronic presence of moisture. Therefore, when erythema is assessed, it is important to "rule out" possible causative factors by (1) protecting the skin from gastric contents, (2) checking the external bumper is not too tight against the skin, and (3) confirming the tube is properly stabilized from mobility.

An infection should be suspected when the erythema persists, increases in size or intensity of color, and is associated with purulent drainage or pain at the site, edema at the site, or fever (Alsunaid et al., 2021). Topical antibiotic ointment may be applied with cotton-tipped application at the exit site, although systemic antibiotics may be needed in select situations. When a peritubular draining or infected wound at the exit site is apparent, hypertonic saline dressings may be applied (Townley, Wincentak, Krong, Schippke, & Kingsnorth, 2017).

BURIED BUMPER SYNDROME

BBS is the condition in which the internal securement device (bumper, balloon, etc.) migrates along the tract and becomes displaced outside the stomach. This develops as a consequence of excessive compression between the internal securement device/bumper and the external securement device/bumper. Risk factors for BBS include immunosuppression, malnutrition, chemotherapy, steroids, and positioning of the external bumper (Wei et al., 2021). As prevention, the excess tension between the internal and external bumpers should be avoided (Alsunaid et al., 2021). Ideally the external bumper is positioned approximately 1 cm away from the skin, although some providers prefer tighter positioning of the external bumper in the few days following initial insertion.

TUBE REMOVAL

Enteral tubes are removed when the patient is able to resume adequate oral nutrition and may need to be removed when they are hopelessly occluded, kinked, or malpositioned. The method of removal will depend on the type of tube, the technique used to insert the tube, and the type of tube tip (Boxes 40.5–40.7). PEG tubes can be removed by external traction, endoscopy, or "cut and push." With the "cut and push" method, the outer bumper is loosened, the tube is rotated and advanced slightly into the stomach (to ensure the internal bumper is mobile and not attached to the gastric mucosa), and, while external traction is applied on the tube, the tube is severed at skin level. The internal portion of the tube will be expelled in the stool. A dressing is applied over the percutaneous tube site and replaced daily. Patients are NPO for 6 hours before the procedure and for 2 hours after the procedure. Performance of these PEG tube removals should be reserved for nurses who have successfully completed a formal competency check, such as nutritional therapist nurses and interventional radiology nurses.

PATIENT EDUCATION

Patient education is a key nursing responsibility and is absolutely critical to the patient with a gastrostomy or

---

BOX 40.5   Traction-Pull Technique for Removal of Standard Nonballoon G-Tubes, Transgastric G/J-Tubes, and Transgastric J-Tubes

Equipment
- Nonsterile gloves
- Towel
- Water-soluble lubricant
- Gauze (4 × 4)

Procedure
1. Note: This traction-pull technique is only appropriate for non-balloon enteral feeding tubes that have a collapsible internal bolster/bumper. If this is not collapsible, an endoscopic removal is required.
2. Confirm order from provider to remove tube and that the tube has a nonballoon, collapsible internal bolster.
3. Patient should be NPO except for sips of water and medications for 4 h prior to removal.
4. Place towel across the patient's abdomen.
5. Lubricate the stoma with water-soluble lubricant or anesthetic jelly.
6. Place one hand flat against the patient's abdomen around the site for counter-traction.
7. Using dominant hand, grasp PEG tubing above bumper and wrap it around your hand to maintain a firm grip.
8. While exerting moderate force, pull on percutaneous tube until inner bumper comes through skin opening. Slight bleeding may occur. If resistance is too great, stop and call physician.
9. Cover opening with gauze until ready to insert replacement gastrostomy tube. Insert tube immediately to prevent closure of the tract.

   Note: Original PEG tube must be at least 2 weeks past time of insertion before nurse performs this procedure.

Lord, L. M. (2018). Enteral access devices: Types, function, care and challenges. *Nutrition in Clinical Practice, 33*(1), 16–38.

BOX 40.6   Instructions for Removal of Balloon Replacement Gastrostomy Tube

Equipment
- 20-mL Luer-Lok syringe
- Gauze (4 × 4)
- Towel
- Water-soluble lubricant
- Nonsterile gloves

Procedure
1. Confirm order from provider to remove tube and that tube has a balloon.
2. Patient should be NPO except for sips of water and medications for 4 h prior to removal.
3. Place towel across the patient's abdomen.
4. Lubricate the stoma with water-soluble lubricant or anesthetic jelly.
5. Connect 20-mL syringe to balloon port of tube and aspirate all water out of balloon. (*Note:* Less than 20 mL may be present as a result of evaporation.)
6. Slowly withdraw tube from abdominal site.
7. Cover opening with gauze until ready to reinsert replacement tube. Insert tube immediately to prevent closure of the tract.

Lord, L. M. (2018). Enteral access devices: Types, function, care and challenges. *Nutrition in Clinical Practice, 33*(1), 16–38.

BOX 40.7 Instructions for Reinsertion of Balloon Replacement Gastrostomy

Equipment
- Replacement gastrostomy tube of correct size
- 60-mL syringe with male tip
- Lubricant (e.g., K-Y jelly)
- Stethoscope
- Nonsterile gloves
- 20-mL Luer-Lok syringe
- 20 mL of sterile water

Procedure
1. Choose replacement gastrostomy tube that is the same size as the previously used tube unless otherwise indicated.
2. Draw up 20 mL of sterile water into syringe. Do not use saline.
3. Insert syringe into balloon port; fill balloon to ensure proper inflation.
4. Withdraw water out of balloon and lubricate distal end of gastrostomy tube.
5. Gently insert gastrostomy tube into existing opening in abdomen. Tube should go in without resistance. If resistance is detected, pull back and attempt to insert again at a slightly different angle. If resistance is met again, stop and call physician.
6. Once gastrostomy tube is inserted into existing tract, gastric contents should return into the tube. To confirm proper placement, instill 30 mL of air into gastrostomy tube and auscultate for sound, which should be heard in the stomach (not the abdomen).
7. Once placement is confirmed, fill balloon with 20-mL water-filled syringe. (Check balloon port to determine exact amount of water needed to fill balloon.)
8. After balloon is inflated, gently pull back on tube until resistance is felt, then slide down external bumper or disk until it rests lightly on the skin.
9. Rotate the catheter 360 degrees to confirm that tube has free rotation.
10. Cleanse skin around tube with soap and water; no dressing is necessary.

BOX 40.8 Key Content for Patient Education

1. Name of procedure
2. Purpose for tube insertion
3. Characteristics of normal tube function
4. Type of tube placed
5. Size of balloon (if present)
6. Tube stabilization (why it is important, how it is achieved)
7. Routine site care (daily)
8. Weekly balloon inflation checks (if present)
9. Signs and symptoms of complications and appropriate response
10. Tube feeding schedule and procedure (when applicable)
11. Name of person to call with questions or problems
12. What to do if tube falls out

jejunostomy tube. Because the hospitalization period after tube placement may be brief to nonexistent, detailed caregiver education is essential, and outpatient follow-up care is imperative. In some situations, percutaneous tube placement may be performed strictly on an outpatient basis. In either case, home health care will be important to facilitate patient and caregiver independence in the process, safety with the procedure, and monitoring for complications. Key content areas to be included in a patient teaching plan are listed in Box 40.8.

MISCELLANEOUS DRAIN TUBES

A drainage tube can be placed to drain an abscess or fluid collection that will not resolve on its own, in which antibiotics are ineffective and the patient is too ill for surgery. These are often placed by the interventional radiologist in a minimally invasive procedure and site care managed by the interventional radiology nurse. For example, a percutaneous cholecystectomy is an example in which a tube is placed in the gallbladder to decompress a distended, inflamed, or infected gallbladder. Although surgery may be performed to manage a fluid collection, surgery may not be appropriate due to local inflammation, the severity or location of the abscess, or the patient's comorbidities. With the assistance of computed tomography or fluoroscopy, a catheter can be placed anywhere in the body where pus accumulates. Once the drain is in place, the abscess may require a few weeks to a few months to resolve. The drain tube will facilitate resolution of inflammation so that a patient who does require surgical intervention will be in a more stable overall condition and therefore at decreased risk for complications associated with surgery. Each drain tube should be labeled so that documentation is clear and consistent among the physicians, nurses, and interventional radiologists. Site care involves tube securement and protection from drainage with foam or hydrocolloid dressings or protective barrier ointments. Excessive peritubular leakage may require pouching. Biliary tubes will require stabilization with a nonabsorbable skin suture and can be expected to develop minor erythema (Padmore, Sutherland, & Ball, 2021). However, peritubular skin care remains essential to maintain integrity and prevent MASD; excessive peritubular drainage may need to be managed with a drainable pouch. Drain tubes should be irrigated only when the provider who inserted the catheter gives specific instructions. Orders to irrigate the drainage tube should specify use of sterile saline, the amount of solution to use, and the frequency of irrigations. Slight force is used to irrigate the drain tube so that debris that has lodged in the lateral holes of the catheter can be dislodged.

In critical care, additional percutaneous tubes that require careful attention to stabilization, site care, and skin protection include the catheters inserted to provide extracorporeal membrane oxygenation, chest tubes, and tracheostomy. Peristomal tracheostomy site care requires keeping the skin clean and dry to reduce the risk of MASD. Sterile water or normal saline-moistened cotton swabs or gauze pads can be used to clean the peristomal skin and to remove dried secretions; dilute hydrogen peroxide can be used to loosen dried secretions but must be rinsed off with saline. Stomal infection and cellulitis is also a risk for the patient with a tracheostomy because of the constant exposure of the tracheostomy site to respiratory flora contaminates present in tracheal secretions (Zouk & Batra, 2021). A peristomal skin inspection and assessment is recommended every 4–8 hours in the newly placed tracheostomy (Alsunaid et al., 2021). Foam dressings and/or skin sealant can be used as needed for protection from moisture as well as the flange of the tracheostomy tube (Ghattas, Alsunaid, Pickering, & Holden, 2021).

CLINICAL CONSULT

A: Referral received to consult with an older adult patient admitted from a long-term care setting who had a PEG tube placed recently. Nurses report they have to change the gauze dressings around the site 4 or 5 times a day due to leakage around the site. Upon examination, the silastic bumper has advanced to 4 cm away from the skin and gauze is taped to the peritubular site. The peritubular skin is erythematous with shallow islands of denudation.
D: Ineffective securement of PEG tube; peritubular MASD secondary to leakage of gastric contents.
P: Instruct nurses on proper technique for securing PEG. Manage skin denudement.

I: (1) Check balloon for proper inflation. (2) Cleanse skin with tap water and dab dry. (3) Dust skin barrier powder over denuded skin and apply thin silicone adhesive border foam with large center cut out to position over skin and around PEG site. (4) Position silastic bumper loosely against thin silicone adhesive border foam dressing. (5) Cleanse site daily with tap water and cotton-tipped applicator.
E: Remove foam dressing after 7 days and discontinue; reposition silicone bumper approximately 1 cm from the skin. Reconsult if peritubular drainage resumes.

SUMMARY

- Percutaneous tubes contribute to both quantity and quality of life for many patients.
- Regardless of who inserts the tube or the purpose of the tube, all percutaneous tubes require stabilization and should be monitored for patency and complications.

- It should not be assumed that nursing staff are familiar with the appropriate care of percutaneous tubes.
- The patient and caregiver should have education for care of the tubes including instructions for follow-up.

SELF-ASSESSMENT QUESTIONS

1. A percutaneous tube that is placed to relieve a high ureteral obstruction is a:
   a. Jackson Pratt drain
   b. gastrostomy tube
   c. Penrose drain
   d. nephrostomy tube
2. The purpose of stabilizing a percutaneous tube is to:
   a. minimize exit site erosion
   b. enhance gastric peristalsis
   c. allow the tube to move with peristalsis and respirations
   d. reduce the length of time the tube will be needed
3. Which of the following is an appropriate initial first step in managing leakage from a gastrostomy site?

   a. Inflate an additional 2 mL of air or saline into the balloon.
   b. Apply an ostomy pouch to contain the drainage and protect the skin.
   c. Cauterize the tract with silver nitrate.
   d. Determine the cause for the leakage.
4. To clean the jejunostomy tube site, the nurse should do which of the following?
   a. Use a cotton-tipped applicator and warm water once daily.
   b. Use a skin cleanser 3 times daily.
   c. Apply bacitracin ointment once daily.
   d. Dab with diluted hydrogen peroxide once daily.

REFERENCES

Alsunaid, S., Holden, V. K., Kohli, A., Diaz, J., & O'Meara, L. B. (2021). Wound care management: Tracheostomy and gastrostomy. *Journal of Thoracic Disease, 13*(8), 5297–5313. https://doi.org/10.21037/jtd-2019-ipicu-13.

Berman, L., Hronek, C., Ravel, M. V., Browne, M. L., Snyder, C. L., Heiss, K. F., et al. (2017). Pediatric gastrostomy tube placement: Lessons learned from high-performing institutions through structured interviews. *Pediatric Quality and Safety, 2*(2), e016. https://doi.org/10.1097/pg9.0000000000000016.

Blumenstein, I., Shastri, Y. M., & Stein, J. (2014). Gastroenteric tube feeding: Techniques, problems and solutions. *World Journal of Gastroenterology, 20*(26), 8505–8524. https://doi.org/10.3748/wjg.v20.i26.8505.

D'Cruz, J. R., & Cascella, M. (2022). Feeding jejunostomy tube. In *StatPearls*. Treasure Island, FL: StatPearls Publishing. Available from: https://www.ncbi.nlm.nih.gov/books/NBK562278/.

DeLegge, M. H. (2018). Enteral access and associated complications. *Gastroenterology Clinics of North America, 47*, 23–37. https://doi.org/10.1016/j.gtc.2017.09.003.

Gauderer, M. W. L., & Stellato, T. A. (1986). Gastrostomies: Evolution, techniques, indications and implications. *Current Problems in Surgery, 23*, 657–719.

Ghattas, C., Alsunaid, S., Pickering, E. M., & Holden, V. K. (2021). State of the art: Percutaneous tracheostomy in the intensive care unit. *Journal of Thoracic Disease, 13*(8), 5261–5276.

Hitawala, A. A., & Mousa, O. Y. (2022). Percutaneous gastrostomy and jejunostomy. In *StatPearls*. Treasure Island, FL: StatPearls Publishing. Available from: https://www.ncbi.nlm.nih.gov/books/NBK559215/.

Jones, D. B. (2004). *Laparoscopic surgery: Principles and procedures, Second Edition, revised and expanded (1st ed.)*. CRC Press. https://doi.org/10.1201/b14143.

Lord, L. M. (2018). Enteral access devices: Types, function, care and challenges. *Nutrition in Clinical Practice, 33*(1), 16–38.

Padmore, G., Sutherland, F. R., & Ball, C. G. (2021). The art and craft of biliary T-tube use. *The Journal of Trauma and Acute Care Surgery, 91*(2), e46–e49.

Rahnemai-Azar, A. A., Rahnemaiazar, A. A., Naghshizakdian, R., Kurtz, A., & Farkas, D. T. (2014). Percutaneous endoscopic gastrostomy: Indications, technique, complications and management. *World Journal of Gastroenterology, 20*(24), 7739–7751. https://doi.org/10.3748/wjg.v20.i24.7739.

Rothrock, J. C., & Alexander, S. M. (2012). *Alexander's surgical procedures*. St. Louis, MO: Elsevier.

Saberi, R. A., Gilna, G. P., Slavin, B. V., Ribieras, A. J., Cioci, A. C., Urrechaga, E. M., et al. (2021). Pediatric gastrostomy tube placement: Less complications associated with laparoscopic approach. *Journal of Laparoendoscopic & Advanced Surgical Techniques, 31*(12), 1376–1383. https://doi.org/10.1089/lap.2021.0347.

Senadhi, V., Emuron, D., Singh, R., et al. (2012). PEG tube placement in morbidly obese patients. *Endoscopy 44*, E53.

Shapiro, D. S., & Montgomery, S. C. (2019). Access and intubation of the stomach and small intestine. In C. J. Yeo, et al. (Eds.), *Shackelford's surgery of the alimentary tract* (8th ed.). St. Louis: Elsevier.

Siow, S. L., Mahendran, H. A., Wong, C. M., Milaksh, N. K., & Nyunt, M. (2017). Laparoscopic T-tube feeding jejunostomy as an adjunct to staging laparoscopy for upper gastrointestinal malignancies: The technique and review of outcomes. *BMC Surgery, 17*, 25. https://doi.org/10.1186/s12893-017-0221-2.

Strong, A. T., Sharma, G., Davis, M., Mulcahy, M., Punchai, S., O'Rourke, C. P., et al. (2017). Direct percutaneous endoscopic jejunostomy (DPEJ) tube placement: A single institution experience and outcomes to 30 days and beyond. *Journal of Gastrointestinal Surgery, 21*, 4460452. https://doi.org/10.1007/s11605-016-3337-2.

Tong, A. (2010). Pancreatic enzyme products update. *Cleveland Clinic Pharmacotherapy Update, 13*(6). http://www.clevelandclinicmeded.com/medicalpubs/pharmacy/pdf/Pharmacotherapy_XIII-6.pdf. Accessed March 5, 2022.

Townley, A., Wincentak, J., Krong, K., Schippke, J., & Kingsnorth, S. (2017). Paediatric gastrostomy stoma complications and treatments: A rapid scoping review. *Journal of Clinical Nursing, 27*, 1369–1380.

Vudayagiri, L., Hoilat, G. J., & Gemma, R. (2021). Percutaneous endoscopic gastrostomy tube. In *StatPearls*. Treasure Island, FL: StatPearls Publishing. Available from: https://www.ncbi.nlm.nih.gov/books/NBK535371/.

Wei, M., Ho, E., & Hegde, P. (2021). An overview of percutaneous endoscopic gastrostomy tube placement in the intensive care unit. *Journal of Thoracic Disease, 13*(8), 5277–5296. https://doi.org/10.21307/jts-19-3728.

Yarmus, L., Gilbert, C., Lechtzin, N., et al. (2013). Safety and feasibility of interventional pulmonologists performing bedside percutaneous endoscopic gastrostomy tube placement. *Chest, 114*(2), 436–440.

Zhu, Y., Shi, L., Hao, T., & Tao, G. (2012). Current considerations in direct percutaneous endoscopic jejunostomy. *Canadian Journal of Gastroenterology, 26*(2), 92–96.

Zouk, A. N., & Batra, H. (2021). Managing complications of percutaneous tracheostomy and gastrostomy. *Journal of Thoracic Disease, 13*(8), 5314–5330. https://doi.org/10.21037/jtd-19-3716.

Tools to Support Skin and Wound Care

POLICY AND PROCEDURE: PREVENTION OF PRESSURE ULCERS/INJURIES

Policy

All patients will have a skin inspection and be assessed for risk of pressure ulcers/injuries (PU/I) on admission (as soon as possible but at least within 8 hours), daily, and with significant change in condition. Appropriate preventive interventions will be implemented.

Risk Assessment Procedure

Risk assessment includes determining a person's risk for PU/I development using the appropriate PU/I Risk Assessment Tool. PU/I preventive interventions will target modifiable risk factors as determined by the pressure PU/I risk assessment. Age-appropriate risk assessment tools will be used.

Over age 15: The Braden Scale for Predicting Pressure Sore Risk
Under age 16: Braden Q Scale

Skin Inspection

A head-to-toe skin inspection, including around and under medical devices, between all skin folds and back of head. During inspection, pressure points are examined and palpated closely for any of the following conditions:

- Alteration in skin moisture
- Change in texture, turgor
- Change in temperature compared to surrounding skin (warmer or cooler)
- Color changes (e.g., red, blue, and purplish hues)
- Nonblanchable erythema
- Consistency (e.g., bogginess [soft] or induration [hard])
- Edema
- Open areas, blisters, rash, drainage
- Pain

Note: Blanching erythema is an early indicator of the need to redistribute pressure. Nonblanching erythema is suggestive that tissue damage has already occurred or is imminent. Indurated or boggy skin is a sign that tissue damage may have occurred.

Preventive Interventions

1. Minimize or Eliminate Friction and Shear

   One or more of the following interventions and observations will be used to minimize or eliminate dragging or sliding the patients' skin against any surface (e.g., bed or chair) if friction/shear has been identified as a risk factor

   - Use safe patient handling methods (e.g., mechanical lifts, HoverMatt, trapeze, surgical slip sheets) to lift rather than drag the patient's body while moving up in a bed/chair or transferring to another surface.
   - Slightly engage knee gatch 20 degrees then limit head of the bed elevation to 30 degrees to prevent sliding in bed unless contraindicated.
   - Place a pad or pillow between skin surfaces that may rub together.
   - Apply commercial protective products or dressings to reduce friction (they do not reduce pressure).
   - Apply creams or lotions frequently to lower surface tension on skin and reduce friction and to keep skin well hydrated and moisturized.
   - Lubricate bedpan with incontinence care lotion or ointment before placing under patient. Position bedpan by rolling patient on and off rather than pushing and pulling bedpan in and out.

2. Minimize Pressure

   Immobility is the most significant risk factor for PU/I development. Patients who have any degree of immobility should be closely monitored for PU/I development. One or more of the following interventions will be used if immobility is identified as a risk factor:

   Patient in Bed
   - Make frequent, small position changes.
   - Use pillows or wedges to reduce pressure on bony prominences.
   - Turn patient a minimum of every 2 hours.
   - Do not position patient lying on side directly on trochanter (hip).
   - Use pressure redistribution mattresses/surfaces.
   - Free-float heels by placing a pillow under calf muscle and keeping heels off all surfaces.
   - Avoid elevating head of the bed more than 30 degrees unless contraindicated.

   Patient in Chair
   - Encourage patient to shift weight every 15 minutes (e.g., perform chair pushups if able to reposition self;

stand and reseat self if able; make small shift changes, such as elevating legs).
- Reposition patient every hour if he or she is unable to reposition self.
- Use chair cushions for pressure redistribution.

3. Minimize/Eliminate Pressure From Medical Devices
   - Follow manufacturer's instructions for appropriate use of medical devices (e.g., oxygen masks and tubing, catheters, cervical collars, casts, intravenous tubing, and restraints).
   - Routinely remove or reposition devices as needed for skin inspection, pressure relief, and pressure redistribution.

4. Manage Moisture

   Management of moisture from perspiration, wound drainage, and incontinence is an important aspect of PU/I prevention. Moisture from incontinence may be a precursor to PU/I development because of skin maceration and increased friction. Fecal incontinence is a greater risk factor than urinary incontinence for PU/I development because the stool contains bacteria and enzymes that are caustic to the skin. In the presence of both urinary and fecal incontinence, fecal enzymes convert urea to ammonia, raising the skin pH. With a more alkaline skin pH, the skin becomes more permeable to other irritants. One or more of the following interventions will be used to minimize or eliminate moisture when it is identified as a risk factor:
   - Contain wound drainage.
   - Keep skin folds dry.
   - Evaluate type of incontinence (urinary, fecal, or both).
   - Implement toileting schedule or bowel/bladder program as appropriate.
   - Check for incontinence a minimum of every 2 hours and as needed.
   - Cleanse skin gently with pH-balanced cleanser at each soiling. Avoid excessive friction and scrubbing, which can further traumatize the skin. Cleansers with non-ionic surfactants are gentler on the skin than are anionic surfactants in typical soaps.
   - Use incontinence skin barriers (e.g., creams, ointments, pastes, film-forming skin protectants) as needed to protect and maintain intact skin or to treat nonintact skin.

- Assess for candidiasis and treat as indicated.
- Use external containment products (such as catheters or collection devices) or indwelling containment devices when appropriate.
  i. Use of indwelling urinary catheters must have provider order and meet CAUTI criteria
  ii. Use of indwelling fecal containment devices must have provider order after all indications, contraindications, and manufacturer's instructions have been followed.

5. Maintain Adequate Nutrition/Hydration

   The patient who is malnourished and/or dehydrated is at increased risk for PU/I development. One or more of the following interventions will be used when nutrition is identified as a risk factor:
   - Provide nutrition compatible with individual's wishes or condition.
   - Encourage hydration, as well as high-protein and high-calorie supplements, for the patient with multiple risk factors for PU/I development.

6. Address Sustainability of Plan of Care and Goals

   The patient's ability to participate in PU/I prevention interventions may be affected by physical and behavioral factors. Declination of care may be related to inability to participate, lifestyle issues, cultural differences, medical condition, physical condition, lack of trust, or knowledge gaps. Possible activities to address include the following:
   - Provide education that increases patient/family knowledge of PU/I risk and appropriate interventions.
   - Identify barriers to patient participation and develop strategies to address those barriers.

7. Patient/Family Education

   The patient, family, and/or caregivers will be educated on risk assessment and skin inspection technique. They will be informed of current status of risk assessment and skin inspection findings and will be involved in planning interventions.

8. Documentation
   - All assessments, plan of care for prevention of skin breakdown, patient engagement and response to interventions, and informed refusals will be described and documented.

POLICY AND PROCEDURE: WOUND ASSESSMENT, DOCUMENTATION, AND QUALITY TRACKING

Policy

All wounds will be assessed upon admission or occurrence, at least weekly, with significant changes, and upon transfer or discharge.

Procedure

The following parameters will be documented:
A. Anatomic location of skin breakdown
B. Etiology (type) of skin breakdown

C. Classification of skin breakdown
- Pressure ulcers/injuries (PU/I) will be classified according to the National Pressure Injury Advisory Panel (NPIAP) staging system.
- All other wounds will be classified as either "partial thickness" or "full thickness."
  - *Partial thickness:* Wounds extend through the first layer of skin (the epidermis) and into, but not through, the second layer of skin (the dermis).
  - *Full thickness:* Wounds extend through both the epidermis and dermis and may involve subcutaneous tissue, muscle, and possibly bone.
  - *Approximated incisions:* Staples, sutures, or Steri-strips are present.

D. Wound measurements in centimeters
Length and width: To ensure consistency, use the clock method for wound measurement. Visualize the wound as if it were the face of a clock. The top of the wound (12 o'clock position) is always toward the patient's head. Conversely, the bottom of the wound (6 o'clock position) is in the direction of the patient's feet. Therefore, length will be measured from the 12 o'clock to the 6 o'clock position, using the head and feet as guides. Width will be measured from side to side, or from the 3 o'clock to the 9 o'clock position.

Depth: The depth of the wound can be described as the distance from the visible surface to the deepest point in the wound, perpendicular to the skin surface. To measure the depth of the wound, use a sterile, flexible, cotton-tipped applicator.
- Put on gloves and gently insert the applicator into the deepest portion of the wound.
- Grasp the applicator with the thumb and forefinger at the point level to the skin surface.
- Withdraw the applicator while maintaining the position of the thumb and forefinger.
- Measure (with a ruler marked in centimeters) from the tip of the applicator to that position.

Tunneling (also known as *sinus tracts*): This is a passageway under the surface of the skin that is generally open at the skin level. However, most of the tunneling is not visible.
- Put on gloves and gently insert the sterile cotton-tipped applicator into the deepest extent of the tunnel.
- Pinch the applicator at the point where it meets the wound edge.
- Hold the pinched length of the applicator next to a centimeter ruler to determine the depth of tunneling.
- Document the length and location of the tunnel using the clock method.

Undermining: Tissue destruction underlies intact skin. Both the direction and extent of undermining should be documented.
- Put on gloves and gently insert the sterile cotton-tipped applicator into the sites where undermining occurs.
- View the wound as though it were the face of a clock (as previously described). The 12 o'clock position corresponds to the wound edge that aligns toward the patient's head.
- Progressing in a clockwise direction, gently probe to determine the extent of undermining (e.g., 2 o'clock to 5 o'clock position).
- Insert the cotton-tipped applicator into the deepest area of the undermining. Grasp the applicator with thumb and forefinger at the point where it is level to the skin surface.
- Withdraw the applicator while maintaining the position of thumb and forefinger. Measure (using a ruler marked in centimeters) from the tip of the applicator to that position.
- Document the extent and deepest measurement of undermining in a manner similar to the following example: "Undermining from 2 o'clock to 5 o'clock position. Deepest point is 2.5 cm at 3 o'clock position."

E. Wound bed appearance (type and percentage of tissue in the wound bed)
F. Wound Edge Appearance (punched out, rolled, attached)
G. Exudate/drainage
- Color
- Amount (percentage saturating dressing and type of dressing)
H. Periwound
- *All wounds:* Assess and document condition of periwound skin condition (maceration, induration, and erythema)
- *Lower extremity wounds:* Assess and document edema and dorsalis pedis and posterior tibial pulses and sensation
I. Presence or absence of overt signs of infection
- New/increased slough
- Drainage excess, change in color/consistency
- Poor granulation tissue (friable, bright red, and exuberant)
- Redness, warmth, induration around wound
- Suddenly high glucose level in patient with diabetes
- Pain or tenderness
- Unusual odor
- Lack of improvement after 2 weeks of optimal management (including elimination or reduction of PU/I risk factors as well as cofactors to impaired wound healing)

J. Pain
  - Assess pain using a visual analog scale or a faces rating scale
K. Patient/family education
  - Signs and symptoms of infection
  - Status or assessment of wound
L. Pressure PU/I reporting

- PU/I that are present on admission will be reported to the provider for evaluation and documentation in the provider's notes.
- Facility acquired PU/I will be reported to the provider, and a quality tracking report will be sent to quality management for possible root-cause analysis.

POLICY AND PROCEDURE: WOUND MANAGEMENT

Policy

A wound treatment plan will be initiated for a patient at the time of admission or upon development of a wound. The patient's treatment plan will be evaluated at least every week thereafter and revised as necessary. The treatment plan will be based on the principles outlined next.

Procedure

A. Establish realistic goals related to wound management in collaboration with the patient, family, caregivers, and providers.
  - If wound healing is *not* a realistic goal, create a plan of care that will minimize pain, odor, and infection while optimizing quality of life.
  - If wound healing *is* a realistic goal, the following interventions should be incorporated into the care plan.
B. Control/eliminate causative factors.
C. Optimize nutrition.
  - Complete a nutritional screening on admission per nutritional assessment policy and procedure.
  - Consult registered dietician (RD) per nutritional assessment policy and procedure.
  - Reassess and consider RD consult if wound does not improve within 1 week of optimal wound management.
D. Assess, prevent, or manage pain.
E. Remove devitalized tissue when appropriate.
  - In the presence of adequate perfusion, remove devitalized tissue through mechanical, autolytic, or enzymatic debridement.
  - Heel ulcers with dry eschar need not be debrided if no signs of infection are present.
  - Sharp debridement by a qualified professional should be conducted when indicated.
F. Cleanse wound.
  - Cleanse wound initially and at each dressing change.
  - Use minimal mechanical force while cleaning a wound.

- Avoid cleaning wounds using abrasive or antiseptic agents. (Normal saline is most often appropriate.)
G. Provide a physiologic wound environment with appropriate dressings.
  - If blood supply to the wound site is adequate, keep the wound bed moist.
  - If blood supply to wound site is *not* adequate, keep the wound clean and dry.
  - Keep periwound skin dry and intact.
  - Control exudate.
  - Consider caregiver time.
  - Eliminate dead space.
  - Avoid overpacking the wound.
H. Manage bacterial colonization and infection.
  - When treating multiple wounds on the same patient, attend to the most contaminated wound last.
  - Clean technique may be used for chronic wounds and PU/I.
  - Perform cleansing and debridement of wounds as appropriate.
  - Consider a 2-week trial of topical antimicrobials as a course of treatment of wounds that are not healing after 2 weeks of optimal care.
  - Protect wounds from exogenous sources of contamination (e.g., feces).
  - Immediately report signs of infection to the provider.
I. Provide patient/family education.
    The patient, family, and/or caregivers will be educated regarding the following:
  - Signs and symptoms of infection
  - Status or assessment of wound
  - Skin inspection and preventive interventions for skin breakdown (see policy on prevention of skin breakdown)
  - PU/I risk assessment findings (see policy on prevention of skin breakdown)
  - Dressing changes (if applicable)

POLICY: NAIL CARE

Purpose

The purpose of this study is to identify patients who need expert nail clipping from a certified or trained specialist after discharge.

Responsibility

Provider (referral for expert nail care)
  Nursing (basic nail trimming)

Policy

- *Expert nail clipping* is required for patients with nail disorders and conditions with risk factors known to lead to significant infection, poor wound healing, excessive bleeding, or limb loss. Expert nail care is not within the scope of nursing and requires a provider referral upon discharge to a podiatrist or trained/certified professional.
- *Basic nail clipping* is considered part of patient hygiene and within the scope of nursing practice.

Process

A. The need for nail clipping is identified by the patient, family, hospital personnel, or provider.
B. The MD evaluates risk factors and determines if patient requires any of the following:
  - *Basic nail trimming* by staff nurses as specified in the *Nursing Procedure Manual*

- *Expert nail clipping* by a trained expert due to nail disorders and conditions with risk factors known to lead to significant infection, poor wound healing, excessive bleeding, or limb loss. Examples include but are not limited to the following:
  1. Onychophosis (incurvated or involuted nails)
  2. Onychogryposis (deformed, hypertrophic nails)
  3. Diabetes
  4. Rheumatoid arthritis
  5. Pernicious anemia
  6. Peripheral vascular disease
  7. Conditions that require warfarin (Coumadin)
  8. Neutropenia (absolute neutrophil count <1000)
  9. Thrombocytopenia (platelet count ≤60,000)
C. The MD orders *basic* nail trimming by nurse or generates a podiatry referral upon discharge if *expert nail clipping* is indicated. (*Note*: Inpatient podiatry consultations remain available for acute needs such as surgical procedures and debridement.)

Related Resources

Howes-Trammel, S. (2023). Foot and nail care. In R. Bryant & D. Nix (Eds.), *Acute and chronic wounds: Interprofessional Novice to Expert* (6th ed.). St. Louis: Mosby/Elsevier.

POLICY: ANTIEMBOLISM STOCKINGS

Purpose

The purpose of this study is to assist health care providers in the appropriate assessment and use of antiembolism stockings (AES) and to delineate patient care requirements to minimize/eliminate risks associated with AES use.

Policy

Use of AES may be indicated in the immobile/bedridden patient as a mechanical means of deep vein thrombosis (DVT) pulmonary embolus (PE) prophylaxis in a patient who is at risk.

Procedure

Adherence to the following assessment, use, and maintenance requirements is required. By definition, AES are elastic stockings that provide between 18- and 25-mm Hg gradient pressure. Medical center use is limited to knee-high stockings.
A. Indications for use:
  1. An order by provider

  2. For DVT/PE prophylaxis in the immobile/bedridden patient
  3. *Contraindications* for use:
    a. Arterial insufficiency (including symptoms of claudication, lower extremity pain with elevation)
    b. Absent peripheral pulses
    c. Anatomic abnormality
    d. Dermatitis or loss of skin integrity
    e. Massive edema of legs or pulmonary edema from congestive heart failure
    f. Suspected or actual acute DVT
    g. Lower extremity ischemia or gangrene
    h. Recent vein ligation
    i. Recent skin graft
    j. Ambulatory patient
B. Assessment, care, and maintenance:
  1. Initial assessment as noted in A, nos. 1–3.
  2. Provide patient education, emphasizing the stocking is to be used only while the patient is immobile or

bedridden. Once he or she is ambulatory, the stocking should be discarded.

3. Measure the patient for knee-high AES only after he or she has been supine for at least 30 minutes.

4. Measure the extremity(ies) for the appropriate size according to the manufacturer's directions and brand being used. (The ankle is the most important measurement.)

5. Ensure the patient's leg is clean and completely dry prior to initial application of the stocking.

6. *Safety check:* Apply the stockings according to nursing procedure and complete a safety check, including the following:

   a. Heel is located in the center of the heel pocket.

   b. Toes are freely mobile, and patient reports no cramping.

   c. Fit is smooth over sensitive areas (toes, heel, anterior foot, ankle).

   d. Knit change at the knee is just below popliteal fossa.

7. Reassess lower extremity circulation within 1–2 hours after initial application. If circulation is diminished (i.e., toes discolored, patient reports numbness, and burning sensation), remove the stockings and notify the ordering practitioner.

8. Remove the stockings for 30–60 minutes every shift and conduct a reassessment. Particular at-risk areas include the patient's toes, heels, malleolus, anterior ankle, and top of stocking (possible tourniquet effect). Once daily, wash the lower extremities and lubricate the skin. Allow the lubricant to absorb before reapplying the stockings. Powder can be used if the extremity is thoroughly dried prior to application.

9. Discontinue and discard the stockings when the patient is ambulatory.

C. Documentation:

1. *Stocking note:* Document as a progress note the initial assessment (including peripheral pulse assessment), measurements, size applied, and education provided.

2. Ongoing q.s. removal, assessment, and hygiene are recorded on the treatment record. Discontinuation of AES is also recorded on the treatment record.

3. Additional progress notes are required only when stockings require discontinuation due to impaired circulation, potential loss of skin integrity, or patient intolerance. Such progress notes will include provider notification.

4. Skin breakdown associated with use of the stockings requires an incident report to be initiated.

D. Special notes:

1. Alternative interventions effective for prevention of DVT/PE:

   a. Dorsal and plantar flexion of the foot at least 10 times every hour while the patient is awake. Such interventions should be documented on the treatment sheet.

   b. Progressing patients to an ambulatory status as soon as clinically and physically indicated is one of the most effective measures for DVT/PE prevention.

   c. AES are not recommended for use with sequential compression devices (SCDs). Rather, absorbent cotton stockings or stockinette is recommended for use.

   d. Mechanical foot pumps or compression therapy increase lower extremity peripheral blood flow.

2. Pharmacologic agents effective for prevention of DVT/PE:

   a. Low-molecular-weight heparin

   b. Warfarin

   c. Subcutaneous heparin

3. Little-known facts:

   a. AES *are not* effective in treating lower extremity edema in the upright patient. Ambulatory compression stockings (e.g., Jobst) can be ordered for this purpose. A variety of gradient pressure models (range 20–50 mm Hg) are available from the prosthetics department.

   b. Treatment of orthostatic hypotension may include ambulatory compression stockings (Jobst).

   c. Ankle–brachial index (ABI) is a noninvasive test that measures the patency of lower extremity arteries. ABI <0.8 indicates arterial occlusion and borderline perfusion. Normal ABI is >0.9–1.3. Use of compression garments when the ABI is less than 0.9 should be under the supervision of a vascular specialist. In these situations, an ankle perfusion pressure (APP) is preferred because it better correlates with tissue perfusion pressure. Modified compression (lower levels of compression) can be applied when the APP is >60 mm Hg and the ABI is greater than 0.6.

E. Patient/family education: Describe the purpose of the stockings before application. Instruct the patient to notify the nurse or provider with burning, tingling, numbness, or pain following application. If patients are discharged with AES, provide review and handout related to application, maintenance, laundering, and problem reporting with the patient.

INTERDEPARTMENTAL HANDOFF

Fairview Southdale Hospital
Communication Tool

Hospital Handoff Information

Date:_____ Time:_____

Discharge/Transport from:

_____

Patient Sticker Here

Primary Patient Problem(s):

| **Allergies:** | **None** | **See Arm Band** | **Latex** |

Safety Risks:
- ☐ **Full CODE**
- ☐ **DNR/DNI**
- ☐ **Fall Risk: Mental Status (orientation/confusion):**
- ☐ **Fall Risk: Functional Status (indep/limited mobility):**
- ☐ **Infection Risk: MRSA   VRE   Other:**
- ☐ **Pressure Ulcer Risk (Braden ≤18)** – See back of sheet for interventions (excluding OR)
  - ○ **Existing Pressure Ulcer   Location:** _____ See back for interventions (excluding OR)
- ☐ **Restraints**
- ☐ **Suicide or Elopement Precautions–72 Hours HOLD (Security w/Patient)**

Special Alert Care Plan: _____

Sensory Risk(s):
- ☐ **HOH   (R)   (L)   Both**
- ☐ **Vision Aids:**_____
- ☐ **Speech/Language difficulties:**_____
   _____
- ☐ **Interpreter Needed: Yes   No**
   Contacted:_____

Equipment & Special Needs:
- ☐ **Needs assistance to transfer X**_____
  people (more than 2, please send on cart)
- ☐ **Only guidance needed**
- ☐ **Uses cane/walker/other:**_____
- ☐ **Special Needs:**

   _____

Able to have water: Yes   No

RN Signature:_____   **Ext:**_____

Note Patient Belongings:

_____Glasses _____Dentures _____Hearing aid _____Clothing _____Other (list)

Sending Department: _____ Initial

Receiving Department: _____ Initial

Discharging Department: _____ Initial

Return from procedural department:

Test #1

Signature:_____ ext:_____

Test #2

Signature:_____ ext:_____

ATTENTION NURSING:_____

_____

_____

The chart should remain with patient whenever possible.
Completion of this form is expected for patient safety, employee safety, tracking of patient belongings, and
communication between inpatient and procedural areas.
A new form is needed each day or anytime greater than two procedures have occurred in one day.
This is not a permanent chart copy.

ALGINATE/HYDROFIBER DRESSING CHANGE PROCEDURE

Purpose

Promote autolysis of nonviable tissue and absorb exudate.

Wound Location: _____   Dressing Change Frequency: _____

Supplies (Circle All That Apply)

a. Alginate or hydrofiber dressing
b. Normal saline or hospital-approved wound cleanser
c. Tape
d. Gauze to dry periwound skin

e. Secondary dressing (ABD transparent dressing, border gauze)
f. Moisture barrier ointment or sealant
g. Cotton-tipped applicators
h. Other: _____

Procedure

1. Wash hands and apply gloves.
2. Remove and discard dressing. Remove gloves and wash hands thoroughly per handwashing policy. Apply new gloves and put on appropriate personal protective equipment.
3. Cleanse with normal saline or hospital-approved wound cleanser.
4. Apply skin barrier to protect periwound skin from exudate.
5. Apply dressing. If the wound has depth, gently fill wound space with dressing.
6. Cover with secondary dressings and secure as needed.

GEL/OINTMENT/PASTE/ENZYME DRESSING CHANGE PROCEDURE

Purpose

Wound enzymes promote enzymatic debridement in a moist environment. Wound ointments, gels, and paste facilitate autolysis of nonviable tissue

Wound Location: _____   Dressing Change Frequency: _____

Supplies (Circle All That Apply)

a. Gel/ointment/enzyme/paste as applicable
b. Normal saline or hospital-approved wound cleanser
c. Secondary nonabsorptive island dressing
d. Tape

e. Sterile gauze
f. Moisture barrier ointment or skin sealant
g. Cotton-tipped applicators
h. Other: _____

Procedure

1. Wash hands and apply gloves.
2. Remove and discard dressing per facility policy. Remove gloves, wash hands, apply new gloves, and put on appropriate personal protective equipment.
3. Cleanse with normal saline or wound cleanser.
4. If needed, apply skin barrier around wound to protect patient's surrounding intact periwound skin from moisture.
5. Apply thin layer of product to wound base.
6. If needed, gently fill wound depth with normal saline moistened gauze.
7. Cover with secondary dressings and secure as needed.
Note: Most enzymes require a moist environment to be effective.

HYDROCOLLOID DRESSING CHANGE PROCEDURE

Indication

Noninfected, minimally exudative wound

Purpose

Promote autolysis of nonviable tissue and provide a moist wound-healing environment.

Wound Location: _____   Dressing Change Frequency: _____

Supplies (Circle All That Apply)

- Hydrocolloid dressing
- Normal saline or hospital-approved wound cleanser
- Gauze to dry around wound

Procedure

1. Wash hands and apply gloves.
2. Carefully remove and discard dressing per facility policy. Carefully remove gloves, wash hands, apply new gloves, and put on appropriate personal protective equipment.
3. Cleanse with normal saline or hospital-approved wound cleanser.
4. Apply hydrocolloid to wound base. Allow 1 additional inch of product to cover and protect surrounding intact periwound skin.
5. Apply paper tape if needed to prevent dressing edges from rolling up.

HYDROGEL-SATURATED GAUZE DRESSING CHANGE PROCEDURE

Indication

Dry to minimally exudative wound

Purpose

Donate moisture to prevent tissue dehydration, promote autolysis of nonviable tissue, and provide a moist wound-healing environment.

Wound Location: _____   Dressing Change Frequency: _____

Supplies (Circle All That Apply)

a. Hydrogel product
b. Normal saline or hospital-approved wound cleanser to clean wounds
c. Tape
d. Gauze to dry around wound

e. Secondary dressing (ABD, 4×4 cover sponge, foam, border gauze)
f. Moisture barrier ointment or skin sealant
g. Cotton-tipped applicators (Q-tips)
h. Other: _____

Procedure

1. Wash hands and apply gloves.
2. Remove and discard dressing. Remove gloves, wash hands, apply new gloves, and put on appropriate personal protective equipment.
3. Cleanse with normal saline or wound cleanser.
4. Apply skin barrier to protect periwound skin from exudate.
5. Spread apart gel-impregnated sterile gauze and gently place or pack in wound base (or saturate gauze with hydrogel from a tube).
6. Follow with additional sterile gauze only if needed to fill depth of wound.
7. Cover with secondary dressing and secure as needed.

WOUND AND SKIN CARE COMPETENCIES

Learner Name: _____

Learner: It is your responsibility to get the individual competencies in front of your preceptor for observation, checking off, and signatures.

Preceptor: It is your responsibility to observe, initial, and date each item only if learner is deemed competent by meeting each criterion.

Pressure Ulcer/Injury Prevention Competency Criteria	Preceptor's Signature/Date
1. Performs head-to-toe skin inspection and palpation, including under medical devices and between skin folds	
2. Documents accurate PU/I risk assessment (e.g., Braden score)	
3. Develops and documents skin safety care plan; links individual risk factors to specific interventions	
4. Places patient *and all tubes* in proper position	
5. Prevents shear injury by keeping head of bed at 30 degrees or less with slight activation of knee gatch (20 degree)	
6. Uses draw sheet and gets assistance to minimize dragging patient against mattress while moving in bed	
7. Floats heels off of bed with use of pillows under legs and identifies alternatives to offloading heels when pillows are not effective	
8. Shifts weight every hour while in the chair	
9. Describes strategies for managing moisture and incontinence; identifies and finds relevant supplies	

Wound Assessment Competency Criteria	Preceptor's Signature/Date
1. Identifies self and explains procedure to patient	
2. Washes hands	
3. Gathers necessary supplies *before* beginning the procedure (measuring guide, cotton-tipped applicators, method for recording measurements, and dressing change supplies)	
4. Follows infection control guidelines for discarding dressings into the red container	
5. Cleans wound prior to assessment using appropriate infection control technique	
6. Notes correct anatomic location of wound	
7. Measures the wound's (in centimeters) height, width, depth, tunneling, and undermining	
8. Notes tissue type (red, granular, yellow, necrotic)	
9. Notes condition of periwound skin	
10. Notes presence or absence of signs of infection	
11. Applies new dressing according to step-by-step instructions	
12. Documents accurate wound assessment	

Wound Care Competency Criteria	Preceptor's Signature/Date
1. Washes hands	
2. Reviews step-by-step instructions for dressing change	
3. Gathers necessary supplies *before* beginning the procedure	
4. Follows infection control guidelines for discarding dressings	
5. Washes hands again after removing the dressing and applies new gloves	
6. Follows step-by-step instructions during dressing change, including a strategy for protecting the periwound skin	
7. Places patient in proper position	

Pouch Change Competency Criteria	Preceptor's Signature/Date
1. Empties ostomy pouch when one-third full of gas or stool	
2. Changes pouch *immediately* if leaking occurs and verbalizes why leakage can and should be prevented	
3. Reviews step-by-step instructions for ostomy pouch change procedure	

Continued

4. Gathers necessary supplies

5. Follows infection control guidelines for discarding pouch

6. Positions patient flat (or ensures no abdominal wrinkles) during procedure

7. Dries the skin completely before applying a new pouch

8. Follows step-by-step instructions during pouch change

Support Surface Competency Criteria   **Preceptor's Signature/Date**

1. Demonstrates use of CPR controls on a low air-loss surface

2. Explains rationale for using the least amount of linen possible under the patient

3. Demonstrates use of max inflate button on a low air-loss surface

4. Explains why max inflate should be used during repositioning on a low air-loss surface

5. Demonstrates appropriate selection of under pads (air permeable for air beds only)

6. Identifies process for selecting and obtaining pressure redistribution support surfaces
   for beds, chairs, and heels

Negative Pressure Wound Therapy (NPWT) Competency Criteria   **Preceptor's Signature/Date**

1. Locates and views video in resource room

2. Reviews step-by-step instructions

3. Identifies self and explains procedure to patient

4. Washes hands

5. Gathers necessary supplies *before* beginning the procedure

6. Follows infection control guidelines for discarding dressings into the red container

7. Washes hands again after removing the dressing and applies new gloves

8. Cuts the foam wound filler to fit the wound without overlapping onto intact skin

9. Ensures that tubing is positioned so that the patient does not lie or sit on the tubing

10. Applies transparent drape to ensure adequate seal

11. Activates prescribed NPWT therapy

12. Demonstrates canister change

13. Verbalizes or demonstrates ability to interpret alarms, ensure correct pressure, and
    operate machine

14. Records number of foam pieces inserted into wound on the outer dressing
    and in the medical record

SAFE SKIN GAP ANALYSIS: OPERATING ROOM

Safe Skin Practice The Following Key Strategies for Preventing OR-Related PU/I Have Been Implemented:	Gap? Y/N	If Yes, Strategies to Meet This Practice	Person Responsible	Timeline
(1a) A thorough preoperative skin inspection is performed the day of the procedure prior to hand-off to the perioperative team.				
(1b) PU/I risk and status is communicated to perioperative staff.				
(1c) Perioperative staff assesses the patient's surgical risk factors for PU/I development.				
(1d) An OR table mattress pad with pressure redistributing properties greater than the standard OR mattress pad is used for patient's at high risk for PU/I development.				
(1e) Facilities have a policy addressing patient transfer processes to prevent shearing of patient's skin during transfers.				
(1f) Patient's PU/I risk, correct patient position, and related equipment are communicated to the full perioperative team through a preoperative briefing or other communication strategy.				
(1g) Responsibility for positioning and repositioning the patient is assigned and well defined.				
(1h) When patient is in a supine position, the patient's heels are suspended off the surface.				
(1i) Perioperative staff is educated on areas of increased risk for PU/I, based on patient position, and strategies for reducing PU/I risk.				
(1j) Patients with expected postoperative hemodynamic instability and medical contraindications to turning are placed on a Group II pressure redistribution surface for postoperative care.				
(1k) The perioperative nurse communicates patient's position in the OR, existing PU/I, and preoperative PU/I risk to the postoperative nurse.				
(1l) Patient's heels are suspended off the bed/surface during postoperative care.				
(1m) Postop patients are repositioned to alternate position than OR position if not medically contraindicated.				

SAFE SKIN GAP ANALYSIS: RESPIRATORY EQUIPMENT

Safe Skin Practice The Following Key Strategies for Preventing Respiratory Device-Related Pressure Ulcers/Injuries (PU/I) Have Been Implemented:	Gap? Y/N	If Yes, Strategies to Meet This Practice	Person Responsible	Timeline
(1a) Respiratory therapy is represented on the organization's PU/I prevention team.				
(1b) The skin beneath and around oxygen administration devices are thoroughly inspected at least every 8–12 hours.				
(1c) Patients and caregivers are educated on the importance of frequent skin inspection beneath and around respiratory devices and of informing staff if they experience discomfort or pain beneath or around the devices.				
(1d) Responsibility is clearly assigned (to a specific clinical discipline) for inspection and documentation of skin integrity around and under oxygen administration devices.				
(1e) Abnormal skin integrity findings, site care, and interventions are documented in the patient's medical record in a location that is accessible to all relevant clinical disciplines.				
(1f) Ear protectors are used on oxygen tubing as appropriate.				
(1g) Strap tension and skin integrity beneath and around life sustaining CPAP and NPPV masks are checked at least every 4 hours, with oral intake, and with oral care.				
(1h) During routine tracheostomy site care (at least every 8–12 hours) skin integrity and tension are checked under the straps, around and in back of the neck, around the stoma, and under the tracheostomy tube flange/faceplate.				
(1i) Commercially available foam/collar type adjustable tracheostomy straps are used rather than ties or twill tape.				
(1j) A standard procedure for management of tracheostomy sutures is in place.				
(1k) The tension and skin integrity under and around ETTs and straps are checked every 2 hours with close attention to the neck, lips, and mouth.				
(1l) When using commercial stabilizers, the position of the ETT (right, middle, left) is rotated at least every 2 hours.				

SAFE SKIN GAP ANALYSIS: CERVICAL COLLAR

Safe Skin Practice The Following Key Strategies for Preventing Cervical Collar-Related PU/I Have Been Implemented:	Gap? Y/N	If Yes, Strategies to Meet This Practice	Person Responsible	Timeline
(1a) Provider order, including frequency of use, is obtained for collar application.				
(1b) Orthotist, or other trained provider, is consulted for appropriate collar fit.				
(1c) Patients are removed from backboard on arrival in emergency department or as soon as possible.				
(1d) Standardized processes are in place to achieve definitive care (e.g., collar removal, change to longer-term collar, within 24 hours or less).				
(1e) If the patient condition permits, the skin is inspected and cleaned during change from transport collar to longer-term collar.				
(1f) Staff is trained in proper technique for cervical collar placement.				
(1g) A neurologic assessment is conducted after initial collar application, then every 8 hours (and as needed), or per provider orders.				
(1h) Cervical collars are removed to cleanse, inspect, and palpate skin every 8–12 hours and removal of device and findings are documented.				
(1i) Patient is log-rolled and repositioned every 2 hours (and as needed).				
(1j) If collar has removable inner pads, pads are changed and washed every 24 hours (and as needed).				
(1k) Staff is trained in proper technique for skin inspection and care of skin related to cervical collars.				
(1l) Orthotists or other trained providers are available for staff questions or concerns.				
(1m) Education provided to patients/family prior to discharge includes information on application, wearing and removal of collar, proper cervical alignment, skin care and inspection, and collar pad cleaning.				

Modified from Minnesota Hospital Association. All Rights Reserved. Accessed November 20, 2022.

SAFE SKIN ICU PLEDGE

OUR ICU SAFE SKIN TEAM PLEDGE

We will:
1. **Keep our ICU patients moving**—Our team will develop a repositioning schedule for each patient (L-R-Center), based on the patient's condition, and will consistently follow the schedule to redistribute pressure for our patients.
2. **Float heels off the bed.**
3. **Immediately evaluate patients for the most appropriate surface** to redistribute pressure.

4. If a patient is not able to be adequately or routinely repositioned, our team will provide:
   - **Written confirmation** that patient cannot be repositioned from the provider with daily reevaluation
   - At least **hourly mini shifts** off the tailbone
5. **Check our patients' skin beneath devices**—Every shift we will use opportunities such as oral care, vital sign checks, and respiratory treatments to look for skin issues.

PRESSURE ULCER PREVENTION PATIENT AND FAMILY EDUCATION

Pressure I.N.J.U.R.Y. Bundle

INSPECT

- Inspect skin and evaluate risk for pressure injury on admission, daily or per hospital standard, and when there is a change in patient condition.
- Evaluate the need for a specialty mattress/bed.
- Initiate an incontinence protocol based on risk assessment findings (Braden subscale score ≤ 3).

NUTRITION

- A nutritional screening is completed within 24 hours of admission.
- Reassess nutritional status daily or per hospital standard, and when there is a change in patient condition.
- If the patient is at risk (Braden subscale score ≤ 2) or a wound is identified, a nutritional consult is ordered.
- Offer additional nutritional nourishment as appropriate to assist with healing.

JUST MOVE

- Evaluate activity, mobility and ability to communicate pain on admission and daily or per hospital standard.
- If the patient is at risk (Braden subscale score ≤ 2) a therapy consult is requested.
- Mobility is continually assessed and encouraged when possible.
- Float the heels of patients with impaired mobility, activity and/or ability to communicate pain.

UNDER AND AROUND DEVICES

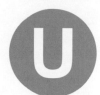

- Medical devices increase the risk of pressure injury development.
- Remove devices (or position nonremoveable devices) to inspect the skin under and around the device.
- Pain assessment is completed on pressure points with nonremovable devices.
- Devices are repositioned with the patient to ensure devices are not pulled, kinked or lodged under the patient or between skin folds.

REPOSITION

- Patients are repositioned every 2 hours limiting supine (or back/center).
- If medically contraindicated hourly microshifts/offloading is recommended.
- Reposition every 30 minutes when up in the chair or when head of bed is greater than 30 degrees.

YOU ARE IMPORTANT

- Patients, families and caregivers are partners in developing the pressure injury prevention plan of care.
- Patients, families and caregivers are encouraged to engage in skin and risk assessment to understand current risk factors and how to address them.
- Tools are available on skin safety for patients at risk for pressure injury development.

Minnesota Hospital Association

PARTNERSHIP FOR PATIENTS ℠

PIEPER ZULKOWSKI PRESSURE ULCER/INJURY KNOWLEDGE ASSESSMENT TOOL (REVISED 2020)

DEMOGRAPHIC SHEET

DIRECTIONS: Please answer each of the following questions about your background by checking the appropriate boxes).

1.   **Where do you primarily work?**   ☐ Hospital   ☐ Long term Care   ☐ Home Care
☐ Private Practice   ☐ Education   ☐ Other (specify)_____

2.   **Age:**_____

3.   **Gender:**   ☐ Male   ☐ Female

4.   **Job Category:**   ☐ Physician (MD/DO)   ☐ Registered Nurse **(**RN)   ☐ Licensed Practical Nurse (LPN)   ☐ Certified Nurse Assistant (CNA)   ☐ Administrator   ☐ Nurse Practitioner (NP)

☐ Physician Assistant (PA)   ☐ Other (specify)_____

5.   **Number of years in practice**:

☐ < 1 year   ☐ 1–5 years   ☐ > 5 years to <10 years

☐ 10 years to < 15 years   ☐ 15 years to < 20 years   ☐ 20 years or more

6.   **Highest** **degree held (check one):** ☐ Diploma   ☐ Associate   ☐ Baccalaureate   ☐ Masters
☐ Doctorate   ☐MD/DO

7.   **Are you certified in any clinical specialty?**   ☐ Yes ☐ No Certification
type_____

8.   **Are you certified as Wound Specialist?**   ☐ Yes ☐ No Certifying
Organization_____

9.   **When was the last time you *listened to a lecture* on pressure ulcers/injuries? (Check one)**

☐ 1 year or less   ☐ Greater than 1 year but less than 2 years

☐ 2–3 years   ☐ 4 years or greater   ☐ Never

10.   **When was the last time you *read an article, book, or guideline* about pressure ulcers/injuries? (Check one)**

☐ 1 year or less   ☐ Greater than 1 year but less than 2 years

☐ 2–3 years   ☐ 4 years or greater   ☐ Never

11.   **Have you sought information about pressure ulcers/injuries on the web within the past year?**

☐ Yes   ☐ No

Pieper-Zulkowski Pressure Ulcers/Injuries Knowledge Test (Revised 2020)
Please answer each of the following by circling your answer. Be truthful; if you don't know, don't guess.
Note: In some countries, the term *Category* is used in place of *Stage*.

1.	Slough is yellow or cream-colored necrotic/devitalized tissue on a wound bed.	TRUE	FALSE	DON'T KNOW
2.	A pressure ulcer/injury is a sterile wound.	TRUE	FALSE	DON'T KNOW
3.	Foam dressings may increase wound pain.	TRUE	FALSE	DON'T KNOW
4.	Alkaline soap products should be used to cleanse soiled skin.	TRUE	FALSE	DON'T KNOW
5.	Seating should be for short periods in an appropriate chair/wheelchair with a pressure redistribution cushion for persons at risk for pressure ulcers/injuries.	TRUE	FALSE	DON'T KNOW
6.	A Stage 3 pressure ulcer/injury is a partial thickness skin loss involving the epidermis and/or dermis.	TRUE	FALSE	DON'T KNOW
7.	Hydrogel dressings should not be used on pressure ulcers/injuries with granulation tissue.	TRUE	FALSE	DON'T KNOW
8.	Reposition individuals with or at risk of pressure ulcer/injury on an individualized schedule regardless of mobility level unless contraindicated.	TRUE	FALSE	DON'T KNOW
9.	A pressure ulcer/injury scar will break down faster than unwounded skin.	TRUE	FALSE	DON'T KNOW
10.	Pressure ulcers/injuries progress in a linear fashion from Stage 1 to 2 to 3 to 4.	TRUE	FALSE	DON'T KNOW
11.	Eschar is healthy tissue.	TRUE	FALSE	DON'T KNOW
12.	Nonblanchable erythema anywhere in the body is a Stage 1 pressure ulcer/injury.	TRUE	FALSE	DON'T KNOW
13.	The goal of palliative care is wound healing.	TRUE	FALSE	DON'T KNOW
14.	A Stage 2 pressure ulcer/injury is a full thickness skin loss.	TRUE	FALSE	DON'T KNOW
15.	Dragging the patient up in bed increases friction.	TRUE	FALSE	DON'T KNOW
16.	Increased body temperature is a risk factor for pressure ulcer/injury.	TRUE	FALSE	DON'T KNOW
17.	Diabetes mellitus does not increase a person's risk for pressure ulcer/injury.	TRUE	FALSE	DON'T KNOW
18.	A comprehensive pain assessment should be done on persons with pressure ulcer/injury.	TRUE	FALSE	DON'T KNOW
19.	High absorbency incontinence products should be used for individuals with pressure ulcers/injuries when incontinence is present.	TRUE	FALSE	DON'T KNOW
20.	A pressure redistribution surface manages tissue load and the microclimate against the skin.	TRUE	FALSE	DON'T KNOW
21.	A Stage 2 pressure ulcer/injury may have slough in its base.	TRUE	FALSE	DON'T KNOW
22.	If necrotic tissue is present and if bone can be seen or palpated, the ulcer is a Stage 4.	TRUE	FALSE	DON'T KNOW
23.	Oral nutritional supplements should be used in addition to usual diet for individuals at high risk for pressure ulcers/injuries.	TRUE	FALSE	DON'T KNOW
24.	To prevent heel pressure ulcer/injury, the weight of the leg should be distributed along the calf during heel elevation.	TRUE	FALSE	DON'T KNOW
25.	When necrotic tissue is removed, an unstageable pressure ulcer/injury will be classified as a Stage 2 ulcer/injury.	TRUE	FALSE	DON'T KNOW
26.	Donut devices/ring cushions help to prevent pressure ulcers/injuries.	TRUE	FALSE	DON'T KNOW
27.	It is the nurse's responsibility to be sure a specialty bed is working properly and document its use.	TRUE	FALSE	DON'T KNOW
28.	ABD pads may be used to protect the skin.	TRUE	FALSE	DON'T KNOW
29.	Persons at risk for pressure ulcers/injuries should be nutritionally assessed (i.e., weight, nutrition intake, blood work, etc.).	TRUE	FALSE	DON'T KNOW
30.	Biofilms may develop in any type of wound.	TRUE	FALSE	DON'T KNOW
31.	Critical care patients may need slow, gradual turning because of being hemodynamically unstable.	TRUE	FALSE	DON'T KNOW
32.	Blanching refers to whiteness when pressure is applied to a reddened area.	TRUE	FALSE	DON'T KNOW
33.	A blister on the heel is nothing to worry about.	TRUE	FALSE	DON'T KNOW
34.	Staff education alone may reduce the incidence of pressure ulcers/injuries.	TRUE	FALSE	DON'T KNOW
35.	Early changes associated with pressure ulcer/injury development may be missed in persons with darker skin tones.	TRUE	FALSE	DON'T KNOW
36.	A footrest should not be used for an immobile patient whose feet do not reach the floor.	TRUE	FALSE	DON'T KNOW
37.	Bone, tendon, or muscle may be exposed in a Stage 3 pressure ulcer/injury.	TRUE	FALSE	DON'T KNOW
38.	A topical opioid may help manage acute pressure ulcer/injury pain.	TRUE	FALSE	DON'T KNOW
39.	Wound biofilm is associated with decreased wound drainage.	TRUE	FALSE	DON'T KNOW

Pieper-Zulkowski Pressure Ulcers/Injuries Knowledge Test (Revised 2020)
Please answer each of the following by circling your answer. Be truthful; if you don't know, don't guess.
Note: In some countries, the term *Category* is used in place of *Stage*.

40. It may be difficult to distinguish between moisture associated skin damage and a pressure ulcer/injury.	TRUE	FALSE	DON'T KNOW
41. Wounds that become chronic are frequently stalled in the proliferative phase of healing.	TRUE	FALSE	DON'T KNOW
42. Dry, adherent eschar on the heels should be removed for the wound to heal.	TRUE	FALSE	DON'T KNOW
43. Deep tissue injury is a localized area of purple or maroon discolored intact skin or a blood-filled blister.	TRUE	FALSE	DON'T KNOW
44. Massage of bony prominences is essential for quality skin care.	TRUE	FALSE	DON'T KNOW
45. Poor posture in a wheelchair may be the cause of a pressure ulcer/injury.	TRUE	FALSE	DON'T KNOW
46. For persons who have incontinence, skin cleaning should occur at the time of soiling and at routine intervals.	TRUE	FALSE	DON'T KNOW
47. Patients who are spinal cord injured need knowledge about pressure ulcers/injuries prevention and self-care.	TRUE	FALSE	DON'T KNOW
48. In large and deep pressure ulcers/injuries, the number of dressings used needs to be counted and documented so that all dressings are removed at the next dressing change.	TRUE	FALSE	DON'T KNOW
49. A mucosal membrane pressure ulcer/injury as the result of medical equipment is a Stage 3.	TRUE	FALSE	DON'T KNOW
50. Pressure ulcers/injuries can occur around the ears in a person using oxygen by nasal cannula.	TRUE	FALSE	DON'T KNOW
51. Persons, who are immobile and can be taught, should shift their weight every 30 minutes while sitting in a chair.	TRUE	FALSE	DON'T KNOW
52. Stage 1 pressure ulcers/injuries are intact skin with nonblanchable erythema over a bony prominence. Same as 12; change stage #.	TRUE	FALSE	DON'T KNOW
53. When the ulcer/injury base is totally covered by slough, it cannot be staged.	TRUE	FALSE	DON'T KNOW
54. Selection of a pressure redistribution surface only considers the person's level of pressure ulcer/injury risk.	TRUE	FALSE	DON'T KNOW
55. Shear injury is not a concern for a patient using a pressure redistribution surface.	TRUE	FALSE	DON'T KNOW
56. It is not necessary to have the patient with a spinal cord injury evaluated for seating.	TRUE	FALSE	DON'T KNOW
57. To help prevent pressure ulcers/injuries, the head of the bed should be elevated at more than a 45-degree angle.	TRUE	FALSE	DON'T KNOW
58. Urinary catheter tubing should be positioned under the leg.	TRUE	FALSE	DON'T KNOW
59. Properly sized equipment may help avoid pressure ulcers/injuries in bariatric patients.	TRUE	FALSE	DON'T KNOW
60. A dressing should keep the wound bed moist, but the surrounding skin dry.	TRUE	FALSE	DON'T KNOW
61. Hydrocolloid and film dressings should be removed quickly to decrease pain.	TRUE	FALSE	DON'T KNOW
62. Nurses should avoid turning a patient onto a reddened area.	TRUE	FALSE	DON'T KNOW
63. Skin tears are classified as Stage 2 pressure ulcers/injuries.	TRUE	FALSE	DON'T KNOW
64. A Stage 3 pressure ulcers/injuries may appear shallow if located on the ear, malleolus/ankle, or heel.	TRUE	FALSE	DON'T KNOW
65. Hydrocolloid dressings should be used on Stage 2 infected ulcer/injury.	TRUE	FALSE	DON'T KNOW
66. Pressure ulcers/injuries are a lifelong concern for a person who is spinal cord injured.	TRUE	FALSE	DON'T KNOW
67. Pressure ulcers/injuries should not be cleansed with drinking water.	TRUE	FALSE	DON'T KNOW
68. Alginate dressings can be used for Stage 3 and 4 pressure ulcers/injuries with moderate exudate.	TRUE	FALSE	DON'T KNOW
69. Deep tissue injury will not progress to another ulcer/injury stage.	TRUE	FALSE	DON'T KNOW
70. Film dressings absorb a lot of drainage.	TRUE	FALSE	DON'T KNOW
71. Nonsting skin prep should be used around a wound to protect surrounding tissue from moisture.	TRUE	FALSE	DON'T KNOW
72. Stage 4 pressure ulcers/injuries always have undermining.	TRUE	FALSE	DON'T KNOW

Pieper-Zulkowski Pressure Ulcers/Injuries Knowledge Test (Revised 2020)
Key

1.	Slough is yellow or cream-colored necrotic/devitalized tissue on a wound bed.	**TRUE**	FALSE	DON'T KNOW
2.	A pressure ulcer/injury is a sterile wound.	TRUE	**FALSE**	DON'T KNOW
3.	Foam dressings may increase wound pain.	TRUE	**FALSE**	DON'T KNOW
4.	Alkaline soap products should be used to cleanse soiled skin.	TRUE	**FALSE**	DON'T KNOW
5.	Seating should be for short periods in an appropriate chair/wheelchair with a pressure redistribution cushion for persons at risk for pressure ulcers/injuries.	**TRUE**	FALSE	DON'T KNOW
6.	A Stage 3 pressure ulcer/injury is a partial thickness skin loss involving the epidermis and/or dermis.	TRUE	**FALSE**	DON'T KNOW
7.	Hydrogel dressings should not be used on pressure ulcers/injuries with granulation tissue.	TRUE	**FALSE**	DON'T KNOW
8.	Reposition individuals with or at risk of pressure ulcer/injury on an individualized schedule regardless of mobility level unless contraindicated.	**TRUE**	FALSE	DON'T KNOW
9.	A pressure ulcer/injury scar will break down faster than unwounded skin.	**TRUE**	FALSE	DON'T KNOW
10.	Pressure ulcers/injuries progress in a linear fashion from Stage 1 to 2 to 3 to 4.	TRUE	**FALSE**	DON'T KNOW
11.	Eschar is healthy tissue.	TRUE	**FALSE**	DON'T KNOW
12.	Nonblanchable erythema anywhere in the body is a Stage 1 pressure ulcer/injury.	TRUE	**FALSE**	DON'T KNOW
13.	The goal of palliative care is wound healing.	TRUE	**FALSE**	DON'T KNOW
14.	A Stage 2 pressure ulcer/injury is a full thickness skin loss.	TRUE	**FALSE**	DON'T KNOW
15.	Dragging the patient up in bed increases friction.	**TRUE**	FALSE	DON'T KNOW
16.	Increased body temperature is a risk factor for pressure ulcer/injury.	**TRUE**	FALSE	DON'T KNOW
17.	Diabetes mellitus does not increase a person's risk for pressure ulcer/injury.	TRUE	**FALSE**	DON'T KNOW
18.	A comprehensive pain assessment should be done on persons with pressure ulcer/injury.	**TRUE**	FALSE	DON'T KNOW
19.	High absorbency incontinence products should be used for individuals with pressure ulcers/injuries when incontinence is present.	**TRUE**	FALSE	DON'T KNOW
20.	A pressure redistribution surface manages tissue load and the microclimate against the skin.	**TRUE**	FALSE	DON'T KNOW
21.	A Stage 2 pressure ulcer/injury may have slough in its base.	TRUE	**FALSE**	DON'T KNOW
22.	If necrotic tissue is present and if bone can be seen or palpated, the ulcer is a Stage 4.	**TRUE**	FALSE	DON'T KNOW
23.	Oral nutritional supplements should be used in addition to usual diet for individuals at high risk for pressure ulcers/injuries.	**TRUE**	FALSE	DON'T KNOW
24.	To prevent heel pressure ulcer/injury, the weight of the leg should be distributed along the calf during heel elevation.	**TRUE**	FALSE	DON'T KNOW
25.	When necrotic tissue is removed, an unstageable pressure ulcer/injury will be classified as a Stage 2 ulcer/injury.	TRUE	**FALSE**	DON'T KNOW
26.	Donut devices/ring cushions help to prevent pressure ulcers/injuries.	TRUE	**FALSE**	DON'T KNOW
27.	It is the nurse's responsibility to be sure a specialty bed is working properly and document its use.	**TRUE**	FALSE	DON'T KNOW
28.	ABD pads may be used to protect the skin.	TRUE	**FALSE**	DON'T KNOW
29.	Persons at risk for pressure ulcers/injuries should be nutritionally assessed (i.e., weight, nutrition intake, blood work, etc.).	**TRUE**	FALSE	DON'T KNOW
30.	Biofilms may develop in any type of wound.	**TRUE**	FALSE	DON'T KNOW
31.	Critical care patients may need slow, gradual turning because of being hemodynamically unstable.	**TRUE**	FALSE	DON'T KNOW
32.	Blanching refers to whiteness when pressure is applied to a reddened area.	**TRUE**	FALSE	DON'T KNOW
33.	A blister on the heel is nothing to worry about.	TRUE	**FALSE**	DON'T KNOW
34.	Staff education alone may reduce the incidence of pressure ulcers/injuries.	TRUE	**FALSE**	DON'T KNOW
35.	Early changes associated with pressure ulcer/injury development may be missed in persons with darker skin tones.	**TRUE**	FALSE	DON'T KNOW
36.	A footrest should not be used for an immobile patient whose feet do not reach the floor.	TRUE	**FALSE**	DON'T KNOW
37.	Bone, tendon, or muscle may be exposed in a Stage 3 pressure ulcer/injury.	TRUE	**FALSE**	DON'T KNOW
38.	A topical opioid may help manage acute pressure ulcer/injury pain.	**TRUE**	FALSE	DON'T KNOW
39.	Wound biofilm is associated with decreased wound drainage.	TRUE	**FALSE**	DON'T KNOW
40.	It may be difficult to distinguish between moisture associated skin damage and a pressure ulcer/injury.	**TRUE**	FALSE	DON'T KNOW
41.	Wounds that become chronic are frequently stalled in the proliferative phase of healing.	TRUE	**FALSE**	DON'T KNOW

Pieper-Zulkowski Pressure Ulcers/Injuries Knowledge Test (Revised 2020)
Key

42.	Dry, adherent eschar on the heels should be removed for the wound to heal.	TRUE	**FALSE**	DON'T KNOW
43.	Deep tissue injury is a localized area of purple or maroon discolored intact skin or a blood-filled blister.	**TRUE**	FALSE	DON'T KNOW
44.	Massage of bony prominences is essential for quality skin care.	TRUE	**FALSE**	DON'T KNOW
45.	Poor posture in a wheelchair may be the cause of a pressure ulcer/injury.	**TRUE**	FALSE	DON'T KNOW
46.	For persons who have incontinence, skin cleaning should occur at the time of soiling and at routine intervals.	**TRUE**	FALSE	DON'T KNOW
47.	Patients who are spinal cord injured need knowledge about pressure ulcers/injuries prevention and self-care.	**TRUE**	FALSE	DON'T KNOW
48.	In large and deep pressure ulcers/injuries, the number of dressings used needs to be counted and documented so that all dressings are removed at the next dressing change.	**TRUE**	FALSE	DON'T KNOW
49.	A mucosal membrane pressure ulcer/injury as the result of medical equipment is a Stage 3.	TRUE	**FALSE**	DON'T KNOW
50.	Pressure ulcers/injuries can occur around the ears in a person using oxygen by nasal cannula.	**TRUE**	FALSE	DON'T KNOW
51.	Persons, who are immobile and can be taught, should shift their weight every 30 minutes while sitting in a chair.	TRUE	**FALSE**	DON'T KNOW
52.	Stage 1 pressure ulcers/injuries are intact skin with nonblanchable erythema over a bony prominence. Same as 12; change stage #	**TRUE**	FALSE	DON'T KNOW
53.	When the ulcer/injury base is totally covered by slough, it cannot be staged.	**TRUE**	FALSE	DON'T KNOW
54.	Selection of a pressure redistribution surface only considers the person's level of pressure ulcer/injury risk.	TRUE	**FALSE**	DON'T KNOW
55.	Shear injury is not a concern for a patient using a pressure redistribution surface.	TRUE	**FALSE**	DON'T KNOW
56.	It is not necessary to have the patient with a spinal cord injury evaluated for seating.	TRUE	**FALSE**	DON'T KNOW
57.	To help prevent pressure ulcers/injuries, the head of the bed should be elevated at more than a 45-degree angle.	TRUE	**FALSE**	DON'T KNOW
58.	Urinary catheter tubing should be positioned under the leg.	TRUE	**FALSE**	DON'T KNOW
59.	Properly sized equipment may help avoid pressure ulcers/injuries in bariatric patients.	**TRUE**	FALSE	DON'T KNOW
60.	A dressing should keep the wound bed moist, but the surrounding skin dry.	**TRUE**	FALSE	DON'T KNOW
61.	Hydrocolloid and film dressings should be removed quickly to decrease pain.	TRUE	**FALSE**	DON'T KNOW
62.	Nurses should avoid turning a patient onto a reddened area.	**TRUE**	FALSE	DON'T KNOW
63.	Skin tears are classified as Stage 2 pressure ulcers/injuries.	TRUE	**FALSE**	DON'T KNOW
64.	A Stage 3 pressure ulcers/injuries may appear shallow if located on the ear, malleolus/ankle, or heel.	**TRUE**	FALSE	DON'T KNOW
65.	Hydrocolloid dressings should be used on Stage 2 infected ulcer/injury.	TRUE	**FALSE**	DON'T KNOW
66.	Pressure ulcers/injuries are a lifelong concern for a person who is spinal cord injured.	**TRUE**	FALSE	DON'T KNOW
67.	Pressure ulcers/injuries should not be cleansed with drinking water.	TRUE	**FALSE**	DON'T KNOW
68.	Alginate dressings can be used for Stage 3 and 4 pressure ulcers/injuries with moderate exudate.	**TRUE**	FALSE	DON'T KNOW
69.	Deep tissue injury will not progress to another ulcer/injury stage.	TRUE	**FALSE**	DON'T KNOW
70.	Film dressings absorb a lot of drainage.	TRUE	**FALSE**	DON'T KNOW
71.	Nonsting skin prep should be used around a wound to protect surrounding tissue from moisture.	**TRUE**	FALSE	DON'T KNOW
72.	Stage 4 pressure ulcers/injuries always have undermining.	TRUE	**FALSE**	DON'T KNOW

DEBRIDEMENT COMPETENCY

Conservative Sharp Wound Debridement: Mentorship Skills Checklist

Name: _____

Date CSWD Education Module Completed: _____

Date Skills Laboratory Completed: _____

Competency	Achieved Date	Follow-up (if needed) Date
1. Demonstrates understanding of relevant anatomy, underlying tissue and structures.		
2. Identifies viable and nonviable tissue.		
3. Conducts a complete wound assessment to determine need for debridement (includes diabetic foot screen, lower limb and vascular assessments).		
4. States precautions and contraindications for CSWD.		
5. Provides rationale for use of CSWD based on client assessment.		
6. Conducts an environmental scan to determine safety to debride (i.e., adequate lighting, equipment and assistance to hold/stabilize limb or position client).		
7. Explains procedure to the client and obtains informed consent.		
8. Positions the client so that they are comfortable and the wound is easily accessible.		
9. Assembles what is needed to address bleeding during the procedure and identifies the process for addressing bleeding.		
10. Uses sterile or no touch technique correctly.		

11. Demonstrates acceptable skills and techniques:
  i. Gathers appropriate instruments to debride the specific wound.
  ii. Selects the appropriate tool (curette, forceps, or scalpel) for the tissue type to be removed.
  iii. Handles instruments appropriately with respect to safety.
  iv. Grasps the tissue to be removed securely with care for the underlying viable tissues.
  v. Removes nonviable tissue is one layer at a time.
  vi. Does not compromise viable tissue.		

12. Manages pain and discomfort prior to, during and following the procedure.		
13. Identifies when to stop the procedure at the appropriate level of tissue.		
14. Applies an appropriate wound dressing once the procedure is completed.		
15. Recognizes skill limitations and the need to involve others if necessary.		
16. Utilizes secondary debridement techniques if needed.		
17. Documents wound assessment and procedure.		
18. Outlines a comprehensive plan of care for reassessment, ongoing debridement and wound healing.		

Mentoring Objectives Achieved

Date:

Mentor Signature:

Mentee Signature:

From Conservative Sharp Wound Debridement (CSWD) in Adults & Children: Evidence Informed Practice Tools, March 2019. Copyright Winnipeg Regional Health Authority.

PAIN ASSESSMENT MODELS AND SCALES

"Carrying on Despite the Pain": Eight Themes	
Responses • Expecting pain with the ulcer • Feeling frustrated	**Common Experiences** • Interfering with the job • Starting pain all over again: painful debridements
Practical Knowledge • Swelling = pain • Not standing	**Shared Meanings** • Having to make significant life changes • Finding satisfaction in new activities

From Krasner, D. (1997). *Carrying on despite the pain: Living with painful venous ulcers: A Heideggerian hermeneutic analysis* (Doctoral dissertation). Ann Arbor: University of Michigan.

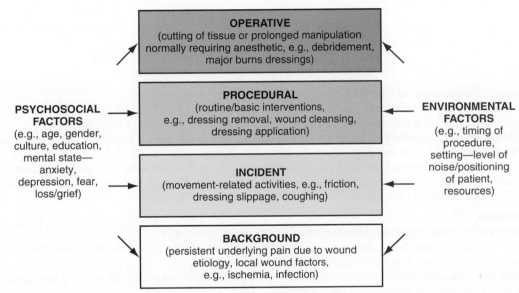

OPERATIVE
(cutting of tissue or prolonged manipulation normally requiring anesthetic, e.g., debridement, major burns dressings)

PROCEDURAL
(routine/basic interventions, e.g., dressing removal, wound cleansing, dressing application)

PSYCHOSOCIAL FACTORS
(e.g., age, gender, culture, education, mental state—anxiety, depression, fear, loss/grief)

ENVIRONMENTAL FACTORS
(e.g., timing of procedure, setting—level of noise/positioning of patient, resources)

INCIDENT
(movement-related activities, e.g., friction, dressing slippage, coughing)

BACKGROUND
(persistent underlying pain due to wound etiology, local wound factors, e.g., ischemia, infection)

Causes of pain. (From IASP Task Force on Taxonomy, Merskey, H., & Bogduk, N. (Eds.), (1994). *Classification of chronic pain: Descriptions of chronic pain syndromes and definitions of pain terms* (2nd ed.). Seattle, WA: IASP Press.)

Pain Assessment in Advanced Dementia (PAINAD) Scale

Items[a]	0	1	2	Score
Breathing independent of vocalization	Normal	Occasional labored breathing Short period of hyperventilation	Noisy labored breathing Long period of hyperventilation Cheyne–Stokes respirations	
Negative vocalization	None	Occasional moan or groan Low-level speech with a negative or disapproving quality	Repeated troubled calling out Loud moaning or groaning	
Facial expression	Smiling or inexpressive	Sad Frightened Frown	Facial grimacing	
Body language	Relaxed	Tense Distressed pacing Fidgeting	Rigid Fists clenched Knees pulled up Pulling or pushing away Striking out	
Consolability	No need to console	Distracted or reassured	Unable to console, distract, or reassure	
			Total[b]	

Breathing

1. Normal breathing is characterized by effortless, quiet, rhythmic (smooth) respirations.
2. Occasional labored breathing is characterized by episodic bursts of harsh, difficult, or wearing respirations.
3. Short period of hyperventilation is characterized by intervals of rapid, deep breaths lasting a short time.
4. Noisy labored breathing is characterized by negative-sounding respirations on inspiration or expiration. They may be loud, gurgling, or wheezing. They appear strenuous or wearing.
5. Long period of hyperventilation is characterized by an excessive rate and depth of respirations lasting a considerable time.
6. Cheyne–Stokes respirations are characterized by rhythmic waxing and waning of breathing, from very deep to shallow respirations with periods of apnea (cessation of breathing).

Negative Vocalization

1. None is characterized by speech or vocalization that has a neutral or pleasant quality.
2. Occasional moan or groan is characterized by mournful or murmuring sounds, wails, or laments. Groaning is characterized by louder-than-usual inarticulate involuntary sounds, often abruptly beginning and ending.
3. Low-level speech with a negative or disapproving quality is characterized by muttering, mumbling, whining, grumbling, or swearing in a low volume with a complaining, sarcastic, or caustic tone.
4. Repeated troubled calling out is characterized by phrases or words being used over and over in a tone that suggests anxiety, uneasiness, or distress.
5. Loud moaning or groaning is characterized by mournful or murmuring sounds, wails, or laments that are much louder than usual volume. Loud groaning is characterized by louder-than-usual inarticulate involuntary sounds, often abruptly beginning and ending.
6. Crying is characterized by an utterance of emotion accompanied by tears. There may be sobbing or quiet weeping.

Facial Expression

1. Smiling is characterized by upturned corners of the mouth, brightening of the eyes, and a look of pleasure or contentment. Inexpressive refers to a neutral, at ease, relaxed, or blank look.
2. Sad is characterized by an unhappy, lonesome, sorrowful, or dejected look. There may be tears in the eyes.
3. Frightened is characterized by a look of fear, alarm, or heightened anxiety. Eyes appear wide open.
4. Frown is characterized by a downward turn of the corners of the mouth. Increased facial wrinkling in the forehead and around the mouth may appear.
5. Facial grimacing is characterized by a distorted, distressed look. The brow is more wrinkled, as is the area around the mouth. Eyes may be squeezed shut.

Body Language

1. Relaxed is characterized by a calm, restful, mellow appearance. The person seems to be taking it easy.
2. Tense is characterized by a strained, apprehensive, or worried appearance. The jaw may be clenched (exclude any contractures).
3. Distressed pacing is characterized by activity that seems unsettled. A fearful, worried, or disturbed element may be present. The rate may be faster or slower.
4. Fidgeting is characterized by restless movement. Squirming about or wiggling in the chair may occur. The person might be hitching a chair across the room. Repetitive touching, tugging, or rubbing body parts may be observed.
5. Rigid is characterized by stiffening of the body. The arms and/or legs are tight and inflexible. The trunk may appear straight and unyielding (exclude any contractures).

Continued

Pain Assessment in Advanced Dementia (PAINAD) Scale—cont'd

Items	0	1	2	Score

6. Fists clenched is characterized by tightly closed hands. They may be opened and closed repeatedly or held tightly shut.
7. Knees pulled up is characterized by flexing the legs and drawing the knees up toward the chest. An overall troubled appearance may be seen (exclude any contractures).
8. Pulling or pushing away is characterized by resistiveness upon approach or to care. The person may try to escape by yanking or wrenching himself or herself free or shoving you away.
9. Striking out is characterized by hitting, kicking, grabbing, punching, biting, or other forms of personal assault.

Consolability

1. No need to console is characterized by a sense of well-being. The person appears content.
2. Distracted or reassured by voice or touch is characterized by a disruption in the behavior when the person is spoken to or is touched. The behavior stops during the period of interaction, with no indication that the person is distressed.
3. Unable to console, distract, or reassure is characterized by the inability to soothe the person or stop a behavior with words or actions. No amount of comforting, verbal or physical, will alleviate the behavior.

[a]See the description of each item in the lower part of the table.
[b]Total scores range from 0 to 10 (based on a scale from 0 to 2 for five items), with a higher score indicating more severe pain (0 = "no pain" to 10 = "severe pain").
From Warden, V., Hurley, A. C., & Volicer, L. (2003). Development and psychometric evaluation of the pain assessment in advanced dementia (PAINAD) scale. *Journal of the American Medical Directors Association, 4,* 9–15, excerpted from Frampton, K. (2004). Vital sign #5. *Caring for the Ages, 5*(5), 26.

FLACC Pain Scale for Children 2 Months to 7 Years

Category	SCORING		
	1	2	3
Face	No particular expression or smile	Occasional grimace or frown, withdrawn, disinterested	Frequent to constant quivering chin, clenched jaw
Legs	Normal position or relaxed	Uneasy, restless, tense	Kicking, or legs drawn up
Activity	Lying quietly, normal position, moves easily	Squirming, shifting back and forth, tense	Arched, rigid or jerking
Cry	No cry (awake or asleep)	Moans or whimpers; occasional complaint	Crying steadily, screams or sobs, frequent complaints
Consolability	Content, relaxed	Reassured by occasional touching, hugging, or being talked to; distractible	Difficult to console or comfort

FLACC, Face, Legs, Activity, Crying, Consolability.
From Merkel, S., Voepel-Lewis, T., Shayevitz, J. R., et al. (1997). The FLACC: A behavioral scale for scoring postoperative pain in young children. *Pediatric Nursing, 23*(3), 293–297.

CRIES Pain Scale for Neonates (0 to 6 Months)

Crying

0	No crying, or crying but not high pitched
1	High pitched but infant consolable
2	Inconsolable

Requires O$_2$

Babies experiencing pain manifest decreased oxygenation. Consider other causes of hypoxemia (e.g., oversedation, atelectasis, pneumothorax).

0	No oxygen required; oxygen saturation >95%
1	≤30% supplemental oxygen required to keep oxygen saturation >95%
2	>30% supplemental oxygen required to keep oxygen saturation >95%

Increased Vital Signs

Take BP last because process may awaken the child, making mean assessments difficult.

0	Both HR and mean BP are unchanged or are less than baseline
1	HR or mean BP is increased ≤20% from baseline level
2	HR or BP is increased >20% over baseline level

Continued

CRIES Pain Scale for Neonates (0 to 6 Months)—cont'd

Expression

Facial expression most often associated with pain is a grimace, which may be characterized by brow lowering, eyes squeezed shut, deepening nasolabial furrow, or open lips and mouth.

0	No grimace present
1	Grimace alone is present
2	Grimace and noncry vocalization grunt is present

Sleepless

Scored based on infant's state during the hour preceding this recorded score.

0	Child has been continuously asleep
1	Child has awakened at frequent intervals
2	Child has been awake constantly

BP, blood pressure; *CRIES,* Crying, Requires O₂, Increasing Vital Signs, Expression, Sleepless; *HR,* heart rate.
From Krechel, S. W., & Bildner, J. (1995). CRIES: A new neonatal postoperative pain measurement score-initial testing of validity and reliability. *Paediatric Anaesthesia, 5,* 53–61.

ASEPSIS SCORING TOOL FOR EVALUATING ACUTE WOUND COMPLICATIONS

Instructions for use: The surgical wound site is observed (if possible for the first 5 postoperative days) and the wound characteristics scored according to the proportion of the wound affected and the presence of the characteristic. Additional points are added based on factors such as antibiotic treatment specifically for wound infection. Daily points for characteristics and any additional factors are added for the final wound score and are interpreted according to the category of infection as shown in the table.

Total Score: Category of Infection

0–10: Satisfactory healing
11–20: Disturbance of healing
21–30: Minor wound infection
31–40: Moderate wound infection
>40: Severe wound infection

ASEPSIS Wound Score

Wound Characteristic	Proportion of Wound Affected (%)					
	0	<20	20–39	40–59	60–79	≥80
Serous exudate[a]	0	1	2	3	4	5
Erythema[a]	0	1	2	3	4	5
Purulent exudate[a]	0	2	4	6	8	10
Separation of deep tissue[a]	0	2	4	6	8	10

	Criteria and Points		Score
A	**A**dditional treatments[b]		
	Antibiotics = 10	Drainage of pus (local anesthesia) = 5	Debridement of wound (general anesthesia) = 10
S	**S**erous discharge = sum of daily scores (0–5 points possible each day)		
E	**E**rythema = sum of daily scores (0–5 points possible each day)		
P	**P**urulent exudate = sum of daily scores (0–10 points possible each day)		
S	**S**eparation of deep tissue = sum of daily scores (0–10 points possible each day)		
I	**I**solation of bacteria[b] = 10		
S	**S**tay as inpatient prolonged over 14 days[b] = 5		
	Total Score		

[a]Indicates factors that are scored only on days 0–5 of the first 7 postoperative days.
[b]Indicates factors that are scored and added to the total score once.
From: Campwala, I., Unsell, K., & Gupta, S. (2019). A comparative analysis of surgical wound infection methods: Predictive values of the CDC, ASEPSIS, and Southampton scoring systems in evaluating breast reconstruction surgical site infections. *Plastic Surgery (Oakville, Ont.), 27*(2), 93–99. https://doi.org/10.1177/2292550319826095. Retrieved 04/27/2023 from https://www.ncbi.nlm.nih.gov/pmc/articles/PMC6505358/.

CDC CRITERIA FOR SURGICAL SITE INFECTION (SSI)

Superficial	Deep Incisional	Organ/Space
Occurs within 30 days after the operation	Occurs within 30-90 days	Occurs within 30-90 days
Involves only skin or subcutaneous tissue of the incision	Involves deep soft tissues (e.g., fascial and muscle layers of the incision	Involves any part of the body deeper than the fascial/muscle layers, which is opened or manipulated during the operative procedure
Involves at least one of the following signs or symptoms of infection: • Pain or tenderness, • Localized swelling, redness or heat • AND superficial incision is deliberately opened by the surgeon unless incision is culture negative • Diagnosis made by surgeon or attending physician	Involves at least one of the following: • Purulent drainage from the deep incision but not from the organ/space component of the surgical site, • Deep incision spontaneously dehisces or is deliberately opened by a surgeon when the patient has at least one of the following signs or symptoms: fever, localized pain, or tenderness, unless site is culture negative • An abscess or other evidence of infection involving the deep incision is found on direct examination, during reoperation, or by histopathologic or radiologic examination. • Diagnosis made by surgeon or attending physician	Involves at least one of the following: • Purulent drainage from a drain that is placed into the organ/space • Organisms are identified from an aseptically obtained fluid or tissue in the organ/space by a culture or nonculture= based microbiologic testing method that is performed for purposed of clinical diagnosis or treatment • An abscess or other evidence of infection involving the organ/space that is detected on direct examination or by histopathologic or radiologic examination • Diagnosis made by surgeon or attending physician

The following conditions are not SSI: stitch abscess, localized stab wound or pin site infection, infected burn wound, infected circumcision. Infection that involved both superficial and deep incision sites is reported as deep incisional SSI; an organ/space SSI that drains through the incision is reported as a deep incision SSI.

From: Campwala, I., Unsell, K., & Gupta, S. (2019). A comparative analysis of surgical wound infection methods: Predictive values of the CDC, ASEPSIS, and Southampton scoring systems in evaluating breast reconstruction surgical site infections. *Plastic Surgery (Oakville, Ont.), 27*(2), 93–99. https://doi.org/10.1177/2292550319826095. Retrieved 04/27/2023 from https://www.ncbi.nlm.nih.gov/pmc/articles/PMC6505358/.

SOUTHAMPTON SSI SCORING SYSTEM

- Grade 0—Normal healing
- Grade I—Normal healing with mild bruising or erythema
  - A—Some bruising
  - B—Considerable bruising
  - C—Mild erythema
- Grade II—Erythema plus other signs of inflammation
  - A—At 1 point
  - B—Around sutures
  - C—Along wound
  - D—Around wound
- Grade III—Clear or hemoserous discharge
  - At 1 point only (<2 cm)
  - Along wound (>2 cm)
  - Large volume
  - Prolonged (>3 days)
- Grade IV—Pus
  - A—At 1 point only (<2 cm)
  - B—Along wound (>2 cm)
- Grade V—Deep or severe wound infection with or without tissue breakdown; hematoma requiring aspiration

From: Campwala, I., Unsell, K., & Gupta, S. (2019). A comparative analysis of surgical wound infection methods: Predictive values of the CDC, ASEPSIS, and Southampton scoring systems in evaluating breast reconstruction surgical site infections. *Plastic Surgery (Oakville, Ont.), 27*(2), 93–99. https://doi.org/10.1177/2292550319826095. Retrieved 04/27/2023 from https://www.ncbi.nlm.nih.gov/pmc/articles/PMC6505358/.

SATISFACTION SURVEY

Wound, Ostomy, Continence, Foot Care Nursing Program

⊘Riverwood HEALTHCARE CENTER

Recently, you have received services of our Wound, Ostomy, Continence, Foot Care Nursing Program. Please take a moment to give us your assessment of the program to aid us in evaluating our services.

Please indicate below the service you received (check only one)

☐ Wound Care   ☐ Ostomy Care   ☐ Continence Care   ☐ Foot & Nail Care

Please indicate the most recent date of service .... [ ][ ]/[ ][ ]/[ ][ ]

Response Definition: P=Poor F=Fair G=Good VG=Very Good E=Excellent

	P	F	G	VG	E
1. Procedures, treatment and care practices were thoroughly explained by staff	☐	☐	☐	☐	☐
2. Professionalism of staff	☐	☐	☐	☐	☐
3. Staff members were friendly and encouraging	☐	☐	☐	☐	☐
4. The space provided for care and education was adequate	☐	☐	☐	☐	☐
5. Comfort and pain issues were addressed appropriately and in a timely manner	☐	☐	☐	☐	☐
6. How would you rate the Wound, Ostomy, Continence, Foot Care Nursing Program?	☐	☐	☐	☐	☐

	Y	N
7. Were your questions regarding your condition answered to your satisfaction?	☐	☐
8. Have you continued with the home instructions regarding care and prevention?	☐	☐
9. Has this program assisted you in changing your self-care habits?	☐	☐
10. Were you provided with appropriate education regarding your condition?	☐	☐
11. Would you recommend the Wound, Ostomy, Continence, Foot Care Nursing program to others?	☐	☐

Is there anything in the program that could be added or changed that would be helpful to you?

Please feel free to make any comments regarding the program inside the box below. Include your name and telephone if you would like someone to contact you regarding the services you received.

Please make no marks below this line

ACTIVITY LOG

Month _____

WOUND/SKIN CARE SERVICES

Daily Activity, Patient Case Mix, and Time Summary (1 unit = 15 minutes)

1. Pressure Ulcer/Injury (PU/I) nosocomial 2. PU/I-present on admission 3. Skin tear 4. Surgical wound 5. Incontinence 6. Venous 7. Arterial 8. Neuropathic 9. Mixed 10. Tube 11. Colostomy 12. Ileostomy 13. Urostomy 14. Committee work 15. Quality management 16. Staff education 17. Research/Trials 18. _____ 19. _____

Patient	Unit #	1	2	3	4	5	6	7	8	9	10	11	12	13	14	15	16	17	18	19	20	21	22	23	24	25	26	27	28	29	30

Self-Assessment Answers

CHAPTER 1

1. c
2. c
3. d
4. a

CHAPTER 2

1. d
2. a
3. False
4. b

CHAPTER 3

1. c
2. d
3. d
4. b
5. a

CHAPTER 4

1. a
2. a

CHAPTER 5

1. a
2. b
3. c

CHAPTER 6

1. e
2. d
3. e
4. e
5. d
6. e
7. e

CHAPTER 7

1. b
2. b
3. d
4. a

CHAPTER 8

1. b
2. c
3. b
4. c

CHAPTER 9

1. Factors known to damage the skin include mechanical, chemical, vascular, allergic, infectious, immunologic, burn, and disease-related types.
2. b
3. a
4. c
5. b
6. d
7. The two phases of an allergic contact dermatitis are the sensitization phase and the elicitation phase.
8. a
9. d

CHAPTER 10

1. a
2. b
3. c
4. a
5. a
6. d
7. d

CHAPTER 11

1. d
2. b
3. a
4. b
5. b
6. d
7. a
8. a
9. c
10. b
11. d

CHAPTER 12

1. a
2. b
3. d
4. c
5. b

CHAPTER 13

1. b
2. d
3. c
4. d
5. b
6. d
7. a
8. d
9. b
10. a

CHAPTER 14

1. c
2. b
3. c
4. d
5. d
6. d

CHAPTER 15

1. A competent venous system includes deep veins, superficial veins, and perforator veins. The perforator veins (communicating veins) connect the deep and superficial veins to transport blood. Veins function by one-way valves to prevent backflow. The calf muscle pump and one-way valves work together to propel venous blood back to the heart. During ambulation, the calf muscle contracts and pumps the blood out of the deep veins, and the one-way valves in the perforator system close to prevent backflow into superficial veins. When the calf muscle relaxes, the valves in the perforator veins open to permit blood flow into the deep veins.

2. c
3. d
4. Elastic compression devices deliver a sustained pressure, regardless of the patient's activity level. Nonelastic compression devices compress the calf muscle during ambulation. The constant compression increases interstitial tissue pressure to reduce leakage of fluid from capillaries. The sedentary patient should be managed with elastic compression devices because he or she has decreased calf muscle pump action.
5. c
6. a
7. a

CHAPTER 16

1. c
2. a
3. d

CHAPTER 17

1. b
2. d
3. d
4. d
5. b

CHAPTER 18

1. d
2. a
3. d
4. d
5. c
6. c
7. b
8. d
9. c
10. d
11. d
12. c

CHAPTER 19

1. d
2. c
3. c
4. b
5. b
6. b
7. a
8. c
9. a

CHAPTER 20

1. d
2. Considerations in the use of enzymatic debridement include the following
   - Enzymes are inactivated by heavy metal ions (chlorine, silver, mercury).
   - Enzymes may be used to debride an infected wound.
   - Enzymatic debridement necessitates dressing changes at least daily.
   - Selection of debriding enzyme is primarily based on clinician preference, cost, availability, and ease of use.
3. a
4. b

CHAPTER 21

1. d
2. d
3. b
4. d
5. b
6. d
7. d
8. Objectives for local wound management are to prevent and manage infection, cleanse the wound, remove nonviable tissue (debridement), maintain an appropriate level of moisture, eliminate dead space, control odor, eliminate or minimize pain, and protect the wound and periwound skin.

CHAPTER 22

1. d
2. c
3. a
4. b
5. a
6. True
7. 1. Address underlying pathology.
   2. Correct systemic factors interfering with wound healing.
   3. Identify and treat clinical infection.
   4. Debride all necrotic tissue, fibrinous slough, and surrounding callus.
   5. Ensure complete contact of product with wound bed.
   6. Fenestrate product (if not already packaged that way) to allow wound fluid to escape and prevent accumulation of fluid under product.
   7. Keep products without synthetic backings moist.
   8. Follow package insert for directions specific to individual products.

CHAPTER 23

1. a
2. d
3. b
4. a

CHAPTER 24

1. c
2. b
3. a
4. a
5. c

CHAPTER 25

1. b
2. c
3. True
4. False
5. e

CHAPTER 26

1. a
2. a
3. True
4. d
5. d
6. b

CHAPTER 27

1. b
2. d
3. c
4. d
5. a

CHAPTER 28

1. True. Patients may benefit from nonpharmacological as well as pharmacological agents or a combination thereof. Identifying the needs of the patient is important to tailoring the type of pain medication.
2. d. All of the above.
3. True. It is important to start with the local anesthetics and then work stepwise to include other blocks and general anesthesia as necessary.
4. e. All interventions can be utilized to minimize patient discomfort depending on the degree of pain elicited by the intervention.

CHAPTER 29

1. c
2. a
3. a

CHAPTER 30

1. b
2. c

3. e
4. d
5. c
6. b
7. d
8. b
9. e
10. d

CHAPTER 31

1. e. All factors listed above can lead to poorer wound healing.
2. True. SSI complications lead to unnecessary return to the operating room, increase length of stay, as well as contribute to morbidity and mortality.
3. e. All of the above.
4. a. The most common tool used for acute wound complication is the CDC criterion.
5. False. Routine use of antibiotics can lead to resistance and does not demonstrate improvement in wound healing.

CHAPTER 32

1. c
2. c
3. b

CHAPTER 33

1. c
2. a
3. d
4. c

CHAPTER 34

1. d
2. d
3. b
4. b

CHAPTER 35

1. b
2. b
3. d

CHAPTER 36

1. d. Multiple factors contribute to pressure injury formation in the obese individual. A combination of limited mobility, excess pressure/weight, friction between skin folds, inappropriately sized equipment, and the difficulty of caregivers to help move the patients.

2. b. Patients with obesity are at higher risk of postoperative wound dehiscence, skin infections, and lung complications after surgery. There is some evidence that obesity is protective after surgery for mortality compared to individuals without obesity.
3. a. An abdominal binder has been shown to decrease the chance of wound dehiscence. Early mobility can help decrease hospital length of stay and other complications like deep vein thrombosis. Fowler's position can improve breathing postoperatively.

CHAPTER 37

1. a
2. False
3. b
4. c
5. c

CHAPTER 38

1. c
2. a
3. c
4. d

CHAPTER 39

1. d
2. c
3. a. Small bowel to skin
   b. Colon to skin
   c. Bladder to vagina
   d. Rectum to vagina
   e. Colon to bladder
4. b
5. a
6. c

CHAPTER 40

1. d
2. b
3. d
4. a

INDEX

Note: Page numbers followed by *f* indicate figures, *t* indicate tables, and *b* indicate boxes.